Frontiers in Healthy Cities: Policy Impacts and Inclusive Governance

Frontiers in Healthy Cities: Policy Impacts and Inclusive Governance

Editors

Jie Chen
Qian Zhou
Ting Zhang

MDPI • Basel • Beijing • Wuhan • Barcelona • Belgrade • Manchester • Tokyo • Cluj • Tianjin

Editors
Jie Chen
School of International and Public Affairs, Shanghai Jiao Tong University,
Shanghai, China

Qian Zhou
Economics School, Zhongnan University of Economics and Law,
Wuhan, China

Ting Zhang
School of International and Public Affairs, Shanghai Jiao Tong University,
Shanghai, China

Editorial Office
MDPI
St. Alban-Anlage 66
4052 Basel, Switzerland

This is a reprint of articles from the Special Issue published online in the open access journal *International Journal of Environmental Research and Public Health* (ISSN 1660-4601) (available at: https://www.mdpi.com/journal/ijerph/special_issues/Frontiers_Healthy_Cities).

For citation purposes, cite each article independently as indicated on the article page online and as indicated below:

LastName, A.A.; LastName, B.B.; LastName, C.C. Article Title. *Journal Name* **Year**, *Volume Number*, Page Range.

ISBN 978-3-0365-6021-2 (Hbk)
ISBN 978-3-0365-6022-9 (PDF)

Contents

About the Editors

Jie Chen

Professor Jie Chen, the Director of Centre for Housing and Urban-Rural Development (CHURD), is a tenured full professor at the School of International and Public Affairs (SIPA) and K. Wah Professor at China Institute for Urban Governance (CIUG) at Shanghai Jiao Tong University (SJTU). He received a PhD from Uppsala University, a master's degree from the University of Oslo, and a bachelor's degree from Fudan University. Before joining SJTU in 2018, he worked as a faculty member at Uppsala University, Fudan University and Shanghai University of Finance and Economics. His research area is urban and housing-related studies. He is on Trustee Board of Urban Studies Foundation, and on the editorial Board of Housing Studies and International Journal of Housing Policy. He is also vice Chairman of China Institute of Real Estate Appraisers and Agents, a steering member of Asia-Pacific Network of Housing Research (APNHR) and vice chairman of the Regional Science Association's (RSA) China Chapter. Professor Chen has received several national-level research grants, including being awarded NSFC-ESRC joint funding.

Qian Zhou

Associate professor Qian Zhou works at the Economics School, Zhongnan University of Economics and Law. She got her PhD degree from Shanghai University of Finance and Economics in 2017. Her research interests are urban economics and environmental economics. She has published 50 papers and received several grants.

Ting Zhang

Dr. Ting Zhang is currently a postdoctoral fellow at the School of International Affairs and Public Administration, Shanghai Jiao Tong University. She received her PhD in earth systems and geographic information science from the Chinese University of Hong Kong in 2020. Her research interests are housing-related environmental health and governance innovation.

Preface to "Frontiers in Healthy Cities: Policy Impacts and Inclusive Governance"

Today, the proportion of human beings residing in cities has exceeded 56 percent, and this number is increasing every year. By 2050, 70 percent of the world's population will live in cities. While cities provide many opportunities for human being development, they also pose unique health risks. The disproportionate effects of the contagious disease COVID-19 on the urban world today has strongly urged policymakers worldwide to place health high up on the social, economic, and political agenda of city governments. As articulated by the World Health Organization (WHO) in a recent statement, a healthy city is defined by a process, not an outcome. The WHO also defines healthy cities as a process to strive to create social and physical environments which empower people to mutually support each other, both in getting on with daily life and reaching their maximum potential. The planning and design of urban space, the built environment, and community structures have been found to be critical elements in the formation of a healthy city. However, to ensure health justice, people's involvement and inclusion in the governance of urban health issues are also crucial. To promote advances in the knowledge on the formation and governance of healthy cities, we organized this Special Issue on "Frontiers in Healthy Cities: Policy Impacts and Inclusive Governance" in the peer-reviewed scientific International Journal of Environmental Research and Public Health. The current collection contains 37 high-quality original papers that drew from a large number of submissions after a rigorous double-blind reviewing process. A broad range of topics are covered in this collection, something which will help to shed light on the improvement directions of the governance of healthy cities for worldwide policy makers and scholars.

Jie Chen, Qian Zhou, and Ting Zhang
Editors

International Journal of
Environmental Research and Public Health

MDPI

Article

How Does Urban Sprawl Affect Public Health? Evidence from Panel Survey Data in Urbanizing China

Yan Yan [1], Hui Liu [2,*] and Canfei He [3]

[1] College of Urban Economics and Public Administration, Capital University of Economics and Business, Beijing 100070, China; yanyan@cueb.edu.cn
[2] School of Government, Central University of Finance and Economics, Beijing 100081, China
[3] College of Urban and Environmental Sciences, Peking University, Beijing 100871, China; hecanfei@urban.pku.edu.cn
* Correspondence: liuhui@cufe.edu.cn

Abstract: This study takes urbanizing China as the research object, employs data from three follow-up surveys conducted by the Harmonized China Health and Retirement Longitudinal Study, and examines the effects of urban sprawl on public health from physical and mental health perspectives. Although urban sprawl does not necessarily increase the risk of each specific type of disease or psychological feeling, it has a significant impact on overall physical and mental health. Further analysis reveals significant heterogeneity in the effects of urban sprawl on the physical and mental health of different groups. Specifically, urban sprawl is detrimental to the physical health of males and females, but only has negative impact on the mental health of females. Younger groups are more vulnerable to physical and mental health damage from urban sprawl relative to middle-aged and older groups. In addition, urban sprawl has a significant negative impact on the health of the low-education group but a very limited impact on the health of the high-education counterpart. From an income perspective, however, the preference for suburban housing among middle- and high-income groups makes their health more vulnerable to the negative effects of urban sprawl than low-income groups living in urban centers.

Keywords: urban sprawl; physical health; mental health

Citation: Yan, Y.; Liu, H.; He, C. How Does Urban Sprawl Affect Public Health? Evidence from Panel Survey Data in Urbanizing China. *IJERPH* **2021**, *18*, 10181. https://doi.org/10.3390/ijerph181910181

Academic Editors: Jie Chen, Qian Zhou and Ting Zhang

Received: 1 September 2021
Accepted: 26 September 2021
Published: 28 September 2021

1. Introduction

Urban sprawl has become a common spatial structure worldwide [1–4]. This phenomenon is characterized by the expansion of urban areas exceeding the growth of the urban population, the dispersal of large numbers of people and economic activities to the suburbs, a decrease in land-use intensity and population density, and a decentralized and polycentric urban form [5–8]. According to the OECD measurements of 1156 cities in 29 OECD countries, many countries and cities have experienced a dramatic increase in urban sprawl since 1990 [9]. Such low-density urban spatial growth pattern resulted in a range of negative impacts on urban economic, social, and environmental aspects, such as lower productivity and labor wage incomes [10,11], higher energy consumption [12,13], decreased air quality [14–16], auto reliance [6,17], and ecosystem fragmentation [18,19]. As a result, urban sprawl has become a hot topic of concern for scholars and policy makers worldwide [1,3,4,20].

Recently, researchers in urban planning and public health have begun to focus on the relationship between urban sprawl and public health, noting that a sprawling urban spatial growth pattern can be harmful to public health [21–27]. One branch of the literature focuses on the effects of urban sprawl on obesity and finds that people living in sprawl areas are more likely to be obese than those living in compact areas [22,25,28–30]. Another stream of literature explores the effects of urban sprawl on mortality and various diseases [25,31] and confirms that residents living in sprawl areas may face higher mortality rates [32,33] and are more likely to develop heart disease [25,34], high blood pressure, and diabetes [25]. By contrast, a compact urban form can reduce cardiovascular mortality [35]. The third branch of the literature examines the impact of urban sprawl on the health care costs of the residents and establishes that urban sprawl increases residents' health care expenditures [36,37]. Accordingly, the World Health Organization (WHO) advocates the use of urban planning as a tool for high public health [38].

Several studies subsequently explore the mechanisms by which urban sprawl affects public health and verify that urban sprawl can affect public health through reduced physical activity [25,36,39], decreased air quality [14–16], pedestrian-unfriendly built environment [1,40,41], pedestrian injuries and fatalities [22,42], and other ways. Urban sprawl can reduce the physical activity of residents, and the lack of physical activity is considered the fourth leading risk factor for death globally and causes 3.2 million deaths annually. Urban sprawl also tends to fragment intra-urban spaces and increases commuting distances for residents, with this occurrence leading to reliance on cars and a reduction in active transport (e.g., such as walking and cycling), which is considered a convenient way to increase physical activity [6,43–45]. Furthermore, urban sprawl tends to create built environments that are not friendly for walking, and this situation can lower the probability of resident engagement in physical activity [1,40]. In addition, urban sprawl can lead to a decrease in air quality, a condition which affects the health of residents [14–16]. Urban sprawl contributes to increased vehicle emissions [12,13] and rising construction dust [46], both of which can further harm the residents' health by causing respiratory diseases, cardiovascular diseases, and liver fibrosis [47,48].

Relatively rich research on urban sprawl and public health is available, but some shortcomings and deficiencies are evident in the literature. First, scholars have mostly studied the effect of urban sprawl on public health from the perspective of physical health. Some discussions regarding mental health have emerged in recent years, but they are still very limited. In fact, urban sprawl also affects mental health directly or indirectly. Air pollution caused by urban sprawl can increase oxidative stress and systemic inflammatory responses in humans, directly contributing to depression and cognitive dysfunction and even causing brain damage and dementia [49,50]. Changes in the built environment because of urban sprawl can also increase the risk of depression among residents [51]. Second, existing studies on the relationship between urban sprawl and public health mainly focused on developed countries such as European nations and the U.S. [27,28], with relatively few studies targeting developing countries. China is a typical case of a developing country for studying this issue. As a developing country undergoing rapid urbanization, China's traditional high-density model of urban spatial development has been disappearing gradually. On the contrary, urban sprawl has become a common phenomenon in its current urban development [4,52]. Although urban sprawl in Chinese cities has been promoted jointly by local states and market forces and simultaneously by real estate developer and industrial manufacturers, both of which are different from western cities, the spatial pattern and its multidimensional impacts are quite similar to those in other countries [53,54]. At the same time, public health has become an important challenge for developing countries. This is the case for China as well. The WHO (2016) reported that mental illness, diabetes, and cardiovascular disease will cause the most economic damage in urbanizing China in the future among all diseases, and this trend is exacerbated by urban sprawl and the lifestyle and the work changes it generates. Third, given the limitation of survey data, most previous research on the relationship between urban sprawl and public health have used cross-sectional data. Nevertheless, cross-sectional data are difficult to control for all unobservable individual differences and are prone to problems such as omitted variables.

Accordingly, this study uses the authoritative data published by the China Health and Retirement Longitudinal Study (CHARLS) to examine the effects of urban sprawl on public health in urbanizing China. The main contributions of this work are as follows. First, this article assesses the effect of urban sprawl on public health from the perspectives of physical and mental health, which are comprehensive viewpoints. Second, this study uses China as a case and thus makes up for the relative lack of such research in developing countries. Third, the data used in this work are tracking survey data, cover three periods (2011, 2013, and 2015), and are comparable between periods. The tracking survey data provide information on the dynamic behavior of individuals and can significantly improve the precision of the estimation. Fourth, this work further explored the heterogeneous characteristics of the effects of urban sprawl on the physical and mental health of different groups in four dimensions: gender, age, education, and income level.

2. Research Methods and Data Sources

2.1. Model

To test the impact of urban sprawl on public health, this study constructs the following model.

$$PH_{ict} = \beta_0 + \beta_1 US_{ct} + \gamma_1 X_{it} + \tau_c + \omega_t + \varepsilon_{ct} \tag{1}$$

$$MH_{ict} = \beta_0 + \beta_1 US_{ct} + \gamma_1 X_{it} + \tau_c + \omega_t + \varepsilon_{ct} \tag{2}$$

where the subscript i represents different individuals, c denotes city, and t denotes waves of survey. τ_c and ω_t refer to the city fixed effects and time fixed effects, respectively. PH_{ict} and MH_{ict} represent the physical and mental health status of respondent i living in city c for the tth waves of survey. US_{ct} represents the degree of urban sprawl in city c in year t. Referring to the previous literature, the control variables mainly include the following three categories. The first category controls individual demographic variables, such as age, gender, marital status, education level, and employment status. The second category controls lifestyle and health behavior variables, including smoking and alcohol consumption. The third category controls family structure variables, including the number of people living in household, whether any child is co-residing with the respondent, and annual household income. As CHARLS involves longitudinal data, this study refers to Lim and Hong [55] and Wang et al. [56] and employs the generalized estimating equations (GEE) method to examine the relationship between urban sprawl and public health.

2.2. Data Sources

The individual-level microdata of middle-aged and older adults used in this paper were obtained from the Harmonized CHARLS database which was provided by the Center for Socioeconomic Research (CESR) at the University of Southern California and has been widely used to study health problems of Chinese residents [57,58]. The raw data for Harmonized CHARLS came from the CHARLS data organized by the National Development Institute of Peking University. CHARLS started the baseline survey in 2011 and conducted follow-up interviews in 2013, 2015, and 2018. CHARLS adopted a multi-stage cluster and stratified probability proportionate to size (PPS) sampling method to conduct the survey to ensure the representativeness and unbiasedness of samples. CHARLS randomly selected residents aged 45 years or older and their spouses for the survey. For ease of use and international comparison, CESR linked the CHARLS data to the variables from the Health and Retirement Study data produced by the RAND Corporation (RAND HRS) and named the outcome as Harmonized CHARLS. The Harmonized CHARLS database combines the CHARLS 2011, CHARLS 2013, and CHARLS 2015 samples, making each wave of survey comparable for easy establishment of panel models. In addition, the Harmonized CHARLS integrates numerous variables on the basis of CHARLS data, with relatively few missing variables and high data quality.

The urban sprawl index was calculated according to the MODIS Global Urban Extent Product (MGUP) data [59] and WorldPop global population density data. To obtain a reliable urban sprawl index, the extent of urban built-up areas and their respective populations needed to be identified. However, the area provided by China's urban economic statistics may vary in standard from time to time and from city to city. Furthermore, China does not have resident population statistics accurate to the neighborhood scale as the United States does. Therefore, a more precise method is required to measure urban built-up areas and their population. In this research, we use MGUP data to identify the largest patches within the administrative boundaries of each city as urban built-up areas, combine the WorldPop data to calculate the population of each built-up area, and finally compute the urban sprawl index accordingly. MGUP data are widely used in the study of global urban areas [59,60]. MGUP has been validated to be more than 90% accurate in identifying urban boundaries in multiple scenarios [61]. As a class of data reflecting the spatial distribution of population, WorldPop data have higher estimation accuracy and longer duration compared to other gridded population spatial distribution data and is ideal for measuring the spatial distribution of urban populations [62].

We linked individual-level survey data for each city with city-level urban sprawl index for further analysis. This study only retains samples that are 45 years old or older and do not have missing dependent and important independent variables. As urban sprawl mainly affects the health of residents living in urban areas, this study removed the sample of respondents living in rural areas. It is worth noting that although the lifestyle and mobility of residents living in the suburb are affected more severely by urban sprawl than those living in the city center, the latter cannot completely escape from the impacts of urban sprawl because their commuting and everyday life are citywide behaviors which cannot be restrained only in the city center.

2.3. Variable Definition

This study used the total number of diseases from which the respondent suffered as a measure of physical health, which is widely used in the previous literature [63,64]. CHARLS asks respondents whether or not a doctor has told them they had a specific disease. The specific diseases include cancer, high blood pressure, diabetes, dyslipidemia, heart problem, stroke, asthma, lung disease, liver disease, kidney disease, stomach/digestive disease, and arthritis. A code of 0 indicates that the respondent does not report having been told by a doctor they have the condition. A code of 1 indicates that the respondent reports having been told by a doctor they have a condition. We summed the respondents' answers to 12 conditions as a measure of physical health. The final value of PH_{ict} ranges from 0 to 12, with larger values representing poorer physical health.

Previous studies have mostly evaluated the mental health in terms of cognitive ability and depression self-assessment [49–51]. Relatively, self-assessment of depression is a more common indicator to measure residents' mental health. Fortunately, CHARLS offers the short form of the Center for Epidemiological Studies Depression scale (CESD-10), which is widely used in mental health research [57,65,66]. Lei et al. examined the reliability and validity of the CESD-10 scale using CHARLS data and confirmed the validity of the scale in the Chinese population studies [57]. The CESD-10 scale contains three depressive mood items, five somatic symptom items, and two positive mood items. The CESD-10 scale contains three depressive mood items, five somatic symptom items and two positive mood items. CHARLS reports the frequency of the respondents' feeling over the week prior to the interview, specifically including whether the respondent was feeling depressed, whether the respondent was feeling that everything was an effort, whether the respondent's sleep was restless, whether the respondent felt happy, whether the respondent felt lonely, whether the respondent bothered by thing that did not usually bother them, whether the respondent felt they could not get going, whether the respondent has trouble keeping their mind on what they are doing, whether the respondent felt hopeful about the future, and whether the respondent felt fearful. When respondents answered to negative mood as "rarely or never (less than once a day)," "some or a little of the time (1–2 days)," "occasionally or a moderate amount of time (3–4 days)," and "most or all of the time (5–7 days)," they were scored 0–3 points. The positive emotions were reverse coded. Referring to the existing literature, this study used the CESD-10 scale to measure the degree of mental health. The score ranges from zero to 30, with higher values representing worse mental health.

Given data limitations, previous literature typically used population density as an approximate measure of urban sprawl. This study adopts the approach from Fulton et al. [67] to reflect the degree of urban sprawl by calculating the ratio of the urban built-up area growth rate and urban population growth rate using the following method. Note that the larger the US_{ct}, the higher the degree of urban sprawl.

$$US_{ct} = \frac{A_{ct} - A_{ct-1}}{A_{ct-1}} / \frac{(P_{ct} - P_{ct-1})}{P_{ct-1}} \quad (3)$$

where A_{ct} refers to the built-up area at time t, and P_{ct} refer to the population within the study area at time t.

The control variables are defined as follows. Age indicates the respondent's age. Gender indicates the respondent's gender which set to 1 for male and 0 for female. Marriage indicates the respondent's reported marital status. Marriage is set to 1 for married and 0 for separated, divorced, widowed, and never married. Education indicates the highest level of education the respondent has attained. Education is defined 1 for upper secondary and vocational training and 0 for less than lower secondary education. Education_2 is defined 1 for tertiary education and 0 for less than lower secondary education. Employment refers to the working status. Employment is set to 1 for currently working and 0 for unemployed, retired, or never worked. Smoke indicates whether the respondent reports ever smoking. Smoke is set to 1 for ever smoking and 0 for never having smoked. Drink indicates whether the respondent has had any alcoholic beverages in the past. Drink is set to 1 for having had an alcoholic drink in the past and 0 for never having an alcoholic drink in the past. Hhincome (for household income) indicates the sum of all income at the household level. To make the data comparable, this work uniformly converts annual household income to 2015 prices according to the consumer price index, excluding the effect of price factors. To eliminate the effect of heteroskedasticity, annual household income is taken in logarithmic form in the regression. Hhcoresd indicates whether any child is co-residing with the respondent. Hhcoresd is set to 1 for any child co-resides with respondent and 0 for no child co-resides with respondent. Hhnum indicates the number of people living in household. Table 1 shows the descriptive statistics of the main variables.

Table 1. Descriptive statistics of the main variables.

Variable Name	Definition	Obs	Mean	SD	Min	Max
Health						
Physical health	Total number of diseases the respondent had	9232	1.718	1.586	0	10
Mental health	Score of the short form of the Center for Epidemiological Studies Depression scale	9435	7.160	5.757	0	30
Urban sprawl						
Urban sprawl	Urban sprawl index	9803	2.581	3.092	−11.813	19.625
Individual demographic characteristics						
Age		9803	60.502	9.439	45	94
Gender	0 for female; 1 for male	9803	0.471	0.499	0	1
Marriage	0 for separated, divorced, widowed, and never married; 1 for married	9803	0.135	0.342	0	1
Education	0 for less than lower secondary education, 1 for upper secondary and vocational training	9803	0.156	0.363	0	1
Education_2	0 for less than lower secondary education, 1 for tertiary education	9803	0.035	0.183	0	1
Employment	0 for unemployed, retired, or never worked; 1 for currently working	9803	0.536	0.499	0	1
Health behavior variables						
Smoke	0 for never having smoked; 1 for ever smoking	9803	0.404	0.491	0	1
Drink	0 for never having an alcoholic drink in the past; 1 for having had an alcoholic drink in the past	9803	0.428	0.495	0	1

Table 1. *Cont.*

Variable Name	Definition	Obs	Mean	SD	Min	Max
Family structure variables						
Ln(Hhincome)	The sum of all income at the household level	9803	9.713	2.379	0	14.863
Hhcoresd	0 for no child co-resides with respondent; 1 for any child co-resides with respondent	9803	0.549	0.498	0	1
Hhnum	The number of people living in household	9803	3.305	1.576	1	12

3. Empirical Analysis

3.1. Benchmark Regression Results

Table 2 shows the results of the benchmark regression of the effect of urban sprawl on public health. Urban sprawl has a significant negative effect on the physical and mental health of respondents. As the level of urban sprawl increases, the total number of specific diseases and the level of psychological depression of the respondents rose significantly. Specifically, each 1-unit increase in the urban sprawl index was associated with a 1.1% rise in the number of specific diseases and a 1.2% rise in the CESD-10 scale score which reflects the degree of depression.

Table 2. Benchmark regression results.

	Physical Health	Mental Health
	(1)	(2)
Urban sprawl	0.011 ***	0.012 ***
	(4.04)	(3.94)
Age	0.033 ***	−0.000
	(25.13)	(−0.34)
Gender	−0.208 ***	−0.244 ***
	(−6.40)	(−8.26)
Marriage	−0.084 **	0.112 ***
	(−2.53)	(3.74)
Education	0.049	−0.240 ***
	(1.27)	(−7.64)
Education_2	0.048	−0.345 ***
	(0.79)	(−5.56)
Employment	−0.024	−0.045 **
	(−1.49)	(−2.40)
Drink	0.058 ***	−0.005
	(3.75)	(−0.24)
Smoke	0.133 ***	0.061 **
	(5.66)	(2.26)
Ln(Hhincome)	−0.008***	−0.022 ***
	(−3.68)	(−7.18)
Hhcoresd	0.012	−0.006
	(0.83)	(−0.28)
Hhnum	−0.032 ***	0.006
	(−5.42)	(0.93)
Constant	−1.342 ***	2.296 ***
	(−14.22)	(26.62)
N	9232	9435

*** and ** indicate significance at the 1% and 5% levels, respectively.

The regression results of other control variables are further observed. As age increases, the physical health of the respondents worsens and the likelihood of getting various diseases increases. However, the effect of age on the mental health is not significant, thereby indicating that the mental health of the respondents has little relationship with their age. Compared to females, males have better physical and mental health, a lower risk of developing diseases, and relatively lower degree of depression. Compared to unmarried, widowed, and divorced respondents, married counterparts had better physical health but relatively poorer mental health. Marriage has a protective effect on health and married individuals have better physical health status [68]. Compared to those with less than lower secondary education, respondents with higher levels of education have relatively better mental health but no significant differences in physical health. Studies confirmed that individuals with higher levels of education are more capable of adjusting their behavior and regulating their psychology amid stressful life events and have higher levels of mental health [69]. Compared to people who are unemployed, retired or have never worked, respondents currently working have better mental health. Respondents with drinking and smoking habits are more likely to have a disease, and smoking also has a significant effect on mental health. The negative health effects of drinking and smoking have been confirmed by numerous studies [70–72]. Respondents with higher household income had relatively better physical and mental health. Higher income groups generally have a relatively higher quality of life and are more likely to access advanced medical resources and healthy nutrition. Moreover, the accumulation of wealth can affect cognitive functioning and mental health, so higher income groups are physically and mentally healthier [73,74]. Whether or not living with children has no significant effect on respondents' physical and mental health. With increasing family size, respondents' physical health rises, but their mental health does not change significantly.

3.2. Robustness Test

To further examine the effect of urban sprawl on physical health, this study investigates that effect on each specific disease. Figure 1 plots the coefficients and 90% confidence intervals of regressions for each specific disease. The black dots in the figure represent the percentage increase in the probability of getting a specific disease when urban sprawl increases by 1 unit. The horizontal lines in the figure represent the 90% confidence intervals of regression results. In general, the respondents' risk of getting stomach/digestive disease and arthritis increases significantly. However, urban sprawl does not have a significant effect on other specific diseases. Although urban sprawl does not necessarily increase the risk of each specific disease, it has a significant effect on the overall level of physical health.

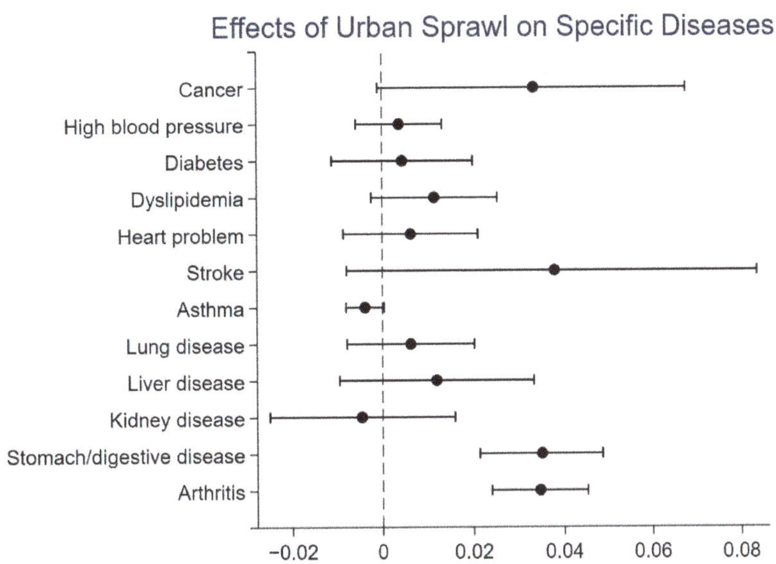

Figure 1. Coefficients and 90% confidence intervals of regressions for each specific disease.

To further examine the effect of urban sprawl on mental health, this study examines that effect on each type of psychological feeling reported by respondents in the CESD-10. Figure 2 plots the coefficients and 90% confidence intervals of regressions for each feeling reported by respondents. As urban sprawl increases, the frequency of negative feelings (e.g., the feeling of depressed, feeling that everything is an effort, feeling lonely, and having trouble keeping their mind on what they are doing) increases significantly as the level of urban sprawl rises. However, the effect of urban sprawl on other feelings is not significant. These feelings include the feeling of sleeping being restless, being happy, being bothered by little things, inability to get going, being hopeful about the future, and being fearful. Similar to the previous findings, urban sprawl does not necessarily increase the risk of each negative psychological feeling but has a significant effect on the overall level of mental health.

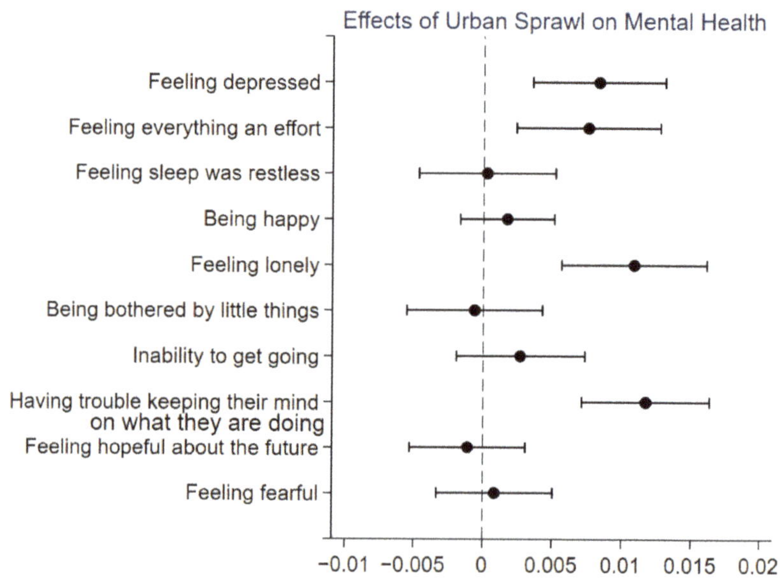

Figure 2. Coefficients and 90% confidence intervals of regressions for each psychological feeling.

3.3. *Heterogeneity Analysis*

Urban sprawl may have differential effect on public health for different groups. In this study, we examine the heterogeneity of the health effects of urban sprawl in four dimensions: gender, age, education, and household income level.

3.3.1. Gender Heterogeneity

Figure 3 shows the regression results of the effect of urban sprawl on public health for different genders. Urban sprawl significantly reduces the physical and mental health of females. Moreover, urban sprawl reduces the physical health of males, but has no significant effect on their mental health.

3.3.2. Age Heterogeneity

Figure 4 shows the regression results of the effect of urban sprawl on public health for groups in different ages. Urban sprawl significantly reduces the physical health of respondents in the 55–74 age group and the mental health of respondents under the age of 75, but has no significant effect on the health of the 75+ age group. This result may be explained by the following reasons. As cities grow, urban spaces mostly expand outward in a circle-like pattern [75]. Most individuals in the older age groups have purchased houses before the massive urban expansion. As cities have expanded, the location of the older group's housing has become the central urban areas. Meanwhile, older groups have a higher demand for medical facilities, which are mostly concentrated in central urban areas in China. For the relatively younger group, the housing prices in the central urban areas have risen by the time they buy their homes, so they proceed to the spreading suburbs where they can afford the housing prices at lower prices. Thus, in terms of the spatial distribution of the population within the city, the older age groups mostly live in the central city and the relatively younger groups live more in the sprawling suburbs [76]. Therefore, urban sprawl has a significant impact on the health of the relatively younger group and has no significant impact on the 75+ age group.

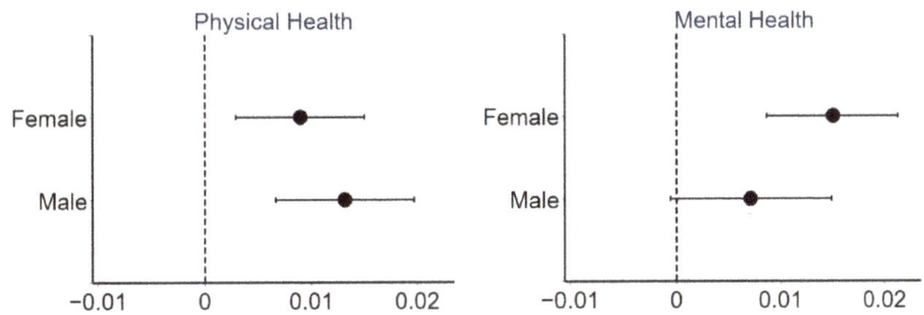

Figure 3. Coefficients and 90% confidence intervals of regressions for different gender group.

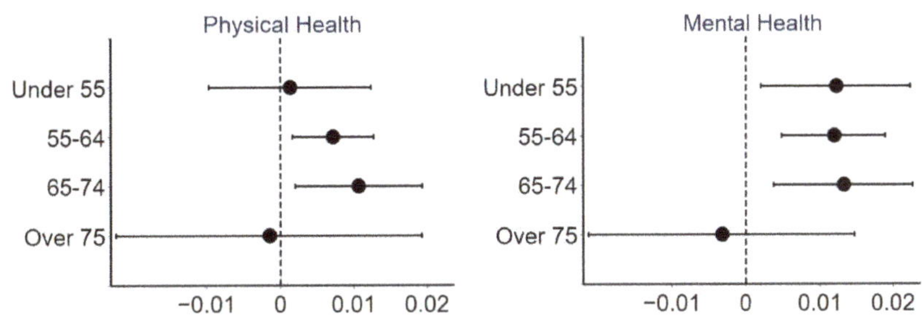

Figure 4. Coefficients and 90% confidence intervals of regressions for different age groups.

3.3.3. Education Heterogeneity

Figure 5 shows the regression results of the effect of urban sprawl on public health for groups with different education levels. This study divides the sample into three categories according to the highest education level of the respondents: less than lower secondary education, upper secondary and vocational training, and tertiary education. Urban sprawl has a negative impact on the health of all groups with different education levels. However, this effect is significant in the less educated group but not in the more educated group. Previous research established that the highly educated group in China tends to work in the civil service or public institutions. Most members of that group have local household registration and enjoy housing benefits, and the majority of such housing is in the residential area of the unit which is relatively close to the workplace, thereby facilitating the achievement of work–life balance [77]. By contrast, individuals in the less educated group mostly need to purchase houses on their own in the market, and most of these houses are located in urban sprawl areas. Therefore, urban sprawl does not have a significant impact on the health of the group with high education but has a significant negative impact on the health of the low education group.

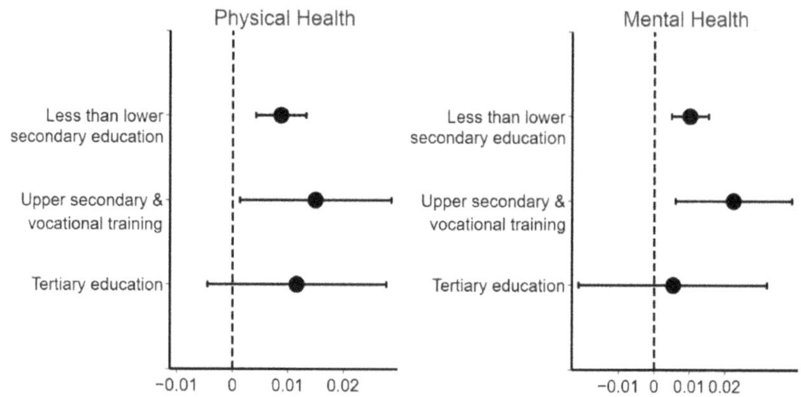

Figure 5. Coefficients and 90% confidence intervals of regressions for different education groups.

3.3.4. Income Heterogeneity

Figure 6 shows the regression results of the effect of urban sprawl on public health for groups with different household income levels. This work trisects the sample according to annual household income and classifies respondents into three categories: low income, middle income, and high income. Urban sprawl has a significant negative impact on the physical health of all groups and mental health of the middle- and high-income groups. Moreover, the effect of urban sprawl on respondents' physical health increases with rising income levels. Most members of the higher income groups are relatively young. As discussed, those individuals generally live in sprawling suburban or new town areas, so urban sprawl has a more significant impact on them. The low-income groups are mostly elderly people who depend on pensions and who mainly live in central or old urban areas where population density is relatively high. Thus, urban sprawl has a significant negative impact on the health of relatively high-income groups but not on the health of relatively low-income.

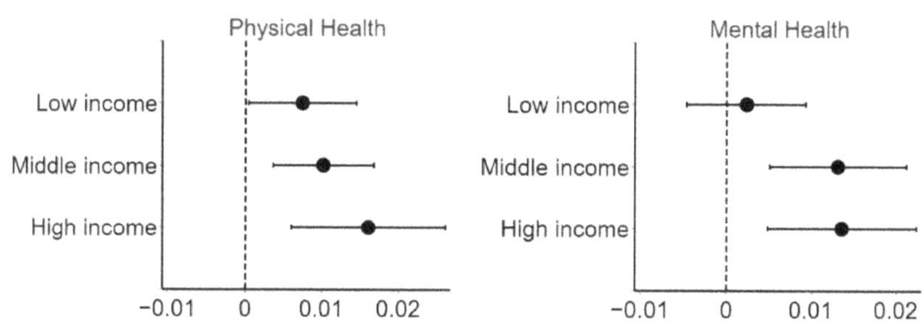

Figure 6. Coefficients and 90% confidence intervals of regressions for different income groups.

4. Conclusions

This study takes urbanizing China as its research object, uses data from three follow-up surveys conducted by Harmonized CHARLS, and examines the effects of urban sprawl on public health from physical and mental health perspectives. Results show that although urban sprawl does not necessarily increase the risk of each specific type of disease or psychological feeling, it has a significant impact on the overall level of physical and mental health. Further analysis reveals significant heterogeneity in the effects of urban sprawl on the physical and mental health of different groups. Specifically, urban sprawl is detrimental to the physical health of males and females but only has a negative impact on the mental health of females. Among the middle-aged and older groups, the physical and mental health of the younger groups are more vulnerable to damage from urban sprawl. In addition, urban sprawl has a significant negative impact on the health of the low-education group but a very limited impact on the health of the high-education group. From an income perspective, however, the preference for suburban housing among middle- and high-income groups makes their health more vulnerable to the negative effects of urban sprawl than low-income groups living in urban centers.

This study has the following limitations, many of which should motivate future research. First, this study is focused merely on the middle-aged and older groups due to the limited data availability. However, the negative effects of urban sprawl are very likely to be severe for other vulnerable groups such as the poor and children whose health and well-being deserve scholarly and public attentions as well. Second, this study briefly explored several possible mechanisms for urban sprawl to affect public health, such as reduced physical activity [25,36], decreased air quality [15,16], pedestrian-unfriendly built environment. Nevertheless, these mechanisms can hardly be confirmed without substantial empirical tests when data are available in future. Third, since CHARLS only reported the city where the respondent resided but not the exact location within the city, this study can only explore the effect of the overall urban sprawl on residents' health, but cannot examine the different effects on people living in the city center and those in the suburb. This comparative study is crucial for further study due to the nature of urban sprawl focusing mainly on the spatial pattern of the suburb rather than the city center. Last but not the least, this study is based mainly on survey data and statistical methods with relatively limited theoretical discussion and qualitative analysis. Although data often tell the truth, qualitative or mixed methods are a must for further in-depth investigation on urban spatial structure and residents' physical and mental health.

Author Contributions: Conceptualization, Y.Y., H.L. and C.H.; methodology, Y.Y., H.L. and C.H.; software, Y.Y.; validation, Y.Y.; formal analysis, Y.Y. and H.L.; data curation, Y.Y. and H.L.; writing—original draft preparation, Y.Y., H.L. and C.H.; writing—review and editing, Y.Y., H.L. and C.H.; visualization, Y.Y.; project administration, Y.Y.; funding acquisition, Y.Y. All authors have read and agreed to the published version of the manuscript.

Funding: This research was funded by the General Project of Social Science of Beijing Municipal Education Commission (SM201810038012), the Social Science Foundation of Beijing, China (20JCC019), the Fundamental Research Funds for the Capital University of Economics and Business (QNTD202009).

Institutional Review Board Statement: Not applicable.

Informed Consent Statement: Not applicable.

Data Availability Statement: The data presented in this study are publicly available as explained in the main text.

Conflicts of Interest: The authors declare no conflict of interest.

References

1. Frenkel, A.; Ashkenazi, M. Measuring urban sprawl: How can we deal with it? *Environ. Plan. B Plan. Des.* **2008**, *35*, 56–79. [CrossRef]
2. Inostroza, L.; Baur, R.; Csaplovics, E. Urban sprawl and fragmentation in Latin America: A dynamic quantification and characterization of spatial patterns. *J. Environ. Manag.* **2013**, *115*, 87–97. [CrossRef]
3. Ewing, R.; Hamidi, S.; Grace, J.B.; Wei, Y.D. Does urban sprawl hold down upward mobility? *Landsc. Urban Plan.* **2016**, *148*, 80–88. [CrossRef]
4. Wang, X.; Shi, R.; Zhou, Y. Dynamics of urban sprawl and sustainable development in China. *Socio-Econ. Plan. Sci.* **2020**, *70*, 100736. [CrossRef]
5. Glaeser, E.L.; Kahn, M.E. Sprawl and Urban Growth. In *Handbook of Regional and Urban Economics*; JV Henderson and J.-F. Thisse: Amsterdam, The Netherlands, 2004; Volume 4. [CrossRef]
6. Aguilera, A.; Mignot, D. Urban sprawl, polycentrism and commuting. A comparison of seven French urban areas. *Urban Public Econ. Rev.* **2004**, *1*, 93–113.
7. Oueslati, W.; Alvanides, S.; Garrod, G. Determinants of urban sprawl in European cities. *Urban Stud.* **2015**, *52*, 1594–1614. [CrossRef]

8. Lv, Y.; Zhou, L.; Yao, G.; Zheng, X. Detecting the true urban polycentric pattern of Chinese cities in morphological dimensions: A multiscale analysis based on geospatial big data. *Cities* **2021**, *116*, 103298. [CrossRef]
9. OECD. *Rethinking Urban Sprawl Moving towards Sustainable Cities*; OECD Publishing: Paris, France, 2018. Available online: https://oe.cd/urban-sprawl (accessed on 20 April 2021).
10. Fallah, B.N.; Partridge, M.D.; Olfert, M.R. Urban sprawl and productivity: Evidence from US metropolitan areas. *Pap. Reg. Sci.* **2011**, *90*, 451–472. [CrossRef]
11. Hamidi, S.; Zandiatashbar, A. Does urban form matter for innovation productivity? A national multi-level study of the association between neighbourhood innovation capacity and urban sprawl. *Urban Stud.* **2019**, *56*, 1576–1594. [CrossRef]
12. Ye, H.; He, X.; Song, Y.; Li, X.; Zhang, G.; Lin, T.; Xiao, L. A sustainable urban form: The challenges of compactness from the viewpoint of energy consumption and carbon emission. *Energy Build.* **2015**, *93*, 90–98. [CrossRef]
13. Navamuel, E.L.; Morollón, F.R.; Cuartas, B.M. Energy consumption and urban sprawl: Evidence for the Spanish case. *J. Clean. Prod.* **2018**, *172*, 3479–3486. [CrossRef]
14. Stone, B., Jr. Urban sprawl and air quality in large US cities. *J. Environ. Manag.* **2008**, *86*, 688–698. [CrossRef] [PubMed]
15. Lu, C.; Liu, Y. Effects of China's urban form on urban air quality. *Urban Stud.* **2016**, *53*, 2607–2623. [CrossRef]
16. Mou, Y.; Song, Y.; Xu, Q.; He, Q.; Hu, A. Influence of urban-growth pattern on air quality in China: A study of 338 cities. *Int. J. Environ. Res. Public Health* **2018**, *15*, 1805. [CrossRef]
17. Sultana, S.; Weber, J. Journey-to-work patterns in the age of sprawl: Evidence from two midsize southern metropolitan areas. *Prof. Geogr.* **2007**, *59*, 193–208. [CrossRef]
18. Miller, M.D. The impacts of Atlanta's urban sprawl on forest cover and fragmentation. *Appl. Geogr.* **2012**, *34*, 171–179. [CrossRef]
19. Canedoli, C.; Crocco, F.; Comolli, R.; Padoa-Schioppa, E. Landscape fragmentation and urban sprawl in the urban region of Milan. *Landsc. Res.* **2018**, *43*, 632–651. [CrossRef]
20. Brueckner, J.K. Urban sprawl: Diagnosis and remedies. *Int. Reg. Sci. Rev.* **2000**, *23*, 160–171. [CrossRef]
21. Frumkin, H. Urban Sprawl and Public Health. *Public Health Rep.* **2002**, *117*, 201–217. [CrossRef]
22. Ewing, R.; Schieber, R.A.; Zegeer, C.V. Urban sprawl as a risk factor in motor vehicle occupant and pedestrian fatalities. *Am. J. Public Health* **2003**, *93*, 1541–1545. [CrossRef]
23. Frumkin, H.; Frank, L.; Frank, L.D.; Jackson, R.J. *Urban Sprawl and Public Health: Designing, Planning, and Building for Healthy Communities*; Island Press: Washington, DC, USA, 2004.
24. Iram, A.; Rasool, L.; Shahzad, F.; Saeed, Y. Impact of Urban sprawl on public health: An Analysis of Lahore-Pakistan. *World Appl. Sci. J.* **2012**, *20*, 80–86. [CrossRef]
25. Ewing, R.; Meakins, G.; Hamidi, S.; Nelson, A.C. Relationship between urban sprawl and physical activity, obesity, and morbidity–Update and refinement. *Health Place* **2014**, *26*, 118–126. [CrossRef]
26. Garrido-Cumbrera, M.; Ruiz, D.G.; Braçe, O.; Lara, E.L. Exploring the association between urban sprawl and mental health. *J. Transp. Health* **2018**, *10*, 381–390. [CrossRef]
27. Hamidi, S.; Ewing, R.; Tatalovich, Z.; Grace, J.B.; Berrigan, D. Associations between urban sprawl and life expectancy in the United States. *Int. J. Environ. Res. Public Health* **2018**, *15*, 861. [CrossRef]
28. Lopez, R. Urban sprawl and risk for being overweight or obese. *Am. J. Public Health* **2004**, *94*, 1574–1579. [CrossRef] [PubMed]
29. Zhao, Z.; Kaestner, R. Effects of urban sprawl on obesity. *J. Health Econ.* **2010**, *29*, 779–787. [CrossRef] [PubMed]
30. Wu, T.; Yang, S.; Liu, M.; Qiu, G.; Li, H.; Luo, M.; Jia, P. Urban sprawl and childhood obesity. *Obes. Rev.* **2021**, *22*, e13091. [CrossRef]
31. Lathey, V.; Guhathakurta, S.; Aggarwal, R.M. The impact of subregional variations in urban sprawl on the prevalence of obesity and related morbidity. *J. Plan. Educ. Res.* **2009**, *29*, 127–141. [CrossRef]
32. Fan, Y.; Song, Y. Is sprawl associated with a widening urban–suburban mortality gap? *J. Urban Health* **2009**, *86*, 708–728. [CrossRef]
33. Berrigan, D.; Tatalovich, Z.; Pickle, L.W.; Ewing, R.; Ballard-Barbash, R. Urban sprawl, obesity, and cancer mortality in the United States: Cross-sectional analysis and methodological challenges. *Int. J. Health Geogr.* **2014**, *13*, 1–15. [CrossRef] [PubMed]
34. Griffin, B.A.; Eibner, C.; Bird, C.E.; Jewell, A.; Margolis, K.; Shih, R.; Slaughter, M.E.; Whitsel, E.A.; Allison, M.; Escarce, J.J. The relationship between urban sprawl and coronary heart disease in women. *Health Place* **2013**, *20*, 51–61. [CrossRef] [PubMed]
35. Shen, Y.S.; Lung, S.C.C. Multiple impacts and pathways of urban form and environmental factors on cardiovascular mortality. *Sci. Total Environ.* **2020**, *738*, 139512. [CrossRef]
36. Trubka, R.; Newman, P.; Bilsborough, D. The costs of urban sprawl–Physical activity links to healthcare costs and productivity. *Environ. Des. Guide* **2010**, 1–13. Available online: https://www.jstor.org/stable/26150804 (accessed on 25 September 2021).
37. Çetin, M.; Bakırtaş, İ. Does Urbanization Induce the Health Expenditures? A Dynamic Macro-Panel Analysis for Developing Countries. *Dumlupınar Üniversitesi Sos. Bilimler Derg.* **2019**, *61*, 208–222.
38. World Health Organization. China-WHO Country Cooperation Strategy 2016–2020. 2016. Available online: https://iris.wpro.who.int/bitstream/handle/10665.1/13088/WPRO_2016_DPM_003_eng.pdf (accessed on 12 May 2021).
39. Garden, F.L.; Jalaludin, B.B. Impact of urban sprawl on overweight, obesity, and physical activity in Sydney, Australia. *J. Urban Health* **2009**, *86*, 19–30. [CrossRef] [PubMed]
40. Tsai, Y.H. Quantifying urban form: Compactness versus' sprawl'. *Urban Stud.* **2005**, *42*, 141–161. [CrossRef]
41. Koprowska, K.; Łaszkiewicz, E.; Kronenberg, J. Is urban sprawl linked to green space availability? *Ecol. Indic.* **2020**, *108*, 105723. [CrossRef]

42. Guerra, E.; Dong, X.; Kondo, M. Do denser neighborhoods have safer streets? population density and traffic safety in the Philadelphia Region. *J. Plan. Educ. Res.* **2019**. [CrossRef]
43. Travisi, C.M.; Camagni, R.; Nijkamp, P. Impacts of urban sprawl and commuting: A modelling study for Italy. *J. Transp. Geogr.* **2010**, *18*, 382–392. [CrossRef]
44. Wanner, M.; Götschi, T.; Martin-Diener, E.; Kahlmeier, S.; Martin, B.W. Active transport, physical activity, and body weight in adults: A systematic review. *Am. J. Prev. Med.* **2012**, *42*, 493–502. [CrossRef] [PubMed]
45. Fishman, E.; Böcker, L.; Helbich, M. Adult active transport in the Netherlands: An analysis of its contribution to physical activity requirements. *PLoS ONE* **2015**, *10*, e0121871. [CrossRef] [PubMed]
46. Sun, L.; Wei, J.; Duan, D.H.; Guo, Y.M.; Yang, D.X.; Jia, C.; Mi, X.T. Impact of Land-Use and Land-Cover Change on urban air quality in representative cities of China. *J. Atmos. Sol. -Terr. Phys.* **2016**, *142*, 43–54. [CrossRef]
47. Zheng, Z.; Zhang, X.; Wang, J.; Dandekar, A.; Kim, H.; Qiu, Y.; Xu, X.; Cui, Y.; Wang, A.; Chen, L.C.; et al. Exposure to fine airborne particulate matters induces hepatic fibrosis in murine models. *J. Hepatol.* **2015**, *63*, 1397–1404. [CrossRef]
48. Liu, C.; Chen, R.; Zhao, Y.; Ma, Z.; Bi, J.; Liu, Y.; Meng, X.; Wang, Y.; Chen, X.; Li, W.; et al. Associations between ambient fine particulate air pollution and hypertension: A nationwide cross-sectional study in China. *Sci. Total Environ.* **2017**, *584*, 869–874. [CrossRef]
49. Calderón-Garcidueñas, L.; Azzarelli, B.; Acuna, H.; Garcia, R.; Gambling, T.M.; Osnaya, N.; Monroy, S.; Tizapantzi, M.D.R.; Carson, J.L.; Villarreal-Calderon, A.; et al. Air pollution and brain damage. *Toxicol. Pathol.* **2002**, *30*, 373–389. [CrossRef] [PubMed]
50. Moulton, P.V.; Yang, W. Air pollution, oxidative stress, and Alzheimer's disease. *J. Environ. Public Health* **2012**, *472751*. [CrossRef] [PubMed]
51. Melis, G.; Gelormino, E.; Marra, G.; Ferracin, E.; Costa, G. The effects of the urban built environment on mental health: A cohort study in a large northern Italian city. *Int. J. Environ. Res. Public Health* **2015**, *12*, 14898–14915. [CrossRef] [PubMed]
52. Adaku, E. Urban sprawl: A view from developing and developed countries. *Afr. J. Geogr. Reg. Plan.* **2014**, *1*, 193–207.
53. Zhou, Y.; Ma, J.C.L. Economic restructuring and suburbanization in China. *Urban Geogr.* **2000**, *21*, 205–236. [CrossRef]
54. Feng, J.; Zhou, Y.; Wu, F. New Trends of Suburbanization in Beijing since 1990: From Government-led to Market-oriented. *Reg. Stud.* **2008**, *42*, 83–99. [CrossRef]
55. Lim, Y.H.; Kim, H.; Kim, J.H.; Bae, S.; Park, H.Y.; Hong, Y.C. Air pollution and symptoms of depression in elderly adults. *Environ. Health Perspect.* **2012**, *120*, 1023–1028. [CrossRef]
56. Wang, Y.; Eliot, M.N.; Koutrakis, P.; Gryparis, A.; Schwartz, J.D.; Coull, B.A.; Mittleman, M.; Milberg, W.P.; Lipsitz, L.A.; Wellenius, G. Ambient air pollution and depressive symptoms in older adults: Results from the MOBILIZE Boston study. *Environ. Health Perspect.* **2014**, *122*, 553–558. [CrossRef]
57. Lei, X.; Smith, J.P.; Sun, X.; Zhao, Y. Gender differences in cognition in China and reasons for change over time: Evidence from CHARLS. *J. Econ. Ageing* **2014**, *4*, 46–55. [CrossRef]
58. Zhao, Y.; Hu, Y.; Smith, J.P.; Strauss, J.; Yang, G. Cohort profile: The China health and retirement longitudinal study (CHARLS). *Int. J. Epidemiol.* **2014**, *43*, 61–68. [CrossRef] [PubMed]
59. Huang, X.; Huang, J.; Wen, D.; Li, J. An updated MODIS global urban extent product (MGUP) from 2001 to 2018 based on an automated mapping approach. *Int. J. Appl. Earth Obs. Geoinf.* **2021**, *95*, 102255. [CrossRef]
60. Mertes, C.M.; Schneider, A.; Sulla-Menashe, D.; Tatem, A.J.; Tan, B. Detecting change in urban areas at continental scales with MODIS data. *Remote Sens. Environ.* **2015**, *158*, 331–347. [CrossRef]
61. Sulla-Menashe, D.; Gray, J.M.; Abercrombie, S.P.; Friedl, M.A. Hierarchical mapping of annual global land cover 2001 to present: The MODIS Collection 6 Land Cover product. *Remote Sens. Environ.* **2019**, *222*, 183–194. [CrossRef]
62. Bai, Z.; Wang, J.; Wang, M.; Gao, M.; Sun, J. Accuracy assessment of multi-source gridded population distribution datasets in China. *Sustainability* **2018**, *10*, 1363. [CrossRef]
63. Cohen-Mansfield, J.; Pawlson, G.; Lipson, S.; Volpato, S. The measurement of health: A comparison of indices of disease severity. *J. Clin. Epidemiol.* **2001**, *54*, 1094–1102. [CrossRef]
64. Wang, Y.; Luo, N. Air Pollution, Health Depreciation and Medical Costs: Research Based on the Three Perspectives of Physical Health, Mental Health and Social Adaptability. *Econ. Res. J.* **2020**, *55*, 80–97. (In Chinese)
65. Cheng, S.T.; Chan, A.C. The center for epidemiologic studies depression scale in older Chinese: Thresholds for long and short forms. *Int. J. Geriatr. Psychiatry A J. Psychiatry Late Life Allied Sci.* **2005**, *20*, 465–470. [CrossRef]
66. Qin, X.; Wang, S.; Hsieh, C.R. The prevalence of depression and depressive symptoms among adults in China: Estimation based on a National Household Survey. *China Econ. Rev.* **2018**, *51*, 271–282. [CrossRef]
67. Fulton, W.B.; Pendall, R.; Nguyễn, M.; Harrison, A. *Who Sprawls Most? How Growth Patterns Differ across the US*; Brookings Institution, Center on Urban and Metropolitan Policy: Washington, DC, USA, 2001.
68. Koball, H.L.; Moiduddin, E.; Henderson, J.; Goesling, B.; Besculides, M. What do we know about the link between marriage and health? *J. Fam. Issues* **2010**, *31*, 1019–1040. [CrossRef]
69. Cutler, D.M.; Lleras-Muney, A.; Vogl, T. Socioeconomic status and health: Dimensions and mechanisms. *NBER Working Paper* **2008**, 14333. [CrossRef]
70. Cutler, D.M.; Glaeser, E. What explains differences in smoking, drinking, and other health-related behaviors? *Am. Econ. Rev.* **2005**, *95*, 238–242. [CrossRef] [PubMed]

71. Bagnardi, V.; Rota, M.; Botteri, E.; Tramacere, I.; Islami, F.; Fedirko, V.; Scotti, L.; Jenab, M.; Turati, F.; Pasquali, E.; et al. Alcohol consumption and site-specific cancer risk: A comprehensive dose–response meta-analysis. *Br. J. Cancer* **2015**, *112*, 580–593. [CrossRef] [PubMed]
72. Garaycoechea, J.I.; Crossan, G.; Langevin, F.; Mulderrig, L.; Louzada, S.; Yang, F.; Guilbaud, G.; Park, N.; Roerink, S.; Nik-Zainal, S.; et al. Alcohol and endogenous aldehydes damage chromosomes and mutate stem cells. *Nature* **2018**, *553*, 171–177. [CrossRef] [PubMed]
73. Kahn, J.R.; Pearlin, L.I. Financial strain over the life course and health among older adults. *J. Health Soc. Behav.* **2006**, *47*, 17–31. [CrossRef] [PubMed]
74. Van Doorslaer, E.; Masseria, C.; Koolman, X. Inequalities in access to medical care by income in developed countries. *CMAJ* **2006**, *174*, 177–183. [CrossRef]
75. Li, G.; Li, F. Urban sprawl in China: Differences and socioeconomic drivers. *Sci. Total Environ.* **2019**, *673*, 367–377. [CrossRef]
76. Tao, L.I. Spatial distribution of the aged population in shanghai and influencing factors. *City Plan. Rev.* **2020**, *6*, 39–46. (In Chinese) [CrossRef]
77. Li, Z.; Yuan, L. Professional intergenerational mobility in entering state owned departments: Family background and education. *S. China J. Econ.* **2019**, *9*, 69–83. (In Chinese) [CrossRef]

International Journal of
Environmental Research and Public Health

MDPI

Article

How Much Are People Willing to Pay for Clean Air? Analyzing Housing Prices in Response to the Smog Free Tower in Xi'an

Haiyong Zhang [1,2], Sanqin Mao [2,*] and Xinyu Wang [3]

1 School of Mathematics and Finance, Chuzhou University, Chuzhou 239000, China; haiyongzhang@chzu.edu.cn
2 School of International and Public Affairs, Shanghai Jiao Tong University, Shanghai 200030, China
3 School of Economics and Management, China University of Mining and Technology, Xuzhou 221116, China; wangxinyu@cumt.edu.cn
* Correspondence: alicemao01@sjtu.edu.cn

Abstract: The Smog Free Tower (SFT) in the city of Xi'an, China, is the world's first outdoor architecture that uses solar energy and filtration technology to purify polluted air. It provides a unique opportunity to explore residents' willingness to pay for air quality and their related behaviors. Drawing on data collected after the establishment of the SFT, this paper reveals the characteristics of changes in people's willingness to pay for clean air. We found that, prior to the release of an assessment report on the SFT, housing prices had an inverted U-shaped relationship with the distance to the SFT, which indicated people tended to purchase houses a certain distance away from the SFT. The threshold value of distance was inversely related to the greening ratio of the residential area. However, after the publication of the experimental report on the SFT, housing prices decreased as the distance to the SFT increased, indicating the closer the house was to the SFT, the more likely people were to buy it. These changes confirmed that people are willing to pay for clean air. The convenience of transportation had a significant moderating effect on the willingness to pay for clean air, however. In other words, people may buy houses with lower air quality if they have better transportation accessibility. The findings of this paper may have practical implications for environmental governance, urban planning, residential satisfaction, and real estate market regulation.

Keywords: Smog Free Tower; air purification; housing price; moderating effect; traffic convenience

Citation: Zhang, H.; Mao, S.; Wang, X. How Much Are People Willing to Pay for Clean Air? Analyzing Housing Prices in Response to the Smog Free Tower in Xi'an. *IJERPH* **2021**, *18*, 10210. https://doi.org/10.3390/ijerph181910210

Academic Editors: María-del-Mar Alonso-Almeida, Pasquale Avino and Paul B. Tchounwou

Received: 4 August 2021
Accepted: 25 September 2021
Published: 28 September 2021

1. Introduction

Air pollution has increasingly become a worldwide public health concern [1,2]. It has been reported that air pollution not only increases the risk of various physical illnesses [2–4], such as respiratory diseases, neurodegenerative diseases, hypertension, cardiovascular diseases, and circulatory diseases, but can also induce severe insomnia and psychological problems [5,6]. Air pollution is more pronounced in metropolitan cities, where urban factors such as heavy automobile traffic and high population density produce more air pollution [6]. To prevent or minimize pollution damage, a series of measures have been taken against air pollution, including adding green spaces, more efficiently reducing emissions, the adjustment of the energy structure, and the development of alternative energy resources [7,8].

In China, air pollution has attracted public attention in recent decades, especially following the release of the documentary "Under the Dome" by Chai Jing in 2015 [9]. People's awareness of air pollution has continued to increase as haze has become more frequent and serious in recent years. To protect themselves from hazardous haze, many citizens use air purifiers indoors and wear anti-smog face masks outdoors. The government has also enacted series of projects to build greener cities for citizens [10]. However, the governance of outdoor air pollution is more difficult than that of indoor pollution.

Therefore, developing an outdoor technical system to absorb haze and purify the air has become an urgent and crucial issue.

To this end, the world's first outdoor air purification building, which is known as the Smog Free Tower (SFT), was built in June 2016 in the city of Xi'an, China. The full name of the tower is the Solar-Assisted Large-Scale Cleaning System (SALSCS in short) [11,12]. It is the first architecture in the world to use solar energy and filtering techniques to clean polluted air [12]. Its basic operation principle is to inhale polluted air from the bottom of the tower first, heat the air by solar energy, then dispose of the air using a filter net and photocatalytic material, before lastly exporting fresh air through the diversion tower. The project group first unveiled an experimental report on the SFT in April 2018. It reported that the SFT was able to improve the air quality in a range of 10 km around the tower. The tower can reduce the concentration of $PM_{2.5}$ particulate pollution by about 11 to 19 percent. Moreover, the neighborhoods closest to the SFT also benefit from the purification treatment, even if affected by polluted air inhaled by the tower clusters in areas near the SFT [13].

Air quality has increasingly become an important factor influencing citizens' residential choices [14]. It has been shown that housing prices are higher in places with better air quality [15,16]. In other words, housing prices can be an important instrument to measure people's willingness to pay for clean air, using the hedonic model [17,18]. As the first outdoor air-purifying tower, the SFT is a completely new concept, which could send divergent messages to residents at different stages. Therefore, the operation of the tower provides a unique opportunity to analyze the impacts of residents' willingness to pay for clean air. However, despite much public attention on the SFT, there have been few published studies on the willingness to pay for clean air in this particular situation, except for one study based on data from January 2016 to June 2017, which revealed that the SFT had increased the housing prices of the purified area by 4% [19]. However, the cited study only focused on the completion period of the SFT. Thus, it may not have fully captured the impacts on housing prices caused by changes in public attitudes. Much more consideration should be given to the public's responses in a longer observation window, especially after the release of the assessment report for the SFT. Did the publication of the test report increase people's willingness to pay for clean air? Before the publication of the test report, to what extent did the risk of the uncertainty around the effectiveness and operation process of the SFT influence residents' housing choices? Moreover, what role do traditional decisive variables, such as the greening ratio and transportation accessibility, play in the relationship between the distance to the SFT and housing prices? This study aimed to answer these questions and provide a renewed understanding of the willingness to pay for clean air based on data before and after the announcement of the assessment report of the SFT. Such research may help environment policymakers to consider the impacts of environmental improvement projects, and also enlighten people around practices related to real estate development, transportation, and urban planning in China and even the world.

In the following sections, the theoretical perspective and hypothesis development are illustrated. Based on the literature review, suitable variables, models, and data are outlined. Then, the housing prices of the affected area before and after the assessment report was released are presented. Further, hedonic models are employed to analyze how much people are willing to pay for clean air. Lastly, the main findings are summarized, and policy implications are also highlighted.

2. Review of the Literature and Hypothesis Development

Housing prices have long been a popular topic in urban studies. Unraveling the determinants of housing prices has attracted a significant amount of research attention. Transportation accessibility and neighborhood and structural characteristics are the key variables in determining housing prices [20–23]. In recent years, the positive effects of air quality on residents' choice of residential location have drawn considerable attention [24]. Its attraction has grown with the rising concern about environment pollution. However, unlike the other three groups of variables, the measurement of residents' willingness to pay for clean air is difficult, in that air quality has no fixed value as a type of public good [19]. Two major perspectives regarding the measurement of the economic value of clean air can be identified [19,25]. First, the stated preference approach posits that residents can accurately pinpoint their willingness to pay for different levels of air quality [26]. The contingent valuation model is generally employed to directly examine willingness to pay. However, the results obtained using this approach are likely to be biased because residents may not present their willingness correctly and objectively [19]. The revealed preference approach gauges the economic value of clean air through market data, mainly based on the hedonic price model. Existing research often used the impact on housing prices to evaluate willingness to pay [27,28]. This approach could also give biased results in view of the spatial self-selecting problem [19].

While a plethora of studies have delved into residents' willingness to pay for clean air in developed countries, intellectual inquiries about the extent people are willing to pay for air quality in developing countries have just begun in recent years [19,29]. China has experienced unprecedented industrialization and urbanization in the past few decades, along with worsening air quality in most cities [30,31]. Scholars have reported on the spatial spillover effects of city-level air pollution on housing prices [32,33]. Nonetheless, there is a relatively small body of micro-data research concerning the willingness to pay for clean air. As an exception, Lan et al. (2020) argued that the extant studies suffer from self-selection bias, and suggested that the SFT provides a unique opportunity to address the self-selection problem [19]. Using the hedonic model, they calculated the net effect of the SFT on housing prices and revealed that the purification area's housing prices have increased after the installment of the SFT. Based on the effectiveness of the SFT on changing housing prices in the above study, our present paper attempted to further explore the dynamics of residents' willingness to pay for clean air and the moderating effects of three groups of variables on the relationship between air quality and housing prices. Specifically, four hypotheses concerning the relationship between the distance to the SFT and housing prices are proposed.

First, we proposed that the actual functioning of the SFT is critical to residents' willingness to pay and related behavior. When the SFT was completed, the news media reported its general situation and function, which attracted wide public attention [34,35]. However, it can take time for people to trust new technology [36]. Before the assessment report of the tower's trial operation was published, positive expectations of the effect of the SFT may not have formed due to residents' concern regarding the potential negative impacts of the SFT. There was some concern that the polluted air absorbed by the SFT would aggregate in areas near the SFT, worsening the air pollution close to the SFT. The noise and radiation were also considered significant potential risks when choosing to live near the SFT. On the other hand, residents may have been interested in the opportunity to maximize access to clean air after the results of the trial operation were published. Thus, they may have tended to choose residential areas a certain distance away from the SFT, while areas within a closer area were of less interest. This means that there could have been a critical distance, rather than the closer the better being the rule, wherein if the distance to the SFT was less than the threshold, the housing prices could be expected to increase as the distance increased. Once beyond the threshold, the housing prices could be expected to decrease as the distance increased. Therefore, Hypothesis 1 of this study was proposed as follows:

Hypothesis 1 (H1). *Before the release of the assessment report of the trial operation, a critical distance would have existed, and housing prices could be expected to rise and then fall with the distance.*

Although people tended to select houses located away from the critical distance, the value of the critical distance was also impacted by the greening ratio of the residential area. The important role of green plants in preventing and controlling air pollution has been well evidenced [37,38]. Green plants offer the absorption and purification of atmospheric pollutants in several ways, such as dust reduction, dust retention, dust absorption, dust fall, and dust prevention [38,39]. Thus, residential areas with plentiful greenery have a strong purifying ability of their own, which may have reduced concerns about the potential negative or limited effects of the SFT. On that account, living closer to the SFT may be more acceptable if the living area has a higher rate of greening. It seems the greening ratio acted as an insurance policy, ensuring maximum access to fresh air. Thus, based on Hypothesis 1, we proposed Hypothesis 2 as follows:

Hypothesis 2 (H2). *Before the release of the assessment report of the trial operation, the value of the critical distance was inversely related to the greening ratio of the residential area.*

The assessment report was published at a press conference on 17 April 2018, by the Chinese Academy of Sciences, and was reported on in detail by the media. Most of the public's questions were addressed at the press conference. The report demonstrated that the SFT effectively alleviated the haze by reducing 11% to 19% of the $PM_{2.5}$ concentration level, and a surrounding area of 10 square kilometers benefited. Moreover, after the polluted air is sucked into the tower for purification, the clean air sinks and circulates from a height of 60 m, so the air is purified in the closest neighborhoods surrounding the SFT [11,12]. That is, polluted air does not accumulate in areas near the SFT. In addition, the report clarified that no radioactive materials were used during the construction and operation processes of the SFT, eliminating any potential radiation risks of living in the area close to the SFT. After the press conference, public uncertainty was reduced, and an understanding that the closer one lives to the SFT, the cleaner the air will be became widespread. Thus, the demand for houses close to the SFT was expected to increase due to the greater access to clean air. Accordingly, we proposed Hypothesis 3 as follows:

Hypothesis 3 (H3). *After the release of the assessment report of the trial operation, housing prices decreased with increasing distance from the SFT.*

The release of the assessment report convinced the public that the closer they were to the SFT, the easier it would be to obtain clean air. However, since residential choice is influenced by many structural and environmental attributes, factors related to housing prices are complicated [22,40]. Locational convenience is one of the most important factors [40]. For example, people may prefer to live further away from the SFT for traffic convenience. Thus, people generally make a trade-off choice between living closer to the SFT and convenience [22]. Thus, it is reasonable to expect convenience to have a moderating role on the impact of clean air on housing prices. Hypothesis 4 in this study was as follows:

Hypothesis 4 (H4). *After the release of the assessment report of the trial operation, the relationship between the distance to the SFT and housing prices was moderated by convenience.*

Figure 1 displays the conceptual model, which includes the four main testable hypotheses.

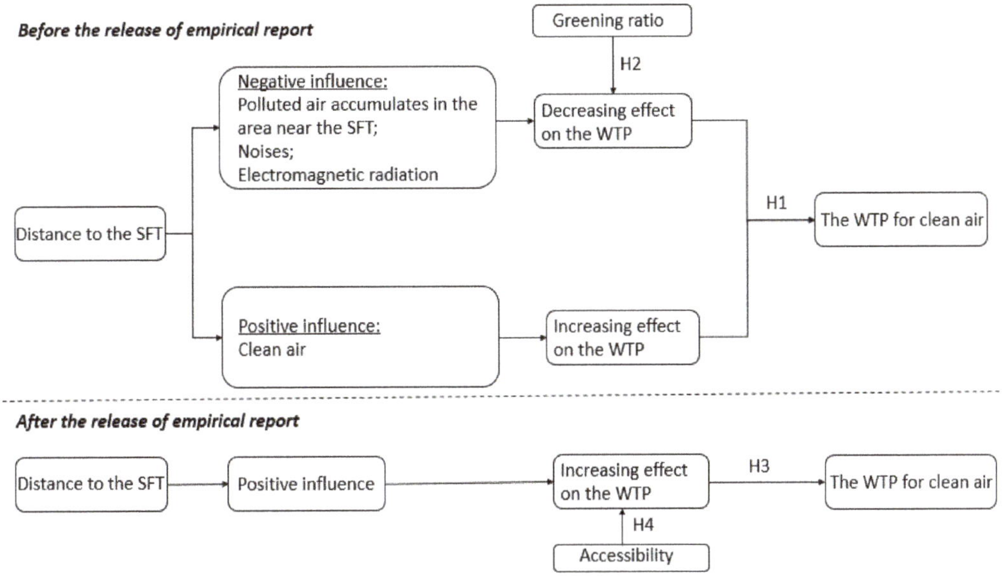

Figure 1. The proposed model (WTP: willingness to pay).

3. Methodology, Variables, and Data

To test the above four theoretical hypotheses, suitable methodologies, variables, and data were needed. In this section, we elaborate on the models used to capture the relationship between housing prices and the distance to the SFT, describe the relevant variables in detail, and show the characteristics of the selected data.

3.1. Model Specifications

As a universal model to capture housing buyers' willingness to pay for various housing characteristics, the hedonic model was employed in this study. Following the literature, housing prices should be a function of a number of variables related to housing features and location [22,41,42].

The baseline hedonic model applied in this paper is given by:

$$\begin{aligned} \mathrm{HOUPRI_{it}} = {} & \alpha + \beta_1 \mathrm{DISTAN}_i + \beta_2 \mathrm{DISTAN}_i^2 + \sum_{j=1}^{k} \gamma_j x_{ijt} + \mathrm{dummy_{circle}} \\ & + \mathrm{dummy_{business}} + \mathrm{dummy_{year}} + \mathrm{dummy_{season}} + \varepsilon_{it} \end{aligned} \quad (1)$$

In Equation (1), $\mathrm{HOUPRI_{it}}$ represents the housing price of neighborhood i at quarter t. $\mathrm{DISTAN_i}$ is the linear distance from neighborhood i to the SFT, and $\mathrm{DISTAN_i}^2$ is the square of the distance. x_{ijt} is the value of the control variable j in neighborhood i at quarter t (the control variables include the number of households in the neighborhood, greening ratio, floor area ratio, number of bus stations, supermarkets, restaurants, banks, parks, schools, and hospitals within a 1 km radius). $\mathrm{dummy_{circle}}$ is the dummy variable for the loop line of the neighborhood, $\mathrm{dummy_{business}}$ is the dummy variable for the business district of the neighborhood, $\mathrm{dummy_{year}}$ is the dummy variable for the built year of the neighborhood, and $\mathrm{dummy_{season}}$ is the dummy variable for the season. α is the constant term, β_i and γ_j are the coefficients to be estimated, and ε_{it} is the error term. Notably, the logarithm of the housing price is applied in the regression models.

Despite the important effect of wind direction on the association between air quality and housing prices, the effect of wind direction could be ignored in the framework of this study for two reasons. First, unlike emissions that are clearly visible or have a pungent odor, clean air is difficult to detect by sight and smell [43]. In this context, residents tend to be more concerned about the distance to the SFT rather than the wind direction. Second, the prevailing wind direction in Xi'an is northeast and southwest, and the frequency of perennial static wind is 29% [44]. Thus, regardless of where a house is located around the SFT, it is difficult for people to balance the seasonal changes in wind direction. Wind direction was therefore not considered in our model specifications.

To capture the moderating effect of the greening ratio before the release of the assessment report, the interaction of distance and the greening ratio was added to Equation (1):

$$\begin{aligned}\mathrm{HOUPRI}_{it} &= \alpha + \beta_1(\mathrm{DISTAN}_i \times \mathrm{GRERAT}_i) + \beta_2(\mathrm{DISTAN}_i \times \mathrm{GRERAT}_i)^2 \\ &+ \sum_{j=1}^{k}\gamma_j x_{ijt} + \mathrm{dummy}_{circle} + \mathrm{dummy}_{business} + \mathrm{dummy}_{year} + \mathrm{dummy}_{season} + \varepsilon_{it}\end{aligned} \tag{2}$$

where GRERAT_i is the greening ratio of neighborhood i. The meanings of the other symbols are the same as those in Equation (1).

To capture the moderating effects of convenience after the release of the assessment report, the interaction terms of the distance and convenience variables were added to the hedonic model:

$$\begin{aligned}\mathrm{HOUPRI}_{it} = \alpha &+ \beta\mathrm{DISTAN}_i + \sum_{j=1}^{k}\eta_j(\mathrm{DISTAN}_i \times x_{ijt}) + \sum_{j=1}^{k}\gamma_j x_{ijt} \\ &+ \mathrm{dummy}_{circle} + \mathrm{dummy}_{business} + \mathrm{dummy}_{year} + \mathrm{dummy}_{season} + \varepsilon_{it}\end{aligned} \tag{3}$$

where $\mathrm{DISTAN}_i \times x_{ijt}$ is the interaction term of the distance and convenience variables, and β and η_j are the coefficients to be estimated. The meanings of the other symbols are the same as those in Equation (1).

3.2. Variables and Data

The SFT was operated in August 2016, and the assessment report was released in April 2018. Therefore, the time frame of March 2017 to March 2018 was selected as the stage before the publication of the assessment report, and May 2018 to December 2018 as the stage after the publication of the assessment report. The research area in this paper included the neighborhoods inside a radius of about 5 km around the SFT, and the housing prices of these neighborhoods were observed during both stages. Figure 2 shows the geography of the research site. The SFT is located in Changan District, which is in the suburbs of the city of Xi'an. The appearance of the SFT and the surrounding environment is shown in Figure 3. This includes residential areas and varied types of neighborhoods, including newly built neighborhoods, old neighborhoods built before 2000, and neighborhoods under construction. After the demarcation of the boundary of the research area, 108 neighborhoods were selected. The data on second-hand housing prices and the control and dummy variables for the 108 neighborhoods were collected from the website Anjuke (https://xa.anjuke.com) (accessed on 20 January 2020), which is a large chain real estate company in China. The linear distance from the neighborhood to the SFT was gauged based on the Baidu electronic map. The definitions and statistics of the variables in this study are shown in Table 1.

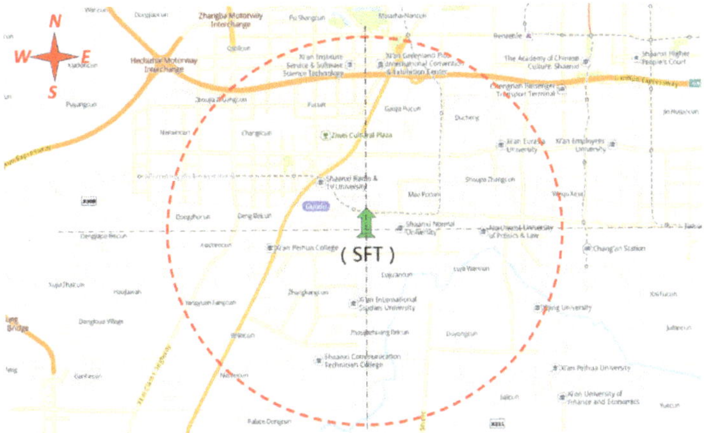

Figure 2. Research site.

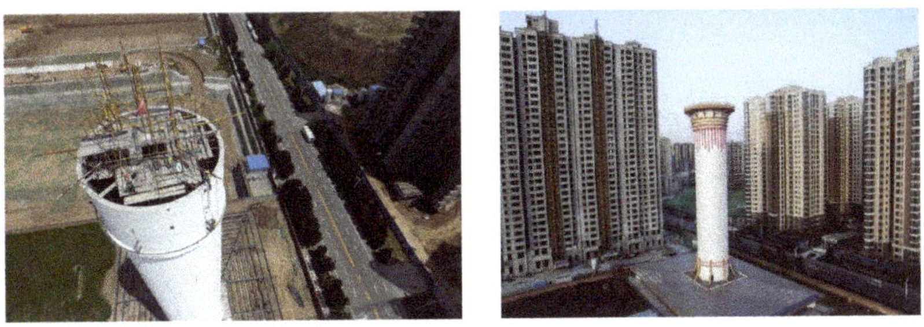

Figure 3. Pictures of the SFT (source: https://image.baidu.com, accessed on 12 July 2021).

Table 1. Definition and descriptive statistics of the variables.

Variable	Definition	Unit or Coding	Mean	St. Dev.	Minimum	Maximum
HOUPRI	Average unit price of the neighborhood	Yuan/m^2	10,353.53	4625.321	1800	32,673
DISTAN	Distance to the SWF	km	3.33	1.325	0.37	5.1
HOUHOL	Neighborhood size	households	1537.99	2038.521	36	12,746
GRERAT	Greening ratio	%	36.64	8.180	16	60
FAR	Floor area ratio	%	3.42	1.309	0.96	10.3
BUSTOP	Number of bus stops	PCs	6.20	1.977	1	13
SUPMAR	Number of supermarkets	PCs	7.21	2.869	1	14
RESTAU	Number of restaurants	PCs	6.67	4.481	0	16
BANK	Number of banks	PCs	6.01	3.929	0	24
PARK	Number of parks	PCs	1.06	1.030	0	4
SCHOOL	Number of schools	PCs	5.21	2.949	0	14
HOSPIT	Number of hospitals	PCs	2.24	2.565	0	11
SECRIN	Whether located within the second ring (Yes = 1, No = 0)	—	0.01	0.096	0	1
SECTHI	Whether located between the second and third ring (Yes = 1, No = 0)	—	0.21	0.410	0	1
BEYTHI	Whether located outside of the third ring (Yes = 1, No = 0)	—	0.77	0.422	0	1

Note: — indicates that the corresponding variable is unitless. Due to limited space, season dummy variables (8), business district dummy variables (19), and built year dummy variables (23) are not included in the table. They can be found in the Appendix A Table A1. The included bus stops, supermarkets, restaurants, banks, parks, schools, and hospitals are all within 1 km of the neighborhoods.

4. Empirical Findings and Discussions

In the subsequent analysis, we first give detailed information on the dynamics of housing prices between March 2017 and December 2018. Then, the hedonic models specified above are applied to test the changes in the effects of distance to the SFT on housing prices before and after the release of the assessment report.

4.1. Descriptive Analysis

Based on the collected data, we calculated the average housing prices within 5 km of the SFT in each observational window. Figure 4 shows how the housing prices changed as the distance to the SFT increased from March 2017 to December 2018. Several observations can be derived from the figure. First, the prices of all neighborhoods show an obvious upward trend, which indicates the rising trend in the housing market in the city. Second, intuitively, housing prices inside the radius of 5 km have rapidly increased since the disclosure of the assessment report, especially in the area within a radius of 2 km. This validates our assumption that residents' housing choice behavior would change due to the assessment report disclosure. Third, the housing prices of neighborhoods located less than 1 km from the SFT experienced complex dynamics; they were the lowest at the start of the observational window, but the highest at the end. This demonstrates how people's willingness to pay for clean air increased with the operation process of the SFT.

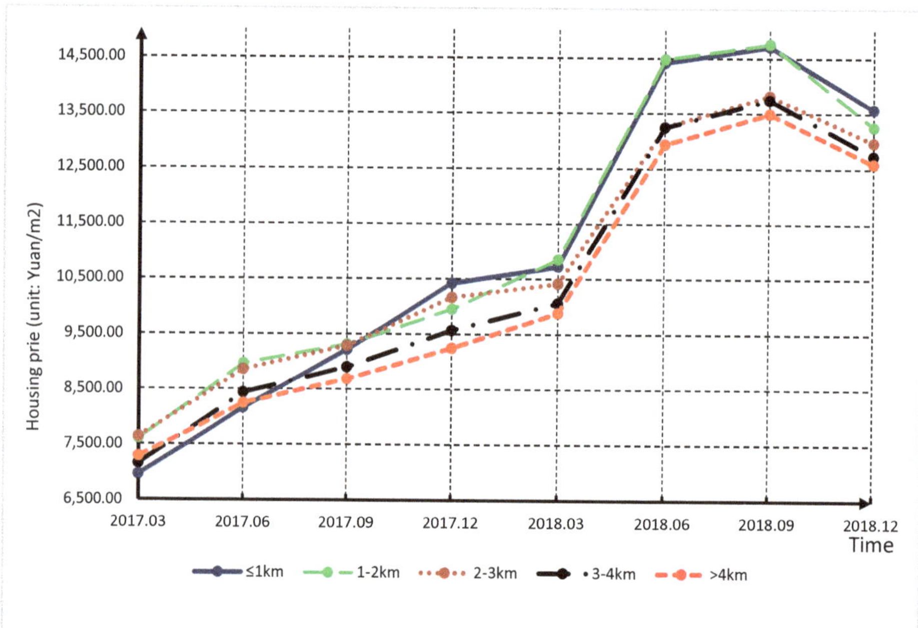

Figure 4. Average housing prices of different radiation areas from March 2017 to December 2018.

4.2. Estimation Results and Discussions

Equations (1)–(3) were used to further test the hypotheses highlighted above. The estimation results of these models are presented in Tables 2–5. In general, the results supported our hypotheses. As predicted, the change in people's expectations regarding the effectiveness of the SFT leads to changes in their willingness to pay for clean air. After the confirmation of the effectiveness of the SFT, the distance to the SFT became a significant variable influencing housing prices. In addition, the ideal distance also depended on the greening ratio and transportation accessibility of the residential area.

Table 2. Link between the distance to the SFT and housing prices before the release of the assessment report.

	Model 1	Model 2	Model 3	Model 4
	HOUPRI	**HOUPRI**	**HOUPRI**	**HOUPRI**
DISTAN	0.09146	0.05124	0.04663	0.06672
	(0.07267)	(0.05297)	(0.05982)	(0.05247)
$DISTAN^2$	−0.14607 ***	−0.19027 **	−0.19397 **	−0.23079 ***
	(0.04452)	(0.08232)	(0.09080)	(0.07987)
HOUHOL		0.08676 ***	0.07006 ***	0.07089 ***
		(0.01225)	(0.01315)	(0.01161)
GRERAT		0.00030	0.00137	0.00238
		(0.00195)	(0.00241)	(0.00215)
FAR		−0.04047 ***	−0.05460 ***	−0.05304 ***
		(0.01059)	(0.01225)	(0.01072)
BUSTOP		0.10697 **	0.12980 ***	0.10775 ***
		(0.04422)	(0.04396)	(0.03915)
SUPMAR		−0.01296 **	−0.00923 *	−0.00985 **
		(0.00521)	(0.00559)	(0.00491)
RESTAU		−0.00082	0.00610	0.00581
		(0.00431)	(0.00479)	(0.00419)
BANK		0.00958 **	0.01448 ***	0.01182 **
		(0.00444)	(0.00517)	(0.00457)
PARK		0.01388	0.03416 **	0.02093
		(0.01518)	(0.01689)	(0.01526)
SCHOOL		−0.01257 **	0.00181	0.00097
		(0.00601)	(0.00678)	(0.00592)
HOSPIT		0.00046	0.01072	0.02143 **
		(0.00921)	(0.00958)	(0.00878)
$dummy_{business}$		Yes	Yes	Yes
$dummy_{year}$			Yes	Yes
$dummy_{season}$				Yes
$dummy_{circle}$				Yes
C	9.10578 ***	8.55806 ***	8.06303 ***	7.73887 ***
	(0.03889)	(0.14620)	(0.19919)	(0.22661)
N	540	540	540	540
F	12.90515	23.53453	18.48574	24.04787
Root MSE	0.39413	0.27077	0.24719	0.21589
R-squared	0.04586	0.57233	0.65893	0.74357

Note: *, **, and *** indicate statistical significance at the 10%, 5%, and 1% levels, respectively. Standard errors are in parentheses.

Table 3. The moderating role of the greening ratio before the release of the assessment report.

	Model 5	Model 6	Model 7	Model 8
	HOUPRI	**HOUPRI**	**HOUPRI**	**HOUPRI**
DISTAN × GRERAT	0.00566 ***	0.00221 *	0.00328 **	0.00299 ***
	(0.00080)	(0.00124)	(0.00131)	(0.00115)
$(DISTAN \times GRERAT)^2$	−0.02955 ***	−0.01698 ***	−0.02256 ***	−0.02216 ***
	(0.00385)	(0.00577)	(0.00607)	(0.00529)
Control Variables		Yes	Yes	Yes
$dummy_{business}$		Yes	Yes	Yes
$dummy_{year}$			Yes	Yes
$dummy_{season}$				Yes
$dummy_{circle}$				Yes
C	8.86052 ***	8.59337 ***	8.38673 ***	8.02393 ***
	(0.04361)	(0.36108)	(0.44121)	(0.39258)
N	540	540	540	540
F	29.41852	23.03047	18.59793	24.76161

Table 3. *Cont.*

	Model 5	Model 6	Model 7	Model 8
	HOUPRI	HOUPRI	HOUPRI	HOUPRI
Root MSE	0.38305	0.26993	0.24520	0.21355
R-squared	0.09875	0.57580	0.66508	0.74911

Note: *, **, and *** indicate statistical significance at the 10%, 5%, and 1% levels, respectively. Standard errors are in parentheses. The control variables are the same as in Table 2.

Table 4. The relationship between the distance and housing prices after the release of the assessment report.

	Model 9	Model 10	Model 11	Model 12
	HOUPRI	HOUPRI	HOUPRI	HOUPRI
DISTAN	−0.03916	−0.13825 **	−0.15634 **	−0.12153 *
	(0.08206)	(0.06156)	(0.06889)	(0.06994)
$DISTAN^2$	−0.00513	0.00113	0.00035	−0.00123
	(0.00534)	(0.00456)	(0.00477)	(0.00484)
Control Variables		Yes	Yes	Yes
$dummy_{business}$		Yes	Yes	Yes
$dummy_{year}$			Yes	Yes
$dummy_{season}$				Yes
$dummy_{circle}$				Yes
C	9.52623 ***	8.56181 ***	8.03078 ***	8.01684 ***
	(0.04537)	(0.17654)	(0.25695)	(0.25425)
N	324	324	324	324
F	5.07284	20.10844	14.87738	14.36817
Root MSE	0.34820	0.21165	0.19605	0.19356
R-squared	0.03064	0.67308	0.74058	0.75084

Note: *, **, and *** indicate statistical significance at the 10%, 5%, and 1% levels, respectively. Standard errors are in parentheses. The control variables are the same as in Table 2.

Table 5. The moderating roles of accessibilities after the release of the assessment report.

	Model 13	Model 14	Model 15	Model 16
	HOUPRI	HOUPRI	HOUPRI	HOUPRI
DISTAN	−0.19616	−0.40333 *	−0.44946 *	−0.62495 **
	(0.20141)	(0.23198)	(0.24382)	(0.25382)
DISTAN × BUSTOP	0.06071	0.15067 *	0.17054 *	0.20703 **
	(0.07273)	(0.08189)	(0.08824)	(0.09046)
DISTAN × SUPMAR	0.06140	−0.04347	−0.05022	0.01202
	(0.07566)	(0.10260)	(0.10270)	(0.10528)
DISTAN × RESTAU	−0.01030	−0.00983	−0.01281	−0.01796 *
	(0.00745)	(0.00802)	(0.00945)	(0.00966)
DISTAN × BANK	0.03497 ***	0.03732 ***	0.03732 ***	0.03154 **
	(0.01145)	(0.01425)	(0.01418)	(0.01428)
DISTAN × PARK	−0.01574	0.03306	0.02737	0.02981
	(0.03286)	(0.03961)	(0.04058)	(0.04123)
DISTAN × SCHOOL	−0.03510 ***	−0.00842	−0.00324	0.00033
	(0.01153)	(0.01516)	(0.01748)	(0.01741)
DISTAN × HOSPIT	−0.02443	−0.02850	−0.02503	−0.00511
	(0.02905)	(0.03624)	(0.03652)	(0.03717)
Control Variables	Yes	Yes	Yes	Yes
$dummy_{business}$	Yes	Yes	Yes	Yes
$dummy_{year}$		Yes	Yes	Yes
$dummy_{season}$			Yes	Yes
$dummy_{circle}$				Yes
C	8.27132 ***	7.98072 ***	8.08150 ***	8.28313 ***
	(0.35942)	(0.40710)	(0.44657)	(0.45350)

Table 5. *Cont.*

	Model 13	Model 14	Model 15	Model 16
	HOUPRI	HOUPRI	HOUPRI	HOUPRI
N	324	324	324	324
F	18.28400	14.14256	13.67857	13.53692
Root MSE	0.20610	0.19352	0.19248	0.19102
R-squared	0.69637	0.75189	0.75732	0.76279

Note: *, **, and *** indicate statistical significance at the 10%, 5%, and 1% levels, respectively. Standard errors are in parentheses. The control variables are the same as in Table 2.

4.2.1. Association between the Distance to the SFT and Housing Prices before the Release of the Assessment Report

Table 2 shows the link between the distance to the SFT and housing prices. In Model 1 of Table 2, housing prices were only regressed on distance and the square of it. To obtain more accurate estimation results, we gradually added control variables in Models 2, 3, and 4. Further, we controlled for the general time trend effect by employing a time dummy for each season ($dummy_{season}$) in Model 4. The four models showed that the square of the distance was significantly and negatively related to housing prices, which indicates that there is an inverted U-shaped relationship between the distance to the SFT and housing prices, and the relationship is robust. Model 4 shows the lowest value of the Root MSE but the highest R-squared, indicating the model with all dummies had the highest estimated accuracy. Then, the critical distance was calculated using the estimated coefficients of distance and the square in Model 4. It was revealed that the distance to the SFT was positively related to housing prices when the distance was shorter than 145 m, whereas it was negatively related to housing prices when the distance was greater than 145 m. This indicates that people tended to choose houses 145 m away from the tower and as close to it as possible, probably because people were worried about the poor purification effects when too close to the tower, but were not willing to lose the opportunity to obtain the maximum amount of clean air before the release of the assessment report. Therefore, Hypothesis 1 was confirmed.

Table 3 presents the moderating effect of the greening ratio on the relationship between the distance to the SFT and housing prices. Model 8 in Table 3 displays the lowest value of the Root MSE and the highest R-squared, indicating the model with all dummies had the highest estimated accuracy in Table 3. According to the coefficients in Model 8, we found that the critical distance is equal to 67.5/GRERAT, which revealed the critical distance was inversely related to the greening ratio. Taking the maximum value of the greening ratio in the sample, the critical distance was about 112.5 m. However, using the minimum value of the greening ratio in the sample, the critical distance was about 421.9 m. This means the ideal threshold of the distance ranges from about 113 to 422 m with changes to the greening ratio. Thus, the greening ratio indeed played a moderating role in the relationship between the distance to the SFT and housing prices. Hypothesis 2 was supported.

4.2.2. Association between the Distance to the SWF and Housing Prices after the Release of the Assessment Report

Table 4 reports the relationship between distance and housing prices after the release of the trial result. It can be seen that the estimates of distance-squared are not significant, while the coefficients of distance are negatively and significantly related to housing prices except in Model 9 in Table 4. This indicates that people's worries reduced and they thought the purifying tower was efficient after the release of the assessment report, which induced an increase in housing prices of neighborhoods located near the tower. Therefore, the closer to the SFT, the higher people's willingness was to pay for clean air. Hypothesis 3 was confirmed.

Table 5 shows the moderating roles of various accessibilities in the relationship between distance and housing prices after the release of the trial result. Model 16 showed the lowest value of the Root MSE but the highest R-squared, which confirmed it had the highest estimation accuracy. It can be seen from Model 16 that the estimate of the distance was significantly negative, and the coefficient of the interaction of distance and the number of bus stops was significantly positive. Further, its value was much higher than the other interaction coefficients. This implies that, compared to air quality, residents are more sensitive to transportation accessibility. The number of bus stops is fewer in residential areas closer to the SFT. On average, the neighborhoods within 1 km from the tower have five bus stations; in comparison, neighborhoods 1 km away have about 6.3 bus stops. Thus, residents were more likely to choose houses with easily accessible transportation than clean air. In other words, people generally place more weight on transportation accessibility than on air quality. This suggests that the government should optimize the transportation conditions around the air purification tower to increase people's residential satisfaction.

4.3. Implications of Results

Air quality has increasingly become an important factor influencing housing choices [18,19,24,45]. In confronting serious air pollution, it is common and efficient to control pollution from the source. While households can obtain clean air by installing indoor air purifiers, there is no mature technical method for the efficient purification of polluted air in outdoor public spaces at a large scale, in a recyclable and sustainable manner. Passive outdoor haze control technology systems do not target the source of pollution, and this needs to be considered in future research. However, the Smog Free Tower (SFT) in Xi'an is the first in the world, and so is considered a novel outdoor haze reduction experiment. Before the publication of the assessment report on the tower, people doubted the new technology. Our analysis evidenced that residents tended to buy houses a certain distance away from the SFT. This attitude changed, however, after the publication of the assessment report, which confirmed the effectiveness of the SFT and alleviated concerns about the potential risks.

The analysis of the responses of residents' housing choice behavior to the SFT in the two stages revealed practical implications for building healthy cities, including for environmental governance, the real estate market, transportation, and urban planning. First, as haze is becoming increasingly serious, environmental protection measures are urgently needed to control it. The present paper confirmed people's increased environmental awareness. It suggests that the public's expectations of environmental governance are likely to change as the intermediate evaluation changes. Second, clean air has a positive capitalization effect on housing prices. In future, appropriate design environment policy, and the associated effects of such a policy on the housing market, should be considered. Third, this study highlighted the persistent importance of transportation accessibility and the greening ratio in housing choices. It suggested that the government should optimize the transportation conditions around air purification facilities to increase people's satisfaction with living there.

5. Conclusions

This study attempted to reveal residents' willingness to pay for clean air by using the unique quasi-natural experiment of the world's first outdoor air purification building in Xi'an, China. This rare experiment not only overcomes self-selection bias, but also provides a valuable opportunity to distinguish dwellers' behavior responses to air quality improvements at different stages. This study captured the changes in residents' attitudes to the SFT, and the characteristics of their willingness to pay for clean air, through comparing the housing data before and after the publication of the assessment report for the tower. Simultaneously, the present study emphasized the moderating roles of the greening ratio and transportation accessibility in people's pursuit of air quality. Hedonic models were employed to quantify the relative importance of the distance to the SFT and depict its changing relationship with housing prices. Specifically, the estimation results showed that before the publication of the assessment report, the distance to the SFT had an inverse

U-shaped relationship with housing prices, and obvious threshold effects. Green plants can be regarded as the community's own air purification facilities, as they have a protective effect against air pollution and can purify polluted air. The greening ratio of the residential area had a moderating effect on the non-linear relationship between the distance to the SFT and housing prices. After the publication of the assessment report, the distance to the SFT was negatively related to housing prices. The tendency of the housing price changes demonstrated that people are willing to pay for clean air. However, we found that transportation accessibility is more significant when selecting a residential location than clean air. That is, residents generally place more weight on transportation accessibility than on air quality when buying houses.

The present study contributes to the understanding of willingness to pay for clean air. We demonstrate how people's expectations of the effectiveness of air purification change this willingness to pay. It is among the first to use a quasi-natural experiment to explain residents' willingness to pay for air quality [19]. It uncovers the behavior dynamic in dwellers' willingness to pay for clean air based on a longer observation window than in many existing studies. This particular experiment was able to overcome the traditional endogenous bias and provide more reliable analysis results. Furthermore, we find that improving transportation accessibility and the greening ratio increases the willingness to pay for clean air. This may help to improve theories on locational attainment. In addition, the moderating effects of transportation accessibility and greening ratio on the willingness to pay might have several implications for urban planners and policymakers.

Several limitations of this work should be acknowledged. First, we used the number of restaurants, supermarkets, banks, hospitals, and schools to measure the convenience of the neighborhood, but did not consider the quality of those surrounding services and facilities [40,41]. Second, important housing structure characteristics, such as the decoration degree and property management level, were not included in this study [40,46]. Third, as the present data were at the neighborhood level, we were not able to infer relationships between individual characteristics (e.g., income, education level, family structure) and willingness to pay for clean air. To overcome such limitations and provide a more complete picture of residents' responses to the SFT and willingness to pay for clean air, we intend to complement the largely quantitative fieldwork by conducting a large-scale survey and qualitative in-depth interviews in the future.

Author Contributions: Conceptualization, H.Z.; methodology, H.Z.; software, H.Z.; validation, S.M.; formal analysis, S.M.; investigation, H.Z.; resources, X.W.; data curation, H.Z.; writing—original draft preparation, H.Z.; writing—review and editing, S.M.; supervision, X.W.; project administration, S.M.; funding acquisition, H.Z. All authors have read and agreed to the published version of the manuscript.

Funding: This research was funded by the National Natural Science Foundation of China, grant number 71871215; Scientific Research Project of National Bureau of Statistics, grant number 2021LY088; Foundation for Cultivating Excellent and Outstanding Talents in Colleges and Universities of Anhui Province, grant number gxbjZD2021011; China Postdoctoral Science Foundation, grant number 2019M651511; Provincial Natural Science Foundation of Anhui, grant number 2008085MG237; and Scientific Research Foundation of Chuzhou University, grant number 2018qd12. The APC was funded by the Provincial Natural Science Foundation of Anhui.

Institutional Review Board Statement: Not applicable.

Informed Consent Statement: Not applicable.

Data Availability Statement: Data that support the findings of this study are available from the corresponding author upon reasonable request.

Conflicts of Interest: The authors declare no conflict of interest.

Appendix A

Table A1. Definition and descriptive statistics of the dummy variables not included in Table 1.

Variable	Definition	Unit or Coding	Mean	St. Dev.	Minimum	Maximum
S20173	Whether it is the first quarter of 2017. (Yes = 1, No = 0)	—	0.13	0.331	0	1
S20176	Whether it is the second quarter of 2017. (Yes = 1, No = 0)	—	0.13	0.331	0	1
S20179	Whether it is the third quarter of 2017. (Yes = 1, No = 0)	—	0.13	0.331	0	1
S201712	Whether it is the fourth quarter of 2017. (Yes = 1, No = 0)	—	0.13	0.331	0	1
S20183	Whether it is the first quarter of 2018. (Yes = 1, No = 0)	—	0.13	0.331	0	1
S20186	Whether it is the second quarter of 2018. (Yes = 1, No = 0)	—	0.13	0.331	0	1
S20189	Whether it is the third quarter of 2018. (Yes = 1, No = 0)	—	0.13	0.331	0	1
S201812	Whether it is the fourth quarter of 2018. (Yes = 1, No = 0)	—	0.13	0.331	0	1
XIZHAI	Whether located in the business district Xizhai (Yes = 1, No = 0)	—	0.06	0.229	0	1
GUODU	Whether located in the business district Guodu (Yes = 1, No = 0)	—	0.22	0.416	0	1
XCAJ	Whether located in the business district Chang'an Street (Yes = 1, No = 0)	—	0.08	0.277	0	1
ZIWU	Whether located in the business district Ziwu (Yes = 1, No = 0)	—	0.01	0.096	0	1
XIFENG	Whether located in the business district Xifeng (Yes = 1, No = 0)	—	0.05	0.210	0	1
DAXUCH	Whether located in the business district Daxue (Yes = 1, No = 0)	—	0.17	0.373	0	1
DIZICH	Whether located in the business district Dianzi (Yes = 1, No = 0)	—	0.05	0.210	0	1
ZWTYDS	Whether located in the business district Ziwei (Yes = 1, No = 0)	—	0.03	0.164	0	1
WEIQU	Whether located in the business district Weiqu (Yes = 1, No = 0)	—	0.17	0.373	0	1
KEJI	Whether located in the business district Keji (Yes = 1, No = 0)	—	0.03	0.164	0	1
JINYE	Whether located in the business district Jinye (Yes = 1, No = 0)	—	0.06	0.229	0	1
CHANSQ	Whether located in the business district Chang'an Square (Yes = 1, No = 0)	—	0.01	0.096	0	1
ZHBAXI	Whether located in the business district Zhangba (Yes = 1, No = 0)	—	0.02	0.135	0	1
DZJIE	Whether located in the business district Dianzi Street (Yes = 1, No = 0)	—	0.01	0.096	0	1
LIMEXICH	Whether located in the business district Lianmeng (Yes = 1, No = 0)	—	0.01	0.096	0	1
XIMEYU	Whether located in the business district Rongchuang (Yes = 1, No = 0)	—	0.01	0.096	0	1
YAHUZH	Whether located in the business district Yanhuan (Yes = 1, No = 0)	—	0.01	0.096	0	1
MINGDE	Whether located in the business district Mingde (Yes = 1, No = 0)	—	0.01	0.096	0	1
GXYIZH	Whether located in the business district Gaoxin (Yes = 1, No = 0)	—	0.01	0.096	0	1
Y1999	Whether the neighborhood was completed in 1999. (Yes = 1, No = 0)	—	0.01	0.096	0	1
Y2000	Whether the neighborhood was completed in 2000. (Yes = 1, No = 0)	—	0.01	0.096	0	1
Y2001	Whether the neighborhood was completed in 2001. (Yes = 1, No = 0)	—	0.02	0.135	0	1
Y2002	Whether the neighborhood was completed in 2002. (Yes = 1, No = 0)	—	0.01	0.096	0	1
Y2003	Whether the neighborhood was completed in 2003. (Yes = 1, No = 0)	—	0.03	0.164	0	1
Y2004	Whether the neighborhood was completed in 2004. (Yes = 1, No = 0)	—	0.04	0.189	0	1
Y2005	Whether the neighborhood was completed in 2005. (Yes = 1, No = 0)	—	0.02	0.135	0	1
Y2006	Whether the neighborhood was completed in 2006. (Yes = 1, No = 0)	—	0.04	0.189	0	1
Y2007	Whether the neighborhood was completed in 2007. (Yes = 1, No = 0)	—	0.05	0.210	0	1
Y2008	Whether the neighborhood was completed in 2008. (Yes = 1, No = 0)	—	0.06	0.246	0	1
Y2009	Whether the neighborhood was completed in 2009. (Yes = 1, No = 0)	—	0.06	0.246	0	1
Y2010	Whether the neighborhood was completed in 2010. (Yes = 1, No = 0)	—	0.10	0.303	0	1
Y2011	Whether the neighborhood was completed in 2011. (Yes = 1, No = 0)	—	0.06	0.246	0	1
Y2012	Whether the neighborhood was completed in 2012. (Yes = 1, No = 0)	—	0.06	0.246	0	1
Y2013	Whether the neighborhood was completed in 2013. (Yes = 1, No = 0)	—	0.05	0.210	0	1
Y2014	Whether the neighborhood was completed in 2014. (Yes = 1, No = 0)	—	0.09	0.290	0	1
Y2015	Whether the neighborhood was completed in 2015. (Yes = 1, No = 0)	—	0.10	0.303	0	1
Y2016	Whether the neighborhood was completed in 2016. (Yes = 1, No = 0)	—	0.02	0.135	0	1
Y2017	Whether the neighborhood was completed in 2017. (Yes = 1, No = 0)	—	0.07	0.262	0	1
Y2018	Whether the neighborhood was completed in 2018. (Yes = 1, No = 0)	—	0.03	0.164	0	1
Y2019	Whether the neighborhood was completed in 2019. (Yes = 1, No = 0)	—	0.03	0.164	0	1
Y2020	Whether the neighborhood was completed in 2020. (Yes = 1, No = 0)	—	0.03	0.164	0	1
Y2021	Whether the neighborhood was completed in 2021. (Yes = 1, No = 0)	—	0.01	0.096	0	1

Note: — indicates that the corresponding variable is unitless.

References

1. Pope, C.A.; Douglas, W.D. Health Effects of Fine Particulate Air Pollution: Lines That Connect. *J. Air Waste Manag. Assoc.* **2006**, *56*, 1368–1380. [CrossRef]
2. Pope, C.A., III; Burnett, R.T.; Thun, M.J.; Calle, E.E.; Krewski, D.; Ito, K.; Thurston, G.D. Lung Cancer, Cardiopulmonary Mortality, and Long-Term Exposure to Fine Particulate Air Pollution. *JAMA* **2002**, *287*, 1132–1141. [CrossRef]
3. Gautam, D.; Bolia, N.B. Air pollution: Impact and interventions. *Air Qual. Atmos. Health* **2020**, *13*, 209–223. [CrossRef]

4. Brunekreef, B.; Holgate, S.T. Air Pollution and Health. *Lancet* **2002**, *360*, 1233–1242. [CrossRef]
5. Heyes, A.; Zhu, M. Air pollution as a cause of sleeplessness: Social media evidence from a panel of Chinese cities. *J. Environ. Econ. Manag.* **2019**, *98*, 102247. [CrossRef]
6. Wang, R.; Xue, D.; Liu, Y.; Liu, P.; Chen, H. The Relationship between Air Pollution and Depression in China: Is Neighbourhood Social Capital Protective? *Int. J. Environ. Res. Public Health* **2018**, *15*, 1160. [CrossRef]
7. Yang, X.; Zhang, J.; Ren, S.; Ran, Q. Can the new energy demonstration city policy reduce environmental pollution? Evidence from a quasi-natural experiment in China. *J. Clean. Prod.* **2020**, *287*, 125015. [CrossRef]
8. Xie, Y.; Wu, D.; Zhu, S. Can new energy vehicles subsidy curb the urban air pollution? Empirical evidence from pilot cities in China. *Sci. Total. Environ.* **2020**, *754*, 142232. [CrossRef] [PubMed]
9. Tan, Z. Smog Free Tower: Studio Roosegaarde, Beijing, September 2016–Present. *Technol. Archit. Des.* **2017**, *1*, 253–254. [CrossRef]
10. Zhou, Q.; Zhang, X.; Shao, Q.; Wang, X. The non-linear effect of environmental regulation on haze pollution: Empirical evidence for 277 Chinese cities during 2002–2010. *J. Environ. Manag.* **2019**, *248*, 109274. [CrossRef] [PubMed]
11. Cao, Q.; Huang, M.; Kuehn, T.H.; Shen, L.; Tao, W.-Q.; Cao, J.; Pui, D.Y. Urban-scale SALSCS, Part II: A Parametric Study of System Performance. *Aerosol Air Qual. Res.* **2018**, *18*, 2879–2894. [CrossRef]
12. Cao, Q.; Kuehn, T.H.; Shen, L.; Chen, S.-C.; Zhang, N.; Huang, Y.; Cao, J.; Pui, D.Y. Urban-scale SALSCS, Part I: Experimental Evaluation and Numerical Modeling of a Demonstration Unit. *Aerosol Air Qual. Res.* **2018**, *18*, 2865–2878. [CrossRef]
13. The Only Smog Free Tower in the world. Available online: http://news.hsw.cn/system/2018/0418/979401.shtml?rand=r8Lx5fEb (accessed on 18 April 2018).
14. Chay, K.Y.; Greenstone, M. Does air quality matter? Evidence from the housing market. *J. Polit. Econ.* **2005**, *113*, 376–424. [CrossRef]
15. Smith, V.K.; Huang, J.C. Hedonic models and air pollution: Twenty-five years and counting. *Environ. Resour. Econ.* **1993**, *3*, 381–394. [CrossRef]
16. Zabel, J.E.; Kiel, K.A. Estimating the Demand for Air Quality in Four U.S. Cities. *Land Econ.* **2000**, *76*, 174–194. [CrossRef]
17. Harrison, D.; Rubinfeld, D.L. Hedonic housing prices and the demand for clean air. *J. Environ. Econ. Manag.* **1978**, *5*, 81–102. [CrossRef]
18. Won, K.C.; Phipps, T.T.; Anselin, L. Measuring the benefits of air quality improvement: A spatial hedonic approach. *J. Environ. Econ. Manag.* **2003**, *45*, 24–39.
19. Lan, F.; Lv, J.; Chen, J.; Zhang, X.; Zhao, Z.; Pui, D.Y. Willingness to pay for staying away from haze: Evidence from a quasi-natural experiment in Xi'an. *J. Environ. Manag.* **2020**, *262*, 110301. [CrossRef]
20. Can, A. Specification and estimation of hedonic housing price models. *Reg. Sci. Urban Econ.* **1992**, *22*, 453–474. [CrossRef]
21. Efthymiou, D.; Antoniou, C. How do transport infrastructure and policies affect house prices and rents? Evidence from Athens, Greece. *Transp. Res. Part A Policy Pract.* **2013**, *52*, 1–22. [CrossRef]
22. Li, H.; Wei, Y.D.; Yu, Z.; Tian, G. Amenity, accessibility and housing values in metropolitan USA: A study of Salt Lake County, Utah. *Cities* **2016**, *59*, 113–125. [CrossRef]
23. Smersh, G.T.; Smith, M.T. Accessibility Changes and Urban House Price Appreciation: A Constrained Optimization Approach to Determining Distance Effects. *J. Hous. Econ.* **2000**, *9*, 187–196. [CrossRef]
24. Jim, C.; Chen, W. Consumption preferences and environmental externalities: A hedonic analysis of the housing market in Guangzhou. *Geoforum.* **2007**, *38*, 414–431. [CrossRef]
25. Adamowicz, W.; Louviere, J.; Williams, M. Combining Revealed and Stated Preference Methods for Valuing Environmental Amenities. *J. Environ. Econ. Manag.* **1994**, *26*, 271–292. [CrossRef]
26. Luechinger, S. Valuing Air Quality Using the Life Satisfaction Approach. *Econ. J.* **2009**, *119*, 482–515. [CrossRef]
27. Cobb, S.A. Site rent, air quality, and the demand for amenities. *J. Environ. Econ. Manag.* **1977**, *4*, 214–218. [CrossRef]
28. Zheng, S.; Kahn, M.; Liu, H. Towards a System of open cities in China: Home prices, FDI flows and air quality in 35 major cities. *Reg. Sci. Urban Econ.* **2010**, *40*, 1–10. [CrossRef]
29. Zheng, S.; Cao, J.; Kahn, M.E.; Sun, C. Real estate valuation and cross-boundary air pollution externalities: Evidence from Chinese cities. *J. Real Estate Financ. Econ.* **2014**, *48*, 398–414. [CrossRef]
30. Rohde, R.A.; Muller, R.A. Air Pollution in China: Mapping of Concentrations and Sources. *PLoS ONE* **2015**, *10*, e0135749. [CrossRef]
31. Xie, Y.; Dai, H.; Dong, H.; Hanaoka, T.; Masui, T. Economic Impacts from PM 2.5 Pollution-Related Health Effects in China: A Provincial-Level Analysis. *Environ. Sci. Technol.* **2016**, *50*, 4836–4843. [CrossRef]
32. Zhang, H.; Chen, J.; Wang, Z. Spatial Heterogeneity in Spillover Effect of Air Pollution on Housing Prices: Evidence from China. *Cities* **2021**, *113*, 103145. [CrossRef]
33. Chen, S.; Jin, H. Pricing for the clean air: Evidence from Chinese housing market. *J. Clean. Prod.* **2018**, *206*, 297–306. [CrossRef]
34. The Smog Free Tower in the City of Xi'an. Available online: http://news.cctv.com/2016/05/17/VIDEM1LWsSImujfeU24PHqUM160517.shtml (accessed on 17 May 2016).
35. The Smog Free Tower in Xi'an Is Rooted. Available online: https://www.sohu.com/a/75289553_119038 (accessed on 13 May 2016).
36. Zhou, H. Difficulties to overcome the adoration of GDP—four conceptual disorder during the development and their errorness nature. *People's Trib.* **2014**, *5*, 76–78. (In Chinese)
37. Morancho, A.B. A hedonic valuation of urban green areas. *Landsc. Urban Plan.* **2003**, *66*, 35–41. [CrossRef]
38. Anderson, L.M.; Cordell, H.K. Influence of Trees on Residential Property Values in Athens, Georgia (USA): A Survey Based on Actual Sales Prices. *Landsc. Urban Plan.* **1988**, *15*, 153–164. [CrossRef]

39. Gromke, C.; Ruck, B. Influence of Trees on the Dispersion of Pollutants in an Urban Street Canyon–Experimental Investigation of the Flow and Concentration Field. *Atmos. Environ.* **2007**, *41*, 3287–3302. [CrossRef]
40. Duan, J.; Tian, G.; Yang, L.; Zhou, T. Addressing the Macroeconomic and Hedonic Determinants of Housing Prices in Beijing Metropolitan Area, China. *Habitat Int.* **2021**, *113*, 102374. [CrossRef]
41. Geng, B.; Bao, H.; Liang, Y. A study of the effect of a high-speed rail station on spatial variations in housing price based on the hedonic model. *Habitat Int.* **2015**, *49*, 333–339. [CrossRef]
42. Sirmans, S.; Macpherson, D.; Zietz, E. The Composition of Hedonic Pricing Models. *J. Real Estate Lit.* **2005**, *13*, 1–44. [CrossRef]
43. Anstine, J. Property Values in a Low Populated Area when Dual Noxious Facilities are Present. *Growth Chang.* **2003**, *34*, 345–358. [CrossRef]
44. Zhao, J.; Wang, Q. The impact of wind projecting angles on energy consumption of buildings—The case from Xi'an. *Urban Probl.* **2010**, *9*, 38–41. (In Chinese)
45. Chen, J.; Hao, Q.; Yoon, C. Measuring the welfare cost of air pollution in Shanghai: Evidence from the housing market. *J. Environ. Plan. Manag.* **2018**, *61*, 1744–1757. [CrossRef]
46. Wen, H.; Zhang, Y.; Zhang, L. Assessing amenity effects of urban landscapes on housing price in Hangzhou, China. *Urban For. Urban Green.* **2015**, *14*, 1017–1026. [CrossRef]

International Journal of
Environmental Research and Public Health

MDPI

Article

Study on the Spatiotemporal Evolution and Influencing Factors of Urban Resilience in the Yellow River Basin

Yu Chen [1], Xuyang Su [1] and Qian Zhou [2,*]

[1] School of Economics and Management, Zhengzhou University of Light Industry, Zhengzhou 450000, China; 2012030@zzuli.edu.cn (Y.C.); suxuyang_123@163.com (X.S.)
[2] Economics School, Zhongnan University of Economics and Law, Wuhan 430073, China
* Correspondence: Z0005072@zuel.edu.cn

Abstract: The outbreak of COVID-19 has prompted consideration of the importance of urban resilience. Based on a multidimensional perspective, the authors of this paper established a comprehensive evaluation indicator system for evaluating urban resilience in the Yellow River basin (YRB), and various methods such as the entropy value method, Theil index, exploratory spatial data analysis (ESDA) model, and geographical detector model were used to measure the spatiotemporal characteristics and influencing factors of urban resilience in the YRB from 2011 to 2018. The results are as follows. (1) From 2011 to 2018, the urban resilience index (URI) of the YRB showed a "V"-shaped dynamic evolution in the time series, and the URI increased by 13.4% overall. The resilience of each subsystem showed the following hierarchical structure: economic resilience > social resilience > ecological resilience > infrastructure resilience. (2) The URI of the three major regions—upstream, midstream, and downstream—increased, and the resilience of each subsystem in the region showed obvious regional characteristics. The comprehensive difference in URI values within the basin was found to be shrinking, and intraregional differences have contributed most to the comprehensive difference. (3) There were obvious zonal differences in the URI from 2011 to 2018. Shandong Peninsula and Hohhot–Baotou–Ordos showed a "High–High" agglomeration, while the southern and southwestern regions showed a "Low–Low" agglomeration. (4) Among the humanist and social factors, economic, fiscal, market, urbanization, openness, and innovation were found to be the factors that exert a high impact on the URI, while the impacts of natural factors were found to be low. The impact of the interaction of each factor is greater than that of a single factor.

Keywords: urban resilience; spatiotemporal differentiation; ESDA; geographical detector model; YRB

Citation: Chen, Y.; Su, X.; Zhou, Q. Study on the Spatiotemporal Evolution and Influencing Factors of Urban Resilience in the Yellow River Basin. *IJERPH* **2021**, *18*, 10231. https://doi.org/10.3390/ijerph181910231

Academic Editor: Xinbin Feng

Received: 5 August 2021
Accepted: 26 September 2021
Published: 28 September 2021

Publisher's Note: MDPI stays neutral with regard to jurisdictional claims in published maps and institutional affiliations.

1. Introduction

The establishment of an urban system is randomly affected by changes in the internal and external environment as a consequence of the nonlinear interaction of multiple factors such as economic and social change, cultural adaptation, and resource integration [1], which forms a complex and interconnected geographic entity [2]. At present, COVID-19 has caused immeasurable economic losses, social impacts, and casualties worldwide. This is not only a major public health crisis but also a test of urban disaster risk emergency management. From the perspective of temporal and spatial scales, factors such as population, capital, information, energy, and resources continuously flow among cities and promote the rapid development of urbanization. The essence of urbanization is population migration [3]; in 2020, 56.2% of the world's population lived in urban areas, and it is expected that this proportion will increase to 62.5% by 2035 [4]. Exponential population growth, sustained economic development, and excessive resource consumption place tremendous pressure on urban systems, making cities extremely vulnerable to human–natural issues such as negative externalities, climate change, and various disasters [2,5]. Uncertainty and unknown risks have gradually become bottlenecks that restrict urban survival and sustainable development and directly or indirectly threaten the safety and quality of life of urban residents. Maintaining the initial core structure and basic functions under various unpredictable disturbances and pressures [1,6], improving the adaptability of the urban system, enhancing resistance to shocks and the ability to recover from disasters, and minimizing the adverse effects of perturbation factors have become urgent issues in the process of urbanization [7]. China's "14th Five-Year Plan" proposed building liveable, innovative, smart, green, humane, and resilient cities; enhancing the capacity of public facilities to cope with storms, droughts, and geological disasters; and improving emergency shelter functions in public facilities and buildings. Resilient city construction has attracted wide attention from academics, social organizations, and government departments, as well as becoming a crucial topic in the field of urban geography and planning.

As a new model and concept of urban disaster prevention and mitigation, many scholars have discussed urban resilience from qualitative and quantitative point of views, and the relevant research has mainly focuses on the following:

(1) Concept definition: The term resilience originated from the Latin "resilio" [8]. In the 1990s, the theory of resilience was creatively introduced into urban planning and construction, expanding the horizons of urban disaster research [7]. Urban resilience is usually recognized as the preparation and planning by urban systems for unfavourable factors, with absorption, recovery, and better adaptability in the face of disturbances [9] and complex and dynamic characteristics in the development process [10]. To enhance the short-term response capacity and long-term adaptability of urban systems [11], resilient cities can mitigate and prevent disaster risks; minimize loss or disadvantage to life, property, infrastructure, economic activities, and the environment from potential threats [12]; effectively guarantee the integrity and liveability of urban systems; and ensure the effective operation of functions in changing socioeconomic and environmental conditions [13]. Although there is no unified and recognized notion of urban resilience in academia, the construction of resilient cities is considered to be a new way to guide the development of sustainable cities [5], which should have three important abilities: the ability to absorb various pressures and maintain a stable state, the ability to self-organize, and the ability to adapt and learn [14]. Urban resilience is also characterized by biodiversity, versatility, multiscale networks, modularity, and adaptive design [15].

(2) Evaluation system and method selection: Building a reasonable evaluation index system based on the multidimensional perspective is the basis of quantitative research on urban resilience. Many scholars have chosen indicators from several dimensions of economy, society, infrastructure, institutions, and natural environment [16–18], using models such as the system dynamics [19,20], performance credit card [10], resilience maturity model [21,22], situation analysis [23], and "Scale–Density–Morphology" evaluation models [14] to measure the level of urban resilience or explore a certain dimension of it, such as economic resilience [24], social resilience [25], ecological resilience [26], or infrastructure resilience [27]. In addition, some scholars have used the propensity score matching and difference in difference model to explore the role of smart city construction in improving resilience [28].

(3) Influencing factors: The improvement of the urban resilience level is subject to the combined effect of multiple factors, and identifying the leading factors behind such resilience is conducive to guiding the planning and construction of resilient cities. From both internal and external perspectives, the factors affecting urban resilience are mainly explored from the human and natural perspectives, and theoretical frameworks of urban resilience such as PEOPLES [22], DROP [29], RCPF [30], and HES [6] have been established through various methods to explore the influence of social [31], economic [32], regime [29], and ecological environment [33] on urban resilience. These empirical studies have systematically analysed the reasons for differences in urban resilience at different scales across the country, urban agglomerations, or provinces, and they have proposed specific resilient city construction paths for different regions.

In summary, scholars have made fruitful achievements in the study of urban resilience, but there remain problems that need to be explored in depth. First, current studies are mostly focused on qualitative research such as concept introduction and theoretical exploration, with less extensive quantitative research focused on certain dimensions of urban resilience, such as urban economic, social, ecological, or infrastructure resilience. Research on comprehensive urban resilience is neither thorough nor systematic. Second, the influencing factors of urban resilience are mainly selected from humanistic and economic factors, and the impact of natural factors on urban resilience has not been fully considered. As a giant system with a complex enmeshment of "economy–society–nature", it is more reasonable to judge the influencing factors from the perspective of humanity and nature. Finally, existing studies are mostly concentrated at the national, provincial, and urban agglomeration levels, while research on watershed areas, which are regions with significant spatial heterogeneity, is relatively insufficient.

The YRB is the birthplace of Chinese civilization. In 2019, the ecological protection and high-quality development of the YRB was determined as a national strategy, and the region has a very important position in the construction of a new domestic and international economic dual-cycle development pattern. Compared with the Yangtze River Basin, the YRB spans multiple natural subregions and is a typical area with rapid changes in economics, society, and environment [34]; multiple fragile ecosystems in the basin have produced a relatively close spatial coupling. The uneven distribution of water and land resources and the shortage of water resources comprise the main contradiction that leads to the tense relationship between man and land, as well as causing the poor navigation conditions of the Yellow River. Most of the regional economic development is organized through a "centre–periphery" structure, and the main trend of industrial population flow and distribution is formed by relying on the main traffic axis. There are obvious differences in urban economic development strength, natural resource endowments, and traffic location conditions in the basin. The construction of urban resilience in this area is relatively insufficient, and its resilience is inadequate in the face of various disasters and risk intrusions. For example, Zhengzhou in the lower reaches of the Yellow River is a national central city and an important transportation hub. The extreme weather on 20 July 2021 caused serious waterlogging, traffic paralysis, and casualties in the city. Water and power outages in some areas caused inconvenience to residents' daily lives. The socioeconomic and ecological system is somewhat fragile, which severely restricts regional coordination and linkage and sustainable development. Therefore, it is necessary to measure the urban resilience level in the basin and clarify its driving factors. Based on this, the authors of this paper used the entropy method to measure the urban resilience index and then analysed the spatial heterogeneity and imbalance of urban resilience development by using spatial autocorrelation and the Theil index. Finally, the geographical detector model was used to explore the influencing factors of urban resilience. The results of this study are expected to provide reference for urban planners and decision makers in the construction of resilient cities.

2. Methods and Data Description

2.1. Construction of Evaluation System

Urban resilience is the extent to which an urban system can withstand and absorb the impact of various uncertain factors, as well as the ability to adapt, recover, and learn when dealing with disturbances. Based on the relevant literature, 24 specific indicators from four dimensions (economic resilience, society resilience, ecological resilience, and infrastructure resilience) were established to measure the URI of the YRB. The index system is attached in Appendix A (Table A1).

Economic resilience is embodied in the adaptability and stability of urban economic systems when facing the impact of unknown risks [24]. A highly resilient urban system requires a similarly strong level of economic development and has the ability to quickly overcome the crisis and resume production in response to external disturbances. Accordingly, six indicators were selected from the aspects of economic aggregate, financial security, economic structure, financial capital, investment intensity, and economic growth to reflect a city's comprehensive economic strength, economic diversity, and stability.

Social resilience reflects a city's health security and emergency management when it suffers short or long-term disturbance, with a focus on creating a high-quality social environment with development potential [25]. We selected six indicators from the aspects of education level, medical investment, residence income, employment structure, unemployment structure, and health protection to reflect a city's human capital and the ability to resolve risks.

Ecological resilience is reflected in the resilience of an urban ecological environment when facing excessive emissions of pollutants and reduction of green space that lead to environmental overload. It is an important factor of urban resilience [35]. For this, we selected six indicators from the aspects of environmental conservation level, urban greening level, waste utilization, environmental remediation, environmental pollution pressure, and waste emission intensity that reflect the service capacity, governance capacity, and pressure of an ecological environment.

Infrastructure resilience reflects the ability of a city to protect people, evacuate, and communicate with others during disasters or risks. It is at the forefront of crises response [36]. Six indicators from the aspects of infrastructure construction, level of transportation facilities, engineering support capability, internet penetration, electricity development level, and communication sophistication were selected to reflect infrastructure resilience.

2.2. Research Methods

2.2.1. Entropy Value Method

The entropy value method is an objective comprehensive evaluation method that can effectively avoid human interference [37] and that many scholars have applied to comprehensive evaluation. To better reflect the role of negative indicators, the extreme value standardization method was used to nondimensionally process the data of various indicators, and the URI was calculated according to the linear fitting formula. The specific calculation steps are as follows [35].

First, according to the positive and negative indicators of urban resilience, the range method was used to standardize the original data:

$$\text{Positive indicator}: \ x'_{ij} = \frac{x_{ij} - \min(x_{ij})}{\max(x_{ij}) - \min(x_{ij})} \tag{1}$$

$$\text{Negative indicator}: \ x'_{ij} = \frac{\max(x_{ij}) - x_{ij}}{\max(x_{ij}) - \min(x_{ij})} \tag{2}$$

where x_{ij} is the original value of the i-th evaluation object corresponding to the j-th index; x'_{ij} is the standardized value; $\max(x_{ij})$ and $\min(x_{ij})$ are the maximum and minimum values of each index, respectively.

Second, the entropy value of the j-th index was calculated:

$$e_j = -k \sum_{i=1}^{n} P_{ij} \ln P_{ij} \tag{3}$$

where $k = 1/\ln(n)$, n is the sample size and $P_{ij} = x'_{ij} / \sum_{i=1}^{n} x'_{ij}$.

Third, the URI and sub-resilience index S_i of each city were calculated:

$$S_i = \sum_{j=1}^{m} w_j \times x'_{ij} \tag{4}$$

where $w_j = \frac{d_j}{\sum_{j=1}^{m} d_j}$, represents the weight of index j; $d_j = 1 - e_j$.

2.2.2. Theil Index

Based on the concept of entropy in information theory, the Theil index was initially applied to the analysis of income gaps among individuals or regions; the total gap can be broken down into intragroup and intergroup gaps to more clearly identify its source [38]. In this paper, the unbalanced characteristics of the URI in the YRB were explored through the Theil index and its decomposition method, which is calculated as follows:

$$T = T_B + T_W = \sum_{k=1}^{K} y_k \ln\left(\frac{y_k}{n_k/n}\right) + \sum_{k=1}^{K} y_k\left(\sum_{i \in g_k} \frac{y_i}{y_k} \ln\left(\frac{y_i/y_k}{1/n_k}\right)\right) \tag{5}$$

where T, T_B, and T_W are the total gap, the intragroup gap, and the intergroup, respectively; n is the sample cities, which are divided into K groups (the authors of this paper divided the cities in the YRB into three groups: upper, middle, and lower reaches); each group is represented by g_k (K = 1, 2, 3); n_k is the number of cities in group K; y_k is the ratio of the URI in group K to that in the YRB; and y_i is the ratio of the URI of city i to the total.

2.2.3. ESDA Model

Global Spatial Autocorrelation

The global autocorrelation analysis was used to verify whether there was a spatial aggregation of variables throughout the region by measuring the spatial interdependencies of observational data, characterized primarily by Moran's I index. Thus, we used the global Moran's I index to explore the spatial agglomeration of the URI in the YRB, and the formula [39] is as follows:

$$I = \frac{n\sum_{i=1}^{n}\sum_{j=1}^{n} W_{ij}(x_i - \overline{x})(x_j - \overline{x})}{\sum_{i=1}^{n}\sum_{j=1}^{n} W_{ij}\sum_{i=1}^{n}(x_i - \overline{x})^2} \tag{6}$$

where n is the number of research cities; i and j are two different research cities in the region; x_i and x_j are the average values of the URI of city i and j, respectively; and $\overline{x}$ is the average value of the URI of all cities. W_{ij} is the spatial weight matrix: if i and j are adjacent, then W_{ij} is 1, but if not, then $W_{ij} = 0$. The range of I is $[-1, 1]$, and when $I > 0$, it indicates positive spatial correlation; the larger the I value is, the stronger the spatial correlation and vice versa. The significance test of I was required, and the formula [40] is:

$$Z(I) = \frac{1 - E(I)}{\sqrt{Var(I)}} \tag{7}$$

where $Z(I)$ is the significance level of Moran's I, and $E(I)$ and $Var(I)$ are the mathematical expectation and variance, respectively. When $Z(I) > 0$ and is significant, it indicates positive spatial autocorrelation; when $Z(I) < 0$ and is significant, it indicates negative spatial autocorrelation.

Local Spatial Autocorrelation

To clarify the specific location of spatial agglomeration of high-value and low-value resilient cities within the YRB, we used the local Moran's I index to identify the local spatial autocorrelation characteristics of urban resilience. The formula [41] is as follows:

$$I_i = \frac{\sum_{i=1,j=1}^{n} W_{ij}(x_i - x)(x_j - x)}{S^2} \tag{8}$$

where I_i is the local Moran's I index of the i-th city and $S^2 = \frac{1}{n}\sum_{i=1}^{n}(x_i - \overline{x})^2$; the results also needed to be Z-tested, as in the formula above. At a certain level of significance, according to the significance level of the Moran's I index and the results of the Z test, the research cities could be divided into four agglomeration relationships: (1) When Moran's I was significant and positive and $Z(I) > 0$, it was a "High–High" (H–H) agglomeration relationship, and the URI of the research city and neighbouring cities is high; (2) when the Moran's I index was significant and positive and $Z(I) < 0$, it was a "Low–Low" (L–L) agglomeration relationship, and the URI of the research city and neighbouring cities was low; (3) when the Moran's I index was significant and negative and $Z(I) > 0$, it was a "High–Low" (H–L) agglomeration relationship, the URI of the research city was high, and the URI of the neighbouring unit was low; (4) when the Moran's I index was significant and negative and $Z(I) < 0$, it was a "Low–High" (L–H) agglomeration relationship, the URI of the research city was low, and the URI of the neighbouring cities was high. When $Z(I) = 0$, it was randomly distributed.

2.2.4. Geographical Detector Model

A geographical detector is a statistical model to distinguish spatial separation and reveal its influencing factors, including those of risk, ecological, and interaction [42]. In practical applications, it does not require too many assumptions, and influencing factor analysis offers advantages such as immune collinearity of multiple independent variables that have been applied in many fields in recent years [14,43]. The basic principle is to divide the total sample into several sub-samples and then use variance to judge spatial heterogeneity and variable relationships. If the sum of the sub-sample variances is less than the total variance of all samples, there is a spatial difference. If the spatial distribution of two variables tends to be consistent, there is a statistical correlation between the two variables. To consider the influence mechanism of urban resilience in the YRB, we constructed an index system that assessed urban resilience and identified the core influencing factors of URIs through factor detection and interaction detection in geographical detectors.

The main purpose of factor detection is to explore the degree of interpretation of the dependent variable y by the influence factor x, which is measured by the q value. The formula is:

$$q = 1 - \frac{1}{N\sigma^2} \sum_{h=1}^{L} N_h \sigma_h^2 \quad (9)$$

where q is the interpretive intensity of the influence factor on the URI with a range of [0, 1], and the larger the q value is, the stronger the spatial divergence of the dependent variable Y; if the spatial divergence is caused by the factor X, the larger the value of q is, so the interpretation of urban resilience is stronger; h is the stratification of factor X or variable Y; N is the sample size and N_h is the number of cities in layer; and σ^2 and σ_h^2 are the variances of the whole area and h area, respectively.

Interaction detection is used to identify the interaction between different influencing factors X_i and X_j. It can evaluate whether the factors X_i and X_j will increase or decrease the interpretation of the dependent variable Y when they work together, or whether the influence of these factors on the dependent variable Y is independent.

2.3. Data

The research data could be divided into three main groups. (1) Socio-economic data: these data were mainly derived from the 2011–2018 "China City Statistical Yearbook", "China City Construction Statistical Yearbook", statistical yearbooks of provinces and cities, statistical bulletins of national economic and social development of cities, and individual missing data supplemented by interpolation or official local official websites. (2) Environmental data: annual precipitation and annual average temperature data were from the China Meteorological Data Network, and the original data were the monthly data from meteorological stations. After the abnormal values were removed, the annual average of the remaining stations was calculated, and the raster data of annual precipitation and annual average temperature were generated by kriging interpolation. MODIS NDVI data came from the Resource, Environment and Data Centre of the Chinese Academy of Sciences. (3) Geographical information data: based on the administrative cities mentioned in the YRB ecological protection and high-quality development strategy, the vector diagram of the administrative boundary of the YRB came from the National Basic Geographic Information

Centre. Considering the integrity and continuity of the data, the authors of this paper excluded the Jiyuan, Zhongwei, Haidong, Linxia, Gannan Tibetan Autonomous, and Alxa regions. To better analyse the spatial heterogeneity and imbalance of urban resilience development in the YRB, the authors of this paper drew on existing research and divided it into three regions: the upstream, midstream, and downstream [44]. The study area is shown in Figure 1.

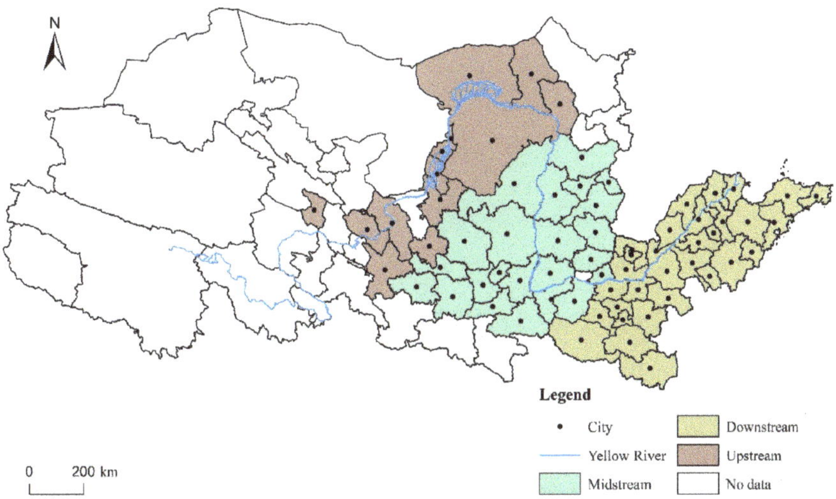

Figure 1. Sample area: the Yellow River Basin.

3. Spatiotemporal Evolution Characteristics of Urban Resilience

3.1. Temporal Evolution of URI

3.1.1. Comprehensive Evolution Analysis

Figure 2 shows that the URI of the YRB showed a "V"-shaped dynamic development trend from 2011 to 2018, with an increase of 13.4%. Its evolution can be characterized in two stages. In the first stage (2011–2012), the URI showed a downward trend from 0.2437 in 2011 to 0.1765 in 2012, a decrease of 27.6%. The reason for this decrease may be that in the post-financial crisis era, the development model oriented by resources and labour led to prominent contradictions in industrial structure, the low level of economic development led to less supply of social public goods, and pressure to "maintain growth" ignored the rational limited development of resources and environmental protection, thereby resulting in a serious ecological and environment problem and a significant decline in the URI. In the second stage (2012–2018), the URI showed a fluctuating upward trend from 0.1765 in 2012 to 0.2763 in 2018, an increase of 41.6%. During this period, the effectiveness of the "12th Five-Year Plan" gradually became apparent. The new round of development in the western region and the rise of the central region were implemented in depth. The construction of the main functional area began; it was proposed to optimize urbanization and significantly improve comprehensive urban carrying capacity, resilience, and risk resistance. Although the URI of the YRB has improved, the value remains relatively small, with obvious volatility and tortuousness. This phenomenon is directly associated with the weak economic strength of the cities in the YRB, their imperfect social systems and mechanisms, and the fragile ecological environment. These results indicate that there is a long road ahead to enhance urban resilience in the YRB.

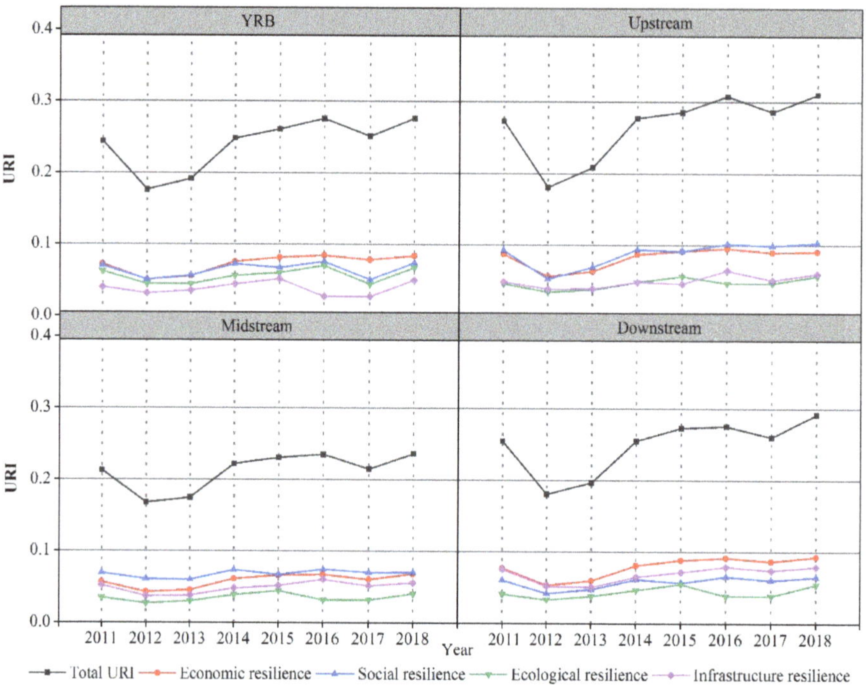

Figure 2. Temporal evaluation of the URI and subsystems in the YRB during 2011–2018.

The subsystems showed obvious volatility and hierarchical characteristics in the YRB from 2011 to 2018. The data distribution showed the characteristics of economic resilience > social resilience > ecological resilience > infrastructure resilience. At this stage, the URI of each subsystem improved, although the increases were quite different. Specifically, infrastructure resilience rose from 0.0399 to 0.0502, an increase of 26%; economic resilience rose from 0.0719 to 0.0841, an increase of 16.9%; ecological resilience rose from 0.0622 to 0.0677, an increase of 8.9%; social resilience rose from 0.0698 to 0.0743, an increase of 6.4%. The economic, social, ecological, and infrastructural resilience development of the YRB is obviously unbalanced, and it has also become an important factor restricting the improvement of comprehensive urban resilience. On the whole, the economic and social resilience index is high, while the infrastructure and ecological resilience index is low. The reason for such differences may be that the emergence of "urban diseases" has prompted the government to pay more attention to the adjustment and transformation of urbanization and industrialization, as well as issues related to social equity and stability such as education, medical care, and employment. However, the extensive resource-based cities in the YRB account for 47% of the total. They have not fundamentally eliminated the "resource curse" [45,46]. The negative environmental externalities caused by the transfer of high-polluting industries, coupled with these cities' own poor ability to restore and purify ecological damage and environmental pollution, can easily transform these developed areas into "pollution refuges".

In general, the coordinated and balanced development of various subsystems is a necessary measure to enhance urban resilience in the YRB. The malleable strategic framework of ecological protection and high-quality development will be able to strengthen the investment in and construction of infrastructure, as well as urban ecological and infrastructure resilience, under the guidance of ecological civilization.

3.1.2. Regional URI Evolution

From 2011 to 2018, the comprehensive and subsystem URI of cities upstream, midstream, and downstream of the YRB increased (Figure 2). The comprehensive URI showed a "V"-shaped development trend, and the development of subsystem resilience significantly differed. The URI of upstream and midstream cities was found to be driven by "economy and society", and the URI of downstream cities was found to be driven by "economy and infrastructure". Specifically, in the upstream region, the comprehensive URI increased from 0.2731 in 2011 to 0.3104 in 2018, an increase of 13.7%, and the economic, social, ecological, and infrastructure resilience indices increased by 4.6%, 11%, 25%, and 24.4%, respectively. After 2013, the social resilience index surpassed the economic resilience index and became the dominant force in urban resilience. After 2016, the infrastructure resilience index surpassed the ecological resilience index. In the midstream region, the comprehensive URI rose from 0.2129 in 2011 to 0.2363 in 2018, an increase of 11%, and the URI of each subsystem had the most obvious hierarchy. The economic, social, ecological, and infrastructure resilience indices increased by 5.5%, 2.6%, 8.7%, and 12.4%, respectively. Unlike the other two regions, the ecological resilience index was lowest in the midstream. A probable reason for this is the midstream flow through the Loess Plateau, where soil erosion is the most serious. The ecological environment in this area is extremely sensitive and fragile, which, coupled with the high intensity of production, life, and resource development in many resource-based cities (as well as a disregard of the general natural laws of environmental protection and inefficient management) has resulted in the worst ecological resilience. In the downstream region, the comprehensive URI increased from 0.2543 in 2011 to 0.2917 in 2018, an increase of 14.7%, and the economic, social, ecological, and infrastructure resilience indices increased by 20.7%, 7.4%, 31.9%, and 4.9%, respectively. The economic resilience index was the highest and demonstrated a large increase. The high level of economic development drives urban infrastructure construction, so the infrastructure resilience index was the highest of the three regions. However, the coordination between economic growth and environmental protection is poor, and ecological resilience construction is insufficient.

3.1.3. Difference Analysis Based on the Theil Index

In general, the Theil index dropped from 0.0877 to 0.0700 from 2011 to 2018 (Table 1), a decrease of 20.1%, indicating that the comprehensive URI gap is shrinking. Across time, in 2011–2012, 2013–2016, and 2017–2018, the difference in comprehensive URI narrowed, reaching a minimum of 0.0700 in 2018. In 2012–2013 and 2016–2017, the difference in comprehensive URI expanded, reaching the maximum of 0.0913 in 2013. The URI showed obvious volatility as a wave-like downward trend in the time series.

Table 1. Theil index measurement and contribution rate of URI in the YRB from 2011 to 2018.

Year	Comprehensive Difference	Intraregional Difference					Interregional Difference	
		Upstream	Midstream	Downstream	Contribution Value	Contribution Rate	Contribution Value	Contribution Rate
2011	0.0877	0.1131	0.0676	0.0791	0.0830	94.69%	0.0047	5.31%
2012	0.0842	0.0861	0.0985	0.0723	0.0836	99.30%	0.0006	0.70%
2013	0.0913	0.0983	0.1141	0.0683	0.0890	97.50%	0.0023	2.50%
2014	0.0788	0.0896	0.0614	0.0780	0.0754	95.63%	0.0034	4.37%
2015	0.0773	0.0911	0.0689	0.0688	0.0735	95.13%	0.0038	4.87%
2016	0.0735	0.0692	0.0601	0.0745	0.0690	93.83%	0.0045	6.17%
2017	0.0788	0.0890	0.0595	0.0738	0.0730	92.57%	0.0059	7.43%
2018	0.0700	0.0745	0.0532	0.0660	0.0641	91.55%	0.0059	8.45%
Mean	0.0802	0.0889	0.0729	0.0726	0.0763	95.02%	0.0039	4.98%

In terms of the decomposition of regional differences, the Theil index in the upstream, midstream, and downstream areas declined during the study period, i.e., the regional differences in URI narrowed, with decreases of 34%, 21.2%, and 16.6%, respectively, and they showed a ladder-like rule of upstream > midstream > downstream. During this period, the mean contribution value and contribution rate of intraregional differences to the comprehensive URI difference were significantly greater than those of interregional differences. Compared with the beginning of the period, the intraregional differences decreased and the interregional differences slightly increased; thus, the differences in URI mainly reflected in intraregional differences. In summary, the comprehensive and intraregional differences in URI have diminished in fluctuations, while the changes in interregional differences are more complex. Therefore, in the construction of resilient cities, more attention should be given to regional coordination, linkage, and integrated development.

3.2. Spatial Pattern of URI

3.2.1. Differentiation Characteristics of Comprehensive URI

According to the results of the URI and referring to the classification standards of urban resilience in existing studies [35], the authors of this paper used 0.2, 0.35, and 0.5 as critical values to visualize the URI in 2011, 2014, 2016, and 2018 (Figure 3). $Y \leq 0.2$ indicates low resilience, $0.2 < Y \leq 0.35$ indicates to mid-low resilience, $0.35 < Y \leq 0.5$ indicates mid-high resilience, and $Y > 0.5$ indicates high resilience.

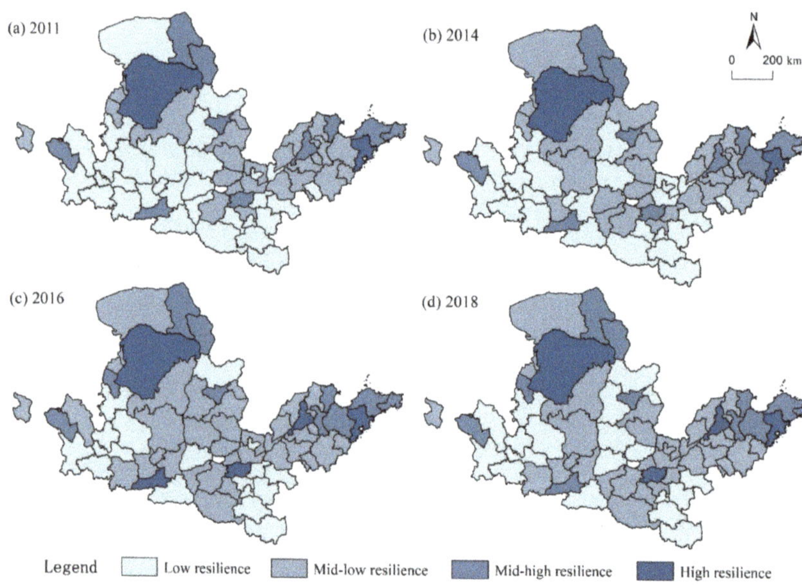

Figure 3. The spatial distribution of URI in the YRB from 2011 to 2018.

On the whole, the URI of the YRB has clustering characteristics, with regional central cities as the core and showing obvious zonal differences, as shown in Figure 4. First, the highly resilient cities are distributed, as indicated by dots in the figure. Before 2016, the cities of Ordos and Qingdao were representative, and Zhengzhou and Jinan also entered the ranks. The reason is that these cities have a significant "siphon effect" in the region. The collection of advantageous resources promotes the improvement of a city's emergency mechanisms, and their considerable economic strength can bear the high cost of urban restoration. Moreover, social maturity and social vitality are high. Both increased labour costs and pressures on resources and the environment force cities to upgrade their industrial structure and technological transformation, which improves their environmental pollution prevention and control capabilities. Consequently, the ecosystem resilience increases, so the pressure URI is relatively high. Second, cities with mid-high resilience are mostly located on the fringes of cities with high resilience, such as Hohhot, Baotou, and Shizuishan in the upper reaches and Zibo, Weifang, and Yantai in the Shandong Peninsula; there are also a small number of cities distributed as indicated by dots in the figure, such as Lanzhou, Xi'an, and Taiyuan. Their resilience pattern was relatively stable during the study period. Finally, mid-low and low resilience cities accounted for 82.1% in 2011 and 77.6% from 2014 to 2018. They are widely distributed in the midwestern and southern regions and show certain spatial solidification characteristics. These are mainly small and medium-sized cities with poor basic conditions, insufficient economic growth momentum, and a low comprehensive URI.

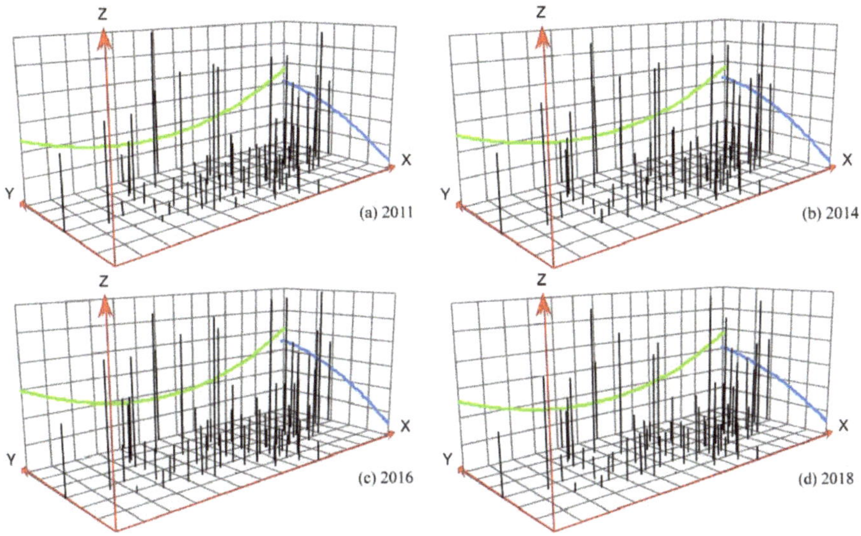

Figure 4. The evolution trend of URI in the YRB.

3.2.2. Spatial Correlation Analysis

Global Spatial Autocorrelation Analysis

The comprehensive URI of cities presents a positive spatial autocorrelation in the regional space; that is, cities with similar comprehensive resilience showed a spatial agglomeration trend. The Moran's *I* index dropped from 0.211 in 2011 to 0.191 in 2018 (Table 2), indicating that the agglomeration trend weakened. From the perspective of subsystem resilience, economic resilience showed a positive spatial correlation, and both the Moran's *I* value and the significance level are higher than other system resilience levels, again highlighting that economic resilience exerts the greatest impact on comprehensive URI while the impact of infrastructure resilience on comprehensive URI is second only to economic resilience. The low significance level and weak agglomeration trend of social and ecological resilience are additional evidence of the imbalanced social and ecological development among cities in the YRB.

Table 2. The Moran's *I* Index of URI in the YRB.

Year	Moran's *I*				
	Comprehensive URI	**Economic Resilience**	**Social Resilience**	**Ecological Resilience**	**Infrastructure Resilience**
2011	0.211 ***	0.423 ***	0.005	0.047	0.210 ***
2012	0.248 ***	0.374 ***	0.069	−0.030	0.240 ***
2013	0.127 *	0.288 ***	−0.025	0.288 ***	0.188 ***
2014	0.221 ***	0.405 ***	0.026	0.118 *	0.167 **
2015	0.167 **	0.384 ***	0.011	0.152 **	0.173 **
2016	0.177 **	0.385 ***	0.015	0.032	0.093
2017	0.159 **	0.371 ***	0.009	0.032	0.129 *
2018	0.191 ***	0.365 ***	0.030	0.067	0.136 **

Note: ***, **, and * represent significance at the levels of 0.01, 0.05, and 0.1, respectively.

Local Spatial Autocorrelation Analysis

The local autocorrelation test showed that in 2011, 2014, 2016, and 2018, 19.4%, 16.4%, 17.9%, and 16.4% of the cities, respectively, showed obvious positive spatial correlation (Table 3). Specifically, the urban resilience in "H–H" agglomeration areas was found to mainly be concentrated in the Shandong Peninsula Blue Yellow Economic Zone and the Hohhot–Baotou–Ordos urban agglomeration, including locations such as Weifang Yantai, Zibo, Hohhot, and Baotou. These cities have the advantages of good regional coordination and linkage. The radiation trickle effect of large cities such as Qingdao and Hohhot will drive economic growth and infrastructure construction. Together with the gradual improvement of the cross-regional coordinated governance pattern, the comprehensive ecological and environmental benefits have improved. The comprehensive resilience in the region is relatively high. Urban resilience in "L–L" agglomeration areas is distributed in the southern and southwestern parts of the YRB, such as Guyuan, Pingliang, Tianshui, Nanyang, Zhoukou, and Zhumadian. These cities have weak basic conditions and insufficient regional development endowments. Constrained by location, transportation, and resources, they have formed "depressions" for urban resilient development. Urban resilience in "L–H" and "H–L" agglomeration areas become fault areas in the radiation conduction of high and low-value areas. "H–L"-type cities such as Lanzhou and Xi'an have a strong siphon effect on the surrounding cities and are in the polarization stage of absorbing the collection of various resources around them, causing the resilience construction of the surrounding underdeveloped cities to comparatively lag. As a result, an "L–H" type of urban resilience development deficit has formed.

Table 3. Local spatial evolution of URI in the YRB.

Year	H–H	L–L	L–H	H–L
2011	Weifang, Yantai, Zibo, Binzhou, Hohhot, Baotou	Guyuan, Pingliang, Tianshui, Qingyang, Nanyang, Zhoukou, Zhumadian	Bayannaoer, Shizuishan, Xinzhou, Rizhao	Lanzhou
2014	Weifang, Yantai, Zibo, Hohhot, Baotou	Guyuan, Pingliang, Tianshui, Luohe, Nanyang, Zhumadian	Bayannaoer, Shizuishan, Xinzhou, Binzhou, Rizhao	Lanzhou, Xi'an
2016	Weifang, Yantai, Zibo, Baotou, Shizuishan	Guyuan, Pingliang, Tianshui, Luohe, Nanyang, Zhoukou, Zhumadian	Bayannaoer, Xinzhou, Binzhou, Laiwu, Rizhao	Lanzhou, Xi'an
2018	Weifang, Yantai, Zibo, Binzhou, Baotou	Guyuan, Pingliang, Tianshui, Nanyang, Zhoukou, Zhumadian	Bayannaoer, Shizuishan, Rizhao	Lanzhou

3.2.3. Evolution Trend Analysis

To more intuitively illustrate the spatial evolution characteristics of URIs, ArcGIS 10.2 software was used to describe the spatial distribution trend of URIs in the YRB in 2011, 2014, 2016, and 2018 (Figure 4). In these visualisations, the Z-axis represents the URI, the line on the X-axis corresponds to the trend of the URI in the east–west direction, and that on the Y-axis indicates the north–south direction. On the whole, the curve of the URI from 2011 to 2018 has a relatively small range, and the overall stability remains steady. In the east–west direction, the curve presents an obvious U-shaped distribution pattern of high east–west and low central. This result indicates that cities in the east and west of the YRB have high resilience, whereas the central area has low urban resilience. In the north–south direction, the "high in the north and low in the south" curve trend is obvious, indicating that the URI of the northern part of the YRB is higher than that of the southern part, which shows significant regional differences.

3.3. Analysis of Influencing Factors of URI

3.3.1. Index Selection

As shown by the analysis, there are significant spatiotemporal differences in URI throughout the YRB, and differences in the development of resilience among different cities and regions coexist with spatial correlation. As this area straddles the three major tectonic plates in China's eastern, middle, and western regions, its socioeconomic development and natural background conditions are strongly imbalanced and the nonlinear interaction of various factors has led to a complicated spatiotemporal pattern of urban resilience. A review of the existing literature revealed that most of the current analysis on factors affecting urban resilience have focused on humanity and society and seldom involved the discussion of the impact of natural factors on urban resilience. The authors of this paper constructed an indicator system for multiple influencing factors of urban resilience in the YRB.

In terms of social and economic factors, the influencing effect of human factors was verified through the eight aspects of economic [47], infrastructure [8], fiscal [48], market [48], urbanization [48], financial [25], openness [48], and innovation factors [48]. According to the literature, we selected GDP/administrative area (x_1), urban municipal public facilities construction/total investment in fixed assets (x_2), fiscal revenue/GDP(x_3), per capita retail sales of consumer goods (x_4), urban population/total population (x_5), financial institution deposit balance/loan balance (x_6), total import and export/GDP (x_7), and technology and education expenditure/GDP (x_8) for characterization. Regarding natural factors, the impact of the natural environment on urban resilience was verified through the three aspects of water, air, and vegetation. The related variables were annual precipitation (x_9), annual average temperature (x_{10}), and vegetation index (x_{11}). Jenks was used to discretize each explanatory variable into a type quantity. Based on factor and interactive detection in the geographical detector model, the main influencing factors of the URI in the YRB and the influence of the interaction of various factors on urban resilience were identified.

3.3.2. Analysis of Influencing Factors

Through the use of factor detection to measure the interpretation strength of each influencing factor (q) (Table 4), the results showed that the influencing forces of each factor significantly varied, with the most influential factors including the economic (0.3891), fiscal (0.3181), market (0.748), urbanization (0.5875), openness (0.3471), and innovation factors (0.3803). Compared with social and economic factors, the significance level of natural factors was found to be low, as was their impact on URI.

Table 4. Detection results of factors affecting urban resilience in the YRB.

Year	2011	2014	2016	2018	Average
x_1	0.4089 ***	0.3382 **	0.4280 ***	0.3811 **	0.3891
x_2	0.3139 *	0.2101	0.1133	0.2031	0.2101
x_3	0.2102 **	0.2535 **	0.3798 ***	0.4288 ***	0.3181
x_4	0.8401 ***	0.7454 ***	0.7889 ***	0.6167 ***	0.7478
x_5	0.4189 ***	0.6586 ***	0.6513 ***	0.6212 ***	0.5875
x_6	0.3042 ***	0.2230 ***	0.1888 **	0.2456 ***	0.2404
x_7	0.2840 **	0.3252 *	0.4511 ***	0.3282 ***	0.3471
x_8	0.4081 ***	0.4115 ***	0.2987 ***	0.4031 ***	0.3803
x_9	0.0846	0.1578	0.0476	0.0579	0.0870
x_{10}	0.1142	0.1194	0.1383	0.0766	0.1121
x_{11}	0.1267 *	0.1335	0.0788	0.1376	0.1191

Note: ***, **, and * represent significance at the levels of 0.01, 0.05, and 0.1, respectively.

Economic factors exert a significant impact on urban resilience. When citizens are attacked by man-made or natural disasters, robust economic strength can provide the necessary economic foundation and material guarantees for a city's post-disaster recovery and development. In the early stages of urban development, excessive reliance on resource input reduced the spatial carrying capacity of the urban system, which weakened its ability to prevent external shocks and unknown risks and resulted in ecological environment system overloaded. Areas such as Changzhi, Xinzhou, Linfen, and Lvliang in Shanxi Province are important coal mine bases. Economic development mainly relies on resource-intensive industries, with low development quality and greater environmental protection pressure. In addition, in some cities such as Ordos, a large number of new district constructions have led to the oversupply of real estate development, imperfect infrastructure, and even "ghost cities", causing great damage and pollution to the natural environment and seriously affecting urban resilience. With the transformation of the urban economic development model to high-quality intensification, technological progress and increased awareness of environmental protection have forced cities to improve their pollution control levels and the ability of urban systems to self-repair has increased. Such transformation has also provided capital accumulation for post-disaster recovery and strengthened cities' resistance to various risk interferences. Therefore, efforts should be made to realize the linkage of the upstream, midstream, and downstream economies and industry synergy; promote the diversification of economic industries; further promote the transformation of economic development from quantitative expansion to qualitative improvement; and build a resilient economic structural system.

Fiscal factors play an important role in influencing urban resilience and exert an impact on the rise of resilience overall. The fiscal role is related to the government macro control. The larger the fiscal scale is, the more able the government is to centrally allocate social resources and provide strong human, material, and fiscal support for cities to resist external risks. The YRB mostly comprises small- and medium-sized cities in the middle of industrialization. The city scale is small, and most of the various elements are close to resource-based industries, which reduces the stability of the urban system and ecosystem in long-term development and leads to path dependence on the government's fiscal support in the construction of urban resilience. However, if the fiscal scale exceeds the total amount of social surplus products, it will cause difficulty in capital turnover in the market, which is adverse for the optimal distribution of various resources in the urban system. Moreover, excessive government regulation is contrary to the general operational law of cities, easily produces rigidity in the process of urban development, and is not conducive to the construction of urban resilience. Therefore, in the future construction of resilient cities, the role of fiscal factors should be fully integrated to build an efficient service-oriented government and to improve the fiscal guarantee mechanism in the daily operation of the urban system.

Market factors exert a significant influence on urban resilience. Increased market capacity can strengthen the degree of regional marketization, stimulate the endogenous growth momentum of the urban economy, and enhance the resilience of local cities while promoting the resilience of surrounding areas through the radiation and driving effect of the market. In most underdeveloped small and medium-sized cities, residents tend to have a strong marginal willingness to consume, whereas their actual spending power is relatively weak. With the improvement of the urban social security level, residents' burdens on medical care, education, and hygiene can be greatly reduced. This alleviation, in turn, can stimulate the conversion of residents' income into production and living consumption, as well as provide a powerful impetus for urban economic development. In the process of building resilient cities, it is important to focus on improving the level of marketization and market activity, deepening the reform of the market-oriented allocation of factors, stimulating market potential, and improving the market's emergency early warning mechanism to respond to disturbance threats.

Urbanization factors exert a significant influence on urban resilience. An increase in the urbanization level means that the degree of urban agglomeration will increase. When a city is hit by disasters, it can quickly realize the allocation and complementation of various resources in the city, as well as reduce the degree of damage to the urban system.

In recent years, the construction of new-type urbanization has intensified, the quality of urbanization has significantly improved, ecological cities and smart cities have improved the effectiveness of urban governance, and the operation of various functions in the urban system has been complemented and enhanced. The increase in urbanization has also strengthened the information communication within cities, avoiding the paralysis of the city system due to poor communication or "information failure", improving the vitality of urban development, and strengthening the city's ability to resist various shocks and threats. Therefore, urban planning and management should be coordinated to form a spatial pattern of urbanization with complete functions and the division of labour and coordination to provide good environmental support for improving urban resilience.

Openness factors exert a significant driving effect on urban resilience. According to the "pollution refuge hypothesis", there are different environmental regulations among regions, and pollution-intensive industries show corresponding comparative advantages in different regions. When environmental regulations are relatively loose, the inflow of these polluting industries will increase the pressure on the local ecological environment, which is not conducive to the construction of ecological resilience. However, increasing the openness level is conducive to accumulating various resource elements and accelerating the diversified development of the industrial structure, with the effect of economies of scale thus becoming increasingly prominent. In the process of opening up, cities should acquire reverse knowledge spillovers, improve local technological innovation capabilities, and accelerate the optimization and upgrading of industrial structure to achieve balanced coordination between economic growth and environmental protection. In the construction of resilient cities, efforts should be made to build inland opening-up heights, actively guide the flow of funds to low-polluting and high-tech industries, and strengthen the introduction of talent and intellectual exchanges.

Innovation factors exert a significant influence on urban resilience. The achievements of scientific and technological innovation not only inject new momentum into economic development but also provide an effective means to solve ecological and environmental problems. From the perspective of science and technology, as localities pay increasing attention to science and technology investment, innovation dividends gradually appear. Technology spillovers are promoted through the network of city cooperation, which improves the efficiency of energy resource utilization and the input–output ratio, promotes the exploration and utilization of new energy, reduces the proportion of fossil energy consumption, improves the ability to control ecological environmental pollution, and reduces pollution emissions from industrial enterprises. In terms of education investment, the talent team is the key to technological innovation. Education investment helps to improve human capital, thereby improving the overall quality of workers, raising awareness of environmental protection, and providing a talent pool for the future development of the city, thereby strengthening the economic system and ecosystem anti-risk ability. All of these factors are highly beneficial to economic and ecological resilience.

From the perspective of other influencing factors: (1) The infrastructure factor (0.2101) showed a trend from significant to insignificant. Excessive government intervention is one possible reason [49]. Unreasonable planning and infrastructure investment have little effect on urban resilience, but the suboptimal allocation of the internal resource elements of a city system reduces the efficiency of resource use. However, this does not mean that infrastructure investment is negligible in the construction of urban resilience. Complete infrastructure is the basic material condition for cities to face various risks and challenges, and it provides basic support for the construction of resilient cities. In future infrastructure construction, more attention should be paid to improving the efficiency of infrastructure investment and building a multifaceted and systematic infrastructure pattern. (2) The financial factor (0.2404) was found to exert less impact on urban resilience than other factors and showed a downward trend, possibly because of the small financial scale of the cities in the YRB and the long-term dual economic structure. Idle funds in society are easily guided by policies to flow to highly resilient cities. Improving financial efficiency will intensify the competition of financial resources between high and low resilience cities, which will easily lead to financial risks. At present, the impact of the financial factor on urban resilience construction is limited.

Based on factor detection, the authors of this paper used interaction detection analysis to detect interaction types for impact factors (Table 5). The results showed that any two factors exerted a greater impact on urban resilience than a single factor, and the interaction types were all revealed to be nonlinear enhancements, indicating that urban resilience is affected by multiple factors. Specifically, the interaction between market factors and other influencing factors, such as infrastructure, fiscal, and urbanization, can better explain urban resilience. Compared to these, the impact of the other two factors is relatively low.

Table 5. Interaction of influencing factors on urban resilience in the YRB.

2011		2014		2016		2018	
Interaction Factor	Value	Interaction Factor	Value	Interaction Factor	Value	Interaction Factor	Value
$x_3 \cap x_1$	0.6304	$x_3 \cap x_1$	0.6274	$x_3 \cap x_1$	0.6679	$x_3 \cap x_2$	0.6490
$x_4 \cap x_2$	0.9326	$x_4 \cap x_3$	0.8677	$x_4 \cap x_1$	0.8375	$x_4 \cap x_1$	0.7714
$x_4 \cap x_3$	0.9393	$x_5 \cap x_1$	0.7629	$x_4 \cap x_2$	0.8247	$x_4 \cap x_3$	0.7264
$x_5 \cap x_1$	0.6862	$x_5 \cap x_2$	0.6895	$x_4 \cap x_3$	0.9154	$x_5 \cap x_1$	0.7160
$x_5 \cap x_2$	0.6324	$x_5 \cap x_3$	0.7912	$x_5 \cap x_1$	0.7444	$x_5 \cap x_2$	0.6429
$x_6 \cap x_1$	0.6045	$x_5 \cap x_4$	0.8273	$x_5 \cap x_3$	0.7969	$x_5 \cap x_4$	0.7069
$x_6 \cap x_5$	0.6240	$x_6 \cap x_4$	0.8022	$x_5 \cap x_4$	0.8367	$x_6 \cap x_4$	0.7295
$x_8 \cap x_1$	0.6924	$x_6 \cap x_5$	0.7378	$x_7 \cap x_3$	0.6698	$x_6 \cap x_5$	0.6770
$x_8 \cap x_2$	0.6141	$x_7 \cap x_3$	0.6112	$x_8 \cap x_1$	0.6387	$x_7 \cap x_3$	0.6085
$x_8 \cap x_3$	0.6917	$x_7 \cap x_5$	0.7491	$x_8 \cap x_3$	0.7827	$x_7 \cap x_4$	0.7099
$x_8 \cap x_5$	0.6853	$x_8 \cap x_4$	0.6445	$x_8 \cap x_5$	0.6901	$x_8 \cap x_3$	0.6054
$x_8 \cap x_7$	0.6299	$x_8 \cap x_5$	0.6945	$x_8 \cap x_7$	0.6538	$x_8 \cap x_5$	0.6578

Note: This table only lists the interaction factors with higher interaction values.

4. Conclusions

Based on the panel data of 67 cities in the YRB from 2011 to 2018, the temporal and spatial differentiation characteristics of urban resilience in the YRB were analysed, and a geographical detector model was used to analyse the influencing factors of urban resilience. The main conclusions are as follows:

(1) From 2011 to 2018, the comprehensive URI of the YRB was at a low-medium level, showed two-stage evolutionary characteristics, and presented a "V"-shaped dynamic fluctuation; it rose from 0.2437 to 0.2763, an increase of 13.4%. The resilience of each subsystem has obvious volatility and hierarchical characteristics, showing the following trend: economic resilience > social resilience > ecological resilience > infrastructure resilience.

(2) From the regional perspective, the comprehensive URI of the upstream, midstream, and downstream regions has somewhat increased, but the development and change of the resilience index of each subsystem in the region show significant regional characteristics. In addition, the comprehensive difference in URI in the basin has shown a shrinking trend. The intraregional differences in the three major sectors have shrunk, while the interregional differences have slightly increased. Intraregional differences are the main source of urban resilience differences.

(3) From the spatial analysis, we found that the URI of the YRB had obvious zonal differences from 2011 to 2018. The global Moran's I index showed that the URI has presented a positive spatial autocorrelation in the regional space. In terms of local agglomeration, the "H–H"-type cities are mostly concentrated in the Shandong Peninsula and the Hohhot–Baotou–Ordos urban agglomeration, and the "L–L"-type cities are distributed in the southern and southwestern parts of the YRB. From the perspective of global trends, the U-shaped distribution trend in the east–west direction indicates that the urban resilience of the eastern and western parts of the YRB is

significantly greater than that of the central region, and the upward trend from north to south indicates that the resilience of northern cities is greater than that in the south.

(4) From the analysis of influencing factors, we found that socioeconomic factors exert a greater influence on urban resilience than natural factors. Factor detection results showed that economic, fiscal, market, urbanization, openness, and innovation factors are the core impacts factors of urban resilience, while infrastructure and financial factors exert low impacts on urban resilience. In terms of interactive detection, the impact of the interaction factor on urban resilience was found to be significantly greater than that of a single factor, the interaction type of each interaction factor is characterized by nonlinear enhancement, and urban resilience in the basin is affected by multiple influencing factors.

5. Implications

The authors of this paper define urban resilience as a city's ability to resist unknown risks and recover after a disaster. We used empirical analysis methods to explore the spatiotemporal evolution and influencing factors of urban resilience. This analysis provides a helpful reference for the prevention and resolution of major risks in the YRB against the background of the new era and provides new ideas for building resilient cities to promote sustainable development. In the process of urban development, the evolution of humanistic and natural elements or coupling with other elements constantly shapes the spatial form within the city, presenting multiscale characteristics within the spatiotemporal differentiation of urban resilience, which also makes the influencing factors of urban resilience more complex. At present, the urban resilience of the YRB is generally at a mid-low level, with large spatial and regional differences. The resilience of subsystems within the basin and among regions shows a clear hierarchical structure, reflecting a significant imbalance of economic, social, ecological, and infrastructure construction in the YRB. Achieving the coordinated development of the resilience of various subsystems has become the key to strengthening urban resilience. For this reason, cities in the YRB should strengthen the strategic top-level design of resilient city construction on the basis of their natural endowments and actual social and economic conditions; build effective economic development, social and public policy coordination, and infrastructure planning and construction mechanisms; strengthen the capacity of ecological and environmental protection; and establish a scientific and reasonable urban resilience system evaluation system. Considering that academia has not yet reached a consensus on the basic connotations of and evaluation criteria for urban resilience, future research will start with basic concepts to analyse the scientific connotation and framework structure of urban resilience and take a diversified and composite perspective on urban resilience development in various regions to find a reasonable and resilient city construction path.

Author Contributions: Conceptualization, Y.C. and Q.Z.; data curation, X.S.; formal analysis, X.S. and Q.Z.; funding acquisition, Y.C.; methodology, X.S. and Q.Z.; software, X.S.; supervision, Q.Z. and Y.C.; writing—original draft, X.S.; writing—review and editing, Q.Z. and Y.C. All authors have read and agreed to the published version of the manuscript.

Funding: This work was supported by grants from Support Plan for Scientific and Technological Innovation Talents in Henan Institutions of Higher Learning (humanities and social sciences) (2018-cx-012); Training Plan for Key Young Teachers in Henan Institutions of Higher Learning (2018GGJS094); Good Scholar in Philosophy and Social Sciences in Henan Institutions of Higher Learning (2019-YXXZ-20); and Philosophy and Social Science Innovation Team Building Program of Henan Universities (2021-CXTD-12); Basic research projects of philosophy and social sciences in Colleges and Universities of Henan Province (2021-JCZD-25).

Institutional Review Board Statement: Not applicable.

Informed Consent Statement: Not applicable.

Data Availability Statement: The data presented in this study are openly available in National Bureau of Statistics, reference number 978-7-5037-9120-8, 978-7-5037-8770-6, 978-7-5037-8432-3, 978-7-5037-8082-0, 978-7-5037-7706-6, 978-7-5037-7350-1, 978-7-5037-7019-7, 978-7-5037-6754-8.

Conflicts of Interest: The authors declare no conflict of interest. The funders had no role in the design of the study; in the collection, analyses, or interpretation of data; in the writing of the manuscript, or in the decision to publish the results.

Appendix A

Table A1. The evaluation index system of urban resilience in the YRB.

Target	Criterion Layer	Index Layer	Nature	Index Meaning	Reference
Urban resilience	Economic resilience	GDP per capita	+	Economic aggregate	Shi et al. [1,50]
		Per capita fiscal expenditure	+	Financial security	Shi et al. [1,50]
		The proportion of tertiary industry in GDP	+	Economic structure	Chen et al. [49]
		Per capita savings deposit balance	+	Financial capital	Chen et al. [49]
		Per capita investment in fixed assets	+	Investment intensity	Shi et al. [1,50]
		Number of industrial enterprises above designated size	+	Economic growth	Chen et al. [49]
	Social resilience	Number of college students per 10,000 people	+	Education level	Chen et al. [49]
		Number of hospital beds per 10,000 people	+	Medical investment	Kammouh et al. [22]
		Average salary of employees	+	Residence income	Shi et al. [1,50]
		Proportion of employment in tertiary industry	+	Employment structure	Shi et al. [1,50]
		Number of registered unemployed persons in urban areas	+	Unemployment structure	Shi et al. [1,50]
		Health technicians per 10,000 people	−	Health protection	Kammouh et al. [22]
	Ecological resilience	Park green area per capita	+	Environmental conservation level	Kammouh et al. [22]
		Green coverage rate in built-up area	+	Urban greening level	Kammouh et al. [22]
		Comprehensive utilization rate of industrial solid waste	+	Waste utilization	Chen et al. [49]
		Harmless treatment rate of urban domestic garbage	+	Environmental remediation	Chen et al. [49]
		Industrial wastewater discharge per unit GDP	−	Environmental pollution pressure	Chen et al. [49]
		Industrial smoke and dust emissions per unit of GDP	−	Waste emission intensity	Chen et al. [49]
	Infrastructure resilience	Road area per capita	+	Infrastructure construction	Chen et al. [49]
		Number of buses per 10,000 people	+	Level of transportation facilities	Kammouh et al. [22]
		Density of urban drainage pipes	+	Engineering support capability	Chen et al. [49]
		Number of Internet broadband users	+	Internet penetration	Kammouh et al. [22]
		Electricity consumption per capita	−	Electricity development level	Shi et al. [1,50]
		Number of mobile phone users at the end of the year	+	Communication sophistication	Kammouh et al. [22]

References

1. Shi, Y.; Zhai, G.; Xu, L.; Zhou, S.; Lu, Y.; Liu, H.; Huang, W. Assessment methods of urban system resilience: From the perspective of complex adaptive system theory. *Cities* **2021**, *112*, 1–9. [CrossRef]
2. Kamila, B.; Peter, N.; Porfirio, G. Urban resilience patterns after an external shock: An exploratory study. *Int. J. Disaster Risk Reduct.* **2018**, *31*, 381–392.
3. Sun, J.; Wang, J.; Wang, T.; Zhang, T. Urbanization, economic growth, and environmental pollution. *Manag. Environ. Qual. Int. J.* **2019**, *30*, 483–494. [CrossRef]
4. United Nations Human Settlements Programme. *World Cities Report 2020: The Value of Sustainable Urbanization*; UN-Habitat: Nairobi, Kenya, 2020; pp. 11–15.

5. Marta, S.; Erik, G.; Javier, B.; Daniella, T. Towards an Urban Resilience Index: A Case Study in 50 Spanish Cities. *Sustainability* **2016**, *8*, 774.
6. Sara, M.; Joshua, P.N.; Melissa, S. Defining urban resilience: A review. *Landsc. Urban Plan* **2016**, *147*, 38–49.
7. Chen, C.; Xu, L.; Zhao, D.; Xu, T.; Lei, P. A new model for describing the urban resilience considering adaptability, resistance and recovery. *Saf. Sci.* **2020**, *128*, 104756. [CrossRef]
8. Kim, D.; Lim, U. Urban Resilience in Climate Change Adaptation: A Conceptual Framework. *Sustainability* **2016**, *8*, 405. [CrossRef]
9. Susan, L.C.; Joseph, A.A.; Bernard, A.; Patrick, C.; Elizabeth, A.E.; Gerald, E.G.; Michael, F.G.; Howard, C.K.; Meredith, L.; Monica, S.; et al. Disaster Resilience: A National Imperative. *Environ. Sci. Policy Sustain. Dev.* **2014**, *55*, 25–29.
10. Sara, M.; Joshua, P.N. Resilience and Complexity: A Bibliometric Review and Prospects for Industrial Ecology. *J. Ind. Ecol.* **2015**, *19*, 236–251.
11. Nathan, L.E.; Ariane, D.B.; Elizabeth, L.M.; Richard, H.M. Towards a resilience indicator framework for making climate-change adaptation decisions. *Mitig. Adapt. Strateg. Glob. Chang.* **2014**, *19*, 1295–1312.
12. Marjolein, S.; Bas, W. Building up resilience in cities worldwide-Rotterdam as participant in the 100 Resilient Cities Programme. *Cities* **2017**, *61*, 109–116.
13. Ayyoob, S.; Yoshiki, Y. *Resilient Urban Form: A Conceptual Framework*; Springer International Publishing: Cham, Switzerland, 2018; pp. 167–179.
14. Feng, X.; Xiu, C.; Bai, L.; Zhong, Y.; Wei, Y. Comprehensive evaluation of urban resilience based on the perspective of landscape pattern: A case study of Shenyang city. *Cities* **2020**, *104*, 102722. [CrossRef]
15. Jack, A.; Sarel, C.; Jari, N. The concept of ecosystem services in adaptive urban planning and design: A framework for supporting innovation. *Landsc. Urban Plan* **2014**, *125*, 254–259.
16. Jonas, J.; Rajib, S.; Yukiko, T.; Ramasamy, K. Action-oriented resilience assessment of communities in Chennai, India. *Environ. Hazards* **2012**, *11*, 226–241.
17. Oto, H.; Aura, R.; Monika, S. Resilience capacity and vulnerability: A joint analysis with reference to Slovak urban districts. *Cities* **2018**, *73*, 24–35.
18. Susan, L.C.; Kevin, D.A.; Christopher, T.E. The geographies of community disaster resilience. *Glob. Environ. Chang.* **2014**, *29*, 65–77.
19. Marta, B.; Giulia, D.; Elena, D.A. A System Dynamics Model and Analytic Network Process: An Integrated Approach to Investigate Urban Resilience. *Land* **2020**, *9*, 1–26.
20. Maksims, F.; Francesco, R. Assessment of Urban Resilience to Natural Disasters with a System Dynamics Tool: Case Study of Latvian Municipality. *Environ. Clim. Technol.* **2020**, *24*, 249–264.
21. Sherrieb, K.; Norris, F.H.; Galea, S. Measuring Capacities for Community Resilience. *Soc. Indic. Res.* **2010**, *99*, 227–247. [CrossRef]
22. Omar, K.; Ali, Z.N.; Gian Paolo, C.; Stephen, A.M. Resilience Assessment of Urban Communities. *Civ. Eng.* **2019**, *5*, 4019002.
23. Doğan, D.; Defne, D.; Ahmet Burak, K. Urban Resilience Assessment of Trabzon. *J. Inst. Sci. Technol.* **2020**, *10*, 1286–1297.
24. James, S.; Ron, M. The economic resilience of regions: Towards an evolutionary approach. *Camb. J. Reg. Econ. Soc.* **2010**, *3*, 27–43.
25. Christian, R.; Thomas, S. Towards social resilience: A quantitative and qualitative survey on citizens' perception of social media in emergencies in Europe. *Technol. Forecast. Soc. Chang.* **2017**, *121*, 168–180.
26. Brian, C.C.; Murray, S. Social-ecological resilience and geomorphic systems. *Geomorphology* **2018**, *305*, 221–230.
27. Cai, B.; Xie, M.; Liu, Y.; Liu, Y.; Feng, Q. Availability-based engineering resilience metric and its corresponding evaluation methodology. *Reliab. Eng. Syst. Saf.* **2018**, *172*, 216–224. [CrossRef]
28. Zhou, Q.; Zhu, M.; Qiao, Y.; Zhang, X.; Chen, J. Achieving resilience through smart cities? Evidence from China. *Habitat. Int.* **2021**, *111*, 102348. [CrossRef]
29. Cutter, S.L.; Barnes, L.; Berry, M.; Burton, C.; Evans, E.; Tate, E.; Webb, J. A place-based model for understanding community resilience to natural disasters. *Glob. Environ. Chang.* **2008**, *18*, 598–606. [CrossRef]
30. Jabareen, Y. Planning the resilient city: Concepts and strategies for coping with climate change and environmental risk. *Cities* **2013**, *31*, 220–229. [CrossRef]
31. Saja, A.M.A.; Teo, M.; Goonetilleke, A.; Ziyath, A.M. An inclusive and adaptive framework for measuring social resilience to disasters. *Int. J. Disaster Risk Reduct.* **2018**, *28*, 862–873. [CrossRef]
32. Martin, R.; Sunley, P. On the notion of regional economic resilience: Conceptualization and explanation. *J. Econ. Geogr.* **2014**, *15*, 1–42. [CrossRef]
33. Joerin, J.; Shaw, R.; Takeuchi, Y.; Krishnamurthy, R. The adoption of a Climate Disaster Resilience Index in Chennai, India. *Disasters* **2014**, *38*, 540–561. [CrossRef] [PubMed]
34. Zhou, L.; Zhou, C.; Che, L.; Wang, B. Spatio-temporal evolution and influencing factors of urban green development efficiency in China. *J. Geogr. Sci.* **2020**, *30*, 724–742. [CrossRef]
35. Xiao, W.; Lv, X.; Zhao, Y.; Sun, H.; Li, J. Ecological resilience assessment of an arid coal mining area using index of entropy and linear weighted analysis: A case study of Shendong Coalfield, China. *Ecol. Indic.* **2020**, *109*, 105843. [CrossRef]
36. Ranasinghe, U.; Jefferies, M.; Davis, P.; Pillay, M. Resilience Engineering Indicators and Safety Management: A Systematic Review. *Saf. Health Work* **2020**, *11*, 127–135. [CrossRef]
37. Wang, M.; Zhao, H.; Cui, J.; Fan, D.; Lv, B.; Wang, G.; Li, Z.; Zhou, G. Evaluating green development level of nine cities within the Pearl River Delta, China. *J. Clean. Prod.* **2018**, *174*, 315–323. [CrossRef]

38. Nosek, V.; Netrdová, P. What values of Moran's I and Theil index decomposition really mean under different conditions: On the issue of interpretation. *Lett. Spat. Resour. Sci.* **2017**, *10*, 149–159. [CrossRef]
39. Moran, P.A.P. Notes on continuous stochastic phenomena. *Biometrika* **1950**, *37*, 17–23. [CrossRef]
40. Cliff, A.D.; Ord, J.K. Spatial Processes: Models and Applications. *Geogr. J.* **1982**, *148*, 383–385.
41. Luc, A. Local Indicators of Spatial Association-LISA. *Geogr. Anal.* **1995**, *27*, 93–115.
42. Wang, J.F.; Xu, C.D. Geodetector: Principle and prospective. *Acta Geogr. Sin.* **2017**, *72*, 116–134. (In Chinese)
43. Ding, Y.; Zhang, M.; Qian, X.; Li, C.; Chen, S.; Wang, W. Using the geographical detector technique to explore the impact of socioeconomic factors on PM2.5 concentrations in China. *J. Clean Prod.* **2019**, *211*, 1480–1490. [CrossRef]
44. Guo, F.Y.; Tong, L.J.; Qiu, F.D.; Li, Y.M. Spatio-temporal differentiation characteristics and influencing factors of green development in the eco-economic corridor of the Yellow River Basin. *Acta Geogr. Sin.* **2021**, *76*, 726–739. (In Chinese)
45. Liu, K.; Jiang, H.; Zhou, Q. Spatial Analysis of Industrial Green Development and Sustainable Cities in the Yellow River Basin. *Discret. Dyn. Nat. Soc.* **2021**, *2021*, 5529153. [CrossRef]
46. Li, H.; Jiang, Z.; Dong, G.; Wang, L.; Huang, X.; Gu, X.; Guo, Y. Spatiotemporal Coupling Coordination Analysis of Social Economy and Resource Environment of Central Cities in the Yellow River Basin. *Discret. Dyn. Nat. Soc.* **2021**, *2021*, 6637631.
47. Bai, L.M.; Xiu, C.L.; Feng, X.H.; Mei, D.W.; Wei, Z. A comprehensive assessment of urban resilience and its spatial differentiation in China. *World Reg. Stud.* **2019**, *28*, 77–87. (In Chinese)
48. Zhu, J.H.; Sun, H.X. Research on Spatial-temporal Evolution and Influencing Factors of Urban Resilience of China's Three Metropolitan Agglomerations. *Soft Sci.* **2020**, *34*, 72–79. (In Chinese)
49. Chen, Y.; Zhu, M.; Zhou, Q.; Qiao, Y. Research on Spatiotemporal Differentiation and Influence Mechanism of Urban Resilience in China Based on MGWR Model. *Int. J. Environ. Res. Public Health* **2021**, *18*, 1056. [CrossRef]
50. Shi, T.; Qiao, Y.; Zhou, Q. Spatiotemporal evolution and spatial relevance of urban resilience: Evidence from cities of China. *Growth Chang.* **2021**. [CrossRef]

International Journal of
Environmental Research and Public Health

MDPI

Article

Neighborhood-Based Social Capital and Depressive Symptoms among Adults: Evidence from Guangzhou, China

Sanqin Mao [1] and Jie Chen [1,2,*]

1 School of International and Public Affairs, Shanghai Jiao Tong University, Shanghai 200030, China; alicemao01@sjtu.edu.cn
2 China Institute for Urban Governance, Shanghai Jiao Tong University, Shanghai 200030, China
* Correspondence: chenjie100@sjtu.edu.cn

Abstract: This study examined the association between neighborhood-based social capital (NSC) and depressive symptoms in the context of urban neighborhoods in China, with special attention given to the association heterogeneity across socioeconomic groups. Drawing on cross-sectional data collected from 39 neighborhoods in Guangzhou, this research demonstrated that adults' depressive symptoms were higher among those with lower cognitive (trustworthiness, reciprocity, and cohesion within a neighborhood) and structural (social network and participation) dimensions of NSC. Further analysis showed that the negative association between NSC and depressive symptoms was significantly heterogeneous across socioeconomic groups. Specifically, this negative relationship was more prominent in the lower socioeconomic classes than in the upper socioeconomic classes, indicating that the lower accumulation of NSC among disadvantaged groups may aggravate depression unequally across social classes. In addition, the negative association between social participation and depressive symptoms was stronger for people who are older or unemployed. The findings of this study not only provide new evidence concerning the significance of the beneficial effects of NSC in the Chinese context, but also, more importantly, highlight that NSC plays a crucial role in creating mental health inequality across social classes. Thus, the relevant social interventions including fostering neighborhood relationships and social activities should be carefully tailored against the backdrop of community building during the urbanization process. The implications of our study for urban governance to promote healthy cities are discussed.

Keywords: social capital; social participation; volunteering; urban China; urban governance

Citation: Mao, S.; Chen, J. Neighborhood-Based Social Capital and Depressive Symptoms among Adults: Evidence from Guangzhou, China. *IJERPH* **2021**, *18*, 11263. https://doi.org/10.3390/ijerph182111263

Academic Editor: Paul B. Tchounwou

Received: 9 September 2021
Accepted: 25 October 2021
Published: 27 October 2021

1. Introduction

Depression has increasingly become a worldwide mental health concern. It has been reported that depression affects 120 million people worldwide [1], and it ranks 15th among the leading contributors to disability-adjusted life years (DALY) [2]. Depression not only adversely affects normal life but also substantially raises the risk of various physical illness, such as addiction, stroke, self-injury, and cardiovascular disorders [3–6]. In order to reduce the occurrence of depression, a growing number of studies have tried to examine the potential contributors to depression. A large body of research has found that depressive symptoms vary across different population groups, such as age cohorts [7,8], gender groups [9], and migration categories [10,11]. Research has also revealed that neighborhood characteristics, such as the neighborhood's physical environment (e.g., built environment, green spaces, and communal spaces) [1,7,10], social environment, including relationships among neighbors (e.g., trustworthiness, social cohesion, and shared norms of reciprocity) [4,12–14], and participation in neighborhood activities (such as volunteering and participation in associations) [8,13,14], have specific links to depressive symptoms.

While a plethora of studies have delved into the linkage between neighborhoods' social environment and mental health in developed countries, intellectual inquiries about how this link works in developing countries has only just begun in recent years [13]. It has been reported that people from developing countries are more likely to be depressed than ever before, and depression has become one of the most important risk factors for disability and morbidity [15,16]. However, little is known about the social environment drivers of depression in these populations. To that end, there is an urgent need to disentangle the mental health benefits of residential social environments in developing countries for future public policies and social interventions. This study contributes to the literature by examining the association between neighborhood-based social capital (hereafter NSC) and depressive symptoms in the Chinese context, where the rates of depressive symptoms and depression have increased rapidly, and have topped 37.9% and 4.1%, respectively [17]. To date, only a few studies have examined the link between NSC and depressive symptoms in Chinese cities [13,18,19]. However, these studies have only focused on people who are older. Furthermore, studies concerned with the association of NSC with depressive symptoms have been left with many questions, considering that social capital is a multi-dimensional concept, and can take various forms. More studies are needed not only to investigate the relationship between NSC and depressive symptoms across population groups of different age cohorts, but also on whether and to what extent different forms of social capital are associated with depression.

Using data from a city-wide survey of 39 neighborhoods completed in early 2013 in Guangzhou, this study attempts to investigate the association between two forms of NSC and depressive symptoms, and further investigate whether this association may vary across socioeconomic groups. This question is of great significance for understanding the role of neighborhoods in preventing and treating mental illness within China's phenomenal urban transformation. This study contributes to the literature in three aspects. First, it makes the first attempt to systematically explore the relationship between NSC and depressive symptoms among adults in the Chinese context. Second, it breaks down the notions of different forms of social capital, and distinguishes between the effects of different forms of NSC. Third, it contributes to the existing literature on depression and to the debate on the significance of neighborhoods by examining the heterogeneous relationship between NSC and depressive symptoms across socioeconomic groups.

In this study, we first review the urban sociology literature on the association of NSC with depressive symptoms, including works pertaining to Chinese cities, and formulate several hypotheses accordingly (Section 2). In Section 3, we present the methodology and data of the study. We then analyze the extent to which different forms of NSC are related to depressive symptoms, and further explore the heterogeneous relationship between NSC and depressive symptoms across socioeconomic groups (Section 4). In Section 5, we discuss implications, limitations, and avenues for future study. Finally, the main findings are highlighted in Section 6.

2. Literature Review and Hypothesis Development

2.1. Association between Neighborhood-Based Social Capital and Depression

Social capital has received much attention in the past decades since Putnam, in his seminal work, *Bowling Alone*, argued that the American society is facing the loss of social capital, which leads to a myriad of social problems [20,21]. Despite the growing number of studies on social capital, we still lack of a precise definition for the term. Existing studies have explored social capital from different sources (e.g., neighborhood, employment, and family social capital) and in different forms (e.g., bridging vs. bonding, structural vs. cognitive, trust vs. reciprocity, individual vs. collective) [10,11,19,22,23]. This study focused on individual-level neighborhood-based social capital, which is one of the most important sources of social capital among adults. It adapts the typical typology of social capital to distinguish between two forms of NSC: neighborhood-based cognitive social capital (hereafter NCSC), and neighborhood-based structural social capital (hereafter NSSC) [19–21,24]. NCSC refers to residents' subjective perceptions and evaluations of social relationships within local neighborhoods, such as perceptions of the trustworthiness of neighbors, solidarity among neighbors, shared norms of reciprocity, and commitment within the neighborhood [10,11,14]. Unlike NCSC, NSSC is objective and measurable, and reflects residents' social behavior in local neighborhoods. Common indicators of NSSC include neighborhood acquaintances, neighbor interactions, and neighborhood participation (primarily social activities and volunteering) [10,14,25].

Previous studies have revealed that NCSC has more powerful protective effects against depressive symptoms than NSSC [24,26]. Residents who perceive their neighborhood to have a high level of mutual trust [27], social cohesion [14,23], and reciprocity [28] were significantly less likely to suffer from depressive symptoms in Western contexts. The main underlying mechanisms are that trust, reciprocity, shared norms, and values within a neighborhood can promote personal information exchange and knowledge transmission, affect the allocation and utilization of resources and services, back up the social credibility of residents, support healthy behaviors, and offer social support [27–30]. As for NSSC, current studies have revealed that social networks and neighborhood participation are significantly negatively associated with depressive symptoms [31–33]. Neighborhood participation, which is also a multidimensional construct in the literature, covers a wide range of activities, such as political, social, leisure, and cultural activities in the neighborhood. Several explanations for the obvious negative link between neighborhood participation and mental health have been proposed. For a start, participation in neighborhood activities provides individuals with opportunities to share information and exchange opinions mutually, which helps people to decrease feelings of loneliness, and to embrace healthier habits and lifestyles [33,34]. Furthermore, joint activities increase social contact, which can foster supportive and caring relationships, and consolidate social integration [8]. People can receive assistance and support more easily through these relationships, thereby reducing the risk of depression. Moreover, participation may make people recognize that they are part of the neighborhood, which promotes confidence, and inspires them to be more enthusiastic about neighborhood affairs [10].

Despite the strong evidence for the inverse relationship between NSC and depressive symptoms, some studies have revealed no significant relation between them [10,14,31]. A 2005 literature review [26] reported that, of the 11 works included in the study, seven revealed significant negative relationships between NCSC and depression, but only three revealed significant negative relationships between NSSC (primarily social engagement) and depression. Cao et al. [24] and Lu et al. [19] summarized the reasons behind these inconclusive findings regarding NSC and depression. First, due to differences in the measures and conceptualization, it is difficult to compare results across relevant works. Second, many studies have only focused on one component of NSC, but have not included measures of both NCSC and NSSC. These issues within the literature pinpoint that further study is needed, and that both levels of measures should be included.

2.2. NSC and Its Association with Depression under China's Unprecedented Urban Spatial Restructuring

Compared with the large volume of empirical evidence focused on Western countries, fewer cases have been located in the context of urban China, where the phenomenal urban transformation has brought about fundamental changes in neighborhoods' physical and social environments during the recent decades [35]. In China, the 40-plus years of reform and opening up have radically changed people's lives, including neighborhood life [36]. The 1998 reform, in particular, aimed to end the welfare allocation of housing, with a view to developing urban real estate as a growth anchor [35,37]. Since then, phenomenal urban expansion into the surrounding countryside and large-scale inner-city regeneration have continually reshaped urban spatial and social structures. In almost every major city, tract after tract of traditional inner-city neighborhoods have given way to high-rise office block towers, new commodity housing neighborhoods, and condominiums [36,37]. In sprawling suburbs, new commodity housing estates and development zones have replaced farmlands at amazing speed [37–39].

Underlying the unprecedented urban transformation is the increased rate of inter-city and intra-urban migration, which were inhibited before the reform. For example, it has been reported that around 10% of the citizens in Guangzhou have experienced at least one move per year from 2000 to 2012, and the city's migrant population has increased from 2.99 million to 8.83 million from 2000 to 2020 [38,40,41]. The prevalent phenomenon of migration has created different imprints in a variety of neighborhoods, which constitute a mosaic of enclaves in Chinese cities [35,39]. Obviously, urban spatial developments and the associated population dynamics have impinged heavily on NSC, and would have undermined the long-established social networks. Unlike traditional compounds, where intensive interactions among peer-neighbors engendered the so-called *dayuan*, or big compound sub-culture, current residential compounds have transformed to a locale comprising strangers who do not readily trust each other [42]. It has been indicated in earlier studies that neighborhoods, especially newer neighborhoods, have seen a decline in social interactions [43,44]. The prevalence of individualization, the pluralization of lifestyles, and advances in online communication tools have further undermined neighborly connections [45]. Meanwhile, the management of the neighborhood rests upon the estate management firm, usually a subsidiary of the developer, which reduces the dependence on neighbors, hence decreasing the intensity of social interaction. In this context, some scholars have indicated that China is facing the demise of neighborhoods, and have shown empirical evidence on the side of the 'community lost' thesis during the urbanization process in the past few decades [46].

Although the reduction in the social capital of the neighborhoods has been explored, few have examined how the neighborhood's social environment is related to depressive symptoms in Chinese cities. A small number of studies have begun to focus on the group of people who are older in China, and have explored the link between NSC and depressive symptoms in this group [18,19,24]. For example, Cao et al. [24] revealed that individual social networks, reciprocal exchange, and mutual trust among neighbors were negatively associated with depressive symptoms among older adults. Similarly, Wang et al. [18] found that reciprocal exchange was significantly related to a lower level of depression among older people. As for the effect of NSSC, Wang et al. [18] focused on a group of older people, and observed significant associations between neighborhood social participation and the risk of geriatric depression. Notably, the literature in the Chinese context has mainly focused on the group of people who are older. This study attempted to empirically analyze the link between NSC and depressive symptoms among adults based on a typology combining the cognitive and structural forms of social capital.

2.3. Hypothesis Development

Based on previous empirical studies, our model includes two main testable hypotheses:

Hypothesis 1 (H1). *neighborhood-based cognitive social capital—neighborhood trust, reciprocity and social cohesion—will be negatively associated with depressive symptoms, after controlling for socioeconomic variables.*

Hypothesis 2 (H2). *neighborhood-based structural social capital—networks and social participation—will be negatively associated with depressive symptoms, after controlling for socioeconomic variables.*

While, according Howley et al. [47], the neighborhood plays a significant role in some groups' daily lives, NSC may have little or no impacts on other groups. Accordingly, we expect the association between NSC and depressive symptoms to differ among population groups. In particular, for residents who spend a considerable amount of their time in their residential neighborhood and are less affluent and have scant personal resources, which makes them reliant more on resources from their neighborhood (including the people who are older, unemployed, and of a lower socioeconomic status), a stronger relationship between NSC and depressive symptoms is expected. In contrast, residents who are more physically mobile and have much personal connection with social networks outside of the neighborhood are expected to be less likely to be influenced by NSC [48]. Thus, we suspect that the neighborhood may be particularly relevant for mental health in populations of people who are older or of lower socioeconomic status. However, there is high uncertainty regarding other socioeconomic factors such as gender, family structure, education level, and marital status. We did not plan to derive a specific hypothesis for the heterogeneous relationships between NSC and depressive symptoms, but have left them for the following empirical investigations.

3. Data and Research Method

3.1. Data Collection

In this research, we analyzed the relationship between NSC and depressive symptoms in the city of Guangzhou, China. Guangzhou is one of the largest cities in the south of China, with a resident population of over 18 million in 2020 [41]. Guangzhou has been considered as a forerunner in urban regeneration, but has been confronted by severe social problems, such as aging and residential segregation [39]. Consequently, the findings of this study have practical implications for policy-makers regarding the construction of healthy cities. The data were derived from a city-wide household survey conducted jointly by a collaboration of Sun Yat-sen University, Hong Kong Baptist University, and Duke University. Conducted from October 2012 to January 2013, this survey was a large-scale, face-to-face investigation on neighborhood-based social capital and neighborhood governance. To obtain a representative sample, the research team used a multistage stratified random sampling method to recruit respondents. The detailed design process was as follows: first, 30 streets (*jiedao*) or sub-districts were sampled from the list of all streets located within the city based on a GIS sampling method; second, two or three neighborhoods (*xiaoqus*) within the selected street were randomly sampled, based on the neighborhood size and location; third, within each neighborhood, respondents were selected based on the interval sampling method, and interviewed by trained interviewers. The exact number of target respondents from each neighborhood depended on the population size of the neighborhood and the addresses of the respondents. Respondents were approached personally by interviewers visiting them at home, and were asked to complete a questionnaire. In total, 39 neighborhoods that varied in location, type, and size were selected for this research. In total, 1771 respondents have successfully completed the survey.

The age, gender, education, and *hukou* status ratios of participants were consistent with the 2010 Population Census of Guangzhou City. Specifically, people aged 20–64 account for 88.03% of the sample, and 81.91% of the entire population. In terms of gender, males constitute 44.32% of the sample, and 52.26% of the entire population. In terms of *hukou* status, the share of people with non-local *hukou* in the sample is 28.23%, whereas the share indicated by the population census is 36.32%. The relatively lower proportion of the migrant sample is possibly due to the informal housing neighborhoods such as urban villages and self-built settlements not being covered. Thus, the group of non-local *hukou* holders need to be considered in future research.

3.2. Measures

3.2.1. Dependent Variable: Depressive Symptoms

Depressive symptoms in the week before the survey were measured by the 20-item Likert scale questionnaire of the CES-D 20 (Center for Epidemiologic Studies Depression Scale) [49]. This measurement instrument has been widely used and verified to have high reliability for adults in many countries [16,18]. Participants were asked to report the frequency of experiencing depressive symptoms such as feeling scared, feeling upset, and feeling lonely. Their answers to each item were rated on a four-point scale. A higher total score indicated greater levels of depressive symptoms. The total CES-D 20 scores were assessed (Cronbach's alpha = 0.85) and used as the dependent variable.

3.2.2. Independent Variables: NCSC, NSSC and Socioeconomic Variables

NCSC, consisting of neighbor trustworthiness, reciprocity, and social cohesion (feelings of commitment and trust) dimensions [19,23,25,50], was calculated from six items (see Table 1). For all six statement, respondents' responses were scored on a 5-point scale from 1 (strongly disagree) to 5 (strongly agree). According to our survey, about 53.28% of respondents agreed or strongly agreed that their neighbors are trustworthy, and 63.26% of respondents agreed or strongly agreed that people in the neighborhood are helpful. The average of the respondents' answers to the six items was 3.59, between the choice of 'neutral' and 'agree'. Considering multicollinearity of these dimensions, the method of principal component analysis was adopted. As shown in Table 1, the method indicated that one single component explained 66.73% of the total variance (Cronbach's alpha = 0.85). Therefore, the overall factor score was used to represent NCSC.

Table 1. Principal component analysis of NCSC.

Statements	'Neutral' (%)	'Agree' (%)	'Strongly Agree' (%)	Mean	Component
					1
(a) People in this neighborhood can be trusted	36.33	48.72	4.56	3.47	0.697
(b) People are willing to help one another in the neighborhood	28.75	57.16	6.10	3.61	0.796
(c) I can rely on my neighbors to help with things such as collecting mail, newspaper, milk, and so on	27.11	49.06	7.59	3.46	0.618
(d) People in the neighborhood can get together to address neighborhood issues	27.57	53.91	8.99	3.61	0.735
(e) People in this neighborhood can get along with one another	13.91	73.23	10.25	3.90	0.694
(f)This is a cohesive community	32.46	48.95	7.21	3.51	0.795

NSSC was measured in two dimensions [14,24]. The first dimension was the discussion network, which was assessed by the logarithm of the number of neighbors with whom respondents could discuss private affairs. The second dimension was social participation. Previous empirical studies in Asian populations have reported that participation in welfare, volunteering, and leisure activities is significantly associated with lower levels of depressive symptoms [14,19,50]. Thus, social participation was measured by attendance at volunteer activities such as donating clothes, money or blood, and leisure activities such as walking, exercising, shopping, and other recreational activities in the communal space with neighbors in past six months. A binary variable was calculated, with respondents who do not take part in any kind of activity having a value of 0, and the rest having a value of 1.

According to existing work on depression [14,19,24], the set of personal variables included age, gender, *hukou* status, presence of children, years of schooling, homeownership, length of residence, self-perceived socioeconomic status, and employment conditions (unemployed or not).

3.3. *Analytic Strategy*

The analysis was based on the complete information provided by 1771 respondents. We began by providing the descriptive statistics of the respondents. The multicollinearity of the independent variables was then checked before running the models. After that, the regression analysis was applied to unravel the relationships between the two types of NSC and depressive symptoms. To further explore the heterogeneous relationship between NSC and depressive symptoms, interaction terms were then added. Only interaction terms which obviously enhanced the goodness of fit of the model were included. Furthermore, because previous studies have highlighted the significant role of neighborhoods in the life of people who are older, the interactions of people who are older and two types of NSC were added to capture the particular effect of NSC for the group of people who are older.

4. Analysis Results

4.1. Descriptive Analysis

Table 2 shows the basic characteristics of the sample. The mean age of the respondents is approximately 45 years. More than half of the total sample is female. Around half of the respondents had completed higher levels of education after high school. As for *hukou* status, 71.77% of the sample have Guangzhou *hukou*. With respect to tenure status, near 80% of respondents are homeowners, reflecting the high rate of homeownership since 1998 [38]. In terms of occupation status, 7.45% were unemployed. Furthermore, 42.02% of participants consider themselves to be middle class or above, whereas 57.98% of participants define themselves as being part of the lower socioeconomic class. Referreing to NSSC, on average, residents have five neighbors with whom they can discuss private affairs. In the survey, 81.25% of the participants reported that they had engaged in at least one activity. On the whole, most respondents' CES-D 20 scores were below 16 (the cut-off point of clinical depression), and the average CES-D 20 score of the total sample is 9.98, with a range from 0 to 44.

Table 2. Sample profile (N = 1771).

	Mean	S.D.	Min.	Max.
Age	45.17	14.66	20.00	86.00
Male	0.45	0.49	0.00	1.00
Married	0.81	0.38	0.00	1.00
Years of education	12.93	3.45	6.00	21.00
Lower class	0.58	0.49	0.00	1.00
Unemployed	0.07	0.27	0.00	1.00
Child in house	0.61	0.49	0.00	1.00
Local *Hukou*	0.72	0.45	0.00	1.00
Homeownership	0.79	0.40	0.00	1.00
Years of residence	7.30	5.42	0.00	50.00
NCSC	0.00	1.00	−4.74	2.65
Discussion network	5.27	10.99	0.00	100.00
Social participation	0.81	0.35	0.00	1.00
Depressive symptoms	9.98	6.75	0.00	44.00

4.2. Model Results

The relationships between the two types of NSC and depressive symptoms are presented in Model 1 (see Table 3). The heterogeneous relationships between NSC and depressive symptoms are further explored in Model 2 and 3. The increased adjusted R^2 indicates that Model 2 and Model 3 have a better predictive value than Model 1, and obtained satisfactory results. As shown in Model 1, the subjective socioeconomic status and employment status are key differentiators of depressive symptoms. This finding is in line with existing studies showing that people who are of a lower socioeconomic status ($\beta = 1.334$, $p < 0.001$) and people who are unemployed ($\beta = 3.499$, $p < 0.001$) are more likely to suffer depressive symptoms and report a high risk of mental illness [51,52].

4.2.1. Association of Cognitive and Structural Social Capital with Depression

The NCSC (interpersonal trust and reciprocity in neighbors and neighborhood cohesion) was associated with lower risks of depressive symptoms, as shown in Model 1 ($\beta = -0.963$, $p < 0.001$), after controlling socioeconomic variables. This is consistent with previous studies in other countries and other studies from China that NCSC benefits to people's mental health [13,19,24]. It is clear that living in a trusting, reciprocal, and close-knit neighborhood could reduce depressive symptoms by generating positive states and emotional support. As for NSSC, social network group ($\beta = -1.176$, $p < 0.01$) and social participation ($\beta = -2.043$, $p < 0.001$) were significantly and negatively associated with levels of depressive symptoms, which is consistent with previous research [13,53]. Resources embedded in social network and social participation, including volunteering, welfare activities, and leisure activities are beneficial to psychological well-being for dealing with life stressors.

Table 3. Relationship between NSC and depressive symptoms.

	Model 1		Model 2		Model 3	
Variable	Coef.	S.E.	Coef.	S.E.	Coef.	S.E.
Age	−0.008	0.016	−0.010	0.016		
Elderly (Ref. The younger)					6.192	1.748
Gender (1 = male)	0.316	0.396	0.448	0.397	0.416	0.396
Marital status (1 = married)	−0.567	0.553	−0.526	0.551	−0.650	0.546
Years of education	0.042	0.069	0.027	0.069	0.045	0.066
Social-economic status (Ref. Middle class or above)						
Lower class	1.334 **	0.400	1.589 *	1.463	1.189 *	1.458
Unemployed	3.499 ***	1.117	15.146 ***	4.634	16.553 ***	4.619
Child						
Hukou (1 = local)	−0.117	0.470	−0.137	0.470	−0.225	0.464
Homeownership	−0.080	0.563	−0.036	0.565	−0.078	0.558
Years of residence	0.003	0.040	0.001	0.040	−0.004	0.039
NCSC	−0.963 ***	0.209	−1.270 ***	0.279	−1.107 ***	0.298
Discussion network	−1.176 **	0.467	−1.769 **	0.597	−1.453 *	0.645
Social participation	−2.043 ***	0.687	−1.421 *	0.855	−0.049	0.934
Lower class × NCSC			−0.597 **	0.422	−0.530 *	0.420
Lower class × Discussion network			−1.497 *	0.926	−1.561 *	0.920
Lower class × Social participation			−0.892	1.450	−1.330	1.446
Unemployed × NCSC			−0.669	1.060	−0.552	1.053
Unemployed × Discussion network			−0.093	2.981	−0.416	2.966
Unemployed × Social participation			−12.301 ***	4.730	−13.509 ***	4.711
Elderly × NCSC					−0.580	0.518
Elderly × Discussion network					−1.363 *	1.065
Elderly × Social participation					−5.616 ***	1.697
Constant	11.584	1.459	11.584	1.531	11.463	1.299
F	6.858 ***		5.371 ***		5.460 ***	
Adj_R^2	0.063		0.071		0.081	

Note: *, **, and *** indicate statistical significance at the 5%, 1%, and 0.1% levels respectively.

4.2.2. Heterogeneity Analysis

As discussed in Section 2, the relationships between NSC and depressive symptoms may obscure various differences across different population groups. On that account, the details of the heterogeneity of the relationships between NSC and depressive symptoms were examined. There were significant differences in age, employment status, and subjective socioeconomic status as presented in Model 2 and 3.

Age

As shown in Model 3, the association between social networks with neighbors and depressive symptoms was more prominent in the older population than in the younger population (β = −1.363, $p < 0.05$). In addition, the significant link between social participation and depressive symptoms is accentuated for the older group (β = −5.616, $p < 0.001$). For ease of presentation, Figure 1 displays how the relationships between both neighborhood discussion networks and social participation, as well as depressive symptoms varied among age groups, after controlling for socioeconomic variables. As shown in Figure 1A, social participation was associated with lower levels of depressive symptoms, and this effect was more notable for people who are older. Similarly, Figure 1B suggested that the larger the neighborhood discussion network, the fewer the depressive symptoms. This effect was stronger in the older than the younger group.

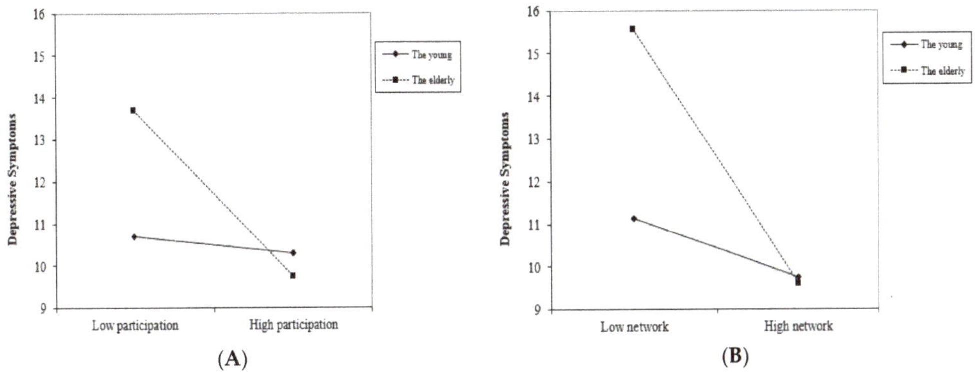

Figure 1. The relationship between NSC and depressive symptoms varied among age groups. (**A**) refers to the relationship between social participation and derpessive symptoms among age groups; (**B**) refers to the relationship between discussion network and depressive symptoms among age groups.

Socioeconomic Status

There was a significant interaction effect between socioeconomic status and NCSC on depressive symptoms ($\beta = -0.597$, $p < 0.01$). This indicates that the negative association between NCSC and depressive symptoms was stronger in lower socioeconomic groups than higher socioeconomic groups. The interaction effect between socioeconomic status and neighborhood discussion networks ($\beta = -1.497$, $p < 0.05$) was also significant. As shown in Figure 2, despite trust, reciprocity, perception of social cohesion, and discussion networks being associated with fewer depressive symptoms for all classes, the effect was more prominent for individuals in a lower socioeconomic class than those in the middle class or above.

Employment Status

Interaction analysis also showed that social participation was significantly more significant for people who are unemployed ($\beta = -12.301$, $p < 0.001$). This suggests that social participation may play an important role for those who have no work. Unemployment has been confirmed as a significant determinant of depression, mainly through threats to individual identity, and economic pressure [54]. As shown in Figure 3, neighborhood social participation may buffer the typically negative link between unemployment and depressive symptoms.

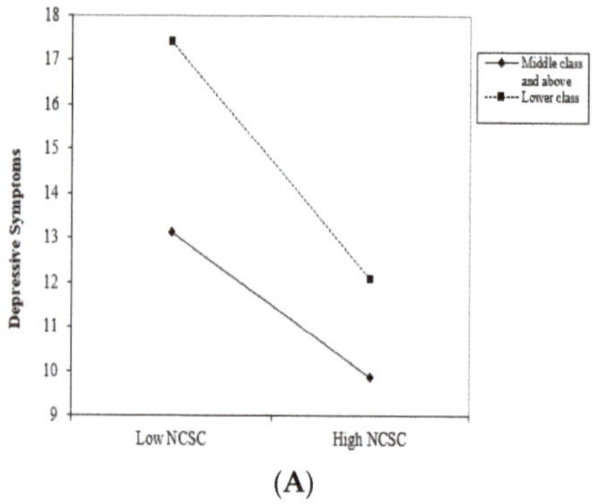

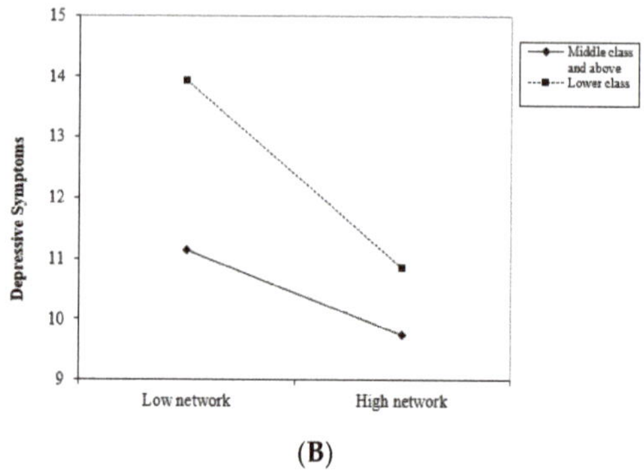

Figure 2. The relationship between discussion network and depressive symptoms varied among socioeconomic groups. (**A**) refers to the relationship between NCSC and derpessive symptoms among socioeconomic groups; (**B**) refers to the relationship between discussion network and depressive symptoms among socioeconomic groups.

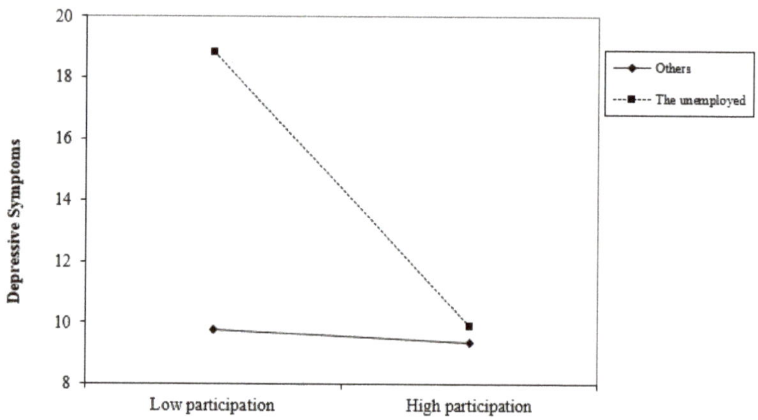

Figure 3. The relationship between neighborhood participation and depressive symptoms varied among people with different types of employment status.

5. Discussion

In line with the findings revealed in developed countries, this study has confirmed the significant inverse association between NSC and depressive symptoms in China. Residents living in neighborhoods that are stronger in mutual trust, reciprocity, and social cohesion, along with those with larger discussion networks and higher levels of social engagement, were more likely to report fewer depressive symptoms than others. The result further revealed that the association between NSC and depressive symptoms was heterogeneous across population groups. Specifically, the association of NSSC (including neighborhood discussion networks and social engagement) was stronger in the older group than in the younger group. People who are older have limited mobility or are restricted in their means of transportation, and they cannot make or are unaccustomed to making use of social media connections. Accordingly, they tend to develop more neighborhood contacts and engage in neighborhood activities. In this context, neighborhood-based discussion networks and neighborhood activities are important for people who are older, as confirmed by a large body of research [13,55].

Our findings have also verified that the association between NSC and depressive symptoms is more prominent in the lower socioeconomic group than in higher socioeconomic groups. This pattern suggests that NSC is still a significant source of support for people who are of lower socioeconomic class. It is understandable that higher-class individuals generally tend to have larger social networks and more social support beyond the boundaries of the neighborhood, compared with individuals in a lower socioeconomic class [54]. Moreover, those in the lower class are more likely to be trapped in the neighborhood, and restricted to spending time in the neighborhood, whereas the upper class are more able to change residence for adjusting their housing consumption [38]. Previous studies have demonstrated that lower socioeconomic status can seriously threaten people's psychiatric health [51,52]. Residents with the lowest incomes in a given location are 1.5 to 3 times as likely to suffer depression or anxiety than those with the highest incomes [55]. Therefore, these interaction effects suggest that a greater accumulation of NSC may help reduce socioeconomic inequality in depressive symptoms. We have also observed that the negative linkage between neighborhood participation and depressive symptoms was stronger in people who are in the unemployed group than in the employed group. One possible explanation is that people who are unemployed have more time in the neighborhood, and leisure activities and volunteering activities help them to alleviate anxiety [56].

These findings suggest the following implications regarding NSC interventions towards depressive symptoms in urban Chinese neighborhoods. First, our findings suggest that residents are in a better mental health position if they live in neighborhoods with a higher level of social capital. Thus, neighborhood governors, social workers, and organization leaders should act jointly to build up trust, reciprocity, and cooperation in the living spaces, and develop volunteering and leisure activities. Second, the marginal groups (people who are of lower socioeconomic class, people who are older, and people who are unemployed) should receive more attention in such interventions. Our results suggest that lower levels of NSC will aggravate socioeconomic inequalities in depressive symptoms, and increase the risks of mental health for people who are older and people who are unemployed. Thus, rebuilding the neighborhood to increase NSC is an important policy implication for an aging society with a continuous rise in socioeconomic inequality [57,58]. In economic terms, it is found that specifically targeting the right group can bring their life and satisfaction substantial improvements [59], and reduce the risk of falling into poverty in view of high healthcare costs [60]. In this regard, targeting at the right group will eventually help mitigate social inequalities [61]. Therefore, policymakers and urban planners are advised to create a more friendly environment for the marginal groups to encourage their interaction and outdoor activities. Promoting social activities (especially volunteering engagement), increasing facilities provision (e.g., sport and entertainment facilities), and the supply of neighborhood communal space (e.g., gardens and residential greenness) should be effective policies for impoverished neighborhoods.

Some limitations to this study should be acknowledged. First, the survey upon which this study was based was conducted from 2012 to 2013, and is somewhat dated. In recent years, the development of communication devices and online technology may have affected the correlation between NSC and depressive symptoms. Nonetheless, this study provides a comprehensive and systematic framework for future studies on the relationship between mental health and neighborhood relationships in China. Second, besides the main kinds of neighborhoods considered in this study, informal housing estates such as old reform housing and urban villages, should be considered in future research. Lastly, this study was based on cross-sectional data, and was not able to infer the causal relationship between NSC and depressive symptoms. Thus, longitudinal studies are needed in future studies to comprehensively reveal the casual relationships between NSC and depressive symptoms.

6. Conclusions

There has been growing research interest in community building in China [42]. However, the effects of these spatial and social changes on residents' mental health have been insufficiently explored. Drawing data from a city-wide survey in Guangzhou, China, the present study explored the relationship between neighborhood-based social capital and depressive symptoms among Chinese adults. The findings of our study not only report new evidence about the consistent beneficial effects of NSC beyond national borders in the Chinese context, but also, more importantly, highlight that NSC is especially important for the marginal population's depressive symptoms. Particularly, our analysis confirmed that perceptions of higher levels of NCSC were negatively associated with depressive symptoms, consistent with what has been found in developed countries. In addition, the NSSC (e.g., neighborhood-based social networks, and participation in leisure, volunteering, and welfare activities) was also linked with having fewer depressive symptoms. Moreover, our analysis found that the relationships between NSC and depressive symptoms were significantly heterogeneous across socioeconomic groups. This indicates that lower levels of NSC among disadvantaged groups may aggravate depression inequalities across social classes. In addition, the association between social participation and depressive symptoms was accentuated for people who are older, and for people who are unemployed. The present study provided evidence to suggesting that NSC plays a significant role in reducing depression for people who are older who spent more time in the neighborhood, and for individuals in a lower socioeconomic class and people who are unemployed who have smaller networks outside of the neighborhood, and who have become neighborhood-dependent [54]. Thus, our study highlights the need for building neighborhoods, especially for the marginal groups.

Author Contributions: Conceptualization, S.M.; methodology, S.M.; software, S.M.; validation, S.M.; formal analysis, S.M.; investigation, S.M.; resources, S.M.; data curation, S.M.; writing—original draft preparation, S.M.; writing—review and editing, J.C.; supervision, J.C.; project administration, J.C.; funding acquisition, J.C. All authors have read and agreed to the published version of the manuscript.

Funding: This research was funded by National Natural Science Foundation of China (grant number NSFC71974125: NSF71573166).

Institutional Review Board Statement: Not applicable.

Informed Consent Statement: Not applicable.

Data Availability Statement: Data that support the findings of this study are available from the Corresponding author upon reasonable request.

Conflicts of Interest: The authors declare no conflict of interest.

References

1. Joshi, S.; Mooney, S.J.; Rundle, A.G.; Quinn, J.W.; Beard, J.R.; Cerdá, M. Pathways from neighborhood poverty to depression among older adults. *Health Place* **2017**, *43*, 138–143. [CrossRef]
2. Kassebaum, N.J.; Arora, M.; Barber, R.M.; Bhutta, Z.A.; Brown, J.; Carter, A.; Casey, D.C.; Charlson, F.J.; Coates, M.; Coggeshall, M.; et al. Global, regional, and national disability-adjusted life-years (DALYs) for 315 diseases and injuries and healthy life expectancy (HALE), 1990–2015: A systematic analysis for the Global Burden of Disease Study 2015. *Lancet* **2016**, *388*, 1603–1658. [CrossRef]
3. Hare, D.L.; Toukhsati, S.; Johansson, P.; Jaarsma, T. Depression and cardiovascular disease: A clinical review. *Eur. Heart J.* **2013**, *35*, 1365–1372. [CrossRef]
4. Wulsin, L.R.; Vaillant, G.E.; Wells, V.E. A systematic review of the mortality of depression. *Psychosom. Med.* **1999**, *61*, 6–17. [CrossRef] [PubMed]
5. Psaltopoulou, T.; Sergentanis, T.N.; Panagiotakos, D.B.; Sergentanis, I.N.; Kosti, R.; Scarmeas, N. Mediterranean diet, stroke, cognitive impairment, and depression: A meta-analysis. *Ann. Neurol.* **2013**, *74*, 580–591. [CrossRef] [PubMed]
6. Vos, T.; Allen, C.; Arora, M.; Barber, R.M.; Bhutta, Z.A.; Brown, A.; Murray, C.J.L. Global, regional, and national incidence, prevalence, and years lived with disability for 310 diseases and injuries, 1990–2015: A systematic analysis for the Global Burden of Disease Study 2015. *Lancet* **2016**, *388*, 1545–1602. [CrossRef]
7. Generaal, E.; Hoogendijk, E.; Stam, M.; Henke, C.E.; Rutters, F.; Oosterman, M.; Huisman, M.; Kramer, S.E.; Elders, P.J.M.; Timmermans, E.J.; et al. Neighbourhood characteristics and prevalence and severity of depression: Pooled analysis of eight Dutch cohort studies. *Br. J. Psychiatry* **2019**, *215*, 468–475. [CrossRef] [PubMed]
8. Aw, S.; Koh, G.; Oh, Y.J.; Wong, M.L.; Vrijhoef, H.J.; Harding, S.C.; Geronimo, M.A.B.; Lai, C.Y.F.; Hildon, Z.J. Explaining the continuum of social participation among older adults in Singapore: From 'closed doors' to active ageing in multi-ethnic community settings. *J. Aging Stud.* **2017**, *42*, 46–55. [CrossRef]
9. Gao, W.; Ping, S.; Liu, X. Gender differences in depression, anxiety, and stress among college students: A longitudinal study from China. *J. Affect. Disord.* **2020**, *263*, 292–300. [CrossRef] [PubMed]

10. Daoud, N.; Haque, N.; Gao, M.; Nisenbaum, R.; Muntaner, C.; O'Campo, P. Neighborhood settings, types of social capital and depression among immigrants in Toronto. *Soc. Psychiatry Psychiatr. Epidemiol.* **2016**, *51*, 529–538. [CrossRef]
11. Yuasa, M.; Ukawa, S.; Ikeno, T.; Kawabata, T. Multilevel, cross-sectional study on social capital with psychogeriatric health among older Japanese people dwelling in rural areas. *Australas. J. Ageing* **2013**, *33*, E13–E19. [CrossRef]
12. Kim, D. Blues from the neighborhood? Neighborhood characteristics and depression. *Epidemiol. Rev.* **2008**, *30*, 101–117. [CrossRef]
13. Wang, R.; Feng, Z.; Liu, Y.; Lu, Y. Relationship between neighbourhood social participation and depression among older adults: A longitudinal study in China. *Health Soc. Care Community* **2020**, *28*, 247–259. [CrossRef] [PubMed]
14. Han, K.-M.; Han, C.; Shin, C.; Jee, H.-J.; An, H.; Yoon, H.-K.; Ko, Y.-H.; Kim, S.-H. Social capital, socioeconomic status, and depression in community-living elderly. *J. Psychiatr. Res.* **2018**, *98*, 133–140. [CrossRef] [PubMed]
15. Harpham, T. Urban health in developing countries: What do we know and where do we go? *HealthPlace* **2009**, *15*, 107–116.
16. Tomita, A.; Burns, J.K. A multilevel analysis of association between neighborhood social capital and depression: Evidence from the first South African National Income Dynamics Study. *J. Affect. Disord.* **2013**, *144*, 101–105. [CrossRef]
17. Qin, X.; Wang, S.; Hsieh, C.-R. The prevalence of depression and depressive symptoms among adults in China: Estimation based on a National Household Survey. *China Econ. Rev.* **2016**, *51*, 271–282. [CrossRef]
18. Wang, R.; Chen, H.; Liu, Y.; Lu, Y.; Yao, Y. Neighborhood social reciprocity and mental health among older adults in China: The mediating effects of physical activity, social interaction, and volunteering. *BMC Public Health* **2019**, *19*, 1–10. [CrossRef] [PubMed]
19. Lu, N.; Peng, C. Community-based structural social capital and depressive symptoms of older urban Chinese adults: The mediating role of cognitive social capital. *Arch. Gerontol. Geriatr.* **2019**, *82*, 74–80. [CrossRef]
20. Etzioni, A.; Putnam, R.D. Is bowling together sociologically lite? Bowling alone: The collapse and revival of American community. *Contemp. Sociol. A J. Rev.* **2000**, *30*, 223. [CrossRef]
21. Putnam, R.D. *Making Democracy Work: Civic Traditions in Modern Italy*; Princeton University Press: Princeton, NJ, USA, 1993.
22. Beaudoin, C.E. Bonding and bridging neighborliness: An individual-level study in the context of health. *Soc. Sci. Med.* **2009**, *68*, 2129–2136. [CrossRef] [PubMed]
23. Cramm, J.M.; van Dijk, H.M.; Nieboer, A.P. The importance of neighborhood social cohesion and social capital for the well being of older adults in the community. *Gerontology* **2013**, *53*, 142–152. [CrossRef]
24. Cao, W.; Li, L.; Zhou, X.; Zhou, C. Social capital and depression: Evidence from urban elderly in China. *Aging Ment. Health* **2015**, *19*, 418–429. [CrossRef]
25. Miao, J.; Wu, X.; Sun, X. Neighborhood, social cohesion, and the Elderly's depression in Shanghai. *Soc. Sci. Med.* **2019**, *229*, 134–143. [CrossRef]
26. De Silva, M.J.; Mckenzie, K.; Harpham, T.; Huttly, S.R.A. Social capital and mental illness: A systematic review. *J. Epidemiol. Community Health* **2005**, *59*, 619–627. [CrossRef]
27. Bassett, E.; Moore, S. Social capital and depressive symptoms: The association of psychosocial and network dimen-sions of social capital with depressive symptoms in Montreal, Canada. *Soc. Sci. Med.* **2013**, *86*, 96–102. [CrossRef]
28. Fujiwara, T.; Kawachi, I. A prospective study of individual-level social capital and major depression in the United States. *J. Epidemiol. Community Health* **2008**, *62*, 627–633. [CrossRef] [PubMed]
29. Blair, A.; Ross, N.A.; Garièpy, G.; Schmitz, N. How do neighborhoods affect depression outcomes? A realist review and a call for the examination of causal pathways. *Soc. Psychiatry Psychiatr. Epidemiol.* **2014**, *49*, 873–887. [CrossRef]
30. Bourdieu, P. The forms of capital. In *Handbook of Theory and Research for the Sociology of Education*; Richardson, J., Ed.; Greenwood Press: New York, NY, USA, 1986; pp. 241–258.
31. Cohen-Cline, H.; Beresford, S.A.; Barrington, W.; Matsueda, R.; Wakefield, J.; Duncan, G.E. Associations between social capital and depression: A study of adult twins. *Health Place* **2018**, *50*, 162–167. [CrossRef]
32. Forsman, A.; Nyqvist, F.; Schierenbeck, I.; Gustafson, Y.; Wahlbeck, K. Structural and cognitive social capital and depression among older adults in two Nordic regions. *Aging Ment. Health* **2012**, *16*, 771–779. [CrossRef] [PubMed]
33. Yamaguchi, M.; Inoue, Y.; Shinozaki, T.; Saito, M.; Takagi, D.; Kondo, K.; Kondo, N. Community social capital and depressive symptoms among older people in Japan: A multilevel longitudinal study. *J. Epidemiol.* **2019**, *29*, 363–369. [CrossRef]
34. Cornwell, B.; Laumann, E.O. The health benefits of network growth: New evidence from a national survey of older adults. *Soc. Sci. Med.* **2013**, *125*, 94–106. [CrossRef]
35. Li, S.-M. Housing inequalities under market deepening: The case of Guangzhou, China. *Environ. Plan. A Econ. Space* **2012**, *44*, 2852–2866. [CrossRef]
36. Chen, J.; Hu, M.; Lin, Z. China's housing reform and labor market participation. *J. Real Estate Financ. Econ.* **2021**, 1–25. [CrossRef]
37. Huang, Y.; Deng, F.F. Residential mobility in Chinese cities: A longitudinal analysis. *Hous. Stud.* **2006**, *21*, 625–652. [CrossRef]
38. Li, S.-M.; Mao, S. Exploring residential mobility in Chinese cities: An empirical analysis of Guangzhou. *Urban Stud.* **2017**, *54*, 3718–3737. [CrossRef]
39. He, S. New-build gentrification in Central Shanghai: Demographic changes and socioeconomic implications. *Popul. Space Place* **2010**, *16*, 345–361. [CrossRef]
40. Guangzhou Statistical Bureau. Guangzhou Statistical Yearbook. 2000. Available online: http://www.tjcn.org/tjgb/19gd/2392_3.html (accessed on 10 January 2010).
41. Guangzhou Statistical Bureau. Guangzhou Statistical Yearbook. 2020. Available online: http://www.gz.gov.cn/zwgk/sjfb/tjgb/content/post_7177238.html (accessed on 10 January 2021).

42. Li, S.-M.; Mao, S.; Du, H. Residential mobility and neighbourhood attachment in Guangzhou, China. *Environ. Plan. A Econ. Space* **2019**, *51*, 761–780. [CrossRef]
43. Forrest, R.; Yip, N.-M. Neighbourhood and neighbouring in contemporary Guangzhou. *J. Contemp. China* **2007**, *16*, 47–64. [CrossRef]
44. Wu, F. Gated and packaged suburbia: Packaging and branding Chinese suburban residential development. *Cities* **2010**, *27*, 385–396. [CrossRef]
45. Urry, J. *Sociology beyond Societies. Mobilities for the Twenty-Frst Century*; Routledge: London, UK, 2012.
46. Xu, Y. The "Community Question" in the State-Led Urbanization Process of Post-Reform China: A Case Study of Shanghai. Ph.D. Thesis, The Hong Kong Polytechnic University, Hong Kong, China, 2010.
47. Howley, P.; Neill, S.O.; Atkinson, R. Who needs good neighbors? *Environ. Plan. A* **2015**, *47*, 939–956. [CrossRef]
48. Ellen, I.G.; Turner, M.A. Does neighborhood matter? Assessing recent evidence. *Hous. Policy Debate* **1997**, *8*, 833–866. [CrossRef]
49. Radloff, L.S. The CES-D scale: A self-report depression scale for research in the general population. *Appl. Psychol. Meas.* **1977**, *1*, 385–401. [CrossRef]
50. De Silva, M.J.; Huttly, S.R.; Harpham, T.; Kenward, M.G. Social capital and mental health: A comparative analysis of four low income countries. *Soc. Sci. Med.* **2007**, *64*, 5–20. [CrossRef]
51. Lorant, V.; Deliège, D.; Eaton, W.; Robert, A.; Philippot, P.; Ansseau, M. Socioeconomic inequalities in depression: A meta-analysis. *Am. J. Epidemiol.* **2003**, *157*, 98–112. [CrossRef] [PubMed]
52. Sareen, J.; Afifi, T.O.; McMillan, K.A.; Asmundson, G.J.G. Relationship between household income and mental disorders: Findings from a population-based longitudinal study. *Arch. Gen. Psychiatry* **2011**, *68*, 419–427. [CrossRef] [PubMed]
53. Wu, Z.; Bies, A. Volunteering and self-rated health in urban China: New evidence from analyses of treatment-effects models. *Appl. Res. Quali. Life* **2020**, *4*, 1–17.
54. Ridley, M.; Rao, G.; Schilbach, F.; Patel, V. Poverty, depression, and anxiety: Causal evidence and mechanisms. *Science* **2020**, *370*, eaay0214. [CrossRef]
55. Hoogerbrugge, M.M.; Burger, M.J. Neighborhood-Based social capital and life satisfaction: The case of Rotterdam, The Netherlands. *Urban Geogr.* **2018**, *39*, 1484–1509. [CrossRef]
56. Tausig, M. The sociology of work and well-being. In *Handbook of the Sociology of Mental Health*, 2nd ed.; Aneshensel, C.S., Phelan, J.C., Bierman, A., Eds.; Springer: New York, NY, USA, 2012.
57. Cai, Y.; Cheng, Y.; Claus, I.; Oxley, L. Pension reform in China: Challenges and opportunities. *J. Econ. Surv.* **2014**, *28*, 636–651. [CrossRef]
58. Huang, J. Income inequality, distributive justice beliefs, and happiness in China: Evidence from a nationwide survey. *Soc. Indic. Res.* **2019**, *142*, 83–105. [CrossRef]
59. Vuong, Q.H. Sociodemographic factors influencing vietnamese patient satisfaction with healthcare services and some meaningful empirical thresholds. *Iran. J. Public Health* **2018**, *47*, 119–126. [PubMed]
60. Vuong, Q.H. Be rich or don't be sick: Estimating Vietnamese patients' risk of falling into destitution. *SpringerPlus* **2015**, *4*, 1–31. [CrossRef] [PubMed]
61. Vuong, Q.-H.; Ho, T.; Nguyen, H.K.; Vuong, T.-T. Healthcare consumers' sensitivity to costs: A reflection on behavioural economics from an emerging market. *Palgrave Commun.* **2018**, *4*, 70. [CrossRef]

International Journal of
Environmental Research and Public Health

MDPI

Article

How Do Chinese National Scenic Areas Affect Tourism Economic Development? The Moderating Effect of Time-Limited Rectification

Yongcuomu Qu [1], Ziqiong Zhang [1], Yanchao Feng [2,*] and Xiaorong Cui [3]

[1] School of Economics and Management, Harbin Institute of Technology, Harbin 150001, China; qycm@hit.edu.cn (Y.Q.); ziqiong@hit.edu.cn (Z.Z.)
[2] Business School, Zhengzhou University, Zhengzhou 450001, China
[3] College of Physics and Electronic Information, Inner Mongolia Normal University, Hohhot 010022, China; 20194016010@mails.imnu.edu.cn
* Correspondence: m15002182995@163.com; Tel.: +86-150-0218-2995

Abstract: Based on panel data on 124 prefecture-level and above cities from 2003 to 2018, this study investigated the impact of CNSAs on tourism economic development and the moderating effect of time-limited rectification by comprehensively using the quasi-DID model, the static spatial Durbin model, and the dynamic spatial Durbin model. The results showed that the impact of CNSAs on tourism economic development has a heterogeneous characteristic in terms of tourists and revenue. In addition, the spatial spillover effect and the path dependence have effectively promoted tourism economic development. Furthermore, the effectiveness of time-limited rectification has been proved in this study, while the "beggar-thy-neighbor" effect has, to some extent, weakened the promotional effect of CNSAs on tourism economic development, especially in terms of international tourists and international tourism revenue. Finally, relevant policy implications for the superior department in charge, local governments, and the management department of CNSAs are outlined to provide a practical reference for promoting the high-quality development of the tourism economy in China.

Keywords: Chinese national scenic areas; tourism economy; moderating effect; time-limited rectification

Citation: Qu, Y.; Zhang, Z.; Feng, Y.; Cui, X. How Do Chinese National Scenic Areas Affect Tourism Economic Development? The Moderating Effect of Time-Limited Rectification. *IJERPH* **2021**, *18*, 11620. https://doi.org/10.3390/ijerph182111620

Academic Editors: Jie Chen, Qian Zhou and Ting Zhang

Received: 27 September 2021
Accepted: 2 November 2021
Published: 5 November 2021

1. Introduction

Faced with the dichotomous challenge of balancing the quest for economic growth and its associated risks for the environment, the tourism economy has taken central stage among scholars and policymakers at home and abroad for its features of cleaner production and sustainability [1–4]. In particular, over the past 40 years, China's tourism industry has stimulated economic activities thereby serving as a great catalyst for economic growth [5]. Furthermore, to achieve the dual goals of protection and development, the Chinese authorities have issued various policies to promote the development of the regional tourism economy based on protecting natural and cultural resources [5,6].

As important support of tourism development, Chinese national scenic areas (hereafter CNSAs) have been acknowledged as an important engine of regional economic growth by driving infrastructure construction, increasing employment opportunities, and promoting industrial structure upgrading [6]. Since the first list of 44 CNSAs was issued in 1982, a total number of nine lists including 244 CNSA have been acknowledged as of 2018. In particular, to show China's major scenic areas conveniently, competent authorities have set CNSAs as top-level scenic spots [7,8].

Generally, the application of a CNSA is submitted by the provincial-, autonomous regional-, and municipal-level government and jointly evaluated by the relevant construction department under the State Council, the relevant Environmental Protection Department under the State Council, the relevant forestry department, and the relevant cultural relics department, and finally approved and announced by the State Council [9].

The clear definition of a CNSA using the assessment of landscape resources, measurement for ecological resources protection, layout of major construction projects, intensity of development and utilization, functional structure, and spatial layout prohibit or restrict development areas, and tourist capacity is necessary for achieving the optimal balance of tourism-focused economic development and conservation of environmental and cultural resources [10,11].

However, CNSAs have been regarded as permanent and unregulated for a long time, and this situation inevitably leads to complex situations of weak impetus, poor planning, destruction of resources, and unreasonable exploitation [7,12,13]. At the same time, the relevant authorities have lacked the corresponding assessment, resulting in the delayed construction and poor service of CNSAs which, in turn, erodes their "brand effect" [14,15]. Moreover, due to the huge benefits that CNSAs bring to local governments, they tend to follow up on applications but fail to follow through after authentication [16].

Against this background, the Ministry of Housing and Urban–Rural Development launched a four-year program to rectify the aforementioned problems during the period of 2012–2015, ordered problematic CNSAs to be rectified within one year, and reviewed the final effect of time-limited rectification in 2016. In particular, the main contents of the program included five aspects: institutional construction, planning management, construction management, service management, and image publicity. In addition, the evaluation results were divided into five grades: excellent, good, qualified, need to be rectified, and unqualified. When categorized as needs to be rectified or unqualified, the CNSA was ordered to make time-limited rectification within one year. If the substandard CNSA still failed to satisfy the standard after time-limited rectification, it would be listed as disqualified by the State Council.

According to the inspection results of the Ministry of Housing and Urban–Rural Development, there were 70 cases (times) where CNSAs were warned and put on the list of needing to be rectified, and there were 29 cases (times) where they failed to meet the standards and were placed on the list of unqualified. Fortunately, from the time-limited rectification results announced in 2016, 42 CNSAs have passed the inspection, while seven CNSAs still failed to pass. In particular, the prominent problems of increasing prices casually, ticket within ticket, compulsory consumption behavior, and natural resource destruction resulted in complaints from tourists, weakened the "advertising effect" of CNSAs, and, thus, need to be rectified.

Nevertheless, as for the moderating effect of time-limited rectification on the nexus between CNSAs and tourism economic development, existing research has not been fully explored, which leaves an incentive and opportunity for this study. In particular, whether or not CNSAs have a spatial spillover effect on tourism economic development, aside from local effects, has yet to be comprehensively studied. In addition, the effects of CNSAs on local tourism economic development before and after time-limited rectification has yet to be explored. Therefore, the aim of this study was to explore the effects of CNSA on tourism economic development and the moderating effect of time-limited rectification by comprehensively and systematically employing a series of econometric methods.

The marginal contributions of this study can be drawn from two aspects. Theoretically, to the best of our knowledge, this study analyzed the effect of CNSAs on tourism economic development for the first time and illustrates the theoretical basis for how time-limited rectification affects tourism economic development at the macroeconomic level. Methodologically, we treated time-limited rectification as a quasi-natural experiment and evaluated its effect on tourism economic development by using panel data on prefecture-level and above cities. More importantly, this study provides a normative theoretical explanation and systematic empirical facts, which aim to drive the sustainable development of tourism economy and provides decision-making guidance for strengthening the reputation of CNSAs.

The remainder of this study proceeds as follows: Section 2 provides a literature review. Section 3 presents the methodology including variables selection, data sources, and models specification. Section 4 reports and analyzes the empirical results based on three different econometric models, followed by an in-depth discussion in Section 5. Concluding remarks, policy implications, and research prospects are provided in Section 6. To vividly illustrate the research steps in this study, we drew them in Figure 1.

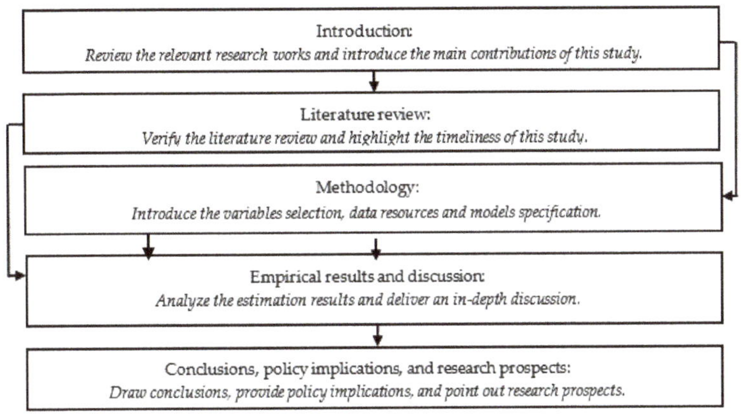

Figure 1. Research steps.

2. Literature Review

Noted as the world's largest service sector, tourism plays an important role in boosting the sustainable development of the entire economy, while disorganized tourism development has aggravated the conflict between tourism economic development and tourism resources protection [17,18]. Against the background of an ecological civilization construction strategy in the new era, plenty of studies have focused on exploring how to realize tourism economic development without destruction of tourism resources [19,20], how to improve the service quality of the tourism industry [21,22], and how to promote the sustainable, healthy, and high-quality development of the tourism economy [23,24].

Until now, both domestic and international scholars have explored the effects of tourism on regional economic development [25,26], the relationship between tourism economic development and ecological environment [27,28], and the influencing factors of tourism efficiency [29,30], which provide ample references for this study. Specifically, although some studies have gradually paid attention to investigate the economic and environmental effects of CNSAs in China [31], there is a paucity of studies investigating how CSNAs affect tourism economic development from the dual perspectives of tourists (i.e., the number of international tourists and the number of domestic tourists) and revenue (i.e., international tourism revenue and domestic tourism revenue), notwithstanding how time-limited rectification moderates the nexus between CNSAs and tourism economic development.

As for the econometric model of policy evaluation, most of the existing literature employed the difference-in-differences (DID) model, which should pass the parallel trend test [32], the placebo test [33], and the counterfactual test [34]. However, the core explanatory variable, that is, the number of CNSAs, is a continuous index and not a binary index; thus, treating the announcement of CNSAs as an unbalanced quasi-experiment, this study aimed to employ the quasi-DID model as the basic model [35]. More importantly, the spatial spillover effect was usually neglected across regions in the empirical analysis of the tourism economy, which may reduce the robustness of the estimation results; thus, it is necessary and important to adopt the spatial econometric model [36,37]. Furthermore, except for the spatial spillover effect, ignoring temporal inertia may also lead to endogenous problems; therefore, the adoption of a dynamic spatial econometric model was also necessary for comparison to ensure the robustness of the empirical results [38].

Therefore, to fill the above-mentioned research gaps and promote the high-quality development of CNSAs simultaneously, this article attempted to explore the impact of CNSAs on tourism economic development and the moderating effect of time-limited rectification by comprehensively using the quasi-DID model, the static spatial Durbin model, and the dynamic spatial Durbin model, which can, to some extent, guarantee the robustness and reliability of the empirical results.

3. Methodology

3.1. Variables Selection

Dependent variables: four indicators were employed to act as the proxy variables of tourism economic development such as the number of international tourists (y_1), the number of domestic tourists (y_2), international tourism revenue (y_3), and domestic tourism revenue (y_4).

Core explanatory variables: The number of CNSAs (d_1) was employed to act as the benchmark independent variable. In addition, a dummy indicator (d_2) was employed to act as the proxy variable of time-limited rectification, which equaled -1 when a CNSA belonged to the list of not up to standard and 1 otherwise.

Control variables: To capture the character of the city where a CNSA was located, several control variables, such as economic development (x_1, measured by per capita gross domestic product), consumption (x_2, measured by per capita retail sales of consumer goods), industrial structure upgrading (x_3, measured by the shares of tertiary industry in the local gross domestic product), infrastructure (x_4, measured by per capita urban road area), green rate (x_5, measured by the green coverage rate of built-up area), the air pollution of sulfur dioxide (x_6, measured by per capita emission of sulfur dioxide), the air pollution of dust (x_7, measured by per capita emission of dust), and the liquid pollution of wastewater (x_8, measured by per capita emission of wastewater), were employed by referring to the studies in [4,7,12].

3.2. Data Sources

The samples used in this study consisted of 124 prefecture-level and above cities that had at least one CNSA in 2018, and the investigation period covered from 2003 to 2018. Several data sources were used, which were the China City Statistical Yearbook (2004–2019), the China Tourism Yearbook (2004–2019), and the website of the Ministry of Housing and Urban–Rural Development in China (www.mohurd.gov.cn, accessed on 3 March 2021). In particular, the original data for the control variables were collected from the China City Statistical Yearbook (2004–2019), the original data for the four dependent variables were collected from the China Tourism Yearbook (2004–2019), while the time-limited rectification information on CNSAs was collected from the website of the Ministry of Housing and Urban–Rural Development in China (www.mohurd.gov.cn, accessed on 12 May 2021). To eliminate the potential interference of heteroscedasticity, all the dependent and control variables incorporated into the regression equation were in the natural logarithm form, and there statistical description are shown in Table 1.

3.3. Models Specification

To investigate the effects of CNSA on tourism economic development and the moderating effect of time-limited rectification comprehensively, this study employed three econometric methods including the quasi-DID model, the spatial Durbin model, and the dynamic spatial Durbin model.

Table 1. The statistical description of relevant variables.

Variables	Meaning	Unit	Count	Mean	SD	Minimum	Maximum
y_1	The number of international tourists	Person	1984	4.637	2.033	−4.711	9.408
y_2	The number of domestic tourists	Person	1984	9.665	1.171	1.099	12.561
y_3	International tourism revenue	10^6 USD	1984	3.713	2.339	−6.238	8.777
y_4	Domestic tourism revenue	10^6 CNY	1984	9.435	1.398	2.890	12.799
d_1	The number of CNSAs	Piece	1984	1.225	0.705	0.000	4.000
d_2	Time-limited rectification	-	1984	0.930	0.367	−1.000	1.000
x_1	Economic development	CNY	1984	10.332	0.671	7.906	12.778
x_2	Consumption	CNY	1984	9.535	0.823	6.011	11.592
x_3	Industrial structure upgrading	%	1984	3.689	0.227	2.484	4.447
x_4	infrastructure	m^2	1984	2.180	0.630	−0.525	4.159
x_5	Green rate	%	1984	3.602	0.320	−0.511	4.541
x_6	The air pollution of sulfur dioxide	Ton	1984	3.851	1.076	−2.115	7.346
x_7	The air pollution of dust	Ton	1984	5.714	1.243	−3.378	8.255
x_8	The liquid pollution of wastewater	Ton	1984	5.014	1.277	−0.779	11.069

Following the study of Yang et al. [35], we first used the quasi-DID method to investigate the impact of CNSAs on tourism economic development. The difference between this method and the standard DID method is that we used a continuous treatment (i.e., the number of CNSAs) to capture the relative impact. In particular, the corresponding econometric model was established as follows:

$$y_{it} = \alpha_0 + \alpha_1 d_1 + \beta x_{it} + f_i + f_t + prov_j * year_t + \varepsilon_{it} \quad (1)$$

where i and t denote the city and the time, respectively; y denotes the dependent variables (i.e., y_1, y_2, y_3 and y_4), α_0 denotes the constant term; d_1 denotes the number of CNSAs; α_1 denotes the coefficient of d_1; x_{it} denotes a vector of control variables; β denotes the coefficients of x_{jt}; f_i denotes the city fixed effect; f_t denotes the time fixed effect; $prov_j * year_t$ denotes the joint fixed effect of province and time to capture the impact of provincial tourism policy; ε_{it} denotes the error term.

To investigate the moderating effect of time-limited rectification on the nexus between CNSAs and tourism economic development, the interactive term $d_1 * d_2$ was incorporated into the equation after being centralized.

$$y_{it} = \alpha_0 + \alpha_2 d_1 * d_2 + \beta x_{it} + f_i + f_t + prov_j * year_t + \varepsilon_{it} \quad (2)$$

where d_2 denotes a dummy variable that is equal to -1 when a CNSA is listed in the time-limited rectification, and 1 otherwise, while the other parameters are consistent with Equation (1).

Since Equations (1) and (2) belong to the nonspatial model, it implicitly assumes that there is no spatial spillover effect. However, the changes in CNSAs in local cities usually affect tourism economic development in surrounding cities, especially in the long term. In addition, tourism economic development usually has the characteristic of spatial correlation. Hence, it was necessary to take into account such a spatial lagged effect to obtain an accurate result. Accordingly, we added the spatial lag term of the dependent variables and the independent variables including the core explanatory variables and the control variables into Equations (1) and (2) to investigate whether there were spatial spillover effects from them. Thus, referring to the study of Elhorst [36], the static spatial Durbin model was employed to carry out the estimation as follows:

$$y_{it} = \rho W * y_{it} + \alpha_1 d_1 + \beta_j x_{jt} + \theta_1 W * d_1 + \varphi_j W * x_{jt} + f_i + f_t + \varepsilon_{it} \quad (3)$$

$$y_{it} = \rho W * y_{it} + \alpha_2 d_1 * d_2 + \beta_j x_{jt} + \theta_2 W * d_1 * d_2 + \varphi_j W * x_{jt} + f_i + f_t + \varepsilon_{it} \quad (4)$$

where W denotes the spatial weight matrix [37]; ρ denotes the spatial coefficient of the dependent variable; θ_1, θ_2, and φ_j denote the spatial lag coefficients to be estimated; the other parameters are consistent with Equation (2).

In addition, considering the possible path dependence of tourism economic development and the possibility of endogenous causality between CNSAs and time-limited rectification and other factors, the lag phase of the dependent variable was introduced into the static spatial Durbin model to formulate the dynamic spatial Durbin model [38].

$$y_{it} = \tau y_{i,t-1} + \rho W * y_{it} + \alpha_1 d_1 + \beta_j x_{jt} + \theta_1 W * d_1 + \varphi_j W * x_{jt} + f_i + f_t + \varepsilon_{it} \quad (5)$$

$$y_{it} = \tau y_{i,t-1} + \rho W * y_{it} + \alpha_2 d_1 * d_2 + \beta_j x_{jt} + \theta_2 W * d_1 * d_2 + \varphi_j W * x_{jt} + f_i + f_t + \varepsilon_{it} \quad (6)$$

where $y_{i,t-1}$ denotes the dependent variables of the first lag phase used to control and examine the time lag effect of their changes; τ denotes the temporal lag coefficient of the dependent variables; the other parameters are consistent with Equation (4).

4. Empirical Results and Analysis

4.1. Nonspatial Results and Analysis

The estimation results of Equations (1) and (2) are shown in Table 2. In Columns (1)–(4), we examined the impacts of CNSAs on tourism economic development; in Columns (5)–(8), we replaced the number of CNSAs (i.e., d_1) with its interactive term and time-limited rectification (i.e., $d_1 * d_2$) and re-estimated the impacts. It can be noted that the coefficients of d_1 in Columns (1) and (3) were significantly positive, while its coefficients in Columns (2) and (4) were positive but insignificant; in other words, without the consideration of time-limited rectification, CNSAs have effectively attracted international tourists and increased international tourism revenue, while the corresponding impacts on attracting domestic tourists and increasing domestic tourism revenue were relatively poor. However, all the coefficients of $d_1 * d_2$ in Columns (5)–(8) were significantly positive; in other words, after the implementation of time-limited rectification, CNSAs have not only effectively attracted domestic tourists and international tourists but also increased domestic tourism revenue and international tourism revenue, that is, time-limited rectification released the vitality of domestic tourism in the nonspatial analysis.

4.2. Static Spatial Results and Analysis

The estimation results of Equations (3) and (4) are shown in Table 3. In Columns (1)–(4), we examined the impacts of CNSAs on tourism economic development; In Columns (5)–(8), we replaced the number of CNSAs (i.e., d_1) with its interactive term and time-limited rectification (i.e., $d_1 * d_2$) and re-estimated the impacts. It can be noted that all spatial lag coefficients (i.e., ρ) were significantly positive, implying that the positive spatial spillover effect of tourism economic development in China was fully established under the formula of the spatial Durbin model. In addition, the coefficients of d_1 were significantly positive in Columns (1)–(4), the spatial lag coefficients of it were significantly positive in Columns (1)–(3) but insignificantly positive in Column (4); in other words, without the consideration of time-limited rectification, CNSAs not only effectively attracted international and domestic tourists in local and surrounding cities but also increased foreign tourism revenue and domestic tourism revenue in the local and surrounding cities, while the impact of it on domestic tourism revenue in surrounding cities was relatively poor. Moreover, the coefficients of $d_1 * d_2$ were significantly positive in Columns (5)–(7) but insignificantly positive in Column (8), while the spatial lag coefficients of it were insignificantly positive in Columns (5) and (7), insignificantly negative in Column (6), and significantly negative in Column (8); in other words, after the implementation of time-limited rectification, the direct and positive impacts of CNSAs on tourism economic development were retained in local cities, while the indirect and positive impacts of it on tourism economic development were no longer supported in surrounding cities, that is, the effectiveness of time-limited rectification was not supported in the static spatial analysis.

Table 2. Results of the nonspatial econometric estimation.

Variables	y_1	y_2	y_3	y_4	y_1	y_2	y_3	y_4
	(1)	(2)	(3)	(4)	(5)	(6)	(7)	(8)
d_1	0.313 **	0.084	0.304 **	0.070				
	(2.392)	(1.344)	(2.213)	(1.515)				
$d_1 \times d_2$					0.053 **	0.024 **	0.069 **	0.021 **
					(1.987)	(2.074)	(2.368)	(2.466)
x_1	−0.010	0.017	0.022	0.022	−0.014	0.016	0.019	0.021
	(−0.130)	(0.356)	(0.256)	(0.624)	(−0.171)	(0.343)	(0.215)	(0.608)
x_2	0.048	0.054	0.143	0.019	0.035	0.051	0.131	0.017
	(0.459)	(0.988)	(1.292)	(0.564)	(0.335)	(0.938)	(1.215)	(0.481)
x_3	−0.419	0.240	−0.534 *	−0.211	−0.401	0.246	−0.514 *	−0.206
	(−1.633)	(1.453)	(−1.871)	(−1.479)	(−1.568)	(1.502)	(−1.828)	(−1.427)
x_4	−0.004	−0.038	0.019	−0.017	−0.014	−0.040	0.011	−0.019
	(−0.050)	(−0.790)	(0.227)	(−0.634)	(−0.181)	(−0.830)	(0.127)	(−0.694)
x_5	−0.129	0.018	0.186	0.040	−0.108	0.023	0.205	0.045
	(−1.221)	(0.498)	(1.390)	(1.042)	(−0.989)	(0.647)	(1.526)	(1.157)
x_6	0.016	−0.017	0.014	0.015	0.020	−0.016	0.017	0.015
	(0.374)	(−0.472)	(0.254)	(0.753)	(0.465)	(−0.460)	(0.306)	(0.751)
x_7	0.017	0.090*	0.017	0.137 ***	0.020	0.091 *	0.019	0.137 ***
	(0.309)	(1.878)	(0.258)	(3.318)	(0.347)	(1.893)	(0.285)	(3.237)
x_8	0.063	0.005	0.079	0.033 *	0.055	0.003	0.072	0.032
	(1.655)	(0.166)	(1.624)	(1.677)	(1.442)	(0.101)	(1.470)	(1.622)
constant	5.426 ***	7.546 ***	2.433	8.614 ***	5.806 ***	7.624 ***	2.760	8.677 ***
	−0.010	0.017	0.022	0.022	(3.489)	(7.239)	(1.593)	(13.017)
N	1936	1936	1936	1936	1936	1936	1936	1936
R^2	0.954	0.940	0.955	0.980	0.953	0.940	0.955	0.980

Note: t statistics are in parentheses; * $p < 0.1$, ** $p < 0.05$, and *** $p < 0.01$.

Table 3. Results of the static spatial econometric estimation.

Variables	y_1	y_2	y_3	y_4	y_1	y_2	y_3	y_4
	(1)	(2)	(3)	(4)	(5)	(6)	(7)	(8)
ρ	0.274 ***	0.395 ***	0.211 ***	0.258 ***	0.281 ***	0.399 ***	0.217 ***	0.259 ***
	(12.190)	(21.588)	(9.224)	(12.249)	(12.588)	(21.882)	(9.509)	(12.265)
d_1	0.452 ***	0.129 ***	0.435 ***	0.047 **				
	(9.310)	(4.941)	(8.105)	(2.076)				
$d_1 \times d_2$					0.076 ***	0.023 **	0.087 ***	0.009
					(3.750)	(2.157)	(3.890)	(1.003)
$W \times d_1$	0.163 **	0.079 **	0.243 ***	0.032				
	(2.305)	(2.094)	(3.119)	(0.990)				
$W \times d_1 \times d_2$					0.044	−0.008	0.040	−0.025 *
					(1.510)	(−0.534)	(1.254)	(−1.905)
Control Variables	Yes	Yes	Yes	Yes	Yes	Yes	Yes	Yes
N	1984	1984	1984	1984	1984	1984	1984	1984
R^2	0.193	0.404	0.181	0.287	0.225	0.343	0.221	0.252

The z-statistics are in parentheses; *** $p < 0.01$, ** $p < 0.05$, and * $p < 0.1$.

4.3. Dynamic Spatial Results and Analysis

The estimation results of Equations (5) and (6) are shown in Table 4. In Columns (1)–(4), we examined the impacts of CNSAs on tourism economic development; in Columns (5)–(8), we replaced the number of CNSAs (i.e., d_1) with its interactive term and time-limited rectification (i.e., $d_1 * d_2$) and re-estimated the impacts. It can be noted that all the spatial lag coefficients (i.e., ρ) were significantly positive, implying that the positive spatial spillover effect of tourism economic development in China was also fully established under the dynamic spatial Durbin model. In addition, all the temporal lag coefficients (i.e., τ) were significantly positive and greater than the corresponding spatial lag coefficients (i.e., ρ), implying that the positive temporal effect of tourism economic development in China was not only fully established under the dynamic spatial Durbin model but also had a greater impact than the spatial spillover effect of it.

Table 4. Results of the dynamic spatial econometric estimation.

Variables	y_1	y_2	y_3	y_4	y_1	y_2	y_3	y_4
	(1)	(2)	(3)	(4)	(5)	(6)	(7)	(8)
τ	0.777 ***	0.677 ***	0.788 ***	0.710 ***	0.795 ***	0.679 ***	0.797 ***	0.711 ***
	(48.497)	(51.667)	(47.947)	(48.790)	(50.001)	(52.129)	(49.059)	(48.822)
ρ	0.152 ***	0.170 ***	0.161 ***	0.165 ***	0.151 ***	0.173 ***	0.155 ***	0.167 ***
	(7.590)	(10.545)	(8.102)	(9.254)	(7.623)	(10.745)	(7.835)	(9.372)
d_1	0.160 ***	0.017	0.155 ***	0.017				
	(4.200)	(0.956)	(3.647)	(1.058)				
$d_1 \times d_2$					0.009	0.008	0.021	0.008
					(0.670)	(1.153)	(1.334)	(1.396)
$W \times d_1$	−0.095 *	0.023	−0.191 ***	0.037				
	(−1.714)	(0.905)	(−3.107)	(1.628)				
$W \times d_1 \times d_2$					−0.034 *	−0.009	−0.050 **	0.001
					(−1.693)	(−0.994)	(−2.227)	(0.073)
Control Variables	Yes	Yes	Yes	Yes	Yes	Yes	Yes	Yes
N	1860	1860	1860	1860	1860	1860	1860	1860
R^2	0.935	0.948	0.939	0.956	0.937	0.948	0.940	0.957

The z-statistics are in parentheses; *** $p < 0.01$, ** $p < 0.05$, and * $p < 0.1$.

In addition, the coefficients of d_1 were significantly positive in Columns (1) and (3), and insignificantly positive in Columns (2) and (4), while the spatial lag coefficients were significantly negative in Columns (1) and (3) but insignificantly positive in Columns (2) and (4); in other words, without the consideration of time-limited rectification, CNSAs have merely attracted international tourists and increased international tourism revenue in local cities, while the insignificant results for domestic tourists and domestic tourism revenue in local and surrounding cities may give evidence of domestic tourists' little interest for the homogeneous service of CNSAs. Moreover, the coefficients of $d_1 * d_2$ were insignificantly positive in Columns (5)–(8), while the spatial lag coefficients of it were significantly negative in Columns (5) and (7), insignificantly negative in Column (6), and insignificantly positive in Column (8); in other words, after the implementation of time-limited rectification, the positive impacts of CNSAs on international tourists and international tourism revenue in local cities were weakened. One possible reason could be that the destination selection of international tourists has the characteristic of a "herd effect", and they are more sensitive to negative information regarding time-limited rectification.

5. Further Discussion

From the estimation results in Tables 2–4, it can be drawn that the results under the dynamic spatial Durbin model, which considers both the spatial and temporal lag effects of independent variables simultaneously, had the best theoretical explanation and practical significance. Therefore, in the following discussion, we focus on the results in Table 4.

After the implementation of time-limited rectification, the services of all CNSAs ought to be improved, while the psychological shadow of international tourists pushes them to choose the tourism destinations which are not listed in the roster of time-limited rectification [39]. Thus, it is not hard to learn why the direct coefficients of $d_1 * d_2$ become insignificant in Columns (5) and (7).

In addition, no matter with or without the consideration of time-limited rectification, the significant negative effects of CNSAs (or the interactive term of CNSAs and time-limited rectification) on tourism economic development were merely supported for international tourists and international tourism revenue; one possible reason may be that compared with domestic tourists, international tourists face the disadvantage of information acquisition, that is, the information asymmetry has restricted their options [40].

Generally, international tourists tend to choose CNSAs as their tourism destination, while their available time for travel is limited, which creates the problem of limited options and causes the "beggar-thy-neighbor" effect of CNSAs, that is, a vicious strategy devoted to attracting more international tourists in one city at the expense of a reduction in surrounding regions [41]. Thus, to eliminate the prevalence of the "beggar-thy-neighbor" effect among CNSAs and win a greater reputation in the world, an in-depth reform of the cooperation mechanism in the Chinese tourism industry is necessary for the future [42].

6. Conclusions, Policy Implications, and Research Prospects

6.1. Conclusions

Based on panel data on 124 prefecture-level and above cities from 2003 to 2018, this study investigated the impacts of CNSAs on tourism economic development and the moderating effect of time-limited rectification by comprehensively using the quasi-DID model, the static spatial Durbin model, and the dynamic spatial Durbin model. The main conclusions can be drawn as below.

Firstly, the impacts of CNSAs on tourism economic development can be attributed to discrete categories in terms of domestic tourists and international tourists and domestic tourism revenue and international tourism revenue. For instance, when comparing domestic versus international tourists, the information asymmetry not only increased the difficulty for international tourists in the selection of a tourism destination but also caused irrational competition among CNSAs, which formed a vicious circle.

Secondly, both the spatial spillover effect and path dependence were the impetus in promoting tourism economic development, which not only highlights the advantage of the dynamic spatial Durbin model compared with the nonspatial and static spatial econometric models but also provides evidence of cherishing the "brand effect" and "advertising effect" of CNSAs so as to achieve their sustainable development in the long run.

Thirdly, the effectiveness of time-limited rectification has been conditionally and partly proved in this study. The existence of the "beggar-thy-neighbor" effect among different cities has, to some extent, weakened the promotion effect of CNSAs on tourism economic development, especially in terms of international tourists and international tourism revenue. The realization of a more effective system in place of a vicious cycle of CNSA remains incomplete.

6.2. Policy Implications

The above-mentioned findings can draw the following policy implications for the related departments.

Firstly, for the superior department in charge, a CNSA is a good choice to promote tourism economic development where the incentive and restraint mechanism is necessary for its high-quality development. In particular, to take advantage of the path dependence, the evaluation criteria and supervision mechanism of CNSAs should be dynamic and normalized.

Secondly, for local governments, CNSAs can improve the reputation of regional tourism destinations in the short term, but it could lead to the problem of inaction or slackness. To win their reputation and attract more tourists in the long term, the service level of CNSAs should be promoted actively rather than rectified passively, and a periodic inspection system should be established.

Thirdly, for the management department of CNSAs, it is important and necessary to clarify the responsibility of each section rather than multi-sector coordinated management, which could reduce the transaction cost and the rent-seeking space. It is also important and necessary to avoid the vicious competition among stakeholders and promote tourism economic development with the aid of the spatial spillover effect.

6.3. Research Prospects

This study initially examined the moderating effect of time-limited rectification on the nexus between CNSAs and tourism economic development, while several limitations should be identified to highlight research prospects. For instance, except for CNSAs and time-limited rectification, other influencing factors, including government cooperation and environmental regulation, may have remarkable effects on tourism economic development [8,10]. In addition, to achieve an optimal balance of economic development and conservation of environmental resources, how the tourism economy affects the local ecological environment, energy consumption, and urbanization may be potential investigation directions, which also has great theoretical and practical significance for similar emerging countries [1,4].

Author Contributions: Y.Q. had the initial idea for the study and interpreted the results. Z.Z. designed the conceptual framework of the methodology, drafted and revised the manuscript. Y.F. conducted the work of data collection and econometric analysis. X.C. conducted the work of draft revision. All of the authors have contributed to the writing and finalizing of the paper. All authors have read and agreed to the published version of the manuscript.

Funding: This research was supported by the National Natural Science Foundation of China (No. 71874042).

Institutional Review Board Statement: Not applicable.

Informed Consent Statement: Not applicable.

Data Availability Statement: The data used to support the findings of this study are available from the corresponding author upon request.

Acknowledgments: Especially, we would like to thank the experts who participated in the improvement of this study. Any remaining errors are the responsibility of the authors.

Conflicts of Interest: The authors declare that they have no conflict of interest.

References

1. Alola, A.; Alola, U.V. Agricultural land usage and tourism impact on renewable energy consumption among Coastline Mediterranean Countries. *Energy Environ.* **2018**, *29*, 1438–1454. [CrossRef]
2. Eluwole, K.K.; Akadiri, S.S.; Alola, A.A.; Etokakpan, M.U. Does the interaction between growth determinants a drive for global environmental sustainability? Evidence from world top 10 pollutant emissions countries. *Sci. Total Environ.* **2020**, *705*, 135972. [CrossRef] [PubMed]
3. Alola, A.A.; Lasisi, T.T.; Eluwole, K.K.; Alola, U.V. Pollutant emission effect of tourism, real income, energy utilization, and urbanization in OECD countries: A panel quantile approach. *Environ. Sci. Pollut. Res.* **2021**, *28*, 1752–1761. [CrossRef]
4. Lasisi, T.; Eluwole, K.; Alola, U.; Aldieri, L.; Vinci, C.; Alola, A. Do Tourism Activities and Urbanization Drive Material Consumption in the OECD Countries? A Quantile Regression Approach. *Sustainability* **2021**, *13*, 7742. [CrossRef]
5. Cao, F.; Huang, Z.; Jin, C.; Xu, M. Chinese national scenic areas' tourism efficiency: Multi-scale fluctuation, prediction and optimization. *Asia Pac. J. Tour. Res.* **2015**, *21*, 570–595. [CrossRef]
6. Chen, Z.; Fu, W.; Konijnendijk van den Bosch, C.C.; Pan, H.; Huang, S.; Zhu, Z.; Qiao, Y.; Wang, N.; Dong, J. National forest parks in china: Origin, evolution, and sustainable development. *Forests* **2019**, *10*, 323. [CrossRef]
7. Cao, F.; Huang, Z.; Jin, C.; Xu, M. Influence of Chinese economic fluctuations on tourism efficiency in national scenic areas. *Tour. Econ.* **2016**, *22*, 884–907. [CrossRef]
8. Du, W.; Penabaz-Wiley, S.M.; Kinoshita, I. Relationships between land use changes, stakeholders, and national scenic area administrations: A case study of Mount Jinfo and its surroundings in China. *Environ. Plan. C Politics Space* **2019**, *37*, 1507–1530. [CrossRef]
9. Wang, F.; Peng, X.; Qin, Y.; Wang, C. What can the news tell us about the environmental performance of tourist areas? A text mining approach to China's National 5A Tourist Areas. *Sustain. Cities Soc.* **2020**, *52*, 101818. [CrossRef]
10. Liu, B.P.; Liu, Q.G. Evaluating water environmental conditionality for tourism of national scenic—A Case of Chaohu Lake, China. *Adv. Mater. Res.* **2013**, *726-731*, 1245–1250. [CrossRef]
11. Xu, B.; Pan, J. Spatial distribution characteristics of national protected areas in China. *J. Geogr. Sci.* **2019**, *29*, 2047–2068. [CrossRef]
12. Lu, C.; Li, W.; Pang, M.; Xue, B.; Miao, H. Quantifying the economy-environment interactions in tourism: Case of Gansu Province, China. *Sustainability* **2018**, *10*, 711. [CrossRef]
13. Shi, F.; Weaver, D.; Zhao, Y.; Huang, M.-F.; Tang, C.; Liu, Y. Toward an ecological civilization: Mass comprehensive ecotourism indications among domestic visitors to a Chinese wetland protected area. *Tour. Manag.* **2019**, *70*, 59–68. [CrossRef]
14. Qin, X.; Li, X. Evaluate on the decoupling of tourism economic development and ecological-environmental stress in China. *Sustainability* **2021**, *13*, 2149. [CrossRef]
15. Chen, H. Complementing conventional environmental impact assessments of tourism with ecosystem service valuation: A case study of the Wulingyuan Scenic Area, China. *Ecosyst. Serv.* **2020**, *43*, 101100. [CrossRef]
16. Xu, J.; Wei, J.; Zhao, D. Influence of social media on operational efficiency of national scenic spots in china based on three-stage DEA model. *Int. J. Inf. Manag.* **2016**, *36*, 374–388. [CrossRef]

17. Zheng, Q.; Kuang, Y.; Huang, N. Coordinated development between urban tourism economy and transport in the Pearl River Delta, China. *Sustainability* **2016**, *8*, 1338. [CrossRef]
18. Ma, D.; Xia, H.L. Analysis of the Impact of water pollution on tourism activities in scenic spots under the concept of eco-logical environment protection. *Fresen. Environ. Bull.* **2021**, *30*, 9966–9971.
19. Cerda, C.; Barkmann, J.; Marggraf, R. Non-market economic valuation of the benefits provided by temperate ecosystems at the extreme south of the Americas. *Reg. Environ. Chang.* **2014**, *14*, 1517–1531. [CrossRef]
20. Mayuzumi, Y. Is meeting the needs of tourists through ethnic tourism sustainable? Focus on Bali, Indonesia. *Asia Pac. J. Reg. Sci.* **2021**, 1–29. [CrossRef]
21. Sadeh, E.; Garkaz, M. Interpretive structural modeling of quality factors in both medical and hospitality services in the medical tourism industry. *J. Travel Tour. Mark.* **2019**, *36*, 253–267. [CrossRef]
22. Hsieh, L.-Y.; Lin, S.-M.; Lee, Y.-H. Benefit analysis of service quality degradation: A case study of the tourism industry. *J. Inf. Optim. Sci.* **2017**, *38*, 1347–1356. [CrossRef]
23. Han, L.; Li, L. Sustainable development of tourism under the background of low-carbon and green economy. *Adv. Mater. Sci. Eng.* **2021**, *2021*, 1–8. [CrossRef]
24. Wang, L.; Zhang, H. The Impact of marine tourism resources development on sustainable development of marine economy. *J. Coast. Res.* **2019**, *94*, 589–592. [CrossRef]
25. Chen, H.B.; Dong, K.; Wang, F.F.; Ayamba, E.C. The spatial effect of tourism economic development on regional ecological efficiency. *Environ. Sci. Pollut. Res.* **2020**, *27*, 38241–38258.
26. Motsa, A.; Rybakova, S.; Shelemetieva, T.; Zhuvahina, I.; Honchar, L. The Effect of Regional Tourism on Economic Development (Case Study: The Eu Countries). *Int. Rev.* **2021**, *1–2*, 58–65.
27. Yang, X.; Jia, Y.; Wang, Q.; Li, C.; Zhang, S. Space–time evolution of the ecological security of regional urban tourism: The case of Hubei Province, China. *Environ. Monit. Assess.* **2021**, *193*, 1–20. [CrossRef]
28. Huang, C.; Wang, J.W.; Wang, C.M.; Cheng, J.H.; Dai, J. Does tourism industry agglomeration reduce carbon emissions? *Environ. Sci. Pollut. Res.* **2021**, *28*, 30278–30293. [CrossRef]
29. Xiao, Z.; Muhtar, P.; Huo, W.; An, C.; Yang, L.; Zhang, F. Spatial and temporal differentiation of the tourism water footprint in mainland China and its influencing factors. *Sustainability* **2021**, *13*, 10396. [CrossRef]
30. Tang, R. The impact of integration policies on tourism industry convergence in the Yangtze River Delta: Theoretical mechanism and empirical test. *Lett. Spat. Resour. Sci.* **2021**, *14*, 141–167. [CrossRef]
31. Li, X.; Ma, B.; Lu, C.; Yang, H.; Sun, M. Spatial Pattern and development of protected areas in the north-south transitional Zone of China. *Chin. Geogr. Sci.* **2021**, *31*, 149–166. [CrossRef]
32. Zhang, Y.J.; Wang, W. How does China's carbon emissions trading (CET) policy affect the investment of CET-covered enterprises? *Energ. Econ.* **2021**, *98*, 105224. [CrossRef]
33. Wang, S.S.; Chen, G.; Han, X. An Analysis of the impact of the emissions trading system on the green total factor productivity based on the spatial difference-in-differences approach: The Case of China. *Int. J. Environ. Res. Public Health* **2021**, *18*, 9040. [CrossRef]
34. Zhou, L.; Tang, L.Z. Environmental regulation and the growth of the total-factor carbon productivity of China's industries: Evidence from the implementation of action plan of air pollution prevention and control. *J. Environ. Manag.* **2021**, *296*, 113078. [CrossRef] [PubMed]
35. Yang, Z.; Fan, M.; Shao, S.; Yang, L. Does carbon intensity constraint policy improve industrial green production performance in China? A quasi-DID analysis. *Energy Econ.* **2017**, *68*, 271–282. [CrossRef]
36. Elhorst, J.P. *Spatial Econometrics: From Cross-Sectional Data to Spatial Panels*; Springer: Heidelberg/Berlin, Germany, 2014.
37. Feng, Y.; Wang, X.; Du, W.; Wu, H.; Wang, J. Effects of environmental regulation and FDI on urban innovation in China: A spatial Durbin econometric analysis. *J. Clean. Prod.* **2019**, *235*, 210–224. [CrossRef]
38. Feng, Y.; Wang, X. Effects of urban sprawl on haze pollution in China based on dynamic spatial Durbin model during 2003–2016. *J. Clean. Prod.* **2020**, *242*, 118368. [CrossRef]
39. Orlov, I.; Popov, A. Imported goods and the spirit of consumerism: Consumption in soviet tourism abroad. *Sov. Post. Sov. Rev.* **2016**, *43*, 182–218. [CrossRef]
40. Bak, S.; Min, C.-K.; Roh, T.-S. Impacts of UNESCO-listed tangible and intangible heritages on tourism. *J. Travel Tour. Mark.* **2019**, *36*, 917–927. [CrossRef]
41. Feng, Y.; He, F. The effect of environmental information disclosure on environmental quality: Evidence from Chinese cities. *J. Clean. Prod.* **2020**, *276*, 124027. [CrossRef]
42. Matveevskaya, A.S.; Pogodin, S.N.; Wang, J.T. Russia and China in the field of international tourism. *Vestnik St. Petersb. Univ. Philos. Confl. Stud.* **2020**, *36*, 384–393. [CrossRef]

International Journal of
Environmental Research and Public Health

MDPI

Article

Have China's Pilot Free Trade Zones Improved Green Total Factor Productivity?

Qingshan Ma [1], Yuanmeng Zhang [2], Kexin Yang [3] and Lingyun He [2,*]

[1] School of Economics, Xiamen University, No. 422 Siming South Road, Xiamen 361005, China; maqingshan@stu.xmu.edu.cn
[2] Economics School, Zhongnan University of Economics and Law, No. 182 Nanhu Avenue, Wuhan 430073, China; yuanmeng_zhang@foxmail.com
[3] Economics and Management School, Wuhan University, No. 299 Bayi Road, Wuhan 430072, China; kexin_yang@whu.edu.cn
* Correspondence: helingyun@zuel.edu.cn

Abstract: Free trade zones (FTZ) are designated areas for promoting trade openness and investment facilitation. In China, FTZs are also regarded as "green areas" in which planning actions and institutional innovations are implemented, and there is a commitment to promoting urban green and healthy development. Given that green total factor productivity (*GTFP*) is an important measure of a city's health and green performance, this study exploits the difference-in-differences method to explore the impact of pilot FTZs on urban *GTFP* in 280 cities in China for the period between 2005 and 2017. The results show that the green areas positively contributed to the growth of *GTFP*. Moreover, the outcome holds with robustness tests. Statistically, the positive effect emerged in cities during the first three years after introducing the initiative, with the effect disappearing afterward. It also had a strong positive impact in the central and western regions and in large and medium-sized cities, while the influence remained insignificant in the remaining areas in China. Furthermore, the paper also reveals that the promotion of foreign direct investment and industrial structure upgrading are the primary channels through which the positive relationship between pilot FTZs and *GTFP* is established.

Keywords: pilot free trade zones; green total factor productivity; green development; difference-in-differences; quasi-natural experiment

Citation: Ma, Q.; Zhang, Y.; Yang, K.; He, L. Have China's Pilot Free Trade Zones Improved Green Total Factor Productivity?. *IJERPH* **2021**, *18*, 11681. https://doi.org/10.3390/ijerph182111681

Academic Editors: Jie Chen, Qian Zhou and Ting Zhang

Received: 7 September 2021
Accepted: 27 October 2021
Published: 7 November 2021

1. Introduction

The Chinese economy has undergone spectacular growth in recent decades, while environmental degradation from traditional extensive economic development is becoming an extremely serious problem. Environmental pollution brings challenges to the sustainable and healthy development of cities [1]. According to "the Report on the State of the Ecology and Environment", in 2020, 40.1% of the 337 cities at or above the prefecture level exceeded air quality standards. Severe environmental pollution endangers people's health [2], which results in inequality [3], aggravates public finance burden [4], and hinders the process of urban renewal [5]. Therefore, the need for urban green and sustainable transition has become inevitable. In this context, the Chinese government has released a series of institutional innovations and policy experiments to control environmental pollution and improve the urban population's health. One of these innovations is the free trade zone (FTZ) policy.

According to Teifenbrun [6] and Akbari et al. [7], an FTZ refers to an area where goods may be landed, handled, manufactured, or reconfigured, and then re-exported without the intervention of customs authorities. In the zones, multiple institutional incentives such as free movement of goods and people and preferential taxation are provided. Since the 1980s, countries such as the United States and Brazil have established FTZs, which are conductive to attract foreign direct investment (FDI), and greatly promote trade development [8–10]. The Chinese government has always been committed to deepening reform and opening wider to the outside world. In 1980, Shenzhen, Zhuhai, Shantou, and Xiamen were approved as special economic zones (SEZ). Then, China established the first bonded zone (BZ) in Shanghai in 1990, and successively set up BZs in Tianjin, Dalian, and other cities. In 2000, China approved 15 pilot export processing zones (EPZs) including Yantai Weihai, Hangzhou, at one time. Since then, China has continuously established some other SEZs, BZs, and EPZs. On 29 September 2013, China's first FTZ, the Shanghai pilot FTZ, was established, which marks a new stage of China's opening-up. After that, more pilot FTZs were built in Tianjin, Chongqing, and other cities by March 2017.

Compared to previous policy zones like SEZs, the opening-up of the service and financial industries has been expanded in pilot FTZs for the first time. The Chinese pilot FTZs have also implemented a series of institutional innovations in addition to possessing functions similar to those of other countries. The institutional innovations mainly include: first, optimizing government functions and improving trade and investment efficiency through one-window service; second, tax holidays and tax regimes such as reduced income tax for some enterprises in pilot FTZs; third, introducing the "Negative List" management model to provide guidance and governs industry sectors in which foreign investment is prohibited or where possible restrictions may apply.

"Green development" is a major development idea of Chinese pilot FTZs. As the concepts emphasized in the "Guiding Opinions on Strengthening Ecological Environment Protection in Pilot Free Trade Zones" issued by the Ministry of Ecology and Environment (MEE) of China, the ideas of green development should penetrate to the entire process of pilot FTZs construction, and pilot FTZs must develop a modern green service industry, green manufacturing, green supply chain, and green trade in the future. Some studies also indicated that pilot FTZs make efforts to become green areas in various ways [11]. Therefore, as green areas, have the pilot FTZs effectively promoted urban green development? This paper attempts to address this question and provide useful policy alternatives.

Numerous studies have examined the economic effects of the policy zones. The literature has indicated that Chinese SEZs, EPZs, and BZs are all conducive to attracting more investors and promoting trade development [12–14]. These special zones gain other benefits such as participation in global value chains and knowledge exchange [15,16]. Some researchers have indicated that FTZs also have effects on attracting FDI and promoting trade development [17]. As suggested by Jiang et al. [18], pilot FTZs can effectively combine domestic production factors with advanced international technology. Moreover, pilot FTZs greatly promote cross-country knowledge spillover and improve China's competitive advantages in global industrial and supply chains [19,20]. Additionally, Song et al. [21] found that the policy advantages of pilot FTZs are beneficial to upgrading the organization and performance of local export-oriented enterprises.

Although few studies have attempted to estimate the impact of policy zones on urban green and healthy development, many studies have explored their impact on economic growth. Most extant studies support that SEZs, EPZs, and BZs positively contribute to innovation stimulation and economic growth [22,23]. However, additional critical findings suggest that these policies also have some dampening effects such as resource mismatches [24], widening the gap between the rich and poor [25], and tax evasion [26]. Concerning FTZs, the existing literature mainly focuses on positive effects. For instance, some studies have found that FTZs play an important role in innovation stimulation and enhancing the competitiveness of enterprises, which promotes economic growth [18,27–30]. From the perspective of Chinese pilot FTZs, Tan et al. [31] focused on the Shanghai pilot FTZ and provided evidence that there is a significant and positive effect on the growth rate of the total imports and exports of Shanghai. Based on the difference-in-differences (DID) method, Zhang et al. [32] found that pilot FTZs drive regional economic growth. Chen et al. [33] also suggested that China's FTZ policy is effective and increases the national economic welfare.

Another emerging stream of literature emphasizes the impact of policy zones on environmental pollution. Some researchers argue that the policy zones promote environmental protection, whereas other researchers find that these zones generate high emissions of metals and other negative products that contaminate the environment [34,35]. Regarding FTZs, it is generally believed that Chinese pilot FTZs have reduced environmental pollution, since various measures such as clean production mechanisms are adopted by the government for pollution prevention and control [36,37].

Based on these two strands of literature, the important question that we focus on is whether the economic growth brought by pilot FTZs is at the expense of the environment or has green characteristics. Currently, green total factor productivity (*GTFP*) has been widely used in the research field of environmental economics to reflect the level of green development [38,39]. Previous literature has regarded total factor productivity (TFP) as an important measure of economic growth [40–42]. These studies conducted related research by taking only the traditional input (e.g., capital and labor) and desirable output (e.g., GDP) into account, while ignoring the green and environmental factors. With the development of society, the constraints of the environment on economic growth have become increasingly prominent. Therefore, it is not sufficient to use the traditional TFP indicator to analyze green and sustainable economic development. *GTFP* is a new productivity indicator that comprehensively incorporates resource and environmental constraints. Specifically, the new indicator adds resource consumption as an input factor to the traditional TFP analysis framework and adds environmental pollution emissions as an undesirable output to the input-output efficiency analysis [25,43,44], which can effectively reflect the level of green and healthy development [45,46].

At present, a small amount of attention has been given to the impact of pilot FTZs in other countries on regional green development [7,47,48]. However, concerning China, regarding pilot FTZs and green development, only a few researchers such as Jiang et al. [18], have conducted research on the Shanghai pilot FTZ and found that pilot FTZ is a great incentive to promote green development. However, Zhuo et al. [49] took the Guangdong pilot FTZ as the research object and concluded that this FTZ operates at the expense of the environment: for every 100 million yuan increase in the GDP, discharged wastewater and waste gas increases by 1.746 million tons and 28.016 tons, respectively.

According to the abovementioned literature, the following problems still need to be remedied. First, current studies mainly explore the impact of pilot FTZs on economic growth, but few studies have focused on the relationship between pilot FTZs and green development. Clarifying the relationship between pilot FTZs and green development is of great significance for providing policy implications to promote urban green development through institutional innovations. Second, the existing literature on pilot FTZs and green development focuses only on the case studies of a special pilot FTZ, and the conclusions remain inconsistent and controversial. Therefore, the relationship between pilot FTZs and urban green development is uncertain, and we do not know whether the effect is of universal significance.

Therefore, the present study takes advantage of the quasi-experiments provided by the policy of FTZ construction and adopts the DID method to explore the impacts of pilot FTZs on urban green development. This study contributes to the existing literature in two ways. First, our article contributes to the literature on the economic and environmental impacts of different policy zones. We discuss the impact of the ideas of green development and institutional innovation measures implemented in pilot FTZs on the relationship between free trade and environmental pollution. Therefore, the research in this paper is helpful for a deeper understanding on how to exert government functions to better promote urban green development. Second, this paper takes the pilot FTZs as research objects and uses the DID and propensity score matching-DID (PSM-DID) methods to investigate the impact of pilot FTZs on urban green development, which can address the endogeneity problem, and ensure the reliability of the research conclusions.

The structure of the rest of paper is as follows. The institutional background and theoretical hypothesis are explained in the second section. The data and methodology are reported in the third section. The empirical results are proposed in the fourth section. Exploring the mediating effect of FTZ policy on *GTFP* is explored in the fifth section. Finally, conclusions are presented in the sixth section.

2. Institution Background and Theoretical Hypothesis

2.1. Institution Background

Since 1978, China has established SEZs. The zones were designed as major platforms that provided preferential policies such as tax reduction for foreign enterprises. In addition, BZs have been successfully constructed since the 1990s. Goods are exempt from duty in these zones. Further, the Chinese government set up EPZs where goods manufactured for export are exempt from tax.

Government's peculiarities and intervention play an important role in the development of these policy zones [50–52]. In the Chinese context, the key experiences of SEZs, EPZs, and BZs can best be summarized as gradualism with an experimental approach; a strong commitment; and the active, pragmatic facilitation of the state [53]. First, the Chinese government provides preferential policies and broad institutional autonomy such as duty-free benefits, which greatly promoted industrial clusters. Second, strong support and proactive participation of governments are provided, especially in the areas of public goods and externalities, which ensure a stable and supportive environment for long-term development. Third, the government continuously promotes technology learning and upgrading by designing policies and foresight activities.

Under the positive impact and intervention of government, most of special zones in China, though differing in characteristics, are quite successful in FDI introduction and trade prosperity. However, there is still considerable room for China to expand the opening of its service industry and attract advanced foreign investment.

To further accelerate the pace of opening to the outside world, on 27 September 2013, the first Pilot FTZ (Shanghai) in mainland China was founded. Up to March 2017, the Chinese government has established a total of 11 pilot FTZs. The policies of pilot FTZs include not just the free entry and exit of goods, zero-tariff policies, and other traditional policies that promote trade liberalization. More importantly, the FTZ policy is China's first policy to expand the service industry and financial opening after joining the WTO. For example, the "Negative List" management model and "pre-entry national treatment" were adopted in pilot FTZs to achieve expanding openness in the fields of the modern services industry, such as banking, insurance, capital markets, and other fields. On the premise of complying with relevant regulations, qualified foreign-funded institutions and organizations are allowed to establish companies to conduct related business in the form of joint ventures or independent forms, while enjoying various preferential policies. In addition, the convertibility of the RMB capital account, the marketization of interest rates in the financial market, the reform of foreign exchange management, the opening of financial institutions, and the construction of international block trading platforms are all piloted in pilot FTZs. Compared with other special policy zones, FTZs are multifunctional areas that gather multiple innovational advantages, as shown in Table 1.

Table 1. Comparison between FTZs and other policy zones.

Policy	Industry	Free Currency	Free Trade	Free Entry and Exit of Goods	Free Storage of Goods	Free Entry and Exit of Personnel
FTZs	√	√	√	√	√	√
SEZs	√	×	×	×	×	×
EPZs	√	×	×	×	×	×
BZs	√	×	×	√	√	×

Source: The author manually compiled according to the relevant policies of China. √ means that the innovative policies such as industry policy, free currency policy, and free entry and exit of goods, etc. were implemented in the policy zones; In contrast, × represents the policies were not implemented in the policy zones.

Different from the FTZs of other countries, pilot FTZs in China have implemented a series of institutional innovations to improve trade efficiency, investment efficiency, and administrative efficiency. Institutional innovation is reflected in the simplified customs clearance procedures for commodities and higher administrative efficiency. For example, pilot FTZs apply the "first entering and then declaring" process and simplify customs clearance documents, and so on. In addition, pilot FTZs have vigorously promoted the reform of e-government, improved the administrative examination and approval efficiency of the enterprises in the zone. Moreover, high-tech enterprises, financial service enterprises, cultural and creative enterprises, and many other industries in the zones can enjoy lower income tax rates. Overseas high-tech talents in pilot FTZs can also enjoy personal income tax relief. These measures have effectively promoted the development of emerging industries and economic growth in pilot FTZs.

FTZs are also set as demonstration zones for protecting the environment and achieving high-quality development [54]. "Opinions of the Ministry of Commerce on Supporting the Innovative Development of Pilot Free Trade Zones 2015" proposes to continuously explore the establishment of a green supply chain management system and encourage the development of green trade. "The Guiding Opinions on Strengthening the Ecological Environment Protection and Promoting High-quality Development in Free Trade Zones" released by the MEE of China highlighted the need to explore institutional innovations related to environmental protection in these green areas. Currently, all planned actions of the 21 existing pilot FTZs include provisions for promoting green development. For instance, "Article 50 of the Regulations of China (Shanghai) Pilot Free Trade Zone" clearly stipulates that pilot FTZs should strengthen environmental protection, improve environmental assessment classification management, and use the advantage of openness to be in line with international environmental and energy system standard certification. Shenzhen is committed to ensuring 100% coverage of green buildings, establishing a green and creative transportation system, and constructing a central cooling project in the zone to reduce pollutant emissions. Other pilot FTZs are also actively engaged in green development, for instance, the Nanjing pilot FTZ develops green finance. Figure 1 shows that the average investment in environmental governance of the provinces where pilot FTZs are located has increased from 66.11 billion yuan in 2003 to 310.44 billion yuan in 2017, and after the FTZ policy emerged, it maintains a continuous upward trend, which fully reflects the green development effects created by FTZs.

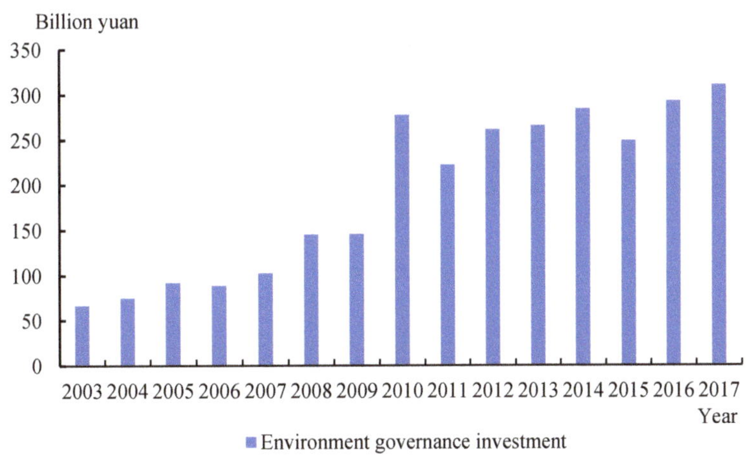

Figure 1. The average value of environmental governance investment in provinces where pilot FTZs are located. Source: China Statistical Yearbook on Environment, 2003–2017.

2.2. Hypotheses

An important influencing mechanism of pilot FTZs on urban *GTFP* is investment facilitation. Yao et al. [55], Qu et al. [56], and Tan and Yan [57] found that pilot FTZs have a strong foreign investment-induced effect. FTZs are committed to attracting the entry of foreign-funded enterprises with high productivity. The preferential policies of pilot FTZs have abolished many of the previous restrictions on the share of FDI, relaxed investment restrictions, and continued to simplify investment procedures. Both the Shanghai pilot FTZ and the Guangdong pilot FTZ have implemented preferential tax policies for high-tech enterprises and access and work convenience policies for high-tech talent. Pilot FTZs have gradually become a gathering place for high-end foreign enterprises. On the one hand, with the expansion of the scale of enterprises that gather in the pilot FTZs, different enterprises can establish connections with one another through resource sharing and the division of labor based on specialization, which effectively reduces transaction costs, and increases productivity [58]. At the same time, the knowledge spillover effect allows the spread of advanced technology and management experience in the agglomeration zone, thereby enabling the enterprises in the zone to learn and use more advanced energy-saving technologies and management methods [59]. The two effects work synergistically to continuously improve the production and environmental efficiency of the enterprises in the zones, which, in turn, has a positive impact on improving urban *GTFP*. On the other hand, the inflow of FDI squeezes the market share of domestic enterprises to a certain extent, intensifies industry competition, and creates a selection mechanism for the survival of the fittest. This phenomenon strongly motivates domestic enterprises to carry out technological innovation, thereby promoting the improvement of urban *GTFP*. Therefore, we put forward the following hypothesis:

Hypothesis 1 (H1). *Pilot FTZs can increase GTFP through the promotion of FDI.*

Industrial upgrading is another influencing mechanism of pilot FTZs on urban *GTFP*. As an innovation in the trade management system, pilot FTZs play an active role in breaking down trade barriers, overcoming obstacles to factor flow, and making advanced resources flow freely on an international scale. On the one hand, the main policy goal for China to set up pilot FTZs is to accelerate the opening of the service and financial industry, which is beneficial to the upgrading of the industrial structure [60]. Upgrading of the industrial structure can not only reduce the emission of pollutants but also accelerate green development [61]. Therefore, it has a considerably positive effect on the growth in urban *GTFP*. On the other hand, the trade facilitation brought by pilot FTZs also brings new opportunities for industrial upgrading. The special policies of pilot FTZs can not only simplify international trade procedures and reduce international trade costs but also improve logistics efficiency, which effectively promotes the flow of high-tech production factors [62,63]. Advanced production factors continuously flow to high value-added industries, which can not only facilitate the development of import, export, and service trade, enhance the competitiveness of related industries, but also optimize the industrial structure and promote industrial upgrading [29,64]. In addition, pilot FTZs can boost the optimization and upgrading of industrial structures by eliminating internal low-efficiency enterprises and absorbing advanced technologies from the outside [65]. With the continuous upgrading of the industrial structure, related enterprises also actively improve their production efficiency and achieve green production, which promotes the improvement of urban *GTFP*. Based on the above analysis, we propose hypothesis 2. In addition, the framework of influencing mechanisms of pilot FTZs on urban *GTFP* is shown in Figure 2.

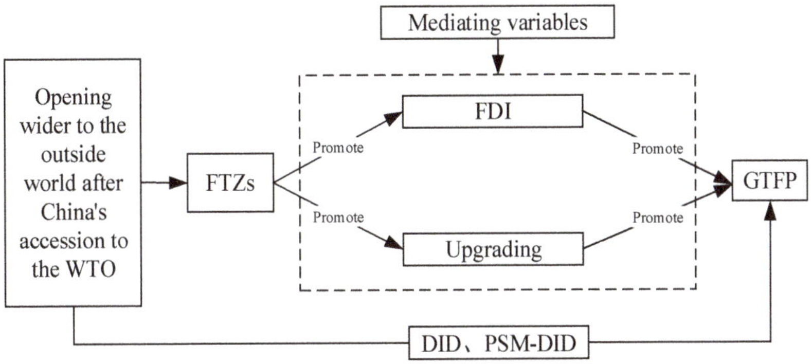

Figure 2. The framework of the influence of pilot FTZs on *GTFP*. Source: Compiled by the author.

Hypothesis 2 (H2). *Pilot FTZs can increase GTFP through the promotion of industrial upgrading.*

3. Data and Methodology

3.1. *The Measurement of* GTFP

Urban *GTFP* can accurately describe and reflect the development efficiency of urban economies under the constraints of resources and the environment [39]. Under the framework of environmental technology analysis, this paper uses the slack-based measure (SBM) model based on undesirable output and the Malmquist index model to measure *GTFP*.

3.1.1. SBM Model

The traditional data envelopment analysis (DEA) model has advantages in managing the problems of multi-input indices and multi-output indices [38,66]; thus, it is widely used in the field of development performance measurement. However, the traditional DEA method only considers economic benefits when measuring efficiency values but does not consider the impact of undesirable output. This fact is not only inconsistent with the actual production process but also ignores the slack problem of input and output factors; accordingly, there is a deviation between the measured value and the actual value [67]. Therefore, to solve this problem, Tone [68] first proposed a nonradial, nonangle SBM model based on slack variables. This model resolves the influence of slack variables on the measured value by incorporating the slacks of the input and output factors directly into the objective function, and it effectively improves the accuracy of the measured values [69,70]. Therefore, in line with the above research, the SBM model proposed in this paper is constructed as follows:

$$\rho = \min_{s^x, s^y, s^b, \lambda} \frac{1 - \frac{1}{M}\sum_{m=1}^{M} \frac{s_m^x}{x_{km}}}{1 + \frac{1}{N+L}\left(\sum_{n=1}^{N} \frac{s_n^y}{y_{kn}} + \sum_{l=1}^{L} \frac{s_l^b}{b_{kl}}\right)} \tag{1}$$

$$s.t. \begin{cases} x_{km} = \sum_{k=1}^{K} \lambda_k x_{km} + s_m^x, m = 1, 2, \ldots, M \\ y_{kn} = \sum_{k=1}^{K} \lambda_k y_{kn} - s_n^y, n = 1, 2, \ldots, N \\ b_{kl} = \sum_{k=1}^{K} \lambda_k b_{kl} + s_l^b, l = 1, 2, \ldots, L \\ s_m^x \geq 0, s_n^y \geq 0, s_l^b \geq 0 \end{cases}$$

where ρ is the efficiency value; x, y, and b represent the vectors of the input factors, desirable outputs and undesirable outputs, respectively, and M, N and L represent the number of the types of input factors, desirable outputs and undesirable outputs, respectively; (x_{km}, y_{kn}, b_{kl}) are the input and output values of the k-th decision-making unit; λ represents the weight of the decision-making unit; and s_m^x, s_n^y, and s_l^b are the slack variables of the input factors, desirable outputs and undesirable outputs, respectively. Among them, s_m^x

and s_l^b represent the redundancy of input and undesirable output, respectively, and s_n^y represents the shortage of desirable output; the objective function ρ is strictly monotonically decreases with respect to s_m^x, s_n^y, and s_l^b, and the value range of ρ is 0–1. If $\rho = 1$, then $s_m^x = s_n^y = s_l^b = 0$, which indicates that the evaluation unit is completely efficient, and there is no redundancy of input or shortage of output. If $\rho = 0$, then the evaluation unit is technically completely inefficient at present.

In addition, Equation (1) represents the SBM model under the assumption of constant returns to scale (CRS). If the constraint condition $\sum_{k=1}^{K} \lambda_k = 1$ is introduced into the SBM model, then Equation (1) can be transformed into the SBM model under the assumption of variable returns to scale (VRS).

The SBM model also has certain shortcomings. For example, its objective function is to minimize the efficiency value, that is, to maximize the inefficiency of input and output. From the perspective of the distance function, the projection point of the evaluated unit is the point on the front surface that is farthest from the evaluated unit. Tone [68] tried to design a method to calculate the shortest distance to the frontier, but it is only suitable for the case where there are fewer units to be evaluated. At present, the SBM model is still the mainstream method of efficiency measurement and has been widely used in the relevant literature [69–72].

3.1.2. Malmquist Index Model

The Malmquist index is based on the distance function proposed by Malmquist in 1953 [73]. The index is calculated based on the quantitative data from inputs and outputs without the need for pricing information [74], and it can provide a breakdown of the change in productivity changes [75]. According to the Malmquist index model, we can accurately measure the dynamic growth trend of the *GTFP* in 280 cities of China. Referring to the practice of Chung et al. [76], the specific equation is set as follows:

$$GTFP = \left[\frac{\rho_k^t(x_k^t, y_k^t, b_k^t)}{\rho_k^t(x_k^{t+1}, y_k^{t+1})} \frac{\rho_k^{t+1}(x_k^t, y_k^t)}{\rho_k^{t+1}(x_k^{t+1}, y_k^{t+1})} \right] \tag{2}$$

where $\rho_k^t(x_k^t, y_k^t)$ is the efficiency value of the decision-making unit in period t, $\rho_k^t\left(x_k^{t+1}, y_k^{t+1}\right)$ is the efficiency value of the decision-making unit in period $t+1$, and $\rho_k^{t+1}(x_k^t, y_k^t)$ $\rho_k^t\left(x_k^{t+1}, y_k^{t+1}\right)$ are the cross-efficiency values in period t and period $t+1$, respectively. *GTFP* represents the green total factor productivity index. If $GTFP > 1$, then the *GTFP* of the decision-making unit increased in the current period, and if $GTFP < 1$, then the *GTFP* of the decision-making unit decreased in the current period.

However, the above indicator calculated according to the Malmquist index model is not the *GTFP* in each year but the rate of change of the *GTFP* relative to the previous year. Therefore, if we set the value of the *GTFP* in the base year to 1 and then multiply it by the *GTFP* of subsequent years, we can obtain the *GTFP* values of 280 sample cities in China from 2005 to 2017.

3.2. DID Method

In this paper, we use the DID method to evaluate the influence of FTZ policy on *GTFP*. The Chinese government established the China (Shanghai) Pilot FTZ in September 2013. To date, China has established pilot FTZs in six batches cover 21 provinces or municipalities. Therefore, we regard FTZ policy as a quasi-natural experiment. Tan and Yan [57] considered integrated FTZs to be the predecessor of pilot FTZs. To reduce the research bias, we regard the cities with integrated FTZs and pilot FTZs as the treatment groups. Other cities belong to the control group. The DID model is set as follows:

$$GTFP_{it} = \alpha_0 + \alpha_1 dt_{it} + \sum \partial_k year_k + \sum \gamma_j X_{it} + \mu_{city} + \lambda_{it} \tag{3}$$

where *dt* represents whether city *i* has a pilot FTZ in year *t* and *GTFP* is the urban green total factor productivity measured by the super-efficiency SBM model of undesirable outputs and the Malmquist index. *X* represents a set of control variables, including the level of informatization of the city (Informatization), population density (Pdensity), the development level of the service industry (Service_sec), the level of science and technology (SciTec), and the scale of fixed assets (Fixed_assets). *year* represents the year fixed effect, μ represents the city fixed effect, and λ represents the random error term.

In addition, the premise of using a DID method is to meet the parallel trend hypothesis; that is, before the impact of the pilot FTZs, the *GTFP* of the experimental group and the *GTFP* of the control group have the same change trend. Referring to Li et al. [77] and Beck et al. [78], this paper uses the event analysis method and presents the dynamic model as follows:

$$GTFP_{it} = \alpha + \sum_{k \geq -5, k \neq -1}^{5} \beta_k {D_{it}}^k + \sum \partial_k year_k + \sum \gamma_j X_{it} + \mu_{city} + \lambda_{it} \tag{4}$$

where ${D_{it}}^k$ is a dummy variable that represents whether the city approved the establishment of a pilot FTZ. The value of ${D_{it}}^k$ is assigned according to the following rules: s_i represents the specific year of the establishment of a pilot FTZ. If $t - s_i < -5$, then define ${D_{it}}^k = 1$; otherwise ${D_{it}}^k = 0$. If $t - s_i = k$, then define ${D_{it}}^k = 1$; otherwise, ${D_{it}}^k = 0$ ($k \in [-5, 5]$ and $k \neq -1$). The process of establishing a pilot FTZ is that the local governments submit an application to the State Council of China after completing the preparations and planning plans for pilot FTZs. The State Council then sends staff to the field to conduct research and perform repeated demonstrations and communication changes involving the specific plan. Only after more than a year of revisions and necessary administrative procedures will the State Council officially approve the establishment of a pilot FTZ. In fact, when the pilot FTZ was established, many service industry and high-tech companies had made preparations in advance. Therefore, we set the year before the pilot FTZ was approved as the base year.

3.3. Variables and Data Description

Dependent variable. As described in Section 3.1, the *GTFP* of 280 cities in China from 2005 to 2017 was estimated through the SBM model and the Malmquist index. The specific input factors, desirable outputs and undesirable outputs are presented in Table 2.

Dependent variable. As described in Section 3.1, *GTFP* is based on the DEA framework. This framework uses the non-radial and non-angle SBM model of undesirable outputs, and measures *GTFP* by constructing the Malmquist productivity index.

Independent variables. The FTZ policy (dt) is set in the form of a dummy variable. For the city with a pilot FTZ, the pilot year and subsequent years are set to 1, and the other years are set to 0. Up to now, China has established six batches of FTZs. the first batch of FTZs established in 2013 include the Shanghai FTZ, the second batch of FTZs established in 2015 include Guangzhou, Shenzhen, Zhuhai, Tianjin, Fuzhou, and Xiamen FTZs, and the third batch of FTZs established in 2017 includes Shenyang, Yingkou, Dalian, Zhoushan, Kaifeng, Luoyang, Zhengzhou, Yichang, Wuhan, Xiangyang, Chongqing, Chengdu, Luzhou and Xi'an FTZs. After that, the Chinese government successively established the fourth, fifth and sixth batches of free trade zones in different cities. Due to data limitations, this paper regards only the cities with pilot FTZs in the first, second, and third batches as the research objects.

Table 2. Explanation of each indicator.

Category	Factor	Explanation
Input factors	Capital stock	Based on the calculation method provided by Shan [79], the perpetual inventory method is used to measure capital stock. The depreciation rate is set to 10.96%, and the fixed asset investment data for each city are deflated by using the fixed asset investment price index of the province. As a result, we adjust it to the actual value of constant prices in 2005.
	Number of laborers	The total number of employees in the secondary and tertiary industries is used as an indicator of the labor input in various cities.
	Energy input	The entire society's electricity consumption and urban water supply are used as measures of energy and resource consumption, respectively, during economic development.
Desirable outputs **	Urban output	Actual regional GDP
	Resident quality of life	Green coverage of the built-up area
Undesirable outputs	Wastewater	Industrial wastewater discharge
	Exhaust gas	Industrial SO_2 emissions ***
	Soot	Industrial soot emissions
	Haze pollution	PM2.5 concentration *

Data source: The above data are mainly from the "China Urban Statistical Yearbook" and the statistical bulletins of provinces and cities over the sample period. * The PM2.5 concentration data for cities come from satellite remote sensing data compiled by the National Aeronautics and Space Administration (NASA) (http://earthdata.nasa.gov (accessed on 1 November 2020). We use the 1.4 million Chinese basic geographic information data provided by the National Basic Geographic Information Center to obtain the average PM2.5 concentration in various cities over the sample period [80]. ** Desirable outputs refer to strong (good) outputs, such as paper or electricity. Undesirable outputs refer to weak (bad) outputs, such as suspended solids or SO_2 [76,81]. *** Since the Chinese official government has not published the city-level CO_2 industrial emissions data, the industrial SO_2 emissions is adopted here.

Control variables. This paper includes the following control variables: the level of informatization of the city (Informatization), as measured by the number of internet users in the city (by taking the logarithm); population density (Pdensity), measured by the number of people per square kilometer; the development level of the service industry (Service_sec), as measured by the proportion of the added value of the service industry in GDP; the level of science and technology (SciTec), as measured by the amount of urban technology investment (by taking the logarithm); and the scale of fixed assets (Fixed_assets), as measured by the amount of fixed asset investment in the city (by taking the logarithm).

The data source is the "China Urban Statistical Yearbook". The sample of this paper consists of 2005–2017 data on 280 prefecture-level cities in China. The descriptive statistics of each variable are presented in Table 3.

Table 3. Descriptive statistics.

	Variables	N	Mean	Std	Min	Max
Dependent variable	*GTFP*	3640	0.369	0.222	0.0138	3.679
Independent variables	dt	3640	0.0555	0.229	0	1
	treated	3640	0.236	0.425	0	1
Mediating variables	FDI	3481	0.761	1.853	0.0003	30.83
	INSU	3591	0.846	0.426	0.0943	4.166
Control variables	Informatization	3606	12.69	1.160	5.466	17.76
	Pdensity	3566	0.436	0.325	0.0047	2.648
	Service_sec	3591	37.56	9.048	8.580	80.23
	SciTec	3623	9.469	1.709	3.526	15.21
	Fixed_assets	3596	15.62	1.148	11.83	18.97

4. Results and Discussion

4.1. Parallel Trend Test and Dynamic Test

Before using the DID method to evaluate the impact of FTZ policy on *GTFP*, we first conducted a parallel trend test based on Equation (4). The changing trend of *GTFP* before and after the implementation of FTZ policy is shown in Figure 3. The figure illustrates that before the construction of pilot FTZs, there was no significant difference between the experimental and control groups. Therefore, the parallel trend hypothesis is met, and it is reasonable to use the DID method to evaluate the impact of FTZ policy on *GTFP*.

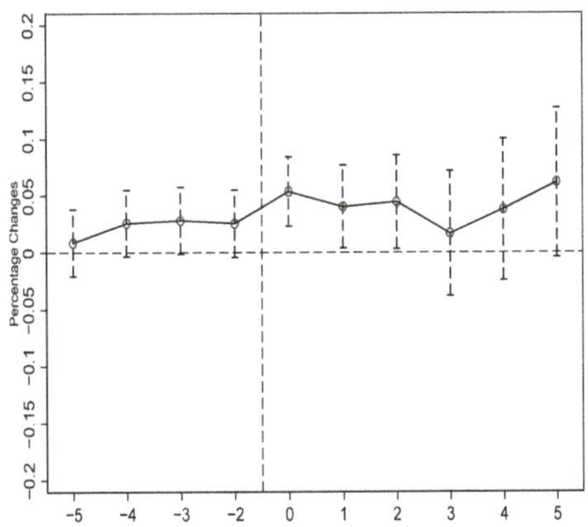

Figure 3. Parallel trend and dynamic effect test of the impact of FTZ policy on *GTFP*.

Figure 3 also allows us to determine the dynamic effect of FTZ policy on *GTFP*. The results illustrate that the driving effect of pilot FTZs on *GTFP* is significant in the first and second years. This indicates that pilot FTZs effectively attracted the agglomeration of environmentally friendly foreign capital in the zones, and supportive policies enabled the development of some high-tech industries and green industries, which, in turn, promoted urban green development. However, we also find that in the third, fourth, and fifth years after the establishment of pilot FTZs, the promotion effect was no longer significant. This may be because imperfect policy guarantee systems, especially the failure to establish an effective intellectual property system, interfered with the positive impact of pilot FTZs on *GTFP* [49]. We can see that the effect of pilot FTZs on *GTFP* shows an upward trend from the third year. Due to the unavailability of data, we are not able to estimate the long-term effect of pilot FTZs on *GTFP*. Since the ideas of green development are continuously applied in the pilot FTZs, we can infer that a long-term positive effect will exist. In the future, the governments should continue to adhere to the ideas of green development in the pilot FTZs so that they can effectively drive urban green development.

4.2. Baseline Regression

Table 4 shows the baseline regression results of the influence of FTZ policy on *GTFP*. In column (1), only the dummy variable (dt) is used as the independent variable for the regression analysis, and the estimated coefficient is positive and significant at the 1% level. There are three possible reasons for this result. First, there is the time trend effect. Second, there is selectivity bias; that is, the cities where pilot FTZs are located have a higher *GTFP*. Third, the FTZ policy significantly improved the *GTFP* of cities. Column (2) adds time dummies to the control variables. The regression coefficient remains significantly positive, and the regression results show that the urban *GTFP* level has a trend of increasing year by year excluding the first reason above. Column (3) further controls for city-specific fixed effects, and the regression coefficient is significantly positive at the 1% level. This result shows that after controlling for the differences between the experimental and control groups, the regression coefficient of *dt* is still significantly positive at the 1% level, which further excludes the second reason and indicates that the pilot FTZ policy has significantly improved *GTFP*. The control variables are added in column (4), and the results do not change substantially.

Table 4. Baseline regression results.

Variables	(1)	(2)	(3)	(4)
	GTFP	*GTFP*	*GTFP*	*GTFP*
dt	0.098 ***	0.053 ***	0.058 ***	0.034 ***
	(0.012)	(0.012)	(0.013)	(0.013)
Informatization				−0.021 ***
				(0.007)
Pdensity				0.319 ***
				(0.071)
Service_sec				0.002 ***
				(0.001)
SciTec				0.016 ***
				(0.005)
Fixed_assets				−0.045 ***
				(0.009)
Year FE	NO	YES	YES	YES
City FE	NO	NO	YES	YES
Constant	0.363 ***	0.390 ***	0.390 ***	0.954 ***
	(0.002)	(0.013)	(0.008)	(0.151)
Observations	3640	3640	3640	3529
R^2	0.0202	0.0568	0.0568	0.0755

***, **, and * indicate statistical significance at the 1%, 5% and 10% levels, respectively. * To save space, this paper does not present the regression results of the year dummy variables in Table 4.

4.3. Regression Analysis Based on PSM-DID

To minimize the systematic differences between the experimental and control groups as much as possible and to reduce the estimation bias of the DID model, referring to Liu and Zhao [82], this paper further uses the PSM-DID approach to test the robustness of the above results. The propensity score is obtained by conducting a logit regression on a series of variables for cities with or without a pilot FTZ. The city with the propensity scores closest to that of the experimental group (the city with a pilot FTZ) is regarded as the control group. After obtaining the matched experimental group and control group cities, it is still necessary to further verify whether the matching results meet the common support assumption. The results after matching are presented in Figure 4 and Table 5, which show the reduced bias in the covariates after matching, and that most samples are successfully matched.

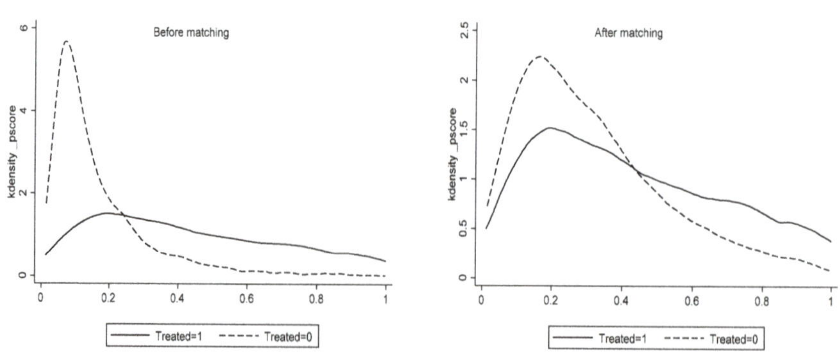

Figure 4. Kernel distribution of the propensity scores before and after matching.

Table 5. Reduced bias in the covariates after matching.

Variables	State	Mean (Treated)	Mean (Control)	% Bias	T	P
Informatization	Unmatched	13.581	12.404	112.3	28.44	0.000
	Matched	13.535	13.527	0.7	0.15	0.880
Pdensity	Unmatched	0.62111	0.37941	75.8	19.75	0.000
	Matched	0.60123	0.67936	−24.5	−3.31	0.001
Service_sec	Unmatched	43.24	35.641	85.0	23.04	0.000
	Matched	42.675	42.239	4.9	0.99	0.320
SciTec	Unmatched	10.711	9.0694	100.9	26.70	0.000
	Matched	10.625	10.56	4.0	0.86	0.389
Fixed_assets	Unmatched	16.565	15.317	125.3	30.94	0.000
	Matched	16.534	16.474	6.0	1.36	0.173

This section describes use of the PSM-DID method as a robustness test to study the effects of the FTZ policy on *GTFP*. The estimated results are presented in Table 6, which illustrates that the impact of the FTZ policy on *GTFP* is still significantly positive after using the PSM-DID method. The differences in the regression coefficients are not substantial, and the significance is almost the same whether using the DID method or using the PSM-DID method, which verifies that the policy is beneficial in improving *GTFP*.

Table 6. PSM-DID estimation results.

Variables	(1)	(2)	(3)	(4)
	GTFP	*GTFP*	*GTFP*	*GTFP*
dt	0.092 ***	0.039 ***	0.045 ***	0.022 *
	(0.012)	(0.013)	(0.013)	(0.013)
Informatization				−0.023 ***
				(0.007)
Pdensity				0.254 ***
				(0.076)
Service_sec				0.002 ***
				(0.001)
SciTec				0.007
				(0.006)
Fixed_assets				−0.048 ***
				(0.011)
Year FE	NO	YES	YES	YES
City FE	NO	NO	YES	YES
Constant	0.355 ***	0.364 ***	0.359 ***	1.088 ***
	(0.002)	(0.014)	(0.009)	(0.177)
Observations	3295	3295	3295	3184
R^2	0.0197	0.0595	0.0595	0.0734

***, **, and * indicate statistical significance at the 1, 5 and 10% levels, respectively.

The present research contributes to the literature on policy zones that are devoted to promoting FDI, international trade, and the environment. Moreover, on the basis of previous research concerning the effect of pilot FTZs on economic growth [31,32] and environmental pollution [36], this paper further shows that the urban economic growth brought by the pilot FTZs is not at the expense of the environment. Using DID and PSM-DID, our findings are consistent with the research conclusion of Jiang et al. [18] based on the case of the Shanghai pilot FTZ. This suggests that the concept of green development applied by the central and local governments in pilot FTZs is effective, which is not just limited to Shanghai, and the FTZs as green zones drive the green development of cities.

4.4. Heterogeneity Analysis

We analyzed the heterogeneity from the aspects of location and city size. There are numerous differences in the level of economic development, marketization, and institutional quality among the various regions in China [83]. As a result, we can expect that pilot FTZ policy may have a different promoting effect on *GTFP* in different regions. Following the research of Gong and Shen [84], we divided the samples into three categories, namely, the eastern, central, and western regions, to explore the heterogeneous effects of the FTZ policy on *GTFP*. The results are shown in Columns 1–3 of Table 7. The construction of pilot FTZs significantly promote the level of *GTFP* in central and western China, but the impact on cities in eastern China is not significant. The levels of trade openness, industrial development, and technological innovation in the eastern region are inherently high; therefore, the marginal effect of the FTZ policy on *GTFP* is not significant. Although the development level is lower in the central region than in the eastern region, the central region has relied on the support of national policies to seek opportunities for development in recent years. The pilot FTZ policy can effectively promote trade facilitation and the entry of high-quality foreign capital in the central region, and thus greatly promote the upgrading of the industrial structure and the green innovation of enterprises. As a region with relatively backward economic development in China, the optimization of trade administration and the facilitation of trade and investment in the pilot FTZs in the western region have released a large institutional dividend, which has a significant marginal effect on *GTFP*.

Table 7. Heterogeneity analysis of the effects of FTZ policy on *GTFP*.

Variables	(1)	(2)	(3)	(4)	(5)
	Location			City Size	
	Eastern	Central	Western	Large and Medium-Sized Cities	Small Cities
dt	0.013	0.036 *	0.085 **	0.032 **	−0.018
	(0.019)	(0.019)	(0.043)	(0.013)	(0.092)
Constant	0.789 ***	0.432 **	1.657 ***	0.993 ***	0.933 ***
	(0.275)	(0.201)	(0.390)	(0.204)	(0.243)
Controls	YES	YES	YES	YES	YES
Year FE	YES	YES	YES	YES	YES
City FE	YES	YES	YES	YES	YES
Observations	1439	1346	744	2415	1114
R^2	0.116	0.069	0.095	0.097	0.071

***, **, and * indicate statistical significance at the 1, 5 and 10% levels, respectively. * The classification of city size comes from the Notice of the State Council on Adjusting the Standards for Categorizing City Sizes, No. 51 [2014], State Council of China.

In general, compared with smaller cities, larger cities tend to have advantages in industrial structure, resource agglomeration, and scientific and technological development [85,86], which may render the policy effect of pilot FTZs on *GTFP* heterogeneous. Therefore, we also carried out a subsample regression according to the different sizes of cities. According to the size of the urban population, we divided the sample into large and medium-sized cities and small cities. If the population of a city is more than 500,000, we defined it as a large and medium-sized city, and if the population of a city is less than 500,000, then we defined it as a small city. The regression results are shown in Columns 4 and 5 of Table 7. In large and medium-sized cities, pilot FTZs have significantly promoted the improvement of *GTFP*, while in small cities, the policy effect has not been significant. This difference may be because large and medium-sized cities have not only good basic conditions for trade and foreign investment but also a high degree of spatial agglomeration of innovation [85]. Therefore, the pilot FTZ policy can significantly promote the development of green technology. However, in small cities, the level of capital stock is weak, the industrial foundation is poor, and the level of scientific and technological development is low. As a result, pilot FTZs fail to have good policy effects in the short term in small cities.

5. Exploring the Mediating Effect of the FTZ Policy on *GTFP*

To explain the potential mechanisms of the green economic growth impacts, we believe that pilot FTZs can enhance *GTFP* by promoting FDI and industrial upgrading. To test this hypothesis, according to Baron and Kenny [87], we constructed a mediating effect model:

$$GTFP_{it} = \beta_0 + \beta_1 dt_{it} + \sum \delta_k year_k + \phi \sum_{N=1}^{N} X_{it} + \mu_{city} + \nu_{it} \quad (5)$$

$$M_{it} = \lambda_0 + \lambda_1 dt_{it} + \sum \delta_k year_k + \theta \sum_{N=1}^{N} X_{it} + \mu_{city} + \xi_{it} \quad (6)$$

$$GTFP_{it} = \gamma_0 + \gamma_1 dt_{it} + \gamma_2 M_{it} + \sum \delta_k year_k + \psi \sum_{N=1}^{N} X_{it} + \mu_{city} + \tau_{it} \quad (7)$$

In Equations (5)–(7), *M* represents the mediating variable, which is defined from the perspective of FDI and industrial upgrading. FDI is measured by the amount of FDI in a city. Referring to Gan et al. [88], industrial structure upgrading (INSU) is measured by the ratio of the output value of the tertiary industry to the output value of the secondary industry.

The steps in testing the mediating effect are as follows. First, urban *GTFP* is considered to be the dependent variable, and the pilot FTZs are taken as the core independent variable for the regression. Second, the mediating variables are considered to be the dependent variables, and the pilot FTZs are taken as the independent variable for the regression. Finally, the pilot FTZs variable and mediating variables are both included in the regression model to observe their impacts on urban *GTFP*. If the coefficients β_1, λ_1, γ_2 are significant and γ_1 decreases or is significantly lower than β_1, then a mediating effect exists.

Column 1 in Table 8 presents the overall effect of the FTZ policy on *GTFP* based on Equation (5), which suggests that pilot FTZs significantly improve *GTFP*. This result might be because the pilot FTZs expand the scale of FDI and promote industrial structure upgrading, thereby enhancing *GTFP*. As shown in Column 2 in Table 8, we find a positive and statistically significant impact of the FTZ policy on FDI. Turning to the results in Column 3, the estimated coefficients of FDI and the pilot FTZs are both statistically significant. Compared with the results in Column 1, the regression coefficient of the pilot FTZs decreases, which implies that this policy has promoted an increase in *GTFP* by expanding the scale of FDI. By the same logic, the regression results in Columns 1, 4 and 5 indicate that pilot FTZs can enhance *GTFP* by promoting industrial structure upgrading.

Table 8. Transmission mechanism of the FTZ policy affecting *GTFP*.

Variables	(1)	(2)	(3)	(4)	(5)
	GTFP	FDI	*GTFP*	INSU	*GTFP*
dt	0.034 ***	0.631 ***	0.021 *	0.049 ***	0.032 **
	(0.013)	(0.072)	(0.013)	(0.009)	(0.013)
FDI			0.018 ***		
			(0.003)		
INSU					0.048 ***
					(0.016)
Constant	0.954 ***	−1.251	0.918 ***	0.813 ***	0.965 ***
	(0.151)	(0.884)	(0.154)	(0.105)	(0.150)
Controls	YES	YES	YES	YES	YES
Year FE	YES	YES	YES	YES	YES
City FE	YES	YES	YES	YES	YES
Observations	3529	3392	3392	3529	3529
R^2	0.075	0.187	0.084	0.788	0.075

***, **, and * indicate statistical significance at the 1, 5 and 10% levels, respectively.

Although several studies, such as Jiang et al. [18], have examined the impact of the Shanghai pilot FTZ on green development, they did not study the underlying mechanism. The present study fills this gap and finds that pilot FTZs promote the green development of cities by promoting FDI and industrial structure upgrading. First, government has implemented a series of institutional innovations that improve investment liberalization and facilitation in the pilot FTZs, which has greatly encouraged the entry of foreign capital. It is worth noting that pilot FTZs have strict environmental requirements for foreign investment; therefore, they mainly attract foreign investment with high-tech, high value-added, and environmentally friendly characteristics, which is conducive to the green development of a city. In addition, the government attaches great importance to the industrial planning and design of pilot FTZs and is committed to prioritizing the development of the high-tech industry, high-end service industry, and financial services industry to promote industrial upgrading and green development.

6. Conclusions

To promote an all-dimensional, multilayered, and wide-ranging opening up to the outside world, China set up pilot FTZs after the establishment of SEZs, EPZs, and BZs. The Chinese pilot FTZs not only facilitate trade and investment liberalization and facilitation through institutional innovation but also take green development as the basic concept in the development of construction plans. For this reason, this research investigates the impact of FTZ policy on the green and healthy development of cities by using the DID and PSM-DID methods. Based on a theoretical analysis, we find that pilot FTZs have strict environmental requirements for foreign investment. In particular, pilot FTZs mainly encourage foreign investment with high-tech, high value-added, and environmentally friendly characteristics, which is beneficial to the green growth of a city. In addition, the industry planning and design sets for pilot FTZs tend to prioritize the development of the high-tech industry, high-end service industry, and financial services industry, which promotes industrial upgrading and further boosts the green development of cities. Consequently, we propose the hypothesis that pilot FTZs promote green development through FDI and industrial upgrading and confirm the mechanism through the mediation model.

The evidence indicates that, first, the pilot FTZs have significantly improved the *GTFP* of cities, and the results are robust to the estimation conclusion of the PSM-DID. Second, pilot FTZs have a positive impact on urban *GTFP* by expanding the scale of FDI and promoting industrial structure upgrading. Third, there are heterogeneous effects according to the region and city size. The impact of FTZ policy on *GTFP* is significant in the central and eastern cities of China but not in the western regions. In addition, pilot FTZs have a positive effect in large- and medium-sized cities, while their effects are not significant in small cities.

The research conclusions of this article suggest that pilot FTZs carry out trade and investment following internationally accepted green trade rules and commercial and ecological environmental management rules. The concept of green development penetrates the entire process of the pilot FTZs construction. In addition, the pilot FTZs vigorously develop the modern green service industry, green manufacturing, and green supply chain, which greatly promotes the green and healthy development of cities. Indeed, the pilot FTZs aim to develop into green areas, which has become a feature that distinguishes them from Chinese policy zones such as SEZs, EPZs, and BZs and the FTZs in other countries [11].

European countries are at the forefront in the fields of green energy, low-carbon technology, and environmental governance technologies [89]. China urgently needs the EU's advanced technical support and experience sharing to takes advantage of the considerable potential in the clean energy market and low manufacturing costs. At present, some pilot FTZs such as the Qingdao pilot FTZ have cooperated with Germany and other countries on sustainable production. In the future, the Chinese pilot FTZs can further relax market access for EU companies in the above fields and attract them to enter China's environmental protection market. More importantly, pilot FTZs should actively use cooperation with European countries in these fields to boost the green development of cities.

Academic research in the future should give attention to how the pilot FTZs can adhere to the concept of green development and continue to transform themselves into green areas in the future. Due to data limitations, our research can only examine the short-term effect of FTZs on urban green development. With more data available, future researchers will have the opportunity to explore the long-term effect of the pilot FTZs on urban green development. Moreover, evaluating the development status of green finance, environmentally conscious manufacturing, and environmental supply chains, etc., in FTZs is also an important research topic in the future.

Author Contributions: Conceptualization, Q.M. and L.H.; methodology, Q.M.; software, Q.M.; validation, Q.M., K.Y. and L.H.; formal analysis, L.H. and Y.Z.; investigation, Y.Z.; resources, L.H.; data curation, Q.M.; writing—original draft preparation, Q.M., K.Y. and L.H.; writing—review and editing, Y.Z. and L.H.; visualization, Y.Z.; supervision, L.H.; project administration, Q.M.; funding acquisition, L.H. All authors have read and agreed to the published version of the manuscript.

Funding: This research was funded by the Ministry of Education of China Youth Program in Humanities and Social Science [grant number: 18YJC790040].

Institutional Review Board Statement: Not applicable.

Informed Consent Statement: Not applicable.

Data Availability Statement: The data presented in this study are available on request from the corresponding author. The data are not publicly available due to privacy.

Conflicts of Interest: The authors declared no potential conflict of interest with respect to the research, authorship, and/or publication of this article.

References

1. Chen, S.; Golley, J. Green productivity growth in China's industrial economy. *Energy Econ.* **2014**, *44*, 89–98. [CrossRef]
2. Maisonet, M.; Correa, A.; Misra, D.; Jaakkola, J.J.K. A review of the literature on the effects of ambient air pollution on fetal growth. *Environ. Res.* **2004**, *95*, 106–115. [CrossRef] [PubMed]
3. Daniels, G.; Friedman, S. Spatial inequality, and the distribution of industrial toxic releases: Evidence from the 1990 TRI. *Soc. Sci. Q.* **1999**, *80*, 244.
4. Yong, Z.; Luo, L.; Gu, Y.; Li, C. Implication of excessive length of stay of asthma patient with heterogenous status attributed to air pollution. *J. Environ. Health Sci. Eng.* **2021**, *19*, 95. [CrossRef] [PubMed]
5. Zhu, G.; Hu, W.; Liu, Y.; Cao, J.; Ma, Z.; Deng, Y.; Sabel, C.E.; Wang, H. Health burdens of ambient PM 2.5 pollution across Chinese cities during 2006–2015. *J. Environ. Manag.* **2019**, *243*, 250–256. [CrossRef] [PubMed]
6. Teifenbrun, S.U.S. Foreign Trade Zones and Chinese Free Trade Zones: A Comparative Analysis. *J. Int. Bus. Law* **2015**, *14*, 1–58.
7. Akbari, M.; Azbari, M.E.; Chaijani, M.H. Performance of the Firms in a Free-Trade Zone: The Role of Institutional Factors and Resources. *Eur. Manag. Rev.* **2019**, *16*, 363–378. [CrossRef]
8. Chauffour, J.P.; Maur, J.C. *Preferential Trade Agreement Policies for Development: A Handbook*; World Bank Publications: Herndon, VA, USA, 2011.
9. Benton, C.N.; Napier, M.; Uelkue, M.A. On Supply Chain Integration to Free Trade Zones: The Case of the United States of America. *Glob. Bus. Rev.* **2016**, *17*, 1–11. [CrossRef]
10. Mohebi, M.; Mirshojaee, F. Microdata analysis of the consequences of free trade port policy: The case of Iran free zones. *Appl. Econ.* **2019**, *52*, 1–11. [CrossRef]
11. An, G.; Zi, W. Research on Green Finance in the Aspect of Promoting the Sustainable Development of the Free Trade Zone. *Public Financ. Res.* **2020**, *5*, 117–129.
12. Hong, C.; Nan, L.; He, Y. Remanufacturing of electronic products in bonded port area across home and foreign markets. *Int. J. Logist. Manag.* **2016**, *27*, 309–334.
13. Yang, J.; Zhou, L.; Zou, H. Evaluation of the Economic Growth Effect of the Establishment of Special Economic Zones in my country—Analysis Based on the Synthetic Control Method. *Econ. Perspect.* **2017**, *1*, 41–51.
14. Zhang, P.; Xu, J.; Liu, H. The Effectiveness of Industrial Policy in Promoting Global Value Chain Upgrading: Based on the Quasi-Experiment of Chinese Export Processing Zones. *J. Financ. Res.* **2019**, *5*, 76–95.
15. Miyagiwa, K.F. A reconsideration of the welfare economics of a free-trade zone. *J. Int. Econ.* **1986**, *21*, 337–350. [CrossRef]
16. Sun, P.; Zhang, Y. Foreign Investment Opening Policy, Export Processing Zone and Export Survival—From the Perspective of Industrial Linkage Effect. *China Econ. Q.* **2019**, *18*, 701–720.

17. Li, S.; Liu, J.; Kong, Y. Pilot Free Trade Zones and Chinese Port-listed companies Performance: An Empirical Research Based on Quasi-Natural Experiment. *Transp. Policy* **2021**, *111*, 125–137. [CrossRef]
18. Jiang, Y.; Wang, H.; Liu, Z. The impact of the free trade zone on green total factor productivity—Evidence from the shanghai pilot free trade zone. *Energy Policy* **2021**, *148*, 112000. [CrossRef]
19. Sheng, B. Tianjin Free Trade Zone: A Comprehensive Experimental Field for Institutional Innovation. *Intertrade* **2015**, *1*, 4–10.
20. Yang, Z.; Xiao, J. Optimized path of regional industrial supply chain development under the background of free trade zone construction. *J. Commer. Econ.* **2021**, *9*, 176–178.
21. Song, M.; Wang, J.; Wang, S.; Zhao, D. Knowledge accumulation, development potential and efficiency evaluation: An example using the Hainan free trade zone. *J. Knowl. Manag.* **2018**, *23*, 1673–1690. [CrossRef]
22. Wu, W.; Hong, C.; Muhammad, A. The Spillover effect of export processing zones. *China Econ. Rev.* **2020**, *63*, 101478. [CrossRef]
23. Ye, X. Bonded Zones, Export Processing Zones and Industrial Structure Upgrading—An Empirical Research Based on DID Method. *Econ. Surv.* **2020**, *37*, 100–107.
24. Zhou, J. The negative impact of China's regional economic differences. *Rev. Econ. Res.* **2017**, *6*, 33.
25. Jones, R.S.; Yoo, B. Korea's green growth strategy: Mitigating climate change and developing new growth engines. *OECD Publ.* **2011**, *798*, 31.
26. Chaisse, J.; Ji, X. The Pervasive Problem of Special Economic Zones for International Economic Law: Tax, Investment, and Trade Issues. *World Trade Rev.* **2020**, *19*, 567–588. [CrossRef]
27. Kouparitsas, M.A. A dynamic macroeconomic analysis of NAFTA. *Econ. Perspect.* **1997**, *21*, 14–35.
28. Feils, D.J.; Rahman, M. Regional economic integration, and foreign direct investment: The case of NAFTA. *Manag. Int. Rev.* **2008**, *48*, 147–163. [CrossRef]
29. Seyoum, B.; Ramirez, J. Foreign trade zones in the United States. *J. Econ. Stud.* **2012**, *39*, 13–30. [CrossRef]
30. Castilho, M.; Menéndez, M.; Sztulman, A. Poverty changes in Manaus: Legacy of a Brazilian FTZ? *Rev. Dev. Econ.* **2018**, *23*, 102–130. [CrossRef]
31. Tan, N.; Zhou, X.; Lin, J. Study on Economic Growth Effect of Shanghai Pilot Free Trade Zone Based on Counterfactual Analysis with Panel Data. *J. Int. Trade* **2015**, *10*, 14–24.
32. Zhang, J.; Yan, D.; Feng, Z.; Li, C. Can free trade zone effectively promote economic growth? a DID model dynamic analysis perspective. *Inq. Econ.* **2018**, *11*, 125–133.
33. Chen, H.; Yuan, B.; Cui, Q. Does the pilot free trade zone policy attract the entering of foreign-invested enterprises? The evidence from China. *Appl. Econ. Lett.* **2021**, *28*, 1–7. [CrossRef]
34. Dong, Z.; Du, Y.; Chen, Y.; Cheng, C. Process and Practical Experience of 40-Year Eco-Environmental Protection in Shenzhen since the Establishment of Shenzhen Special Economic Zone. *Chin. J. Environ. Manag.* **2020**, *12*, 65–72.
35. Hidayat, S.; Negara, S.D. Special Economic Zones, and the Need for Proper Governance: Empirical Evidence from Indonesia. *Contemp. Southeast Asia* **2020**, *42*, 251–275. [CrossRef]
36. Wang, Y. Environmental Protection Review in the Free Trade Zone. *Chin. Econ.* **2017**, *50*, 291–296.
37. Liu, X.; Liu, W. The Foreign Investment Policy and Industry Pollution—Based on Traditional Investment Policy and the Negative List of Free trade zone. *Int. Bus.* **2017**, *2*, 62–71.
38. Cooper, W.; Seiford, L.M.; Tone, K. *Data Envelopment Analysis: A Comprehensive Text with Models, Applications, References and DEA-Solver Software*; Kluwer Academic Publishers: Dordrecht, The Netherlands, 2007.
39. Fare, R.; Grosskopf, S.; Pasurka, C.A. Accounting for Air Pollution Emissions in Measures of State Manufacturing Productivity Growth. *J. Reg. Sci.* **2010**, *41*, 381–409. [CrossRef]
40. Neiman, B.; Gopinath, G. Trade Adjustment and Productivity in Large Crises. *Am. Econ. Rev.* **2011**, *104*, 793–831.
41. Wu, S.; Li, B.; Nie, Q.; Chen, C. Government Expenditure, Corruption and Total Factor Productivity. *J. Clean. Prod.* **2017**, *168*, 279–289. [CrossRef]
42. Mattsson, P. The impact of labour subsidies on total factor productivity and profit per employee. *Econ. Anal. Policy* **2018**, *62*, 325–341. [CrossRef]
43. Jefferson, G.H.; Rawski, T.G.; Zhang, Y. Productivity growth and convergence across China's industrial economy. *J. Chin. Econ. Bus. Stud.* **2008**, *6*, 121–140. [CrossRef]
44. Zhu, X.; Chen, Y.; Feng, C. Green total factor productivity of China's mining and quarrying industry: A global data envelopment analysis. *Resour. Policy* **2018**, *57*, 1–9. [CrossRef]
45. Tian, P.; Lin, B. Promoting green productivity growth for China's industrial exports: Evidence from a hybrid input-output model. *Energy Policy* **2017**, *111*, 394–402. [CrossRef]
46. Liu, Z.; Xin, L. Has China's Belt and Road Initiative promoted its green total factor productivity?—Evidence from primary provinces along the route. *Energy Policy* **2019**, *129*, 360–369. [CrossRef]
47. Neumayer, E. A blueprint for making the prospective Mediterranean free trade zone an environmental role model. *Eur. Environ.* **2001**, *11*, 173–184. [CrossRef]
48. Aloise, P.G.; Macke, J. Eco-innovations in Developing Countries: The case of Manaus Free Trade Zone (Brazil). *J. Clean. Prod.* **2017**, *168*, 30–38. [CrossRef]
49. Zhuo, C.; Mao, Y.; Rong, J. Policy dividend or "policy trap"? Environmental welfare of establishing free trade zone in China. *Sci. Total Environ.* **2021**, *756*, 143856. [CrossRef]

50. Vernay, A.-L.; D'Ippolito, B.; Pinkse, J. Can the government create a vibrant cluster? Understanding the impact of cluster policy on the development of a cluster. *Entrep. Reg. Dev.* **2018**, *30*, 901–919. [CrossRef]
51. Aritenang, A.F.; Chandramidi, A.N. The Impact of Special Economic Zones and Government Intervention on Firm Productivity: The Case of Batam, Indonesia. Bull. Indones. *Econ. Stud.* **2019**, *56*, 1–40. [CrossRef]
52. Sosnovskikh, S.; Cronin, B. The effects of culture, attitudes, and perceptions on industrial cluster policy: The case of Russia. *Compet. Chang.* **2021**, *25*, 350–381. [CrossRef]
53. Zeng, D.Z. How do special economic zones and industrial clusters drive China's rapid development? *Policy Res. Work. Pap.* **2011**, *5*, 1–53.
54. Li, Y. The Green Ecological Environment in Shanghai Free Trade Area. *Nat. Environ. Pollut. Technol.* **2016**, *15*, 755–760.
55. Yao, D.; Whalley, J. The China (Shanghai) Pilot Free Trade Zone: Background, Developments and Preliminary Assessment of Initial Impacts. *World Econ.* **2016**, *39*, 2–15. [CrossRef]
56. Qu, T.; Qu, R.Y. Research on the Induced Effect of Foreign Investment in China's Pilot Free Trade Zone and Its Influence Path. *Int. Econ. Trade Explor.* **2018**, *9*, 17–30.
57. Tan, J.; Yan, L. On Establishment of Free Trade Zone and Corporate Technology Innovation. *J. Zhongnan Univ. Econ. Law* **2020**, *2*, 48–56.
58. Lei, X.; Han, B. Study on Industrial Agglomeration Level of China's Manufacturing Industry Based on EG Index Model. *Sci. Technol. Prog. Policy* **2012**, *29*, 43–46.
59. Kim, H.; Lee, H.; Lee, J. Technology diffusion and host-country productivity in South-South FDI flows. *Jpn. World Econ.* **2015**, *33*, 1–10. [CrossRef]
60. Hamilton, C.; Svensson, L.E.O. On the Welfare Effects of a "Duty-Free" Zone. *J. Int. Econ.* **1982**, *13*, 45–64. [CrossRef]
61. Chen, J.; Zheng, W.; Zhang, F.; Park, N.K.; Zheng, A.; Zhao, J. Evaluation and comparison of the development performances of typical free trade port zones in China. Transp. *Res. Part A Policy Pract.* **2018**, *118*, 506–526.
62. Helpman, E.; Krugman, P.R. *Market Structure and Foreign Trade*; The MIT Press: Cambridge, MA, USA, 1985.
63. Sun, Y.; Yan, K. Inference on Difference-in-Differences average treatment effects: A fixed-b approach. *J. Econom.* **2019**, *211*, 560–588. [CrossRef]
64. Chen, Z.; Zhang, J.; Zhang, W. Import and innovation: Evidence from Chinese firms. *Eur. Econ. Rev.* **2017**, *94*, 205–220. [CrossRef]
65. Melitz, M.J. The Impact of Trade on Intra-Industry Reallocations and Aggregate Industry Productivity. *Econometrica* **2003**, *71*, 1695–1725. [CrossRef]
66. Hu, J.L.; Wang, S.C. Total-factor energy efficiency of regions in China. *Energy Policy* **2006**, *34*, 3206–3217. [CrossRef]
67. Seiford, L.M.; Zhu, J. Modeling undesirable factors in efficiency evaluation. *Eur. J. Oper. Res.* **2002**, *142*, 16–20. [CrossRef]
68. Tone, K. A slacks-based measure of efficiency in data envelopment analysis. *Eur. J. Oper. Res.* **2001**, *130*, 498–509. [CrossRef]
69. Pongpanich, R.; Peng, K.-C.; Maichum, K. The performance measurement of listed companies of the agribusiness sector on the stock exchange of Thailand. *Agric. Econ.* **2017**, *63*, 234–245.
70. Huang, Q.; Hu, J.; Chen, X. Environmental regulation, and green total factor productivity: Dilemma or win-win? *China Popul. Resour. Environ.* **2018**, *28*, 140–149.
71. Zhou, P.; Ang, B.W.; Poh, K.L. Slacks-based efficiency measures for modeling environmental performance. *Ecol. Econ.* **2007**, *60*, 111–118. [CrossRef]
72. Chang, Y.; Zhang, N.; Danao, D.; Zhang, N. Environmental efficiency analysis of transportation system in China: A non-radial DEA approach. *Energy Policy* **2013**, *58*, 277–283. [CrossRef]
73. Malmquist, S. Index numbers and indifference surfaces. *Trab. De Estad.* **1953**, *4*, 209–242. [CrossRef]
74. Fuentes, R.; Lillo-Banuls, A. Smoothed bootstrap Malmquist index based on DEA model to compute productivity of tax offices. *Expert Syst. Appl.* **2015**, *42*, 2442–2450. [CrossRef]
75. Grifell-Tatje, E.; Lovell, C. Deregulation, and productivity decline: The case of Spanish bavings banks. *Eur. Econ. Rev.* **1996**, *40*, 1281–1303. [CrossRef]
76. Chung, Y.; Fare, R. Productivity and Undesirable Outputs: A Directional Distance Function Approach. *Microeconomics* **1997**, *51*, 229–240. [CrossRef]
77. Li, P.; Lu, Y.; Wang, J. Does Flattening Government Improve Economic Performance? *Soc. Sci. Electron. Publ.* **2016**, *123*, 18–37. [CrossRef]
78. Beck, T.; Levine, R.; Levkov, A. Big Bad Banks? The Winners and Losers from Bank Deregulation in the United States. *J. Financ.* **2010**, *65*, 1637–1667. [CrossRef]
79. Shan, H. Reestimating the Capital Stock of China: 1952~2006. *J. Quant. Tech. Econ.* **2018**, *10*, 17–31.
80. Zhou, L.; Zhou, C.; Yang, F.; Wang, B.; Sun, D. Spatio-temporal evolution and the influencing factors of PM2.5 in China between 2000 and 2011. *Acta Geogr. Sin.* **2017**, *72*, 2079–2092.
81. Färe, R.; Grosskopf, S.; Noh, D.-W.; Weber, W. Characteristics of a polluting technology: Theory and practice. *J. Econom.* **2005**, *126*, 469–492. [CrossRef]
82. Liu, R.; Zhao, R. Western Development: Growth Drive or Policy Trap—An Analysis Based on PSM-DID Method. *China Ind. Econ.* **2015**, *6*, 32–43.
83. Wang, Q.; Dong, Y. Research on the Regional Difference and Distributional Dynamic Evolution of Real Economy Development. *J. Quant. Tech. Econ.* **2018**, *35*, 77–94.

84. Gong, J.; Shen, K. Regional Distribution and Environment Pollution of Energy—Intensive Industries in China. *J. Quant. Tech. Econ.* **2011**, *28*, 20–36.
85. Lu, M.; Chen, Z. Urbanization, Urban-Biased Economic Policies and Urban-Rural Inequality. *Econ. Res. J.* **2004**, *39*, 50–58.
86. Pflüger, M.; Tabuchi, T. Comparative Advantage, Agglomeration Economies and Trade Costs. *J. Urban Econ.* **2019**, *109*, 1–13. [CrossRef]
87. Baron, R.M.; Kenny, D.A. The moderator-mediator variable distinction in social psychological research: Conceptual, strategic, and statical consideration. *J. Personal. Soc. Psychol.* **1986**, *51*, 1173–1182. [CrossRef]
88. Gan, C.; Zheng, R.; Yu, D. An Empirical Study on the Effects of Industrial Structure on Economic Growth and Fluctuations in China. *Econ. Res. J.* **2011**, *46*, 4–16.
89. Tutak, M.; Brodny, J.; Bindzár, P. Assessing the Level of Energy and Climate Sustainability in the European Union Countries in the Context of the European Green Deal Strategy and Agenda 2030. *Energies* **2021**, *14*, 1767. [CrossRef]

International Journal of
Environmental Research and Public Health

MDPI

Article

Land Use Evolution and Land Ecological Security Evaluation Based on AHP-FCE Model: Evidence from China

Yong Zhu [1], Shihu Zhong [2,*], Ying Wang [3] and Muhua Liu [1,4,*]

1 School of Business, Hunan University of Science and Technology, Xiangtan 411201, China; 160115030001@mail.hnust.edu.cn
2 Shanghai National Accounting Institute, Shanghai 201799, China
3 School of Computer Science and Engineering, Hunan University of Science and Technology, Xiangtan 411201, China; 1050060@hnust.edu.cn
4 Hunan Engineering Research Center for Intelligent Decision-Making and Big Data on Industrial Development, Hunan University of Science and Technology, Xiangtan 411201, China
* Correspondence: zhongshihu@163.sufe.edu.cn (S.Z.); muhualiu@hnust.edu.cn (M.L.)

Abstract: China experienced rapid urbanization and socioeconomic development at an unusual rate during the past four decades. Against such background, land use evolution and land ecological security have both been affected in a volatile way. Therefore, it is necessary to investigate the land use and the land ecological security in China. However, the traditional assessment approaches have paid more attention to the environmental and economic factors than the sustainable development of ecology, which cannot comprehensively assess the land ecological security. From the perspective of ecological sustainable development, this study identifies 3 main factors and 17 sub-factors. We also construct a model to integrate the FCE approach with the AHP. The results show that from 2004 to 2017, China's land use structure was unbalanced. The construction land, mining land, and cultivated land increased rapidly, leading to the shrinkage of ecological land. Moreover, the weight of the sustainable development of resources and the environment, economic sustainable development, social sustainable development are 0.3341, 0.3780, and 0.2879, respectively, demonstrating that economic sustainable development is the most important factor affecting land ecological security. Finally, although the value of comprehensive land ecological security in China has been on the rise from 2004 to 2017, it remains at an unsecured level. Moreover, the value of the sustainable development of resources and the environment has been declining since 2011 and is lower than the values of economic sustainable development and social sustainable development. This study demonstrates that more attention should be paid to enhancing land ecological security, especially promoting the sustainable development of resources and the environment.

Keywords: land use evolution; land ecological security; AHP-FCE model; evaluation; China

Citation: Zhu, Y.; Zhong, S.; Wang, Y.; Liu, M. Land Use Evolution and Land Ecological Security Evaluation Based on AHP-FCE Model: Evidence from China. *IJERPH* **2021**, *18*, 12076. https://doi.org/10.3390/ijerph182212076

Academic Editor: Xiaowei Chuai

Received: 7 September 2021
Accepted: 15 November 2021
Published: 17 November 2021

1. Introduction

Land is the fundamental resource and physical condition which humanity depends on for survival and development. Whereas land use and land cover change (LUCC) reflect human activities such as socioeconomic development in the most direct way [1], land ecological security plays a key role in sustainable development for the future of humanity. China is a good research object for studying land ecological security. During the past four decades, China has experienced the rapid urbanization and socioeconomic development at an unusual rate. Against such background, the land use structure in China has witnessed drastic change, giving rise to the contradiction between land ecological security and enormous land demand caused by urban expansion [2–4]. Neglectedecological land and its protection, together with the irrational use of land resources, exacerbate ecological imbalance in land. Therefore, as the foundation and key to the sustainable use of land resources [5–7], land ecological security maintains the long-term balance in the compound ecosystem of the nature, economy, and society. Dynamic land use change and regional land ecological security and its structure have become vital topics in regional sustainable development [8].

The existing research has mainly focused on the socioeconomic and environmental impacts of land use. Humanity changes the outlook of the world through such ways as expanding agricultural production, increasing urban area, and reducing ecological land, including forest, grassland, and woodland. Land use in different parts of the world may be varied in specific usages. However, the ultimate outcome is similar: The natural environment and ecological security often pay the cost due to the exploitation of natural resources to meet the urgent and insatiable human demand [9,10]. For example, Foley et al. (2005) and Liu et al. (2019) pointed out that land use alters the surface of the earth and disrupts the natural ecosystem, particularly on the land administration, where humans play the dominant role [11,12]. Salvati et al. (2018) indicated that land use change and urban expansion directly affect urban structure and socioeconomic function [7]. Some studies have further unrvaled the impact of land use on climate change, the global ecosystem, the disturbance on global carbon cycle and water resources, and the degradation of biodiversity [13,14]. Studies have echoed the opinion that land use change damages the integrity of ecosystem, which calls for the protection of land and sustainable administration over land use [14,15].

At present, five categories of methods are often employed to the evaluate regional LUCC and the land ecological security: comparative analysis, Geographic Information Systems tools (GIS), regressions, AHP, and the fuzzy comprehensive evaluation (FCE) approach [16–23]. Martínez-Fernández et al. (2019) and Mezősi et al. (2019) compared the land use data of regions in different times, and analyzed their ecological security evolution and trend. They found that regional land use changed dramatically over time, and there was a significant difference in the land ecological security among regions [16,17]. Using Geographic Information Systems tools such as the Corine Land Cover, Castanho et al. (2019) reviewed the land use evolution and characteristics in Poland; examined its development model, future orientation, and impact on economic development; and found that land use plays an essential role in long-term sustainable development [18]. Similarly, Wen et al. (2021) employed a geographic detector to assess the spatiotemporal patterns of land ecological security at both the administrative district scale and grid scale in Chaohu Lake Basin [19]. Feng et al. (2018) used the GIS and generalized additive model to assess the land ecological security in Ningbo city on the southeast coast of China [20]. In addition, Yang et al. (2019) applied the stepwise regression and geographically weighted regression (GWR) to quantify the effects of land use change and urban expansion intensity on landscape patterns [21]. They found that land uses have different contributions to the changes of landscape patterns in the downtown area, suburban plain area, and mountainous suburban areas. Although comparative analysis, GIS, and regressions have certain advantages in accuracy, the results are uncertain, with low accuracy and reliability, and are difficult to widely use.

Further, Han et al. (2015) employed the FCE method to evaluate the land ecological security in several Chinese cities [22]. The results indicated that the socioeconomic indicator contributes more to the improvement of land ecological security. Similarly, Cheng (2022) used the PSR framework and FCE method to evaluate the ecological security of land resources in China [23]. The FCE method processes fuzzy evaluation objects through precise digital means and can provide a more scientific, reasonable, and realistic quantitative evaluation of the data with the hidden information presenting fuzziness. In addition, AHP is more often used in solving complex multi-decision problems [24,25]. Liao (2018) combined the fuzzy comprehensive evaluation method and the analytic hierarchy process to explore the environmental conflict risk in Xiangtan of China [26]. Zhang et al. (2020) used the improved group AHP and FCE methods to investigate the ecological environment impact in highway construction activities. They pointed out that the AHP-FCE model has good applicability and popularization value in the ecological environment assessment [27]. Therefore, this study integrates fuzzy comprehensive evaluation with the analytic hierarchy process to evaluate the land ecological security in China. Our study aims to offer theoretical reference and science-based evidence for the sustainable use of land resources and improvement of land ecological security.

This study contributes to the existing literature in the following aspects. First, our study employs a model integrating the FCE approach with the AHP to provide the empirical evaluation on the land use and the land ecological security in China, which could highlight the complementary advantages of different evaluation methods. Previous literature regarding the land ecological security of China has generally focused on qualitative research, such as concept introduction and comparative analysis, while less quantitative research has focused on the use of the GIS, regression, AHP, and FCE methods alone. As a multi-index compound model, the AHP-FCE method combines quantitative weighting and qualitative indicators, which can comprehensively assess the land ecological security.

Second, this study constructs a resources and environment-economic-social sustainable development analytical framework on understanding the comprehensive status of land ecological security. The existing studies have mainly selected indicators such as environmental factors and economic factors as the main indicators of land ecological security, and the resources and social factors have not been fully considered. However, land ecological security is a complex system, which includes not only the status of land resource utilization itself and the impact of land resource utilization on the economic environment, but also the impact of social development on land use and changes in land carrying capacity. Compared with a single-dimensional or less-dimensional assessment of land ecological security, using the resources and environment-economic-social sustainable development analytical framework is more objective and convincing.

Third, this study measures the status and evolution of China's ecological security at the national level from a macro perspective. Ecological security assessments related to land often only examine a certain province, city, or river basin in China. Few national-level empirical work has been described in the literature to date. China is a centralized country, and land use in different provinces or cities is strongly related. Therefore, analyzing China's land ecological security issues at the national level will help to internalize the externalities of land use.

2. Methodology

2.1. Establishing Indicators System

Based on the theory of sustainable development [28,29], combined with the characteristics of statistical data, the practical operation principles of land ecological security assessment, and the practice of existing literature [30,31], this paper constructs the index system of land ecological security evaluation.

From the perspective of ecological sustainable development, the sustainable development of society and the economy should be equivalent to the sustainable capacity of the natural ecological environment. To ensure the development of human society, we should be within the range that the land ecological environment can carry, and we cannot seek development at the cost of destroying the environment. Only by taking sustainable development as the core, research on land ecological security can highlight its value. Then, combined with the definition of land ecological security, we point out that: (1) Land ecological security emphasizes the sustainability of land ecosystem itself (i.e., the sustainable development of resources and the environment). (2) Land ecological security emphasizes the sustainability of the land ecosystem, providing economic value for human development (i.e., economic sustainable development). (3) Land ecological security emphasizes that human social development should be within the carrying range of the land ecosystem (i.e., social sustainable development).

Further, this paper constructs the index system of land ecological security evaluation from three aspects: the sustainable development of resources and the environment, economic sustainable development, and social sustainable development. Specifically, the sustainable development of resources and the environment indicators related to land mainly include the area of agricultural land, cultivated land, orchard, forest, pastureland, and land for other agricultural use and other indicators that can reflect the sustainable state of the ecosystem. Economic sustainable development related to land mainly contain the land use intensity of non-agricultural land, environmental pollution issues, and environmental pollution abatement and other indicators that can reflect the quantity of economic growth and the quality of economic development. Social sustainable development mainly include the national territorial land area, socioeconomic status, urban development status, food supply pressure, population growth rate, and other indicators that can reflect the harmonious development of man and nature. So far, we have built a land ecological security assessment index system with clear levels and clear goals. The specific index system structure is shown in Figure 1.

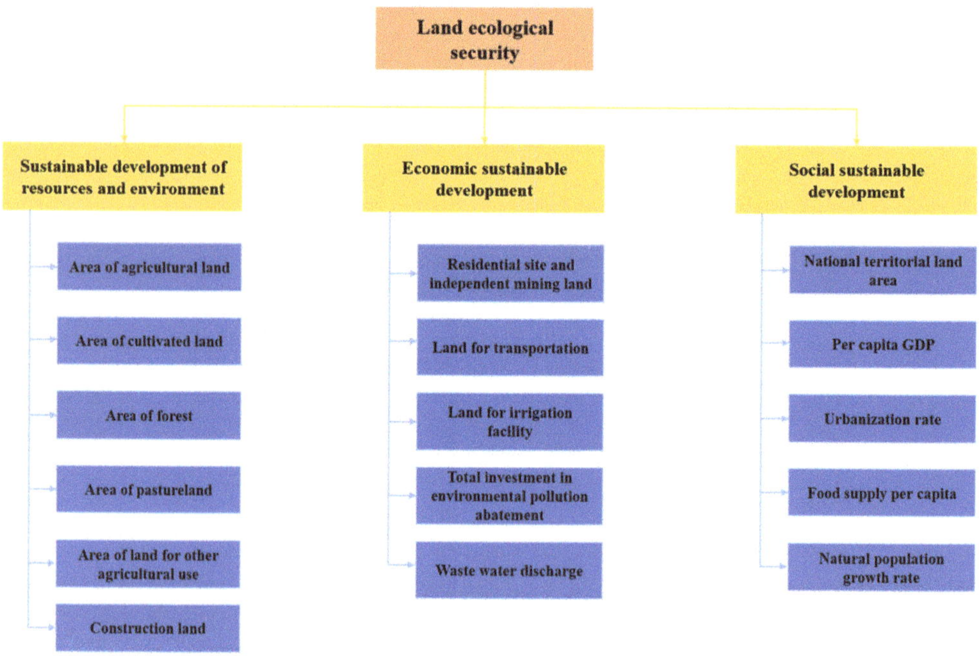

Figure 1. Evaluation framework for land ecological security.

Data for land use indicators were derived from the China Land and Resources Statistical Yearbook from 2004 to 2017. Indicator data for the total investment in environmental pollution abatement, total waste water discharge, per capita GDP, urbanization rate, food supply per capita, and natural population growth rate were derived from China Statistical Yearbook (from 2004 to 2017). The missing data in the statistical yearbook were complemented by relevant statistical reports.

2.2. *Establishing the AHP-FCE Approach*

Appendix A (Figure A1) shows the various steps of the analytic hierarchy process-fuzzy comprehensive evaluation (AHP-FCE) approach used to evaluate the land ecological security in China.

2.2.1. Non-Dimensionalizing Assessment Indicator

The evaluation indicators included in this article differ greatly in units. To eliminate the adverse effects caused by oddity sample data, this study used the linear dimensionless method to normalize the values of the assessment indicators [27]. The evaluation indicators in this article can be divided into two categories: the large-value category and small-value category. The large-value indicators are the maximum values that represents the optimal results, such as the area of orchard (S13), area of forest (S14), area of pastureland (S15), land for transportation (S23), land for irrigation facility (S24), total investment in environmental pollution abatement (S25), national territorial land area (S31), per capita GDP (S32), urbanization rate (S33), and food supply per capita (S34). The small-value indicators are the minimum values that represent the optimal results, such as the area of agricultural land (S11), area of cultivated land (S12), area of land for other agricultural use (S16), construction land (S21), residential site and independent mining land (S22), wastewater discharge (S26), and natural population growth rate (S35). Please refer to Appendix B for the specific calculation equation of the large-value category and small-value category.

2.2.2. Establishing the Analytic Hierarchy Process-Fuzzy Comprehensive Evaluation (AHP-FCE) Approach

The AHP-FCE approach was established based on a five-step process [27,32,33].

Step 1: Establishing the evaluation factors set S.

Each element in the evaluation factors set S represents an index related to land ecological security, as shown in Equations (1)–(4).

$$S = \{S1, S2, S3\} \tag{1}$$

$$S1 = \{S11, S12, S13, S14, S15, S16\} \tag{2}$$

$$S2 = \{S21, S22, S23, S24, S25, S26\} \tag{3}$$

$$S3 = \{S31, S32, S33, S34, S35\} \tag{4}$$

where S1, S2, S3, respectively, represent sustainable development of resources and the environment, economic sustainable development, and social sustainable development. S11, S12, S13, S14, S15, S16, respectively, represent the area of agricultural land, cultivated land, orchard, forest, pastureland, and land for other agricultural use. S21, S22, S23, S24, S25, S26, respectively, represent construction land, residential site and independent mining land, land for transportation, land for irrigation facility, total investment in environmental pollution abatement, and wastewater discharge. S31, S32, S33, S34, S35, respectively, represent the national territorial land area, per capita GDP, urbanization rate, food supply per capita, and natural population growth rate.

Step 2: Establishing the assessment set V.

The assessment set was a collection of various evaluation results. Referring to the practice of Wang et al. (2016) and Wu et al. (2021) [32,34], the assessment set V is described as V = {V1, V2, V3, V4}, in which V1 is safe (S), V2 is relatively safe (RS), V3 is relatively unsafe (RU), and V4 is unsafe (U).

Step 3: Calculating the single factor membership.

The triangular membership function method was used to determine the membership degree of evaluation index to realize the fuzzy mapping from the evaluation factors set S to the assessment set V. The {r1, r2, ⋯, ri} is the set of assessment levels, and the membership function was achieved as Equations (5).

$$f(x) = \begin{cases} 0, \ x \le r_{min} \\ \frac{x - r_{min}}{r_i - r_{min}}, \ r_{min} < x \le r_i \\ \frac{r_{max} - x}{r_{max} - r_i}, \ r_i < x < r_{max} \\ 0, \ x \ge r_{max} \end{cases} \tag{5}$$

Then, according to the calculation of the single factor membership, the single-factor evaluation matrix was achieved as Equation (6).

$$R = \begin{bmatrix} r_{11} & \cdots & r_{1m} \\ \vdots & \ddots & \vdots \\ r_{n1} & \cdots & r_{nm} \end{bmatrix} \quad (6)$$

The value of r_{ij} is judged by expert opinion method (Delphi method). In this study, the assessment set V was divided into four levels. Thus, for $i = 1, 2 \cdots n$, there is:

$$r_{i,j} = \frac{V_{i,j}}{\sum_{j=1}^{4} V_{i,j}} \quad (7)$$

To check the consistency of judgment matrix with different order n, based on the practice of Zhang et al. (2018) [35], this study employed the random consistency index (RI) to judge the matrix consistency. The results are shown in Appendix A (Table A1).

Step 4: Determination of indicator weight.

The AHP approach was employed to measure the relatively importance of each index factor. This method combines the advantages of qualitative analysis and quantitative analysis. This study used the 1 to 9 comparable scale method to compare the impact degree of the index and establish the judgment matrix. The specific meaning of the 1–9 ratio method is attached in Appendix A (Table A2).

Then, after the consistency test, the weight set of index factor W was achieved as Equation (8).

$$W = \{W1, W2, W3, \cdots, W17\} \text{ and } \sum_{i=1}^{17} w_i = 1 \quad (8)$$

where W1, W2, W3, W4, W5, W6, W7, W8, W9, W10, W11, W12, W13, W14, W15, W16, and W17 are the weights for S11, S12, S13, S14, S15, S16, S21, S22, S23, S24, S25, S26, S31, S32, S33, S34, S35, respectively.

Step 5: Multi-level fuzzy comprehensive operation.

According to the principle of fuzzy transform, this study used the weighted average model to synthesize the single-index evaluation matrix (R) and the weight matrix (W) and obtain the multi-index comprehensive evaluation result-matrix (X), as shown in Equation (9).

$$X_i = W_i * R_i \quad (9)$$

3. Results

3.1. Land Use Type Evolution Analysis

As exhibited in Figure 2, in terms of the evolution trend of agricultural land and ecological land, pastureland displayed a large decline, followed by land for other agricultural use. Agricultural land declined slightly. In terms of ecological land, pastureland decreased drastically. Forestry increased, while orchards experienced fluctuation. Cultivated land, forestry, and orchards showed an upward trend. Figure 3 displays the evolution of non-agricultural land. Different kinds of non-agricultural land increased in lockstep. The increase of construction land was the largest, followed by that of residential sites and independent mining land.

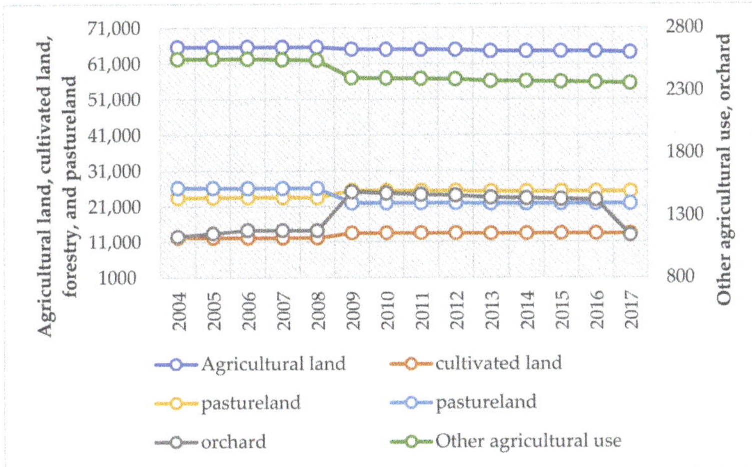

Figure 2. Evolution trend of agricultural and ecological land (2004–2017).

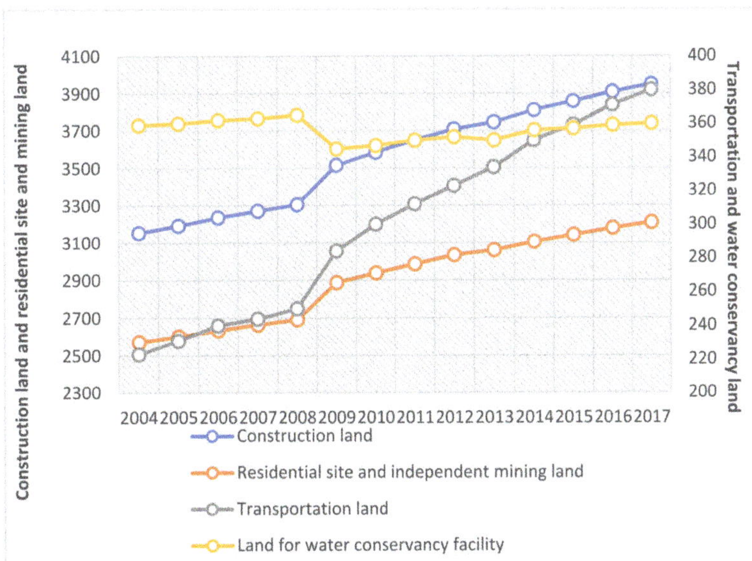

Figure 3. Evolution trend of non-agricultural land (2004–2017).

Overall, since 2007, the proportion of non-agricultural land has continued to increase at an accelerated growth rate while agricultural and ecological land have declined. Construction land, mining land, and cultivated land witnessed the largest increase, with an increase of 25.20%, 24.76%, and 10.18%, respectively. Pastureland and land for other agricultural use experienced a downturn, with a decrease of 16.52% and 7.56%, respectively. The growth rate of non-agricultural land, particularly construction land, far outpaced the decline rate of the proportion of agricultural and ecological land.

3.2. Weight Values of Land Ecological Security Evaluation Indicator

As described in Section 2, this study employed the Analytic Hierarchy Process and Fuzzy Comprehensive Evaluation model (AHP-FCE model) to assess the land ecological security in China. According to the steps of the model, we established the sample set of land ecological security evaluation indicators and normalized the evaluation indicators, as shown in Table 1.

Table 1. Normalized value of the index.

Sub-Factors	S11	S12	S13	S14	S15	S16	S21	S22	S23	S24	S25	S26	S31	S32	S33	S34	S35
2004	0.9997	0.8999	0.7582	0.9210	1.0000	0.9996	0.7987	0.8016	0.5868	0.9836	0.1994	0.6561	1.0000	0.2109	0.7136	0.7992	0.9966
2005	0.9998	0.8973	0.7757	0.9237	0.9978	0.9996	0.8084	0.8106	0.6079	0.9863	0.2494	0.7133	1.0000	0.2427	0.7346	0.8192	1.0000
2006	1.0000	0.8950	0.7938	0.9252	0.9970	1.0000	0.8195	0.8209	0.6316	0.9918	0.2680	0.6997	1.0000	0.2827	0.7577	0.8382	0.8964
2007	0.9997	0.8948	0.7931	0.9252	0.9968	0.9980	0.8284	0.8302	0.6421	0.9945	0.3537	0.7573	1.0000	0.3462	0.7842	0.8398	0.8778
2008	0.9995	0.8946	0.7918	0.9250	0.9967	0.9961	0.8370	0.8386	0.6579	1.0000	0.5156	0.7775	1.0000	0.4071	0.8030	0.8807	0.8625
2009	0.9906	1.0000	1.0000	1.0000	0.8405	0.9409	0.8904	0.8997	0.7474	0.9452	0.5492	0.8011	1.0000	0.4422	0.8260	0.8797	0.8268
2010	0.9899	0.9991	0.9926	0.9993	0.8404	0.9393	0.9078	0.9156	0.7895	0.9507	0.7950	0.8394	1.0000	0.5204	0.8536	0.9017	0.8132
2011	0.9892	0.9989	0.9859	0.9985	0.8401	0.9385	0.9241	0.9305	0.8211	0.9589	0.7429	0.8965	1.0000	0.6132	0.8761	0.9381	0.8132
2012	0.9886	0.9983	0.9812	0.9978	0.8399	0.9370	0.9390	0.9455	0.8500	0.9644	0.8619	0.9312	1.0000	0.6735	0.8983	0.9631	0.8404
2013	0.9832	0.9934	0.9704	0.9923	0.8356	0.9311	0.9484	0.9536	0.8789	0.9589	0.9438	0.9458	1.0000	0.7379	0.9181	0.9785	0.8353
2014	0.9826	0.9927	0.9657	0.9916	0.8354	0.9307	0.9648	0.9676	0.9211	0.9753	1.0000	0.9740	1.0000	0.7940	0.9359	0.9819	0.8846
2015	0.9822	0.9922	0.9617	0.9913	0.8352	0.9287	0.9770	0.9791	0.9447	0.9781	0.9197	1.0000	1.0000	0.8451	0.9586	1.0000	0.8421
2016	0.9816	0.9916	0.9584	0.9909	0.8350	0.9268	0.9899	0.9903	0.9763	0.9836	0.9629	0.9671	1.0000	0.9067	0.9800	0.9863	0.9949
2017	0.9769	0.9915	0.7670	0.9905	0.8348	0.9240	1.0000	1.0000	1.0000	0.9863	0.9962	0.9515	1.0000	1.0000	1.0000	0.9808	0.9032

Then, we established the fuzzy evaluation matrix based on the normalized value of indicators and constructed the judgment matrix. In addition, we checked the consistency of judgment matrix and calculated the weight. The result show that the consistency coefficient was 0. Therefore, the judgment matrix was considered as consistent. The weights of the indicators were calculated by the AHP method. The specific values are shown in Table 2.

Table 2. Weight values of the land ecological security evaluation indicators in China.

Object	Main Factors	Weight	Sub-Factors	Unit	Security Trend	Weight	Weight Rank
Land ecological security evaluation S	Sustainable development of resources and environment S1	0.3341	Area of agricultural land S11	thousand hectares	Negative	0.1176	4
			Area of cultivated land S12	thousand hectares	Negative	0.0994	5
			Area of orchard S13	thousand hectares	Positive	0.0343	9
			Area of forest S14	thousand hectares	Positive	0.0408	8
			Area of pastureland S15	thousand hectares	Positive	0.0205	15
			Area of land for other agricultural use S16	thousand hectares	Negative	0.0207	14
	Economic sustainable development S2	0.3780	Construction land S21	thousand hectares	Negative	0.1185	3
			Residential site and independent mining land S22	thousand hectares	Negative	0.1233	2
			Land for transportation S23	thousand hectares	Positive	0.0304	10
			Land for irrigation facility S24	thousand hectares	Positive	0.041	7
			Total investment in environmental pollution abatement S25	hundred million yuan	Positive	0.0111	16
			Waste water discharge S26	hundred million ton	Negative	0.009	17
	Social sustainable development S3	0.2879	National territorial land area S31	ten thousand hectares	Positive	0.1836	1
			Per capita GDP S32	yuan	Positive	0.0739	6
			Urbanization rate S33	%	Positive	0.0301	11
			Food supply per capita S34	kg/person	Positive	0.023	12
			Natural population growth rate S35	%	Negative	0.0227	13

Table 2 shows the weight values of the land ecological security evaluation indicators of China and their ranks. First, for the main factors, the weight of the sustainable development of resources and the environment, economic sustainable development, and social sustainable development was 0.3341, 0.3780, and 0.2879, respectively, demonstrating that economic sustainable development was the most important factor affecting land ecological security. Second, for the sub-factors, the weight of the national territorial land area, residential site and independent mining land, construction land, agricultural land, cultivated land, per capita GDP, land for irrigation facility, and forest was above 0.04. The eight indicators play a leading role in the land ecological security of China. The weight of the orchard, land for transportation, urbanization rate, food supply per capita, natural population growth rate, land for other agricultural use, and pastureland was above 0.02, showcasing a relatively important on land ecological security. The weight of the total investment in environmental pollution abatement and total wastewater discharge was below 0.02, exhibiting little impacts on the land ecological security. This demonstrates that the investment in environmental pollution abatement and wastewater discharge are less important factors affecting land ecological security.

3.3. The Multi-Index Comprehensive Evaluation on Land Ecological Security

The comprehensive evaluation value of the land ecological security of China was determined by the value of the sustainable development of resources and the environment, economic sustainable development, and social sustainable development. This study employed Equation (9) to calculate the evaluated value of the sustainable development of resources and the environment, economic sustainable development, and social sustainable development. Based on this, we summed the evaluated value of the main factors to obtain the comprehensive evaluation value of land ecological security from 2004 to 2017. The details are shown in Table 3. We found the land ecological security remained at the unsafe level from 2004 to 2017. Limited by resources and the environment and affected by human activity, land ecological security improvement was obstructed. The land ecological system suffered certain degrees of damage. However, the gradual growth of the comprehensive evaluation value of the land ecological security showed signs of the continuous improvement in land resource protection and in the health of the ecosystem.

Table 3. The multi-index comprehensive evaluation results of the land ecological security from 2004 to 2017.

Year	Ecological Security Comprehensive Value	Natural Coordination Value	Economic Sustainability Value	Social Stability Value	Security Level	Security Status
2004	0.2973	0.1038	0.0947	0.0988	U	Unsafe
2005	0.2997	0.1040	0.0958	0.0999	U	Unsafe
2006	0.3024	0.1041	0.0971	0.1012	U	Unsafe
2007	0.3047	0.1041	0.0982	0.1024	U	Unsafe
2008	0.3066	0.1040	0.0992	0.1034	U	Unsafe
2009	0.3255	0.1091	0.1055	0.1109	U	Unsafe
2010	0.3295	0.1090	0.1076	0.1129	U	Unsafe
2011	0.333	0.1088	0.1095	0.1147	U	Unsafe
2012	0.3366	0.1087	0.1113	0.1166	U	Unsafe
2013	0.3381	0.1081	0.1124	0.1176	U	Unsafe
2014	0.3416	0.1080	0.1143	0.1193	U	Unsafe
2015	0.3444	0.1079	0.1158	0.1207	U	Unsafe
2016	0.3472	0.1078	0.1173	0.1221	U	Unsafe
2017	0.3472	0.1054	0.1185	0.1233	U	Unsafe

Note: "U" denotes unsafe.

To intuitively display the evolution of the land ecological security of China, we drew Figure 4. The results show that, from 2004 to 2017, the comprehensive evaluation value of land ecological security in China experienced little fluctuation and grew gradually. The evaluation value of economic sustainable development and social sustainable development increased to some extent and showed a stable upward trend, while the natural coordination value declined. However, the evaluation value of the sustainable development of resources and the environment showed a downward trend from 2004 to 2017. This may have been caused by the unreasonable use of land by human activities.

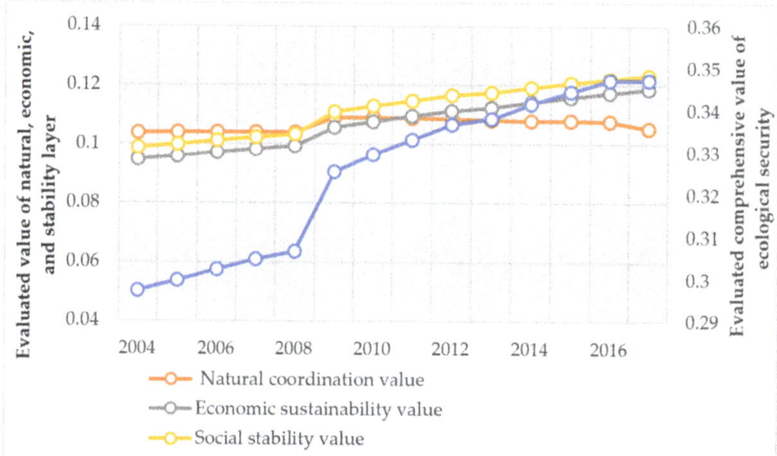

Figure 4. Evolution of land ecological security in China from 2004 to 2017.

In general, the change trend of land ecological security in China is in line with the trend of the sustainable development of resources and the environment, economic sustainable development, and social sustainable development in 2009 and preceding years. However, after 2010, the evaluated value of the sustainable development of resources and the environment began to fall. In addition, its value was continually lower than the value of economic sustainable development and social sustainable development. Affected by this, the rise of the comprehensive evaluation value of land ecological security also slowed. This indicates that sustainable development of resources and environment gradually became the major factor restraining the land ecological security.

4. Conclusions and Discussion

China experienced the rapid urbanization and socioeconomic development at an unusual rate during the past four decades. Against such background, land use structure in China has witnessed drastic change, giving rise to the contradiction between land ecological security and enormous land demand caused by urban expansion. Therefore, it is necessary to investigate the land use and the land ecological security in China. Previous studies have used different methods examine the land use and land ecological security in different regions and time dimensions in China, and the conclusions are also quite different. Moreover, these studies have paid more attention to the environmental and economic factors than the sustainable development of ecology, and lacked a systematic analysis framework and composite evaluation system, which cannot comprehensively assess the land ecological security. By constructing the resources and environment-economic-social sustainable development analytical framework, this study identified 3 main factors and 17 sub-factors. We also constructed a model to integrate the FCE approach with the AHP, making the overall weight ratio distribution more reasonable and objective. This study aimed to explore the land use evolution and evaluate the land ecological security in China from 2004 to 2017.

First, we analyzed the evolution characteristics of land use in China. We found that China's land use structure was unbalanced from 2004 to 2017. The construction land, mining land, and cultivated land increased rapidly, leading to the shrinkage of ecological land. Specifically, construction land, mining land, and cultivated land witnessed the largest increase, with an increase of 25.20%, 24.76%, and 10.18%, respectively. Pastureland and land for other agricultural use experienced a downturn, with a decrease of 16.52% and 7.56%, respectively. The growth rate of non-agricultural land, particularly construction land, far outpaced the decline rate of the proportion of agricultural and ecological land. This may be because, on the one hand, as population continues to grow and urbanization keeps advancing, under limited land resources, construction land and mining land crowd out ecological land. On the other hand, economic development and population growth increase humanity's demand for cultivated land and energy resources. Driven by the expansion of cultivated land and mining land, economic development continues to increase, leading to the shrinkage of ecological land. In addition, the increase in construction land, cultivated land and mining land will, in turn, promote social and economic development and population urbanization. Under the action of this double-helix mutually reinforcing mechanism, cultivated land, mining land, and construction land have increased rapidly, leading to the further shrinkage of ecological land. Overall, land use is closely related to land ecological security. The decrease in agricultural land and the gradual increase in non-agricultural land, especially the increase in construction land, have had a negative impact on China's land ecological security.

Second, we analyzed the influencing factors and weight of land ecological security in China. The results showed that the weight of the sustainable development of resources and the environment, economic sustainable development, and social sustainable development was 0.3341, 0.3780, and 0.2879, respectively, demonstrating that economic sustainable development was the most important factor affecting land ecological security. Moreover, the weight of the national territorial land area, residential site and independent mining land, construction land, agricultural land, cultivated land, per capita GDP, land for irrigation facility, and forest was above 0.04, which plays a leading role in land ecological security of China. The eight indicators play a leading role in the land ecological security of China. The weight of the orchard, land for transportation, urbanization rate, food supply per capita, natural population growth rate, land for other agricultural use, and pastureland was above 0.02, showcasing a relatively important on land ecological security. However, the weight of the total investment in environmental pollution abatement and total wastewater discharge was below 0.02, exhibiting little impacts on land ecological security. This shows that a stable land area is the foundation of national land ecological security. In addition, reasonable planning of residential site and independent mining land, construction land, agricultural land, cultivated land, land for irrigation facility, and forest also plays an important role in improving land ecological security.

Finally, we used the AHP-FCE model to obtain the comprehensive evaluation value of land ecological security from 2004 to 2017. We find that, although the value of comprehensive land ecological security in China has been on the rise from 2004 to 2017, it remains at an insecure level. In addition, the change trend of land ecological security in China was in line with the trend of sustainable development of resources and the environment, economic sustainable development, and social sustainable development in 2009 and preceding years. However, after 2010, the evaluated value of the sustainable development of resources and the environment began to fall. In addition, the value was continuously lower than the values of economic sustainable development and social sustainable development. Affected by this, the rise of the comprehensive evaluation value of land ecological security also slowed. It indicates that the sustainable development of resources and the environment gradually became the major factor restraining the land ecological security. In general, although China's land ecological security has improved, it is still in an unsafe state, especially considering that the level of the sustainable development of resources and the environment has declined rapidly.

The conclusion of this study carries some policy implications. First, efforts should be made to optimize land use structure to reduce the negative impact on land ecological security. It is necessary to increase the area of ecological land and moderately control the construction land, mining land, and cultivated land. Second, we need to continuously improve the level of economic sustainability because it is the most important factor affecting land ecological security. Third, at present, the overall level of land ecological security in China is still low. Therefore, we need to strengthen the protection of land ecological security. More attention should be given to promoting the sustainable development of resources and the environment. However, it is worth noting that, considering the correlation and interdependence between the various subsystems of the land ecological security, improving a single subsystem in the short term may help improve the land ecological security. However, in the long term, this is not sustainable.

There are still several areas for improvement in our study. First, there were limitations in the scope of research. This paper only analyzed the land ecological security of China due to the limitations of data, but it will be very meaningful to extend this research to a wider global scope and conduct comparative analysis. Second, there was insufficiency in measuring the resources and environment-economic-social sustainable development system. We only selected 17 indicators from 3 aspects: the sustainable development of resources and the environment, sustainable development of the economy, and sustainable development of society. It would be of great value to select more corporate- or individual-level indicators from the micro dimensions.

Author Contributions: Conceptualization, Y.Z., S.Z. and M.L.; Methodology, Y.Z., S.Z. and M.L.; Validation, Y.Z., Y.W. and M.L.; Formal Analysis, Y.Z., S.Z. and M.L.; Data Curation, Y.Z., Y.W. and M.L.; Writing—Original Draft Preparation, Y.Z. and M.L.; Writing—Review & Editing, Y.Z. and S.Z.; Visualization, Y.Z. and S.Z.; Supervision, Y.Z. and S.Z.; Funding Acquisition, Y.Z., S.Z. and M.L. All authors have read and agreed to the published version of the manuscript.

Funding: This work was supported by the Social Science Fund of Hunan Province (20YBQ048), the National Statistical Science Research Project of China (2020LY008), the National Social Science Foundation of China (20BGL201), and the National Natural Science Foundation of China (72104109).

Institutional Review Board Statement: Not applicable.

Informed Consent Statement: Not applicable.

Data Availability Statement: Publicly available datasets were analyzed in this study. This data can be found here: https://data.stats.gov.cn.

Conflicts of Interest: The authors declare no conflict of interest.

Appendix A

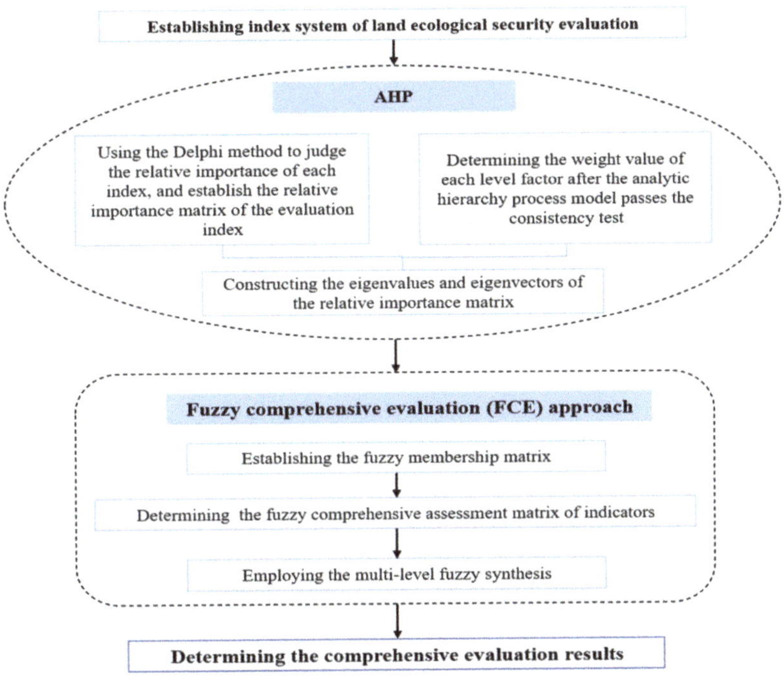

Figure A1. The evaluation process of the AHP-FCE model.

Table A1. Random consistency index (RI) of the judgment matrix.

Matrix Order	1	2	3	4	5	6	7	8	9
RI	0	0	0.52	0.89	1.12	1.26	1.36	1.41	1.46

Table A2. The specific meaning of the 1–9 ratio method.

Score	Connotation
1	The two factors are equally important
3	The factor is slightly more important than the other factor
5	The factor is obviously more important than the other factor
7	The factor is significantly more important than the other factor
9	The factor is extremely more important than the other factor
2,4,6,8	Median values of the above adjacent judgments
Reciprocal	If the importance ratio of factor i to factor j is b_{ij}, the importance of factor j is $1/b_{ij}$ as compared to factor i.

Appendix B

The specific calculation equation of the large-value category and small-value category.

The dimensionless value of assessment indicator is $r_{i,j}$, $r_{i,j} \in [0, 1]$. The assessment index set is set to V, and the assessment indicator is $V_{I,j} \in V$. The indicator attribute value is xi, j. The maximum value of indicator is x_{max}, and the minimum value is x_{min}. The calculations are shown in Equations (A1)–(A3).

$$r_{i,j} = V_{i,j}(x_{i,j}) \quad \text{(A1)}$$

The calculation equation for the judgment where the maximum value represents the optimal result is shown below.

$$r_{i,j} = \frac{x_{i,j}}{x_{max} + x_{min}} \quad \text{(A2)}$$

The calculation equation for the judgment where the minimum value represents the optimal result is shown as follows.

$$r_{i,j} = \frac{x_{max} + x_{min} - x_{i,j}}{x_{max} + x_{min}} \quad \text{(A3)}$$

References

1. Al-Shamiri, A.; Ziadat, F.M. Soil-Landscape Modeling and Land Suitability Evaluation: The Case of Rainwater Harvesting in a Dry Rangeland Environment. *Int. J. Appl. earth Obs. Geoinf.* **2012**, *18*, 157–164. [CrossRef]
2. Liu, S.; Wang, D.; Li, H.; Li, W.; Wang, Q. Ecological Land Fragmentation Evaluation and Dynamic Change of a Typical Black Soil Farming Area in Northeast China. *Sustainability* **2017**, *9*, 300. [CrossRef]
3. Ye, C.; Feng, Y. Ecological Risk Assessment for Pearl River Delta Based on Land Use Change. *Trans. Chin. Soc. Agric. Eng.* **2013**, *29*, 224–232.
4. Li, Y.; Huang, S. Landscape Ecological Risk Responses to Land Use Change in the Luanhe River Basin, China. *Sustainability* **2015**, *7*, 16631–16652. [CrossRef]
5. Watson, S.J.; Luck, G.W.; Spooner, P.G.; Watson, D.M. Land-Use Change: Incorporating the Frequency, Sequence, Time Span, and Magnitude of Changes into Ecological research. *Front. Ecol. Environ.* **2014**, *12*, 241–249. [CrossRef]
6. Recatalá, L.; Ive, J.R.; Baird, I.A.; Hamilton, N.; Sánchez, J. Land-Use Planning in the Valencian Mediterranean Region: Using Lupis to Generate Issue Relevant Plans. *J. Environ. Manag.* **2000**, *59*, 169–184. [CrossRef]
7. Salvati, L.; Zambon, I.; Chelli, F.M.; Serra, P. Do Spatial Patterns of Urbanization and Land Consumption Reflect Different Socioeconomic Contexts in Europe? *Sci. Total Environ.* **2018**, *625*, 722–730. [CrossRef]
8. Jansen, L.J.; Di Gregorio, A. Obtaining Land-Use Information from a Remotely Sensed Land Cover Map: Results from a Case Study in Lebanon. *Int. J. Appl. Earth Obs. Geoinf.* **2004**, *5*, 141–157. [CrossRef]
9. Tao, B.; Yang, Y.; Yang, J.; Smith, R.; Fox, J.; Ruane, A.C.; Liu, J.; Ren, W. Recent Shrinkage and Fragmentation of Bluegrass Landscape in Kentucky. *Remote Sens.* **2020**, *12*, 1815. [CrossRef]
10. Carbutt, C.; Henwood, W.D.; Gilfedder, L.A. Global Plight of Native Temperate Grasslands: Going, Going, Gone? *Biodivers. Conserv.* **2017**, *26*, 2911–2932. [CrossRef]
11. Foley, J.A.; DeFries, R.; Asner, G.P.; Barford, C.; Bonan, G.; Carpenter, S.R.; Chapin, F.S.; Coe, M.T.; Daily, G.C.; Gibbs, H.K. Global Consequences of Land Use. *Science* **2005**, *309*, 570–574. [CrossRef]
12. Liu, J.; Coomes, D.A.; Gibson, L.; Hu, G.; Liu, J.; Luo, Y.; Wu, C.; Yu, M. Forest Fragmentation in China and Its Effect on Biodiversity. *Biol. Rev.* **2019**, *94*, 1636–1657. [CrossRef]
13. Zhao, J.; Tsutsumida, N. Mapping Fragmented Impervious Surface Areas Overlooked by Global Land-Cover Products in the Liping County, Guizhou Province, China. *Remote Sens.* **2020**, *12*, 1527. [CrossRef]
14. Alipbeki, O.; Alipbekova, C.; Sterenharz, A.; Toleubekova, Z.; Makenova, S.; Aliyev, M.; Mineyev, N. Analysis of Land-Use Change in Shortandy District in Terms of Sustainable Development. *Land* **2020**, *9*, 147. [CrossRef]
15. Alipbeki, O.; Alipbekova, C.; Sterenharz, A.; Toleubekova, Z.; Aliyev, M.; Mineyev, N.; Amangaliyev, K. A Spatiotemporal Assessment of Land Use and Land Cover Changes in Peri-Urban Areas: A Case Study of Arshaly District, Kazakhstan. *Sustainability* **2020**, *12*, 1556. [CrossRef]
16. Martínez-Fernández, J.; Ruiz-Benito, P.; Bonet, A.; Gómez, C. Methodological Variations in the Production of CORINE Land Cover and Consequences for Long-Term Land Cover Change Studies. The Case of Spain. *Int. J. Remote Sens.* **2019**, *40*, 8914–8932. [CrossRef]
17. Mezősi, G.; Meyer, B.C.; Bata, T.; Kovács, F.; Czúcz, B.; Ladányi, Z.; Blanka, V. Integrated Approach to Estimate Land Use Intensity for Hungary. *J. Environ. Geogr.* **2019**, *12*, 45–52. [CrossRef]
18. Castanho, R.A.; Naranjo Gómez, J.M.; Kurowska-Pysz, J. Assessing Land Use Changes in Polish Territories: Patterns, Directions and Socioeconomic Impacts on Territorial Management. *Sustainability* **2019**, *11*, 1354. [CrossRef]

19. Wen, M.; Zhang, T.; Li, L.; Chen, L.; Hu, S.; Wang, J.; Zhang, Y.; Yuan, L. Assessment of Land Ecological Security and Analysis of Influencing Factors in Chaohu Lake Basin, China from 1998–2018. *Sustainability* **2021**, *13*, 358. [CrossRef]
20. Feng, Y.; Yang, Q.; Tong, X.; Chen, L. Evaluating Land Ecological Security and Examining Its Relationships with Driving Factors Using GIS and Generalized Additive Model. *Sci. Total Environ.* **2018**, *633*, 1469–1479. [CrossRef]
21. Yang, J.; Li, S.; Lu, H. Quantitative Influence of Land-Use Changes and Urban Expansion Intensity on Landscape Pattern in Qingdao, China: Implications for urban sustainability. *Sustainability* **2019**, *11*, 6174. [CrossRef]
22. Han, B.; Liu, H.; Wang, R. Urban Ecological Security Assessment for Cities in the Beijing-Tianjin-Hebei Metropolitan Region Based on Fuzzy and Entropy Methods. *Ecol. Model.* **2015**, *318*, 217–225. [CrossRef]
23. Cheng, H.; Zhu, L.; Meng, J. Fuzzy evaluation of the ecological security of land resources in mainland China based on the Pressure-State-Response framework. *Sci. Total Environ.* **2022**, *804*, 150053. [CrossRef]
24. Saaty, T.L. A Scaling Method for Priorities in Hierarchical Structures. *J. Math. Psychol.* **1977**, *15*, 234–281. [CrossRef]
25. Saaty, T.L. How to Make a Decision: The Analytic Hierarchy Process. *Eur. J. Oper. Res.* **1990**, *48*, 9–26. [CrossRef]
26. Liao, Y.; Yu, G.; Liao, Y.; Jiang, L.; Liu, X. Environmental Conflict Risk Assessment Based on AHP-FCE: A Case of Jiuhua Waste Incineration Power Plant Project. *Sustainability* **2018**, *10*, 4095. [CrossRef]
27. Zhang, D.; Yang, S.; Wang, Z.; Yang, C.; Chen, Y. Assessment of Ecological Environment Impact in Highway Construction Activities with Improved Group AHP-FCE Approach in China. *Environ. Monit. Assess.* **2020**, *192*, 1–18. [CrossRef] [PubMed]
28. Brundtland, G.H. Our Common Future—Call for Action. *Environ. Conserv.* **1987**, *14*, 291–294. [CrossRef]
29. Meadows, D.H.; Randers, J.; Meadows, D.L. *The Limits to Growth*; Yale University Press: New Haven, CT, USA, 2013.
30. Xu, L.; Yin, H.; Li, Z.; Li, S. Land Ecological Security Evaluation of Guangzhou, China. *Int. J. Environ. Res. Public Health* **2014**, *11*, 10537–10558. [CrossRef]
31. Zhang, D.; Wang, X.; Qu, L.; Li, S.; Lin, Y.; Yao, R.; Zhou, X.; Li, J. Land Use/Cover Predictions Incorporating Ecological Security for the Yangtze River Delta region, China. *Ecol. Indic.* **2020**, *119*, 106841. [CrossRef]
32. Wang, W.; Dong, C.; Dong, W.; Yang, C.; Ju, T.; Huang, L.; Ren, Z. The Design and Implementation of Risk Assessment Model for Hazard Installations Based on AHP–FCE Method: A Case Study of Nansi Lake Basin. *Ecol. Inform.* **2016**, *36*, 162–171. [CrossRef]
33. Xie, Q.; Ni, J.Q.; & Su, Z. Fuzzy Comprehensive Evaluation of Multiple Environmental Factors for Swine Building Assessment and Control. *J. Hazard. Mater.* **2017**, *340*, 463–471. [CrossRef] [PubMed]
34. Wu, J.; Wu, M.; & Zang, C. Assessment of Land Use Change and Land Ecological Security in China's the Northwest Rivers Basin. *Arid. Land Geogr.* **2021**, *10*, 380.
35. Zhang, X.; Yang, J.; Zhao, X. Optimal Study of the Rural House Space Heating Systems Employing the AHP and FCE Methods. *Energy* **2018**, *150*, 631–641. [CrossRef]

International Journal of
Environmental Research and Public Health

MDPI

Article

Direct and Indirect Effects of Business Environment on BRI Countries' Global Value Chain Upgrading

Shengbing He [1], Huilin Yao [1] and Zhou Ji [2,*]

[1] School of Business, Hunan University of Science and Technology, Xiangtan 411201, China; heshengbing@163.com (S.H.); 190115010002@mail.hnust.edu.cn (H.Y.)
[2] Shanghai National Accounting Institute, Shanghai 201702, China
* Correspondence: zhouji@snai.edu

Abstract: This study incorporates business environment, foreign direct investment (FDI), and the global value chain upgrading into a unified analysis framework to unravel the effects of business environment and FDI on the Belt and Road Initiative (BRI) countries' status elevation on the global value chain. The panel data of 112 BRI countries from 2007 to 2017 are employed for empirical tests on the trilateral relationship through the panel data regression model. The results show: (1) business environment improvement and FDI inflow significantly promote BRI countries' status elevation on the global value chain. Business environment not only elevates BRI countries' status on the global value chain directly, but indirectly lifts their status through the intermediate effects of FDI; (2) business environment and FDI significantly promote the status elevation on the global value chain for industries that are intensive on varied factors, especially for labor-intensive industry; (3) the test results of the panel threshold model further verify the positive effect of the business environment and FDI inflows on BRI countries' status elevation on the global value chain.

Keywords: business environment; FDI; BRI countries; status elevation the global value chain

Citation: He, S.; Yao, H.; Ji, Z. Direct and Indirect Effects of Business Environment on BRI Countries' Global Value Chain Upgrading. *IJERPH* **2021**, *18*, 12492. https://doi.org/10.3390/ijerph182312492

Academic Editors: Jie Chen, Qian Zhou and Ting Zhang

Received: 14 October 2021
Accepted: 24 November 2021
Published: 27 November 2021

1. Introduction

In recent years, as trade liberalization deepens and technological innovation progresses, an increasing number of countries participate in the division of labor on the global value chain based on their own economic development, factor variety, and resource endowment. In September 2013, Chinese President Xi Jinping coined the Belt and Road Initiative and incorporated the countries involved in the Belt and Road Initiative (hereinafter referred to as BRI countries) into a regional economic cooperation framework characterized by consultation, contribution, and shared benefits, pushing forward new progress in economic globalization. Due to the difference in product advantages of BRI countries, their status, and roles in the division of labor on the global value chain are also varied. Developed countries dominate the high-end section on the global value chain thanks to their leading technologies and essential roles on key links. However, the majority of BRI countries are developing countries with relatively low level of economic development. The products which they produce or export contain little technology, locking themselves in the low end on the global value chain. Furthermore, Asian countries are losing their advantages in product costs, and developed countries are implementing reindustrialization and reshoring manufacturing strategies. BRI countries are therefore facing the dual challenges of backflow of high-end industries and outflow of low-end industries. It has become a focus of BRI countries to resolve their bottlenecks in manufacturing, to improve their competitiveness in international division of labor, and ultimately to move up to the medium and high range on the global value chain.

As research on the global value chain digs deeper, scholars from China and other countries narrow their interest on the factors affecting division of labor on the global value chain. Specifically, the factors affecting division of labor on the global value chain include environmental regulation [1,2], factor endowment [3,4], human capital [5], R&D intensity [6,7], industrial agglomeration [8], financing restriction [9], and business environment etc. Under current complex and changeable domestic situation, the State Council of China emphasizes that improvement of business environment is more important than preferential policies granted by governments at all levels for the development of manufacturing industry. Business environment refers to the total sum of factors and conditions which affects, to some extent, the behavior of market entities within the region, including factors such as political environment, economic and market environment, legal environment, financing environment, and social service environment. Studies on the role of business environment draw a unanimous conclusion that business environment is the key factor in economic development of countries and exerts significant impacts on sustained growth in economic competitiveness [10]. The reason for the importance of business environment is that favorable business environment effectively lowers transaction costs for companies and helps companies explore the international market [11]. Researchers believe business environment affects the efficiency of contract enforcement by companies in a country, making itself a vital factor impacting the country's integration into the division of labor on the global value chain [12]. System environment is an essential part of business environment. Supportive system environment helps increase the sophistication level of export technologies, contributing to status elevation on the global value chain of the country [13]. Improvement of system significantly elevates the status in the division of labor on the global value chain. Favorable system environment is beneficial to the improvement of technology level and product quality. Unleashing system dividend is a vital strategic choice for China to move up on the global value chain [13]. In particular, the improvement of economic system significantly propels economic growth in BRI countries and affects their participation and status in division of labor on the global value chain [14]. Dai (2020) investigates the relation between business environment and division of labor on the global value chain [15]. He reveals improvement of business environment delivers positive effects on improvement and elevation of status in division of labor on the global value chain. In fact, foreign direct investment also plays a vital role in status elevation on the global value chain [16]. Although significantly promoting high-quality growth of the Chinese economy [17], FDI also affects the status of China's manufacturing industry on the global value chain through technological advancement, import of intermediate goods, and embedment into the global value chain [18,19]. FDI restrains the influence of industrial conglomeration on status elevation for manufacturing industry on the global value chain. Research results indicate the influence of industrial conglomeration on manufacturing status elevation on the global value chain is different due to varied levels of FDI. When FDI is below the threshold value, industrial conglomeration suppresses status elevation of manufacturing industry on the global value chain. However, when FDI surpasses the threshold value, industrial conglomeration significantly elevates manufacturing industry's status on the global value chain. However, business environment, FDI, and global value chain are seldom put into a unified framework for comprehensive consideration. Do business environment and FDI affect BRI countries' status elevation on the global value chain? If yes, what is the mechanism through which business environment and FDI affect BRI countries' status elevation on the global value chain? Is there a heterogeneity in the impacts of business environment and FDI due to different factor intensity among industries?

To unravel the above questions, this study put business environment, FDI, and status elevation on the global value chain under a unified analysis framework. From a theoretical and empirical perspective, this study examines the impact of business environment and FDI on BRI countries' status elevation on the global value chain. Compared with existing research, this study contributes in the following aspects: (1) against the backdrop of the Belt and Road Initiative, this study focuses on business environment to investigate its direct impacts on status elevation on the global value chain, which serves as a supplement to current research; (2) combing FDI's role in status elevation on the global value chain, this study employs intermediate effect model to explore the indirect effect of business environment on status elevation on the global value chain. It is a new way to illustrate the mechanism through which business environment affects countries' status on the global value chain; (3) this study uses threshold effects to determine the tipping point of the impact of business environment improvement and FDI inflow on countries' status elevation on the global value chain. Industry-specific heterogeneity is also investigated in an in-depth manner. Such practice not only enriches the study on factors affecting countries' status on the global value chain but offers policy suggestions on elevating BRI countries' status on the global value chain by improving business environment.

2. Theoretical Analysis and Hypothesis

2.1. Direct Effect of Business Environment on Status Elevation on the Global Value Chain

Business environment is the breeding ground for market economy and is the life-giving oxygen for market entities. Only by further improving business environment can productivity be emancipated, and competitiveness enhanced. Improvement in business environment significantly increases domestic value added in gross exports [20]. Investment facilitation helps improve total factor productivity in BRI countries [21,22]. Enhancing companies' innovation capability is the most important in lifting the status in international division of labor on the global value chain, and improvement of business environment stimulates innovation vitality [23,24]. Innovation activities require motivation and basic system support from desirable innovation environment to lower innovation costs [25]. Desirable business environment decreases, on the one hand, the cost of starting a business, offering convenience and support for market entry or exit by companies. On the other hand, it also lowers the operation costs of companies [26]. The transaction cost and system cost are also eased, leaving companies unshackled for technological innovation. Humphrey (2014) points out technological advancement is the key factor in elevating the status on the global value chain [27]. As companies continue to innovate technologies, improve product quality, and upgrade product function, products gain stronger competitiveness at the market, leading to status elevation on the global value chain. Therefore, this study proposes the following hypothesis:

Hypothesis 1. *Improvement in business environment elevates BRI countries' status on the global value chain.*

2.2. FDI's Impact on the Host Country's Status Elevation on the Global Value Chain

FDI plays a vital role in companies' participation in the global value chain [28] and technological progress [17]. For BRI countries to move up on the global value chain, the most important way lies in promotion of technological progress. FDI helps the host country climb up the global value chain through the following three mechanisms. First, FDI inflow increases the value added of domestically produced products for export. FDI inflow offers capital for production at the host country and promotes expansion of production scale, which attracts more multinationals to provide quality intermediate input products and supporting services, leading to increase of value added of domestically produced products for export. Meanwhile, the intermediate product brought by FDI inflow increases the production supply by local upstream companies, which expands export scale of domestic companies, improves product use efficiency, and makes companies further embedded into the global value chain. FDI increases domestic value added in gross export by attracting inflow of intermediate products and embedment into the global value chain [19]. Second, FDI inflow significantly promotes product quality improvement. FDI inflow generates demonstration effects on companies in the host country and drives local companies to improve and innovate by drawing from production mode and management model of foreign-invested companies based on their own conditions. The productivity efficiency at local companies is therefore improved. The methods and models proven effective for local companies help them move up on the global value chain. Third, FDI inflow effectively facilitates technological innovation. Continuous FDI inflow brings about fierce competition for companies at the host country and urges them to make innovation and breakthrough in key technologies, which becomes the driving forces for technological innovation at local companies. To win the competition with foreign companies, local companies must strengthen technological learning and innovation by increasing R&D input. As a result, technological level of the host country is elevated, and productivity and export product quality are improved, leading to status elevation on the global value chain.

Hypothesis 2. *FDI inflow elevates BRI countries' status on the global value chain.*

2.3. Indirect Effect of Business Environment on BRI Countries' Status Elevation on the Global Value Chain

Creating favorable business environment is one of the vital factors in maintaining fast and sustained economic growth. We believe business environment affects countries' status elevation on the global value chain through FDI by the following two channels. First, a country can effectively lower the entry costs and operation risks for FDI by optimizing market and business environment such as renovating infrastructure, enhancing system transparency and bettering financial service system [21]. In such cases, FDI can be channeled into the host country at a rapid pace and stimulate market competition and innovation. Specifically, improvement in business environment at the host country brings down barriers preventing FDI from entering, which shortens the time needed for FDI to access the market and lowers the entry costs and risks for foreign-invested companies substantially. The spillover of advanced management philosophies and technologies from foreign-invested companies also delivers demonstration effects on the host country. Companies at the host country would imitate and replicate the best practice, leading to productivity improvement at the host country. Second, a country can improve export product quality by optimizing market and business environment to attract more FDI [29,30]. As BRI countries improve their openness and business environment, FDI inflow will continue to grow and promote market competition. Under the huge pressure brought by FDI, domestic companies seek collaboration with well-established domestic counterparts to upgrade technologies and enhance their competitiveness. Market competition and productivity improvement decrease the product price under the same category. Technological progress maintains product quality at a reasonable range, further improving the competitiveness of export intermediate products. Quality improvement of export products represents the core competitiveness for companies to move up on the global value chain, making themselves fully embedded into the global value chain and improving their status. Overall, in terms of the sub-indicators of business environment, deregulation, enhancing intellectual property rights protection, and improving cross-border trade facilitation help attract FDI inflow, optimize industrial mix, and promote high-quality development. Fair and just factor market at the mature market economy environment can attract FDI inflow and relax financing restrains, offering more capitals for companies in R&D [31]. Improving the innovation capability of manufacturing industry can accelerate its upgrading and transformation and contribute to quality development [32], which will ultimately elevate the country's status on the global value chain. This study therefore proposes the third hypothesis.

Hypothesis 3. *Improvement in business environment elevates, by attracting FDI inflow, BRI countries' status on the global value chain.*

3. Data and Statistical Model

We incorporate business environment, FDI, and status elevation on the global value chain into a unified analysis framework to examine the impact of business environment and FDI on status elevation on the global value chain.

3.1. Data

Data employed in this study come from three sources. The first is the business environment data of 190 economies from *Doing Business Project* by the World Bank (Washington,

DC, USA). We sift out 134 countries involved in the Belt and Road Initiative. However, due to availability of data, only 112 BRI countries are selected as the research subject and their characteristic variables are controlled. The second type of data are control variable data from *Worldwide Governance Indicators* and *World Development Indicators* by the World Bank. The third type is trade data from UN Comtrade Database. The five-digit category data of the Standard International Trade Classification Revision 3 (SITC Rev.3) which covers 2780 types of commodities are used for the calculation of export technology sophistication. FDI data are from database of the United Nations Conference on Trade and Development (UNCTAD). This study adopts the panel data of 112 countries from 2007 to 2017 to investigate the impact of FDI and business environment on the status elevation on the global value chain.

3.2. Variables

1. Dependent variable: BRI countries' status on the global value chain (GVCs). Koopman (2012) decomposes the total exports of China and the U.S. to measure the status of manufacturing industries on the global value chain [33]. This study adopts sophistication level of exports, coined by Hausmann et al. (2007) [34], as the substitution indicator for status on the global value chain. However, according to the methods by Schott (2008), export similarity index among two countries can be measured by the following equation [35]:

$$ESI_i = \sum_j Min(S_{j,i}, S_{j,r}) \tag{1}$$

where j represents the export product, r is the reference country and i is the sample country. $S_{j,r}$ is the share of product j in the total export of country r. *Min* refers to the smallest number in an interval. If the export in a sample country showcases a high degree of similarity with a developed country with advanced technologies, it means the sophistication level of export in the sample country is relatively high. In other words, the sample country holds a relatively high status on the global value chain. To minimize the impact of intermediate product import, this study constructs the net export similarity index among two countries as follows.

$$NESI_i \sum_j min\left(\frac{NE_{j,i}}{\sum_j NE_{j,i}}, \frac{NE_{j,r}}{\sum_j NE_{j,r}}\right), \text{ and } NE_{j,i} = \begin{cases} E_{j,i} - M_{j,i}, \ if \ j \in B \\ E_{j,i}, if \ other \end{cases} \tag{2}$$

In Equation (2), $E_{j,i}$ denotes the export value of product j in country i, $M_{j,i}$ is the share of product j import, B represents the set of intermediate products. According to the classification of broad economic categories by the United Nations, trade products are divided into primary products, intermediate products, and final products. Intermediate products include semi-finished products and parts and components. Based on the five-digit product category of the Standard International Trade Classification (SITC Rev.3) and BEC, this study makes the following treatment while calculating *NESI*. If product j is an intermediate product. It will be calculated by its net export value. If its net export value is negative, the observation will be scored as 0, meaning country i is incapable of export this kind of intermediate product; if product j is not an intermediate product, its export value will just be calculated by its total export value. The value of *NESI* falls into the range [0,1]. The bigger the value, the higher the similarity among the two countries in export structure and sophistication level of export, and the higher their status on the global value chain. When two countries export completely different products, the value of *NESI* is 0. On the other way round, its value is 1. For the convenience in comparison, this study adopts the average coefficients of net export similarity between Germany, the U.S., and Japan as the reference value to examine the evolution of and difference in sophistication level of export of BRI countries and to measure their manufacturing industries' status on the global value chain. The calculation results based on the data of 112 BRI economies from 2007 to 2017 demonstrate that *NESI* of developed countries are generally higher than the others. *NESI* of China continues to grow with each passing year.

2. Key independent variables: (1) business environment (dtf). Business environment is an important indication of economic soft power of a country. Premier Li Keqiong once noted that business environment is in itself productivity. Business environment in China has been improving on the whole. According to *Doing Business 2019 Report* by the World Bank, business environment in China was ranked 46, elevated by 32 places compared with 2018. Significant progress has also been made in multiple sub-indicators of business environment. Electricity indicator improved by 84 places, starting businesses indicator grew by 65 places, and protection for minority investors increased by 55 places. Djankovetal (2010) attests that the indicator representing business environment of a country in the ease of doing business index by the World Bank is consistent with theories about FDI [36]. Pinheiro-Alves and Zambujal-Oliveira (2012) demonstrate the efficacy of the ease of doing business index in interpreting business environment through factor analysis and Cronbach's alpha [37]. Referring to Li (2018), this study adopts ease of doing business score to measure the overall business environment of an economy [38]. Five sub-category indicators are used to investigate the specific category of business environment, including facilitation for construction permission (construct), facilitation for paying taxes (tax), facilitation for protection over investors (protect), facilitation for contract enforcement (contract), and facilitation for insolvency. The five sub-indicators accurately reflect the specific changes in business environment at each economy over time. The impact of business environment change on economies can also be detected in an accurate manner. The higher the business environment indicator, the more convenient the conditions for operation activities in the country. (2) foreign direct investment (FDI). In recent years, thanks to continuous efforts in opening-up and consistent improvement in business environment, the use of FDI in China has been kept in a good momentum, forming a stark contrast with the downward trend of FDI globally. China ranked third, behind the U.S. and the U.K., in terms of FDI use in 2016. One year later, China secured the second place in FDI use. According to the statistics of United Nations Conference on Trade and Development (UNCTAD), global FDI experienced a four-year downturn with a decline of 31.5% in 2019 from the 2015 level. In 2019, the total FDI in China, with banks, securities, insurances, and other fields included, reached 141.2 billion USD, increased by 2.1% over the preceding year. China's share of FDI in global FDI grew from 6.7% in 2015 to 10.1% in 2019, up by 3.4 percentage points. Tang and Zhang (2017) reveals FDI inflow boosts inflow of foreign intermediate products and introduction of advanced technologies, which improves quality of export products, increases the domestic value added in gross export, and ultimately elevates the status on the global value chain [19]. However, FDI may also impede the status elevation on the global value chain due to the competition brought by imported intermediate products and lock-in on low end of the value chain. This study adopts FDI stock of countries to measure FDI level at different countries. Data are from the database of UNCTAD.
3. Control variables. In reference to existing research, this study selects the following control variables which relates to BRI countries' status on the global value chain. (1) export scale. This study uses the logarithm of the export value in the database of World Development Indicators by the World Bank; (2) resource endowment. The share of the sum of historical export of ores, metals, and fuels in GDP is adopted as its substitution variable; (3) intellectual property rights protection. It is measured by the intellectual property right payment with relevant data derived from World Development Indicators (WDI) of the World Bank; (4) interest rate. High interest rate affects return on investment and investment cost of multinationals, which is a vital impacting factor for FDI. Data are from WDI; (5) per capita wealth (wealth). It is denoted by the logarithm of per capita GDP, and data come from WDI; (6) domestic average level of production (level). It is denoted by the ratio of value added of industry to sales value of industry. Data are from WDI; (7) industrial openness (open).

It is measured by the ratio of trade volume to sales value of industry with data derived from WDI. The descriptive statistics of key variables are shown in Table 1.

Table 1. Descriptive statistics of variables.

	Variable	Code	Mean	SD	Minimum	Maximum
Dependent variable	Status on global value chain	chain	8.207649	4.898577	0	23.34099
Independent variable	Business environment	dtf	5.893868	0.2909366	4.906891	6.483816
	Foreign direct investment	FDI	4.162892	0.9984578	−5	6.894549
Control variable	Per capita wealth	wealth	17.51375	14.57597	0	70.59955
	Intellectual property rights protection	iprp1	6.463159	3.167798	0	10.72787
	Resource endowment	resource	16.07034	26.81276	0	99.98649
	Industrial openness	open	85.21757	46.78791	0	437.3267
	Export scale	exscade1	9.50821	2.439018	0	12.35098
	Interest rate	rate	5.543384	37.4895	−31.9229	1158.026
	Domestic average level of production	Level	27.7054	12.73778	0	74.8123

3.3. Econometric Model

Based on the above analysis, this study starts by constructing the econometric model on the impact of business environment on BRI countries' status elevation on the global value chain.

$$lnGVCs_{it} = \alpha + \beta lndtf_{it} + \delta X_{it} + \gamma_t + \epsilon_{it} \tag{3}$$

where i refers to the country and t represents the year. Dependent variable $GVCs$ denotes BRI countries' status on the global value chain. Independent variable dtf is business environment, X_{it} is the vector of relevant control variables, γ_t is the year fixed effect. ϵ_{it} is the stochastic disturbance term.

In addition, to identify the impact of FDI on the status on the global value chain, we add FDI variable into Equation (3) and obtain the following equation.

$$lnGVCs_{it} = \alpha + \beta lndtf_{it} + \varphi lnFDI_{it} + \delta X_{it} + \gamma_t + \epsilon_{it} \tag{4}$$

Furthermore, this study adds the interaction between business environment and FDI into Equation (4) to investigate the role of business environment in FDI's impact on the statue on the global value chain. The specific model is shown below.

$$lnGVCs_{it} = \alpha + \beta lndtf_{it} + \varphi lnFDI_{it} + \tau lndtf_{it} * FDI_{it} + \delta X_{it} + \gamma_t + \epsilon_{it} \tag{5}$$

This study also divides industries, based on their production factor, into labor-intensive industry, resource intensive industry, capital intensive industry, and technology intensive industry to explore the heterogeneity of the impact of business environment on the statue on the global value chain due to factor difference among industries. The model is constructed as follows:

$$lnGVCs_{it} = \theta_1 zy_{it} + \theta_2 zb_{it} + \theta_3 ld_{it} + \theta_4 js_{it} \tag{6}$$

where *zy* denotes resource intensive industry. *zb* is resource intensive industry, *ld* represents labor-intensive industry, *js* represents technology intensive industry.

4. Empirical Results

4.1. Benchmark Regression Results

We first conduct Hausman tests to identify model setting. The Hausman test result shows that $p = 0.0000$, so the null hypothesis is rejected, which is indicating the fixed-effects model is preferred. Therefore, unless specifically noted, a fixed-effects model is employed in the following sections. We first analyze the relation between business environment and BRI countries' status on the global value chain. Model (1) is the benchmark model for the impact of business environment on the status on the global value chain. Model (2) is constructed by adding the impact of foreign direct investment (FDI) into model (1). Model (3) is constructed by adding the interaction between business environment (dtf) and foreign direct investment into model (2), which means model (3) considers whether spillover effect of business environment is restrained by FDI. The results are presented in Table 2.

Table 2. Business environment's impact on BRI countries' status elevation on the global value chain.

VARIABLES	(1) GVCs	(2) GVCs	(3) GVCs
dtf	8.2060 ***	6.8436 ***	6.2188 ***
	(16.195)	(13.885)	(13.276)
FDI		1.4064 ***	1.8610 ***
		(10.804)	(14.230)
Dtf * FDI			3.1334 ***
			(9.988)
wealth	0.0436 ***	0.0391 ***	0.0476 ***
	(4.498)	(4.315)	(5.548)
resource	0.0177 ***	0.0196 ***	0.0212 ***
	(3.090)	(3.645)	(4.178)
iprp1	0.4248 ***	0.3026 ***	0.2319 ***
	(8.207)	(6.081)	(4.894)
open	−0.0052 *	−0.0045 *	−0.0063 ***
	(−1.944)	(−1.825)	(−2.665)
exscade1	0.3426 ***	0.2657 ***	0.2133 ***
	(4.565)	(3.805)	(3.233)
rate	−0.0318 *	0.0134	0.0106
	(−1.920)	(0.850)	(0.713)
level	−0.0354 ***	−0.0576 ***	−0.0646 ***
	(−2.805)	(−4.863)	(−5.775)
Constant term	−44.9620 ***	−40.7077 ***	38.5919 ***
	(−16.053)	(−15.455)	(4.639)
Year fixed effect	YES	YES	YES
Observation	805	793	793
R-squared	0.556	0.620	0.663
Number of countries	112	112	112

Note: The t value in the parentheses is calculated using the prefecture-level clustering robust standard error. *YES* means corresponding fixed effect is controlled. ***/* indicates the significance at the 1%/10% levels, respectively.

Empirical results reveal when FDI is not taken into consideration the coefficient of business environment in model (1) is 8.2060, which is significant at the 1% level. Once percentage point increase in business environment elevates the status on the global value chain by 8.2060 on average. This demonstrates business environment delivers positive effects on status elevation on the global value chain. One possible explanation is that favorable business environment lowers, to a large extent, entry costs and operation costs, which reduces investment risks, improves expectation on investment benefits, and is beneficial to independent innovation of companies. Therefore, Hypothesis 1 is proved. The impact of FDI and business environment on status elevation on the global value chain is considered in model (2). The empirical results show the estimate coefficient of FDI, and business environment is positive at the 1% significance level, meaning improvement of business environment and promotion of FDI contribute to elevation on the global value chain. The main reason is that FDI enables technological progress and innovation, improves the quality of export product, and increases the value added of export product, leading to status elevation on the global value chain. Thus, Hypothesis 2 is demonstrated. Results of model (3) show, when the interaction between business environment and FDI is added, the coefficient of business environment, FDI, and the interaction is 6.2188, 1.8610, and 3.1334 respectively, all of which are significant at the 1% level. The results indicate the improvement of the business environment can strengthen the positive effect of FDI inflows on the BRI countries' global value chain upgrading.

To corroborate the above-mentioned mechanisms, this study further performs an intermediate model (Baron and Kenny, 1986) to test how the improvement of business environment attracts FDI to promote BRI countries' global value chain upgrading [39]. We choose foreign direct investment (FDI) as mediators. We follow their method in four steps (Baron and Kenny, 1986). In the first step, we run the regression of business environment on the BRI countries' global value chain upgrading to calculate the total effect. In the second step, we show the correlation between mediators and the business environment by running regression models of mediators on the business environment, individually. In the third step, we include both the business environment and mediators in a regression. By doing the second and third steps, we can successfully separate the direct effect of the business environment on BRI countries' global value chain upgrading from the indirect intermediate effect. If both the business environment and mediator variables in the third step are significant, then the mediator is a partial transmission channel for the impact of the business environment on BRI countries' global value chain upgrading. If only the mediators are significant in the third step, then it is a complete transmission channel. The results are shown in detail in Table 3.

Table 3. Estimate Results of FDI's Intermediate Effect.

Dependent Variables	GVCs	FDI	GVCs
dtf	4.7046 ***	2.7787 ***	4.0875 ***
	(0.3227)	(0.2949)	(0.3273)
FDI			1.0654 ***
			(0.1171)

Note: The t value in the parentheses is calculated using the prefecture-level clustering robust standard error. *** indicates the significance at the 1% levels, respectively.

The Sobel test can be used to judge the significance of the intermediate effects. The p value of Sobel test is close to 0, demonstrating the significance of FDI's intermediate effects. The estimate results of main independent variables show optimizing business environment delivers positive effects on elevation on the global value chain at a significant level. FDI promotes status elevation on the global value chain at the 1% significance level. Such results demonstrate FDI's intermediate effects are significant with the value being 2.9604 (2.7787×1.0654). The estimate results of FDI's intermediate effects reveal FDI inflow promotes, to some extent, status elevation on the global value chain. Improvement of business environment means more favorable operation environment and system for foreign-invested companies, which lowers operation costs and risks. Increasing number of premium foreign companies and technologies is therefore channeled into the domestic market, which improves FDI quality, drives domestic technological innovation, and increases value added of export product. It is through improving FDI quality that progress in business environment promotes status elevation on the global value chain. Thus, Hypothesis 3 is proved. Last, the estimate results of control variables are consistent with those of the benchmark model, which are then not repeated here due to limitation of space.

4.2. Industry Heterogeneity Analysis

As shown in model (6), this study also divides the global value chain of different industries, based on the method of Wang (2017) [40], into labor-intensive industry (*ld*), resource intensive industry (*zy*), capital intensive industry (*zb*), and technology intensive industry (*js*) to explore the heterogeneity of the impact of business environment on the statue on the global value chain due to factor difference among industries. According to the empirical results, the estimate coefficients of business environment (dtf) are positive at the 1% significance level and their value is smaller than the coefficients in the benchmark model. The value change in the estimate coefficients of business environment demonstrate the impact of business environment on status elevation on the global value chain is heterogeneous among varied industries. Business environment significantly promotes status elevation on the global value chain for different industries. However, compared with the coefficient of labor-intensive industry, those of resource intensive industry and technology intensive industry are higher, meaning the effects of resource or technology intensive industry are stronger. Meanwhile, the coefficients of foreign direct investment (FDI) are positive at the 1% significance level for the four types of industries. FDI promotes status elevation on the global value chain for industries with varied factor intensity, and its promotion effects on resource intensive industry are the highest with its coefficient being 0.0416. The reason may be that resource intensive countries need to attract foreign direct investment for advanced and new technologies to promote resource exploitation and improve productivity. Similarly, FDI companies are the ones with advanced technologies and need to lower production costs through cheap labor, which in return increases domestic value added in gross export and elevates the status on the global value chain. Therefore, FDI also promotes status elevation for labor-intensive countries. As for technology intensive countries, FDI may enable integration and innovation of new technologies and therefore help them move up to the medium and high range on the global value chain. The results are shown in detail in Table 4.

Table 4. Heterogeneity analysis.

VARIABLES	(1) *ld*	(2) *zy*	(3) *zb*	(4) *js*
dtf	0.1828 ***	0.2039 ***	0.1132 ***	0.2253 ***
	(12.835)	(13.442)	(8.294)	(12.091)
FDI1	0.0412 ***	0.0416 ***	0.0353 ***	0.0407 ***
	(10.950)	(10.397)	(9.792)	(8.270)
wealth	0.0019 ***	0.0000	0.0000	0.0010 ***
	(7.217)	(0.090)	(0.136)	(3.036)
resource	−0.0000	−0.0006 ***	−0.0003 **	−0.0005 ***
	(−0.098)	(−3.844)	(−2.176)	(−2.660)
iprp1	0.0069 ***	0.0092 ***	0.0051 ***	0.0089 ***
	(4.827)	(6.029)	(3.714)	(4.731)
open	0.0001	0.0001	−0.0003 ***	−0.0001
	(0.887)	(1.304)	(−4.957)	(−1.062)
exscade1	0.0063 ***	0.0066 ***	0.0074 ***	0.0104 ***
	(3.100)	(3.079)	(3.838)	(3.922)
rate	−0.0008 *	−0.0012 **	−0.0003	−0.0006
	(−1.751)	(−2.506)	(−0.680)	(−1.059)
level	−0.0009 ***	−0.0000	−0.0002	−0.0015 ***
	(−2.729)	(−0.059)	(−0.677)	(−3.443)
Constant term	−1.1744 ***	−1.3156 ***	−0.7652 ***	−1.3863 ***
	(−15.430)	(−16.232)	(−10.491)	(−13.922)
Year fixed effect	YES	YES	YES	YES
Observation	793	793	793	793
R-squared	0.632	0.599	0.434	0.548
Number of countries	112	112	112	112

Note: The t value in the parentheses is calculated using the prefecture-level clustering robust standard error. *YES* means corresponding fixed effect is controlled. ***/**/* indicates the significance at the 1%/5%/10% levels, respectively.

4.3. Robustness Checks

Referring to Li (2018) [38], this study adopts the five sub-category indicators of business environment to conduct the robustness checks on the effects of business environment on BRI countries' global value chain upgrading, including facilitation for construction permission (construct), facilitation for paying taxes (tax), facilitation for protection over investors (protect), facilitation for contract enforcement (contract), and facilitation for insolvency (insolvency). The five sub-indicators accurately reflect the specific changes in business environment at each economy over time. The higher the business environment indicator, the more convenient the conditions for operation activities in the country. The estimate results are shown in Table 5, which are basically consistent with the previous results, so Hypotheses 1 and 2 are further demonstrated.

Table 5. Robustness checks.

VARIABLES	(1) GVCs	(2) *ld*	(3) *zy*	(4) *zb*	(5) *js*
FDI1	1.2641 ***	0.0403 ***	0.0421 ***	0.0290 ***	0.0359 ***
	(11.602)	(12.869)	(12.474)	(9.793)	(8.661)
construct	0.0085	0.0007 ***	0.0012 ***	0.0005 ***	0.0007 ***
	(1.550)	(4.393)	(7.066)	(3.211)	(3.188)
protect	0.0145 **	−0.0001	−0.0001	−0.0003 *	0.0005 **
	(2.370)	(−0.403)	(−0.701)	(−1.696)	(2.053)
tax	0.0117 **	0.0003 *	0.0003	0.0000	0.0009 ***
	(2.150)	(1.842)	(1.486)	(0.216)	(4.528)
insolvency	0.0824 ***	0.0026 ***	0.0025 ***	0.0023 ***	0.0029 ***
	(13.656)	(14.990)	(13.504)	(13.795)	(12.693)
contract	0.0564 ***	0.0012 ***	0.0013 ***	0.0012 ***	0.0017 ***
	(7.066)	(5.146)	(5.207)	(5.759)	(5.760)
Constant term	−8.7577 ***	−0.3272 ***	−0.3769 ***	−0.2390 ***	−0.3327 ***
	(−13.274)	(−17.270)	(−18.429)	(−13.330)	(−13.256)
Year fixed effect	YES	YES	YES	YES	YES
Observation	1103	1103	1103	1103	1103
R-squared	0.661	0.675	0.638	0.525	0.591
Number of countries	112	112	112	112	Number of countries

Note: The t value in the parentheses is calculated using the prefecture-level clustering robust standard error. *YES* means corresponding fixed effect is controlled. ***/**/* indicates the significance at the 1%/5%/10% levels, respectively.

5. Further Analysis

According to the above econometric test results, business environment and FDI significantly change the status on the global value chain. However, when the business environment and FDI are at different levels, their role in the promotion of the status of the BRI countries' global value chain upgrading may be different, i.e., the role of the business environment and FDI in the promotion of the BRI countries' global value chain upgrading may have a threshold effect. At this time, the traditional linear model assumes that the influence of the business environment and FDI on the BRI countries' global value chain upgrading is fixed, so we need to re-design a model, when the independent variables are in different ranges, the impact on the dependent variable is different. Therefore, this study adopts business environment and FDI as the threshold variable respectively for threshold tests. The results are shown in Tables 6 and 7.

Table 6. Threshold Test and estimation results.

Threshold Variable	Test	F Value	*p* Value
FDI	Single threshold	6.565 **	0.021
	Double threshold	197.688 ***	0.000
	Triple threshold	−0.921 **	0.020
Business environment	Single threshold	5.997	0.443
	Double threshold	102.379 ***	0.000
	Triple threshold	−48.971	1.000

Note: ***/** indicates the significance at the 1%/5% levels, respectively. *p* value and threshold value are obtained by 1000 times of Bootstrap sampling with replacement.

Table 7. Estimation results of threshold model.

Variable	Business Environment (dtf)	Foreign Direct Investment (FDI)
wealth	0.0149 *	0.0308 ***
	(1.94)	(2.93)
iprp1	0.402 ***	0.194 ***
	(10.92)	(3.52)
resource	0.0269 ***	0.0326 ***
	(6.38)	(5.78)
open	0.00284	−0.00320
	(1.00)	(−1.28)
exscade1	0.331 ***	0.365 ***
	(6.31)	(4.92)
rate	0.00908 **	−0.0148
	(2.27)	(−1.13)
level	−0.0499 ***	−0.0215
	(−5.27)	(−1.61)
Dtf (L ≤ r1)		0.0595 ***
		(3.75)
dtf (r1 < L ≤ r2)		0.125 ***
		(8.87)
Dtf (L > r2)		0.155 ***
		(11.05)
FDI (L ≤ r1)	0.776 ***	
	(6.34)	
FDI (r1 < L ≤ r2)	1.165 ***	
	(9.20)	
FDI (L > r2)	1.338 ***	
	(10.80)	
Threshold	Double threshold	Double threshold
Constant	−1.765 ***	−4.153 ***
	(−3.00)	(−4.58)

Note: The t value in the parentheses is calculated using the prefecture-level clustering robust standard error. ***/**/* indicates the significance at the 1%/5%/10% levels, respectively.

Table 6 shows that the F value of the single threshold, double threshold, and triple threshold of FDI is 6.565, 197.688, and−0.921 respectively. The results of single threshold test and triple threshold test are significant at the 5% level while those of the double threshold test is positive at the 1% significance level. Therefore, these demonstrate business environment delivers significant double threshold effects on the status elevation on the global value chain with the estimate threshold value being 3.305 and 4.903, respectively. According to the empirical results of the panel threshold model, when FDI is lower than 3.305 the spillover effect of business environment is significant, and the elastic coefficient is positive at a statistically significant level. A 1% improvement in business environment leads to status elevation on the global value chain by 0.0595%. This indicates spillover of business environment significantly promotes status elevation on the global value chain.

When FDI is higher than 3.305 and is lower than 4.903, business environment promotes status elevation on the global value chain more significantly. The elastic coefficient is 0.125. It is, therefore, identified that there is significant difference in the impact of business environment on status elevation on the global value chain at varied threshold ranges.

Generally, when FDI continues to increase, the positive impact of business environment on status elevation on the global value chain becomes increasingly significant. The main reason is that improvement in business environment promotes status elevation on the global value chain more significantly along with continuous FDI inflow. On the one hand, improving business environment makes capital registration more convenient and cuts costs and time. Companies can enter the market quickly, take preemptive actions, and seize beneficial export opportunities. On the other hand, improving business environment helps protect the legitimate rights and interests of investors and offers favorable and market-based financing conditions. Investors are therefore motivated, and more social capital can be mobilized, leading to rapid development, improvement of export product quality, technological innovation, and status elevation on the global value chain.

According to Table 6, F value of business environment (dtf) double threshold test is 102.379, respectively. which is significant at the 1% level. However, the single threshold test and triple threshold test is not statistically significant. Therefore, foreign direct investment (FDI) delivers double threshold effects on the status elevation on the global value chain. Its threshold value is 56.100 and 65.600, respectively. Based on the empirical results of the threshold model, when business environment (dtf) is below 41.800 the impact of FDI on the status elevation on the global value chain is not statistically significant with the elastic coefficient being 0.143. In another word, when business environment (dtf) is lower than 56.100, FDI does not promote status elevation on the global value chain. When business environment ranges from 56.100 to 65.600, FDI's spillover effect is still significant at the 1% level. The elastic coefficient is 0.774. When business environment is higher than 65.600, FDI promotes status elevation on the global value chain more significantly. A 1% increase in FDI elevates status on the global value chain by 1.338%. Therefore, FDI delivers varied promotion effects on status elevation on the global value chain in different threshold interval of business environment (dtf). Though FDI's impact remains positive, its impact intensity is different.

The reasons for the above phenomenon are explained as follows. Along with the improvement of business environment, FDI's promotion effect on status elevation on the global value chain becomes increasingly significant. Favorable business environment attracts large number of foreign companies to establish close cooperation ties through FDI. The integration and introduction of technologies improve product quality and productivity, leading to status elevation on the global value chain. When business environment reaches certain level, desirable conditions for business and legal support attract more foreign companies to increase investment. In such cases, FDI's positive role in promoting technological innovation is in full play. While bringing in fierce competition, FDI also enables technological upgrading at local companies, helping companies move from the low end to the medium and high end of the global value chain.

6. Conclusions and Policy Implication

With the gradual expansion of the influence of the Belt and Road Initiative, BRI countries are also facing some new challenges, such as backflow of high-end industries and outflow of low-end industries. Solving the manufacturing bottleneck, enhancing the competitiveness of the international division of labor, and finally moving towards the mid to high end of the global value chain, has become an urgent problem for BRI countries. Therefore, this article attempts to discuss the issue of global value chain upgrading in the BRI countries from the perspective of business environment.

This study incorporates business environment, foreign direct investment (FDI), and the global value chain upgrading into a unified analysis framework to unravel the effects of business environment and FDI on BRI countries' status elevation on the global value chain.

The panel data of 112 BRI countries from 2007 to 2017 are employed for empirical tests on the trilateral relationship through the panel data regression model. The results show: (1) business environment improvement and FDI inflow significantly promote BRI countries' status elevation on the global value chain. Business environment not only elevates BRI countries' status on the global value chain directly but indirectly lifts their status through the intermediate effects of FDI; (2) business environment and FDI significantly promote the status elevation on the global value chain for industries that are intensive on varied factors, especially for labor-intensive industry; (3) the test results of the panel threshold model further verify the positive effect of the business environment and FDI inflows on BRI countries' status elevation on the global value chain.

The conclusion of this study carries rich policy implications. New generation of information technology is fully integrated into manufacturing industry, triggering far-reaching industrial revolution. After the global financial crisis in 2008, there has been a trend of deglobalization at the world economy. Developed countries implemented reindustrialization and reshoring manufacturing strategies, which accelerates the formation of the new global trade and investment pattern. Although it is a good opportunity to move up the global value chain, evolution of the global value chain brings higher requirements for a business environment. BRI countries should focus on the following two aspects to construct the business environment which fits in the new situation of and changes in globalization to attract premium FDI inflow. First, the government of BRI countries should make more efforts in improving business environment to strengthen the supporting role of business environment in elevating the status on the global value chain. Efforts should be made in streamlining administrative approval system, deregulation, delegation of power to governments at lower levels, improvement of operational and post-operation oversight mechanism, improvement of government service efficiency, burden-easing for market entities, and improvement of public services. The government ought to improve business environment by resolving the problems for companies, enforcing favorable policies, and eliminating obstacle restraining companies' development to strengthen their confidence and competitiveness. Second, the government should promote FDI inflow and give full play to the complementary role of business environment and FDI inflow.

Author Contributions: Conceptualization, S.H., H.Y. and Z.J.; Methodology, H.Y. and Z.J.; Data Curation, H.Y.; Writing—Original Draft Preparation, S.H., H.Y. and Z.J.; Writing—Review and editing, H.Y. and Z.J.; Visualization, H.Y. and Z.J.; Supervision, S.H.; Funding Acquisition, S.H. and Z.J. All authors have read and agreed to the published version of the manuscript.

Funding: This work was supported by the National Natural Science Foundation of China (71973041) and the Humanities and Social Sciences Foundation of Ministry of Education of China (19YJA790026).

Institutional Review Board Statement: Not applicable.

Informed Consent Statement: Not applicable.

Data Availability Statement: Publicly available datasets were analyzed in this study. This data can be found here: http://data.worldbank.org.

Conflicts of Interest: The authors declare no conflict of interest.

References

1. Ambec, S.; Coria, J. Prices vs quantities with multiple pollutants. *J. Environ. Econ. Manag.* **2013**, *66*, 123–140. [CrossRef]
2. Hu, D.; Jiao, J.; Tang, Y.; Han, X.; Sun, H. The effect of global value chain position on green technology innovation efficiency: From the perspective of environmental regulation. *Ecol. Indic.* **2021**, *121*, 107195. [CrossRef]
3. Antràs, P. Conceptual aspects of global value chains. *World Bank Econ. Rev.* **2020**, *34*, 551–574. [CrossRef]
4. Dallas, M.P. 'Governed' trade: Global value chains, firms, and the heterogeneity of trade in an era of fragmented pro-duction. *Rev. Int. Political Econ.* **2015**, *22*, 875–909. [CrossRef]
5. Caselli, F.; Coleman, W.J. The world technology frontier. *Am. Econ. Rev.* **2006**, *96*, 499–522. [CrossRef]
6. Pietrobelli, C.; Rabellotti, R. Global value chains meet innovation systems: Are there learning opportunities for developing countries? *World Dev.* **2011**, *39*, 1261–1269. [CrossRef]

7. Ge, J.; Fu, Y.; Xie, R.; Liu, Y.; Mo, W. The effect of GVC embeddedness on productivity improvement: From the per-spective of R&D and government subsidy. *Technol. Forecast. Soc. Chang.* **2018**, *135*, 22–31.
8. Humphrey, J.; Schmitz, H. *Governance and Upgrading: Linking Industrial Cluster and Global Value Chain Research*; Institute of Development Studies: Brighton, UK, 2015; Volume 120.
9. Chen, L.; Luo, S.; Zhao, T. Financial constraints, trade mode transition, and global value chain upgrading of Chinese firms. *Sustainability* **2019**, *11*, 4527. [CrossRef]
10. Witkowska, J. Foreign direct investment in the changing business environment of the European Union's new member states. *Glob. Econ. J.* **2007**, *7*, 4. [CrossRef]
11. Bah, E.-H.; Fang, L. Impact of the business environment on output and productivity in Africa. *J. Dev. Econ.* **2015**, *114*, 159–171. [CrossRef]
12. Acemoglu, D.; Johnson, S.; Robinson, J.A. The colonial origins of comparative development: An empirical investigation. *Am. Econ. Rev.* **2001**, *91*, 1369–1401. [CrossRef]
13. Pipkin, S.; Fuentes, A. Spurred to upgrade: A review of triggers and consequences of industrial upgrading in the global value chain literature. *World Dev.* **2017**, *98*, 536–554. [CrossRef]
14. Wu, Z.; Hou, G.; Xin, B. Has the belt and road initiative brought new opportunities to countries along the routes to participate in global value chains? *SAGE Open* **2020**, *10*, 2158244020902088. [CrossRef]
15. Dai, X. Business Environment and GVC Upgrading. *Econ. Theory Bus. Manag.* **2020**, *39*, 47. (In Chinese)
16. Gereffi, G.; Humphrey, J.; Sturgeon, T. The governance of global value chains. *Rev. Int. Political Econ.* **2005**, *12*, 78–104. [CrossRef]
17. Li, X.; Zhou, W.; Hou, J. Research on the impact of OFDI on the home country's global value chain upgrading. *Int. Rev. Financ. Anal.* **2021**, *77*, 101862. [CrossRef]
18. Kee, H.L.; Tang, H. Domestic value added in exports: Theory and firm evidence from China. *Am. Econ. Rev.* **2016**, *106*, 1402–1436. [CrossRef]
19. Tang, Y.H.; Zhang, P.Y. FDI, Global value chain embeddedness and domestic value added in exports. *Stat. Res.* **2017**, *34*, 36–49. (In Chinese)
20. Dai, X.; Qin, S.J. How does optimization of business environment increase the domestic value-added of enterprise's export. *J. Int. Trade* **2020**, *11*, 15–29. (In Chinese)
21. Chen, J.; Liu, Y.; Liu, W. Investment facilitation and China's outward foreign direct investment along the belt and road. *China Econ. Rev.* **2020**, *61*, 101458. [CrossRef]
22. Wang, J.B. The China–Indochina Peninsula economic corridor. In *Routledge Handbook of the Belt and Road*; Routledge: London, UK, 2019; pp. 213–217, 573.
23. Morrison, A.; Pietrobelli, C.; Rabellotti, R. Global value chains and technological capabilities: A framework to study learning and innovation in developing countries. *Oxf. Dev. Stud.* **2008**, *36*, 39–58. [CrossRef]
24. Bi, K.; Huang, P.; Wang, X. Innovation performance and influencing factors of low-carbon technological innovation under the global value chain: A case of Chinese manufacturing industry. *Technol. Forecast. Soc. Chang.* **2016**, *111*, 275–284. [CrossRef]
25. Van Waarden, F. Institutions and innovation: The legal environment of innovating firms. *Organ. Stud.* **2001**, *22*, 765–795. [CrossRef]
26. Yu, W.; Ramanathan, R. Business environment, employee competencies and operations strategy: Anempirical study of retail firms in China. *IMA J. Manag. Math.* **2013**, *24*, 231–252. [CrossRef]
27. Humphrey, J.; Schmitz, H. Governance in global value chains. *IDS Bull.* **2001**, *32*, 19–29. [CrossRef]
28. Adarov, A.; Stehrer, R. Implications of foreign direct investment, capital formation and its structure for global value chains. *World Econ.* **2019**, *44*, 3246–3299. [CrossRef]
29. Li, R.; Liu, Y.; Bustinza, O.F. FDI, service intensity, and international marketing agility: The case of export quality of Chinese enterprises. *Int. Mark. Rev.* **2019**, *36*, 213–238. [CrossRef]
30. Contractor, F.J.; Dangol, R.; Nuruzzaman, N.; Raghunath, S. How do country regulations and business environment impact foreign direct investment (FDI) inflows? *Int. Bus. Rev.* **2020**, *29*, 101640. [CrossRef]
31. Hall, B.H.; Moncada-Paternò-Castello, P.; Montresor, S.; Vezzani, A. Financing constraints, R&D investments and innovative performances: New empirical evidence at the firm level for Europe. *Econ. Innov. New Technol.* **2016**, *25*, 183–196. [CrossRef]
32. Wu, N.; Liu, Z. Higher education development, technological innovation and industrial structure upgrade. *Technol. Forecast. Soc. Chang.* **2021**, *162*, 120400. [CrossRef]
33. Koopman, R.; Wang, Z.; Wei, S.-J. Estimating domestic content in exports when processing trade is pervasive. *J. Dev. Econ.* **2012**, *99*, 178–189. [CrossRef]
34. Hausmann, R.; Hwang, J.; Rodrik, D. What you export matters. *J. Econ. Growth* **2007**, *12*, 1–25. [CrossRef]
35. Schott, P. The relative dophistication of Chinese exports. *Econ. Policy* **2006**, *23*, 6–49. [CrossRef]
36. Djankov, S.; Ganser, T.; McLiesh, C.; Ramalho, R.; Shleifer, A. The effect of corporate taxes on investment and entrepreneurship. *Am. Econ. J. Macroecon.* **2010**, *2*, 31–64. [CrossRef]
37. Pinheiro-Alves, R.; Zambujal-Oliveira, J. The Ease of Doing Business Index as a tool for investment location decisions. *Econ. Lett.* **2012**, *117*, 66–70. [CrossRef]
38. Li, T.T. *Business Environment of the Host Country and the Location Selection of Outward FDI Enterprises: Evidence from Chinese Micro Data*; Jinan University: Jinan, China, 2018.

39. Baron, R.M.; Kenny, D.A. The moderator–mediator variable distinction in social psychological research: Conceptual, strategic, and statistical considerations. *J. Personal. Soc. Psychol.* **1986**, *51*, 1173. [CrossRef]
40. Wang, J.B. Analysis on trade potentiality of "b&r" economic corridors: Based on trade competitiveness, complementarities and industrial international competitiveness. *Asia-Pac. Econ. Rev.* **2017**, *4*, 93–100. (In Chinese)

International Journal of
Environmental Research and Public Health

MDPI

Article

Green TFP Heterogeneity in the Ports of China's Pilot Free Trade Zone under Environmental Constraints

Zongbiao Hu [1], Feng Lan [1] and Han Xu [2,*]

[1] Department of Economics and Trade, School of Business Administration, Zhongnan University of Economics and Law, 182 Nanhu Avenue, Wuhan 430073, China; zbhu@zuel.edu.cn (Z.H.); lannnnnfeng@foxmail.com (F.L.)
[2] Department of Business Administration, School of Management, Wuhan College, 333 Huangjiahu Avenue, Wuhan 430212, China
* Correspondence: coldxu520@163.com

Abstract: In the context of China's Pilot Free Trade Zone (FTZ), ports have a new opportunity to realize high-quality development. Based on the analysis of the current situation of pollutant emissions from ports in China's Pilot Free Trade Zones (FTZs), this paper introduces environmental factors into the analysis framework of the total factor productivity (TFP) of ports in China's FTZs, and uses the Global Malmquist–Luenberger index method to analyze the evolution trend and heterogeneity of green TFP in 28 ports of China's 19 FTZs from 2011 to 2017. The results show that firstly, the emissions of sulfur dioxide (SO_2), nitrogen oxides (NO_X) and other pollutants in China's FTZs have been decreasing year by year. Secondly, both the green TFP and the traditional TFP of the ports in FTZs are on the rise. The absence of environmental factors leads to the underestimation of the TFP of ports. For the green TFP, the main source of its growth is technological progress. Thirdly, there is obvious port heterogeneity in the green TFP of FTZ ports. Nanjing Port has the highest green TFP growth rate, with an average annual growth rate of 21.95%. Ningbo Port, which ranks 14th, has an average annual growth rate of 5.46%. Fuzhou Port, which is rated last, has negative growth. Fourthly, there is also obvious types and regional heterogeneity in the green TFP of FTZ ports. When categorized by type, the average annual growth rate of green TFP in inland ports is significantly higher than that of coastal ports. When categorized by region, the descending order of the average annual growth rate of green TFP is the western region, the eastern region and the central region. Fifthly, the green TFP differences among the eastern, central, and western regions, as well as between inland ports and coastal ports, are shrinking. Moreover, the green TFP differences within inland ports and coastal ports and within central ports and eastern ports are also shrinking, implying there may be σ convergence. The conclusions of this paper have important implications for the scientific understanding of the heterogeneity of green TFP growth in ports in China's FTZs, and how to promote the green development of ports in China's FTZs under environmental constraints.

Keywords: pilot free trade zone; port; green TFP; environmental constraints; regional heterogeneity

Citation: Hu, Z.; Lan, F.; Xu, H. Green TFP Heterogeneity in the Ports of China's Pilot Free Trade Zone under Environmental Constraints. *IJERPH* **2021**, *18*, 12910. https://doi.org/10.3390/ijerph182412910

Academic Editor: Paul B. Tchounwou

Received: 23 September 2021
Accepted: 3 December 2021
Published: 7 December 2021

1. Introduction

With the continuous strengthening of economic globalization, the impact of the economic crisis is more likely to spread all over the world [1]. Affected by the economic crisis to varying degrees, the economic growth trend of developed countries and emerging economies are gradually divided. To maintain its dominant position in the global economic system, regional free trade agreements such as bilateral investment agreements, Trans-Pacific Partnership Agreements, Transatlantic Trade and Investment Partnership Agreements led by developed countries continue to emerge. Compared with the multilateral trade rule system, the economic conditions and needs of countries in the same region are more similar, and regional free trade agreements dominated by bilateral agreements are easier to achieve. Therefore, more and more countries and regions began to sign regional free trade agreements and establish free trade areas (FTA). Consequently, bilateral and free trade pilot areas expanded rapidly in quantity and depth [2]. In recent years, the decline of China's exports has had an impact on the domestic economy; the growth of domestic demand is slow, the contradiction of overcapacity is prominent, and the structural transformation has a long way to go. China's economy urgently needs a "booster", to improve China's economic recovery and move towards a new stage of a higher-energy level. In this context, in order to meet the urgent needs of economic globalization and regional economic integration, and to achieve the goal of high-quality and sustainable economic growth, China's pilot free trade zone (FTZ) was materialized.

Unlike the international traditional free trade area (FTA), which focuses on multinational participation and in which rules are jointly formulated by many countries, a FTZ is a regional special economic zone, established in its own country (region) according to its own (regional) laws and regulations. FTZ strategy requires institutional innovation as the core, accelerating the construction of an institutional framework in line with the general rules of international investment and trade, and accumulating experience for China to gain more voice in international economic cooperation. It is an important strategy for China to actively integrate into the world economic development trend, improve international competitive strength and actively participate in global governance. With the establishment of FTZ, the port, as one of the cores of FTZ, has developed rapidly. According to the statistics of the National Bureau of Statistics of China, the cargo throughput of coastal ports above the designated size increased from 6.16 billion tons in 2011 to 9.19 billion tons in 2019, and the number of 10,000-ton berths of inland ports above the designated size also increased from 340 in 2011 to 444 in 2019, showing rapid development in terms of volume. However, the increase in port input and output does not equate to the improvement of port efficiency. The low efficiency of ports in FTZs and the lack of market competitiveness may still exist. In the context of China's supply-side structural reform, emphasizing high-quality development, it is contrary to the development concept to promote the port development in FTZs by relying only on the input of production factors. Therefore, incremental reform should be used to promote the stock adjustment, correct the distortion of port factor allocation, and promote development by relying on the improvement of total factor productivity (TFP).

At the same time, China's FTZ ports adhere to the concept of green development in the development process. As one of the five development concepts first proposed at the fifth plenary session of the 18th CPC Central Committee, the green development concept emphasizes taking a green low-carbon cycle as the main principle, and ecological civilization construction as the basic starting point of development. This is undoubtedly significant for the sustainable development and high-quality development of ports in FTZs. In fact, as early as November 2002, the report of the 16th CPC National Congress put forward the specific objectives of ecological construction, which emphasized the protection of the environment and resources as the basic national policy, and began to realize that "good ecology" is one of the symbols of "civilization". The report of the 17th CPC National Congress put forward the scientific concept of "ecological civilization", which outlined that "establishing the concept of green and low-carbon development, focusing on energy conservation and emission reduction, improving the incentive and restraint mechanism, accelerating the construction of resource-saving and environment-friendly production and consumption modes, and enhancing the ability of sustainable development" was taken as the general requirement for the development of the national economy. In the report of the 18th CPC National Congress, China incorporated the construction of ecological civilization into the "five-pronged strategy" (economic, political, cultural, social and ecological progress), established the status of a "long-term plan" for the construction of ecological civilization, and clarified its internal relationship with economic construction, political construction, cultural construction, social construction. On this basis, the construction of ecological civilization was highlighted again in the report of the 19th CPC National Congress, which proposed to "establish and improve the economic system of green and low-carbon circular development, build a market-oriented green technology innovation system, develop green finance, expand energy conservation and environmental protection industry, clean production industry, clean energy industry, and build a clean, low-carbon, safe and efficient energy system". It can be seen that the concept of green development has been consistently emphasized in economic development, including FTZ ports.

However, although China's FTZ ports adhere to the concept of green development and promote sustainable development, the operation of port ships still brings much air pollution. In the era of low-carbon economy and green cycle sustainable development, reducing energy consumption and pollution emissions is the top priority of port construction, and also an important standard to evaluate the efficiency of port operation. Moreover, in the "ecological construction" of the 14th five-year plan, it is also emphasized that both economically developed and underdeveloped regions must take "green development" as the precondition of a series of construction requirements, and follow the road of sustainable development unswervingly. Therefore, in the process of promoting economic development through FTZ port development, the concept of green and sustainable development should also be upheld, to reduce the impact on the environment as much as possible. Achieving the green development of ports in FTZs is a difficult problem for China in developing FTZs, and one of the most effective ways to solve this problem is to improve the green TFP of ports. In this context, the main research question of this paper is of the changing trends and heterogeneity of green TFP of the ports in China's FTZs, from the perspective of environmental constraints. Based on this research question, this paper mainly includes three research purposes: (1) analyze the current situation of the port environment in China's FTZs by using pollution emission data such as SO_2 and NO_X; (2) introduce environmental factors into the measurement framework of the TFP of the ports in FTZs, to measure green TFP and compare it with traditional TFP; (3) empirically analyze the port heterogeneity, type heterogeneity and regional heterogeneity of TFP changes, as well as the evolution trend characteristics of port and regional differences. This study is not only conducive to the assessment of the performance of green growth in the ports of FTZs, but also conducive to the analysis of regional differences and evolution trends of green TFP growth in the ports of FTZs. It is of great practical significance for China to formulate appropriate policies for the development of ports in FTZs, to promote the green and sustainable development of ports in FTZs.

The main conclusions of this paper are as follows: first, pollutants such as SO_2 and NO_X emitted by ports in China's FTZs are decreasing year by year, but there are heterogeneous characteristics in pollutant emissions that change these trends. Second, the green TFP and traditional TFP of ports in FTZs are rising. Introducing environmental factors will have a significant impact on the estimation of the TFP of ports in FTZs; thereby, not introducing environmental factors will lead to the underestimation of TFP on the whole. The main source of traditional TFP growth is technical efficiency, and green TFP is technical progress. Third, there is great port heterogeneity in the growth of green TFP in the ports of FTZs. Nanjing Port has the highest green TFP growth rate, with an average annual growth rate of 21.95%. Ningbo Port which ranks 14th has an average annual growth rate of 5.46%. Fuzhou Port, which is rated at the bottom, has negative growth. After the introduction of environmental factors, the green TFP of most ports (except Fuzhou Port, Harbin Port and Yangpu Port) has increased, compared with the traditional TFP, and the main source of growth has changed from technical efficiency to technical progress. Fourth, the green TFP growth of FTZ ports also has large range of types and regional heterogeneity. Taking the type as the division standard, the average annual growth rate of green TFP for inland ports is significantly higher than for those of coastal ports. Taking the region as the division standard, the average regional annual growth rates of green TFP in descending order are: the western region, the eastern region and the central region. Fifth, the green TFP differences among the eastern, central, and western regions, as well as between inland ports and coastal ports, are shrinking. Moreover, the green TFP differences within inland ports and coastal ports, and within central ports and eastern ports, are also shrinking, implying there may be σ convergence.

2. Literature Review

During the 12th five-year plan period, China proposed the strategic adjustment of economic development, and to pay attention to the deep-seated structural problems of the economy. Therefore, during 2011–2015, China's economic development entered a period of deep adjustment, and the economic growth rate has changed from the previous high-speed growth to medium and low-speed growth. For China, higher requirements were put forward in terms of economic structure transformation and the degree of opening to the outside world [3]. China's new stage of "opening-up" is essentially a transition from the border opening-up, to domestic institutional opening-up. The consequent expansion of this opening-up through service trade promotes domestic institutional reform [4]. Therefore, the implementation of the FTZ strategy is the "second quarter" of China's open economy [5]. The main types of FTZs are entrepot distribution type, trade–industry combination type, export-processing type, and bonded-storage type. Different types of FTZs have played an important role in the process of China's foreign trade liberalization [6]. These different types of FTZs are also the basis for the construction of a new round of FTZs in China [7–9].

Overall, the implementation of the FTZ strategy is conducive to accelerating the pace of China's opening to the outside world, optimizing the foreign trade structure, and strengthening the economic and trade relations with other countries [10–12]. The establishment of FTZ is conducive to reducing regional transaction costs, and legally filtering the political forces of trade protection [13,14]. It also plays an important positive role in promoting the construction of the Belt and Road Initiative [15]. However, without an effective coordination mechanism, this positive role will also be affected [16,17]. Previous studies have shown that FTZs in different regions have different policy effects on promoting economic growth, upgrading industrial structure and capital flow [18–22]. In order to further achieve high-quality economic development through the construction of FTZs, we must make full use of the relationship between FTZs and various industries, policies and related infrastructure. Vigorously exploring FTZs is conducive to strengthening the role of FTZs in serving national strategies [23–25].

Scholars have also carried out multi-dimensional research on ports, mainly including the following aspects: first, the research on port cities, such as the port city evolution model [26,27], port city interactive development [28,29], port city interface and spatial planning [30]; second, the research on port logistics, such as the relationship between port logistics and regional economy [31], and port logistics efficiency evaluation [32,33]; third, the research on the port system, such as the evolution model of the port system [34,35] and the impact of new technologies on the port system [36]; fourth, the research on port hinterland, such as the division of port hinterland, and the port hinterland relationship with evolution law [37]; fifth, the research on port transportation, such as the complexity of the shipping network [38,39], and spatial connections and regional differences of the shipping network [40,41]. Among them, the research on port logistics efficiency evaluation is most relevant to this paper.

At present, there are many evaluation methods for port efficiency, which are mainly divided into nonparametric and parametric methods. Data Envelopment Analysis (DEA) is one of the most widely used nonparametric methods. Seth and Feng [42] used the DEA method to evaluate the efficiency changes of 15 container ports in the United States. Barros [43] introduced the Malmquist index on the basis of the DEA to analyze the technical efficiency of five Portuguese seaports in 1999–2000. González et al. [32] used the DEA–Malmquist index to calculate the changes to port efficiency in Spain from 2011 to 2018. Wu and Liang [44] and Li et al. [45] also used the same method to calculate the port efficiency in different regions. Wang and Meng [46] compared the efficiency of China's inland and coastal ports based on the meta-frontier and the sequential SBM-DEA method, and concluded that the overall efficiency of China's ports was low. Some scholars also calculate the port efficiency from the perspective of port managers (port-listed companies) [47].

In recent years, more and more scholars have begun to pay attention to the environmental problems caused by port development. When examining port development, environmental factors are often introduced to measure whether green and sustainable development has been achieved. Teixeira et al. [48] carried out a bibliometric and a structured analysis of the literature focusing on the connection between lean, green, and sustainability concepts. Ikram et al. [49] constructed a corresponding green assessment framework for the goal of sustainable development. Lin et al. [50] used the MDAM model to evaluate the improvement strategy of green infrastructure to support urban sustainable environmental construction. Parida [51] and Ranjbar et al. [52] discussed the interactive relationship between green building and the sustainable development of the environment. Xie and Zhu [53] studied how manufacturing enterprises broke through the dilemma of system and efficiency with the help of green innovation to achieve the sustainable development of enterprises. Scholars have carried out in-depth research on how to incorporate environmental factors into port efficiency measurements in different countries and regions, such as the research on China's ports by Luo et al. [54], Qi et al. [55], and Liu et al. [56], and the research on European and Spanish ports by Quintano et al. [57] and Tovar and Wall [58]. In the study of China's ports, Luo et al. [54] used the SBM-DEA model to set the annual CO_2 emissions of China's eight major container ports as undesirable output to evaluate their environmental efficiency. Qi et al. [55] used the RAM-DEA model to empirically test the statistical data of 10 coastal ports in Jiangsu Province and evaluated the port efficiency from two aspects of port operation performance and environment. Liu et al. [56] refined the research perspective to the ports of FTZs, took the air pollution emitted by ship operation as the undesirable output of the ports and combined this with the expected output to measure the port efficiency. However, they only considered the coastal ports of FTZs, and did not do in-depth research on the changing trends and convergence degrees of green TFP. In the research on ports in other countries and regions around the world, Quintano et al. [57] used the SBM model and REBUS-PLS unit segment detection procedures to detect greenhouse gases such as CO_2, and NO_2 into the output indicators of ports and made a comparative analysis on the ecological efficiency of 24 major container ports in Europe. Tovar and Wall [58] defined CO_2 as "bad output", and used the DEA model to calculate the eco-environmental efficiency of port operations of 28 port administrations in Spain, in 2016.

The previous literature has provided the research basis for this study, but there are still some deficiencies in the following aspects. Firstly, although the existing literature has calculated port efficiency, the research on the calculation of the port efficiency of China's FTZs is still insufficient. With the rapid development of China's FTZs, it is necessary to study the efficiency of ports in FTZs. Secondly, the existing studies on port efficiency mainly focus on the changes of traditional TFP, and lack research on port green TFP calculation under environmental constraints. Furthermore, port operation has caused serious environmental problems. Therefore, the traditional TFP can't truly reflect the actual situation of the current port TFP. Thirdly, the existing literature about productivity convergence rarely involves ports. In order to more objectively and scientifically evaluate the differences of TFP among different regions and types of ports in China, it is necessary to further study the convergence or evolution trend of green TFP in ports.

In view of the above problems, the marginal contribution of this study is as follows. Firstly, to conduct in-depth research on the efficiency of ports in China's FTZs, this paper takes 19 of the current 21 FTZs (except the Shaanxi and Beijing FTZs, due to data availability) as the source of ports, and selects a total of 28 ports as the objects of efficiency measurement. Secondly, we use the Global Malmquist–Luenberger index method to estimate the green TFP of 28 ports in China's 19 FTZs from 2011 to 2017, and compare this with the traditional TFP without considering environmental constraints. We also study the impact of environmental factors on port efficiency evaluation by comparison. Thirdly, we investigate port heterogeneity, port-type heterogeneity and regional heterogeneity of green TFP on the basis of the overall analysis, and explore the internal causes of the heterogeneity. Fourthly, when analyzing the evolution trend of port green TFP in FTZs, the ports are divided into two types (inland and coastal), and three major regions (east, central and west), and the TFP evolution trend of port types and regional differences are deeply analyzed.

3. Analysis on the Current Situation of the Port Environment in China's FTZs

Since the establishment of China's first FTZ in 2013, China has established a total of 21 FTZs through "1 + 3 + 7 + 1 + 6 + 3" wild goose array, and gradually expanded from coastal to inland after six rounds of construction. The first batch was the Shanghai FTZ; the second batch included the Guangdong, Tianjin, Fujian FTZs; the third batch included the Shaanxi, Sichuan, Chongqing, Hubei, Henan, Zhejiang, Liaoning FTZs; the fourth batch was the Hainan FTZ; the fifth batch comprised the Heilongjiang, Yunnan, Hebei, Guangxi, Jiangsu and Shandong FTZs; and the sixth batch were the Hunan, Anhui and Beijing FTZs. This means that more than half of China's provinces have set up FTZs. The new pattern of "no gap along the coast and focus on the mainland" has been formed. Some FTZs are located in the deep inland, with few and small-scale ports (Shaanxi FTZ). Some FTZs have no ports, due to their own special administrative planning (Beijing FTZ), so there are many statistical deficiencies in the ports of these FTZs. Therefore, this paper finally selects 28 ports from 19 FTZs (excluding Shaanxi and Beijing FTZ) as research samples. Before measuring the green TFP and traditional TFP of the ports in FTZs, this paper focuses on the analysis of the environmental pollution of the ports.

3.1. Comparison of Pollutant Emission between Inland Ports and Coastal Ports

Figure 1 shows the SO_2 emissions of inland ports and coastal ports. It can be found that during 2011–2017, the SO_2 emissions of inland and coastal ports continued to decline year by year, to a certain extent, indicating that the concept of green development has gradually been implemented in the construction and operation of ports in FTZs. According to the comparison of port types, it is not difficult to see that most of the coastal ports in the study sample emit SO_2, probably because the majority of ocean-going ships in coastal ports emit more SO_2. From the perspective of the decline rate of SO_2 emissions, both inland ports and coastal ports have generally shown a process of gradually acceleration and then deceleration. For example, the decline rate sharply increased from 2015 to 2016 and then began to slow down. This shows that the goal of energy conservation and emission reduction has been achieved to a certain extent, and now other measures may be needed to further promote green development.

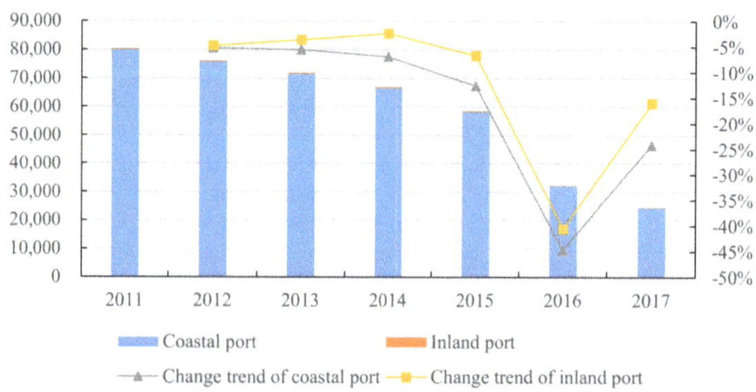

Figure 1. SO_2 emissions from inland and coastal ports (unit: ton). Note: The 2014 SO_2 emission data of coastal and ocean-going ships and inland ships in the Air Pollutant Emission Inventory of Marine in China (2017) calculate their proportion in China's SO_2 emission in 2014 as a fixed proportion value from 2011 to 2017; then, by multiplying by the fixed proportion value according to the SO_2 emission data in the China Statistical Yearbook and Statistical Yearbooks of each province, the SO_2 emission data of each port can be obtained.

Figure 2 shows the NO_X emissions of inland and coastal ports. It can be found that the total NO_X emissions of ports are decreasing, and that the NO_X emissions from coastal ports account for the vast majority of the total emissions; however, compared with the emissions of inland ports, the difference is shrinking. From the range of change, for both the inland ports or coastal ports, the NO_X emission has always been a negative growth, showing a phased downward trend, and the fluctuation degree is basically the same. In addition to 2013, the reduction rate of NO_X emission in coastal ports was lower than that in inland ports, and it was slightly higher than that in inland ports in other years.

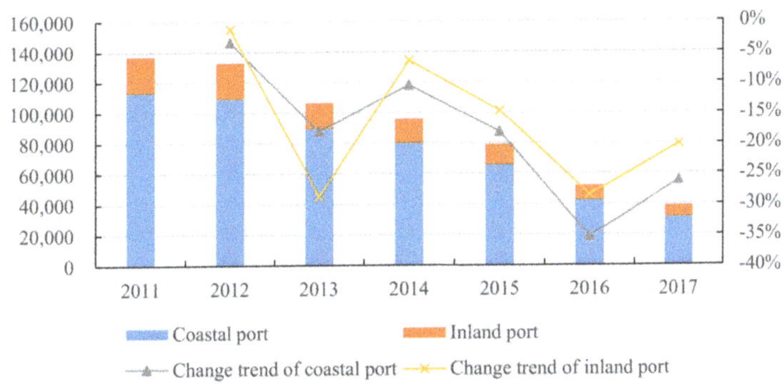

Figure 2. NO_X emission of inland and coastal port (unit: ton). Note: The 2014 NO_X emission data of coastal and ocean-going ships and inland ships in the Air Pollutant Emission Inventory of Marine in China (2017) calculate their proportion in China's NO_X emission in 2014 as a fixed proportion value from 2011 to 2017; then, by multiplying the fixed proportion value according to the NO_X emission data in the China Statistical Yearbook and Statistical Yearbooks of each province, the NO_X emission data of each port can be obtained.

3.2. Comparison of Pollutant Emissions among Eastern, Central and Western Ports

Furthermore, the comparison of pollutant emission in different regions was carried out. Figure 3 shows the SO_2 emissions of the ports in East, Central, and West China shows the specific division of ports in the eastern, central and western regions. It can be seen that the eastern ports account for the vast majority of SO_2 emissions. This is because most of the eastern ports are coastal ports, where ocean-going ships are in the majority and SO_2 emissions are large. The SO_2 emissions of eastern ports showed a downward trend, year by year, and the decline rate has remained stable, except for 2016. The variation range of SO_2 emissions in western ports were basically consistent with those in the eastern ports, but the decrease range was slightly lower than those in the eastern ports. The variation range of SO_2 emissions in central ports were quite different from those in the other two regions; its SO_2 emissions increased in 2013, then kept a slow downward trend until 2016, and turned to a positive growth in 2017.

Figure 4 shows the NO_X emissions of the ports in the eastern, central, and western regions. It can be seen from Figure 4 that the NO_X emissions of the eastern ports account for the vast majority of the total. Under the declining trend of the overall and three regional emissions, year by year, the difference between the NO_X emissions of the eastern ports and those of the other two regions has shrunk. From the perspective of the variation trend, NO_X emissions of the eastern ports have shown a fluctuating decline, whereas the decline rate of the central and western ports has remained basically the same during 2012–2014. During 2015–2016, the decline rate of the NO_X emissions of central ports was significantly lower than those of western ports, which then reversed in 2017. However, the NO_X emissions of the two ports have also shown a fluctuating downward trend, as a whole.

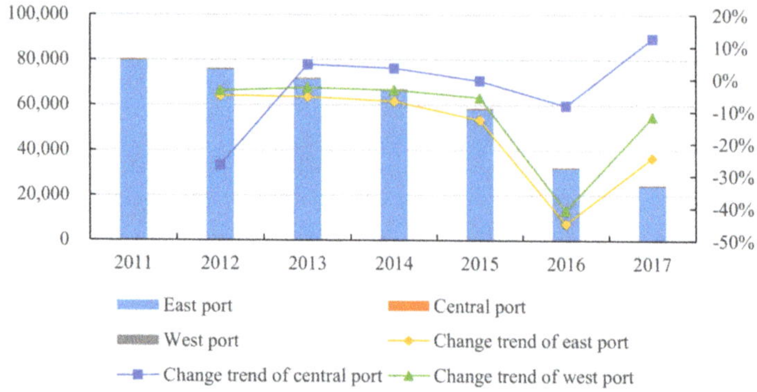

Figure 3. SO_2 emissions from the eastern, central and western ports (unit: ton).

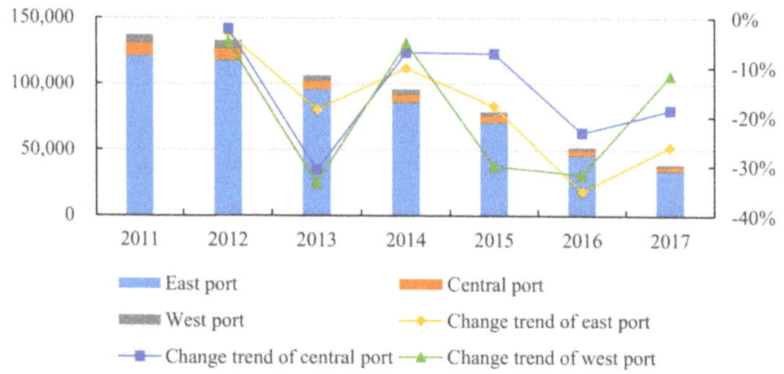

Figure 4. NO_X emissions from ports in East, Central and West China (unit: ton).

To summarize, according to the analysis results of the two major port types of the three regions, the emissions of SO_2 and NO_X from the ports of China's FTZs have decreased year by year. The port environment is gradually improving, and the concept of green development has been thoroughly implemented. However, the pollutant emission and its variation trend have certain heterogeneous characteristics. Most of the pollutants were emitted from coastal ports and eastern ports, especially SO_2. On the downward trend, no matter by type or by region, the reduction of NO_X emission was higher than that of SO_2 emission. Therefore, although the pollutant emissions of the ports in FTZs have been decreasing year by year, it is necessary to investigate whether they affect the calculation results of TFP, in the case that there are still a large number of pollutant emissions. Therefore, it is necessary to introduce environmental factors into the study of TFP in FTZ ports for scientific assessment.

4. Measurement Methods, Variables and Data

4.1. Measurement Methods

4.1.1. Current and Global Production Possibilities Set

First, we needed to build a set of production possibilities, called environmental technologies. This production probabilities set included both "good" outputs, such as GDP, and "bad" outputs, such as CO_2 emissions. We supposed that in different periods $t(t = 1, \ldots, T)$, the port $k(k = 1, \ldots, K)$ used N kinds of inputs $x = (x_1, \ldots, x_N) \in R_N^+$ to produce M kinds of "good" outputs $y = (y_1, \ldots, y_M) \in R_M^+$ and I kinds of "bad" outputs $b = (b_1, \ldots, b_I) \in R_I^+$. For each input vector x, environmental technologies can produce a combination of expected and undesirable outputs simultaneously (y, b). Based on the hypothesis of Wang et al. [59], we used the data envelopment analysis method (DEA) to convert the current environmental technology into Equation (1):

$$P^t\left(x^t\right) = \left\{ \begin{array}{c} \left(y^t, b^t\right) : \sum_{k=1}^{K} z_k^t y_{km}^t \geq y_{km}^t, m = 1, \ldots, M; \\ \sum\limits_{k=1}^{K} z_k^t b_{ki}^t = b_{ki}^t, i = 1, \ldots, I; \\ \sum\limits_{k=1}^{K} z_k^t x_{kn}^t \leq x_{kn}^t, n = 1, \ldots, N; \\ z_k^t \geq 0, k = 1, \ldots, K \end{array} \right\} \quad (1)$$

In Equation (1), z_k^t is the weight measurement index of the observed values of each cross-section, and $z_k^t \geq 0$ means the constant return to scale. When measuring the GML index, the current production possibility set $P^t\left(x^t\right)$ was replaced by the global production possibility set $P^G(x)$, which can be expressed as Formula (2) with the DEA method:

$$P^t\left(x^t\right) = \left\{ \begin{array}{c} \left(y^t, b^t\right) : \sum_{t=1}^{T} \sum_{k=1}^{K} z_k^t y_{km}^t \geq y_{km}^t, m = 1, \ldots, M; \\ \sum_{t=1}^{T} \sum\limits_{k=1}^{K} z_k^t b_{ki}^t = b_{ki}^t, i = 1, \ldots, I; \\ \sum_{t=1}^{T} \sum\limits_{k=1}^{K} z_k^t x_{kn}^t \leq x_{kn}^t, n = 1, \ldots, N; \\ z_k^t \geq 0, k = 1, \ldots, K \end{array} \right\} \quad (2)$$

4.1.2. SBM Directional Distance Function

According to Fukuyama and Weber [60], the global SBM directional distance function incorporated into SO_2 and NO_X emissions on China's FTZ ports is expressed as:

$$\begin{array}{c} S_V^G\left(x^{t,k'}, y^{t,k'}, b^{t,k'}, g^x, g^y, g^b\right) = \max\limits_{s^x, s^y, s^b} \dfrac{\frac{1}{N}\sum_{n=1}^{N} \frac{s_n^x}{g_n^x} + \frac{1}{M+I}\left(\sum_{m=1}^{M} \frac{s_m^y}{g_m^y} + \sum_{i=1}^{I} \frac{s_i^b}{g_i^b}\right)}{2} \\ \text{s. t. } \sum_{t=1}^{T} \sum_{k=1}^{K} z_k^t x_{kn}^t + s_n^x = x_{k'n}^t, \forall n; \\ \sum_{t=1}^{T} \sum_{k=1}^{K} z_k^t y_{km}^t - s_m^y = y_{k'm}^t, \forall m; \\ \sum_{t=1}^{T} \sum_{k=1}^{K} z_k^t b_{ki}^t + s_i^b = x_{k'i}^t, \forall i; \\ \sum_{k=1}^{K} z_k^t = 1, z_k^t \geq 0, \forall k; \\ s_n^x \geq 0, \forall n; \\ s_m^y \geq 0, \forall m; \\ s_i^b \geq 0, \forall i \end{array} \quad (3)$$

In Equation (3), $\left(x^{t,k^t}, y^{t,k^t}, b^{t,k^t}\right)$ is the input and output vector of ports. $\left(g^x, g^y, g^b\right)$ is a direction vector, which represents the decrease in input, the increase in "good" output, and the decrease in "bad" output. $\left(s_n^x, s_m^y, s_i^b\right)$ is a relaxation vector, reflecting the input and output. If the relaxation vectors of both inputs and outputs are positive numbers greater than 0, this means that the actual input and carbon emission of ports are larger than the input-output value of the boundary, whereas the actual output value is smaller than the boundary output value. To summarize, s_n^x, s_m^y, s_i^b represents the situation of excessive input, relatively insufficient "good" output, and excessive pollution emissions of each port [59].

4.1.3. Global Malmquist–Luenberger Productivity Index

After the construction of the SBM directional distance function, we constructed an output-oriented GML index, to measure green TFP. According to Oh [61], the GML index can be expressed as:

$$GML_t^{t+1} = \frac{1 + S_C^G(x^t, y^t, b^t; g)}{1 + S_C^G(x^{t+1}, y^{t+1}, b^{t+1}; g)} \quad (4)$$

Furthermore, the GML index can be divided into two parts: the efficiency change index (GEC) and the technology change index (GTC):

$$GML_t^{t+1} = \frac{1 + S_C^t(x^t, y^t, b^t; g)}{1 + S_C^{t+1}(x^{t+1}, y^{t+1}, b^{t+1}; g)} \times \left[\frac{\frac{1+S_C^G(x^t, y^t, b^t; g)}{1+S_C^t(x^t, y^t, b^t; g)}}{\frac{1+S_C^G(x^{t+1}, y^{t+1}, b^{t+1}; g)}{1+S_C^{t+1}(x^{t+1}, y^{t+1}, b^{t+1}; g)}} \right] \quad (5)$$

When the GML_t^{t+1} (GEC or GTC) index is greater than 1, the green TFP (technical efficiency or technical progress) of the port shows an increasing trend. When the index is equal to (or less than) 1, the green TFP (technical efficiency or technical progress) remains unchanged (or decreases).

4.1.4. Global Malmquist Productivity Index

In order to more intuitively reflect the constraints of environmental factors, such as pollution emissions on China's FTZ ports, we also estimated the traditional TFP of the ports, and applied the DEA–Malmquist productivity index method (Global Malmquist index method) based on the Global technology, and compared it with the GML index. The Global Malmquist index can be expressed as:

$$GM\left(y^{t+1}, x^{t+1}, y^t, x^t\right) = \frac{D^{t+1}(x^{t+1}, y^{t+1})}{D^t(x^t, y^t)} \left[\left(\frac{D^g(x^{t+1}, y^{t+1})}{D^{t+1}(x^{t+1}, y^{t+1})} \times \frac{D^t(x^t, y^t)}{D^g(x^t, y^t)} \right) \right] = EC \times TC \quad (6)$$

4.2. Variable Selection and Data Sources

A total of 21 FTZs have been set up since the first one was established in 2013. Due to the lack of ports in some FTZs or the lack of data in some ports, this paper has collected the input and output data of 28 ports in 19 FTZs in China. The production berth and wharf length are taken as input indicators, the cargo and container throughput as "good output", and SO_2 and NO_X as "bad output". The basic data were mainly from the China Port Yearbook, the China Statistical Yearbook and the China City Statistical Yearbook.

4.2.1. Ports Output—"Good Output"

As an important hub of land and water transportation, the port's basic function is cargo transportation. The existing literature mainly calculates the port efficiency from three perspectives: the input-output perspective of the port itself, the operation perspective of port enterprises, and the consideration of undesirable outputs (Table 1). Among them, most works of literature take the cargo and container throughput as the output indicators, because the cargo and container throughput can directly reflect the output level of the ports. Although some scholars [62–64] used financial indicators, such as net profit, main business income and earnings per share, such indicators need to be obtained from the financial data of the ports group, or the ports company that manages the ports. Due to the large number of ports selected in this paper, it is difficult to obtain financial data of some ports. Therefore, the cargo and container throughput were used as the index to measure the "good output" of the ports.

Table 1. Port input-output literature review.

Author	Input indicator	Output indicator
	Port's Own Input-Output Perspective	
Author	Input indicator	Output indicator
Du et al. (2021) [65]	Length of wharf, number of berths for production, amount of loading and unloading equipment	Cargo throughput, container throughput
Zheng and Yang (2021) [66]	Length of wharf, number of berths for production	Cargo throughput, container throughput
Zhu et al. (2021) [67]	Length of wharf, number of berths for production	Cargo throughput, container throughput
Lu and Li (2018) [68]	Length of wharf, number of berths for production	Port throughput
	Port Enterprise Operation Perspective	
Author	Input indicator	Output indicator
Kuang (2007) [62]	Main business cost, number of employees, fixed assets	Net profit, main business revenue, earnings per share
Wang and Wu (2016) [63]	Number of employees	Net profit, main business revenue, earnings per share
Feng et al. (2017) [64]	Main business cost, fixed assets	Net profit, main business revenue
Han et al. (2021) [69]	Number of employees, number of bridge cranes	Net profit, main business revenue
	Undesirable Output Perspective	
Author	Input indicator	Output indicator
Liu et al. (2021) [56]	Number of berths for production, length of wharf, number of employees, net assets	Port throughput, net profit, SO_2, NO_Xemissions
Liu and Wang (2018) [70]	Length of berths for production, energy consumption (standard coal), production berth above 10,000 tons	Container throughput, CO_2 emissions
Luo et al. (2014) [54]	Berth length, port area, shore jib crane, pusher crane	Container throughput, CO_2 emissions
Sun et al. (2017) [71]	Number of employees, fixed asset, operating costs	Cargo throughput, net profit, NO_X emissions
Wang and Liang (2018) [72]	Number of berths for production, number of employees, oil consumption, electric consumption	Cargo throughput, CO_2 emissions

4.2.2. Ports Output—"Bad Output"

At present, there is no unified definition of "bad output" in the academic circle, and the "bad output" used in the measurement of green TFP is also different. In the course of the operation of port ships, SO_2 and NO_X were the two atmospheric pollutants with the largest emissions and the highest pollution degrees. In this paper, they were regarded as undesirable "bad outputs", and the practice of Liu et al. [56] was used for reference. According to the 2014 SO_2 and NO_X emission data of coastal and ocean-going ships, and inland ships in the Air Pollutant Emission Inventory of Marine in China (2017), the proportion of SO_2 and NO_X in China's two types of pollutant emissions in 2014 is calculated as the fixed proportion value from 2011 to 2017. Subsequently, according to the emission data of two types of pollutants in the China Statistical Yearbook and the Statistical Yearbooks of each province, multiplied by the fixed proportion value, the SO_2 and NO_X emission data of each port can be obtained.

4.2.3. Ports Input

According to Table 1, from the perspective of the port's input, the port's input indicators mainly included the number of berths for production, the length of the wharf, and the amount of loading and unloading equipment [65,66]. These indicators directly reflect the port's scale and infrastructure construction level; from the perspective of the port enterprise operation, port input indicators focus on financial indicators, mainly including main business cost, number of employees, fixed assets, etc. [62,69]. These indicators can reflect the scale and operation level of port operation companies; from the perspective of undesirable output, energy indicators such as oil consumption and electric consumption can also be selected as port input indicators [70,72]. There are two problems in the actual collection of the latter two types of indicators: first, many ports operating enterprises in FTZs are not listed and their financial status is not disclosed, resulting in great difficulty in data collection of financial input indicators; second, in the process of collecting energy input indicators, it is found that there are many missing values in the relevant data of ports in FTZs. Therefore, based on the principle of data availability, this paper mainly selected the number of berths for production and the length of the wharf as input indicators from the perspective of the port's own input. The longer the wharf length, the more berths can be built. The more berths for production, the stronger the ship carrying capacity of the port. The two can reflect the infrastructure construction level of the port from the perspective of actual investment, and represent the scale and production capacity of the ports to a large extent. Table 2 reports the descriptive statistical results of each variable.

Table 2. Descriptive statistical results of input-output variables.

Variable Type	Variable Name	Unit	Obs.	Mean	Median	S.D.	Min	Max
"Good output"	Cargo Throughput	10,000 Tons	196	21,793	14,236.5	19,223.41	348	70,542
	Container throughput	10,000 TEUs	196	675	136.54	1441.51	0	16,602
"Bad output"	SO_2	Ton	196	2097	187.64	3499.4	1.98	17,028
	NO_x	Ton	196	3281	1555.95	4780.1	19.68	24,075
Ports investment	Number of berths for production	Unit	196	225	151	231.39	22	1402
	Length of Wharf	Meter	196	25,585	22,674	18,892	2084	76,469

5. Time Series Characteristics and Heterogeneity Analysis of Green TFP in FTZ Ports

5.1. Overall Temporal Characteristics

Table 3 reports the TFP index of China's FTZ ports and their decomposition results. When the environmental factors were not introduced, the annual growth rate of TFP (TFPC) in FTZ ports from 2011 to 2017 was 1.25%, in which the technical efficiency (TEC) increased by 5.95% annually, whereas the technical progress (TPC) showed negative growth, with an annual decline of 4.44%. After the introduction of environmental factors, the annual growth rate of green TFP of the ports in FTZs increased to 4.43%, of which the annual growth rate of technical efficiency decreased to 0.57%. The technological progress showed positive growth, with an annual growth rate of 3.84%. Through comparison, it was found that after the introduction of environmental factors, technical efficiency decreased by 5.38%, whereas the technical progress and TFP growth rate increased by 8.28% and 3.18%, respectively. This indicated that after the introduction of environmental factors, the technological transition and the decreasing factor utilization rate of the port coexist. Although the decline of technical efficiency is large, the improvement of TFP brought by technological progress is enough to counter for the loss caused by the lack of factor utilization. Therefore, the TFP growth rate can still achieve positive growth after the introduction of environmental factors, and the average annual growth rate can be further improved. It can be seen that the TFP estimation of China's FTZ ports will be affected by environmental factors. Ignoring these environmental factors will lead to the underestimation of the TFP growth rate and technological progress growth rate, and the overestimation of the technical efficiency growth rate.

Table 3. Port TFP index and its decomposition term (2011–2017).

Year	No Environmental Factors Were Introduced			Environmental Factors Were Introduced		
	TEC	TPC	TFPC	TEC	TPC	TFPC
2012	1.0560	0.8232	0.8693	0.9385	0.9271	0.8701
2013	1.0570	1.0161	1.0740	1.0064	1.0965	1.1035
2014	1.0414	0.9765	1.0170	1.1400	0.9005	1.0265
2015	1.1115	0.9140	1.0159	0.9952	1.0254	1.0205
2016	1.0200	0.9856	1.0054	0.9392	1.1678	1.0968
2017	1.0733	1.0350	1.1109	1.0280	1.1439	1.1758
Mean value	1.0595	0.9556	1.0125	1.0057	1.0384	1.0443

In addition to 2012, the green TFP and the traditional TFP of China's FTZ ports have both shown positive growth, which may be due to the fact that since the establishment of the first batch of FTZs in 2013, ports, as an important hub of a region, undertake the functions of trade exchanges and cargo transportation with other countries and regions. To give full play to the role of FTZs in promoting foreign exchanges and economic development, their respective trade zone governments and port groups can pay more attention to port management and technological progress. From 2014 to 2015, the TFP index of the two categories continued to decline, which may be due to the increase in the number of FTZs, or some inefficient FTZ ports pulling down the overall growth rate. On the other hand, it may also be due to the fact that in the early days of the establishment of FTZs, some regions excessively pursued the port's infrastructure construction and blindly expanded, resulting in repeated construction. In the environment of a shrinking market, there is a lack of overall planning awareness and management capacity, which gives some ports excess capacity and low operational efficiency. Since 2011, the green TFP index has been higher than the traditional TFP index. Combination Färe et al. [73] reveal that the reduction in the "bad" output of ports in China's FTZs has exceeded the growth rate of the "good" output, and the technological progress rate of ports in China's FTZs are constantly improving, and moving towards the direction of green development.

According to the decomposition, when it comes to the TFP index, without the introduction of environmental factors, the technical efficiency index is significantly greater than 1, and the technical progress index is less than 1 in most years, showing a negative growth. This indicates that without considering environmental factors, TFP growth mainly depends on the improvement of factor allocation and usage efficiency. By comparison with the results without the introduction of environmental factors, the technical efficiency index decreased significantly after the introduction of environmental factors; on the contrary, the technological progress index, especially in 2016 and 2017, showed significant growth. It may be that under the macro environment of energy conservation and the emission reduction, the RD of new energy and new technology has gradually passed the stage of cost investment, and its dividend has begun to emerge. It can be seen that the introduction of environmental factors has had a crucial impact on the estimation of the TFP of China's FTZ ports. At the same time, this also reveals that the port efficiency of China's FTZs has not fully reached its potential of existing resources and technologies, and there is still much room to promote the performance growth of ports by improving their operation and production efficiency.

5.2. Investigation of Port Heterogeneity

Table 4 reports the TFP index of each port and its decomposition results. It can be found that the TFP of ports in China's FTZs are different. Without considering the environmental factors, Hangzhou port has the highest TFP growth rate (with an average annual growth rate of 15.97%), followed by Changsha Port and Luzhou port, and Fuzhou port has the lowest TFP growth rate. After the introduction of environmental factors, Nanjing port has the highest TFP growth rate (with an average annual growth rate of

21.95%), followed by Hangzhou port and Chongqing port. Fuzhou port's TFP growth rate was still the lowest. From the numerical comparison of the TFP index, we can see that after the introduction of environmental factors, except for Fuzhou port, Harbin Port and Yangpu Port, the TFP index of other ports has increased, with Nanjing port and Xiamen Port increasing by 13.23% and 13.49%, respectively. This also indicates that the TFP ranking of the two ports has significantly improved, ranking first and fifth respectively. Overall, environmental factors have a significant impact on the TFP index of each port.

Table 4. TFP index of each port and its decomposition term (2011–2017).

Port	Type	Region	No Environmental Factors Were Introduced				Environmental Factors Were Introduced			
			TEC	TPC	TFPC	TFP Ranking	TEC	TPC	TFPC	TFP Ranking
Changsha	inland	central	1.1822	0.9621	1.1374	2	1.1098	1.0336	1.1471	4
Dalian	coastal	eastern	1.0602	0.9615	1.0194	13	0.9255	1.1061	1.0237	18
Fuzhou	coastal	eastern	0.8200	0.9616	0.7885	28	0.7870	0.9999	0.7869	28
Guangzhou	coastal	eastern	1.0887	0.9607	1.0459	8	1.0754	1.0333	1.1112	9
Harbin	inland	central	1.0011	0.9615	0.9625	23	0.9317	1.0297	0.9593	25
Haikou	coastal	eastern	0.9682	0.9620	0.9313	27	1.0000	1.0000	1.0000	20
Hangzhou	inland	eastern	1.2062	0.9615	1.1597	1	1.1301	1.0325	1.1668	2
Hefei	inland	central	0.9880	0.9624	0.9508	24	0.9429	1.0332	0.9742	24
Lianyungang	coastal	eastern	1.0275	0.9645	0.9910	19	0.9496	1.0567	1.0034	19
Luzhou	inland	western	1.1632	0.9619	1.1188	3	1.0043	1.1199	1.1248	6
Nanjing	inland	eastern	1.1301	0.9620	1.0872	5	1.1790	1.0343	1.2195	1
Nanning	inland	central	1.0429	0.9615	1.0027	18	1.0299	1.0228	1.0533	15
Ningbo	coastal	eastern	1.0782	0.9437	1.0175	14	1.0555	0.9991	1.0546	14
Qinzhou	coastal	central	0.9802	0.9626	0.9435	26	0.8180	1.1619	0.9504	26
Qingdao	coastal	eastern	1.0209	0.9661	0.9863	20	1.0000	1.0000	1.0000	21
Shanghai	coastal	eastern	1.1261	0.9150	1.0304	11	1.1188	1.0014	1.1204	7
Shenzhen	coastal	eastern	1.1795	0.8584	1.0125	16	1.0000	1.0712	1.0712	11
Suzhou	inland	central	1.0674	0.9623	1.0271	12	1.0000	1.0323	1.0323	17
Tangshan	coastal	eastern	1.0000	0.9802	0.9802	21	1.0000	1.0000	1.0000	22
Tianjin	coastal	eastern	1.0463	0.9684	1.0132	15	1.0315	1.0044	1.0361	16
Wuhu	inland	central	1.0908	0.9625	1.0499	7	1.0142	1.0415	1.0564	13
Wuhan	inland	central	1.0967	0.9620	1.0551	6	1.0413	1.0359	1.0787	10
Xiamen	coastal	eastern	1.0833	0.9298	1.0073	17	1.0158	1.1244	1.1422	5
Yantai	coastal	eastern	1.0113	0.9623	0.9731	22	0.9726	1.0066	0.9791	23
Yangpu	coastal	eastern	0.9825	0.9622	0.9454	25	0.9110	1.0089	0.9191	27
Yueyang	inland	central	1.0743	0.9623	1.0338	10	1.0000	1.0663	1.0663	12
Chongqing	inland	western	1.1545	0.9625	1.1112	4	1.1191	1.0342	1.1574	3
Zhuhai	coastal	eastern	1.0839	0.9618	1.0425	9	1.1066	1.0084	1.1159	8
Mean value			1.0595	0.9556	1.0125		1.0057	1.0384	1.0443	

According to the decomposition term of TFP, for most ports, whether environmental factors are introduced or not determines whether the leading factor of TFP growth is technical efficiency or technical progress. Without the introduction of environmental factors, the technical efficiency index of most ports exceeds the technical progress index (except for Fuzhou port). After the introduction of environmental factors, the comparison of the decomposition terms of most ports is reversed. This shows, once again, that ignoring environmental factors leads to errors in the measurement results of the TFP of ports in China's FTZs. It also means that there is a large space for the vast majority of ports to further promote the growth of TFP, through the improvement of technical efficiency.

5.3. Analysis on Port Types and Regional Heterogeneity

In order to investigate the types and regional heterogeneity of the TFP changes in China's FTZ ports, the FTZ ports were divided into two types (inland ports and coastal ports) and three regions (eastern, central and western regions). It can be seen from Table 5 that there are great differences in the TFP index and its decomposition terms between inland ports and coastal ports. From the regional point of view, the differences between the eastern ports and the central ports are minor, but there are significant differences between them and the western ports.

Table 5. TFP index of port type and region and its decomposition mean (2011–2017).

Port	No Environmental Factors Were Introduced			Environmental Factors Were Introduced		
	TEC	TPC	TFPC	TEC	TPC	TFPC
Overall average	1.0595	0.9556	1.0125	1.0057	1.0384	1.0443
Inland	1.0977	0.9620	1.0561	1.0393	1.0427	1.0837
Coastal	1.0317	0.9508	0.9810	0.9812	1.0352	1.0157
Eastern	1.0509	0.9520	1.0005	1.0103	1.0282	1.0388
Central	1.0551	0.9621	1.0151	0.9824	1.0523	1.0337
Western	1.1588	0.9622	1.1150	1.0601	1.0762	1.1410

Under the classification standard of port types, the TFP annual growth rate of inland ports was significantly higher than those of coastal ports, without the introduction of environmental factors. The TFP annual growth rate of inland ports was 5.61%, whereas for coastal ports this was 1.9%. This difference was mainly determined by technical efficiency. This represents that the difference between coastal ports and inland ports is mainly reflected in factor utilization efficiency, when environmental factors are not considered. It may be that with the opening of the FTZ, coastal areas expand port investment in cases with a more advantageous geographical location, resulting in different degrees of congestion in the number of berths and berth length investment [46]. This leads to low efficiency. After the introduction of environmental factors, the annual growth rate of the TFP of inland ports was still higher than those of coastal ports. Compared with the results without the introduction of environmental factors, the technical efficiency index decreased by different degrees, indicating that in terms of port operation and management, the two types of ports had deficiencies in resource consumption and environmental contamination emission management. Moreover, the technical efficiency of coastal ports had a negative growth. This shows that both inland ports and coastal ports have input in clean technology, green operation and environmental protection technology, and the corresponding input has brought different degrees of income, which lead to the leading factor of TFP growth from the technical efficiency without environmental factors, to the technical progress after the introduction of environmental factors.

Under the regional division standard, without the introduction of environmental factors, the annual growth rate of port TFP from high to low is in the order of western, central and eastern regions. After the introduction of environmental factors, the western region still ranked first, whereas the eastern and central regions alternated. According to the decomposition in terms of the TFP index, compared with the non-introduction of environmental factors, the average annual growth rate of technological progress increased significantly, whereas the average annual growth rate of technical efficiency decreased significantly. Firstly, this shows that the regional ranking of TFP annual growth rate was also affected by environmental factors. Secondly, due to data reasons, ports in the western region solely included Chongqing port and Luzhou port, which may be due to the relatively concentrated population in Chongqing and Luzhou, strong demand for cargo transportation, developed water systems, a long history of ship transportation businesses, rich experience in management and operation, and small pollution emissions from inland ships. Therefore, both traditional TFP and green TFP were ranked first. After the introduction of environmental factors, the ranking of the TFP average annual growth rate in the eastern and central regions alternated, which was mainly affected by the sharp decline in the technical efficiency of the ports in the central region. This reveals that compared with the ports in the eastern region, the ports in the central region still have a certain gap in geographical location, scientific and technological environment, and the concentration of cargo transportation points.

5.4. Analysis on Evolution Trend of Port Types and Regional Differences

Since green TFP can better reflect the green growth performance of the ports in FTZs, we only analyzed the change trend of port types and regional differences of green TFP. Referring to the practice of Teng et al. [74], we used the coefficient of variation to measure the degree of regional difference.

Figure 5 depicts the evolution characteristics of the type difference degree of the green TFP index of the whole sample, inland and coastal ports. It can be found that the difference degree of port type of the green TFP index decreased as time went on, meaning that the green TFP of ports in China's FTZs may exist on whole σ convergence. From the evolution of the internal differences of green TFP between the two types of ports, the evolution trajectory was basically consistent with the whole sample, which indicated that the differences of green TFP between the two types of ports are shrinking, and may also exist on σ convergence. From the mean value of the coefficient of variation, the inland ports were significantly higher than the coastal ports in most years. Regarding the differences between port types, the difference of coefficient of variation between the two types of ports in 2017 was smaller than that in 2012, indicating that the differences between port types are narrowing.

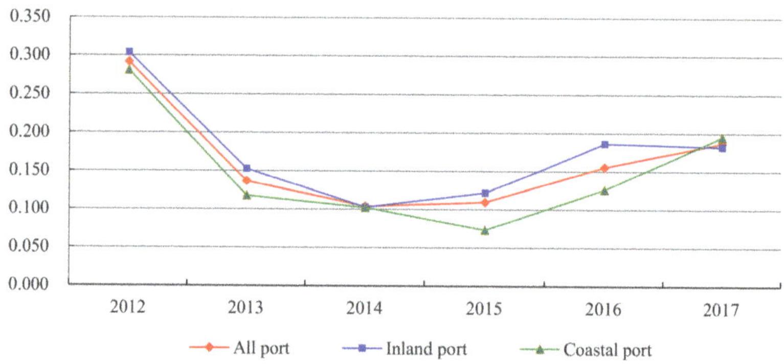

Figure 5. Variation trend of green TFP difference degree in general, inland and coastal ports.

Figure 6 depicts the evolution characteristics of regional differences in the green TFP index of eastern, central and western ports. From the evolution of the internal differences of green TFP of ports in the three regions, the coefficient of variation of central ports decreased significantly, from 0.4469 in 2012 to 0.161 in 2017, with the largest declines in 2012 and 2013; the coefficient of variation of eastern ports decreased from 0.2452 in 2012 to 0.207 in 2017, which was less than those of central ports. It can be seen that the differences of green TFP between the central and eastern ports are shrinking, and there may be some problems with σ convergence. However, the coefficient of variation of western ports remained stable during 2012–2017, and there was no convergence trend. From the mean value of coefficient of variation, except for 2017, the coefficient of variation of the three regions from large to small was central, eastern and western, meaning that the difference of green TFP within the central ports was the largest, followed by eastern and western. From the perspective of regional differences, the difference of the coefficient of variation of the three major regional ports in 2017 was smaller than that in 2012, which indicates that the differences between regions are narrowing.

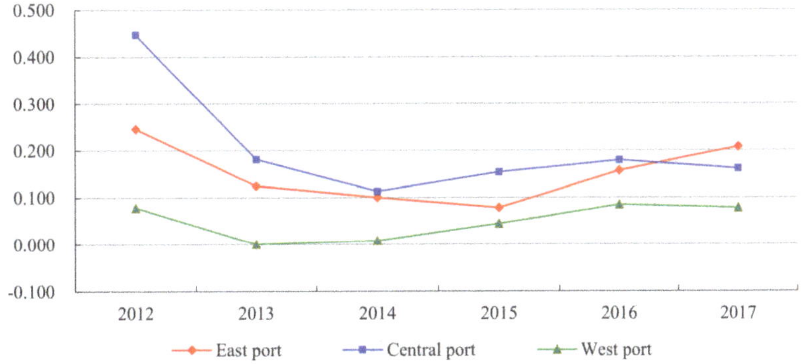

Figure 6. Variation trend of green TFP difference degree in eastern, central and western ports.

6. Conclusions

This paper introduces environmental factors into the measurement framework of TFP in China's FTZs, and compares it with the traditional TFP, without considering environmental factors. The main conclusions are as follows.

Firstly, the emissions of SO_2, NO_X and other pollutants from the ports of China's FTZs have decreased year by year. The port environment has gradually improved, and the concept of green development has been thoroughly implemented. However, there are some heterogeneous characteristics in pollutant emissions and their changing trends, and the pollutant emission of coastal ports and eastern ports account for the vast majority. In the downward trend, the reduction of NO_X emission was generally higher than that of SO_2 emission.

Secondly, both the green TFP and traditional TFP of FTZ ports showed an upward trend, with an average annual growth rate of 4.43% and 1.25%, respectively. It can be seen that the introduction of environmental factors has a significant impact on the estimation of TFP in FTZ ports, which means the non-introduction of environmental factors will lead to the overall underestimation of TFP. The main source of traditional TFP growth is technical efficiency, whereas for green TFP it is technical progress. There is still a large space to further improve the green TFP of FTZ ports through the improvement of technical efficiency.

Thirdly, the growth of green TFP in FTZ ports has great port heterogeneity. Nanjing port has the highest growth rate of green TFP, with an average annual growth rate of 21.95%. Ningbo Port ranked 14th, with an average annual growth rate of 5.46%. At the end of the list, the green TFP of Fuzhou Port showed negative growth. After the introduction of environmental factors, the green TFP of most ports (except for Fuzhou port, Harbin Port and Yangpu Port) increased, compared with the traditional TFP, and the main source of growth changed from technical efficiency without the introduction of environmental factors, to technical progress. The conclusion was the same as the overall time series conclusion.

Fourthly, the growth of ports green TFP in FTZs had great type and regional heterogeneity. Under the classification standard, the annual growth rate of green TFP in inland ports was significantly higher than that in coastal ports. According to the three regional classification standards, the annual growth rate of green TFP from high to low was in the order of: the western region, the eastern region and finally the central region. The central region was more restricted by environmental factors. After the introduction of environmental factors, the TFP growth rate of the central region was lower than that of the eastern and western regions.

Fifthly, from the evolution trend of the internal differences of green TFP between the two types of ports, the differences of green TFP between inland ports and coastal ports are shrinking, and there may be σ convergence. The difference between the two has also narrowed. From the evolution trend of the internal differences of green TFP in the three regional ports, only the differences of green TFP in the central and eastern ports have narrowed, which may exist due to σ convergence. The differences among the three regions are also narrowing.

Based on the above research conclusions, the main enlightenment of this paper is as follows.

Firstly, under the background of economic globalization and regional economic integration, as one of the cores of FTZs, ports in FTZs should pay more attention to the positive impact of TFP on the green and sustainable development of FTZs, and incorporate environmental factors into the evaluation and management system of port TFP. They should also promote the transformation of port growth mode from factor driven to green TFP driven, and further promote the green development of ports in FTZs.

Secondly, it is necessary to maintain the contribution level of technological progress of the TFP of the ports in FTZs, as well as continuously improve the independent innovation ability and technical level of the ports, strictly control pollution emissions, build ecological green ports and strive to improve their core competitiveness. At the same time, the green TFP growth can be promoted through the improvement of technical efficiency, reasonable planning of the port layout, and clear port positioning according to their actual situation, in addition to a focus on the construction of professional and large-scale wharfs, and avoiding the repeated construction and redundant investment of ports. At the same time, we should make full use of the policy advantages of FTA to increase port throughput, improving the carrying capacity of wharfs, and further tapping the potential of existing resources and technologies.

Thirdly, although the regional differences of green TFP growth in ports are shrinking, the government should still formulate corresponding regional difference policies according to the factor endowments of various regions, establish a flexible environmental response system to improve the environmental adaptability of the port industry, and guide ports to make full use of and allocate resources effectively. By promoting the research, development and introduction of environmental protection and clean technologies, strengthening regional green technology exchange and cooperation, we can further narrow the regional differences of port's green TFP growth, and ultimately promote the overall improvement of port's green TFP in China's FTZs.

This study is helpful to scientifically understand the growth trend and heterogeneity of the green TFP of ports in China's FTZs under environmental constraints, and is of great significance in promoting the green development of ports in China's FTZs. However, this work is not over yet. In the future, we can continue to study it from at least the following three aspects: first, this study can be further connected with the theme of sustainable development. We can perform research on the sustainable development of FTZ ports from the perspective of green TFP, meaning that green TFP will be regarded as one of the important factors affecting the sustainable development of ports. By constructing a model to quantitatively evaluate the impact of green TFP on port sustainable development under environmental constraints, we can then put forward the port emission reduction strategy from the perspective of sustainable development. Second, we can perform research on the influencing factors of green TFP of FTZ ports. As an important factor affecting the sustainable development of ports, green TFP is an endogenous variable, determined by a series of economic activities. As a continuation of this study, we can further analyze which factors have an important impact on port green TFP. For example, the city's green infrastructure and comprehensive development level are closely related to the city's TFP and sustainable development. The port is located in a city, so we can focus on identifying the causal impact of the city's green infrastructure and comprehensive development level on the port's green TFP. Third, we can scientifically evaluate the green TFP effect of China's FTZ strategy. Considering that the ports studied in this paper belong to the ports in China's FTZs, there may be differences in policy impact between them and non-FTZ ports. Therefore, we can take the establishment of China's FTZs as a quasi-natural experiment, and scientifically evaluate the real effect of the implementation of China's FTZ strategy on the port pollutant emission and green TFP of FTZs, by using time-varying difference in difference (DID) and other methods.

Author Contributions: Conception and leadership, Z.H.; analysis, Z.H. and F.L.; writing—original draft preparation, Z.H. and F.L.; writing—review and editing, H.X. All authors have read and agreed to the published version of the manuscript.

Funding: This work was funded by the Projects of Ministry of Education Humanities and Social Sciences Foundation (Grant No. 21YJC790051) and National Natural Science Foundation of China (Grant No. 71503273).

Institutional Review Board Statement: Not applicable.

Informed Consent Statement: Not applicable.

Data Availability Statement: The data presented in this study are available on request from the corresponding author (coldxu520@163.com).

Conflicts of Interest: The authors declare no conflict of interest.

References

1. Tuca, S. The relationship between globalization and the economic crisis. *USV Ann. Econ. Public Adm.* **2014**, *14*, 120–126.
2. Horn, H.; Mavroidis, P.; Sapir, A. Beyond the WTO? An anatomy of EU and US preferential trade agreements. *World Econ.* **2010**, *33*, 1565–1588. [CrossRef]
3. Qiao, Z.; Xu, Y.K. Opportunities and challenges brought to China by the new round of world economic transformation. *Contemp. Econ. Res.* **2013**, *12*, 50–55.
4. Pei, C.H. A new round of open scale from the perspective of global governance: An observation from Shanghai Free Trade Zone. *Reformation* **2013**, *12*, 30–40.
5. Chen, A.Z.; Liu, Z.B. Free trade zone: China's open economy "second quarter". *Acad. Mon.* **2014**, *1*, 20–28.
6. Zhang, H.L.; Gai, X.Z. Free trade zone, context, functional orientation and contingent strategy. *Reformation* **2013**, *9*, 98–105.
7. Guo, X.H. Construction of China-ASEAN free trade area: Current situation and prospect. *People's Forum-Acad. Front.* **2016**, *19*, 36–43.
8. Xu, L.P.; Wang, J. Efficiency evaluation of foreign processing export zones, special economic zones and free trade zones and its reference to China. *Shanghai Financ. Res.* **2015**, *11*, 104–112.
9. Meng, G.W. Theoretical basis and model selection of political geography for the establishment of China's free trade zone. *Sci. Geogr. Sin.* **2015**, *35*, 19–29.
10. Cui, X.J.; Ouyang, H.M. A literature study on China's utilization of foreign-invested industrial policies: Based on the quantitative-qualitative-evolutionary three-dimensional framework. *J. Cent. Univ. Financ. Econ.* **2021**, *1*, 96–108.
11. Chen, Y.; Liang, S. The impact of the establishment of Shanghai free trade zone on Shanghai's service trade and its countermeasures. *North. Econ. Trade* **2018**, *1*, 10–12.
12. Shen, G.B. The impact of the establishment of Shanghai pilot free trade zone on China's economic and trade development. *Soc. Sci.* **2013**, *12*, 61–68.
13. Wang, Y.Z.; Luo, Z.; Hu, Z.G. The influence of policy pilot on regional economic development—Evidence from China pilot free trade zone. *J. Hunan Univ. (Soc. Sci.)* **2021**, *35*, 54–62.
14. Yang, X.D. On the relationship between economic and political effects of China (Shanghai) pilot free trade zone—From the perspective of national treatment. *J. Shanghai Univ. Financ. Econ.* **2014**, *16*, 97–104.
15. Li, M. One belt, one road, China's free trade zone, and the strategic relationship. *Economist* **2017**, *5*, 50–57.
16. Chen, T.; Ni, W.H. Research on logistics efficiency of relevant regions under the interaction of free trade zone and the belt and road initiative. *Sci. Technol. Econ.* **2020**, *6*, 71–75.
17. Chen, H.; Cheng, J. Thinking on one belt, one road construction and China's free trade zone strategy. *Contemp. Econ. Manag.* **2019**, *41*, 62–66.
18. Ye, X.Q. Pilot free trade zone and economic growth—An empirical study based on quasi natural experiment. *Econ. Rev.* **2018**, *4*, 18–29.
19. Cui, G.R. Research on the policy effect of service industry growth in Shanghai free trade zone of China. *J. Liaoning Univ.* **2020**, *48*, 28–39.
20. Kang, J.J.; Zheng, W.W. Trade creation effect of China's inland free trade zone: Expanding imports or stimulating exports. *Int. Trade Issues* **2021**, *2*, 16–31.
21. Lv, X.W.; Liu, B.L. The empirical test of the influence of free trade zone on human capital investment under the new development concept—Quasi-natural experiment based on free trade zone establishment. *Soft Sci.* **2021**, *35*, 1–6.
22. Gu, L.L.; Li, Q.I. Research on the impact of China's free trade zone on futures market—Evidence from the development of Zhengzhou futures exchange. *J. Dalian Univ. Technol.* **2020**, *41*, 63–67.

23. Yin, W.W.; Zhang, C. The connotation and upgrade path of free trade port with Chinese characteristics. *Theory Mon.* **2021**, *6*, 54–64.
24. Chen, L.; Yuan, S. Multidimensional policy dividends for free trade port from the perspective of global comparison: National governance effect, economic effect and social effect. *Ind. Econ. Rev.* **2019**, *10*, 134–147.
25. Tong, J.D. Deepening reform of China's pilot free trade zone and establishment of free trade port. *Int. Bus. Stud.* **2018**, *1*, 13–18.
26. Guo, J.K.; Han, Z.L. The port-city spatial system evolution theory and empirical study of Chinese seaport city. *Sci. Geogr. Sin.* **2013**, *33*, 1285–1292.
27. Nugraha, A.T.; Waterson, B.J.; Blainey, S.P.; Nash, F.J. Unravelling the dynamics behind the urban morphology of port-cities using a LUTI model based on cellular automata. *Comput. Environ. Urban Syst.* **2022**, *92*, 101733. [CrossRef]
28. Li, D.S.; Zhang, H.; Gao, A.Y. Spatial layout of port bulk commodity market in China. *Sci. Geogr. Sin.* **2019**, *30*, 541–549.
29. Gurzhiy, A.; Kalyazina, S.; Maydanova, S.; Marchenko, R. Port and city integration: Transportation aspect. *Transp. Res. Procedia* **2021**, *54*, 890–899. [CrossRef]
30. Yang, M.J.; Lin, J.; Li, Y.C. Harbor city pattern and development strategies of harbor cities: A case study of coastal development zone of Weifang. *City Plan. Rev.* **2010**, *34*, 80–85.
31. Li, T.; Wang, L.; Wang, Y. Research on synergetic development between efficiency of port logistics and its hinterland economy in Liaoning. *Econ. Geogr.* **2012**, *32*, 108–113.
32. González, L.F.; Martín, B.F.; Javier, P.D.A. Are Spanish ports efficient and profitable? A quantitative analysis. *Util. Policy* **2021**, *70*, 101195.
33. Tsakiridis, A.; Mateo-Mantecón, I.; O'Connor, E.; Hynes, S.; O'Donoghue, C. Efficiency benchmarking of Irish and North Atlantic Spanish ports: Implications for blue growth. *Util. Policy* **2021**, *72*, 101268. [CrossRef]
34. Cao, Y.H.; Cao, W.D.; Jin, S.S.; Li, H.J.; Wang, L.M. The evolution mechanism of the coastal container port system of China. *Acta Geogr. Sin.* **2003**, *58*, 424–432.
35. Wilmsmeier, G.; Monios, J.; Farfán, A.F.B. Port system evolution in Ecuador—Migration, location splitting or specialisation? *J. Transp. Geogr.* **2021**, *93*, 103042. [CrossRef]
36. Wu, Q.T.; Zhang, H.O.; Ye, Y.Y.; Chen, F.G.; Chen, W.L. Factors and driving mechanism of the port system evolution. *Hum. Geogr.* **2011**, *26*, 106–110.
37. Li, Z.F.; Tang, X.W. The hinterland plume model of port hinterland segmentation. *Sci. Geogr. Sin.* **2014**, *34*, 1169–1175.
38. Guo, J.K.; He, Y.; Hou, Y.J. Spatial connection and regional difference of the coastal container port shipping network of China. *Prog. Geogr.* **2018**, *37*, 1499–1509.
39. Monios, J.; Wilmsmeier, G. Between path dependency and contingency: New challenges for the geography of port system evolution. *J. Transp. Geogr.* **2016**, *51*, 247–251. [CrossRef]
40. Wang, L.H.; Zhu, Y. The evolution of China's international maritime network based on the "21st Century Maritime Silk Road". *Acta Geogr. Sin.* **2017**, *72*, 2265–2280.
41. Karsten, C.V.; Pisinger, D.; Ropke, S.; Brouer, B.D. The time constrained multi-commodity network flow problem and its application to liner shipping network design. *Transp. Res. Part E* **2015**, *76*, 122–138. [CrossRef]
42. Seth, S.; Feng, Q. Assessment of port efficiency using stepwise selection and window analysis in data envelopment analysis. *Marit. Econ. Logist.* **2020**, *22*, 536–561. [CrossRef]
43. Barros, C.P. The measurement of efficiency of Portuguese sea port authorities with DEA. *Int. Transp. Econ.* **2003**, *30*, 335–354.
44. Wu, J.; Liang, L. Performances and benchmarks of container ports using data envelopment analysis. *Int. J. Shipp. Transp. Logist.* **2009**, *1*, 295–310. [CrossRef]
45. Li, L.B.; Liu, J.; Li, C.H. Dynamic efficiency evaluation of the main coastal ports in the mainland, Taiwan and China—Based on DEA-Malmquist total factor productivity index. *Soft Sci.* **2011**, *25*, 80–84.
46. Wang, L.; Meng, H. Efficiency comparison between inland ports and coastal ports in China—Based on common boundary and sequence SBM-DEA. *Soft Sci.* **2013**, *27*, 90–95.
47. Gao, L.; Sun, Q. Operation efficiency evaluation of listed port companies in China. *J. Coast. Res.* **2020**, *111*, 67–79. [CrossRef]
48. Teixeira, P.; Sá, J.C.; Silva, F.J.G.; Ferreira, L.P.; Santos, G.; Fontoura, P. Connecting lean and green with sustainability towards a conceptual model. *J. Clean. Prod.* **2021**, *322*, 129047. [CrossRef]
49. Ikram, M.; Ferasso, M.; Sroufe, R.; Zhang, Q.Y. Assessing green technology indicators for cleaner production and sustainable investments in a developing country context. *J. Clean. Prod.* **2021**, *322*, 129090. [CrossRef]
50. Lin, S.H.; Zhao, X.F.; Wu, J.X.; Liang, F.C.; Li, J.H.; Lai, R.J.; Hsieh, J.C.; Tzeng, G.H. An evaluation framework for developing green infrastructure by using a new hybrid multiple attribute decision-making model for promoting environmental sustainability. *Socio-Econ. Plan. Sci.* **2021**, *75*, 100909. [CrossRef]
51. Xie, X.M.; Zhu, Q.W. How can green innovation solve the dilemmas of "Harmonious Coexistence"? *Manag. World* **2021**, *37*, 128–149.
52. Parida, S.; Ananthram, S.; Chan, C.; Brown, K. Green office buildings and sustainability: Does green human resource management elicit green behaviors? *J. Clean. Prod.* **2021**, *329*, 129764. [CrossRef]
53. Ranjbar, N.; Balali, A.; Valipour, A.; Yunusa-Kaltungo, A.; Edwards, R.; Pignatta, G.; Moehler, R.; Wei, S. Investigating the environmental impact of reinforced-concrete and structural-steel frames on sustainability criteria in green buildings. *J. Build. Eng.* **2021**, *43*, 103184. [CrossRef]

54. Luo, J.H.; Cui, E.Y.; Ji, J.H. Study on environmental efficiency evaluation of China's eight container ports considering CO_2 emission—Based on SBM-DEA model. *Sci. Technol. Manag. Res.* **2014**, *21*, 66–69.
55. Qi, Q.; Jiang, Y.; Wang, D. Evaluation of port unified efficiency based on RAM-DEA model for port sustainable development. *J. Coast. Res.* **2020**, *104*, 724–729. [CrossRef]
56. Liu, J.G.; Wang, X.; Guo, J. Port efficiency and its influencing factors in the context of pilot free trade zones. *Transp. Policy* **2021**, *105*, 67–79. [CrossRef]
57. Quintano, C.; Mazzocchi, P.; Rocca, A. Examining eco-efficiency in the port sector via non-radial data envelopment analysis and the response based procedure for detecting unit segments. *J. Clean. Prod.* **2020**, *259*, 120979. [CrossRef]
58. Tovar, B.; Wall, A. Environmental efficiency for a cross-section of Spanish port authorities. *Transp. Res. Part D Transp. Environ.* **2019**, *75*, 170–178. [CrossRef]
59. Wang, B.; Wu, Y.R.; Yan, P.F. Environmental efficiency and environmental total factor productivity growth in China's regional economies. *Econ. Res. J.* **2010**, *45*, 95–109.
60. Fukuyama, H.; Weber, W.L. A directional slacks—Based measure of technical inefficiency. *Socio-Econ. Plan. Sci.* **2009**, *4*, 274–287. [CrossRef]
61. Oh, D.H. A Metafrontier approach for measuring an environmentally sensitive productivity growth index. *Energy Econ.* **2010**, *32*, 146–157. [CrossRef]
62. Kuang, H.B. Cost efficiency evaluation of China's port listed companies based on super efficiency CCR-DEA. *Manag. Sci. China* **2007**, *3*, 142–148.
63. Wang, Y.; Wu, M. Research on the efficiency of China's port listed companies—Based on two-stage network data envelopment analysis model. *China's Circ. Econ.* **2016**, *30*, 53–61.
64. Feng, F.; Chen, L.; Huang, H. Measurement and improvement path of operational efficiency of China's port listed companies—Based on SBM-DEA model. *China's Circ. Econ.* **2017**, *31*, 106–112.
65. Du, H.; Zhou, L.T.; Kuang, H.B. Research on port operation efficiency based on three-stage super efficiency DEA. *Tech. Econ.* **2021**, *40*, 22–35.
66. Zheng, B.Y.; Yang, H.F. One belt, one road, China coastal city port efficiency evaluation based on DEA game cross efficiency-Tobit model. *Math. Stat. Manag.* **2021**, *40*, 502–514.
67. Zhu, P.Y.; Huang, X.H.; Wang, S.; Lin, C.Y. Comparative study on port efficiency of China's pilot free trade zone. *Asia-Pac. Econ. Rev.* **2017**, *5*, 98–104.
68. Lu, J.; Li, Y.X. Port efficiency, trade liberalization and transaction scale distribution of China's imports. *Int. Econ. Trade Explor.* **2018**, *34*, 35–54.
69. Han, B.; Liu, F.M.; Kuang, H.B. Evaluation of enterprise value-added efficiency in the context of homogeneous competition-a case study of listed port enterprises in China. *Sci. Res. Manag.* **2021**, *42*, 55–64.
70. Liu, Y.; Wang, C.X. Efficiency evaluation of container port group based on undesirable output network DEA. *Syst. Eng.* **2018**, *36*, 121–126.
71. Sun, J.; Yuan, Y.; Yang, R.; Ji, X.; Wu, J. Performance evaluation of Chinese Port Enterprises under significant environmental concerns: An extended DEA-based analysis. *Transp. Policy* **2017**, *60*, 75–86. [CrossRef]
72. Wang, T.; Liang, J. Evaluation of port energy efficiency based on undesirable output super efficiency SBM model. *J. Wuhan Univ. Technol. (Gen. Sci. Eng. Ed.)* **2018**, *42*, 637–641.
73. Färe, R.; Grosskopf, S.; Pasurka, C. Accounting for air pollution emissions in measuring state manufacturing productivity growth. *J. Reg. Sci.* **2001**, *41*, 381–409. [CrossRef]
74. Teng, Z.W.; Hu, Z.B.; Jiang, X.Y. Study on the difference and convergence of carbon productivity in China's service industry. *J. Quant. Tech. Econ.* **2017**, *34*, 78–94.

International Journal of
Environmental Research and Public Health

MDPI

Article

Air Pollution, Health Shocks and Labor Mobility

Yi Zhang [1], Tao Shi [2,*], Ai-Jun Wang [3,*] and Qi Huang [4]

1 School of Business, Jiangsu Normal University, Xuzhou 221116, China; zy2021@jsnu.edu.cn
2 Economics Institute, Henan Academy of Social Science, Fengchan Road 21, Zhengzhou 450002, China
3 Economics School, Zhongnan University of Economics and Law, Nanhu Avenue 182, Wuhan 430073, China
4 Zhengzhou Central Sub-Branch of People's Bank of China, Shangwu Road 21, Zhengzhou 450000, China; huangqixl@163.com
* Correspondence: taoshi_ccp@163.com (T.S.); aijunwang123@zuel.edu.cn (A.-J.W.)

Abstract: The health shocks caused by air pollution seriously interfere with people's economic life. Based on the air pollution index and health shock index calculated by the principal component entropy weight method, this article analyzes the impact of air pollution on labor mobility, and adopts the mediation effect model to test the mediation effect of health shocks, using the threshold model to analyze the time and the health shocks threshold effect of air pollution on labor mobility. Its conclusions are as follows: (1) Air pollution has a negative impact on the net inflow of labor mobility, and the net inflow of labor mobility decreases between 24.9% and 44.7% on average for each unit increase in the health shocks of air pollution. (2) The impact of air pollution on labor mobility is all caused by health shocks; the health shocks are also an important factor influencing the decrease in the labor mobility supply across provinces, and the different health levels of the migrating individuals due to air pollution. (3) The health shocks of air pollution have a single-time threshold effect on labor mobility, and the health shocks of air pollution in China have intensified after 2010, confirming that China's Lewis turning point was 2010. (4) The attraction effect of stable and higher regional real income will partially offset the repulsion effect of health shocks of air pollution on labor mobility, when the health-shocks index of air pollution exceeds the threshold value of 1.9873. Finally, the policy implications of the health shocks of air pollution on labor mobility are also formulated.

Keywords: air pollution; health shocks; labor mobility; mediating effect; threshold effect

Citation: Zhang, Y.; Shi, T.; Wang, A.-J.; Huang, Q. Air Pollution, Health Shocks and Labor Mobility. *IJERPH* **2022**, *19*, 1382. https://doi.org/10.3390/ijerph19031382

Academic Editors: Jie Chen, Qian Zhou, Ting Zhang and Petri Böckerman

Received: 3 November 2021
Accepted: 21 January 2022
Published: 26 January 2022

1. Introduction

The environment, health and reasonable labor mobility are currently hot social topics. Since 1949, the scale of labor mobility has been unprecedented, and it has become an important factor for promoting social and economic development [1]. From 1982 to 2015, China's labor mobility scale first increased and then decreased, with the total population migration across counties enlarging 4.1 times from 1982 to 2010, and decreasing 9.59% from 2010 to 2015 [2], becoming the main labor force for China's economic development, especially in developed regions such as Guangdong, Shanghai and Beijing. Indeed, the characteristics of labor mobility in China can be divided into three stages. Firstly, the early stage of labor mobility (1949–1978). In this stage, only a small number of migrant workers can be migrated to another place, especially to the cities, and labor mobility is mainly based on the government's planned policies to serve social stability and economic development. Secondly, the middle stage of labor mobility (1979–2010). In this stage, laborers begin to flee their regulated workplace for a better income, and the labor mobility scale across regions is growing. Both China's labor mobility index and the annual average inflow of the mobile population are continuously increasing before 2010, as shown in Figure 1. Thirdly, the transition stage of labor mobility (after 2011). In this stage, the characteristics of health-type mobility appeared, and health demands come to be a more important factor influencing labor's mobility.

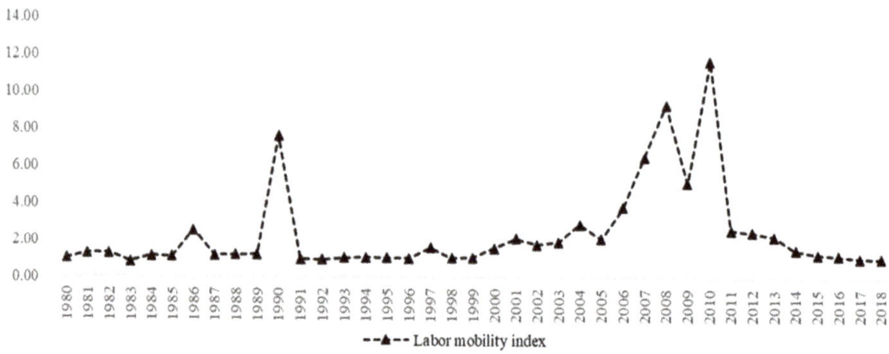

Figure 1. The trend of the labor mobility index and the annual average inflow of floating population in China from 1980 to 2018. Note: According to the calculation formula of net mobility rate in the Section 3.2.2, the annual results of each province were taken as the natural index, and then the annual average value of the whole country was calculated to represent the inflow index.

In the third stage, the deaths caused by air pollution increased. According to the Lancet's "Global Burden of Disease Report 2019," China's PM2.5 caused 1.2 million early deaths and 25 million disabled-adjusted life-year losses in 2019. As the threat of air pollution and health damage continues to increase, the average annual labor mobility index (net labor inflow rate) in each province of China has continued to decline, and this indicates increased labor fleeing as shown in Figure 2(the graph is consistent with Zhang and Wang (2020) [3]). Based on this phenomenon, scholars believe that air pollution has a significant negative impact on labor mobility [4–6].

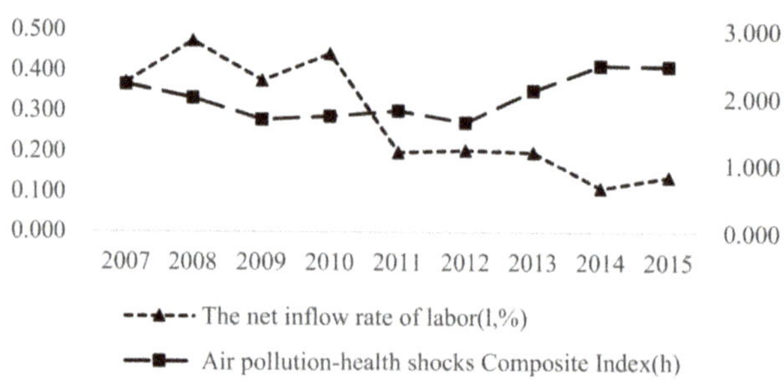

Figure 2. The trend of the net inflow rate of labor mobility and the air pollution-health shocks composite index from 2007 to 2015. Note: (1) The net inflow rate of labor mobility is calculated according to Formula (7) below, which is the average value of each year. (2) The air pollution-health shocks composite index is calculated in Section 3.2.2.

The negative relationship between air pollution and labor mobility refutes the view of surplus labor depletion under the "Lewis Turning Point" from the perspective of exogenous influence. Especially in the developed and eastern coastal regions in China, people decide their own labor supply on facts as health and social investment, the labor income, the leisure replacement and healthy life, and we can also see the counter-urbanization phenomenon known as "fleeing Beijing, Shanghai and Guangzhou" [6]. However, there are few empirical studies on the relationship between air pollution, health and labor mobility. Most studies do not provide direct evidence to confirm air pollution's influence on labor mobility through damaging health, and focus especially on the healthy migration effect and the salmon bias effect after the self-selection of Latin immigrants (also known as the Hispanic paradox) and are limited to using the pollution amount or concentration and other related variables to construct indicators for indirect analysis [5,7]. The health paradox of Latino immigrants (the Hispanic paradox) refers to the fact that Latino immigrants with lower socioeconomic status in the United States who have limited access to healthcare generally have a higher health level than non-Hispanic whites [8,9]. Indeed, facing the health shocks caused by air pollution, the probability of labor migration across provinces is higher than that across counties, and health shocks on labor mobility are more sensitive in larger geographical regions [10]. Therefore, this article focuses on providing direct evidence of air pollution's impact on labor mobility, anchoring the health shocks perspective in provincial samples. The potential contributions of this article are as follows: Firstly, using the principal component-entropy weight combination method, this article calculated the air pollution index and the health shocks effect index, and provided a direct provincial sample for empirical analysis. Second, using the mediation effect model, we found that labor will be impacted by health shocks when it suffers from air pollution. Labor mobility will be promoted to change migration decisions, and the inflow rate of labor mobility across provinces will decrease. These findings will provide additional evidence for the debate on the Lewis turning point and the exploration of the health paradox of Latin immigrants.

The remaining sections of this article are as follows: Section 2 is the literature review, summarizing the methods and conclusions about the relationship between air pollution, health shocks and labor mobility, and providing related hypotheses. Section 3 is the methodology, introducing the mediation effect method and data resources and description. Section 4 reveals the result, showing the impact of air pollution on labor mobility, and the mediation effect of health shocks and the threshold effect. Section 5 is the discussion, focusing on the study's results and their limitations. Finally, in Section 6, the conclusions and policy implications are provided.

2. Literature Review

2.1. The Impact of Air Pollution on Health

Scholars have studied the relationship between different air pollutants and health, and found that air pollution has a significantly positive relationship with the death rate [11], the infant mortality rate [12], respiratory diseases [13], cardiovascular diseases [14], dermatology [15], ocular surface diseases (Jung et al., 2018) [16], neurological diseases [17], cancer [18] and other chronic diseases [19]. For example, Chay and Greenstone (2003) [20] asserted that with a 1% decrease in the total suspended particulate (TSP) the infant mortality would decrease 0.35–0.45%, and indicated a non-linear relationship between air pollution and infant mortality at the county level. Based on a sample of 88 large cities in the United States, Dominici et al. (2002) [21] argued that the mortality rate would increase 0.5% if the PM10 concentration rate on the previous day increased about 10 $\mu g/m^3$, and indicated a linear relationship between concentration and response. Song et al. (2019) [14] further found that hospitalized patients with hypertension increased by 0.56%, 0.31%, 1.18%, 0.40% and 0.03%, while the PM2.5 (lag06), PM10 (lag06), NO_2 (lag03), O_3 (lag06) and CO (lag04) increased by 10 $\mu g/m^3$, respectively.

2.2. The Impact of Health on Labor Mobility

In the 19th century, based on the law of population migration, E. G. Ravenstein first proposed the population movement theory [22]. In the 1960s, E. S. Lee (1966) [23] further perfected R. Herberle's push–pull theory and argued that population migration could be attributed to the joint action of push and pull forces. Poor living conditions and various reasons push people away from their hometown, and good expectations pull people to new places. At the level of occupation, Thomas et al. (2006) [24] studied an intervention experiment in Indonesia, and the results showed that the improved health status significantly increased the probability of male rural residents participating in migrant work. Adhvaryu and Nyshadham (2017) [25] further suggested that most people with long-term illness experienced a shift from agricultural labor to enterprise labor, and sick people are more productive in business than on farms, and confirmed that disease is a push force for labor mobility. However, other scholars have opposite views. Jing et al. (2018) [26] found that health status had little impact on rural migrants' choice of self-employment and employment.

In addition, based on the population migration theory, other scholars have explored the impact of health on labor mobility from the perspective of the Latino health paradox. The health paradox of Latin immigrants can be described as immigrants with lower socioeconomic status and fewer medical resources having better health outcomes than the local residents [27]. Many scholars generally believe that individual health status will significantly affect labor migration or mobility decisions, and have proposed the health depletion effect, the health migration effect [28,29] and the salmon bias effect [30]. The health migration effect suggests that workers with a good health status are more likely to leave home, and the salmon bias effect suggests that workers in poorer health status are more likely to return home.

However, scholars do not fully support the viewpoints above. Indeed, when the labor supply is subjected to a health shock such as an epidemic, there is a temporary or permanent reduction in the labor supply due to the direct and indirect effects of illness and death. At the same time, the fear of being infected by others can lead to a decline in labor participation, and the closure of employment places [31]. If labor suffers a health shock such as COVID-19, this is likely to reduce the mobility inflow rate of different regions [32].

2.3. The Impact of Environmental Pollution on Labor Mobility

Since the early 1990s, scholars have been increasingly concerned about the relationship between environmental pollution and labor mobility. Among them, based on the dual economic structure framework, Harris and Todaro (1970) [33] proposed the classical Harris–Todaro model ("H–T model"), and discussed the relationship between labor transfer and environmental pollution. Based on the H–T model, some scholars have studied the relationship between the pollution and labor mobility from the industry sector perspective [34] and have confirmed that pollution in the industrial sector will affect the marginal income of the labor transfer, and further affect the labor mobility scale between urban and rural regions. Several scholars have studied the relationship between pollution and labor mobility from the population migration and the spatial mobility perspective [35] and have argued that a better quality of environment, including solid waste, the air, water, noise pollution and other factors, is the main factor in the interregional migration of individuals. That is different from the traditional view that economic factors are the dominant contributor to labor mobility.

Focusing on China's labor mobility problem, most scholars have explored the influence of environment on labor mobility at a geo-space level. Their conclusions have shown that the natural environment has gradually become an attractive factor for labor immigrants [36], and air pollution exerts an important influence on labor mobility, especially for male people of a younger age with higher education, high skills or high-income [6]. However, they used air pollution or environmental pollution variables, such as haze and exhaust emissions, to explain the main impacts on labor mobility, and ignored the impact mechanism of the health shocks caused by air pollution on labor mobility. For example, using micro-survey samples in the Beijing-Tianjin-Hebei region, Lu et al. (2018) [7] argued that haze pollution has caused the technical talent loss in the Beijing-Tianjin-Hebei region. Few scholars have paid attention to the impact of environmental pollution on labor mobility between industries. The impact of environmental pollution on the employment scale shows an inverted U-shaped relationship, and the degree of environmental pollution also has an obvious impact on the employment structure of the industry [37].

To sum up, there are many studies on the relationship between air pollution and the health, the health and labor mobility, or air pollution and labor mobility, respectively. However, there are few studies on the relationship between air pollution, the health and labor mobility simultaneously. Meanwhile, studies on the relationship between air pollution and health lack the health-risk-generation perspective at the macro level, and the studies on the relationship between health and labor mobility do not further explain the health paradox of Latino immigrants due to the influence of air pollution. Finally, most studies on labor mobility involving the Lewis turning point are from the perspective of marginal productivity changes [38], and do not consider the impact of exogenous factors. Therefore, this article will focus on the relationship between air pollution, health and labor mobility at a macro level. The theoretical framework is shown in Figure 3.

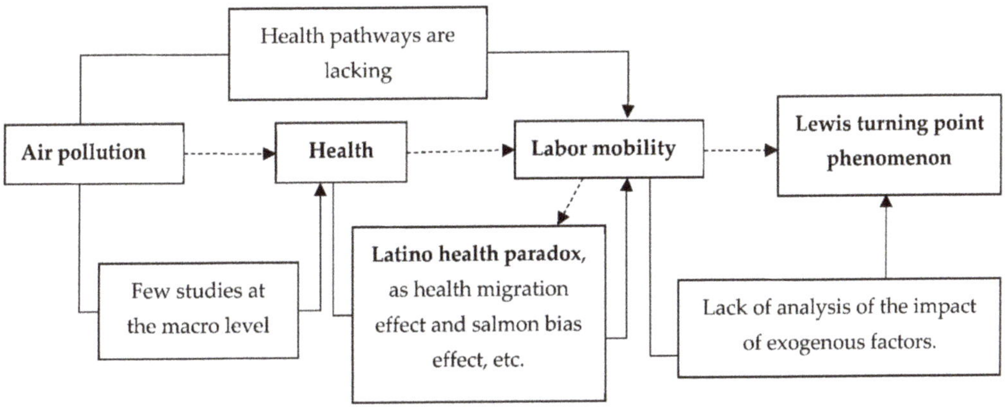

Figure 3. The theoretical framework.

2.4. Research Hypothesis

Indeed, China's labor mobility index has declined, which is especially obvious in the labor force fleeing Beijing, Shanghai and Guangzhou, and labor shortages have restricted the high-quality development of the eastern region. However, areas such as eastern China and north of the Huai River are heavily polluted [11]. According to the reference above, there is a significant functional relationship between air pollution, health shocks and labor mobility. Therefore, we propose hypothesis H1 and H2:

Hypothesis 1 (H1). *Air pollution restricts labor mobility across provinces, and health shocks play a mediating role in that process.*

Hypothesis 2 (H2). *The impact of the health shocks of air pollution on labor mobility varies significantly in different regions. The severely polluted areas in eastern China and north of the Huai River, etc., perform more prominently.*

Furthermore, as mentioned above, China's labor mobility index and the annual average inflow of floating population fluctuated upward before 2010 and then downward. Since the reform and opening up, the continuous advancement of industrial priority and the eastern priority development strategy in China have not only accelerated the development of industrialization and urbanization, but also widened the income gap between different industries and regions, and created large-scale market-oriented spontaneous labor mobility, and the cross-regional scale of labor mobility is growing continuously. The nature of labor mobility is mainly affected by the inequality of development between regions and income equality. Subsequently, although income inequality has been slowly decreasing, the income gap is still obvious, and the average level of health shocks has changed only modestly after 2010, and health inequality between regions has further increased (Figure 4), while the labor mobility index has dropped significantly. Generally, we can conclude that the health shocks of air pollution on labor mobility have time differences, which mainly originated from the income inequality and air pollution [39]. Therefore, we propose hypothesis H3:

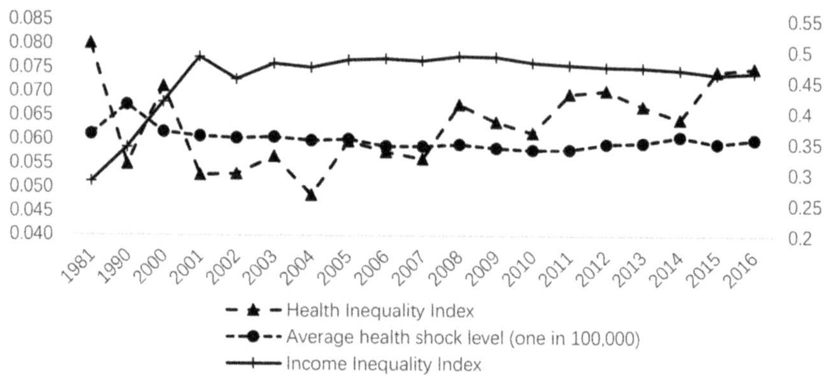

Figure 4. The annual development trend of residents' income and health in China. Note: We used the geometric mean of the mortality rates in each province to represent the average health level, and adopted the annual income Gini coefficient to represent the income inequality index, and calculated the health inequality index in the sample using the Gini coefficient method.

Hypothesis 3 (H3). *The health shocks of air pollution that hinder the inflow of labor mobility across provinces became more significant after 2010, indicating a threshold effect, and the threshold effect mainly originates from income and air pollution.*

3. Materials and Methods

3.1. The Econometric Model

Entropy Method

Firstly, we analyze whether the interaction between the air pollution index and health factors has a significant impact on labor mobility, and the benchmark model is as follows:

$$l_{it} = \rho_0 + \rho_1 pol_{it} + \rho_2 d_{it} + \rho_3 pol_{it} * d_{it} + B * contr + \omega_i + \delta_t + \varepsilon_{it} \quad (1)$$

$$l_{it} = \beta_0 + \beta_1 h_{it} + B_0 * contr + \omega_i + \delta_t + \varepsilon_{it} \quad (2)$$

In Equations (1) and (2), *i*, *t* refers to the province and the year, respectively. The value *l* represents the labor mobility index, pol represents the composite index of air pollution, *d* denotes the health shock index, *pol*∗*d* is the interaction term, *h* represents the coupling index of air pollution and the health shock and ω, δ and ε refer to the individual effect, the time effect and the random effect, respectively. *B* and B_0 represent the coefficient parameter vector of the control variables, ρ_0 and β_0 are the constants, ρ_1, ρ_2, ρ_3 and β_1 represent the coefficient parameters, and contr represents the control variables.

Secondly, we analyze the mediating effect of health shock in the impact of the air pollution on labor mobility, and model as follows:

$$l_{it} = \alpha_0 + \alpha_1 pol_{it} + B_1 * contr + \omega_i + \delta_t + \varepsilon_{it} \quad (3)$$

$$d_{it} = \gamma_0 + \gamma_1 pol_{it} + B_2 * contr1 + \omega_i + \delta_t + \varepsilon_{it} \quad (4)$$

$$l_{it} = \lambda_0 + \lambda_1 pol_{it} + \lambda_2 d_{it} + B_3 * contr + \omega_i + \delta_t + \varepsilon_{it} \quad (5)$$

In Equations (3)–(5), B_1, B_2, B_3, α_1, β_1, γ_1, λ_1 and λ_2 represent the coefficient parameters, respectively. α_0, γ_0, and λ_0 are the constants. *contr*1 represents the control variables. When α_1 in Equation (3) is significant, it indicates that air pollution has an overall influence on labor mobility. Subsequently, Equations (4) and (5) test whether the γ_1, λ_1 and λ_2 are significant, indicating that air pollution affects labor mobility partly by a health shock; if γ_1 and λ_2 are significant on the test, while λ_1 is not, the effect of air pollution on labor mobility is entirely due to a health shock. Finally, if γ_1 or λ_2 show only one or none of the tests to be significant, a Sobel or bootstrap test is required to further determine the mediating effect.

Lastly, we adopt the threshold effect model, to further explore to what level the health shock of air pollution influences labor mobility, and the model as follows:

$$l_{it} = \mu_0 + \mu \times M \times I(\cdot) + \omega_i + \varepsilon_{it} \tag{6}$$

In Equation (6), μ_0 refers to the constant, μ refers to the coefficient and M is the vector set of explanatory variables in Equation (1). $I(\cdot)$ represents the indicative functions of each threshold condition. The time effect is not controlled here, as the threshold condition contains a time variable.

3.2. The Variable Measurement

3.2.1. The Dependent Variables

Referring to Lin and Wang (2006) [40], the population changes caused by the natural population growth were excluded from the total population changes in each region, and the working population aged 15–64 was retained to obtain the net population change scale as the net inflow of labor mobility. Indeed, according to China's Sixth National Census in 2010, 90% of the floating population are of working age [3]. Thus, the net inflow of population multiplied by 90% is an estimate of the net inflow of labor mobility, and can be regarded as the labor mobility index l, and the index l_{it} in region i from time t to t + 1 can be calculated as:

$$l_{it} = \frac{(p_{it+1} - p_{it} \times (1 + n_{it})) \times 90\%}{(p_{it-1} + p_{it})/2} \tag{7}$$

In Equations (7), p refers to the year-end population in one region. $l_{it} > 0$ denotes the net inflow and $l_{it} < 0$ denotes the net outflow.

3.2.2. The Explanatory Variables

The index of health shock effect (d) and the index of air pollution (pol), measured by Zhang and Wang (2020) [3] represent the health shock level (referring to the combined impact level including the air pollution impact and the impact of other factors) and the air pollution level, respectively. h is the coupling measure index of air pollution and health shocks, directly representing or specifically referring to the health shock index of air pollution.

To overcome the different dimensional effects, the multicollinearity and the subjective empowerment arbitrariness of one complex system with more indicators, and avoid the information loss caused by the individual effect and the time effect, we adopt the principal component-entropy weight method. This article analyzes the time and the space value of the selected variables after standardization, and the relative risk values of the two dimensions are, respectively, q and r in the final measure. Meanwhile, in order to better reflect the individual differences among the different samples, the composite index g containing the time and space dimensions is:

$$g = e^q * e^r = e^{(q+r)} \tag{8}$$

Based on the above, to calculate the *pol*, d and h value, the specific measurement steps are as follows:

Firstly, the samples were extracted after standardization, and the principal component dimension reduction analysis was performed to extract the principal components for air pollution and health shock subsystems.

Secondly, the standardized score of the extracted principal components is calculated in each subsystem. Then, using the entropy weight method, the entropy information is extracted from samples, and the weight of each index in the time and the space dimensions is determined.

Finally, using the obtained weight, the relative index values *q*(*pol*), *r*(*pol*), *q*(*d*), *r*(*d*), *q*(*h*) and *r*(*h*) of the spatial and temporal dimensions were calculated, and then the air pollution index (*pol*), the health shock index (*d*), and the coupling index *h* of the air pollution system and the health shock system is calculated as follows:

$$pol = e^{(q(pol)+r(pol))} \tag{9}$$

$$d = e^{(q(d)+r(d))} \tag{10}$$

$$h = e^{(q(h)+r(h))} \tag{11}$$

3.2.3. The Control Variables

The set (contr) of control variables in Equations (1)–(3) and (5) includes:

(1) The real per capita income (gp). The gp is calculated by the proportion of the real per capita GDP on the commodity housing price. Some scholars believe that air pollution is one of the important factors affecting the housing price, and the regional housing price is also one of the important factors influencing labor mobility [41], and the regional housing price factors should be excluded from the regional per capita income. After excluding the regional housing price factors, the region with the higher per capita real income level will be more likely to attract labor inflow [42];

(2) The regional openness (iemport). The iemport is calculated by the proportion of the total imports and exports on GDP, and the region with higher openness will have more job opportunities to attract labor inflow [42];

(3) The regional education level (pere). Education has an important impact on labor migration [43]. The pere is calculated by the weighted education level per capita, and the region with the higher education level is more likely to be a developed region, and to attract labor inflow (the specific calculation formula of per capita education level is as follows: the average number of years of education for the labor force =the proportion of illiterate and semi-illiterate in the employed population *1.5+ the proportion of the employed population receiving primary education);

(4) The industrial structure (thr). Industrial structure is also an important variable affecting labor mobility [44]. The thr is calculated by the proportion of the tertiary industry on GDP. The more developed the tertiary industry is, the more likely it is to attract labor inflow;

(5) The average daily precipitation (rain). The precipitation is also an important factor affecting labor mobility [44]. The rain is calculated by the ratio of annual precipitation to the number of days in the corresponding year. The more the average daily precipitation, the less sunshine there will be, and the more likely it is not conducive to labor inflow;

(6) The per capita road area (perroad). The perroad is calculated by the road area divided by the number of people at the end of the year. The higher the per capita road area, the better urban transportation and infrastructure in one region, the more likely it is to attract labor inflow [45].

The set (contr1) of control variables in Equation (4) includes:

(1) The per capita GDP (pergdp). The pergdp represents the regional economic development level. It is generally believed that the higher the economic level is, the better it is able to resist health shocks [46];

(2) The regional openness (iemport). The higher openness in one region, the more likely it is to acquire new technologies and improve health [47]. However, other scholars have confirmed that higher pollution in one region is always correlated with higher openness [48], which will be worse for resisting health shocks;

(3) The per capita education level (pere). The education level is an important variable affecting the health level [30]. In a region with higher per capita education level, people's health awareness will be stronger than in others, and the better they will be able to resist health shocks;
(4) The average temperature (temp). The temp is substituted by the average temperature of major cities in each province, and it is an important exogenous factor affecting people's health or disease [14];
(5) The number of health technicians per 1000 population (tec). The medical level is also an important variable affecting health level [30]. The higher medical care level in a region, the better it is able to resist health shocks.

3.3. The Sources of Materials

Without special statements, the data used in this article are from provincial statistical yearbooks of China, China Stock Market and Accounting Research Database (CSMAR), China Economic Network Statistical Database, China Statistical Yearbook, China Health Statistics Yearbook, China Environmental Statistics Yearbook and the meteorological monitoring data of Columbia University, etc. In this paper, the sample time ranges from 2007 to 2015; most health indicators' statistic values start from 2007, and this can avoid the exogenous interference of related policies before 2016, as China implemented the Healthy China 2030 Development Strategy in 2016. We also establish panel data from 30 provinces (excluding Hong Kong, Macau, Tibet and Taiwan) from 2008 to 2015, and adjust some variables, such as GDP per capita imports and exports, to avoid influence from inflation. Table 1 shows the descriptive statistics of the variables.

Table 1. The descriptive statistics of the variables.

Variable	Description	Unit	Mean	Std.Dev.	Min	Max
l	The index of labor mobility	%	0.279	1.163	−5.360	5.077
h	The health shocks composite index of air pollution		2.012	0.797	1.085	7.389
pol	Air pollution index		2.029	0.563	1.164	4.552
d	Health shock index		2.206	0.715	1.284	6.185
pergdp	Per capita GDP	yuan/person	33,514.940	19,462.150	6915.000	106,184.200
gp	Per capita real income level	m^2/person	6.467	2.013	2.300	14.075
iemport	The ratio of total imports and exports to GDP	%	0.146	0.224	0.000	1.101
pere	Average years of education	year/person	10.864	1.128	8.267	14.610
thr	Ratio of output value of tertiary industry to GDP	%	41.342	8.823	28.600	79.653
rain	Average daily precipitation	100 million m^3	4.954	3.467	0.151	13.965
perroad	Road area per capita	m^2/person	13.543	4.289	4.040	25.820
temper	Average temperature	Celsius	14.474	5.045	4.300	25.333
tec	Number of health technicians per 1000 population		5.094	1.912	2.140	15.460

Note: The sample size is 270.

4. Results

4.1. Characterization of Main Variables

Based on the measurement results of the above methods, from the annual average of the past three years (see Figure 5), the air pollution index (*pol*), health shock index (*d*) and the health shocks composite index of air pollution (*h*) vary greatly among provinces, and the index of labor mobility (*l*) is generally low.

Furthermore, the annual average growth rate of the labor mobility index (l_z, $l_{zt} = (l_t/l_{t-1}) - 1$), the annual average value of air pollution index (*pol*), the annual average value of the health shock index (*d*) and the annual average value of the health shocks composite index of air pollution (*h*) of each province are shown in Figure 6. We can see that the l_z line shows a positive tendency, and other three lines are showing a negative trend, indicating that the growth in the health shocks of air pollution may be closely related to the decline of the net inflow rate of labor mobility. We will confirm this in the next section.

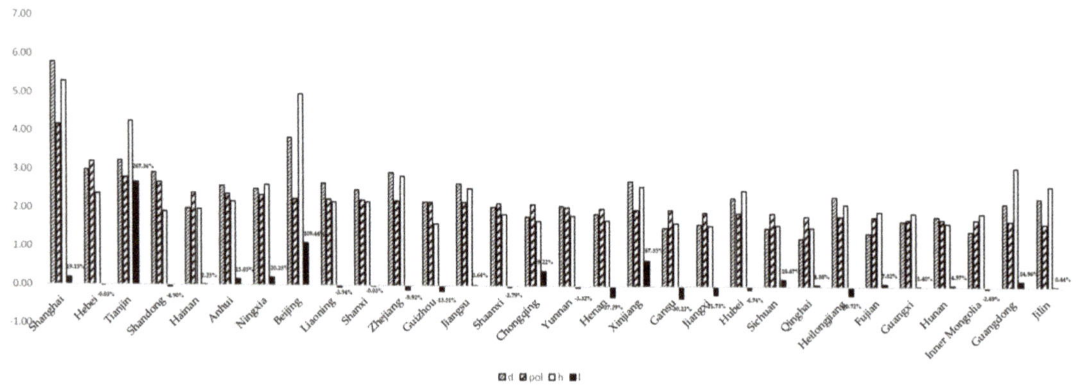

Figure 5. The changes of key variables in 30 provinces in recent years (average value in recent three years). Note: Because the labor mobility index is generally low, numerical labels have been added to show the results clearly; others have not been added.

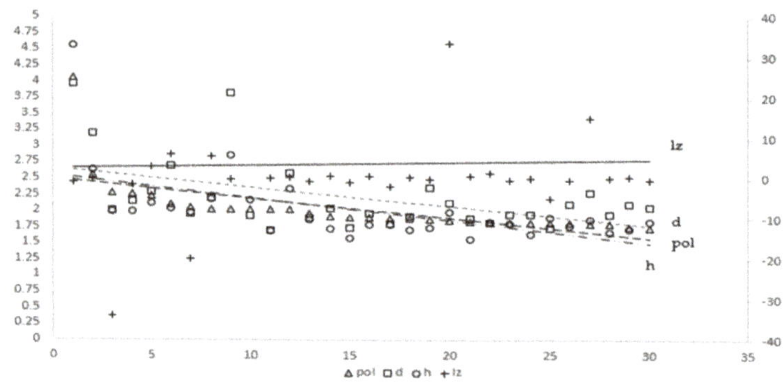

Figure 6. The annual average value and trend of several index measurement results in various provinces. Note: The serial numbers 1–30 on the x-axis represent Shanghai, Tianjin, Hebei, Jiangsu, Ningbo, Guangdong, Shanxi, Liaoning, Beijing, Shandong, Guizhou, Zhejiang, Chongqing, Hainan, Sichuan, Yunnan, Henan, Qinghai, Fujian, Guangzhou, Gansu, Anhui, Shaanxi, Inner Mongolia, Hunan, Hubei, Xinjiang, Jiangxi, Heilongjiang and Jilin.

4.2. The Baseline Results

A fixed or random model is adopted according to the Hausman test. A dynamic system GMM model was adopted to estimate the first-order hysteresis effect and to reduce the endogenous problem, such as the potential autocorrelation effect of the net inflow rate of labor mobility, and the potential impact of the agglomeration effect formed by labor mobility on environmental pollution [49], and Table 2 shows the estimation results.

In column (1), the coefficient of the air pollution index is significantly negative at the 5% confidence level, indicating that air pollution will reduce the net inflow of labor mobility, and the negative impact is further confirmed in column (4). As shown in column (4), for each 1% increase in the air pollution index, the net inflow of labor mobility will drop by 47.6%, significant at a 1% confidence level. Using a sample of 285 cities in China, Zhang (2019) [50] suggested that the number of employed workers will be reduced 33.45% with the SO_2 emissions increasing 1%, and our results further confirm the negative impact of air pollution on labor mobility. Using the comprehensive calculated air pollution, not a single pollutant, as the air pollution index, the negative impact in our article is larger than others. In column (2), the coefficient of the interaction term between air pollution and health shocks is significantly negative at the 5% confidence level. This implies that the net inflow of labor mobility will be reduced by the interaction of air pollution and health shocks, and the endogenous problem underestimates the negative impact shown in column (5). In column (5), when controlling other conditions, for each 1% increase in the interaction item of air pollution and health shocks, the net labor inflow of labor mobility will drop by 15.7%, significant at the 1% confidence level. In column (3), the coefficient of the health shock index of air pollution is significantly negative at the 5% confidence level, indicating that the net inflow of labor mobility will be decreased 24.9%, with a 1% increase in the health shock index of air pollution. In column (6), a dynamic system GMM model is adopted that confirms the negative impact of the health shock index of air pollution on the net inflow of labor mobility. Therefore, we can see that the health shocks of air pollution are a significant hindrance to the net inflow of labor mobility, and confirm the related hypothesis in H1.

Table 2. The baseline main results of OLS and GMM models.

Var.	(1)	(2)	(3)	(4)	(5)	(6)
	OLS(FE)	OLS(RE)	OLS(FE)	GMM	GMM	GMM
L.l				0.338 **	0.379 **	0.287 **
				(2.23)	(2.46)	(2.25)
pol	−0.308 **	−0.100		−0.476 ***	−0.207	
	(−2.50)	(−0.92)		(−3.13)	(−1.49)	
d		−0.358*			−0.165	
		(−1.75)			(−0.76)	
pol∗d		−0.172 **			−0.157 ***	
		(−2.19)			(−2.87)	
h			−0.249 **			−0.429 ***
			(−2.58)			(−4.67)
lngp	1.415 **	0.446	1.148 **	0.334 *	0.309	0.496 ***
	(2.46)	(1.60)	(2.10)	(1.87)	(1.15)	(2.95)
iemport	3.811 ***	1.539 ***	2.844 ***	1.068 **	1.166 **	0.938 **
	(4.36)	(3.36)	(3.81)	(2.46)	(2.02)	(2.31)
lnpere	4.529 **	3.714 ***	3.486 **	0.546	0.752	1.016
	(2.72)	(2.97)	(2.27)	(0.66)	(0.95)	(1.11)
lnthr	0.193	0.982	0.038	0.496	0.549	0.973 *
	(0.22)	(1.16)	(0.04)	(1.21)	(1.09)	(1.80)
lnrain	−0.253	−0.377 ***	−0.297	−0.275 ***	−0.281 **	−0.289 **
	(−0.92)	(−2.62)	(−1.09)	(−2.58)	(−2.12)	(−2.53)
perroad	0.134 *	0.000	0.132 *	−0.013	−0.016	−0.020
	(1.98)	(0.00)	(2.00)	(−0.85)	(−1.00)	(−0.96)
Constant	−14.601 **	−11.485 ***	−11.040 *	−2.270	−3.023	−5.413 **
	(−2.43)	(−2.86)	(−2.04)	(−0.80)	(−1.19)	(−2.06)
Time effect	Y	Y	Y	Y	Y	Y
Observations	270	270	270	240	240	240
Number of provinces	30	30	30	30	30	30
R2	0.172	0.5574	0.183			
F/Wald	3.490	548.56	2.847	115.33	386.24	137.56
AR(1)				0.047	0.041	0.042
AR(2)				0.133	0.147	0.176
Hansen				0.996	1.000	0.987

Note: *, **, *** refers to significance at the level of 10%, 5% and 1%, respectively. The number in parentheses is t value. The Wald values in the GMM model are shown by F/Wald, and the others shown by F values. The same below.

4.3. The Mediation Effect Results

Based on Equations (3) to (5), the mechanism effect results are shown in Table 3. The variable pol has a significant negative impact on the net inflow of labor mobility at the 5%

confidence level in column (7). In column (8), the coefficient of the air pollution index is significantly positive at the 10% confidence level, indicating that there is a negative impact of the air pollution index on health shocks, and health shocks will be increased 16.5% with an air pollution index increase of 1%. The coefficient of health shocks is significantly negative at the 1% confidence level in column (9). However, the coefficient of the air pollution index is not significant in column (9), which means that it exerted a full mediation effect. Therefore, it can be concluded that the impact of air pollution on the labor inflow is all caused by health shocks, and that rectifying health shocks is also an important factor influencing the decrease in the labor supply and migrating individuals with different health levels under different air pollution conditions.

Table 3. The estimation results of the mediation effect.

Var.	(7)	(8)	(9)
	Labor Mobility	**Health Shocks**	**Labor Mobility**
pol	−0.308 **	0.165 *	−0.139
	(−2.50)	(1.97)	(−1.11)
d			−0.546 ***
			(−3.16)
lngp	1.415 **		0.872 *
	(2.46)		(1.87)
iemport	3.811 ***	−2.052 ***	1.956 **
	(4.36)	(−2.92)	(2.34)
lnpere	4.529 **	−2.472	−1.836
	(2.72)	(−1.50)	(−1.43)
lnthr	0.193		−0.436
	(0.22)		(−0.77)
lnrain	−0.253		−0.157
	(−0.92)		(−0.76)
perroad	0.134 *		0.081
	(1.98)		(1.66)
lnpergdp		−2.406 *	
		(−1.78)	
lntemper		0.155	
		(0.32)	
lntec		−1.236 ***	
		(−3.52)	
Constant	−14.601 **	32.794 **	4.974
	(−2.43)	(2.52)	(1.24)
Number of observations	270	270	270
Adjusted R2	0.172	0.492	0.234
F	3.490 ***	9.484 ***	4.991 ***
Individual effect	Y	Y	Y
Time effect	Y	Y	N

Note: *, **, *** refers to significance at the level of 10%, 5% and 1%, respectively. The number in parentheses is t value. The Wald values in the GMM model are shown by F/Wald, and the others shown by F values. The same below.

In order to further ensure the reliability of mediating effect results, the Sobel test is used in this paper. In accordance with Sobel statistics [51], the Sobel values and the p values were directly calculated using the coefficients of each major effect, and the Sobel 95% confidence interval was [1.616, 1.738], with a significant value of $-1.67 < -0.97$ at the 5% confidence level, confirming the mediating effect. As mentioned above, the health shocks of air pollution restrict the net inflow of labor mobility, and the hypothesis H1 has been verified.

4.4. The Robustness Test

Based on the current study, we adopt two main ways to test the robustness of the results above, and Table 4 shows the result. Firstly, we use one lagging term based on the main explanatory variables, and the results are displayed in column (10) to column (13). We can see that the coefficients of the variables pol*d and h are significantly negative at the 10% (or less) confidence level, and confirm the stability of the results above. Secondly, according to the idea of hedonic price, the housing price can measure the labor inflow in one region [52]. However, the housing price does not reflect the real market demand in China influenced by the housing market bubble. Therefore, Xi and Liang (2015) [53] used the idea of choosing a housing sales area as a proxy variable to analyze the effect of environmental migration. Meanwhile, to weaken the scale effect of the provincial population and the influence of natural growth, again referring to Zhang and Wang (2020) [3], we use the natural logarithm of the commodity housing sales area per (lniv6) as the proxy variable of the labor mobility index, and the results are shown in column (14) to column (17). We can find that most coefficients of the variables h, pol and d are significantly negative at the 10% (or less) confidence level, indicating that the conclusion above is robust.

Table 4. The robustness test results of the baseline model.

Var.	(10)	(11)	(12)	(13)	(14)	(15)	(16)	(17)
	Test Model of Lag Term				Test Model of Tool Variable (lniv6)			
	OLS(RE)	GMM	OLS(FE)	GMM	OLS(FE)	GMM	OLS(RE)	GMM
L.l		0.160 (1.24)		0.218 (1.39)				
L.lniv6						0.679 *** (6.03)		0.705 *** (5.63)
L.pol	−0.147 (−0.83)	−0.109 (−0.79)						
L.d	−0.454 * (−1.80)	−0.295 * (−1.66)						
L.(pol∗d)	−0.278 ** (−2.06)	−0.338 *** (−3.28)						
L.h			−0.428 * (−2.02)	−0.378 ** (−2.00)				
pol					0.038 (0.84)	−0.129 * (−1.74)		
d					−0.163 *** (−3.22)	−0.069 (−1.36)		
pol∗d					−0.051 * (−1.79)	0.052 ** (2.32)		
h							−0.083 *** (−2.72)	−0.146 *** (−2.69)
Control variables	Y	Y	Y	Y	Y	Y	Y	Y
Time effect	Y	Y	Y	Y	Y	Y	Y	Y
Observations	240	240	240	240	270	240	270	240
Number of daima	30	30	30	30	30	30	30	30
r2_a	0.5272		0.204		0.509		0.3546	
F/Wald	509.95	167.75	3.066	68.80	38.98	382.38	141.13	297.09
AR(1)		0.045		0.048		0.002		0.001
AR(2)		0.192		0.090		0.062		0.367
Hansen		0.441		0.160		0.999		0.891

Note: *, **, *** refers to significance at the level of 10%, 5% and 1%, respectively.

In addition, we use the lagged term of the air pollution index and the health shock index to test the medication effect, and Table 5 shows the results. In Table 5, we can see that the impact of air pollution on the net inflow of labor mobility is mainly caused by the mediating effect of health shocks. Thus, the reliability of the mediating effect above is rectified (MacKinnon et al. (1995) [54] set 0.97 as the boundary value at the 5% significance level for testing distribution).

4.5. Results of Regional Conditions

Furthermore, from the regional perspective, we analyze the impact of the health shocks of air pollution (h) on the index of labor mobility (l). Since the Seventh Five-Year Plan, China has been strategically divided into four economic development zones in the east, center, west and northeast. Now, these have been redivided into five major economic belts of "two horizontal and three vertical." In order to find the regional differentiates of the samples, we choose the eastern, central and western economic belts and the Yangtze River economic belt as the heterogenous conditions. Scholars believe that the difference in air pollution on the Huai River between the north and south is large, and the health-damaging effects are also accordingly different [6,11]. Therefore, it is necessary to analyze the regional differentiates according to the boundary of the Huai River. The results are shown in Table 6.

Table 5. The robustness test results of the mediation model.

Var.	(18)	(19)	(20)
	Labor Mobility	Health Shocks [1]	Labor Mobility
L.pol	−0.363 * (−1.77)		−0.226 (−1.36)
pol		0.165 * (1.97)	
L.d			−0.684 *** (−3.91)
Adjust the R^2	0.157	0.492	0.276
F	3.774	9.484	6.690
Individual fixation effect	Y	Y	Y
Time fixation effect	Y	Y	Y
Control variables	Y	Y	Y

Note: *, *** refers to significance at the level of 10% and 1%, respectively. [1] According to the mediation model in Equation (2), the pollution index and the health-shocks index should both be regressed at the same time with a lag, but there are still one-to-one correspondences in the same period. Therefore, the actual operation does not use a lag period.

Table 6. Estimated results of heterogeneous conditions.

Var.	(21)	(22)	(23)	(24)	(25)	(26)
	The Eastern Region	The Central Area	The Western Region	Yangtze River Economic Belt	North of Huai River	South of Huai River
h	−0.331 ** (−2.61)	0.072 (0.54)	0.055 (0.59)	−0.346 *** (−5.43)	−0.318 * (−1.89)	−0.218 (−1.33)
R-squared	0.718			0.363		
Control variables	Y	Y	Y	Y	Y	Y
Individual fixed effect	Y	N	N	Y	N	N
Time fixed effect	Y	Y	N	N	N	N
Observations	99	72	99	99	135	135

Note: *, **, *** refers to significance at the level of 10%, 5% and 1%, respectively.

The health shocks of air pollution in the east have significantly hindered the index of labor mobility. When other conditions remain unchanged, for every unit of the health shocks composite index of air pollution, the net inflow rate of labor mobility drops significantly by 33.1%, while the impact in the central and western regions is not significant. This result indicates that the labor force in the eastern region has fled, facing severe health shocks from air pollution. According to the sample, compared with 2007, in 2015, the net inflow rate of labor mobility in the eastern region declined by 86.35%, while that in the central and western regions increased by 85.24% and 196.44%, correspondently.

The impact of the health shocks of air pollution on labor mobility in the Yangtze River economic belt is significantly negative. When other conditions remain unchanged, for each unit increase in the health shocks of air pollution, the net inflow rate of labor mobility drops significantly by 34.6%. This is in line with the fact that there were 12,158 chemical enterprises above the designated size in the Yangtze River economic belt in 2016, accounting for 46% of those in China, with 41% heavy industry among them, forming a "chemical industry surrounding the river" with high pollution emissions. This result implies that in the process of promoting high-quality development, the negative impact of health shocks from air pollution on labor mobility cannot be ignored in the Yangtze River economic belt. Indeed, the rectification of chemical enterprises in the Yangtze River economic belt also took place after 2015, and this effectively avoided the exogenous effects of labor "flight."

The impact of the health shocks of air pollution on labor mobility in the northern part of the Huai River is significantly negative, while not being significant in the southern part. When other conditions remain unchanged, for each unit increase in the health shocks of air pollution, the net inflow rate of labor mobility in the northern Huai River drops significantly by 31.8 %. Because the heating supply has increased more than air pollution only in the northern part of the Huai River, the impact of health shocks of air pollution on labor mobility in north is accordingly obvious [6]. Therefore, the hypothesis H2 has been verified.

4.6. The Threshold Effect Results

According to the current study, the health shocks caused by air pollution changed greatly after 2010 [39]. We chose 2010 as the time threshold variable, to confirm the impact of the health shock of air pollution on the Lewis inflection point theory. We also chose the health shocks of air pollution as a threshold variable to explore the level of the health shocks of air pollution's influence on labor mobility, and the results are shown in Table 6. In Table 6, whether time or the health shocks of air pollution are the threshold variable, the null hypothesis cannot be accepted without a threshold in the single threshold situation, and the alternative hypothesis test with two or three thresholds fails, indicating that there is one threshold. Tables 7 and 8 show the estimated results with a single threshold variable, and Table 9 shows the impact effect estimation of threshold points.

Table 7. Indicators of driving forces of urban resilience.

Time Threshold Test	RSS	MSE	Fstat	Prob	Crit10	Crit5	Crit1
Single ***	94.515	0.362	34.140	0.000	10.361	12.291	17.772
Double	94.052	0.360	1.280	0.713	7.364	11.480	18.015
Triple	93.761	0.359	0.810	0.673	3.383	4.187	6.473
The threshold test of air pollution-health shocks	RSS	MSE	Fstat	Prob	Crit10	Crit5	Crit1
Single **	101.840	0.390	12.910	0.037	9.811	11.732	16.100
Double	99.492	0.381	6.160	0.360	9.479	11.367	14.554
Triple	90.635	0.347	25.510	0.100	25.442	37.189	60.642

Note: **, *** refers to significance at the level of 5% and 1%, respectively.

Table 8. The estimation of single threshold point.

Th-1	Threshold	Lower	Upper
Time threshold	2010	2009	2011
The threshold of air pollution-health shocks	1.9873	1.9577	2.001

Table 9. The impact effect estimation of threshold points.

Var.	(27)	(28)
	Time Threshold	The Threshold of Air Pollution-Health Shocks
0b._cat#c.h	0.051	−0.523 ***
	(0.54)	(−3.25)
1._cat#c.h	−0.366 ***	−0.389 ***
	(−4.92)	(−3.90)
Control variables	Y	Y
F	11.51	7.281
R-squared	0.284	0.201
Observations	270	270

Note: *** refers to significance at the level of 1%, respectively.

In Table 8, the time threshold value is 2010 at the 5% confidence level. In column (27), the coefficient of the time threshold before 2010 is not significant, and the coefficient of the time threshold after 2010 is significantly negative at the 1% confidence level, indicating that the negative effect of the health shocks of air pollution on labor mobility is not significantly obvious before 2010, and the negative effect is obvious after 2010. This result shows that the health shocks of air pollution in China have intensified since 2010.

In Table 8, the threshold value of the health shocks of air pollution is 1.9873 at the 5% confidence level. In column (28), the coefficient of the variable h is −0.523 and −0.389 at the 1% confidence level, respectively. This indicates that the health shocks composite index of air pollution has one threshold effect on the net inflow of labor mobility, and the impact will decrease when the health shocks of air pollution cross the threshold value. In order to explore this interesting phenomenon, Figure 7 shows the sample distribution of real income level under the two risk types of the health shocks of air pollution (there are two reasons to choose the variable of real income. First, since the reform and opening up, one of the main purposes of labor mobility between urban and rural areas in China is to increase family income, and improve family economic conditions. Second, the persistence of severe air pollution in China has been accompanied with extensive economic growth over a long period, and this growth can be reflected in real income factors. Therefore, we chose the real income as the representative factor of the gravity effect for analysis.). The average per capita real income level in type one and two regions is 6.656 and 6.339, respectively, and the percentage of the value is more than 7.106 (the threshold value of 7.106 is obtained by the clustering per capita real income (gp) according to the K-means). The proportion obtained by contingency table analysis is 31.2% and 31.1%, and the standard deviation value is 1.860 and 2.106, respectively, among them. We can find that the average per capita real income, and its percentage, with a value of more than 7.106 in type two is larger than in type one, while the standard deviation value corresponding to type two is less than type one, indicating that the stable and higher real income plays a strong attracting role on the net inflow of labor mobility when the health shocks of air pollution crosses the threshold value, and the attracting effect partially offsets the repulsion effect of the health shocks of air pollution on the inflow of labor mobility.

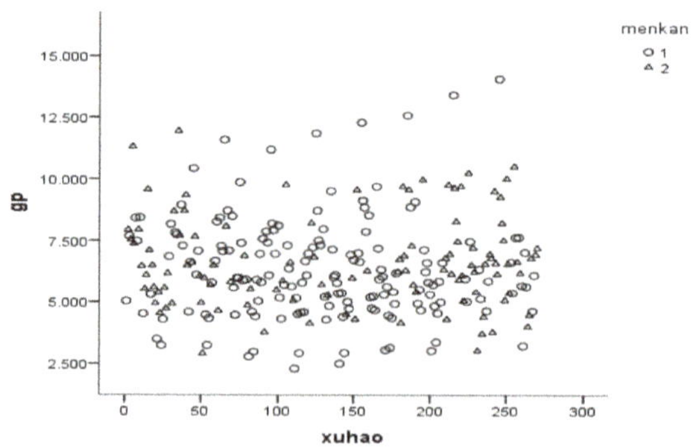

Figure 7. The sample distribution of the real income level under the two risk types of the health shocks of air pollution. Note: Level 1 represents the health shocks of the air pollution risk <1.9873, and level 2 represents ≥1.9873.

In addition, Figure 8 shows the LR statistics value trend estimated for the threshold variable. We can find that the LR values in 4(a) and 4(b) are less than the critical value 7.35 at the 5% confidence level (the dashed line), further confirming the validity of the threshold effect (due to space limitations, other threshold LR test results are omitted). Therefore, hypothesis H3 has been verified, and labor mobility in China is currently simultaneously affected by income and the health shocks of air pollution.

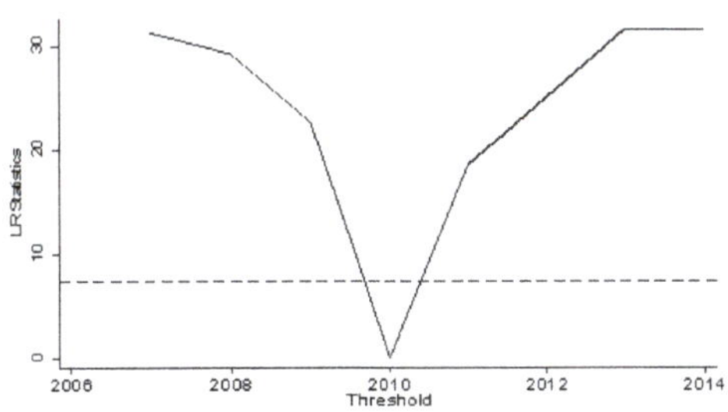

(a) Time

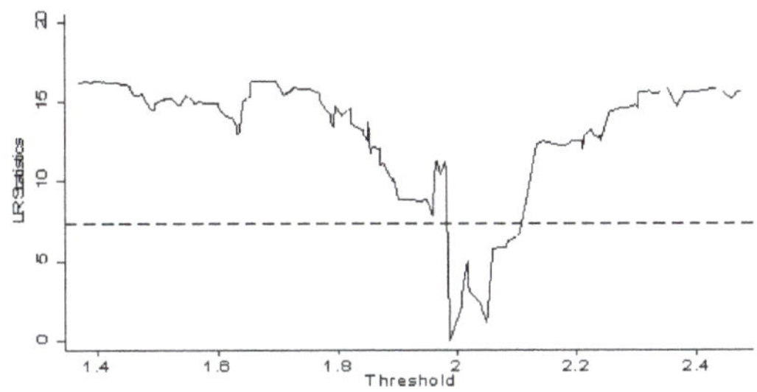

(b) Air pollution-health shocks

Figure 8. The LR statistics value trend estimated for the threshold variable.

5. Discussion

This article used the principal component entropy weighted method to calculate the air pollution composite index and health shock index. Most studies have chosen the AQI or the PM2.5, alternative variables of air pollution, to analyze the impact of air pollution on labor mobility [5,6], but one pollutant, such as in the PM2.5, cannot fully represent the total air pollution, and the calculation process of the AQI index does not eliminate the correlation between different pollutants. The principal component entropy weighted method can identify the most important information of air pollution and health shocks, and avoid the defect of the AQI index and the single air pollutant, to make the conclusion more reliable.

Based on the air pollution composite index and the health shock index above, this article analyzes the impact of air pollution on labor mobility, and the results show that labor mobility is affected by the health shocks of air pollution. Similar results were found by Cropper (1981) [55] and Sun et al. (2019) [39]. However, most studies focused on the impact factors such as the housing price or environmental regulation [56,57] and ignored the impact of health shocks. Adopting the mediation effect model, our results further imply that the impact of air pollution on labor mobility is all caused by health shocks, and health shock is a very important factor of air pollution's impact on labor mobility at the macro level. We can explain these results from two angles: firstly, although individuals have the motivation to invest in their health and human capital, they will display mobility behavior to avoid air pollution, and show more as a moderating effect to avoid health shock [58]. Secondly, when one region faces a serious health shock caused by environmental pollution, it will firstly exclude migrant labor in a poor health condition, and eventually extract the migrant population in a good health condition, resulting in the health level of the migrated population being higher than that of the locals, as described in the Latino health paradox. This phenomenon is similar to the health paradox of Latino immigrants with a health self-screening mechanism [59].

Using the threshold model, our results further show that the health shocks of air pollution on labor mobility across provinces became more significant after 2010, and we confirm the view that China's Lewis turning point was 2010 [60]). However, compared with most current views [61], our results more strongly emphasize health shocks in China's Lewis turning process and its avoidance effect, and argue that the health shocks of air pollution are also an important reason for the decline of labor mobility supply across provinces. It has an obvious difference with the impact of different wages caused by the urban–rural dual structure. Indeed, the impact of the health shocks of air pollution on labor mobility will increase the labor's burden of medical expenses, and decrease the labor's expected income and life expectancy [62]. In addition, when the labor anticipates that there may be a large health shock in one region with severe environmental pollution, the labor will reduce its mobility intention, and the regional labor inflow rate will decline.

Finally, based on the push–pull theory, we conclude that the attraction effect of regional stability and high real income will partially offset the repulsion effect of the health shocks of air pollution on labor mobility, when the health shock index of air pollution exceeds the threshold value of 1.9873, similar to the view of Li et al. (2020) [63]. However, most studies focus only on the negative impact of air pollution on labor mobility. Environmental pollution has null jointness. It is not only a byproduct of production, but also an important input of production [64], especially in developing countries or regions, and the regional economy can quickly achieve extensive growth with a corresponding improvement in pollution levels.

Compared with the empirical conclusions of previous studies, we found similar conclusions, with some differences. We confirm the negative impact of air pollution on labor mobility that Chen et al. found (2017) [5,6]. However, we find the impact of air pollution on labor mobility is all caused by health shocks, and this result is obviously different from most studies, such as that of Kahn and Mansur (2013) [56]. In addition, we find the threshold effect of time and health shocks of air pollution, and confirm China's Lewis turning point was 2010, in a manner similar to Kwan et al. (2018) [60]. However, our study has several limitations. Firstly, the study period ranged from 2008 to 2015. For policy effect interference and data limitation, we did not extend the data to 2020 or 2021, and the statistical bias may underestimate the negative impact of air pollution on labor mobility. Second, the air pollution index and health shock index were calculated by the principal component entropy weight method, and do not consider the weight valued by related experts. This might have resulted in the underestimation of the mediation effect of health shocks. Thirdly, this article did not use the geographical method to display the spatial labor mobility and spatiotemporal impact of air pollution on labor mobility. Therefore, we may have to empirically analyze these in a further study.

6. Conclusions and Policy Implications

6.1. Conclusions

This paper anchors the perspective of health shocks, and discusses the relationship between air pollution, health shocks and labor mobility based on China's macro panel samples. The main conclusions are as follows:

1. Air pollution can have a negative impact on the net inflow of labor mobility, air pollution will reduce the net inflow of labor mobility, the net inflow of labor mobility will be reduced by the coaction with air pollution and health shocks and the net inflow rate of labor mobility will decrease between 24.9% and 44.7% with each unit increase in the health shocks of air pollution. The robustness tests confirm the reliability of these conclusions;
2. The impact of air pollution on labor mobility is entirely caused by health shocks; health shocks are also an important factor influencing the decrease in labor mobility supply across provinces and the different health levels of the migrating individuals with respect to different air pollution;
3. The health shocks of air pollution have a single time threshold effect on labor mobility, and the health shocks of air pollution in China have intensified since 2010. This result confirms China's Lewis turning point was 2010, and health shocks play an important role in China's Lewis turning process and the avoidance effect, similar to the phenomenon of the Latino immigrants' health paradox;
4. When the index of health shocks from air pollution exceeds the threshold value of 1.9873, the attraction effect of regional stability and higher real income will partially offset the repulsion effect of the health shocks of air pollution on labor mobility.

6.2. Policy Implications

Based on the conclusions above, the policy implications are as follows:

1. Increase the investment in air pollution control to reduce the risk of the health shocks caused by air pollution. Although tackling pollution will decrease the economic

growth rate, the higher the health shocks of air pollution, the more they will hamper labor mobility. Therefore, a reasonable increase in investment in air pollution control can reduce the risk of health shocks, stabilize the labor supply and promote high-quality development.

2. Continuously increase the related public expenditure for labor mobility and health protection. This should provide more public expenditure on the floating population, especially. It should highlight the priority development of people's health and pay special attention to environmental health education and training for the floating population. Additionally, improve the public expenditure on medicine and education, to improve the labor's environmental and health awareness, and establish a health shock defense and guarantee mechanism for the floating population to facilitate the rational labor mobility.
3. Implement and strengthen the evaluation of attracting factors, and establish a mechanism to guide labor mobility and work assessment. These results show that the attracting factors, such as stable and higher real income, can partially offset the negative impact of the health shocks of air pollution on labor mobility, and it is necessary for local government to establish an income improving scheme, and especially to control the stability of the housing price and enlarge the supply of the public rental housing to attract more people with a higher education level.

Author Contributions: Conceptualization, Y.Z. and A.-J.W.; data curation, Y.Z. and A.-J.W.; formal analysis, Y.Z., Q.H. and T.S.; funding acquisition, Y.Z. and T.S.; methodology, Y.Z.; software, Y.Z.; supervision, Y.Z. and T.S.; writing—original draft, Y.Z. and T.S.; writing—review and editing, Y.Z. and T.S. All authors have read and agreed to the published version of the manuscript.

Funding: This work was supported by grants from Youth Project of High-end Science and Technology Innovation Think Tank of China Association for Science and Technology "Study on Economic Effect and Optimization Path of 'Air Pollution—Health' in China" (Approval Number: CXY-ZKQN-2019-006); National Social Science Foundation of China (20CJY064).

Institutional Review Board Statement: Not applicable.

Informed Consent Statement: Not applicable.

Data Availability Statement: The data presented in this study are openly available in provincial statistical yearbooks of China, the China Statistical Yearbook, China Health Statistics Yearbook, China Environmental Statistics Yearbook, available at website: https://data.cnki.net/Yearbook/Navi?type=type&code=A, (accessed on 10 November 2021) or http://olap.epsnet.com.cn (accessed on 10 November 2021); China Stock Market and Accounting Research Database, available at website: http://www.gtarsc.com.bbb.hejiantv.cn/#/index (accessed on 10 November 2021); China Economic Network Statistical database, available at website: https://db--cei--cn--dwjj.h.gou5juan.com/ (accessed on 10 November 2021); meteorological monitoring data of Columbia University (Socioeconomic Data and Applications Center (sedac)), available at website: https://sedac.ciesin.columbia.edu/data/set/sdei-global-annual-gwr-pm2-5-modis-misr-seawifs-aod/data-download (accessed on 10 November 2021).

Conflicts of Interest: The authors declare no conflict of interest. The funders had no role in the design of the study; in the collection, analyses, or interpretation of data; in the writing of the manuscript, or in the decision to publish the results.

References

1. Lewis, W.A. Economic development with unlimited supplies of labor. *Manch. Sch.* **1954**, *22*, 139–191. [CrossRef]
2. Ma, Z. Trends of Migration in China in Four-decades of Economic Reform: An Analysis based on Censuses and 1% National Population Surveys. *Chin. J. Popul. Sci.* **2019**, *33*, 16–28. (In Chinese)
3. Zhang, Y.; Wang, A. Health Damage of Air Pollution, Labor Mobility and Economic Growth. *J. Shanxi Univ. Financ. Econ.* **2020**, *42*, 17–30. (In Chinese)
4. Xu, X.; Sylwester, K. Environmental Quality and International Migration. *Kyklos* **2016**, *69*, 157–180. [CrossRef]
5. Chen, S.; Oliva, P.; Zhang, P. *The Effect of Air Pollution on Migration: Evidence from China*; Working Paper No. 24036; National Bureau of Economic Research: Cambridge, MA, USA, 2017.

6. Li, D.; Zhang, Y.; Ma, S. Would smog lead to outflow of labor force? Empirical evidence from China. *Emerg. Mark. Financ. Trade* **2017**, *53*, 1122–1134. [CrossRef]
7. Lu, H.; Yue, A.; Chen, H.; Long, R. Could smog pollution lead to the migration of local skilled workers? Evidence from the Jing-Jin-Ji region in China. *Resour. Conserv. Recycl.* **2018**, *130*, 177–187. [CrossRef]
8. Tong, Y.; Piotrowski, M. Migration and health selectivity in the context of internal migration in China, 1997–2009. *Popul. Res. Policy Rev.* **2012**, *31*, 497–543. [CrossRef]
9. Andersson, G.; Drefahl, S. Long-distance migration and mortality in Sweden: Testing the salmon bias and healthy migrant hypotheses. *Popul. Space Place* **2017**, *23*, e2032. [CrossRef]
10. Ning, G. Self-selection and Regional Employment Income Differentials of Rural Surplus Labor in China: With Reference to the Coming of Lewis Turning Point. *Econ. Res. J.* **2012**, *47*, 42–55. (In Chinese)
11. Chen, Y.; Ebenstein, A.; Greenstonec, M.; Li, H. Evidence on the impact of sustained exposure to air pollution on life expectancy from China's Huai River policy. *Proc. Natl. Acad. Sci. USA* **2013**, *110*, 12936–12941. [CrossRef]
12. Arceo-Gomez, E.O.; Hanna, R.; Oliva, P. *Does the Effect of Pollution on Infant Mortality Differ Between Developing and Developed Countries? Evidence from Mexico City*; Working paper No.18349; National Bureau of Economic Research: Cambridge, MA, USA, 2012.
13. Gauderman, W.J.; Urman, R.; Avol, E.; Berhane, K.; McConnell, R.; Rappaport, E.; Chang, R.; Lurmann, F.; Gilliland, F. Association of Improved Air Quality with Lung Development in Children. *N. Engl. J. Med.* **2015**, *372*, 905–913. [CrossRef] [PubMed]
14. Song, J.; Lu, M.; Lu, J.; Chao, L.; An, Z.; Liu, Y.; Xu, D.; Wu, W. Acute effect of ambient air pollution on hospitalization in patients with hypertension: A time-series study in Shijiazhuang, China. *Ecotoxicol. Environ. Saf.* **2019**, *170*, 286–292. [CrossRef] [PubMed]
15. Krutmann, J.; Liu, W.; Li, L.; Pan, X.; Crawford, M.; Sore, G.; Seite, S. Pollution and skin: From epidemiological and mechanistic studies to clinical implications. *J. Dermatol. Sci.* **2014**, *76*, 163–168. [CrossRef] [PubMed]
16. Jung, S.J.; Mehta, J.S.; Tong, L. Effects of environment pollution on the ocular surface. *Ocul. Surf.* **2018**, *16*, 198–205. [CrossRef] [PubMed]
17. Perera, F.P. Multiple Threats to Child Health from Fossil Fuel Combustion: Impacts of Air Pollution and Climate Change. *Environ. Health Perspect.* **2017**, *125*, 141–148. [CrossRef]
18. Pedersen, M.; Andersen, Z.J.; Stafoggia, M.; Weinmayr, G.; Galassi, C.; Sørensen, M.; Eriksen, K.T.; Tjønnelan, A.; Loft, S.; Jaensch, A.; et al. Ambient air pollution and primary liver cancer incidence in four European cohorts within the ESCAPE project. *Environ. Res.* **2017**, *154*, 226–233. [CrossRef]
19. Tran, H.; Kim, J.; Kim, D.; Choi, M.; Choi, M. Impact of air pollution on cause-specific mortality in Korea: Results from Bayesian Model Averaging and Principle Component Regression approaches. *Sci. Total Environ.* **2018**, *636*, 1020–1031. [CrossRef]
20. Chay, K.Y.; Greenstone, M. The impact of air pollution on infant mortality. *Q. J. Econ.* **2003**, *118*, 1121–1167. [CrossRef]
21. Dominici, F.; Daniels, M.J.; Zeger, S.L.; Samet, J.M. Air Pollution and Mortality: Estimating Regional and National Dose-Response Relationships. *J. Am. Stat. Assoc.* **2002**, *97*, 100–111. [CrossRef]
22. Ravenstein, E.G. The Laws of Migration. *J. Stat. Soc. Lond.* **1885**, *48*, 167–235. [CrossRef]
23. Lee, E.S. A theory of migration. *Demography* **1966**, *3*, 47–57. [CrossRef]
24. Thomas, D.; Frankenberg, E.; Friedman, J.; Habicht, J.; Hakimi, M.; Ingwersen, N.; Jaswadi; Jones, N.; McKelvey, C.; Pelto, G.; et al. *Causal Effect of Health on Labor Market Outcomes: Experimental Evidence*; Population Working Papers; California Center for Population Research, UCLA: Los Angeles, CA, USA, 2006.
25. Adhvaryu, A.; Nyshadham, A. Health, Enterprise, and Labor Complementarity in the Household. *J. Dev. Econ.* **2017**, *126*, 91–111. [CrossRef] [PubMed]
26. Jing, Z.; Chen, J.; Yang, X. Self-employed or Employed: Mechanism and Empirical Test of Human Capital in Rural Floating Population: Analysis of Experience Based on CGSS Data. *Issues Agric. Econ.* **2018**, *462*, 87–97. (In Chinese)
27. Karno, M.; Edgerton, R.B. Perception of Mental Illness in a Mexican-American Community. *Arch. Gen. Psychiatry* **1969**, *2*, 233–238. [CrossRef] [PubMed]
28. Fuller-Thomson, E.; Brennenstuhl, S.; Cooper, R.; Kuh, D. An investigation of the healthy migrant hypothesis: Pre-emigration characteristics of those in the British 1946 birth cohort study. *Can. J. Public Health* **2015**, *106*, e502–e508. [CrossRef] [PubMed]
29. Salas-Wright, C.P.; Vaughn, M.G.; Goings, T.C.; Miller, D.P.; Schwartz, S.J. Immigrants and mental disorders in the United States: New evidence on the healthy migrant hypothesis. *Psychiatry Res.* **2018**, *267*, 438–445. [CrossRef] [PubMed]
30. Yi, Y.; Liao, Y.; Zheng, L.; Li, M.; Gu, J.; Hao, C.; Hao, Y. Health Selectivity and Rural-Urban Migration in China: A Nationwide Multiple Cross-Sectional Study in 2012, 2014, 2016. *Int. J. Environ. Res. Public Health* **2019**, *16*, 1596. [CrossRef]
31. World Bank. *The Economic Impact of the 2014 Ebola Epidemic: Short and Medium-Term Estimates for West Africa*; World Bank Group Publishing: Washington, DC, USA, 2014. Available online: http://documents.worldbank.org/curated/en/2014/10/20270083/economic-impact-2014-ebola-epidemic-short-medium-termestimates-west-africa (accessed on 11 October 2021).
32. Mok, K.H.; Xiong, W.; Ke, G.; Cheung, J.O.W. Impact of COVID-19 pandemic on international higher education and student mobility: Student perspectives from mainland China and Hong Kong. *Int. J. Educ. Res.* **2021**, *105*, 101718. [CrossRef]
33. Harris, J.R.; Todaro, M.P. Migration, Unemployment and Development: A Two-sector Analysis. *Am. Econ. Rev.* **1970**, *60*, 126–141.
34. Jhar, R.; Whalley, J. *The Environmental Regime in Developing Countries*; University of Chicago Press: Chicago, IL, USA, 2001.
35. Germani, A.R.; Scaramozzino, P.; Castaldo, A.; Talamo, G. Does air pollution influence internal migration? An empirical investigation on Italian provinces. *Environ. Sci. Policy* **2021**, *120*, 11–20. [CrossRef]

36. Cao, Z.; Zheng, X.; Liu, Y.; Li, Y.; Chen, Y. Exploring the changing patterns of China's migration and its determinants using census data of 2000 and 2010. *Habitat Int.* **2018**, *82*, 72–82. [CrossRef]
37. Wang, L. Analysis of the Impact of Environmental Pollution Level and Economic Development Level on Employment. *Conf. Ser. Mater. Sci. Eng. IOP Publ.* **2018**, *394*, 052085. [CrossRef]
38. Zhang, Y.; Shao, T.; Dong, Q. Reassessing the Lewis turning point in China: Evidence from 70,000 rural households. *China World Econ.* **2018**, *26*, 4–17. [CrossRef]
39. Sun, W.; Zhang, X.; Zheng, S. Air Pollution and Spatial Mobility of Labor Force: Study on the Migrants' Job Location Choice. *Econ. Res. J.* **2019**, *54*, 102–117. (In Chinese)
40. Lin, L.S.; Wang, Y.Q. Transport Cost, Labor Mobility and the Spatial Distribution of Manufacturing Industries. *Econ. Res. J.* **2006**, *41*, 115–125. (In Chinese)
41. Currie, J.; Davis, L.; Greenstone, M.; Walker, R. *Do Housing Prices Reflect Environmental Health Risks? Evidence from More Than 1600 Toxic Plant Openings and Closings*; Working Paper No. w18700; National Bureau of Economic Research: Cambridge, MA, USA, 2013.
42. Xiao, T. Whether the Environmental Quality Is the Leading Factor of Labor Mobility? *Econ. Rev.* **2016**, *198*, 3–17. (In Chinese)
43. Istudor, N.; Dinu, V.; Gogu, E.; Prada, E.; Petrescu, I. Impact of Education and Economic Growth on Labour Migration in the European Union. A Panel Data Analysis. *EaM Ekon. A Manag.* **2020**, *23*, 55–67. [CrossRef]
44. Liu, Z.; Yu, L. Stay or leave? The role of air pollution in urban migration choices. *Ecol. Econ.* **2020**, *177*, 106780. [CrossRef]
45. Chen, S.; Chen, D. Air Pollution, Government Regulations and High-quality Economic Development. *Econ. Res. J.* **2018**, *53*, 20–34. (In Chinese)
46. Kawachi, I.; Adler, N.E.; Dow, W.H. Money, schooling, and health: Mechanisms and causal evidence. *Ann. N. Y. Acad. Sci.* **2010**, *1186*, 56–68. [CrossRef]
47. Jawadi, F.; El Gouddi, S.; Ftiti, Z.; Kacem, A. Assessing the effect of trade openness on health in the MENA region: A panel data analysis. *Open Econ. Rev.* **2018**, *29*, 469–479. [CrossRef]
48. Jun, W.; Mahmood, H.; Zakaria, M. Impact of trade openness on environment in China. *J. Bus. Econ. Manag.* **2020**, *21*, 1185–1202. [CrossRef]
49. Gan, T.; Yang, H.; Liang, W.; Liao, X. Do economic development and population agglomeration inevitably aggravate haze pollution in China? New evidence from spatial econometric analysis. *Environ. Sci. Pollut. Res.* **2021**, *28*, 5063–5079. [CrossRef] [PubMed]
50. Zhang, H. The Effect of Environmental Pollution on Labor Employment: Evidence from the Policy of Environmental Protection Accountability System. *J. Financ. Econ.* **2019**, *45*, 42–56. (In Chinese)
51. MacKinnon, D.P.; Dwyer, J.H. Estimating mediated effects in prevention studies. *Eval. Rev.* **1993**, *17*, 144–158. [CrossRef]
52. Chay, K.Y.; Greenstone, M. Does Air Quality Matter? Evidence from the Housing Market? *J. Political Econ.* **2005**, *113*, 376–424. [CrossRef]
53. Xi, P.; Liang, R. Urban air quality and environmental migration: An empirical study based on the fuzzy breakpoint model. *Econ. Sci.* **2015**, *37*, 30–43. (In Chinese)
54. MacKinnon, D.P.; Warsi, G.; Dwyer, J.H. A simulation study of mediated effect measures. *Multivar. Behav. Res.* **1995**, *30*, 41–62. [CrossRef]
55. Cropper, M.L. Measuring the benefits from reduced morbidity. *Am. Econ. Rev.* **1981**, *71*, 235–240.
56. Kahn, M.E.; Mansur, E.T. Do local energy prices and regulation affect the geographic concentration of employment? *J. Public Econ.* **2013**, *101*, 105–114. [CrossRef]
57. Walker, W.R. Environmental regulation and labor reallocation: Evidence from the Clean Air Act. *Am. Econ. Rev.* **2011**, *101*, 442–447. [CrossRef]
58. Zhang, Y. The Role of Air Pollution Risk Perception in Labor Migration: The Perspective of Healthy Human Capital Investment. *Popul. Dev.* **2021**, *27*, 51–64. (In Chinese)
59. Agyemang, C. Comfy zone hypotheses in migrant health research: Time for a paradigm shift. *Public Health* **2019**, *172*, 108–115. [CrossRef] [PubMed]
60. Kwan, F.; Wu, Y.; Zhuo, S. Surplus agricultural labour and China's Lewis turning point. *China Econ. Rev.* **2018**, *48*, 244–257. [CrossRef]
61. Zhang, X.; Yang, J.; Wang, S. China has reached the Lewis turning point. *China Econ. Rev.* **2011**, *22*, 542–554. [CrossRef]
62. Hill, T.D.; Jorgenson, A.K.; Ore, P.; Balistreri, K.S.; Clark, B. Air quality and life expectancy in the United States: An analysis of the moderating effect of income inequality. *SSM—Popul. Health* **2019**, *7*, 100346. [CrossRef]
63. Li, X.; Chen, H.; Li, Y. The effect of air pollution on children's migration with parents: Evidence from China. *Environ. Sci. Pollut. Res.* **2020**, *27*, 12499–12513. [CrossRef]
64. Färe, R.; Grosskopf, S.; Pasurka, C.A., Jr. Environmental production functions and environmental directional distance functions. *Energy* **2007**, *32*, 1055–1066. [CrossRef]

International Journal of *Environmental Research and Public Health*

MDPI

Article

Spatial Transformation Characteristics and Conflict Measurement of Production-Living-Ecology: Evidence from Urban Agglomeration of China

Yu Chen [1], Xuyang Su [1] and Xuekai Wang [2,*]

[1] School of Economics and Management, Zhengzhou University of Light Industry, Science Avenue 136, Zhengzhou 450000, China; 2012030@zzuli.edu.cn (Y.C.); suxuyang_123@163.com (X.S.)
[2] National Academy of Economic Strategy, Chinese Academy of Social Sciences, No.1 Dongchanghutong, Beijing 100006, China
* Correspondence: wangxuekaihappy@163.com

Abstract: The land development by human beings has changed from the initial small-scale and low-level transformation to the comprehensive utilization of large-scale and high-intensity implementations. The contradiction between production-living-ecology space (PLES) has become increasingly prominent while drawing land dividends. As one of the important birthplaces of Chinese civilization and the ecological barrier in the northern region, the rapid urbanization and industrialization of the Yellow River Basin (YRB) make the ecological environment very fragile, and the imbalance of land and space development is extremely serious. Therefore, according to the multifunctional characteristics of land use, this paper establishes a classification system of production space (PS), living space (LS) and ecology space (ES), and discusses the spatiotemporal evolution and conflict distribution characteristics of the PLES with the help of the transfer matrix and spatial conflict index (SCI). The results are as follows. In 1990–2020, agricultural production space (APS), grassland ecology space (GES) and other ecology space (OES) yielded the largest proportion of PLES in the YRB. However, compared with 1990, the area of these spatial types decreased in 2020, while the urban living space (ULS) expanded rapidly. The distribution pattern of PLES was generally consistent, and the transformation between PLES in Ningxia, central Inner Mongolia, Loess Plateau and downstream areas was relatively intense. The conflict index of PLES showed an upward trend, but it was generally in a controllable range. The stable and controllable areas were concentrated in the upstream of the urban agglomeration, and the midstream and downstream were basic out of control and seriously out of control, respectively.

Keywords: production-living-ecology; spatial transformation characteristics; spatial conflicts; urban agglomeration

Citation: Chen, Y.; Su, X.; Wang, X. Spatial Transformation Characteristics and Conflict Measurement of Production-Living-Ecology: Evidence from Urban Agglomeration of China. *IJERPH* **2022**, *19*, 1458. https://doi.org/10.3390/ijerph19031458

Academic Editors: Jie Chen, Qian Zhou and Ting Zhang

Received: 27 December 2021
Accepted: 24 January 2022
Published: 27 January 2022

1. Introduction

Territorial space is the carrier of socioeconomic development, as well as the support of human survival and development, and the evolution of its pattern and function is the result of the continuous interaction between humans and land [1,2]. The imbalance between the supply and demand of land resources is increasingly fierce with the construction of modernization, and limited land resources are reallocated quantitatively and spatially in the game among various interests. This dynamic process is known as land use transformation, which reveals the transformation of land use patterns corresponding to the stage of economic and social development in a certain period driven by various internal and external factors [3,4]. However, a healthy land use system has not only structural integrity, but also functional continuity and additivity [5]. Since the beginning of the new century, China's rapid population urbanization and land urbanization process have accelerated the demand for land resources [6–8], and urban and rural construction land has continuously encroached on agricultural and ecological land, causing increasing land use conflicts in space. In essence, land use conflict is the competition for resource elements in time and space among land-using subjects [9], which is manifested as the uncoordinated development of the human-land relationship. Once the conflict level is intensified or out of control, it will lead to a series of problems such as the waste of spatial resources, destruction of ecosystem, weakening of the stability of the landscape pattern and imbalance of social development [10–15].

Since the beginning of the new era, China has attached great importance to land planning to address a series of negative problems caused by the overexploitation of land resources. The report of the 18th National Congress put forward the overall construction goal of "Intensive and efficient in the production space, livable and moderate in the living space, beautiful in the ecological space", and made optimizing the spatial development pattern of the country the first step in the construction of ecological civilization. In 2017, the National Land Planning Outline was released to make specific arrangements for regional development, the construction of the main functional areas and development goals, and in the report of the 19th National Congress, it was further proposed to carry out the delineation of three control lines, namely the "ecological protection red line, permanent basic agricultural land and urban development boundary".

The YRB is a typical region of rapid economic and social transmutation [16–18]; has the PLES spatial pattern in the YRB changed significantly in recent decades? Will the spatial conflict index increase with socioeconomic development? Therefore, the YRB is used as the research object of PLES transformation characteristics and conflict measurement mainly based on the following considerations: (1) Important strategic positioning: The Outline of the Plan for Ecological Protection and High-Quality Development of the YRB regards this region as an important benchmark for the management of large rivers, an important benchmark for ecological safety, an important test area for high-quality development, and an important carrying area for the preservation, inheritance and promotion of Chinese culture. Research on the spatial pattern of PLES in this region is conducive to practicing the concept of ecological civilization construction and building a new pattern of land space development. (2) The unique geographical location: The YRB straddles three major steps in China, with a variety of terrain and landforms crisscrossing the basin and a weak resources and environment carrying capacity. The study of the spatiotemporal patterns and conflict levels of the PLES is conducive to the implementation of refined management, and to solving the outstanding problems of land grabbing for economic and social development in the YRB. (3) The intricate economic and social environment: After decades of reform and opening up, the level of urbanization and industrialization has improved significantly. However, problems such as uncoordinated urban and rural development, unbalanced regional development, the contradiction between economic growth and ecological protection, etc. are more serious. In addition, the ecological environment is fragile, and water resources are extremely scarce. The interaction and coupling system of land relationships demonstrates strong incoordination. Research on the conflict of PLES in this region is helpful to understand the current situation of land use conflict, optimize land use function and improve land use quality.

The structure of this paper is as follows: Section 2 is a literature review on the study of PLES; Section 3 is a presentation of data and methods; Section 4 is an analysis of the evolution, patterns and conflicts of PLES; and Section 5 is a conclusion and suggestions. Abbreviations attached at the end of this paper (Table A1). The research framework is shown in Figure 1.

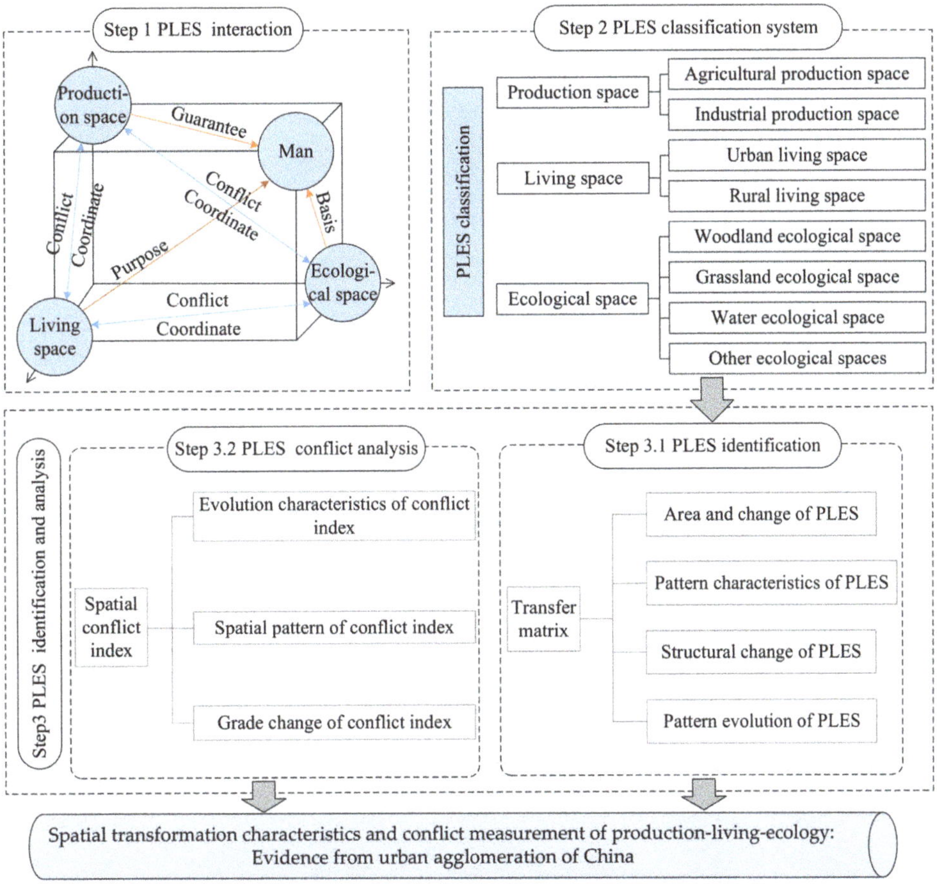

Figure 1. Research framework. Source: The authors.

2. Literature Review

In the 1980s, western countries launched a number of spatial planning research programs. By establishing evaluation models and using GIS and other methods, the suitability and mode of land spatial development were evaluated from the perspective of environmental protection [19]. As research progresses, the multifunctionality of land use is further subdivided into economic, social and ecological functions [20–22]. The study of PLES originated from agriculture in the Taiwan Province, which was originally aimed at balancing agricultural production and protecting the ecological landscape, but later evolved into the study of dividing the whole national space into production, living and ecology space. At present, from the perspective of land use, ecosystem and landscape value, research on PLES mainly focuses on identification and classification, the analysis of spatiotemporal evolution characteristics and influencing factors, spatial optimization and spatial conflict.

2.1. Identification and Classification of the PLES

The quantitative identification of the PLES is mainly based on the measurement of spatial quantity or quality, and the common measurement methods include land use type consolidation and the comprehensive index evaluation. On the one hand, from the existing research results, the method of land use consolidation is the most widely used, and it is based on the functions carried by each land use type to identify the pattern characteristics of the PLES intuitively and quickly [23,24]. However, scholars differ in their understanding of land-bearing functions, which are mainly divided into single spatial division and composite spatial division. Among them, scholars who hold a single spatial view believe that each land use type only considers its dominant function, and the division results in three spatial categories including production, living and ecology space, with no overlapping areas between the spaces [9,13,25]. Some scholars also believe that land can carry multiple functions at the same time, in addition to the single function of production, living and ecological, but also, has three spatial types of composite functions [26], for example, cultivated lands have both production and ecological functions, so the land is divided into production-ecological, living-production, etc., which is a composite spatial division. On the other hand, the method of the evaluation and measurement of the index system is mainly based on the economic, social and environmental factors related to production, living and ecological, and the construction of a comprehensive evaluation index system, such as the general evaluation index [27], coupling and coordination evaluation index [28], spatial suitability evaluation index [29] and resource and environmental carrying capacity evaluation index [30], etc., to evaluate the PLES. In summary, the division of composite space is complicated, and some plots are difficult to merge into a certain type due to their multiple functions at the same time. Evaluation indexes selected by the index system method are mostly biased towards social and economic indicators, which is difficult to reflect the change and coupling coordination of the PLES truly.

2.2. The Spatial and Temporal Evolution of the PLES

Most studies on the spatiotemporal evolution of the PLES have been conducted with the help of the ArcGIS platform and combined with econometric models for quantitative analysis. In the literature, most of the existing studies analyzed the spatial evolution characteristics of PLES in terms of quantity, speed and direction of change, as well as pattern, equilibrium and patch change [27,31–33] based on the theoretical connotation and established the classification system of the PLES, through the land use dynamics, transfer matrix, Gini coefficient and landscape pattern analysis. The scale of the study is divided into national, regional, urban agglomeration, provincial, municipal and county areas. Since the natural environment and socioeconomic conditions of different regions differ greatly, the factors influencing the PLES are also different.

2.3. Study on the Conflict of the PLES

The study of "conflict" originated from sociology, and refers to the psychological or behavior contradictions caused by the incompatibility or opposition of different actors in goals [34–36]. With the increasing contradiction between economic and social development and resource and environmental protection, conflict analysis was introduced into land use and ecological protection, and the concepts of land conflict, land use conflict and space conflict were also put forwards. Among them, spatial conflict originates from the scarcity of spatial resources and spillover of spatial functions, and is a phenomenon of distribution opposition resulting from the competition of spatial resources in the process of man-land relationships [37,38]. Studies on spatial conflicts mainly focus on potential conflict identification, conflict level measurement, analysis of influencing factors, disclosure of evolutionary processes and coordinated governance [26,39–41]. The methods adopted include interview investigation methods [42], multicriteria decision analysis methods [43], pressure-state-response models [35] and adaptability evaluations [44]. Most studies believe that spatial conflict is the result of multiple factors [9,14]. In the early stage when human disturbance intensity is low, natural factors play a major role, while with the increase in population and the acceleration of urbanization and industrialization, human activities gradually play a leading role in shaping the landscape.

In summary, many scholars adopt a variety of methods to carry out research on territorial space or PLES, with diverse research perspectives and rich research results. However, due to the interdisciplinary nature and diversified research standpoint, a unified research route has yet to be formed. Prominent problems such as the contradiction between humans and land caused by the continuous improvement of the utilization intensity of space resources have become increasingly prominent. Research on the spatial conflict of the basin combined with land use conflict and PLES is still rare. The contributions of this paper mainly focus on the following aspects: First, land use conflicts and PLES are combined to reclassify land use types and construct the PLES classification system. Second, taking the YRB as the research object, the spatiotemporal evolution of production, living and ecology space is described, and a conflict model is established to analyze the regional differences in spatial conflicts. Finally, this study provides a scientific basis and decision-making reference for the coordinated and healthy development of PLES, and provides a theoretical basis, technical support and typical case analysis for the management and regulation of land use spatial conflicts in the basin.

3. Methods and Data

3.1. Research Area

The Yellow River is located at 31°31′–43°31′ N, 89°19′–119°39′ E, starting from the Bayan Har Mountains on the Qinghai-Tibet Plateau and flowing eastward through nine provinces (regions): Qinghai, Sichuan, Gansu, Ningxia, Inner Mongolia, Shaanxi, Shanxi, Henan and Shandong (Figure 2). The total length of the Yellow River is 5464 km, and the total area of the basin is approximately 795,000 km^2 (including an influx area of 42,000 km^2). The Yellow River runs across the three strategic regions of East, Central and West China, and is a giant ecological corridor connecting the four geomorphic units of the Qinghai-Tibet Plateau, Inner Mongolia Plateau, Loess Plateau and North China Plain. The overall terrain of the basin is high in the west and low in the east. The average altitude of the western source region is over 4000 m, with numerous mountains and large topographic fluctuations. The elevation of the central region is 1000–2000 m; the geological structure is broken; and the soil texture is loose. Most of the eastern elevation does not exceed 50 m, and is mainly formed by the Yellow River sediment alluvial plain.

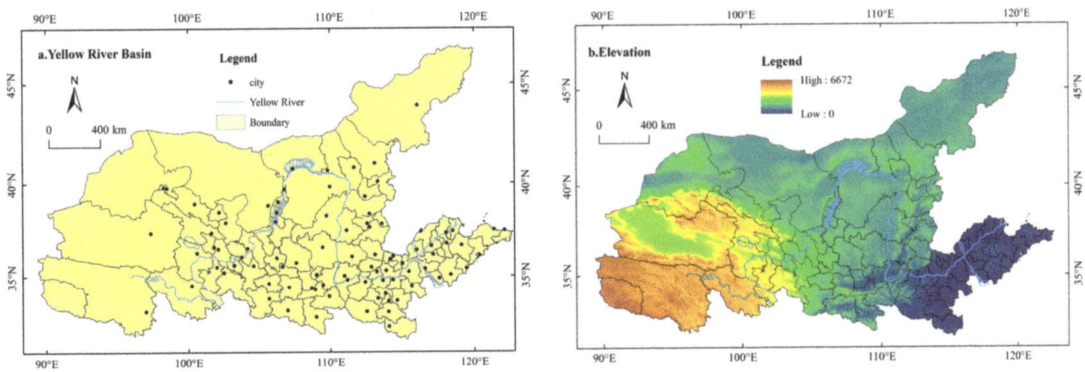

Figure 2. Administrative division of the Yellow River Basin (a) and elevation (b). Source: Developed by authors.

The YRB is a complex area of China's "economy-society-environment" system. By the end of 2018, the total population of the YRB was 420 million, accounting for about 30% of the total population of China, and the regional GDP was 23.9 trillion yuan, accounting for more than a quarter of China. As the foundation and lifeblood of the development of northern China, it formed an obvious ladder development pattern of backwards upstream, rising midstream and developed downstream. In industrial and agricultural production, coal, oil, natural gas and mineral resources are abundant. Resource-based cities relying on the exploitation and processing of energy resources account for 47% of the total number of cities in the basin, and are important energy, chemical, raw materials and basic industrial bases.

Agricultural and animal husbandry production also plays a pivotal role in the national economic pattern. The corresponding human living space is mainly concentrated in some river valleys in the upstream and plain areas in the midstream and downstream. Driven by natural environmental constraints and economic factors, the population distribution is dense in the middle and east, and sparse in the west. The ecological environment of the YRB is very fragile; the ecological functions of natural grasslands in the upper reaches are severely degraded; the middle reaches are faced with severe soil erosion problems; and urban life, industry and agriculture cause pollution to water resources. In recent decades, due to the rapid development of urbanization and industrialization, coupled with the complex geographical and climatic characteristics, the competition between production, living and ecology space has become an important factor restricting the sustainable development of this region.

3.2. Research Methods

3.2.1. Construction of the PLES Classification System

PLES is the reflection of humans' diversified demands for various products and services in daily work and life. It is the result of the interaction of different spatial environments and spatial scale elements, and is manifested in different utilization structures and ways in land use [2]. With the continuous deepening of research on PLES, many scholars divide land use into ecology space, production-ecology space, ecology-production space and living-production space from the perspective of the dominant and secondary functions of land use [9,25]. On the basis of exploring the connotation of PLES theory, some scholars established a spatial classification and evaluation system of PLES based on land use classification according to the national standard of land use classification [45]. Generally, a certain type of land space may have multiple functions at the same time. For example, cultivated land can not only be used for grain production, but also plays an important ecological role, but we usually think of arable land use primarily for food production. This paper draws lessons from the existing ideas and schemes of PLES spatial classification. According to the subjective intention of land use subjects and the dominant function of a certain type of land use, three spatial types of production, living and ecological are adopted to cover different land use patterns. The conflict and coordination among different land use patterns and the classification system are shown in Figure 3 and Table 1.

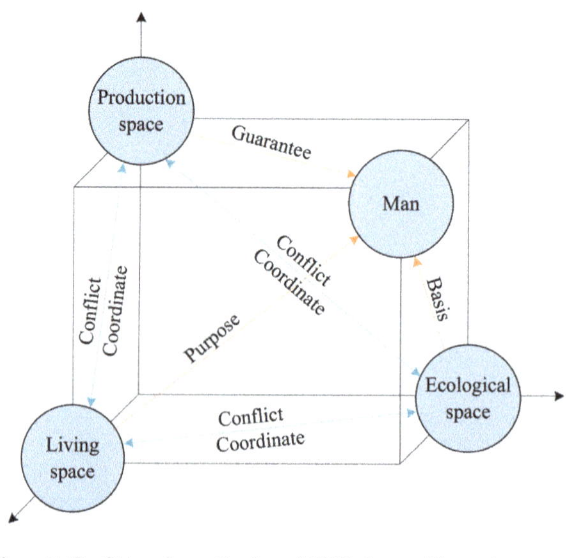

Figure 3. Conflict and coordination of PLES. Source: The authors.

Table 1. Classification system of PLES.

First-Level Classification	Second-Level Classification	Third-Level Classification
Production space	Agricultural production space	Paddy field, Dry land
	Industrial production space	Industrial, mining and transportation construction land
Living space	Urban living space	Urban land
	Rural living space	Rural residential area
Ecology space	Forestland ecology space	Forestland, shrubbery forest, Sparse woodland, Other woodlands
	Grassland ecology space	High, Medium and Low coverage grassland
	Water ecology space	Canal, Lakes, Reservoir pit, Permanent glacier snow, tidal flat
	Other ecology spaces	Sand land, Gobi, Saline-alkali land, Everglade, Bare land, Bare rock texture, Other

Source: The authors.

PS refers to the type of land use space that provides people with various products and services. This space takes land as the carrier to serve the most basic survival needs of human beings. It is the output of production and operation activities of the land use system, providing economic sources for most human beings and achieving the long-term goal of maintaining survival and development. [13]. Among them, dry land and paddy field are the main places for farmers to produce grain by providing agricultural products such as food and raw materials. Industrial, mining and transportation construction land mainly provides industrial products such as goods and service production, which is the main source of human mineral resources, and also includes transportation construction land serving transportation. Therefore, the production space is subdivided into APS and industrial production space (IPS).

LS refers to the type of land use space used by human beings for living, entertainment, science, education, culture and health, and some special purposes. This space aims to provide basic living conditions and security, and further meets the spiritual and cultural needs of human beings, which is the ultimate goal of the land use system [12]. As the current urban-rural dual structure is still relatively obvious, the living space is basically concentrated in urban and rural residential areas. Therefore, the living space is further subdivided into ULS and rural living space (RLS).

ES refers to the type of land use space that regulates the atmospheric environment, protects biodiversity, maintains soil and provides ecological products. This space is the foundation and support of production and living space, and is closely related to local natural resource endowment [9]. It can effectively promote regional sustainable development and ecological balance, and maintain the ecological stability of the natural environment. Therefore, the ecology space is further subdivided into forest ecology space (FES), grassland ecology space (GES), water ecology space and other ecology space (OES).

The essence of PLES evolution is a complex process of land use change. Under the influence of various driving factors such as the social economy and natural environment, it is manifested in the competition of various stakeholders for land use structure and form. In this dynamic process, PS guarantees various products and services produced and developed by human beings; LS meets the purpose of human habitation and social needs; and ES provides the basic material basis for human survival. Taking human beings as the center, various spatial types form the basic relationship of conflict and coordination with their unique functions. For example, ES meets people's ecological needs and provides raw materials for PS. However, if human activities in PS and LS exceed the ecological carrying capacity, this will lead to environmental problems such as ecological pollution. Therefore, the evolution of PLES is a complex dynamic process, and its driving factors are mainly expressed in two aspects. In terms of social factors, the level of economic development, policies and regulations, residents' life, population, industrial development, transportation and education all inevitably have an impact on the evolution of the PLES. Population factors, for example, population growth, distribution, age structure, comprehensive quality and migration will directly or indirectly promote the PLES evolution. In terms of natural factors, topography and climate characteristics are the basic factors affecting the distribution and change of PLES, such as slope, elevation and soil. In addition, the conversion of cropland to forest and grassland, land reclamation and deforestation can also affect the quantitative change of PLES.

3.2.2. Land Use Transfer Matrix

The transformation of the PLES type and structure is realized by a land use transfer matrix model. The transfer matrix is a two-dimensional matrix that lists the transfer area of land use change according to the status quo of land cover in the same area and different phases, which serves as the basis of structural analysis and change direction analysis. It can not only reflect the area of each space type in a fixed region and at a fixed time statically, but also describe the area transfer of each space type at the beginning of the period and the area transfer of each space type at the end of the period [46,47]. This method is derived from the quantitative description of the system state and state transition in system analysis, and the formula is as follows:

$$S_{ij} = \begin{vmatrix} S_{11} & S_{12} & \cdots & S_{1n} \\ S_{21} & S_{22} & \cdots & S_{2n} \\ \cdots & \cdots & \cdots & \cdots \\ S_{n1} & S_{n2} & \cdots & S_{nn} \end{vmatrix} \quad (1)$$

where S is the land area; n is the total number of land types; and i and j are land use types at the beginning and end of the study period, respectively. In this paper, ArcGIS10.2 software is used to calculate the statistics of PLES space types in different periods, and then an Excel pivot table is used to establish the PLES transfer matrix.

3.2.3. Spatial Conflict Index

Land use systems are complex, dynamic, and fragile, so spatial conflicts need to be considered from the three aspects of system complexity, stability and fragility [26]. To avoid excessive fragmentation of the spatial units in the study area, and taking into account factors such as the research scope, data type, spatial resolution, and patch conditions, under comprehensive testing and comparison, a 30 km × 30 km spatial grid was selected as the evaluation unit. The spatial plates that do not cover the entire grid in the boundary of the study area are calculated as a complete grid to calculate the landscape ecological index in each spatial unit to evaluate the degree of spatial conflict quantitatively. The calculation of SCI is [9]:

$$\mathrm{SCI} = \mathrm{CI} + \mathrm{FI} - \mathrm{SI} \quad (2)$$

where SCI is the comprehensive index of spatial conflict, and CI, FI and SI are the spatial complexity index, vulnerability index and stability index, respectively.

The PLES complexity index reflects the gradual increase in the scale and intensity of land use due to rapid urbanization, and the continuous shaping of the surface morphology, resulting in the fragmentation of patches and the intensification of contradictions in space use. The area-weighted mean patch fractal dimension (AWMPFD) reflects the degree of interference of the domain plate on the measured patch, and to a certain extent reflects the impact of human activities on the spatial pattern. The higher the value is, the greater the external pressure on the patch. The AWMPFD in the landscape ecological index is used to characterize the spatial complexity index of PLES to measure the shape complexity of spatial patches. The formula is:

$$\mathrm{AWMPFD} = \sum_{i=1}^{m}\sum_{j=1}^{n}\left[\frac{2\ln(0.25P_{ij})}{\ln(a_{ij})}\left(\frac{a_{ij}}{A}\right)\right] \quad (3)$$

where P_{ij} is the perimeter of the patch; a_{ij} is the area of the patch; A is the total area of the space types in the landscape; i and j are the j-th spatial types in the i-th spatial unit;

m is the total number of spatial evaluation units in the YRB; and n is the total number of PLES types.

The PLES vulnerability index reflects the ability of space patches to withstand external pressure. At different stages, various land use types have different responses to external disturbances. The weaker the resistance is, the more vulnerable it is to external influences, and the higher the level of spatial conflict. Therefore, from the perspective of landscape ecology, using the vulnerability of various landscapes inside the space to calculate the PLES vulnerability index, the formula is as follows:

$$\mathrm{FI} = \sum_{i=1}^{n} F_i \times \frac{a_i}{A} \quad (4)$$

where n is the total number of space types; F_i is the vulnerability index of different space types, referring to existing research results [9,26]. Values are assigned to each space type: PS = 3, ES = 2, LS = 1; a_i is the patch area; and A is the total area of the space type in the landscape.

The PLES stability index refers to the phenomenon where the regional spatial pattern fragments landscape patches under the interference of external pressure; the linear patches are "fishing nets", and the dot-shaped patches show an agglomeration state, with increased density and separation, resulting in a decrease in the proportion of planar patches in the spatial unit. The more fragmented and complex the spatial form, the worse the stability within the spatial unit, the greater the spatial risk and the higher the intensity of spatial conflict. Therefore, the fragmentation degree of the landscape ecology is selected to represent the spatial stability index, and the formula is as follows:

$$SI = 1 - PD\ PD = \frac{n_i}{A} \quad (5)$$

where SI represents the stability index of PLES. PD is patch density, and the larger the patch density is, the higher the degree of spatial fragmentation and the lower the stability of its spatial landscape; n_i is the number of patches of the i-th space type in each space unit; A is the total area of the space type in the landscape.

Using the moving window method in Fragstats 4.2 software to measure the spatial conflict level of the PLES in the YRB, taking into account the characteristics of the research scale, data type, data volume and spatial patch conditions, comparing different size window units (including 1 km × 1 km, 4 km × 4 km, 7 km × 7 km, 10 km × 10 km) and referring to related research, it is found that the 4 km × 4 km window can better express the spatial conflict distribution characteristics. If the patch in the boundary area of the study area does not cover the entire unit area, the calculation is performed based on a complete unit area to calculate the index in each spatial unit mentioned above. Finally, the spatial conflict index is standardized to (0,1). According to the inverted "U"-shaped spatial conflict trajectory model, the space conflict index is divided into four categories: stable and controllable (0, 0.5) and basically controllable (0.5, 0.7), basically out of control (0.7, 0.9) and seriously out of control (0.9, 1).

3.3. Data

The PLES data of the YRB evolved from the land use type. These data come from the Resource and Environmental Science and Data Center of the Chinese Academy of Sciences. Among them, land use data include grid datasets of 1 km × 1 km in 1990, 2000, 2010 and 2020. The data are based on Landsat 8 remote sensing images, generated by the human-computer interaction visual interpretation and interpretation, including 6 primary types and 25 secondary types of cultivated land, forestland, grassland, water, residential land and unused land. Using ArcGIS 10.2 software, the land use types of the YRB were extracted based on the administrative division vector file; the PLES was divided by reclassification and other methods, and this software was used for mapping and data analysis.

4. Results and Discussion

4.1. Analysis of Evolution Characteristics of PLES

4.1.1. Spatiotemporal Evolution Characteristics of PLES

With the help of ArcGIS 10.2 software, the area of the PLES of the YRB in 1990, 2000, 2010 and 2020 was extracted, and the changes in the spatial area of each category were calculated. The results are shown in Table 2. From 1990 to 2020, the PLES of the YRB was dominated by APS, FES, GES and OES. From 1990 to 2000, the overall ES showed a decreasing trend, with a decrease of 0.37%. The decrease in GES and OES was the most obvious. The expansion of PS and LS was 0.87% and 6.75%, respectively. Compared with other spaces, APS and ULS increased greatly. From 2000 to 2010, PS and ES decreased to varying degrees, among which APS and OES decreased significantly. In contrast, the LS expanded rapidly, with an increase of 16.25%, and the ULS expanded more rapidly than the RLS. From 2010 to 2020, with the continuous advancement of urbanization and industrialization, LS continued to expand, with an increase of 10.64%, and the IPS in the PS has an obvious increasing trend, while the ES continued to decrease, and the rate of decrease is 0.33%; thus, the reduction in GES and OES is the most obvious.

Table 2. The area and changes in the PLES of the YRB from 1990 to 2020 (km^2).

Year	PS		LS		ES			
	APS	IPS	ULS	RLS	FES	GES	WES	OES
1990	475,388	3926	7356	43,377	209,919	1,043,018	56,220	710,624
2000	479,304	4166	9544	44,613	209,381	1,035,888	57,123	709,888
2010	469,323	5440	16,226	46,734	211,935	1,039,876	58,748	701,656
2020	461,927	12,768	19,826	49,835	212,412	1,035,644	62,179	695,437
Change between 1990 and 2000	3916	240	2188	1236	−538	−7130	903	−736
Change between 2000 and 2010	−9981	1274	6682	2121	2554	3988	1625	−8232
Change between 2010 and 2020	−7396	7328	3600	3101	477	−4232	3431	−6219
Change between 1990 and 2020	−13,461	8842	12,470	6458	2493	−7374	5959	−15,187

Source: The authors.

Overall, during the study period, the APS, GES and OES showed a shrinking trend, and the other four types of land use space had different degrees of expansion. Among them, ULS has the fastest growth rate, and the rest are IPS, RLS, WES and FES. The reason is that since the reform and opening up, the rich land and natural resources of the YRB gradually entered a stage of rapid development, coupled with its large population, rapid advancement of economic, social and cultural undertakings, rural surplus labor flows to cities and towns, urban land and transportation, and industrial and mining land rapidly increased, leading to the expansion of the ULS and IPS [48]. In addition, the increase in the population of rural Mesozoic families led to an increase in the demand for residential land. Coupled with the relaxation of rural land management and control, the phenomenon of "building new and not dismantling old" appeared in rural residential land, which in turn promoted the expansion of rural living space [49]. The increase in FES and WES was mainly due to the implementation of policies such as returning farmland to forests and ecological restoration. In contrast, while the economy and society are highly developed, a series of unreasonable economic behaviors, such as excessive grazing, reclamation and the mining of mineral resources continue to encroach on agricultural land and ecological land. Coupled with the extremely fragile ecological environment of the YRB and the impact of climate change [50], the GES and OES are gradually reduced.

Based on the above analysis of temporal evolution characteristics, the spatial pattern characteristics of PLES in the YRB are further analyzed, as shown in Figure 4. From 1990 to 2020, the distribution pattern of PLES was basically consistent, and there was no significant indigenous change. The main characteristics are as follows: (1) The PS is dominated by APS, which is concentrated in traditional main grain producing areas such as Henan and Shandong downstream of the Yellow River. In addition, the Guanzhong Plain, Hetao

Plain and Ningxia Plain are important agricultural production bases. The main reason is that these areas are suitable for agricultural production due to their superior human and natural environment, and strict farmland protection policies play a better role in protecting traditional agricultural areas. (2) The distribution of LS corresponds to the location of agricultural and industrial production space. The density of LS in the downstream area was significantly greater than that in the upstream and midstream areas, while the ULS showed a significant expansion trend, and the patch area increased significantly. The reason is that the vast midstream and upstream are mainly continental or plateau climates, with little precipitation and rugged terrain. The flat terrain of the downstream alluvial plain is more suitable for human habitation, and the excellent natural conditions breed the vast agricultural production areas. Due to the low traditional agricultural production technology, a large number of labors gather here to form dense rural settlements. In recent years, although the level of agricultural mechanization was greatly improved, and the demand for agricultural labor declined, due to the huge population base, rural settlements are still the main agricultural population. (3) The ecological spatial distributions are greater in the west and lower in the east. Among them, the FES is mainly distributed in southern Henan, Qinling Mountains and Taihang Mountains; the GES is widely distributed in arid and semiarid areas such as Qinghai, Gansu and eastern Inner Mongolia. Restricted by topography and climate differences, the WES and OES are mostly concentrated upstream of the Yellow River.

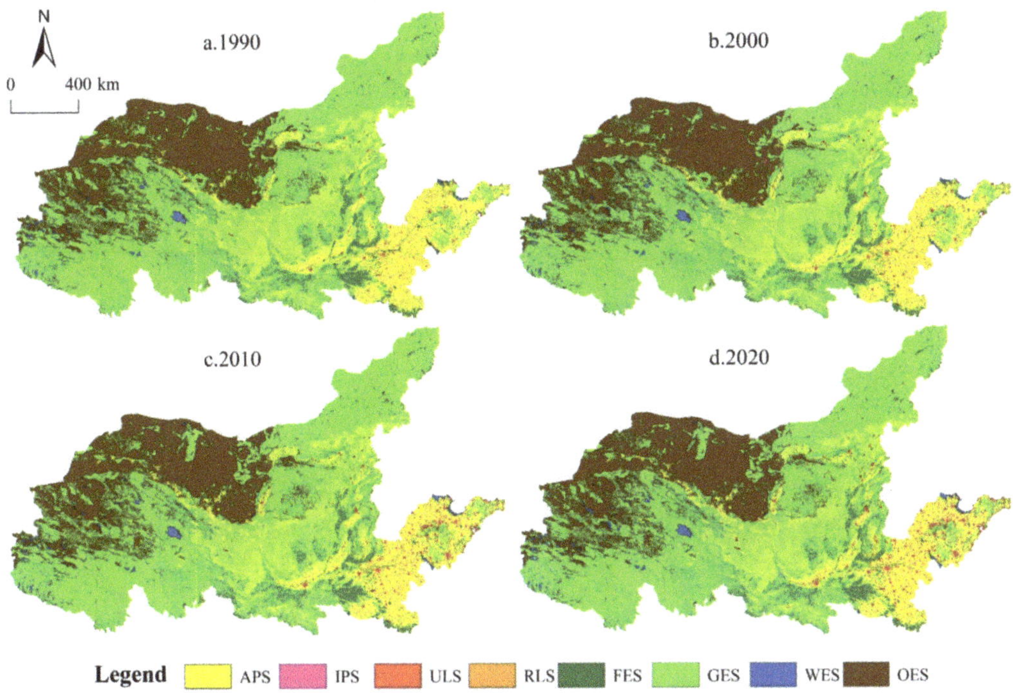

Figure 4. Spatial pattern characteristics of PLES in the YRB from 1990 to 2020: 1990 (**a**), 2000 (**b**), 2010 (**c**) and 2020 (**d**). Source: Developed by authors.

4.1.2. The Structural Transformation Characteristics of PLES

To explore the internal transformation characteristics of the PLES in the YRB, based on the distribution map of the PLES in Figure 3, the spatial analysis function in ArcGIS is used to superimpose the distribution maps of the PLES in different periods to obtain the transfer model of PLES in the study area from 1990 to 2020 to clarify the direction and quantity of the conversion of land use types (Tables 3 and 4). From 1990 to 2020, except for the reduction in APS, GES and OES, the structural space of other land types increased. Compared with the base period area, the IPS and UPS increased by a large margin, by 8828 km^2 and 12,439 km^2, respectively, during the period, and the growth rates were 225.22% and 169.52%. In internal conversion, from the perspective of roll-in structure, in terms of PS, APS is mainly converted from RLS and GES, and IPS is mainly converted from APS and GES; in terms of LS, both ULS and RLS are mainly converted from APS; in terms of ES, FES is mainly converted from APS and GES, and GES is mainly converted from APS and OES. The WES is mainly converted from APS, GES and OES, and OES is mainly converted from GES. From the perspective of roll-out structure, in terms of PS, APS is mainly transformed into ULS, RLS and GES, and IPS is most transferred to OES. In terms of LS, the transformation of ULS to other types of space is not obvious, and RLS is mainly turned to APS. In terms of ES, FES is mainly transformed into GES; GES is transformed into APS and OES; and OES is mainly transformed into GES.

Table 3. The transition matrix of the spatial structure of the PLES from 1990 to 2020 (km^2).

1990	2020								Roll-Out
	APS	IPS	ULS	RLS	FES	GES	WES	OES	
APS	-	4104	9509	10,647	3826	10,929	2432	1363	42,810
IPS	157	-	188	103	39	330	268	402	1487
ULS	238	14	-	214	22	70	6	5	569
RLS	4118	171	1944	-	57	208	69	40	6607
FES	2476	496	245	292	-	3286	205	305	7305
GES	16,653	3473	665	1400	5031	-	2821	17,407	47,450
WES	1998	434	300	139	116	832	-	1537	5356
OES	3704	1623	157	270	705	24,420	5367	-	36,246
Roll-in	29,344	10,315	13,008	13,065	9796	40,075	11,168	21,059	-

Source: The authors.

Table 4. Statistics on the changes and characteristics of the PLES utilization from 1990 to 2020.

Type	Area/km^2					
	Roll-In Rate	Roll-Out Rate	The Total Variation	Exchange Variation	Net Increase	Rate of Increase and Decrease
APS	6.35%	9.01%	72,154	58,688	−13,466	−2.83%
IPS	80.88%	37.88%	11,802	2974	8828	225.22%
ULS	65.71%	7.74%	13,577	1138	12,439	169.52%
RLS	26.22%	15.23%	19,672	13,214	6458	14.89%
FES	4.61%	3.48%	17,101	14,610	2491	1.19%
GES	3.87%	4.55%	87,525	80,150	−7375	−0.71%
WES	18.01%	9.53%	16,524	10,712	5812	10.60%
OES	3.03%	5.10%	57,305	42,118	−15,187	−2.14%

Source: The authors.

Based on the above analysis, the spatial distribution of land conversion in different periods is further discussed (Figure 5). Overall, the conversion areas of 1990–2000 and 2010–2020 were lower than those of 2000–2010. Specifically, from 1990 to 2000, the conversion of ES to PS was concentrated in central Inner Mongolia and Ningxia, and a small amount of PS to ES was also concentrated in central Inner Mongolia. The Henan and Shandong Province downstream of the YRB was dominated by PS to LS, and the distribution was more dispersed. From 2000 to 2010, the distributions of PS to ES and LS were the most extensive. Among them, PS to ES was distributed in the northwestern area of Shanxi, central Inner Mongolia and the Loess Plateau, and ES and PS to LS were mainly in the lower reaches of the YRB. At the same time, there was a small amount of ES to PS in the Shandong Peninsula and the Hexi Corridor of Gansu. From 2010 to 2020, the PS and ES transferred to LS, and were widely distributed in the whole basin, while the PS transferred to ES in the Shanxi Province and was the most prominent. In summary, from 1990 to 2020, the change of PLES in the YRB was dominated by the transformation between ES and PS, which was widely distributed upstream, midstream and downstream of the region. At the same time, the downstream region shows obvious characteristics of mutual transformation between PS and LS, and the transformation of ES and LS is sporadically distributed in various regions.

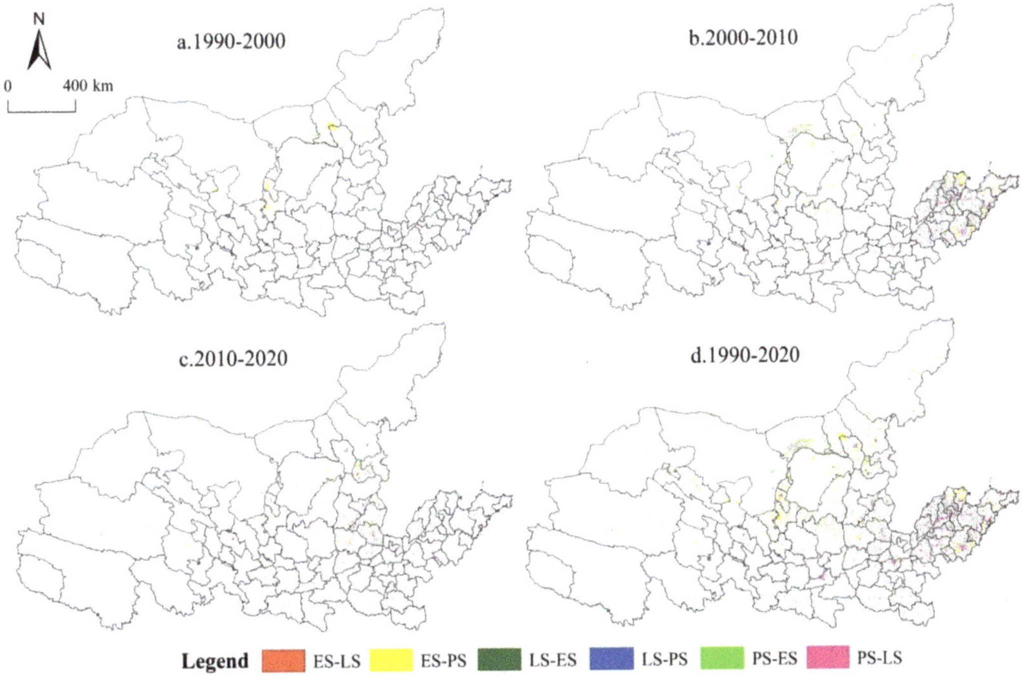

Figure 5. Spatial pattern evolution map of PLES in the YRB from 1990 to 2020: 1990 (**a**), 2000 (**b**), 2010 (**c**) and 2020 (**d**). Source: Developed by authors.

4.2. Analysis of Conflict and Change of PLES

4.2.1. Time Evolution Characteristics

By calculating the spatial conflict index of four periods in the YRB, it is found that the average values of the spatial conflict index in 1990, 2000, 2010 and 2020 are 0.41, 0.43, 0.53 and 0.57, respectively (Table 5). With the rapid development of industrialization and urbanization, the intensity of spatial conflict in the YRB is on the rise, but still belongs to the basic controllable level. The proportion of space conflicts at the controllable level (stable controllable and basic controllable) remained between 74.17% and 81.70%, accounting for more than half of the total space units in the study area, and played an important role in controlling ecological risks and maintaining ecological security. The proportion of space units at stable and controllable levels continued to decline, falling by 17.23% in 2020 compared with 1990, while the proportion of space units at basic controllable levels increased by 31.34% at the end of the period compared with the beginning. The proportion of space units at the basic out of control conflict level showed a rapid growth trend and the largest increase, which increased by 46.29% in 2020 compared with 1990. The proportion of space units at the seriously out of control conflict level showed a wave-like rise, and decreased slightly from 1990 to 2000, but increased rapidly from 2000 to 2020, with an increase of 33.04%. In addition, the gap in the number of spatial units between the controllable level and the out of control level tended to narrow, and the gap between the basic controllable and basic out of control spatial units expanded rapidly. From the perspective of change trends, stable and controllable, basic controllable and basic out of control all showed linear changes, while the number of seriously out of control space units first decreased and then increased. Thus, with the gradual expansion of production and living space, out of control conflicts in some areas tend to expand, and the control over these regions should be strengthened to achieve the coordinated development of PLES in the YRB.

Table 5. Statistics of the PLES Conflict Index in the YRB from 1990 to 2020.

Level of Conflict	Number of Space Units				Percentage (%)			
	1990	2000	2010	2020	1990	2000	2010	2020
Stable and Controllable	2112	2069	1866	1748	68.2	66.81	60.25	56.44
Basic Controllable	418	436	516	549	13.5	14.08	16.66	17.73
Basic Out of Control	445	480	577	651	14.37	15.5	18.63	21.02
Seriously Out of Control	122	112	138	149	3.94	3.62	4.46	4.81
Average	0.41	0.43	0.53	0.57	-	-	-	-
Total	3097	3097	3097	3097	100	100	100	100

Source: The authors.

The spatial conflict index of each spatial unit was further calculated, and the spatial distribution of the conflict index of PLES in the YRB from 1990 to 2020 was visualized by using ArcGIS 10.2 software (Figure 6). In general, the distribution of spatial units with different conflict levels from 1990 to 2020 is relatively fragmented, except that the basic controllable types are concentrated; the basic controllable ones, the basic uncontrollable ones and the severe uncontrollable ones are all fragmented. In addition, the changes in spatial units with different conflict types during the study period show different characteristics. Longitudinally, the change degree of spatial units of different conflict levels was small before 2000, but the change after 2000 was characterized by fast speed and a wide range. Laterally, the stable and controllable areas were mainly concentrated upstream of the Yellow River, and the midstream and downstream were mainly out of control or seriously out of control. Specifically, stable and controllable spatial units are mainly distributed in the west and north of the YRB, and most are concentrated in Qinghai, Gansu and Inner Mongolia. The number of stable and controllable spatial units decreases significantly in the Hexi Corridor, southern Inner Mongolia, Shanxi and WeiHe River Basin. Basic controllable areas are mainly distributed in the midstream of the YRB, and the overall distribution of spatial units has a trend of transformation from fragmentation to centralized contiguous, which is mainly due to the transformation of stable controllable types to basic controllable, resulting in a basic controllable spatial unit distribution to expand outward. The basic out of control space units are widely distributed in the midstream and downstream parts of the Loess Plateau. With the passage of time, the basic out of control space in the Loess Plateau rapidly expands, while the basic out of control space in the downstream is stable and mainly distributed in the periphery of the seriously out of control space. The seriously out of control spatial units were scattered in the midstream and downstream of the YRB. The seriously out of control spatial units in the HeTao Plain changed to the basic out of control level from 2000 to 2020, and the seriously out of control spatial units in southern Henan and northern Shandong continued to spread, indicating that the PLES conflict downstream of the Yellow River increased.

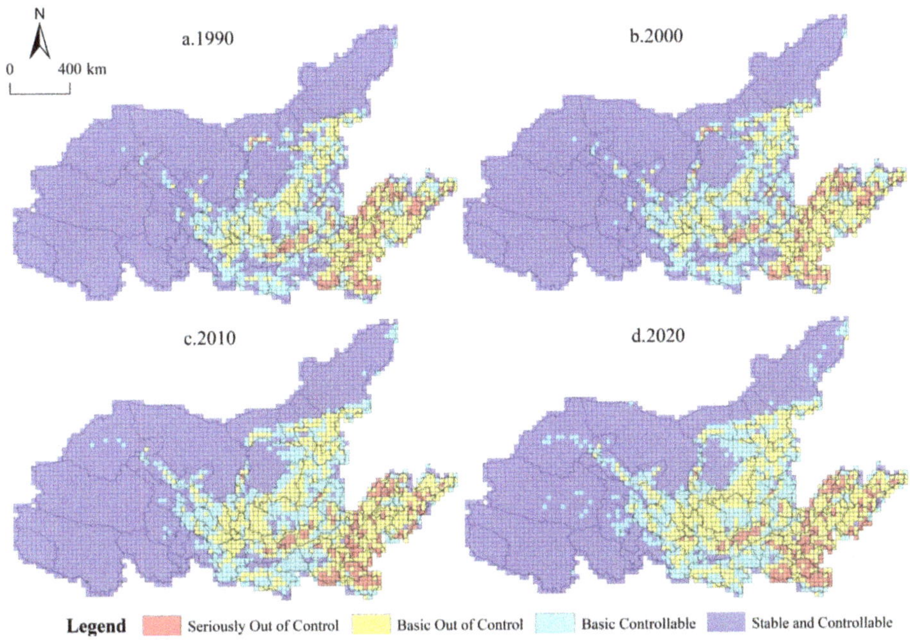

Figure 6. Changes in the PLES conflict index from 1990 to 2020: 1990 (**a**), 2000 (**b**), 2010 (**c**) and 2020 (**d**). Source: Developed by authors.

4.2.2. Conflict Differentiation Characteristics of PLES

The spatial conflict levels of the three spatial types in the YRB were calculated and statistically analyzed (Figure 7), and the results showed that there were differences in the composition of spatial conflict levels among different spatial types, and the level of out of control gradually increased, but all of them remained at the controllable level. The spatial conflict of PS is mainly controllable, accounting for more than 55%. The basic controllable conflict unit decreases year by year, while the stable controllable and basic out of control conflict unit increases year by year, and the serious out of control conflict unit shows a rising trend of fluctuation. PS is mainly concentrated in the midstream and downstream parts of the YRB. These areas have a high level of social and economic development, intensity of human development and construction activities, and the rapid development of urbanization and industrialization has led to prominent contradictions between people and land, increasing external pressure on space and increasing the intensity of space conflicts. The variation range of LS is similar to that of PS, and the spatial conflict is still controlled. The stable and controllable conflict units gradually decreased, with the largest decrease of 29.6% from 2000 to 2010. The basic controllable, basic out of control and serious out of control units increased by 29.3%, 42.4% and 22.5%, respectively. Compared with PS and LS, the variation range of conflict units in ES was smaller. Although stable controllable conflict units showed a slow downwards trend, controllable units remained above 70%. Basic controllable and basic out of control units showed a slight upwards trend, while seriously out of control units had the smallest variation range.

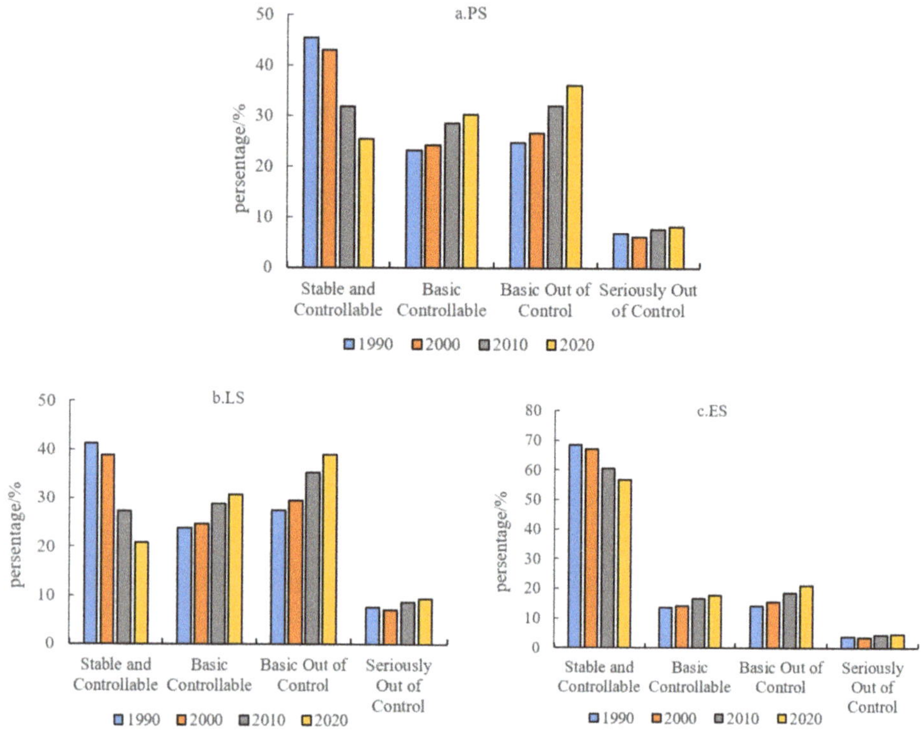

Figure 7. Spatial conflict levels of different spatial types in the YRB from 1990 to 2020: PS (**a**), LS (**b**), ES (**c**). Source: The authors.

5. Conclusions and Suggestions

5.1. Conclusions

(1) From 1990 to 2020, PS and LS expanded by 0.87% and 6.75%, respectively, while ES decreased by 0.37%. In terms of spatial distribution, the APS of PS is concentrated in the traditional agricultural production area downstream, while the APS of the midstream and upstream is scattered. The distribution of LS corresponds to the agricultural and industrial production space. The density of LS in the downstream is significantly higher than that in the midstream and upstream, while the distribution of ecology space is more in the west and less in the east.

(2) APS, GES and OES decreased, and the rest of the space types showed a trend of expansion. IPS and ULS expanded rapidly. In terms of transition and transition structure, each space type has different transformation directions, but the transformation between ES and PS is the main transformation direction. In the downstream area, the transformation between PS and LS is mainly reflected in the mutual transformation of PS and LS, and the transformation distribution of ES and LS is scattered.

(3) From 1990 to 2020, the intensity of conflicts in PLES gradually increased, but it was still controllable. Stable and basic controllable space units accounted for more than 70%, and basic and seriously out of control space units gradually increased. In terms of space, the basic controllable space units are mainly distributed in the upstream region and relatively concentrated, while in the downstream region, they are mainly basic out of control and seriously out of control, and their distribution is relatively fragmented. Specifically, the variation range of conflict units in PS and LS is the same, while the variation range of conflict units in ES is smaller.

5.2. Suggestions

Based on the PLES perspective, this paper constructed a land use classification system in the YRB, and revealed the evolution characteristics and conflict index of PLES from 1990 to 2020. Strengthening spatial governance and improving land use efficiency is a complex system project that is affected by natural and human factors in various regions. Therefore, it is necessary to promote the scientific demarcation of the boundary of PLES in the YRB, strengthen the control and supervision of the boundary of various spatial types and divide the boundary of production, living and ecological spaces scientifically and reasonably according to the resource and environmental carrying capacity, spatial conflict level, spatial development suitability and social and economic development status of each region.

(1) Although most of the upstream areas are in a stable and controllable state, as China's Water Tower and ecological spatial agglomeration area, ecological protection should be considered in the first place; the relationship between the production, living and ecological environment should be correctly handled, promote the construction of water conservation capacity, strengthen regional desertification control and strictly implement the principle of ecological access. The construction of nature reserves should promote ecological restoration, adhere to local conditions, comprehensively utilize engineering measures and biological measures to manage the ecosystem, control the ecology space at different levels and scales, delimit the rigid core elements and elastic space of ecological protection, reduce the frequency of human social and economic activities and alleviate the contradiction between human activities in the ecology space and the ecological environment.

(2) The midstream region should be committed to the spatial governance of soil erosion. On the one hand, it is important to protect forestland, grassland and unused land, enhance the soil and water conservation capacity, prevent the fragmentation of ecology space caused by urbanization and industrialization and take into account the economic and ecological benefits of land use. On the other hand, ecological restoration should be actively promoted to improve the management efficiency in the middle reaches. For irrigated agricultural areas, excessive consumption of water resources in agriculture and industry should be prevented; the proportion of ecological water should be increased; the intensity of land development should be strictly controlled; industries related to ecological environment protection should be developed; and the coupling and coordination level of PLES should be improved.

(3) The downstream region, as the region with the most serious conflict, is densely populated and has high industrial and agricultural production intensity. First, it is necessary to improve the quality of the population while reasonably controlling the size of the population, with land efficient and intensive use as the development goal, optimize the industrial layout, focus on cultivating new industrial systems, strictly control the disorderly expansion of urban and rural construction land, improve the utilization efficiency of existing construction land and alleviate the contradiction between industrial and agricultural production and ecological protection to create a green ecological corridor in the lower reaches of the Yellow River. Second, for the vast agricultural production space, the level of agricultural mechanization should be improved, protect high-quality cultivated land resources, improve land output income and reduce dependence on land resources. Finally, the concept of green development was combined with technical means, using the theory and technology of sponge cities, green buildings and ecological materials to promote the construction of urban ecological civilizations and strengthen the positive impact of land invisible forms on the ecological environment.

Author Contributions: Conceptualization, Y.C. and X.W.; data curation, X.S.; formal analysis, X.S. and X.W.; funding acquisition, Y.C.; methodology, X.S. and X.W.; software, X.S.; supervision, X.W. and Y.C.; writing—original draft, X.S.; writing—review and editing, X.W. and Y.C. All authors have read and agreed to the published version of the manuscript.

Funding: This work was supported by grants from the Support Plan for Scientific and Technological Innovation Talents in Henan Institutions of Higher Learning (humanities and social sciences) (2018-cx-012); Training Plan for Key Young Teachers in Henan Institutions of Higher Learning (2018GGJS094); Good Scholar in Philosophy and Social Sciences in Henan Institutions of Higher Learning (2019-YXXZ-20); and Philosophy and Social Science Innovation Team Building Program of Henan Universities (2021-CXTD-12,2022-CXTD-05). Philosophy and Social Science planning project of Henan Province (2021BJJ112).

Institutional Review Board Statement: Not applicable.

Informed Consent Statement: Not applicable.

Data Availability Statement: The data presented in this study are openly available in the Resource and Environmental Science Data Center of the Chinese Academy of Sciences.

Conflicts of Interest: The authors declare no conflict of interest. The funders had no role in the design of the study; in the collection, analyses or interpretation of data; in the writing of the manuscript; or in the decision to publish the results.

Appendix A

Table A1. Abbreviation table.

Full Name	Abbreviation	Full Name	Abbreviation
Production-living-ecology space	PLES	Rural living space	RLS
Yellow River Basin	YRB	Forestland ecology space	FES
production space	PS	Grassland ecology space	GES
living space	LS	Water ecology space	WES
ecology space	ES	Other ecology spaces	OES
Agricultural production space	APS	Spatial conflict index	SCI
Industrial production space	IPS	area-weighted mean patch fractal dimension	AWMPFD
Urban living space	ULS	patch density	PD

Source: The authors.

References

1. Tian, F.; Li, M.; Han, X.; Liu, H.; Mo, B. A Production–Living–Ecological Space Model for Land-Use Optimisation: A Case Study of the Core Tumen River Region in China. *Ecol. Model.* **2020**, *437*, 109310. [CrossRef]
2. Zhou, D.; Xu, J.; Lin, Z. Conflict or Coordination? Assessing Land Use Multi-Functionalization Using Production-Living-Ecology Analysis. *Sci. Total Environ.* **2017**, *577*, 136–147. [CrossRef]
3. Zou, L.; Liu, Y.; Wang, J.; Yang, Y. An Analysis of Land Use Conflict Potentials Based on Ecological-Production-Living Function in the Southeast Coastal Area of China. *Ecol. Indic.* **2021**, *122*, 107297. [CrossRef]
4. Liu, K.; Qiao, Y.; Zhou, Q. Spatiotemporal Heterogeneity and Driving Force Analysis of Innovation Output in the Yangtze River Economic Zone: The Perspective of Innovation Ecosystem. *Complexity* **2021**, *2021*, 8884058. [CrossRef]
5. Schluessel, V.; Bennett, M.B.; Bleckmann, H.; Blomberg, S.; Collin, S.P. Morphometric and Ultrastructural Comparison of the Olfactory System in Elasmobranchs: The Significance of Structure–Function Relationships Based on Phylogeny and Ecology. *J. Morphol.* **2008**, *269*, 1365–1386. [CrossRef] [PubMed]
6. Liu, Y. Introduction to Land Use and Rural Sustainability in China. *Land Use Policy* **2018**, *74*, 1–4. [CrossRef]
7. Zhang, W.; Zhang, M.; Wu, S.; Liu, F. A Complex Path Model for Low-Carbon Sustainable Development of Enterprise Based on System Dynamics. *J. Clean. Prod.* **2021**, *321*, 128934. [CrossRef]
8. Zhou, Q.; Zhu, M.; Qiao, Y.; Zhang, X.; Chen, J. Achieving Resilience through Smart Cities? Evidence from China. *Habitat Int.* **2021**, *111*, 102348. [CrossRef]
9. Lin, G.; Fu, J.; Jiang, D. Production–Living–Ecological Conflict Identification Using a Multiscale Integration Model Based on Spatial Suitability Analysis and Sustainable Development Evaluation: A Case Study of Ningbo, China. *Land* **2021**, *10*, 383. [CrossRef]
10. Yang, G.; Chen, Z. Rs-Based Fuzzy Multiattribute Assessment of Eco-Environmental Vulnerability in the Source Area of the Lishui River of Northwest Hunan Province, China. *Nat. Hazards* **2015**, *78*, 1145–1161. [CrossRef]
11. Gao, C.; Zhou, P.; Jia, P.; Liu, Z.; Wei, L.; Tian, H. Spatial Driving Forces of Dominant Land Use/Land Cover Transformations in the Dongjiang River Watershed, Southern China. *Environ. Monit. Assess.* **2016**, *188*, 84. [CrossRef] [PubMed]
12. Yang, Y.; Bao, W.; Liu, Y. Coupling Coordination Analysis of Rural Production-Living-Ecological Space in the Beijing-Tianjin-Hebei Region. *Ecol. Indic.* **2020**, *117*, 106512. [CrossRef]

13. Li, J.; Sun, W.; Li, M.; Meng, L. Coupling Coordination Degree of Production, Living and Ecological Spaces and Its Influencing Factors in the Yellow River Basin. *J. Clean. Prod.* **2021**, *298*, 126803. [CrossRef]
14. Zhou, H.; Chen, Y.; Tian, R. Land-Use Conflict Identification from the Perspective of Construction Space Expansion: An Evaluation Method Based on 'Likelihood-Exposure-Consequence'. *ISPRS Int. J. Geo-Inf.* **2021**, *10*, 433. [CrossRef]
15. Zhang, W.; Zhang, M.; Zhang, W.; Zhou, Q.; Zhang, X. What Influences the Effectiveness of Green Logistics Policies? A Grounded Theory Analysis. *Sci. Total Environ.* **2020**, *714*, 136731. [CrossRef]
16. Chen, Y.; Su, X.; Zhou, Q. Study on the Spatiotemporal Evolution, and Influencing Factors of Urban Resilience in the Yellow River Basin. *Int. J. Environ. Res. Public Health* **2021**, *18*, 10231. [CrossRef]
17. Chen, Y.; Zhu, M.; Lu, J.; Zhou, Q.; Ma, W. Evaluation of Ecological City and Analysis of Obstacle Factors under the Background of High-Quality Development: Taking Cities in the Yellow River Basin as Examples. *Ecol. Indic.* **2020**, *118*, 106771. [CrossRef]
18. Liu, K.; Qiao, Y.; Shi, T.; Zhou, Q. Study on Coupling Coordination and Spatiotemporal Heterogeneity between Economic Development and Ecological Environment of Cities Along the Yellow River Basin. *Environ. Sci. Pollut. Res.* **2021**, *28*, 6898–6912. [CrossRef]
19. Liu, H.; Fan, J.; Wang, C. Progress in the Study of European Spatial Planning, and the Inspiration to China. *Geogr. Anal.* **2008**, *6*, 1381–1389.
20. Bach, P.M.; Staalesen, S.; McCarthy, D.T.; Deletic, A. Revisiting Land Use Classification and Spatial Aggregation for Modelling Integrated Urban Water Systems. *Landsc. Urban Plan.* **2015**, *143*, 43–55. [CrossRef]
21. Verstegen, J.A.; Karssenberg, D.; van der Hilst, F.; Faaij, A.P. Detecting Systemic Change in a Land Use System by Bayesian Data Assimilation. *Environ. Model. Softw.* **2016**, *75*, 424–438. [CrossRef]
22. Chen, Y.; Zhu, M.; Zhou, Q.; Qiao, Y. Research on Spatiotemporal Differentiation and Influence Mechanism of Urban Resilience in China Based on Mgwr Model. *Int. J. Environ. Res. Public Health* **2021**, *18*, 1056. [CrossRef] [PubMed]
23. Wu, Y.J.; Yang, Y.Z.; Yang, L.; Zhang, C.; You, Z. Land Spatial Development and Suitability for City Construction Based on Ecological-Living-Industrial Space: Take Ningbo City as an Example. *Resour. Sci.* **2016**, *38*, 2072–2081.
24. Liu, J.L.; Liu, Y.S.; Li, Y.R. Classification Evaluation and Spatial-Temporal Analysis of Production-Living-Ecological Spaces in China. *Acta Geogr. Sin.* **2017**, *72*, 1290–1304.
25. Yang, Y.; Bao, W.; Li, Y.; Wang, Y.; Chen, Z. Land Use Transition and Its Eco-Environmental Effects in the Beijing–Tianjin–Hebei Urban Agglomeration: A Production–Living–Ecological Perspective. *Land* **2020**, *9*, 285. [CrossRef]
26. Lin, G.; Jiang, D.; Fu, J.; Cao, C.; Zhang, D. Spatial Conflict of Production–Living–Ecological Space and Sustainable-Development Scenario Simulation in Yangtze River Delta Agglomerations. *Sustainability* **2020**, *12*, 2175. [CrossRef]
27. Zhu, Y.Y.; Yu, B.; Zeng, J.X.; Han, Y. Spatial Optimization from Three Spaces of Production, Living and Ecology in National Restricted Zones: A Case Study of Wufeng County in Hubei Province. *Econ. Geogr.* **2015**, *35*, 26–32.
28. Chan, R.C.; Shimou, Y. Urbanization and Sustainable Metropolitan Development in China: Patterns, Problems and Prospects. *GeoJournal* **1999**, *49*, 269–277. [CrossRef]
29. Wang, J.P.; Yu, D.; Lu, Y.; Zhang, T.; Zheng, Y.P. Recognition and Analysis of Land Use Conflicts at County Level Based on Production-Living-Ecological Suitability. *J. Nat. Resour.* **2021**, *36*, 1238–1251. [CrossRef]
30. Xiong, J.; Chen, D.; Peng, B.; Deng, S.; Xie, X. Spatio-Temporal Difference of Coupling Coordinative Degree of Ecological Carrying Capacity in the Dongting Lake Region. *Sci. Geogr. Sin.* **2014**, *34*, 1108–1116.
31. Yu, L.; Song, A.; Zheng, Y.; Jian, Q.; Zhang, P. The Ecological-Livingindustrial Land Classification System and the Analysis of Its Spatial Distribution: Case of Changli County. *Chin. J. Agric. Resour. Reg. Plan.* **2017**, *38*, 89–96.
32. Jin, X.; Lu, Y.Q. Research on the Evolution of Spatiotemporal Patterns of Production-Livingecological Space in an Urban Agglomeration in the Fujian Delta Region, China. *Acta Ecol. Sin.* **2018**, *38*, 4286–4295.
33. Mingwei, L.; Yuhan, Y.; Weiqiang, C. Classification and Spatial-Temporal Analysis of Productionliving-Ecological Spaces in Henan Province. *Chin. J. Agric. Resour. Reg. Plan.* **2018**, *39*, 13–20.
34. Tan, S. An Outline of Research on Land Conflicts and Their Administration in Foreign Academe. *China Land Sci.* **2007**, *4*, 74–80.
35. Yang, Y.F.; Qian, A.N.; Zhu, L.Q. Diagnosis Based on the Psr Model of Rural Land-Use Conflicts Intensity. *Prog. Geogr.* **2012**, *31*, 1552–1560.
36. Zhou, D.; Xu, J.; Wang, L. Process of Land Use Conflict Research in China During the Past Fifteen Years. *China Land Sci.* **2015**, *29*, 21–29.
37. Zhou, G.H.; Peng, J.J. The Evolution Characteristics and Influence Effect of Spatial Conflict: A Case Study of Changsha-Zhuzhou-Xiangtan Urban Agglomeration. *Prog. Geogr.* **2012**, *31*, 717–723.
38. Liu, K.; Xie, X.; Zhou, Q. Research on the Influencing Factors of Urban Ecological Carrying Capacity Based on a Multiscale Geographic Weighted Regression Model: Evidence from China. *Land* **2021**, *10*, 1313. [CrossRef]
39. Henderson, S.R. Managing Land-Use Conflict around Urban Centres: Australian Poultry Farmer Attitudes Towards Relocation. *Appl. Geogr.* **2005**, *25*, 97–119. [CrossRef]
40. Iojă, C.I.; Niţă, M.R.; Vânău, G.O.; Onose, D.A.; Gavrilidis, A.A. Using Multi-Criteria Analysis for the Identification of Spatial Land-Use Conflicts in the Bucharest Metropolitan Area. *Ecol. Indic.* **2014**, *42*, 112–121. [CrossRef]
41. Karimi, A.; Hockings, M. A Social-Ecological Approach to Land-Use Conflict to Inform Regional and Conservation Planning and Management. *Landsc. Ecol.* **2018**, *33*, 691–710. [CrossRef]

42. Peerzado, M.B.; Magsi, H.; Sheikh, M.J. Land Use Conflicts and Urban Sprawl: Conversion of Agriculture Lands into Urbanization in Hyderabad, Pakistan. *J. Saudi Soc. Agric. Sci.* **2019**, *18*, 423–428. [CrossRef]
43. Zou, L.; Liu, Y.; Wang, J.; Yang, Y.; Wang, Y. Land Use Conflict Identification and Sustainable Development Scenario Simulation on China's Southeast Coast. *J. Clean. Prod.* **2019**, *238*, 117899. [CrossRef]
44. Qiu, C.H.; Li, Y.B.; Feng, Y.S. Ecological Suitability Assessment and Optimization of Urban Land Expansion Space in Guiyang City. *Yingyong Shengtai Xuebao* **2015**, *26*, 9.
45. Liao, G.; He, P.; Gao, X.; Deng, L.; Zhang, H.; Feng, N.; Zhou, W.; Deng, O. The Production–Living–Ecological Land Classification System and Its Characteristics in the Hilly Area of Sichuan Province, Southwest China Based on Identification of the Main Functions. *Sustainability* **2019**, *11*, 1600. [CrossRef]
46. Liu, W.; Zhan, J.; Zhao, F.; Yan, H.; Zhang, F.; Wei, X. Impacts of Urbanization-Induced Land-Use Changes on Ecosystem Services: A Case Study of the Pearl River Delta Metropolitan Region, China. *Ecol. Indic.* **2019**, *98*, 228–238. [CrossRef]
47. Zhou, Y.; Li, X.; Liu, Y. Land Use Change and Driving Factors in Rural China During the Period 1995-2015. *Land Use Policy* **2020**, *99*, 105048. [CrossRef]
48. Wang, S.Y.; Liu, J.S.; Ma, T.B. Dynamics and Changes in Spatial Patterns of Land Use in Yellow River Basin, China. *Land Use Policy* **2010**, *27*, 313–323. [CrossRef]
49. Kong, D.Y.; Chen, H.G.; Wu, K.S. The Evolution of Production-Living-Ecological Space, Eco-Environmental Effects and Its Influencing Factors in China. *J. Nat. Resour.* **2021**, *36*, 1116–1135. [CrossRef]
50. Yin, D.; Li, X.; Li, G.; Zhang, J.; Yu, H. Spatio-Temporal Evolution of Land Use Transition and Its Eco-Environmental Effects: A Case Study of the Yellow River Basin, China. *Land* **2020**, *9*, 514. [CrossRef]

International Journal of
Environmental Research and Public Health

MDPI

Article

Decoupling between Economic Development and Carbon Emissions and Its Driving Factors: Evidence from China

Xiaochun Zhao [1], Mei Jiang [1] and Wei Zhang [2,*]

[1] School of Management, Anhui University, Hefei 230601, China; 14006@ahu.edu.cn (X.Z.); l21201016@stu.ahu.edu.cn (M.J.)
[2] School of Public Administration, Sichuan University, Chengdu 610065, China
* Correspondence: hbue_wb@163.com; Tel.: +86-180-6200-9973

Abstract: Analyzing the relationship between economic development and carbon emissions is conducive to better energy saving and emission reduction. This study is based on the panel data of China's carbon emissions, from 2009 to 2019, and quantitative analysis of the relationship between carbon emissions and economic development through the Tapio decoupling model and the Logarithmic Mean Divisia Index (LMDI) decomposition model. The results show that: First, carbon emission and economic development are increasing year by year, and the development trend of economic growth rate and carbon emission growth rate presents the characteristics of consistency and stage. Second, China's carbon emissions and economic development are basically in a weak decoupling state, and carbon emissions and economic development are positively correlated. Third, there are significant differences in decoupling indices among the four regions, mainly in that the central region is better than the eastern region, the eastern region is better than the northeast region, the northeast region is better than the western region, and the development of provinces in the region is unbalanced. Fourth, from the perspective of driving factors, the elasticity of population size and economic intensity can restrain the decoupling of carbon emissions, while the elasticity of energy intensity and carbon intensity have a positive effect. Finally, according to the results of empirical analysis, this paper focuses on promoting China's emission reduction and energy sustainable development from the aspects of developing low-carbon and zero carbon technology, supporting new energy industries and promoting the construction of a carbon emission trading market.

Keywords: carbon emissions; Tapio decoupling; LMDI model; provincial level; low-carbon economy

Citation: Zhao, X.; Jiang, M.; Zhang, W. Decoupling between Economic Development and Carbon Emissions and Its Driving Factors: Evidence from China. *IJERPH* **2022**, *19*, 2893. https://doi.org/10.3390/ijerph19052893

Academic Editors: Jie Chen, Qian Zhou and Ting Zhang

Received: 5 January 2022
Accepted: 25 February 2022
Published: 2 March 2022

Publisher's Note: MDPI stays neutral with regard to jurisdictional claims in published maps and institutional affiliations.

1. Introduction

In recent years, global warming has led to increasingly frequent extreme weather, which seriously threatens human survival and development. For example, in July 2021, the extreme rainstorm in Henan Province caused 302 people to lose their lives and a direct economic loss of CNY 53.2 billion. Therefore, global warming caused by carbon dioxide emissions has become a topic of increasing concern [1]. As early as the First World Climate Conference held in Geneva in 1979, the issue of global climate warming was raised for the first time. People realized that the global climate change caused by carbon emissions in the industrial era has already threatened human development; thus, measures must be taken to reduce carbon emissions. At present, as the world's largest energy consumer [2], China ranks first in the world in terms of carbon emissions and faces tremendous pressure to reduce emissions. At the same time, as an active participant in emission reduction, the development of a low-carbon economy has always been of great concern for the Chinese government. Based on the basic national conditions and the status quo of social development, the Chinese government has been active in promoting its carbon neutral action plan, and has made certain achievements in reducing the intensity of carbon emissions [3], but the carbon emission growth rate remains fast as a result of rapid economic growth. From 2009 to 2019, China's gross domestic product (GDP) increased by 2.6 times, and its carbon emissions increased by 1.5 times. In order to increase emission reduction efforts, the Chinese government announced that it would realize the peak carbon dioxide emissions by 2030 and carbon neutrality by 2060. Since carbon dioxide emissions are mainly produced in the process of economic development, this paper believes that we should first clarify the relationship between economic development and carbon emissions in order to achieve carbon neutralization more efficiently. Only by clarifying the relationship between them can we take targeted policy to achieve carbon neutrality at a faster speed.

Therefore, this study takes China as an example, which is divided into four regions: eastern, northeast, central and western. From the perspective of decoupling analysis, it makes an empirical analysis of the relationship between economic development and carbon emissions in four regions of China. Combined with the LMDI driving factor decomposition model, it studies which factors play the main role in decoupling carbon emissions, and on this basis, it takes targeted measures to provide intellectual support for further promotion of the sustainable development of China's green economy. As the largest developing country in the world, the analysis of the relationship between China's economic development and carbon emissions can provide some inspiration for other countries in the world to better reduce carbon emissions.

The arrangement of this paper is as follows: It first sorts out the related research results of economic development and carbon emissions. Afterwards, it introduces the research methods and data sources of this paper. Next, it displays and discusses the specific research results. Finally, it mainly puts forward the research findings and corresponding policy recommendations and summarizes the shortcomings of this paper.

2. Literature Review

2.1. Relationship between Carbon Emission and Economic Development

Scholars have performed considerable research on the relationship between carbon emissions and economic development [4]. According to the literature review, it was found that the existing literature mainly focuses on the application of research methods and commonly uses research methods including the Granger causality test analysis, EKC hypothesis and decoupling model. First, Granger causality is used to analyze the correlation between two variables; it can play a certain role in economic forecasting. For example, Kofi et al. (2017) found that there was a long-term one-way causal relationship between energy consumption and economic growth in China using the Granger causality analysis and proposed that China should transform its trade growth mode [5]. Melike et al. (2019) studied Granger causality between carbon dioxide emissions and economic growth in China and the United States and found that there was a one-way causal relationship between carbon emissions and economic growth in China, but it has not been the case in the United States. The results showed that different regions should adopt different policy recommendations [6]. Second, by analyzing the relationship between economic development and carbon emissions, scholars use the Environmental Kuznets Curve (EKC) as an analytical perspective [7]. EKC reveals that there is an inverted U-shaped relationship between the environment and the economy, which is a powerful tool for studying environmental problems and economic development. For example, Abdul et al. (2018) selected BRICS countries as research objects and analyzed the relationship between financial development, globalization, economic growth, energy consumption, urbanization and carbon emissions of BRICS countries based on the existence of the EKC hypothesis and supported the EKC hypothesis in BRICS countries [8]. Subsequently, the academic circle has conducted many studies on whether the hypothesis of an inverted U-shaped curve is correct. Awaworyi et al. (2018) analyzed the curves of the relationship between environmental pollution and economic development of 20 Organization for Economic Cooperation and Development (OECD) countries through the panel data estimator, and found that only nine countries were in line with the EKC hypothesis. Moreover, there appeared multiple shapes of the relationship curve such as an inverted U, an inverted N and N-shape, but no single shape was applicable to all regions [9]. Pan et al. (2017), based on the data of India and China from 1971 to 2012, discussed the cointegration relationship among carbon emissions and economic activities and tested the EKC hypothesis, thus discovering that the relationship between economic growth and carbon emissions was N-shaped, which deviated from the EKC hypothesis [10]. Finally, in order to clarify the state between economic development and carbon emissions in different regions at different times, academic circles generally use decoupling model for empirical analysis [11]. To analyze the relationship between the European Union (EU) and Finland road traffic flow, carbon dioxide emissions, and GDP from 1970 to 2001, Petri Tapio (2005) introduced decoupling elasticity into decoupling research for the first time, and further subdivided the concepts of decoupling, coupling and negative decoupling, so as to set eight decoupling indicators according to the ratio of carbon emission change to economic development change. The study showed that the relationship between carbon dioxide produced by transportation and GDP was weakly decoupled [12]. Karmellos et al. (2021), based on decoupling theory, analyzed the decoupling state between carbon emissions generated by electricity and economic growth in the EU and discovered that most countries were in a strong decoupling state from 2013 to 2018 [13]. Smbi et al. (2021) used the gravity model, LMDI model and Tapio decoupling model to study the decoupling state between economic development and carbon emissions in Africa, and the results showed that many countries in Africa showed obvious negative decoupling and weak decoupling [14]. Xin et al. (2021) used the two-dimensional decoupling model to explore the dynamic decoupling relationship between economic development and carbon emissions in Gansu Province from 2000 to 2017. The results showed that the two-dimensional decoupling state of Gansu Province was low-level weak decoupling [15].

2.2. Decomposition of Carbon Emission Drivers

In terms of analyzing the decomposition of carbon emission driving factors, scholars have carried out many studies, and the current research methods include the structural decomposition model and exponential decomposition model [16]. The structural decomposition model is used to analyze the change in dependent variables by the change of independent variables. Wang et al. (2017) decomposed the carbon emissions of Guangdong Province based on the structural decomposition model and found that economic and population growth had positive effects on carbon emissions, and the intensity of carbon emissions was the main factor in restraining carbon emissions [17]. Vries et al. (2017) used the structural decomposition model to analyze the decoupling between carbon emissions and economic growth in developed and emerging economies, and decomposed the driving factors into global supply chain participation, consumption and technology [18]. Ninpanit et al. (2019) carried out the structural decomposition analysis (SDA) to study the factors that led to the change in carbon emissions in Thailand, and found that the increase in per capita consumption in Thailand and abroad had obvious influences on the growth of carbon emissions, but the improvement of energy efficiency was not enough to reduce emissions [19].The exponential decomposition model is a method of decomposing the change of the independent variable into the change of the dependent variable [20]. Román et al. (2018) constructed the Index Decomposition Analysis–Logarithmic Mean Divisia Index (IDA-LMDI) model to analyze the driving factors of carbon emissions in Colombia, and pointed out that income and population are the main driving factors affecting carbon emissions [21]. Yang et al. (2021) used the exponential decomposition model to analyze the driving factors of carbon emissions based on the carbon emission panel data of 78 regions and found that the production efficiency and energy-saving technology had positive effects on reducing global carbon emissions, while the growth of per capita GDP and population growth had inhibitory effects on global carbon emissions [22]. Liu et al. (2021) proposed that seven factors had driving effects on carbon emissions based on the decoupling relationship between carbon emissions and economic growth in China's transportation industry [23], and technical effects were the main factors in restraining carbon emissions. To sum up, scholars have conducted in-depth discussions on the research of carbon emission drivers, but most of them are confined to a certain sub-sector, such as transportation, non-ferrous metal industry, and the agriculture and industrial sectors, or are limited to a certain province or region. Little research has been performed on China's overall carbon emission drivers, and to ensure that the results are reliable and have no residuals [24], this paper mainly uses the LMDI model to analyze China's carbon emission drivers.

The research results of these studies are beneficial to reduce carbon emissions, but they still have shortcomings. First, most scholars' analyses of decoupling between carbon emissions and economic development is limited to grade assessment, without analyzing the deep causes of decoupling. Second, the literature analyzing the driving factors of carbon emissions focuses only on a certain industry or region, and there is a lack of research on the driving factors of carbon emissions in China as a whole. Therefore, in order to fill the above research gap, based on the carbon emission panel data of 30 provinces in China, this paper decided to study the decoupling status of economic development and carbon emissions using the Tapio decoupling model and constructs of the LMDI model to explore the driving factors that affect the decoupling of carbon emission, so as to analyze the underlying reasons of China's current decoupling state, with a view to providing policy inspirations for China to realize peak carbon dioxide emissions and carbon neutrality.

3. Research Methods and Data Sources

3.1. Research Methods

3.1.1. Carbon Emission Measurement

Since the China Energy Statistics Yearbook does not have official data on carbon emissions of Chinese provinces, this study refers to the carbon emission coefficient method of energy consumption described by the United Nations Intergovernmental Panel on Climate Change (IPCC) and draws on the research results of Fan et al. (2019) to choose eight carbon sources such as coal, coke, kerosene and natural gas to calculate carbon emissions in combination with the carbon emission coefficient of each energy source [25]. The specific formula is as follows:

$$C = \sum_{j=1}^{8} E_j \times \alpha_j \times \xi_j \tag{1}$$

where C represents carbon emission, E_j represents the physical consumption of the j-th energy, α_j represents the coefficient of standard coal, and ξ_j represents the carbon emission coefficient.

3.1.2. Tapio Decoupling Model

"Decoupling" refers to the trend that the relationship between economic development and environmental pollution is constantly separated. This concept was gradually extended from agricultural policy research to environmental field by OECD. In this study, "decoupling" is used to describe the gradual reduction of carbon emissions with economic growth. Currently, widely used decoupling models mainly include the Organization for Economic Co-operation and Development (OECD) decoupling index method and Tapio decoupling index method. Compared with the OECD decoupling model, the Tapio decoupling index method can better reflect the decoupling state between economic development and carbon emissions without considering the limitation of base period [26]. Therefore, this study uses the Tapio decoupling model to measure China's decoupling elasticity, and the specific formula is as follows:

$$\beta = \frac{\Delta C/C}{\Delta GDP/GDP} \tag{2}$$

where β represents the decoupling index, C and GDP represent the base period values of carbon emissions and GDP, respectively, while $\triangle C$ and $\triangle GDP$ represent the difference between current period and base period of carbon emissions and GDP. The Tapio decoupling model is specifically divided into eight decoupling states, as shown in Figure 1.

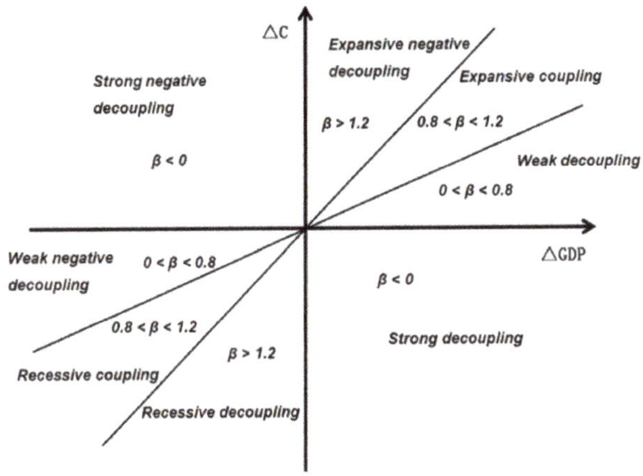

Figure 1. Decoupling state division.

3.1.3. LMDI Driving Factor Decomposition Model of Carbon Emission

The factor decomposition method includes the structure decomposition method and exponential decomposition method. The exponential decomposition method has the advantages of no residual error and strong applicability and can enhance the reliability of the results [27]; thus, the LMDI exponential decomposition method is adopted in this paper. Drawing on the basic principle of Kaya identity, the formula for carbon emission can be expressed as:

$$C = P \times \frac{G}{P} \times \frac{E}{G} \times \frac{C}{E} = p \times g \times e \times s \tag{3}$$

where P represents the population, G represents the gross domestic product, E represents the energy consumption, C represents the carbon emissions, p represents population size, g represents per capita GDP, e represents energy intensity and s represents carbon emission intensity. According to LMDI addition decomposition, the carbon emission change ΔC in the target year relative to the base year can be decomposed into:

$$\Delta C = \Delta C^t - \Delta C^o = \Delta C_p + \Delta C_g + \Delta C_e + \Delta C_s \tag{4}$$

where $\triangle C_p$ represents population effect, $\triangle C_g$ represents economic intensity effect, $\triangle C_e$ represents energy intensity effect and $\triangle C_s$ represents carbon intensity effect. Among them:

$$\begin{gathered} \Delta C_p = \sum W \times \ln \frac{C_p^t}{C_p^o} \\ \Delta C_g = \sum W \times \ln \frac{C_g^t}{C_g^o} \\ \Delta C_e = \sum W \times \ln \frac{C_e^t}{C_e^o} \\ \Delta C_s = \sum W \times \ln \frac{C_s^t}{C_s^o} \\ W = \frac{(C^t - C^o)}{\ln(C^t / C^o)} \end{gathered} \tag{5}$$

By combining Equations (2) and (4), it can be concluded that:

$$\begin{aligned} \beta = \Delta C \times \tfrac{GDP}{C \times \Delta GDP} = (\Delta C_p + \Delta C_g + \Delta C_e + \Delta C_s) \times \tfrac{GDP}{C \times \Delta GDP} = \tfrac{\Delta C_p \times GDP}{C \times \Delta GDP} \\ + \tfrac{\Delta C_g \times GDP}{C \times \Delta GDP} + \tfrac{\Delta C_e \times GDP}{C \times \Delta GDP} + \tfrac{\Delta C_s \times GDP}{C \times \Delta GDP} = f_p + f_g + f_e + f_s \end{aligned} \tag{6}$$

where f_p represents the decoupling index of population, f_g represents the decoupling index of economic intensity, f_e represents the decoupling index of energy intensity and f_s represents the decoupling index of carbon intensity.

3.2. Data Sources

This paper selects the national data from 2009 to 2019 for the empirical analysis. Economic growth is expressed by gross domestic product (GDP). GDP data and population data come from the China Statistical Yearbook (2010–2020), and energy consumption data come from the China Energy Statistical Yearbook (2010–2020). There are eight types of energies in statistics, which are uniformly converted into ten thousand tons of standard coal. Based on the availability of data, this paper takes 30 provinces, cities and municipalities in China as the research object, not including Tibet, Hong Kong, Macao and Taiwan.

4. Results

4.1. Characteristics of Economic Development and Carbon Emissions

According to Equation (1), this study can calculate China's annual carbon emissions from 2009 to 2019. The specific calculation results are shown in Figure 2. In order to better understand the differences in carbon emissions among Chinese provinces, the specific calculation results are shown in Figure 3.

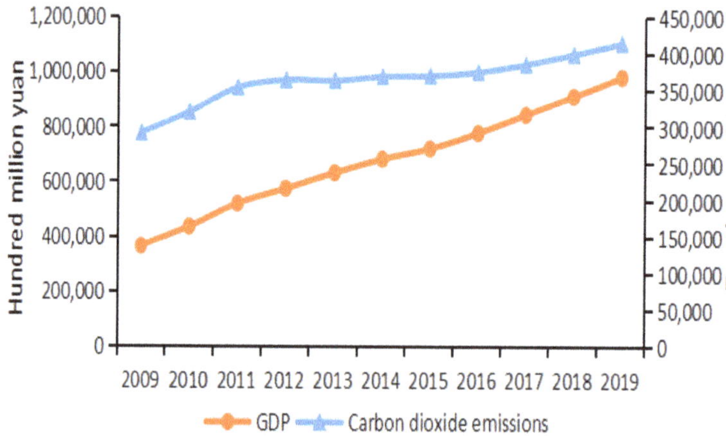

Figure 2. Carbon emissions and economic growth trend (2009–2019).

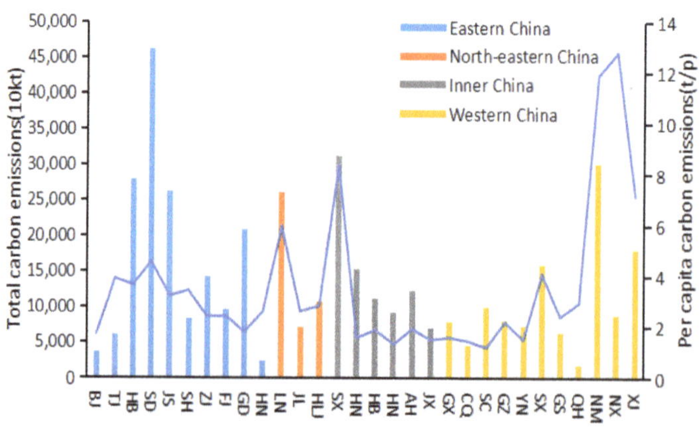

Figure 3. Total carbon emissions and per capita carbon emissions of province.

On the whole, from 2009 to 2019, China's carbon emissions and economic development level increased year by year. This shows that in China, the largest energy consumer, a large amount of energy consumption not only brings rapid economic development, but also leads to an increase in carbon emissions [28]. It can be seen that the level of economic development is closely related to the growth rate of carbon emissions. However, Figure 2 also shows that the growth trend of carbon emission has tended to level off in the past decade under the rapid growth of the economy, showing that China's low-carbon development has achieved some results in recent years. According to the situation of carbon emissions in Figure 2, it can be divided into two stages: the first stage from 2009 to 2012 and the second stage from 2012 to 2019. In the first stage, carbon emissions increased rapidly, while in the second stage, carbon emissions tended to flatten out. The reason for the rapid growth in the first stage may be that the Chinese government strengthened energy consumption after the world financial crisis in 2008 in order to promote economic recovery. The reason for the slowing of carbon emissions in the second phase is that the eighteenth national congress of the Chinese government in 2012 put forward a strategic decision to vigorously promote the construction of ecological civilization. As the basis of the Overall Plan for Development in Five Areas, the building of an eco-civilization has become the focus of the Chinese government. Following the concept of "lucid waters and lush mountains are invaluable assets", China has made great improvement in cutting carbon emissions by implementing effective policies [29].

In order to better understand the characteristics of China's carbon emissions, China's 30 provinces are divided into eastern, northeastern, central and western regions (see Figure 3). The average carbon emissions of eastern China were higher than the northeast, central and western regions, and the economic development level of the eastern region was also higher than the other three regions, indicating that there is a positive correlation between economic development and carbon emissions. According to the provincial data, Hebei, Shandong and Jiangsu provinces have the highest carbon emissions, and the economic development level of these three provinces ranks the top ten in China. Among these three provinces, Jiangsu's carbon emissions are relatively low, but the economic development level is the highest. The main reason is that Jiangsu province is committed to improving energy efficiency and developing emerging industries such as information technology to promote economic development [30], while Shandong and Hebei provinces rely on heavy industry to develop their economy [30], and infrastructure construction is imperfect, industrial energy consumption is large, and the introduction rate of energy-saving technology is low. Therefore, it is urgent that the two provinces increase the policy support. Among them, Beijing, Hainan and Qinghai provinces have the lowest carbon emissions. The main reason is that the population sizes in these three provinces are much smaller than that of other regions. Moreover, Beijing ranks first in terms of the economic development level among these three provinces. As the political center of China, Beijing responds quickly to the green and low-carbon policy and has a great advantage in transportation [31]. It has adopted many effective measures to cut emissions and speed up the transformation and upgrading of the economy. From Figure 3, there are differences between the results of per capita carbon emissions and total carbon emissions in each province. The per capita carbon emissions in Liaoning, Shanxi, Inner Mongolia and Ningxia provinces are much higher than those in Hebei, Shandong and Jiangsu provinces, where the total carbon emissions are relatively high. The reason is that the regional carbon emissions are affected by the population [32]. To sum up, China's carbon emissions not only exist as regional imbalances, but also, the provinces within the region have significant differences due to reasons such as population size and economic development level [33].

It can be seen from Figure 4 that from 2009 to 2019, China's economic growth rate was higher than the growth rate of carbon emissions, and the economic growth rate was consistent with the growth rate of the carbon emissions. Since 2012, the growth rate of carbon emissions has been below 5% (see Figure 4). It can be seen that the concept of green and low carbon has played a certain role in restraining carbon emissions, and the Chinese government has also made great efforts to reduce carbon emissions [34]. From 2011 to 2013 and from 2014 to 2015, the growth rate of carbon emissions decreased significantly, showing that the Chinese government complied with the theme of scientific development and the main line of accelerating the transformation of economic development mode in the 12th Five-Year Plan to effectively solve the problems between the economy and environment [35]. The results also show that the vigorous progress made in the 12th Five-Year Plan has become an important turning point on China's emission reduction road [36], laying a foundation for the slowdown of carbon emissions growth and the improvement of economic development efficiency.

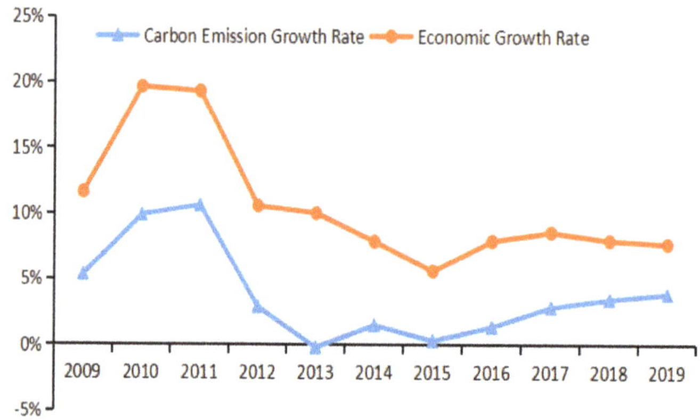

Figure 4. General trend chart of carbon emission growth rate and economic growth rate (2009–2019).

4.2. Decoupling Analysis of China's Economic Growth and Carbon Emissions

The above section analyzes the overall characteristics of carbon emissions in different regions of China and has a systematic understanding of carbon emissions and economic development in different regions of China. Next, this paper uses the Tapio decoupling model, namely Equation (2), to analyze the decoupling between China's economic growth and carbon emissions from 2009 to 2019, and the results are shown in Table 1.

Generally speaking, from 2009 to 2019, China's 30 provinces were basically in a weak decoupling state, and carbon emissions were positively correlated with economic development. During this period, the average growth rate of carbon emissions was 3.6%, while the average growth rate of economic development level was 10.5%. As the economic growth rate was higher than that of carbon emissions, carbon emissions and economic development were in a weak decoupling state, which showed that China, as a big energy country, still has a high dependence on energy consumption to developed economy. According to the fluctuation of the decoupling index, it can be seen that China's decoupling index gradually decreased from 2009 to 2019, which was mainly due to the active measures taken by the Chinese government to transform industrial structures [34], actively developing a green and low-carbon circular development industrial system under the high attention of the international environment to climate issues.

There are significant differences in China's decoupling situation (see Table 1), which mainly shows that the central region is better than the eastern region, the eastern region is better than the northeast region, the northeast region is better than the western region, and the decoupling elasticity of carbon emissions and economic development in the western region was always lower than the average decoupling elasticity in China. The six central provinces share similar conditions of economy and population, and their average decoupling index shows little diverseness. However, Shanxi Province has the highest decoupling index, mainly because Shanxi, as an energy-based province and major coal producer, has a slow rate of economic growth and a strong dependence on energy, and is still at the exploration stage of energy transformation [37]. From 2017 to 2019, Henan Province was in a strong decoupling state. The reason is that the economic development level of Henan has been in the forefront of the country and the industrial structure has continuously been optimized, achieving economic growth while improving environmental benefits [38]. However, there are significant differences in the decoupling situation among the eastern provinces, and the high difference in the decoupling index inhibits the average carbon emission index in the eastern region. Among them, Beijing has been in a strong decoupling type at all stages (see Table 1). The decoupling index between Tianjin and Shandong was relatively high, because Shandong Province, as an industrial city, has large demand for energy that has led to carbon emissions. It can be seen that there are significant internal differences in the decoupling elasticity of carbon emissions in the eastern region. Northeast China is rich in coal resources, with heavy industry as the pillar industry causing carbon emissions [39]. Due to the relatively backward economic development in the western region, the application of energy-saving technologies was relatively rare. Ningxia is the most prominent example in this region, and the decoupling state is expansive coupling. The reason for the expansive coupling may be that Ningxia is well positioned in the field of new energy development with its the utilization rate of new energy taking the lead nationwide [40]. The complete infrastructures in the energy industry and the good trend of economic development have caused the rapid increase in carbon emissions.

Table 1. Decoupling between carbon emissions and economic growth.

Area	Province	2009–2011		2011–2013		2013–2015		2015–2017		2017–2019	
		β	Decoupling	β	Decoupling	β	Decoupling	β	Decoupling	β	Decoupling
Eastern China	Beijing	−0.157	Strong	−0.193	Strong	−0.105	Strong	−0.114	Strong	−0.064	Strong
	Tianjin	0.731	Weak	0.459	Weak	0.295	Weak	0.198	Weak	0.407	Weak
	Hebei	0.513	Weak	0.36	Weak	0.231	Weak	0.149	Weak	0.264	Weak
	Shandong	0.481	Weak	0.307	Weak	0.425	Weak	0.417	Weak	0.532	Weak
	Jiangsu	0.666	Weak	0.471	Weak	0.38	Weak	0.297	Weak	0.248	Weak
	Shanghai	0.466	Weak	0.398	Weak	0.166	Weak	0.128	Weak	0.081	Weak
	Zhejiang	0.349	Weak	0.177	Weak	0.137	Weak	0.135	Weak	0.112	Weak
	Fujian	0.639	Weak	0.304	Weak	0.355	Weak	0.241	Weak	0.257	Weak
	Guangdong	0.594	Weak	0.314	Weak	0.231	Weak	0.231	Weak	0.19	Weak
	Hainan	0.54	Weak	0.231	Weak	0.395	Weak	0.239	Weak	0.235	Weak
	Mean	0.482	Weak	0.283	Weak	0.251	Weak	0.192	Weak	0.226	Weak
Northeast China	Liaoning	0.369	Weak	0.203	Weak	0.147	Weak	0.324	Weak	0.6	Weak
	Jilin	0.609	Weak	0.264	Weak	0.13	Weak	0.095	Weak	0.125	Weak
	Heilongjiang	0.338	Weak	0.199	Weak	0.192	Weak	0.201	Weak	0.224	Weak
	Mean	0.439	Weak	0.222	Weak	0.157	Weak	0.207	Weak	0.317	Weak
Central China	Shanxi	0.349	Weak	0.371	Weak	0.392	Weak	0.421	Weak	0.573	Weak
	Henan	0.502	Weak	0.157	Weak	0.127	Weak	0.04	Weak	−0.032	Strong
	Hubei	0.587	Weak	0.143	Weak	0.106	Weak	0.097	Weak	0.089	Weak
	Hunan	0.369	Weak	0.152	Weak	0.13	Weak	0.136	Weak	0.074	Weak
	Anhui	0.264	Weak	0.311	Weak	0.279	Weak	0.224	Weak	0.165	Weak
	Jiangxi	0.525	Weak	0.429	Weak	0.394	Weak	0.325	Weak	0.279	Weak
	Mean	0.433	Weak	0.26	Weak	0.238	Weak	0.207	Weak	0.191	Weak
Western China	Guangxi	1.058	Expansive	0.791	Weak	0.517	Weak	0.562	Weak	0.545	Weak
	Chongqing	0.482	Weak	0.081	Weak	0.121	Weak	0.086	Weak	0.039	Weak
	Sichuan	0.092	Weak	0.123	Weak	0.084	Weak	0.018	Weak	0.012	Weak
	Guizhou	0.25	Weak	0.249	Weak	0.126	Weak	0.11	Weak	0.067	Weak
	Yunnan	0.201	Weak	0.124	Weak	−0.088	Weak	−0.035	Weak	0.05	Weak
	Shaanxi	0.565	Weak	0.585	Weak	0.532	Weak	0.426	Weak	0.381	Weak
	Gansu	0.573	Weak	0.405	Weak	0.317	Weak	0.239	Weak	0.223	Weak
	Qinghai	0.355	Weak	0.571	Weak	0.284	Weak	0.352	Weak	0.264	Weak
	Inner Mongolia	0.782	Weak	0.537	Weak	0.512	Weak	0.791	Weak	1.197	Expansive
	Ningxia	1.015	Expansive	0.893	Expansive	0.786	Weak	0.862	Expansive	1.007	Expansive
	Xinjiang	0.597	Weak	0.742	Weak	0.79	Weak	0.757	Weak	0.637	Weak
	Mean	0.498	Weak	0.425	Weak	0.332	Weak	0.347	Weak	0.368	Weak
Whole country	Mean	0.49	Weak	0.339	Weak	0.28	Weak	0.265	Weak	0.293	Weak

Note: Strong represents strong decoupling, weak represents weak decoupling, expansive represents expansive coupling.

4.3. Decomposition Analysis of Driving Factors of Carbon Emission in China

According to the LMDI-driven decomposition model, namely Equation (3), Equation (4), Equation (5), and Equation (6), the elasticity of carbon emission driving factors in China's 30 provinces from 2009 to 2019 was measured. It was divided into five stages: 2009–2011, 2011–2013, 2013–2015, 2015–2017, and 2017–2019. The results are shown in Table 2, and the results of the contributions to the four driving factors are shown in Figure 5.

Table 2. Elasticity of Carbon emission driving factors.

Area	Province	Year									
		2009–2011	2011–2013	2013–2015	2015–2017	2017–2019	2009–2011	2011–2013	2013–2015	2015–2017	2017–2019
		f_p					f_g				
Eastern China	Beijing	0.404	0.278	0.227	0.150	0.101	0.434	0.449	0.454	0.440	0.424
	Tianjin	0.230	0.236	0.225	0.184	0.321	0.722	0.614	0.543	0.517	0.519
	Hebei	0.076	0.071	0.080	0.073	0.083	0.846	0.786	0.732	0.674	0.693
	Shandong	0.056	0.048	0.053	0.059	0.071	0.874	0.801	0.793	0.756	0.786
	Jiangsu	0.059	0.043	0.037	0.031	0.028	0.887	0.830	0.777	0.708	0.656
	Shanghai	0.772	0.553	0.360	0.237	0.162	0.167	0.345	0.447	0.494	0.481
	Zhejiang	0.140	0.098	0.082	0.076	0.078	0.757	0.718	0.680	0.626	0.559
	Fujian	0.066	0.056	0.060	0.055	0.048	0.875	0.766	0.737	0.648	0.603
	Guangdong	0.273	0.186	0.153	0.132	0.119	0.672	0.672	0.640	0.604	0.552
	Hainan	0.032	0.042	0.053	0.049	0.050	0.881	0.740	0.747	0.648	0.605
Northeast China	Liaoning	0.035	0.022	0.017	0.023	0.014	0.856	0.773	0.745	0.845	0.900
	Jilin	0.008	0.006	0.005	−0.008	−0.031	0.926	0.806	0.743	0.725	0.841
	Heilongjiang	0.005	0.004	−0.005	−0.012	−0.036	0.879	0.809	0.803	0.796	0.874
Central China	Shanxi	0.098	0.090	0.104	0.085	0.086	0.777	0.760	0.749	0.735	0.770
	Henan	−0.030	−0.013	−0.001	0.006	0.009	0.956	0.821	0.754	0.653	0.549
	Hubei	0.015	0.016	0.019	0.020	0.016	0.908	0.740	0.668	0.608	0.537
	Hunan	0.063	0.052	0.051	0.047	0.040	0.820	0.711	0.654	0.613	0.545
	Anhui	−0.055	−0.021	0.002	0.014	0.017	0.915	0.828	0.761	0.677	0.570
	Jiangxi	0.027	0.027	0.031	0.032	0.030	0.883	0.818	0.773	0.708	0.646
Western China	Guangxi	−0.109	−0.044	−0.014	0.006	0.017	1.119	0.989	0.861	0.843	0.806
	Chongqing	0.044	0.041	0.041	0.040	0.036	0.857	0.687	0.635	0.558	0.481
	Sichuan	−0.035	−0.012	0.002	0.009	0.010	0.868	0.770	0.699	0.595	0.517
	Guizhou	−0.209	−0.086	−0.048	−0.027	−0.016	1.079	0.853	0.695	0.597	0.506
	Yunnan	0.031	0.029	0.029	0.029	0.024	0.834	0.720	0.592	0.544	0.489
	Shaanxi	−0.017	−0.003	0.006	0.013	0.017	0.934	0.884	0.843	0.765	0.713
	Gansu	−0.064	−0.027	−0.015	−0.003	0.003	0.989	0.867	0.813	0.750	0.697
	Qinghai	0.039	0.048	0.051	0.061	0.061	0.834	0.831	0.709	0.706	0.643
	Inner Mongolia	0.061	0.050	0.052	0.082	0.087	0.902	0.839	0.821	0.873	0.959
	Ningxia	0.050	0.068	0.081	0.089	0.104	0.952	0.903	0.853	0.862	0.898
	Xinjiang	0.048	0.065	0.107	0.122	0.114	0.873	0.863	0.828	0.791	0.732
Area	Province	f_e					f_s				
Eastern China	Beijing	−0.941	−0.860	−0.713	−0.639	−0.537	−0.055	−0.061	−0.072	−0.067	−0.051
	Tianjin	−0.207	−0.388	−0.455	−0.481	−0.387	−0.013	−0.003	−0.017	−0.022	−0.045
	Hebei	−0.411	−0.495	−0.572	−0.591	−0.505	0.002	−0.003	−0.009	−0.008	−0.007
	Shandong	−0.424	−0.528	−0.405	−0.375	−0.314	−0.025	−0.013	−0.017	−0.024	−0.011
	Jiangsu	−0.283	−0.398	−0.428	−0.434	−0.429	0.003	−0.003	−0.006	−0.009	−0.008
	Shanghai	−0.465	−0.484	−0.617	−0.578	−0.546	−0.008	−0.015	−0.024	−0.025	−0.016
	Zhejiang	−0.535	−0.623	−0.608	−0.551	−0.512	−0.014	−0.015	−0.018	−0.016	−0.013
	Fujian	−0.276	−0.495	−0.428	−0.451	−0.388	−0.026	−0.024	−0.013	−0.011	−0.006
	Guangdong	−0.389	−0.566	−0.572	−0.509	−0.484	0.039	0.022	0.009	0.004	0.002
	Hainan	−0.341	−0.532	−0.402	−0.453	−0.419	−0.032	−0.019	−0.002	−0.005	−0.001
Northeast China	Liaoning	−0.508	−0.580	−0.604	−0.525	−0.300	−0.014	−0.012	−0.010	−0.018	−0.014
	Jilin	−0.327	−0.546	−0.616	−0.615	−0.675	0.002	−0.001	−0.003	−0.007	−0.009
	Heilongjiang	−0.539	−0.619	−0.603	−0.585	−0.614	−0.007	0.005	−0.002	0.002	0.001
Central China	Shanxi	−0.525	−0.473	−0.453	−0.391	−0.278	−0.001	−0.006	−0.009	−0.008	−0.005
	Henan	−0.419	−0.633	−0.615	−0.605	−0.573	−0.005	−0.019	−0.011	−0.014	−0.016
	Hubei	−0.364	−0.613	−0.575	−0.524	−0.456	0.028	0.000	−0.005	−0.005	−0.007
	Hunan	−0.502	−0.600	−0.560	−0.511	−0.495	−0.011	−0.012	−0.015	−0.014	−0.015
	Anhui	−0.581	−0.482	−0.470	−0.453	−0.411	−0.014	−0.014	−0.014	−0.014	−0.011
	Jiangxi	−0.370	−0.394	−0.391	−0.399	−0.382	−0.015	−0.022	−0.019	−0.017	−0.015
Western China	Guangxi	0.038	−0.171	−0.330	−0.286	−0.282	0.009	0.016	0.000	0.000	0.003
	Chongqing	−0.408	−0.619	−0.531	−0.491	−0.456	−0.011	−0.028	−0.024	−0.020	−0.021
	Sichuan	−0.722	−0.621	−0.597	−0.563	−0.494	−0.020	−0.014	−0.020	−0.023	−0.021
	Guizhou	−0.616	−0.513	−0.511	−0.451	−0.412	−0.004	−0.005	−0.009	−0.009	−0.011
	Yunnan	−0.643	−0.617	−0.690	−0.593	−0.452	−0.020	−0.008	−0.018	−0.015	−0.010
	Shaanxi	−0.358	−0.308	−0.326	−0.356	−0.351	0.006	0.011	0.008	0.004	0.002
	Gansu	−0.351	−0.423	−0.467	−0.493	−0.467	0.000	−0.013	−0.013	−0.015	−0.011
	Qinghai	−0.502	−0.303	−0.460	−0.394	−0.418	−0.016	−0.004	−0.015	−0.020	−0.022
	Inner Mongolia	−0.184	−0.362	−0.372	−0.175	0.135	0.004	0.010	0.010	0.012	0.016
	Ningxia	0.010	−0.083	−0.151	−0.092	0.001	0.003	0.004	0.003	0.003	0.004
	Xinjiang	−0.332	−0.188	−0.142	−0.160	−0.214	0.007	0.002	−0.003	0.004	0.005

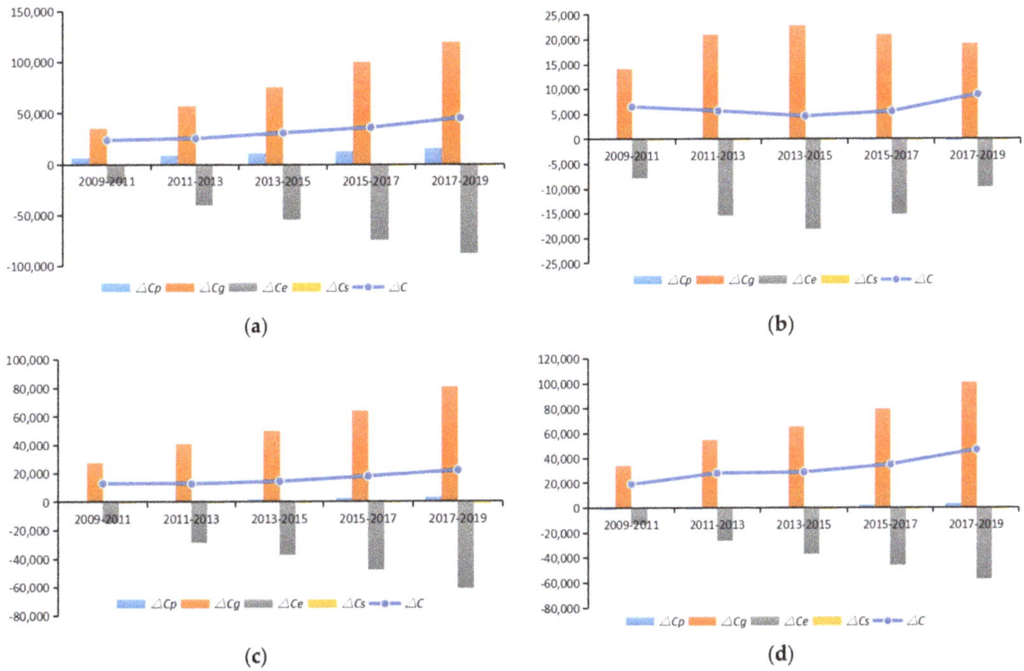

Figure 5. Contribution of various influencing factors of carbon emissions (2009–2019): (**a**) eastern China; (**b**) northeastern China; (**c**) inner China; (**d**) western China.

It can be analyzed from Table 2 that the elasticity of population size and elasticity of economic intensity are basically positive, and these two factors have an inhibition effect on the decoupling state of carbon emissions in various regions of China, and on the whole, the elasticity of economic intensity has the highest value; that is, the elasticity of economic development is the most important inhibition factor for the decoupling of carbon emissions and plays a dominant role in the increase in carbon emissions. It can be seen that various regions of China need to accelerate the transformation of economic development mode. Among the driving factors, energy intensity elasticity and carbon intensity elasticity are negative as a whole, which play major roles in promoting the decoupling of carbon emissions. Among them, carbon intensity elasticity has little influence on the decoupling of carbon emissions, and energy intensity elasticity is the main driving force for restraining carbon emissions. It can be seen that all regions in China need to improve the utilization rate of energy, expand the scope of introducing energy-saving technologies and exert the important influence of energy intensity on the decoupling of carbon emissions. The elasticity of economic intensity of 30 provinces has gradually decreased, and the inhibitory effect on carbon emission decoupling has also decreased. In summary, the Chinese government has made some progress in changing the mode of economic development, which has effectively alleviated the economy's excessive dependence on energy. Energy intensity elasticity is increasingly important, and the Chinese government also provided great support in improving energy efficiency.

From the contribution of driving factors, the economic intensity of the four regions as a whole contributes greatly to the increase in carbon emissions, while the energy intensity contributes to the reduction of carbon emissions, and the contribution of economic intensity was higher than the contribution of incremental carbon emissions. The contribution has risen year by year, which shows that the economy still has a strong dependence on energy. As it is shown in Figure 5, the population size in the eastern region also plays a role in promoting carbon emissions, while the population size in the other three places has no significant influence. The reason may be that the eastern region has a high level of economic development and large population mobility, forming in a certain population size [41]. The increase in carbon emissions in northeast China shows a trend of first rising and then falling and generally shows a slow upward trend, while an increase in carbon emissions in the other three regions shows an increasing trend year by year. Comparing the contribution values of the four regions' economic intensity, the research can find that the eastern region is better than the central region, central region is better than the western region, and the western region is better than the northeast region. To sum up, the energy intensity factors can promote the emission reduction, and there are significant regional differences in the contribution values of the influencing factors of carbon emissions in the four regions.

5. Conclusions and Discussion

This paper estimates the carbon emissions of 30 provinces in China from 2009 to 2019, applying the Tapio decoupling model to analyze the decoupling state of economic development and carbon emissions and the LDMI model to discuss the driving factors behind carbon emissions. Based on China's provincial panel data, we can draw the following conclusions: First, from the perspective of the characteristics of economic development and carbon emissions, both carbon emissions and GDP are increasing year by year, and the economic growth rate is relatively fast and the growth trend of carbon emissions is relatively flat, which is consistent with the policy goal of low-carbon economic development. Second, China's carbon emissions and economic development are basically in a weak decoupling state, and the decoupling index shows a downward trend, from 0.49 to 0.293, which indicates that China's low-carbon economy has achieved certain results, but overall, there is still much room for improvement in China's emission reduction. Third, there are significant differences in the decoupling state between carbon emissions and economic development in different regions of China, and the development of provinces in the region is unbalanced. It mainly shows that the central region is better than the eastern region, the eastern region is better than the northeast region, and the northeast region is better than the western region, and only Beijing Province and Henan Province among the 30 provinces and cities have entered a strong decoupling state. Fourth, the elasticity of economic intensity and the elasticity of population size inhibit the decoupling of China's carbon emissions, while the elasticity of energy intensity and the elasticity of carbon intensity promote it. At the same time, the role of energy intensity in inhibiting carbon emissions is significantly enhanced. Wang and others also found that energy intensity is an important factor in promoting the decoupling process [42], which indicates that China needs to make efforts to improve energy efficiency.

Based on the above research conclusions, in order to promote the construction of China's low-carbon economic development system, the following suggestions are put forward:

(1) Accelerate the development of energy-saving technologies and improve energy utilization [43]. From the panel data of 30 provinces in China, it is concluded that the energy intensity has a positive effect on the decoupling of carbon emissions. Therefore, the Chinese government should pay attention to the application of green technologies to improve energy efficiency [44].
(2) Adjust measures to local conditions and strengthen regional cooperation. In actively exploring the new path of low-carbon development, we should promote the economically developed areas to reach peak carbon dioxide emissions first, and at the same time strengthen regional cooperation [45]. The economically underdeveloped areas should learn from the experience of carbon reduction and promote the sustainable development of energy.
(3) Promote the optimization and upgrading of industrial structure and support the new energy industry. China focuses on the secondary industry, and it is more feasible to develop clean energy than to reduce coal consumption. In recent years, new energy

sources such as solar energy and wind energy have been widely used. The Chinese government can optimize the industrial structure by expanding the proportion of clean energy [46].

(4) Promote the building of the carbon emission trading market. Carbon emission trading market is a powerful tool to reduce carbon emissions by market mechanism and a platform for green and low-carbon economic development. The trading market can effectively reduce the carbon-emission cost, establish a voluntary emission reduction mechanism, and actively promote the regional carbon emission reduction responsibility. Conversely, it is necessary to strengthen the institutional construction of the carbon emission trading market, improve the legal support for the trading market, ensure the standardized operation of the trading market, and promote the strong decoupling between China's economic development and carbon emissions.

The conclusions drawn from the panel data of China's economic development and carbon emissions from 2009 to 2019 can provide a reference for China's low-carbon economic development, but there are still some shortcomings that need to be further improved. First, this study is based on the panel data of 30 provinces only and pays little attention to the characteristics of carbon emissions in different regions within each province; therefore it is limited by the lack of more detailed data, which provide a direction for future research. Second, the driving factors of carbon emissions are diverse and complex, and only four factors are considered in this study. In the future, the research should be further deepened, and other important factors, such as industrial structure and economic structure, should be selected to further improve the research.

Author Contributions: Conceptualization, X.Z.; methodology, M.J.; software, X.Z.; writing—original draft preparation, X.Z.; writing—review and editing, W.Z.; supervision, W.Z. All authors have read and agreed to the published version of the manuscript.

Funding: This work was supported by the National Natural Science Foundation of China (Grant #71804056), Humanities and Social Sciences Research Project of the Ministry of Education of China (#18YJC630250), China Postdoctoral Science Foundation (#2018M642033).

Institutional Review Board Statement: Not applicable.

Informed Consent Statement: Not applicable.

Data Availability Statement: Data available in a publicly accessible repository that does not issue DOIs. Publicly available datasets were analyzed in this study. This data can be found here: [https://navi.cnki.net/knavi/yearbooks/YINFN/detail, accessed on 4 January 2022] [https://navi.cnki.net/knavi/yearbooks/YCXME/detail, accessed on 4 January 2022].

Conflicts of Interest: The authors declare no conflict of interest.

References

1. Chen, J.; Wang, P.; Cui, L.; Huang, S.; Song, M. Decomposition and decoupling analysis of CO2 emissions in OECD. *Appl. Energy* **2018**, *231*, 937–950. [CrossRef]
2. Pan, X.; Guo, S.; Xu, H.; Tian, M.; Pan, X.; Chu, J. China's carbon intensity factor decomposition and carbon emission decoupling analysis. *Energy* **2022**, *239*, 122175. [CrossRef]
3. Wu, Y.; Chau, K.W.; Lu, W.; Shen, L.; Shuai, C.; Chen, J. Decoupling relationship between economic output and carbon emission in the Chinese construction industry. *Environ. Impact Assess. Rev.* **2018**, *71*, 60–69. [CrossRef]
4. Zhou, J.; Guang, F.; Du, S. Decomposing the Decoupling of Carbon Emissions and Economic Growth in China's Power Industry. *Pol. J. Environ. Stud.* **2017**, *26*, 2407–2418. [CrossRef]
5. Boamah, K.B.; Du, J.G.; Bediako, I.A.; Boamah, A.J.; Abdul-Rasheed, A.A.; Owusu, S.M. Carbon dioxide emission and economic growth of China-the role of international trade. *Environ. Sci. Pollut. Res.* **2017**, *24*, 13049–13067. [CrossRef]
6. Bildirici, M.E. Cement production, environmental pollution, and economic growth: Evidence from China and USA. *Clean Technol. Environ. Policy* **2019**, *21*, 783–793. [CrossRef]
7. Rasli, A.M.; Qureshi, M.I.; Isah-Chikaji, A.; Zaman, K.; Ahmad, M. New toxics, race to the bottom and revised environmental Kuznets curve: The case of local and global pollutants. *Renew. Sustain. Energy Rev.* **2018**, *81*, 3120–3130. [CrossRef]
8. Haseeb, A.; Xia, E.; Baloch, M.A.; Abbas, K. Financial development, globalization, and CO2 emission in the presence of EKC: Evidence from BRICS countries. *Environ. Sci. Pollut. Res.* **2018**, *25*, 31283–31296. [CrossRef]

9. Churchill, S.A.; Inekwe, J.; Ivanovski, K.; Smyth, R. The Environmental Kuznets Curve in the OECD: 1870–2014. *Energy Econ.* **2018**, *75*, 389–399. [CrossRef]
10. Pal, D.; Mitra, S.K. The environmental Kuznets curve for carbon dioxide in India and China: Growth and pollution at crossroad. *J. Policy Modeling* **2017**, *39*, 371–385. [CrossRef]
11. Chen, J. Dynamic relationship between urban carbon dioxide emissions and economic growth. *Glob. Nest J.* **2020**, *22*, 632–641. [CrossRef]
12. Tapio, P. Towards a theory of decoupling: Degrees of decoupling in the EU and the case of road traffic in Finland between 1970 and 2001. *Transp. Policy* **2005**, *12*, 137–151. [CrossRef]
13. Karmellos, M.; Kosmadakis, V.; Dimas, P.; Tsakanikas, A.; Fylaktos, N.; Taliotis, C.; Zachariadis, T. A decomposition and decoupling analysis of carbon dioxide emissions from electricity generation: Evidence from the EU-27 and the UK. *Energy* **2021**, *231*, 120861. [CrossRef]
14. Simbi, C.H.; Lin, J.; Yang, D.; Ndayishimiye, J.C.; Liu, Y.; Li, H.; Xu, L.; Ma, W. Decomposition and decoupling analysis of carbon dioxide emissions in African countries during 1984-2014. *J. Environ. Sci.* **2021**, *102*, 85–98. [CrossRef] [PubMed]
15. Xin, L.; Jia, J.; Hu, W.; Zeng, H.; Chen, C.; Wu, B. Decomposition and Decoupling Analysis of CO2 Emissions Based on LMDI and Two-Dimensional Decoupling Model in Gansu Province, China. *Int. J. Environ. Res. Public Health* **2021**, *18*, 6013. [CrossRef] [PubMed]
16. Zha, J.; Dai, J.; Ma, S.; Chen, Y.; Wang, X. How to decouple tourism growth from carbon emissions? A case study of Chengdu, China. *Tour. Manag. Perspect.* **2021**, *39*, 100849. [CrossRef]
17. Wang, C.J.; Wang, F.; Zhang, X.L.; Den, H.J. Analysis of influence mechanism of energy-related carbon emissions in Guangdong: Evidence from regional China based on the input-output and structural decomposition analysis. *Environ. Sci. Pollut. Res.* **2017**, *24*, 25190–25203. [CrossRef]
18. Vries, G.D.; Ferrarini, B. What accounts for the growth of carbon dioxide emissions in advanced and emerging economies? The role of consumption, technology and global supply chain participation. *Ecol. Econ.* **2017**, *132*, 213–223. [CrossRef]
19. Ninpanit, P.; Mali, A.; Wakiyama, T.; Geschke, A.; Lenzen, M. Thailand's energy-related carbon dioxide emissions from production-based and consumption-based perspectives. *Energy Policy* **2019**, *133*, 110877. [CrossRef]
20. Chen, J.; Xu, C.; Song, M. Determinants for decoupling economic growth from carbon dioxide emissions in China. *Reg. Environ. Change* **2020**, *20*, 1–12. [CrossRef]
21. Román, R.; Cansino, J.M.; Rodas, J.A. Analysis of the main drivers of CO2 emissions changes in Colombia (1990–2012) and its political implications. *Renew. Energy* **2018**, *116*, 402–411. [CrossRef]
22. Yang, J.; Hao, Y.; Feng, C. A race between economic growth and carbon emissions: What play important roles towards global low-carbon development? *Energy Econ.* **2021**, *100*, 105327. [CrossRef]
23. Liu, M.; Zhang, X.; Zhang, M.; Feng, Y.; Liu, Y.; Wen, J.; Liu, L. Influencing factors of carbon emissions in transportation industry based on CD function and LMDI decomposition model: China as an example. *Environ. Impact Assess. Rev.* **2021**, *90*, 106623. [CrossRef]
24. Longhofer, W.; Jorgenson, A. Decoupling reconsidered: Does world society integration influence the relationship between the environment and economic development? *Soc. Sci. Res.* **2017**, *65*, 17–29. [CrossRef] [PubMed]
25. Fan, J.S.; Zhou, L. Impact of urbanization and real estate investment on carbon emissions: Evidence from China's provincial regions. *J. Clean. Prod.* **2019**, *209*, 309–323. [CrossRef]
26. Hang, Y.; Wang, Q.; Zhou, D.; Zhang, L. Factors influencing the progress in decoupling economic growth from carbon dioxide emissions in China's manufacturing industry. *Resour. Conserv. Recycl.* **2019**, *146*, 77–88. [CrossRef]
27. Wu, Y.; Tam, V.W.; Shuai, C.; Shen, L.; Zhang, Y.; Liao, S. Decoupling China's economic growth from carbon emissions: Empirical studies from 30 Chinese provinces (2001–2015). *Sci. Total Environ.* **2019**, *656*, 576–588. [CrossRef]
28. Zou, S.; Zhang, T. CO_2 emissions, energy consumption, and economic growth nexus: Evidence from 30 provinces in China. *Math. Probl. Eng.* **2020**, *2020*, 8842770. [CrossRef]
29. Huo, T.; Ma, Y.; Yu, T.; Cai, W.; Liu, B.; Ren, H. Decoupling and decomposition analysis of residential building carbon emissions from residential income Evidence from the provincial level in China. *Environ. Impact Assess. Rev.* **2020**, *86*, 1–12. [CrossRef]
30. Zhang, P.; He, J.; Hong, X.; Zhang, W.; Qin, C.; Pang, B.; Li, Y.; Liu, Y. Carbon sources/sinks analysis of land use changes in China based on data envelopment analysis. *J. Clean. Prod.* **2018**, *204*, 702–711. [CrossRef]
31. Ma, M.; Cai, W. Do commercial building sector-derived carbon emissions decouple from the economic growth in Tertiary Industry? A case study of four municipalities in China. *Sci. Total Environ.* **2018**, *650*, 822–834. [CrossRef] [PubMed]
32. Liu, J.; Li, M.; Ding, Y. Econometric analysis of the impact of the urban population size on carbon dioxide (CO2) emissions in China. *Environ. Dev. Sustain.* **2021**, *23*, 18186–18203. [CrossRef]
33. Wang, B.; Sun, Y.F.; Chen, Q.X.; Wang, Z.H. Determinants analysis of carbon dioxide emissions in passenger and freight transportation sectors in China. *Struct. Change Econ. Dyn.* **2018**, *47*, 127–132. [CrossRef]
34. Liu, Y.; Chen, Z.M.; Xiao, H.W.; Yang, W.; Liu, D.H.; Chen, B. Driving factors of carbon dioxide emissions in China: An empirical study using 2006-2010 provincial data. *Front. Earth Sci.* **2017**, *11*, 156–161. [CrossRef]
35. Qiang, W.; Min, S. The effects of urbanization and industrialization on decoupling economic growth from carbon emission–A case study of China. *Sustain. Cities Soc.* **2019**, *51*, 101758. [CrossRef]

36. Liang, W.; Gan, T.; Zhang, W. Dynamic evolution of characteristics and decomposition of factors influencing industrial carbon dioxide emissions in China: 1991–2015. *Struct. Change Econ. Dyn.* **2019**, *49*, 93–106. [CrossRef]
37. Li, C.; Li, X.; Zhu, X. Examining Economic Development and Carbon Emissions in China's Low-Carbon Pilot Provinces. *Polish J. Environ. Stud.* **2017**, *26*, 2619–2631. [CrossRef]
38. Zhao, H.; Guo, S.; Zhao, H. A panel co-integration analysis for economic development, energy consumption, urbanization, and carbon dioxide emissions in China's six provinces. *Environ. Prog. Sustain. Energy* **2019**, *38*, e13247. [CrossRef]
39. Wang, Y.L. Research on the Relationship Between Green Energy Use, Carbon Emissions and Economic Growth in Henan Province. *Front. Energy Res.* **2021**, *9*, 701551. [CrossRef]
40. Wei, Y.G.; Zhu, X.H.; Li, Y.; Yao, T.; Tao, Y. Influential factors of national and regional CO2 emission in China based on combined model of DPSIR and PLS-SEM. *J. Clean. Prod.* **2019**, *212*, 698–712. [CrossRef]
41. Sheng, P.; Li, J.; Zhai, M.; Majeed, M.U. Economic growth efficiency and carbon reduction efficiency in China: Coupling or decoupling. *Energy Rep.* **2021**, *7*, 289–299. [CrossRef]
42. Wang, M.; Feng, C. Towards a decoupling between economic expansion and carbon dioxide emissions in resources sector: A case study of China's 29 non-ferrous metal industries. *Resour. Policy* **2021**, *74*, 102249. [CrossRef]
43. Wang, Q.; Han, X. Is decoupling embodied carbon emissions from economic output in Sino-US trade possible? *Technol. Forecast. Soc. Change* **2021**, *169*, 120805. [CrossRef]
44. Lin, B.; Wang, M. Dynamic analysis of carbon dioxide emissions in China's petroleum refining and coking industry. *Sci. Total Environ.* **2019**, *671*, 937–947. [CrossRef]
45. Du, L.; Wei, C.; Cai, S. Economic development and carbon dioxide emissions in China: Provincial panel data analysis. *China Econ. Rev.* **2012**, *23*, 371–384. [CrossRef]
46. Meng, L.; Huang, B. Shaping the relationship between economic development and carbon dioxide emissions at the local level: Evidence from spatial econometric models. *Environ. Resour. Econ.* **2018**, *71*, 127–156. [CrossRef]

International Journal of
Environmental Research and Public Health

MDPI

Article

Public Rental Housing and Obesogenic Behaviors among Adults in Hong Kong: Mediator Role of Food and Physical Activity Environment

Ting Zhang [1,2], Bo Huang [2,3,4,*], Hung Wong [5,6], Samuel Yeung-shan Wong [6,7] and Roger Yat-Nork Chung [6,7]

1 School of International and Public Affairs, Shanghai Jiao Tong University, Shanghai 200030, China; tingzhang@sjtu.edu.cn
2 Institute of Space and Earth Information Science, The Chinese University of Hong Kong, Hong Kong 999077, China
3 Department of Geography and Resource Management, The Chinese University of Hong Kong, Hong Kong 999077, China
4 Shenzhen Research Institute, The Chinese University of Hong Kong, Shenzhen 518057, China
5 Department of Social Work, The Chinese University of Hong Kong, Hong Kong 999077, China; hwong@cuhk.edu.hk
6 CUHK Institute of Health Equity, The Chinese University of Hong Kong, Hong Kong 999077, China; yeungshanwong@cuhk.edu.hk (S.Y.-s.W.); rychung@cuhk.edu.hk (R.Y.-N.C.)
7 Jockey Club School of Public Health and Primary Care, The Chinese University of Hong Kong, Hong Kong 999077, China
* Correspondence: bohuang@cuhk.edu.hk; Tel.: +852-3943-6536

Abstract: Public rental housing (PRH) for low-income families has been shown in several studies to be associated with poor health status and obesity. However, the causes of this health disparity are controversial, and the associations and pathways between PRH and obesogenic behaviors remain unknown. Using cross-sectional survey data of 1977 adults living in Hong Kong (aged or over 18) together with multi-source GIS-based environmental data, we examined the associations between PRH and obesogenic behaviors and the extent to which those associations can be explained by neighborhood food and physical environment. The unhealthy food environment, which relates with infrequent fruit and vegetables consumption, was calculated based on the relative density of fast food restaurants and convenience stores to grocery stores. The physical activity environment, which relates to physical inactivity and prolonged sitting, was assessed in terms of density of sports facilities and street greenery, separately. Regressions and mediation analyses show that PRH was negatively associated with physical inactivity directly and also indirectly via higher sports facilities density; however, PRH was positively associated with unhealthy diet largely directly and positively associated with prolonged sitting indirectly via less street greenery. We advanced the international literature of PRH health impact assessment and its environmental health pathways by providing evidence from the least housing-affordable city in the world. The findings provide planning implications in formulating a healthier PRH community for these low-income PRH households and mitigating health disparities induced by housing type.

Keywords: physical inactivity; prolonged sitting; unhealthy diet; sports facilities; street greenery

Citation: Zhang, T.; Huang, B.; Wong, H.; Wong, S.Y.-s.; Chung, R.Y.-N. Public Rental Housing and Obesogenic Behaviors among Adults in Hong Kong: Mediator Role of Food and Physical Activity Environment. *IJERPH* **2022**, *19*, 2960. https://doi.org/10.3390/ijerph19052960

Academic Editor: Paul B. Tchounwou

Received: 6 February 2022
Accepted: 2 March 2022
Published: 3 March 2022

1. Introduction

Public rental housing (PRH), one of the most effective housing solutions for low-income families, has been employed in many countries around the world to improve living conditions of those needy families. Goal 11 of the United Nation's 2030 Agenda for Sustainable Development reflects the significance of inclusive and healthy cities: "making cities inclusive, safe, resilient and sustainable" [1]. Rapid urbanization exerts enormous pressure on housing, due to shortages of land resources and an expanding population.

People with low socio-economic status (SES) tend to live in terrible environments. They are more vulnerable to negative health impacts from their living environments [2,3]. The increasing number of slum dwellers in cities and metropolitan areas, especially in Eastern and Southeastern Asia, has led local governments to take actions such as PRH to safeguard the basic human right of adequate housing. The research on the health impacts of PRH is of particular importance in the context of rapid urbanization, especially in Asia.

There is a systematic review of a total of 14 articles, including 4 prospective studies, 8 cross-sectional studies, and 2 retrospective cohort studies on the relationship between staying in PRH in Singapore and health status [4]. Staying in PRH was found to be associated with all-cause mortality in Singapore and increases hospital utilization [4,5]. Similar to the findings in the United States, whereby the low-income housing policy and poor health has been linked for more than a century [6]. Although residing in PRH appears to be a risk marker of poorer health, the causes of health disparity are controversial. The argument is over if residents entered PRH already ill or if PRH may cause the poor health of its resident [7]. A mixed-methods study in Atlanta, USA, found that the majority of PRH residents entered PRH already ill, and the long tenure in PRH was not associated with an increased poor health after entry into PRH [7]. However, another study using a nationally representative survey in the large cities in the USA found that PRH residency increases obesity and worsens mothers' overall health status by minimizing the selection effect with controls and instrumental variables [6]. The mixed results suggest the urgent need for more research to find out the pathways from residing in PRH to related health outcomes.

From the perspective of the paradigm of traditional housing health research, both interior housing condition and external neighborhood environment could affect residents' health [8]. If PRH residence leads to poor health outcomes, the pathways could be related with poor housing and neighborhood environment in PRH. However, a related study, which leveraged a natural experiment created by PRH redevelopment in Los Angeles, found that there was no significant change in weight-related outcomes during the two years of baseline after the improvements to housing and the built and social environments in PRH communities [9]. Yet, weight-related outcomes, such as body mass index, are relatively long-term health consequences and need to be observed over time. In addition, they are complex, with multiple possible pathways, including both eating and physical activity. The short-term influences include health-related behaviors, attitudes, and health-seeking behaviors [10].

Therefore, more studies are needed to assess the short-term health impact of PRH residence, such as obesogenic behaviors, to help understand the pathways of the health disparities induced by housing type. Surprisingly, such research is scarce. A natural experimental study aimed to assess whether enhancing the physical and social environment could reduce obesity among PRH residents via improving diet and physical activity or not [11]. From baseline to one-year follow-up, they found that the intervention participants significantly changed their eating and activity behaviors, while control participants reported no significant change in any studied variables [12]. However, the associations and pathways linking PRH residence to obesogenic behaviors still need to be further explored.

In Hong Kong, PRH is the primary housing solution to achieve the vision of helping all households gain access to adequate and affordable housing based on the Long Term Housing Strategy (2014), and it was introduced in 1954, after the Shek Kip Mei fire [13]. Approximately 2.13 million persons (29.1%) live in PRH according to the Hong Kong By-census (2016), and the average waiting time for PRH was 4.7 years in 2016 [14]. PRH is not for sale and provides a safety net for low-income families with the eligibility criteria of income and assets. Some studies explored associations between residential environment and health among Hong Kong's PRH residents [15,16]. However, whether there were disparities in the residential environment and health behaviors among PRH and non-PRH residence remains unknown in Hong Kong, as Hong Kong has a different PRH governance from Western cites or other Asian areas such as Singapore. Studies on the associations and environmental pathways between PRH residence and health-related outcomes are very meaningful in one of the least housing-affordable cities in the world. Meanwhile, obesity has become a global problem, spreading rapidly across Asia in the setting of urbanization. In Hong Kong, about 30% of adults are obese and 20% are overweight [17].

To fill the above gaps, this paper examined the associations and pathways linking PRH residence to obesogenic behaviors via food and physical activity environment among adults in a Hong Kong context. We used GIS-based environmental variables together with a representative cross-sectional survey data among Hong Kong adults from 2014 to 2015. Two aspects were analyzed with regression and mediation models: (1) associations of PRH with food and physical activity environment and (2) the direct and indirect associations from PRH to obesogenic behaviors via corresponding food and physical activity environmental exposures. This study aims to not only verify the association among PRH, food, and physical activity environments and obesogenic behaviors but also to highlight the importance of neighborhood environments in mitigating health disparities induced by housing type. The findings in this study advanced the international literature of PRH health impact assessment and its environmental health pathways in the context of a representative world city, which provided governance implications for healthy PRH communities.

2. Theoretical Foundation and Hypothesis Development

Generally, we assumed that PRH residence is associated with obesogenic behaviors via residential environment (summarized in Figure 1) with three detailed hypotheses in a Hong Kong context: (1) PRH residence → unhealthy food environment → infrequent fruits and vegetables (FV) eating; (2) PRH residence → less sports facility density → less physical inactivity; (3) PRH residence → less street greenery → prolonged sitting. These hypotheses include two parts: (1) PRH residence → neighborhood environmental exposures and (2) neighborhood environmental exposures → health behavior outcomes.

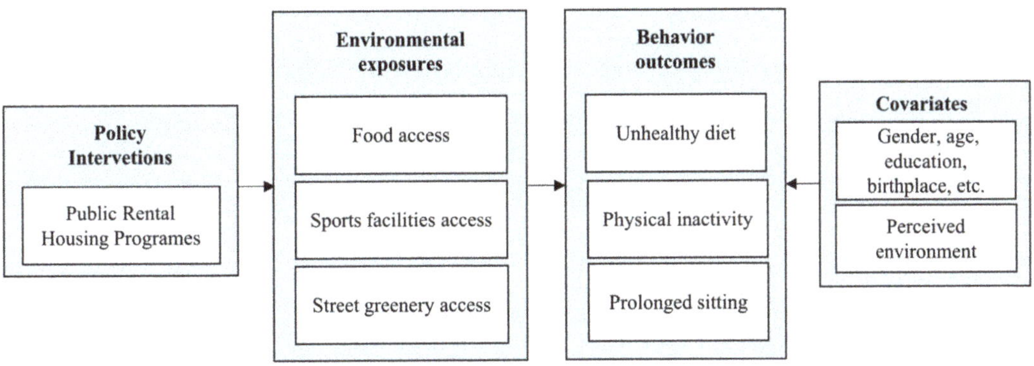

Figure 1. Conceptual framework of direct and indirect pathways through which public rental housing programs influence obesogenic behaviors.

The latter (neighborhood environmental exposures → health behavior outcomes) could be derived from extensive literature on built environmental health [18–21], consistent with the classical Bronfenbrenner's socio-ecological model, which made environmental-level health interventions popular [22]. Specific to obesity-related environmental intervention research, the improvement of food and physical activity environments has been proven to contribute to healthier eating and physical activity behaviors by a large number of studies [23–25]. Sports facility density was found to be related to physical activity behavior, and greenery correlated with sedentary behavior [26,27]. The local retail food environment was also found to be related with dietary behaviors in Hong Kong by one of our former studies [28]. Therefore, the food and physical activity environment in terms of the relative density of fast-food restaurants and convenience stores compared to grocery stores, sports facility density, and street greenery were included in this study [26,28].

Next, we state the theoretical foundation and the logical inference of the former part (PRH residence → neighborhood environmental exposures) and the related hypotheses (PRH residence → unhealthy food environment/higher sports facility density/less street greenery) in the context of Hong Kong. Many studies have explored the environmental determinants of residential satisfaction with PRH in many cities [29–31]. However, studies on systematic disparities of residential environment in PRH and non-PRH are limited despite the stereotype of PRH being associated with poor living conditions. In Hong Kong, one study reveals that people living in public and private housing have significantly different built environments such as population density, the percentage of people living and working in the same district, PRH density, and a gravity-based accessibility [32]. Another study also found a significant difference in the satisfaction levels of the living environment, environmental quality, security, and urban renewal among residents from different housing types in Hong Kong [33]. These results follow the concept of "housing classes" developed by Rex and Moore (1967) that proposes different housing types are characterized by different physical and social settings [33,34]. PRH and non-PRH often distribute different places with their own neighborhood characteristics. Additionally, from the perspective of governance disparities, PRH in Hong Kong, as well as facilities and services in PRH communities, were provided and managed by the Hong Kong Housing Authority under the Hong Kong Government, while those in private housing were provided by private companies. Therefore, in this study, we assumed that PRH communities had different neighborhood food and physical activity environments than non-PRH communities. Specifically, PRH was assumed to be related to poor food and physical environments in terms of a higher relative density of fast-food restaurants and convenience stores compared to grocery stores, less sports facility density, and less street greenery.

3. Materials and Methods

3.1. Study Area

This study was conducted in Hong Kong, a special administrative region of the People's Republic of China. As one of the most densely populated areas in the world, Hong Kong covers approximately 1080 square kilometers of land and had a population of 7,336,585 people at the end of June 2016, with 7,116,829 usual residents and 219,756 mobile residents [14]. Hong Kong is one of the cities with the highest inequality in the world, with an income Gini coefficient of 0.524 in 2016, and 1 in 5 people lived below the poverty line in 2017 [14]. Approximately 2.13 million persons (29.1%) lived in PRH, 1.16 million persons (15.8%) lived in subsidized home ownership housing, and 3.9 million persons (53.2%) lived in private permanent housing with a median monthly mortgage payment of HKD 10,500 (Hong Kong Dollar) [14].

The housing problem is worsened due to a lack of housing land, and Hong Kong has been ranked the least housing-affordable city in the world for a decade since 2011 by an international housing organization, Demographia [35]. An insufficient supply of land also leads to inadequate sites for community facilities. Even after planning for land supply, Hong Kong will still face a land shortage of at least 1200 hectares by 2046 [36]. In 2014, the Government of Hong Kong Special Administrative Region adopted a supply-led housing strategy with a commitment to continuously increase the housing supply, which strengthens the role of public housing and keeps an interchangeable ratio between PRH and subsidized sale flats. As a part of its long-term housing strategy, it adopted a 60:40 public–private split for new housing from 2015–2016 to 2024–2025, with 280,000 public housing units (200,000 PRH and 80,000 subsidized sale flats). In 2018, it revised the public–private split to 70:30 for the next 10-year period due to the strong social demand of public housing [37].

3.2. Data Collection

We used a representative sample of 1977 Hong Kong adults (aged or over 18) derived from a two-stage stratified sampling design by geographical area and housing type. Survey data of the 1977 adults were part of the first wave of the Strategic Public Research (SPPR) project, "Trends and Implications of Poverty and Social Disadvantages in Hong Kong: A Multi-disciplinary and Longitudinal Study" (for methodology details, see references) [38,39]. This was conducted by the Department of Social Work, the Chinese University of Hong Kong. The Survey and Behavioral Research Ethics Committee of the Chinese University of Hong Kong reviewed and approved of the study procedures and materials. The detailed verbal and written information on the study was given to participants. Because of the statistical treatment of data, personal data arising from the study are kept in strictly confidential ways. This sample has detailed information on the latitude and longitude of the respondents' homes, and the cross-sectional survey data were acquired via face-to-face interviews conducted between May 2014 and July 2015. In this study, the following variables were collected: individual variables, such as housing type, sociodemographic variables, and variables of health behaviors, and perceived environmental variables.

Multi-source objective environmental data were also collected in this paper. To measure the local retail food environment, data on different food outlets were collected from Hong Kong's Food and Environmental Hygiene Department [28]. To measure physical activity environment, data on sports facilities were collected from Hong Kong's Leisure and Cultural Service Department. Data on street greenery were collected from Google Street View Images, using an object-based images classification algorithm. All objective environmental measures in this paper were constructed within a buffer around each respondent's residence, using the Geographic Information System (GIS).

3.3. Independent Variable

The independent variable is PRH residence. Housing type of PRH was coded as 1 while housing type of non-PRH including subsidized sale flats and private housing was coded as 0.

3.4. Mediating Variables

Three measures of environmental exposures (Retail Food Environment Index (RFEI), sports facility density, and street view greenness (SVG)) were used as potential mediators. ArcGIS 10.4.1 was used to construct objective environmental measures. The objective environmental measures were standardized with a mean of 0 and a standard deviation of 1. We defined each respondent's neighborhood as the area within a 1 km of Euclidean circular buffer from their home, which was considered as a walkable distance. RFEI was adopted from our previous study to characterize the unhealthy food environment [28]. It was calculated based on the relative density of fast-food restaurants and convenience stores to grocery stores. A higher RFEI indicates an unhealthier food environment.

For characterizing physical activity environment, we used sports facility density and SVG. Data on sports facilities were collected from the Leisure and Cultural Service Department, Hong Kong (https://www.lcsd.gov.hk (accessed on 12 December 2021). Sports facilities were defined as sports center, recreation grounds, water sports centers, swimming pools, or sports grounds [26]. We did not use individually listed sports facilities because they are provided by relevant place. The addresses of the public sports facilities were geocoded to obtain the latitude and longitude using Google Maps application programming interface (API). The density of public sports facilities was calculated in ArcGIS 10.4.1 using the Buffer and the Count Points in Polygon analysis tools.

Street greenery was characterized by SVG-derived street view images using an object-based images classification algorithm. For measuring SVG, we requested a series of images using the Google Street View application programming interface. Referring to the method used in previous studies, the sampling points along the road network were at 100-m intervals, and images were taken in 6 main directions (i.e., 0°, 60°, 120°, 180°, 240°, and 300°) [40,41]. The images were downloaded at each sampling point to cover the full horizontal field of view. To reduce computational time and to consider the actual needs of this study, we only used sampling points that fell within the respondent's neighborhood (i.e., a 1-km Euclidean distance around their home). We obtained 48,250 street-view images in total. We used the object-based image classification algorithm pymeanshift to classify greenery in the images [40]. We calculated the average percentage of greenery in street-view images in six horizontal directions at the sample site and averaged greenness within the neighborhood to represent the SVG of each respondent. We used modified Python scripts based on an open source python library (https://github.com/mittrees/Treepedia_Public (accessed on 24 May 2020).

3.5. Dependent Variables

Three variables of obesogenic behaviors, including infrequent FV eating, physical inactivity, and prolonged sitting, were constructed as outcomes. Infrequent FV eating was defined as not having fruit or vegetables every day. FV consumption frequency data of respondents were collected in the cross-sectional survey. Respondents were asked "How many days a week do you usually have: (1) fruits and (2) vegetables". Response options were continuous number from 1 to 7 (days). For analysis here, we dichotomized the outcome: infrequent FV eating (<7 days/week) and frequent FV eating (=7 days/week) since daily FV consumption is recommended by WHO.

Physical inactivity was defined as lack of vigorous physical activities such as heavy lifting, digging, aerobics, or fast bicycling for at least 10 min at a time during the last week and lack of moderate physical activities such as carrying light loads, bicycling at a regular pace, or doubles tennis during the last week (do not include walking). Prolonged sitting was defined as over six hours of sitting on a weekday. Physical inactivity and prolonged sitting were assessed by the International Physical Activity Questionnaire short form (IPAQ short) [39]. They were dummy variables based on the responses to the following questions: "During the past week, did you do vigorous physical activities such as heavy lifting, digging, aerobics, or fast bicycling for at least 10 min at a time? and did you do moderate physical activities, not including walking, such as carrying light loads, bicycling at a regular pace, or playing doubles tennis?", and "During the past week, did you spend longer than 6 h sitting on a weekday?". Affirmative responses were coded as 1.

3.6. Covariates

Socio-demographic variables and perceived environmental variables extracted from the cross-sectional survey data were covariates, including age, gender, marital status, subjective poverty ("Do you think you are poor now"), and monthly income (equivalized household income; this study used an equivalence scale which divided household income by square root of household size) [38], educational attainment, birthplace, having under-school-aged children, being a Hong Kong permanent resident, area problems, and accommodation problems.

Area problems and accommodation problems were used to characterize the perceived community and housing environment. To measure perceived community environment, residents were asked 12 items in relation to the question "Do you think that any of the things are a problem in this area?": poor street lighting or broken pavement; noise (e.g., traffic, businesses); air pollution; lack of open public spaces; risk from traffic for pedestrians and cyclists; illegal parking; people being drunk or rowdy in the street/park; criminal activity; problems with communal areas (e.g., rubbish in corridors); rats or insects; and others (please specify). To measure perceived housing environment, residents were asked 12 items following the question "Do you have any of these problems with your accommodation?": shortage of space; lack of privacy (within the household or between neighbors); too dark; not enough light; too hot in summer/too cold in winter; damp walls, ceilings, floors, etc.; poor ventilation; rats or insects; light pollution (too bright in the evening); and others (please specify). The number of area problems and the number of accommodation problems were summed for respondents.

3.7. Statistical Analyses

This study investigates the associations among PRH, food and physical activity environments, and obesogenic behaviors among adults in Hong Kong. As the objective environmental variables are continuous variables (Z-score) and the outcomes of interest are binary variables, we used the maximum likelihood method to estimate the parameters of our regression models. In addition, logistic regression was used since it is a useful analysis method for classification problems, and it often models a binary outcome or other two possible discrete outcomes. The statistical analyses were conducted using Mplus Version 8.3 (1998–2017 Muthen & Muthen). The statistical tests were two-tailed, with a significance level of 0.05. Unstandardized regression coefficients (B), standard errors (SE), 95% confidence intervals (CIs), and probability (P) were obtained.

First, to test the associations of PRH with food and physical environment, we regressed RFEI, sports facility density, and SVG on PRH, controlling for socio-demographic and perceived environment covariates.

Second, to test direct and indirect effects from PRH to obesogenic behaviors via food and physical environment, mediation analyses were conducted with several regressions based on the conceptual framework we developed in Figure 1. Three pathways were tested separately: (1) PRH residence → RFEI → infrequent FV eating; (2) PRH residence → sports facility density → physical inactivity; and (3) PRH residence → SVG → prolonged sitting. All the mediation models were adjusted for significant socio-demographic and perceived neighborhood and housing environmental covariates. The Hosmer and Lemeshow test (p) was used to test the fitting degree of the models. If $p > 0.05$, the fit of the model is good. The direct and indirect effects via corresponding food and physical environments were calculated. The proportion of the effect that is mediated was calculated as indirect effect/(direct effect + indirect effect) and presented as a percentage. The Sobel test was applied to test whether the indirect effect was significant.

4. Results

4.1. Decriptive Statistics

Table 1 shows the sample characteristics. Over half (57.1%) of the sample lived in PRH. This sample included 477 (24.1%) young adults (aged 18–39), 804 (40.7%) middle-aged persons (aged 40–59), and 696 (35.2%) older persons (aged 60 or over). Over half of the 1977 adults (51.6%) were not born in Hong Kong, but 95.1% of the 1977 adults had permanent Hong Kong residence. Over half (58.9%) of the participants were female, 24.1% were in subjective poverty, and 26.7% had equivalized household monthly income under HKD 3500. Among the respondents, 85.4% had not attended university, 38.2% were unmarried, and 91.7% did not have under-school-aged children.

Table 1. Characteristics of participants (n = 1977).

	Sample (n = 1977)
Independent variable: RRH residence	n (%)
Code = 1	1129 (57.1)
Code = 0	848 (42.9)
Mediating variables: food and physical activity environment	Mean (SD)
RFEI	0 (1)
Sports Facility Density	0 (1)
SVG	0 (1)
Dependent variables: obesogenic behaviors	%
Infrequent FV eating	36.1%
Physical Inactivity	36.8%
Prolonged Sitting	43.1%
Covariates	n (%)
Gender (n (%))	
Female	1164 (58.9)
Male	813 (41.1)
Age (n (%))	
18–39	477 (24.1)
40–59	804 (40.7)
60+	696 (35.2)
Monthly income (n (%))	
Not low income	1449 (73.3)
Low income (<HK$ 3500)	528 (26.7)
Self-reported poverty b (n (%))	
No	1500 (75.9)
Yes	477 (24.1)
Educational attainment (n (%))	
Higher education	289 (14.6)
Education attainment under college	1688 (85.4)
Marital status (n (%))	
Non-single	1221 (61.8)
Single	756 (38.2)
Birthplace (n (%))	
Non-Hong Kong	1020 (51.6)
Hong Kong	957 (48.4)
Having under-school-aged children (n (%))	
Yes	165 (8.3)
No	1812 (91.7)
Hong Kong permanent residence (n (%))	
Yes	1881 (95.1)
No	96 (4.9)
Area Problems (Mean (SD))	0.87 (1.277)
Accommodation Problems (Mean (SD))	1.30 (1.748)

Note: PRH = public rental housing; RFEI = Retail Food Environment Index; SVG = street-view greenness; FV = fruit and vegetable. Housing type of PRH was coded as 1 while housing type of non-PRH including subsidized sale flats and private housing was coded as 0.

Table 2 shows descriptive statistics of the objective environmental characteristics and obesogenic behaviors among adults with PRH and non-PRH residence. PRH residence had higher averages of sports facility density, but higher RFEI and less SVG than non-PRH residence, indicating better sports environment and unhealthier food environment and worse street greenery environment in PRH communities.

Table 2. Descriptive statistics of environmental exposures and obesogenic behaviors among adults with PRH and non-PRH residence.

	PRH $n = 1129$	Non-PRH $n = 848$
Environmental Exposures	Mean (SD)	Mean (SD)
RFEI	**0.123 (1.091)**	**−0.163 (0.836)**
Sports Facilities Density	**0.135 (1.022)**	**−0.180 (0.941)**
SVG	**−0.073 (0.981)**	**0.097 (1.017)**
Obesogenic behaviors	Positive Rate (%)	
Infrequent FV eating	**40.1%**	**30.8%**
Physical inactivity	**32.9%**	**42.1%**
Prolonged sitting	43.3%	42.9%

Note: PRH = public rental housing; RFEI = Retail Food Environment Index; SVG = street-view greenness. Bold number indicating significant different distributions with non-parametric test ($p < 0.05$). Positive rate was calculated by the proportion of affirmative response.

Non-parametric tests among PRH and non-PRH residences for environmental exposures and obesogenic behaviors were conducted to compare their distributions. Bold numbers indicate significantly different distributions with the non-parametric test ($p < 0.05$). The food and physical activity environment of PRH residence is significantly different from non-PRH residence. The obesogenic behaviors of infrequent FV eating and physical inactivity among residents in PRH are significantly different from those in non-PRH. Specifically, residents in PRH had significantly higher rates of infrequent FV eating and lower rates of physical inactivity than those in non-PRH.

4.2. Results of Regressions

Table 3 shows the associations of PRH residence with food, sports, and greenery environments. PRH residence was significantly associated with RFEI, sports facility density, and SVG, indicating that people living in PRH had very different food and physical activity environments from those living in non-PRH. Specifically, PRH residence was positively associated with RFEI and sports facility density and negatively associated with SVG, suggesting that PRH residence provided a better sports environment, but an unhealthier food environment and less greenery than non-PRH residence.

Table 3. Regression model results of RPH residence on food, sports, and greenery environment.

Independent Variable: PRH Residence	B (S.E.)
Dependent variable: RFEI	0.268 (0.048) ***
Dependent variable: Sports facility density	0.314 (0.047) ***
Dependent variable: SVG	−0.161 (0.048) ***

Notes: *** $p < 0.001$; PRH = public rental housing; RFEI = Retail Food Environment Index; SVG = street-view greenness. Models adjusted for significant socio-demographic and perceived environmental covariates.

4.3. Results of Mediation Models

Table 4 shows the results of mediation models, which estimate the direct and indirect effects from PRH residence to obesogenic behaviors via food and physical activity environment, controlling for socio-demographic and perceived environmental variables. For the direct associations from PRH to obesogenic behaviors, PRH residence showed significantly negative association with physical inactivity but significantly positive association with infrequent FV consumption among adults in Hong Kong. For the indirect associations via food and physical activity environments, PRH residence showed a positive indirect association with infrequent FV eating via RFEI, a negative indirect association with physical inactivity, and a positive indirect association with prolonged sitting. The findings suggested that PRH residence was negatively associated with physical inactivity directly, as well as indirectly, via better sports environment. However, PRH residence was positively associated with unhealthy diet largely directly and positively associated with prolonged sitting indirectly via worse greenery environments.

Table 4. Mediation results of direct and indirect effect from PRH residence to obesogenic behaviors via food environment and physical activity environment among adults in Hong Kong.

Independent Variable: PRH	Direct Effect	Indirect Effect	Hosmer and Lemeshow Test	Mediation Proportion
	B (S.E.)	B (S.E.)	(*p*)	(%)
Direct effect on infrequent FV eating	0.432 (0.112) ***			
Indirect effect via RFEI		0.030 (0.015) *	> 0.05	6.49
Direct effect on physical inactivity	−0.417 (0.124) ***			
Indirect effect via sports facilities density		−0.213 (0.040) ***	> 0.05	33.81
Direct effect on prolonged sitting	0.038 (0.105)			
Indirect effect via SVG		0.043 (0.016) **	> 0.05	53.09

Notes: * $p < 0.05$, ** $p < 0.01$, *** $p < 0.001$; PRH = public rental housing; RFEI = Retail Food Environment Index; SVG = street-view greenness; FV = fruit and vegetables. The proportion of the effect that is mediated (mediation proportion) was calculated as indirect effect/(Direct effect + indirect effect), and presented as percentage. Mediation models were adjusted for significant socio-demographic and perceived environmental covariates. The Sobel test was applied to test whether the indirect effect was significant. Hosmer and Lemeshow test (p) was used to test the fitting degree of the models. If $p > 0.05$, the fit of the model is good.

5. Discussion

To the best of our knowledge, this is the first study to examine the associations between PRH and obesogenic behaviors as well as the mediator role of food and physical activity environment. It was conducted in the world's least housing-affordable city with the data from a representative sample of residents aged 18 or over. Overall, PRH residence was positively associated with infrequent FV eating and negatively associated with physical inactivity among adults in Hong Kong, and these associations were partially mediated by worse neighborhood food environments and better sports environments, separately. The empirical findings in the paper also provide local governments implications for creating healthy residential environments for PRH residents and emphasizing the importance of neighborhood environment in mitigating health disparities induced by housing type. Below, we discuss and explain the results in more details.

Firstly, we found that residents in PRH had significantly higher rates of infrequent FV eating and lower rates of physical inactivity than those in non-PRH. Residing in PRH was not directly associated prolonged sitting. Our results also partly explain the mixed results of previous literature on the association between PRH residence and obesity [9,12]. They were possibly caused by the competition of the two forces, including eating and physical activity behaviors. From the current evidence, it is difficult to extrapolate the association between housing type and obesity in Hong Kong, since PRH residents showed unhealthier eating behavior on the one hand and healthier physical activity behavior on the other hand. The lower rate of physical inactivity in PRH residents could be a breakthrough in improving the health of low-income households and alleviating health disparities.

Secondly, contrary to our preconceived assumption, PRH was positively associated with higher sports facilities density. This result also explained the unexpected significantly lower rate of physical inactivity in PRH residence in Hong Kong. Although the result was surprising at first glance, it was a happy ending and could be explained by the logic behind sports facility planning in Hong Kong. Different from the local retail food environment, which was dominated by the capital market, public sports facilities were provided and distributed by the government. The Planning Department's Hong Kong Planning Standards and Guidelines (2021) list three types of sports facilities including regional, district, and local sports facilities [42]. Local sports facilities in PRH communities were provided by the Housing Authority and were improved timely by "Estate Improvement Program". In addition, the Housing Authority especially provides sports facilities suitable for older persons in PRH due to the concentration of elderly persons in PRH communities caused by the older-person-first PRH allocation policy. Furthermore, while other regional and district sports facilities provided by the Leisure and Cultural Service Department were planned based on population density, PRH in Hong Kong was proved to be associated with higher population density [32]. Therefore, PRH residents have more accesses to sports facilities which could be the reason leading to lower rate of physical inactivity than non-PRH residents.

Thirdly, PRH was positively associated with unhealthier food environment and negatively associated with street greenery indicating a worse food and greenery environment in PRH, which partially explained the significantly higher rate of infrequent FV eating and fully explained the non-significant but higher rate of prolonged sitting in PRH residents. These results also contribute the international review of PRH's health impact and are consistent with the previously reported inverse association between PRH residence and poor health outcomes in developed Western societies and developed Asian countries such as Singapore [4–6]. Additionally, our results provide the cross-sectional evidence of environmental pathways linking PRH residence to potential health-related outcomes, such as obesity and chronic disease. These results correspond with another study conducted in Hong Kong, which indicated that positive associations between residing in PRH and premature mortality risk could be attenuated or even reversed after controlling for neighborhood characteristics [43]. Furthermore, we need to notice that only a small part of the association between PRH and infrequent FV eating could be explained by unhealthier GIS-based objective food environment. These results suggest that despite the objective food environment, there were other unshown factors that mediate the association between PRH residence and eating behaviors. A previous study summarized five dimensions of "food access", including availability, accessibility, affordability, accommodation, and acceptability that affect residents' eating behaviors [44]. Therefore, in addition to food accessibility, we need to pay more attention to other dimensions of "food access", especially affordability. For example, the relative price of other foods to FV near the PRH residential areas could make a difference in eating FV behavior.

The findings in this study advanced international review in several ways including health impact assessment of PRH, environmental pathways linking PRH residence to health, and the association between residential environment and health outcomes. In addition, these findings contribute to the possible solutions of health disparities induced by housing type by improving neighborhood environment in health disadvantaged communities. Hong Kong has a rich experience in PRH governance. The PRH practice in Hong Kong provides a reference for other cities with housing problems. This is first study in Hong Kong linking PRH residence to health-related behaviors. More studies need to be conducted in Hong Kong and compared with other cities for creating a healthy and inclusive residential environment for low-income households.

This study also had several limitations. First, we were unable to establish a causal association between PRH residence, neighborhood environment, and behaviors due to the cross-sectional nature of the study. In addition, the mediation analysis we used comes with several assumptions and considerations about causal mechanisms that might bias the estimation of mediation effects when one or more assumptions are violated (e.g., exposure-induced mediator–outcome confounding) [45,46]. In future studies, we could make use of policy interventions to cleverly design experiments and use natural experiments to explore the causal relationship of housing and health. Second, we did not consider the subjective perceived factors of food and physical activity environments. Although we included perceived environmental covariates in this paper, the variables were rude and do not finely reflect the perceived food and physical activity environments. Further studies could be conducted to compare the difference of objective food and physical activity environment with perceived food and physical activity environment. Third, we need to note that only the density of sports facilities was considered. Even though there were more sports facilities positioned near PRH communities, the type of sports facilities could affect different sports behaviors. Lastly, the self-reported measures of behavior outcomes could be another limitation. More studies should be conducted to assess behaviors more comprehensively and objectively (e.g., accelerometry).

6. Conclusions

We found that residing in PRH was associated with higher rate of infrequent FV eating and lower rate of physical inactivity in the context of Hong Kong. The associations between residing in PRH and obesogenic behaviors were mediated by neighborhood food and physical activity environments. More targeted interventional studies directed at PRH communities need to be carried out to address the health inequalities induced by housing type and understand the causal associations among PRH, neighborhood environment, and health outcomes. These will aid policy makers in formulating better policies to improve health for low-income residents living in PRH and mitigate their health disparities with residents living private housing.

Author Contributions: Conceptualization, T.Z. and B.H.; methodology, T.Z.; software, T.Z.; validation, T.Z.; writing—original draft preparation, T.Z.; writing—review and editing, T.Z., B.H., H.W., S.Y.-s.W. and R.Y.-N.C.; visualization, T.Z.; supervision, B.H.; project administration, H.W.; funding acquisition, H.W. All authors have read and agreed to the published version of the manuscript.

Funding: The work described in this article was fully supported by a grant from the Central Policy Unit of the Government of the Hong Kong Special Administrative Region and the Research Grants Council of the Hong Kong Special Administrative Region, China (Project 4003-SPPR-11).

Institutional Review Board Statement: The Survey and Behavioral Research Ethics Committee of the Chinese University of Hong Kong has granted approval for conducting this research (13 October 2011).

Informed Consent Statement: Informed consent was obtained from all subjects involved in the study.

Data Availability Statement: Not publicly available.

Conflicts of Interest: The authors declare no conflict of interest.

References

1. GA, U.N. *Transforming Our World: The 2030 Agenda for Sustainable Development*; Division for Sustainable Development Goals: New York, NY, USA, 2015.
2. Molina-García, J.; Queralt, A.; Adams, M.A.; Conway, T.L.; Sallis, J.F. Neighborhood built environment and so-cio-economic status in relation to multiple health outcomes in adolescents. *Prev. Med.* **2017**, *105*, 88–94. [CrossRef] [PubMed]
3. Sugiyama, T.; Villanueva, K.; Knuiman, M.; Francis, J.; Foster, S.; Wood, L.; Giles-Corti, B. Can neighborhood green space mitigate health inequalities? A study of socio-economic status and mental health. *Health Place* **2016**, *38*, 16–21. [CrossRef] [PubMed]
4. Chan, C.Q.H.; Lee, K.H.; Low, L.L. A systematic review of health status, health seeking behaviour and healthcare utilisation of low socioeconomic status populations in urban Singapore. *Int. J. Equity Health* **2018**, *17*, 39. [CrossRef]
5. Seng, J.J.B.; Kwan, Y.H.; Goh, H.; Thumboo, J.; Low, L.L. Public rental housing and its association with mortality—A retrospective, cohort study. *BMC Public Health* **2018**, *18*, 665. [CrossRef] [PubMed]
6. Fertig, A.R.; Reingold, D.A. Public housing, health, and health behaviors: Is there a connection? *J. Policy Anal. Manag. J. Assoc. Public Policy Anal. Manag.* **2007**, *26*, 831–860. [CrossRef] [PubMed]
7. Ruel, E.; Oakley, D.; Wilson, G.E.; Maddox, R. Is public housing the cause of poor health or a safety net for the un-healthy poor? *J. Urban Health* **2010**, *87*, 827–838. [CrossRef] [PubMed]
8. Bonnefoy, X. Inadequate housing and health: An overview. *Int. J. Environ. Pollut.* **2007**, *30*, 411–429. [CrossRef]
9. Datar, A.; Shier, V.; Braboy, A.; Jimenez-Ortiz, M.; Hernandez, A.; King, S.E.; Liu, Y. Assessing impacts of redeveloping public housing communities on obesity in low-income minority residents: Rationale, study design, and baseline data from the Watts Neighborhood Health Study. *Contemp. Clin. Trials Commun.* **2022**, *25*, 100879. [CrossRef]
10. Ellen, I.G.; Mijanovich, T.; Dillman, K.-N. Neighborhood Effects on Health: Exploring the Links and Assessing the Evidence. *J. Urban Aff.* **2001**, *23*, 391–408. [CrossRef]
11. Quintiliani, L.M.; DeBiasse, M.A.; Branco, J.M.; Bhosrekar, S.G.; Rorie, J.-A.L.; Bowen, D.J. Enhancing physical and social environments to reduce obesity among public housing residents: Rationale, trial design, and baseline data for the Healthy Families study. *Contemp. Clin. Trials* **2014**, *39*, 201–210. [CrossRef]
12. Bowen, D.J.; Quintiliani, L.M.; Bhosrekar, S.G.; Goodman, R.; Smith, E. Changing the housing environment to reduce obesity in public housing residents: A cluster randomized trial. *BMC Public Health* **2018**, *18*, 883. [CrossRef] [PubMed]

13. Long Term Housing Strategy. 2014. Available online: https://www.thb.gov.hk/eng/policy/housing/policy/lths/LTHS201412.pdf (accessed on 12 December 2021).
14. Hong Kong By-census. 2016. Available online: https://www.bycensus2016.gov.hk/en/ (accessed on 12 December 2020).
15. Lu, Y.; Chen, L.; Yang, Y.; Gou, Z. The Association of Built Environment and Physical Activity in Older Adults: Using a Citywide Public Housing Scheme to Reduce Residential Self-Selection Bias. *Int. J. Environ. Res. Public Health* **2018**, *15*, 1973. [CrossRef] [PubMed]
16. Huang, J.; Chen, Y.; Jones, P.; Hao, T. Heat stress and outdoor activities in open spaces of public housing estates in Hong Kong: A perspective of the elderly community. *Indoor Built Environ.* **2020**, 1–17. [CrossRef]
17. Hong Kong Demographic Health Survey 2014/15. Available online: https://www.chp.gov.hk/tc/static/51256.html (accessed on 12 December 2021).
18. Frank, L.D.; Iroz-Elardo, N.; MacLeod, K.; Hong, A. Pathways from built environment to health: A conceptual framework linking behavior and exposure-based impacts. *J. Transp. Health* **2019**, *12*, 319–335. [CrossRef]
19. Giles-Corti, B.; Vernez-Moudon, A.; Reis, R.; Turrell, G.; Dannenberg, A.L.; Badland, H.; Owen, N. City planning and population health: A global challenge. *Lancet* **2016**, *388*, 2912–2924. [CrossRef]
20. Wang, J.; Huang, B.; Zhang, T.; Wong, H.; Huang, Y. Impact of housing and community conditions on multidimensional health among middle-and low-income groups in Hong Kong. *Int. J. Environ. Res. Public Health* **2018**, *15*, 1132. [CrossRef]
21. McCormack, G.R.; Cabaj, J.; Orpana, H.; Lukic, R.; Blackstaffe, A.; Goopy, S.; Hagel, B.; Keough, N.; Martinson, R.; Chapman, J.; et al. Evidence synthesis A scoping review on the relations between urban form and health: A focus on Canadian quantitative evidence. *Health Promot. Chronic Dis. Prev. Can.* **2019**, *39*, 187–200. [CrossRef]
22. Kilanowski, J.F. Breadth of the socio-ecological model. *J. Agromed.* **2017**, *22*, 295–297. [CrossRef]
23. MacMillan, F.; George, E.S.; Feng, X.; Merom, D.; Bennie, A.; Cook, A.; Sanders, T.; Dwyer, G.; Pang, B.; Guagliano, J.M.; et al. Do Natural Experiments of Changes in Neighborhood Built Environment Impact Physical Activity and Diet? A Systematic Review. *Int. J. Environ. Res. Public Health* **2018**, *15*, 217. [CrossRef]
24. Crane, M.; Bohn-Goldbaum, E.; Grunseit, A.; Bauman, A. Using natural experiments to improve public health evidence: A review of context and utility for obesity prevention. *Health Res. Policy Syst.* **2020**, *18*, 48. [CrossRef]
25. Sallis, J.F.; Glanz, K. Physical Activity and Food Environments: Solutions to the Obesity Epidemic. *Milbank Q.* **2009**, *87*, 123–154. [CrossRef] [PubMed]
26. Zhang, T.; Huang, B.; Wong, H.; Wong, S.Y.-S.; Chung, R.Y.-N. Built Environment and Physical Activity among Adults in Hong Kong: Role of Public Leisure Facilities and Street Centrality. *Land* **2022**, *11*, 243. [CrossRef]
27. Dadvand, P.; Villanueva, C.; Font-Ribera, L.; Martinez, D.; Basagaña, X.; Belmonte, J.; Vrijheid, M.; Grazuleviciene, R.; Kogevinas, M.; Nieuwenhuijsen, M.J. Risks and Benefits of Green Spaces for Children: A Cross-Sectional Study of Associations with Sedentary Behavior, Obesity, Asthma, and Allergy. *Environ. Health Perspect.* **2014**, *122*, 1329–1335. [CrossRef]
28. Zhang, T.; Huang, B. Local Retail Food Environment and Consumption of Fruit and Vegetable among Adults in Hong Kong. *Int. J. Environ. Res. Public Health* **2018**, *15*, 2247. [CrossRef]
29. Byun, G.; Ha, M. The Factors Influencing Residential Satisfaction by Public Rental Housing Type. *J. Asian Arch. Build. Eng.* **2016**, *15*, 535–542. [CrossRef]
30. Gan, X.; Zuo, J.; Baker, E.; Chang, R.; Wen, T. Exploring the determinants of residential satisfaction in public rental housing in China: A case study of Chongqing. *J. Hous. Built Environ.* **2019**, *34*, 869–895. [CrossRef]
31. Huang, Z.; Du, X. Assessment and determinants of residential satisfaction with public housing in Hangzhou, China. *Habitat Int.* **2015**, *47*, 218–230. [CrossRef]
32. Wang, D.; Lin, T. Built environments, social environments, and activity-travel behavior: A case study of Hong Kong. *J. Transp. Geogr.* **2013**, *31*, 286–295. [CrossRef]
33. Ng, S.L.; Zhang, Y.; Ng, K.H.; Wong, H.; Lee, J.W.Y. Living environment and quality of life in Hong Kong. *Asian Geogr.* **2017**, *35*, 35–51. [CrossRef]
34. Rex, J.; Moore, R. *Race, Community and Conflict*; Oxford University Press: London, UK, 1967.
35. Demographia International Housing Affordability Survey. Available online: http://www.demographia.com/db-dhi-index.htm (accessed on 12 December 2021).
36. Report of the Task Force on Land Supply. 2018. Available online: https://www.devb.gov.hk/en/boards_and_committees/task_force_on_land_supply/index.html (accessed on 12 December 2021).
37. Long Term Housing Strategy Annual Progress Report. 2019. Available online: https://www.legco.gov.hk/yr19-20/english/panels/hg/papers/hg20200106cb1-278-3-e.pdf (accessed on 12 December 2021).
38. Lau, M.; Bradshaw, J. Material well-being, social relationships and children's overall life satisfaction in Hong Kong. *Child Indic. Res.* **2018**, *11*, 185–205. [CrossRef]
39. Chung, R.Y.-N.; Chung, G.K.-K.; Gordon, D.; Wong, S.Y.-S.; Chan, D.; Lau, M.; Tang, V.M.-Y.; Wong, H. Deprivation is associated with worse physical and mental health beyond income poverty: A population-based household survey among Chinese adults. *Qual. Life Res.* **2018**, *27*, 2127–2135. [CrossRef]
40. Li, X.; Zhang, C.; Li, W.; Ricard, R.; Meng, Q.; Zhang, W. Assessing street-level urban greenery using Google Street View and a modified green view index. *Urban For. Urban Green.* **2015**, *14*, 675–685. [CrossRef]

41. Liu, Y.; Wang, R.; Lu, Y.; Li, Z.; Chen, H.; Cao, M.; Zhang, Y.; Song, Y. Natural outdoor environment, neighbour-hood social cohesion and mental health: Using multilevel structural equation modelling, streetscape and remote-sensing metrics. *Urban For. Urban Green.* **2020**, *48*, 126576. [CrossRef]
42. Hong Kong Planning Standards and Guidelines. Available online: https://www.pland.gov.hk/pland_en/tech_doc/hkpsg/index.html (accessed on 12 December 2021).
43. Kandt, J.; Chang, S.-S.; Yip, P.; Burdett, R. The spatial pattern of premature mortality in Hong Kong: How does it relate to public housing? *Urban Stud.* **2016**, *54*, 1211–1234. [CrossRef]
44. Caspi, C.E.; Sorensen, G.; Subramanian, S.V.; Kawachi, I. The local food environment and diet: A systematic review. *Health Place* **2012**, *18*, 1172–1187. [CrossRef]
45. VanderWeele, T.J.; Chiba, Y. Sensitivity analysis for direct and indirect effects in the presence of exposure-induced mediator-outcome confounders. *Epidemiol. Biostat. Public Health* **2014**, *11*, e9027. [CrossRef] [PubMed]
46. Nguyen, T.Q.; Schmid, I.; Stuart, E.A. Clarifying causal mediation analysis for the applied researcher: Defining effects based on what we want to learn. *Psychol. Methods* **2021**, *26*, 255–271. [CrossRef]

International Journal of
Environmental Research and Public Health

MDPI

Article

Evaluations of Spatial Accessibility and Equity of Multi-Tiered Medical System: A Case Study of Shenzhen, China

Meng Tian [1], Lei Yuan [1,*], Renzhong Guo [2,3,4], Yongsheng Wu [5] and Xiaojian Liu [5]

1 Lab for Optimizing Design of Built Environment, School of Architecture and Urban Planning, Shenzhen University, Shenzhen 518060, China; meng.tian.c@hotmail.com
2 Research Institute for Smart Cities, School of Architecture and Urban Planning, Shenzhen University, Shenzhen 518060, China; guorz@szu.edu.cn
3 Guangdong Key Laboratory of Urban Informatics, Shenzhen University, Shenzhen 518060, China
4 MNR Technology Innovation Centre of Territorial & Spatial Big Data, Shenzhen University, Shenzhen 518060, China
5 Shenzhen Centre for Disease Control and Prevention, Shenzhen 518055, China; cdc@szcdc.net (Y.W.); xjliu@szcdc.net (X.L.)
* Correspondence: yuanlei@szu.edu.cn

Abstract: The Chinese government has implemented a medical system reform to improve the equity of healthcare resources since 2009. We selected Shenzhen as our study area and evaluated the accessibility and equity of the multi-tiered medical system in China using a novel multi-tiered two-step floating catchment area (MT2SFCA) method. We proposed the benchmark and applied the independent variables of travel time and facility attractiveness, along with a combination of the two factors, as tolerances to determine the new logistic cumulative distribution decay functions. Community health centers (CHCs) and hospitals were included while integrating their features. Results revealed that the MT2SFCA method was able to determine the particular advantages of CHCs and hospitals in the multi-tiered medical system. The CHCs offset the lower accessibility of hospitals in suburban areas and hospitals balanced the regional inequity caused by the CHC. Travel time is the main consideration of patients who have access to CHCs, whereas facility features are the main considerations of patients who have access to hospitals. Notably, both CHCs and hospitals are crucial for the whole multi-tiered medical system. Finally, we suggested modifications in different travel modes, weights of contributing factors, and the validation of decay functions to improve the MT2SFCA method.

Keywords: spatial accessibility; medical system; multi-tiered two-step floating catchment area (MT2SFCA) method; equity; healthcare

Citation: Tian, M.; Yuan, L.; Guo, R.; Wu, Y.; Liu, X. Evaluations of Spatial Accessibility and Equity of Multi-Tiered Medical System: A Case Study of Shenzhen, China. *IJERPH* **2022**, *19*, 3017. https://doi.org/10.3390/ijerph19053017

Academic Editors: Jie Chen, Qian Zhou and Ting Zhang

Received: 24 January 2022
Accepted: 2 March 2022
Published: 4 March 2022

1. Introduction

1.1. Spatial Equity and Accessibility to Health Services

In terms of accessing public facilities, spatial equity may be defined as the degree to which facilities are distributed in an equal way, corresponding to the requirements of facilities over different areas. It is a critical problem that must be considered by urban planners and policymakers to determine the under-provisioned areas and then, make decisions to allocate the public services more effectively [1]. People experiencing easily-accessed and adequately-resourced facilities are generally reported to have higher happiness levels and better health status [2–4]. Achieving equity in healthcare services is one of the fundamental goals of Universal Health Coverage (UHC) [5]. The equity of access to healthcare facilities has become one of the most crucial objectives of healthcare systems in many countries, with the aim of achieving social equity by promoting the livelihood and health conditions of people. In the development targets of the 14th Five-Year Plan, the Chinese government mentioned the equity of healthcare facilities, while highlighting the means of de-centralization of healthcare facilities in city centers [6].

Being the most popular factor used for evaluating the spatial equity of public service facilities, accessibility reflects the demand–supply relations and spatial distributions of facilities along road networks [7,8]. The 2SFCA method has become one of the most popular methods to analyze the accessibility of various infrastructures. The basic model of the 2SFCA method [9] originated from the dichotomous transformation of the gravity model [10]. Subsequently, many advanced versions have been proposed to improve the basic model. Luo and Qi [11] firstly proposed using several travel time zones with various weights to denote the distance decay effects. Continuous gradual decay functions were exploited in Gaussian-based 2SFCA (G2SFCA) [12] and Kernel density-based 2SFCA (KD2SFCA) [13] methods. Wan et al. [14] proposed the three-step-floating catchment area (3SFCA) method, which further explains the supply–demand relation by considering the competitive effects from nearby facilities. Delamater [15] indicated that all the traditional 2SFCA and 3SFCA methods have the shortcoming of container-like systems; therefore, he introduced the modified 2SFCA (M2SFCA) method, while considering the suboptimal conditions of healthcare distributions. Luo and Whippo [16] applied dynamic catchment sizes to balance the discrepant allocations of healthcare facilities in urban and rural areas. Bauer and Groneberg [17] integrated the M2SFCA method with a logistic-based decay function that replaced the impedance coefficients (using available distribution parameter) so that the catchment sizes would vary independently, based on the distributions of facilities within the catchment areas.

Except travel distance, accessibility is also suggested to consider other effects, such as medical management, service quality, consumer income, and cultural factors. Penchansky and Thomas [18] proposed a comprehensive definition of 'access to healthcare' that described the fit between the patient and the healthcare system in a series of aspects, including availability, accessibility, accommodation, affordability, and acceptability. Recently, some studies have considered the characteristics of healthcare when evaluating the spatial accessibility and equity of a health system to obtain results that are much closer to the realistic situation. Luo [19] innovatively applied the Huff model to the 3SFCA method to describe the two factors that affect the decisions of patients to select healthcare facilities, which are the travel distance and the attractiveness of facility. Shin and Lee [20] utilized the number of patient visits normalized by hospital capacity to substitute the travel time in the distance decay function, to calculate the accessibility of emergency medical services in South Korea.

Because the medical system is one of the most important livelihood projects of a country, during the urbanization in China, scholars have paid significant attention to the equity and accessibility of healthcare facilities. Rong et al. [21] evaluated the accessibility of comprehensive hospitals in Zhengzhou, Henan Province, China, and observed that the medical facilities demonstrated a concentric structure in the central area of the city. Lu et al. [22] compared the accessibility before and after the referral reform of the hierarchical health system of China, and deduced that the referral reform significantly improved the accessibility of health services. Wang et al. [23] investigated the accessibility of community/township health centers in Sichuan Province and revealed that the spatial disparity was associated with population density and ethnic minority. Chen et al. [24] evaluated the accessibility of secondary and tertiary hospitals in Shenzhen, based on the big data of taxi trajectory. Similar to all other cities in China, the accessibility of hospitals in Shenzhen also illustrated uneven distributions, and notably, the central area has better access to healthcare services.

1.2. Research Aims and Objectives

According to the literature, we were able to deduce that most studies only concentrated on the accessibility of hospitals; these studies overlooked the benefits of primary healthcare facilities such as community health stations and clinics. Moreover, in most cities in China, the multi-tiered medical system only includes hospitals, among which the primary hospitals are responsible for providing basic, preventive, and rehabilitation healthcare services to the communities; however, there are only a few primary hospitals. For example, in the research focusing on the equity of healthcare resources in Beijing, Lu et al. [22] found that the patients in two remote towns cannot reach any primary hospital within 30 min. Because Shenzhen is a special zone and owing to the early and relatively successful implementation of health system reform in the city, the multi-tiered medical system in Shenzhen has more advantages compared to other cities. It now incorporates three-tier hospitals as well as hundreds of community health centers (CHCs).

The aim of our study is to provide a reliable and viable method to analyze spatial data to reveal possible inequity and inaccessibility of healthcare facilities in Shenzhen, based on the numbers of real outpatient visits to healthcare facilities. In this study, we investigated the accessibility and equity of the multi-tiered medical system in China after the health system reform was implemented. First, we explained the multi-tiered medical system in Shenzhen, China, including the system structure and relevant policies. Then, we introduced the multi-tiered two-step floating catchment area (MT2SFCA) method to determine the accessibility and equity of the multi-tiered medical system. We proposed the independent variables of travel time and facilities attractiveness, along with a combination of the two factors as the benchmark, Scenario 1 and Scenario 2 of tolerance to determine the new logistic cumulative distribution decay function. Finally, we discussed the reasons that affected people's selection of healthcare facilities by comparing the two scenarios used with the benchmark in MT2SFCA model. The results can then be used by policy makers and scholars to address the limitations in accessible healthcare and thus, promote the equity and accessibility of the multi-tiered medical system.

2. Multi-Tiered Medical System in China

To achieve the global goals of UHC, the strategy of Healthy China 2020 was proposed, with the aim of providing basic healthcare coverage to all residents living in urban and rural areas by the year 2020. A new round health system reform was launched in 2009 [25]. The objectives of this reform included improving the accessibility and equity of healthcare services, providing well-rounded health services, and improving the medical insurance system [26].

The healthcare system in China is a multi-tiered medical system having a two-way patient referral mechanism, in which the healthcare facilities are categorized into three tiers. The first-tier includes primary hospitals, CHCs, and clinics to provide healthcare services for common diseases, disease prevention, and rehabilitation. In addition, CHCs also provide services, such as vaccination, health promotion, family planning, medical education, family doctor, home healthcare, and chronic diseases detection and treatment. The second-tier and third-tier hospitals (also known as secondary hospitals and tertiary hospitals) are regional/district hospitals and municipal hospitals, both of which provide specialized and high-level healthcare services. In addition to these services, the tertiary hospitals offer medical research and education.

The two-way patient referral mechanism aims to optimize the allocation of healthcare resources. Patients are freely but encouraged to seek health services in primary healthcare institutions, and then, they are referred to secondary and tertiary hospitals if needed. Other than the referrals that may be generated from primary to secondary and tertiary healthcare facilities, they can also be referred in the reverse direction, that is, the hospitals in higher tiers can generate referrals to CHCs for subsequent treatments such as rehabilitation and chronic diseases management at an affordable cost.

Shenzhen has experienced rapid urbanization for decades and has become one of the most populated Tier 1 cities in China. Therefore, Shenzhen is ideal as a case study for the analysis of urban problems in developing countries [27]. Because it is a new and high-density city with rapid population growth, allocating healthcare resources properly is a tough challenge in Shenzhen. Shenzhen government has moved forward on a healthcare reform program by implementing various actions, including financial and policy supports, and made some achievements. In 2018, the densities of hospital beds, physicians, nurses, and health professionals achieved 3.65, 2.79, 3.09, and 8.82 per 1000 of the population, respectively, for long-term residents in Shenzhen [28]; more than 95% families can reach the nearest healthcare facilities within 15 min [29].

The process of the outpatient service of the multi-tiered medical system in Shenzhen is shown in Figure 1. The system consists of community health centers (CHCs) and hospitals. Hospitals are ranked into three categories, which are primary, secondary, and tertiary hospitals, according to their capacities and service qualities. Each category is subdivided into A, B, and C levels with respect to its medical service level. The outpatient services of local residents depend on the types of their medical insurances. Three ranks of medical insurance can be selected for the residents in Shenzhen. The Tier 1 insurance is the best, followed by Tier 2 and Tier 3. Better insurance also entails more monthly fees and larger proportions of reimbursements while in use. During the outpatient services, the patients with the Tier 1 insurance are free to choose any medical services including CHCs and hospitals. To encourage people to visit CHCs, the government implemented a policy that 30% of the patient's expenses would be covered by the local government when they visit CHC for the first-time outpatient service. The patients with Tier 2 and Tier 3 medical insurances are first asked to visit CHCs for outpatient service and then, the step-by-step referral process (from lower to higher ranked facilities) is followed if needed. In addition, they are still free to choose healthcare facilities for serious illnesses. If patients need subsequent or long-term rehabilitation, they may be transferred to the lower-level facilities. Except for the policies implemented for the patients, some policies are put forward to improve the competitiveness of the lower-tier facilities. The prices of medicines and therapies in tertiary hospitals follow the referenced price-level of the province. The prices of secondary and primary hospitals are set as 95 and 90% of the reference prices, respectively. Notably, the prices of CHCs are set as low as 80% of the reference prices. As stated before, after the Shenzhen government provided sufficient support for primary-care infrastructure construction, personnel training, financial support, and policy implementation, the acceptance of CHCs by local residents has grown. In 2018, about 40% of first-time outpatient services were completed by CHCs for the whole city [30].

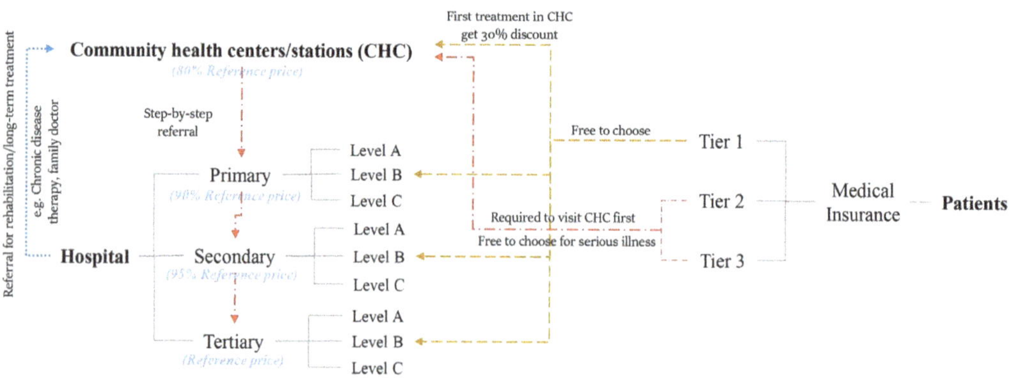

Figure 1. Introduction of multi-tiered medical system in Shenzhen, China.

3. Methods

3.1. *Study Area and Data Sources*

Shenzhen (22°32′ N, 114°30′ E) is located on the central coast of the southern Guangdong Province. As a special economic zone with fast-growing economy, it has become one of the biggest cities in China. The long-term residents have exceeded 12 million [31]. Shenzhen comprises of 10 districts and 74 subdistricts (Figure 2a) that cover an area of ~2000 km^2. Three districts, namely, Luohu, Futian, and Nanshan, are considered as the central areas of the city.

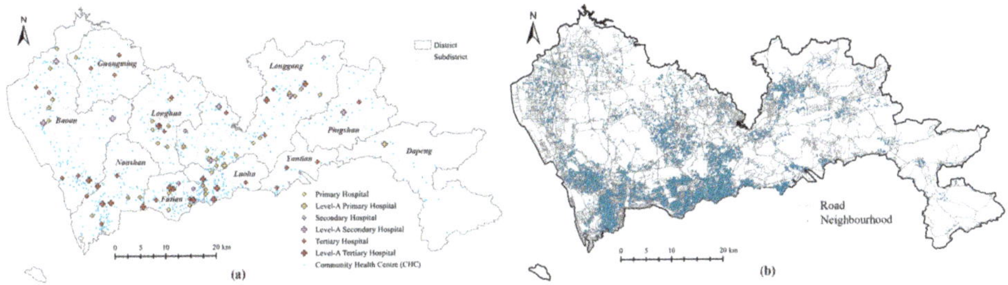

Figure 2. Introduction of research area and objects: (**a**) locations of healthcare facilities in Shenzhen; (**b**) locations of neighborhoods in Shenzhen.

The multi-tiered medical system in Shenzhen consists of hospitals and CHCs. In this study, all 84 general hospitals (including 6 Chinese general hospitals) and 692 CHCs were applied to investigate the accessibility of the multi-tiered medical system through the MT2SFCA method. The numbers of outpatient visits and physicians for each hospital and CHC were obtained from the Statistics Bureau of the Shenzhen Municipality and the 2018 Annual Health Statistics of Shenzhen Municipality [28]. The locations of healthcare facilities were extracted from Open Maps [32] using geocoding (Figure 2a). The catchment areas of hospitals and CHCs were 30 min of driving and 30 min of walking, respectively [33]. According to the Shenzhen Traffic Performance Index System [34], the driving speeds were determined by the average value in peak hours, which were 75 km/h for highways, 45 km/h for arterial roads, 30 km/h for city roads, and 20 km/h for local streets. The walking speed was set as 5 km/h. The road network was obtained from OpenStreetMap [35]. Information about 6328 neighborhoods (Figure 2b) was obtained from the public data of the most popular real estate website [36] in China. The population was estimated using the average values of 2017 and 2018, as reported by the Shenzhen Centre for Disease Control and Prevention. The accessibility was calculated using ArcGIS 10.7 [37].

3.2. *Calculating Accessibility of Multi-Tiered Medical System*

3.2.1. Attractiveness of Health Facilities

The designed capacity of a hospital depends on the potential demand of surrounding neighborhoods, which is reflected by the final size of the hospital, including the numbers of beds, physicians, nurses, and health professionals. Generally, these numbers have strong correlations with each other. For the general hospitals in Shenzhen, the coefficients of determination (R^2) of the linear relationships between the numbers of physicians and nurses, numbers of physicians and health professionals, and numbers of physicians and beds were 0.97, 0.99, and 0.80, respectively. The reason of the lower R^2 of the correlations between the numbers of physicians and beds is that the number of beds is also determined by the specialties of the hospitals. Therefore, the number of physicians represents the designed capacity of the hospital more accurately. Notably, the real demand of the hospital is represented by the annual actual outpatient visits to the hospital. The attractiveness of the hospital can be expressed by Equation (1), which is determined by the ratio of the number of actual visits to the number of physicians in the hospital.

$$q_{ij} = \frac{V_j}{S_j} \quad (1)$$

where j is the healthcare location, i is the population location, q_{ij} is the attractiveness of health facility, V_j is the annual actual outpatient visits of the facility, and S_j is the number of physicians of the facility.

By being divided by the number of physicians, the number of visits was normalized by the hospital capacity, so that the attractiveness due to the hospital itself could be evaluated to portray the high quality of services and expert skills of health professionals. The definitions of attractiveness were discussed in detail under two scenarios in Section 3.2.2.

3.2.2. Tolerance Decay Function

A tolerance decay function $f_i(w_{ij})$ is proposed as a substitute for the distance decay function applied in the 2SFCA method to consider both the attractiveness of the healthcare facility and the distance between the supply and demand points. Therefore, before any other analysis, we first determined the tolerance.

In this study, we analyzed and compared two scenarios of tolerance, as follows:

Scenario 1. *Tolerance was regarded as being affected by the attractiveness* (q_{ij}) *of the health facility including facility features and distance.*

In this scenario, we assumed that the actual outpatient visits of health facilities were affected by the distance and service quality [20]. Thus, the attractiveness (q_{ij}) included the effects by both the facility itself and its distance. The tolerance of residents who visited the healthcare facilities was calculated by Equation (2).

$$w_{1ij} = Norm(-q_{ij}) \tag{2}$$

where w_{1ij} is the tolerance of residents who visited the healthcare facilities under the conditions of Scenario 1, and $Norm(-q_{ij})$ is the normalization of $-q_{ij}$.

Scenario 2. *The attractiveness* (q_{ij}) *of the health facility was considered to only represent the effects of the facility features, such as service quality, physician level, and crowdedness.*

The tolerance of the visitors was considered as the comprehensive assessment of residents visiting a healthcare facility, which consisted of two factors, the distance between the population and healthcare facility and the attractiveness of the healthcare facility. There are several ways to conduct a comprehensive assessment of a criteria affected by several factors, and multiplying or adding weighted factors are the most common methods [38,39]. Compared to multiplication weighted factor, addition weighted factors can obtain a dataset having lower dispersion and smaller fluctuations. Therefore, the addition formula was chosen to determine the tolerance of the patients visiting a healthcare facility (Equation (3)). Notably, we assumed that the attractiveness of the facility and the distance of the facility from the residents' locations had equal influences on the tolerance.

$$w_{2ij} = Norm(t_{ij}) + Norm(-q_{ij}) \tag{3}$$

where w_{2ij} is the tolerance of residents visiting health facilities in Scenario 2, t_{ij} is the travel time from the population location to the supply service, $Norm(t_{ij})$ and $Norm(-q_{ij})$ are the normalizations of the datasets t_{ij} and $-q_{ij}$. They were normalized to [0,1] to eliminate the influence of their numerical values.

The tolerance decay function $f_i(w_{ij})$ was determined by the logistic cumulative distribution function (CDF) [Equation (4)], which is a downward sigmoid function (S-shape) based on a logistic distribution method [17]. Because the CDF used the median and standard deviation (SD) of the tolerance dataset (w_{ij}), a uniquely shaped decay function, $f_i(w_{ij})$, was obtained for every population location i.

Figure 3 illustrates an example of the changes in $f_i(w_{ij})$ with various medians and SDs of w_{ij}. We observed that the median shifted the function in horizontal direction, and the SD changed the steepness. For a fixed SD, a larger median value resulted in stronger tolerance for longer distances and lower attractiveness. For a fixed median, a smaller SD resulted in a steeper curve, indicating that the residents were more sensitive to the tolerance factors.

$$f_i(w_{ij}) = \frac{1 + \exp\left(-\frac{\mu\pi}{\sigma\sqrt{3}}\right)}{1 + \exp\left(\frac{(w_{ij}-\mu)\pi}{\sigma\sqrt{3}}\right)} \tag{4}$$

where μ is the median of w_{ij}, and σ is the SD of w_{ij}.

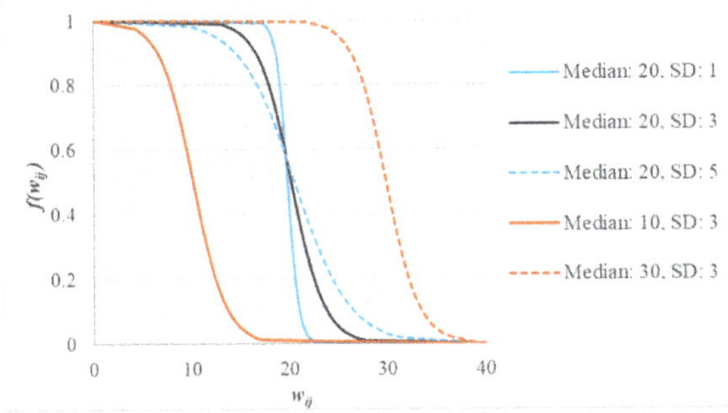

Figure 3. Effects of median and standard deviation (SD) on tolerance decay function; x axis represents the tolerance (w_{ij}) and y axis represents tolerance decay function $f_i\left(w_{ij}\right)$.

3.2.3. Accessibility

The accessibility of healthcare facilities was determined based on the M2SFCA model [15], which considers the supply–demand relations, along with suboptimal configurations, as shown in Equation (5). In this accessibility equation, the traditional distance decay function was substituted by the tolerance decay function, which considered the attractiveness and distance of the health facilities. As discussed in Section 3.2.2, the tolerance decay function, $f_i\left(w_{ij}\right)$, varied for each catchment area. The suboptimal configuration was evaluated by $f_G\left(w_{ij}\right)$, which represented the general benchmark tolerance of patients who visited the healthcare facilities, and it was calculated using all the tolerance values calculated for the entire study area regardless of catchment area [Equation (6)].

$$A_i = \sum\nolimits_{j\in\{t_{ij}\le t_0\}} \frac{S_j f_i\left(w_{ij}\right) f_G\left(w_{ij}\right)}{\sum_{i\in\{t_{ij}\le t_0\}} P_i f_i\left(w_{ij}\right)} \tag{5}$$

where S_j is the number of physicians of the facility, P_i is the population of the demand location, $f_G\left(w_{ij}\right)$ is the global tolerance decay function, t_{ij} is the travel time between the residents and the healthcare locations, t_0 is the maximum travel time of the catchment area, and A_i is the accessibility of the demand location.

$$f_G\left(w_{ij}\right) = \frac{1+\exp\left(-\frac{\mu_G \pi}{\sigma_G \sqrt{3}}\right)}{1+\exp\left(\frac{\left(w_{ij}-\mu_G\right)\pi}{\sigma_G\sqrt{3}}\right)} \tag{6}$$

where μ_G and σ_G are the medians and SDs of all the w_{ij} values calculated for the entire study area regardless of catchment area; it is a constant value.

3.2.4. Accessibility of Multi-Tiered Health System

The multi-tiered health system consists of two main types of healthcare facilities, i.e., hospitals and CHCs. To calculate the accessibility of the multi-tiered health system, we proposed the MT2SFCA method to adapt to the system. The process of evaluating accessibility is demonstrated in Figure 4. First, the respective accessibilities of CHCs and hospitals were calculated separately, and then, the results were compared to the accessibility of the multi-tiered health system (CHCs and hospitals).

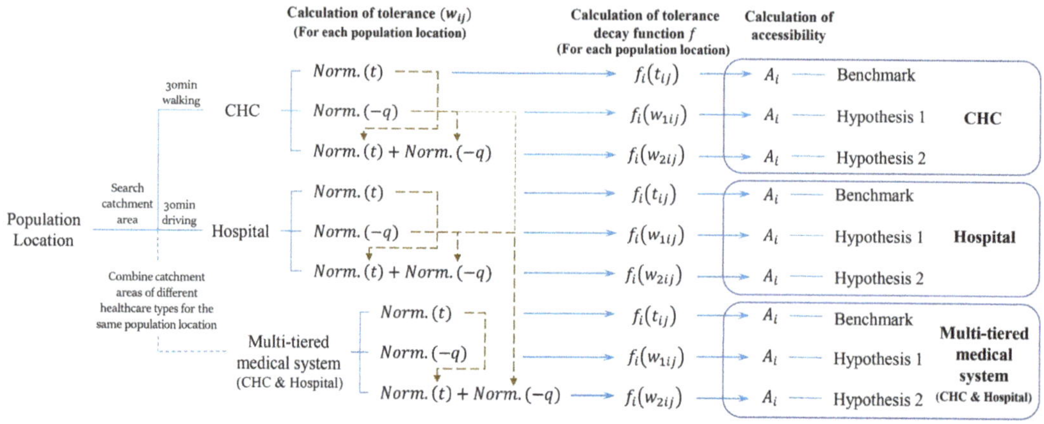

Figure 4. Flowchart explaining the process of calculating the accessibility of CHC, hospital, and the multi-tiered medical system.

For each of the three healthcare configurations, the accessibilities are determined in three ways by varying the tolerance decay function $f_i(w_{ij})$. First, we determined the benchmark value of accessibility by using the travel time, t_{ij}, as the tolerance in Equation (5), which is similar to the traditional 2SFCA method. Then, another two methods consider the attractiveness and travel time of healthcare as tolerance as indicated by Equations (2) and (3) of Scenarios 1 and 2. It is important to note that the catchment areas of CHC and hospital were different, which are determined by '30 min by walking' and '30 min by driving'. When we calculated the accessibility of the multi-tiered medical system, the catchment areas of both the CHCs and hospitals were summed up for each neighborhood, referring to the 2SFCA method with various catchment areas [14].

In terms of the multi-tiered medical system, the normalization of the parameters in tolerance should be carried out after aggregating all the CHCs and hospitals together within their catchment areas for each neighborhood. For Scenario 1, the tolerance was calculated by the normalization of $-q_{ij}$ for the combined dataset of the CHCs and hospitals, because q_{ij} represented the attractiveness of the facility, while considering all the influencing factors. For Scenario 2, the minus attractiveness, $-q_{ij}$, of healthcare facilities within each catchment area was normalized for CHCs and hospitals respectively, and the travel time, t_{ij}, was normalized for the combined dataset of the CHCs and hospitals. Then, the tolerance was calculated by the sum of the normalized $-q_{ij}$ and normalized t_{ij} as indicated by the yellow dashed line in Figure 4. It is important to mention that the combined dataset of CHCs and hospitals was used when the t_{ij} was normalized because travel time is one of the main reasons for patients to prefer a healthcare facility, which is the core competitiveness of CHCs. However, the respective datasets of CHCs and hospitals were used for the normalization of $-q_{ij}$, because the attractiveness of the healthcare facilities in Scenario 2 mainly represented the characteristics of the healthcare facilities themselves. The CHCs and hospitals have their own specialties and drawbacks. CHCs mainly deal with common diseases and hospitals are skilled in treating specialized diseases. Generally, people spend lesser time in CHCs than hospitals. Thus, it is not suitable to normalize the attractiveness of CHC and hospital together.

3.2.5. Gini Index of Accessibility

Gini index is one of the most common measurements to evaluate social inequity [40]. In economics, Lorentz curves are plotted to obtain the Gini index, which presents the cumulative percentage of total wealth against the cumulative of population (possessing the wealth), beginning with the poorest recipient [41]. The equality line represents the situation that each recipient has equal wealth. Gini index is calculated by the area between Lorentz curve and the line of absolute equality, being divided by the triangle area under the equality line, which is independent of the measure unit. The Gini index value of 0 refers to the perfect equality circumstances, in which the Lorentz curve and the straight line of absolute equality are coincident. More unequal conditions are indicated by higher Gini index.

In recent years, Gini index has also been applied to evaluate the spatial equity of health services. In this study, Gini index was used to evaluate the spatial equity of healthcare facilities at the subdistrict level. The Gini index was calculated by the variables of accessibility. The Lorentz curve was plotted using the cumulative percentage of accessibility against the fraction of total population at the subdistrict level, which was arranged in ascending order of accessibility. The Gini index was calculated using RStudio [42].

4. Results

For the ~11.7 million long-term residents living in 6328 neighborhoods in Shenzhen, the average number of physicians per 1000 people were 2.76 and 0.38 for hospitals and CHCs, respectively. The results of accessibility calculated using the MT2SFCA method are illustrated in Figures 5–7 for the CHCs, hospitals, and the entire multi-tiered medical system (including both CHC and hospital), respectively. In each figure, the subpart (a) represents the benchmark value of accessibility. The subparts (b) and (c) of accessibility were obtained for the Scenarios 1 (w_{1ij}) and 2 (w_{2ij}), respectively, using the MT2SFCA method proposed in this study.

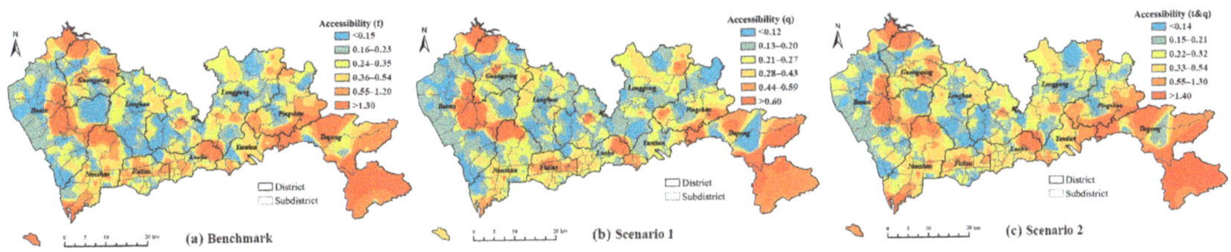

Figure 5. Accessibility of CHCs: (**a**) benchmark of accessibility; (**b**) accessibility calculated for Scenario 1; (**c**) accessibility calculated for Scenario 2.

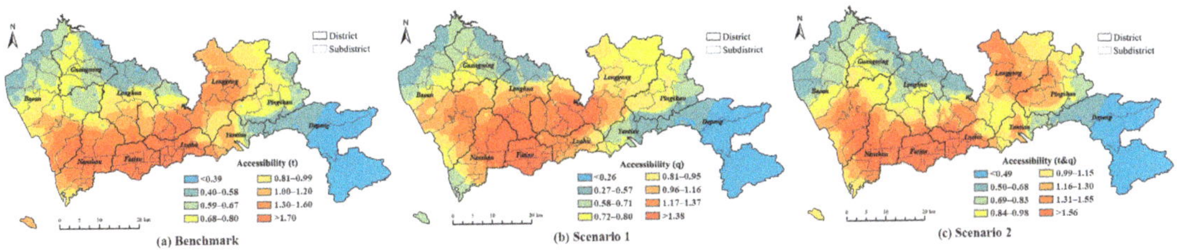

Figure 6. Accessibility of hospitals: (**a**) benchmark of accessibility; (**b**) accessibility calculated for Scenario 1; (**c**) accessibility calculated for Scenario 2.

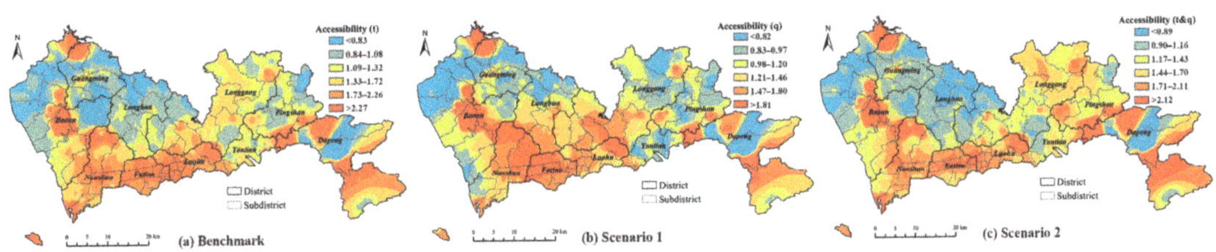

Figure 7. Accessibility of multi-tiered medical system: (**a**) benchmark of accessibility; (**b**) accessibility calculated for Scenario 1; (**c**) accessibility calculated for Scenario 2.

In terms of CHCs, the accessibility determined for Scenario 1 was obviously smaller than the benchmark value, and the results of Scenario 2 were close to the benchmark, based on the values of quantiles (Figure 5). In these three methods, the spatial distributions of the values in sextiles were similar, and only smaller differences could be found. For example, in Scenario 1, the areas of the highest and the lowest quantiles were smaller compared to benchmark, e.g., in Longhua, Longgang, and Nanshan districts. The results showed that the attractiveness and travel time affected the willingness of residents to visit the CHCs in the same way, which implied that the main reason for people choosing CHCs was travel time for both scenarios.

The accessibility of the hospitals calculated using three methods illustrated the apparent discrepancies. The values of the quantiles of the benchmark were higher than those obtained for Scenario 1, and similar for Scenario 2. The spatial distributions of the accessibility values were also different for the three methods. For the benchmark result shown in Figure 6a, the healthcare facilities in the central areas of Shenzhen had better accessibility, that is, the districts of Nanshan, Futian, and Luohu, where the hospitals were densely located. Notably, the distribution of higher accessibility followed the distribution of tertiary hospitals. For the result of Scenario 1 [Figure 6b], the highest quantile of accessibility expanded from the city center to the Longhua and Longgang districts. Compared to the benchmark, the distribution of higher accessibility in Scenario 1 was similar to the distributions of tertiary and primary hospitals. The distribution pattern of accessibility obtained by Scenario 2 indicated similar results to the benchmark. It also implied that in Scenario 1, the attractiveness of the hospitals due to other factors, such as hospital level and service quality, was more important than the travel time when the residents preferred a hospital, whereas in Scenario 2, the travel time indicated a more significant effect compared to the attractiveness of the healthcare facility.

The accessibility of the multi-tiered medical system is demonstrated in Figure 7. The results combined the respective results of the CHCs and hospitals given in previous sections. The higher accessibilities were found not only in the central areas of the city in the Nanshan, Futian, and Luohu districts as the results of hospitals, but also in suburban areas, such as Baoan, Pingshan, and Dapeng districts, similar to the results of CHCs. In terms of the quantile values and spatial distributions, compared to Scenario 1, the result of Scenario 2 was closer to the result of benchmark.

Figure 8 demonstrates how the results of Scenarios 1 and 2 deviated from that of the benchmark. The positive and negative deviations indicated obvious spatial clusters. For Scenario 1, in which we assumed that the healthcare attractiveness, including both travel time and facility features, was calculated by normalized outpatient visits; the accessibility declined mainly in the central areas of Shenzhen (Nanshan, Futian, and Luohu districts). The increments of accessibility were located in suburban areas (Longhua, part of Longgang, and part of Baoan districts). The negative deviations of accessibility occupied more than half the area of the whole city. In terms of Scenario 2, the accessibility decreased mainly in the city center, similar to Scenario 1 and also in some suburban areas, such as the Longhua and Longgang districts. The positive deviations were found in the western and eastern suburban areas.

The Gini indexes of subdistricts in Shenzhen were obtained based on the accessibility of the CHCs, hospitals, and the entire multi-tiered medical system as demonstrated in Figure 9. In general, the accessibility of the CHCs indicated obvious disparities, compared with the accessibility of hospitals, especially in northern areas. The Gini indexes of most subdistricts were 0.4 or higher. Owing to the larger service area, the residents living far from the city center were able to reach the hospitals, and thus, their equity of hospital accessibility provided better results. By considering both the CHCs and hospitals in the multi-tiered medical system, we were able to deduce that the number of the subdistricts that offered unequal health services was small. Only several remote regions indicated an equity problem. Compared to the accessibility distributions, we were able to deduce that the regions having higher accessibility (city center) generally experienced better equity.

However, the more homogeneous distributions of accessibility resulted in lower values of the Gini index, although the values of accessibility may not be high for the hospital accessibility in northern areas, i.e., the Longhua and Longgang districts. The subdistricts having both low and high values of accessibility indicated low equity, e.g., the subdistricts in the Dapeng district.

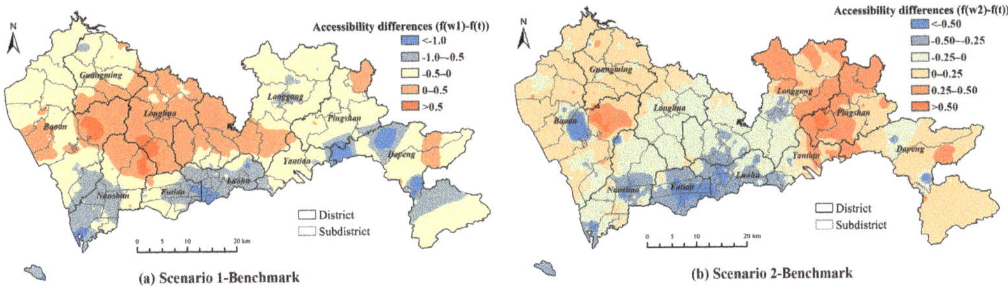

Figure 8. Accessibility differences between: (**a**) Scenario 1 and the benchmark; (**b**) Scenario 2 and the benchmark.

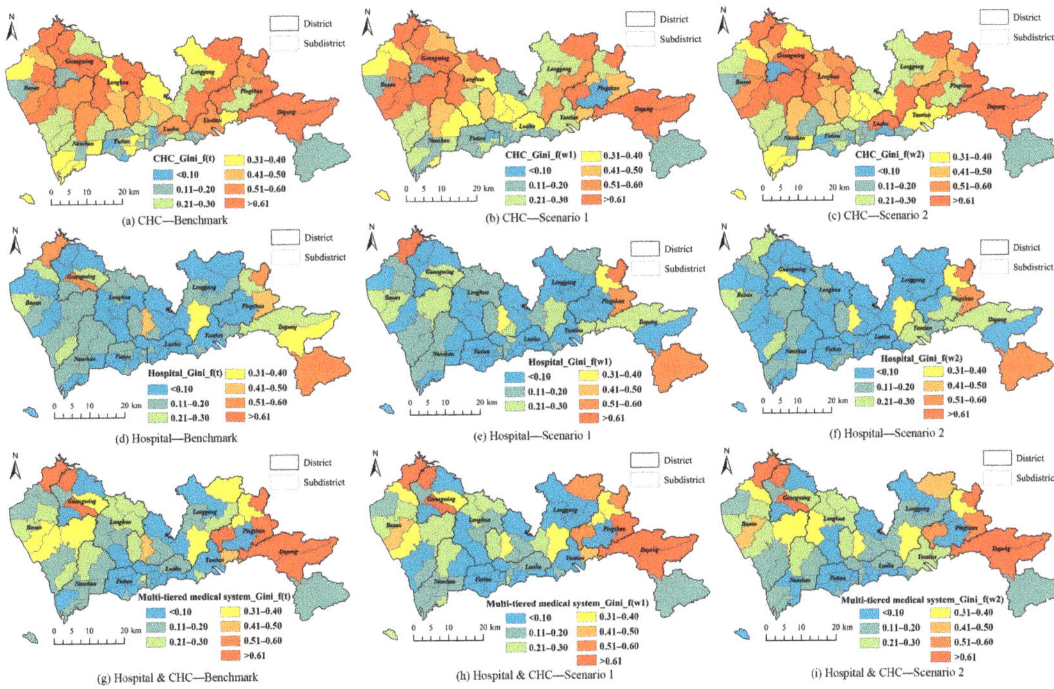

Figure 9. Gini indexes of CHCs, hospitals, and the entire multi-tiered medical system for subdistrict in Shenzhen, China: (**a**) Benchmark of Gini index for CHC; (**b**) Gini index of CHC calculated for Scenario 1; (**c**) Gini index of CHC calculated for Scenario 2; (**d**) Benchmark of Gini index for hospital; (**e**) Gini index of hospital calculated for Scenario 1; (**f**) Gini index of hospital calculated for Scenario 2; (**g**) Benchmark of Gini index for multi-tiered medical system; (**h**) Gini index of multi-tiered medical system calculated for Scenario 1; (**i**) Gini index of multi-tiered medical system calculated for Scenario 2.

The discrepancies in the Gini indexes calculated for the benchmark, Scenario 1, and Scenario 2 are portrayed in Figure 10. Different from accessibility, the discrepancies did not show obvious spatial aggregations. The results of both the scenarios in most subdistricts were lower than the benchmark results. The results of Scenario 2 indicated more subdistricts having discrepancies higher than 0.1 or lower than −0.1, compared to Scenario 1. The results implied that travel time was not the only factor that affected the people's decisions to visit a healthcare facility. Factors, such as facility features and financial conditions of patients, affected the competitiveness of the facilities. Thus, the equity of the healthcare accessibilities of Scenarios 1 and 2 offered better results than the benchmark, which only considered travel time as a major influencing factor.

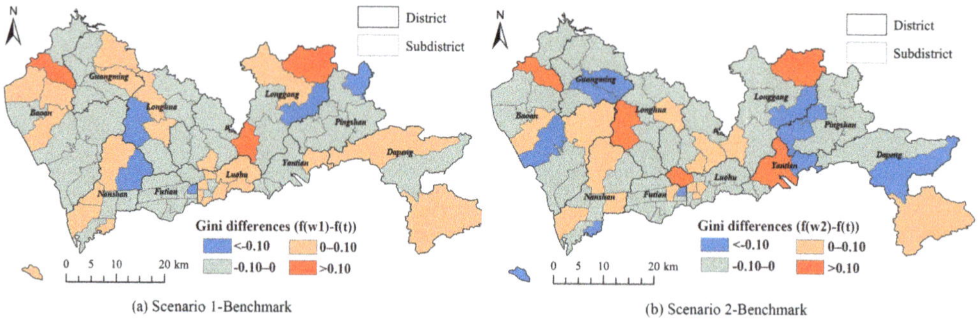

Figure 10. Differences between Gini indexes of: (**a**) Scenario 1 and benchmark; (**b**) Scenario 2 and benchmark of the multi-tiered medical system.

5. Discussion

By considering the time and attractiveness, along with a combination of the two factors, the MT2SFCA method described the supply–demand relations of medical resources in multiple aspects. The results distinguished the main factor that affects the decisions of patients to select different healthcare facilities. The accessibilities of the multi-tiered medical system calculated under the Scenarios 1 and 2 are plotted against the benchmark value in Figure 11. Similar to the spatial distribution, more than half the results were smaller than the benchmark values in Scenario 1. In Scenario 2, the points were above or underneath the 1:1 line, which indicated that travel time played a more predominant role in Scenario 2, compared to Scenario 1.

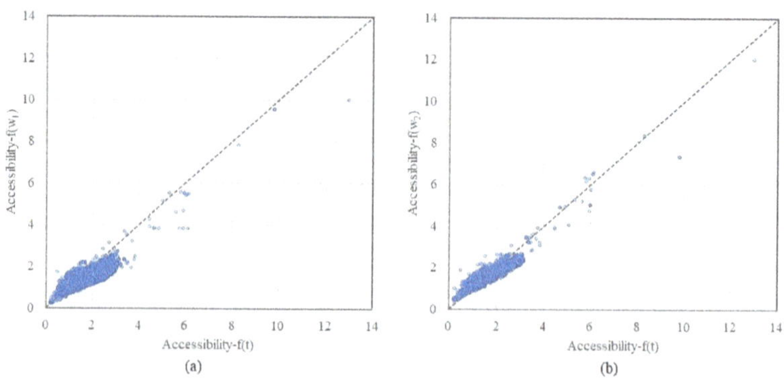

Figure 11. Comparisons of benchmark with (**a**) Scenario 1 and (**b**) Scenario 2, plotted along with a dashed 1:1 line for reference.

The density plots of the MT2SFCA results are illustrated in Figure 12. The results of CHCs, hospitals, and the entire multi-tiered medical system presented unique distributions. The accessibility indicated similar shapes for the benchmark $f(t)$, Scenario 1 $f(w_1)$, and

Scenario 2 $f(w_1)$, in terms of the CHCs. Scenario 1 portrayed the largest peak value, followed by Scenario 2. Due to the lower number of physicians in the CHCs (compared to the hospitals), the accessibility of CHCs was aggregated between 0 to 1. The density plot of the hospital accessibility presented different distributions in Scenario 1 compared to those for the benchmark and Scenario 2. The accessibility of Scenario 1 was mostly clustered between 1 and 1.5, whereas it was mainly distributed around 2 and 2.5 for Scenario 2 and the benchmark, respectively. The accessibility of the entire multi-tiered medical system was the combination of the individual results of the CHCs and hospitals. Notably, the peak values of the neighborhood numbers were lower than those of CHCs, but higher than those of the hospitals. The results of Scenario 2 were consistent at the middle level, among all the results of benchmark, Scenario 1, and Scenario 2 for each healthcare configuration.

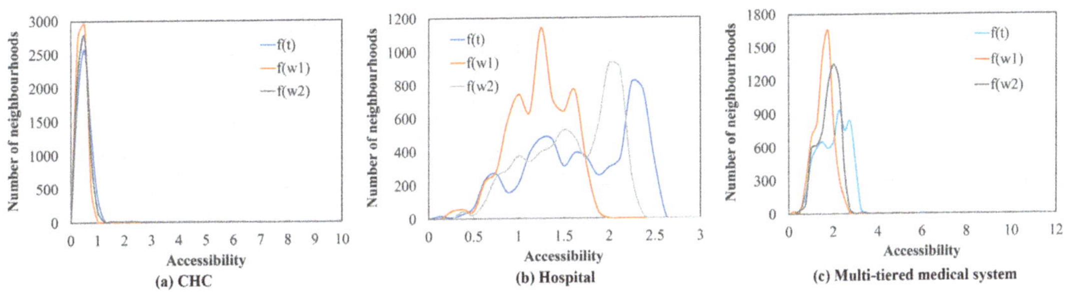

Figure 12. Density plots of MTSFCA results for (**a**) CHCs, (**b**) hospitals, and (**c**) the multi-tiered medical system in Shenzhen, China.

The results also highlighted the importance of primary healthcare facilities including CHCs and primary hospitals. With the increment of referral rate, they played critical roles in improving the accessibility and equity of the multi-tiered medical system, especially for the suburban area. Similar results were also found in the study of Beijing [22]. Thus, increasing the number of primary healthcare facilities was a main solution to solve the inequity of medical services in China [23,43].

For the benchmark, Scenario 1, and Scenario 2, the distance between healthcare facilities and patients was a critical factor that cannot be ignored when patients choose facilities, especially for CHCs. A study focusing on the primary healthcare in Sweden also found that distance is the most important factor in choosing a primary healthcare provider [44]. The distance effect also applicable to online therapy. By investigating a third-party online healthcare platform in China, Chen et al. found that the distance between doctors and patients is negatively associated with online service utilization [45]. In addition, distance has become more important due to the lockdown restrictions during COVID-19. Palm et al. found that many residents in Toronto and Vancouver defer medical care because the healthcare and pharmacy services are too far to reach by walking after stopping riding public transit during COVID-19 [46].

Although the travel distance is important, results revealed that the facility features were considered more when patients were going to choose hospitals. In research in Italy, it was found that many patients are willing to travel far and wait longer for seeking better healthcare services [47]. The better services hospitals offer, the more likely patients will choose [48]. This circumstance also occurs not only in intra-city healthcare, but in cross-city healthcare in China [49].

The accessibility and equity of the multi-tiered medical system consisting of CHCs and hospitals in Shenzhen were investigated in this study. Several advantages of the MT2SFCA method were highlighted. First, the MT2SFCA method was developed based on the M2SFCA method, which settled the limitation of traditional E2SFCA and 3SFCA methods by evaluating the overall effectiveness caused by any system change, i.e., increasing or removing any supply location [15]. Second, the uniquely shaped tolerance decay function for each catchment area solved the distinct allocations of healthcare resources. Other than the multiple attempts of applying various impedance coefficient when using Gaussian function and inverse function as the distance decay function, the logistic cumulative distribution function used in this study adjusted the curve shape by the distribution of dataset values. Moreover, it considered the specific distributions of the travel time or attractiveness of the CHCs and hospitals when evaluating the accessibility of the multi-tiered medical system. In terms of the benchmark, the greater the median travel time to the facilities within the catchment area, the more likely the patients were to travel further. If the healthcare facility provided spatial aggregations, which resulted in smaller standard deviations, the patients preferred to spend less time traveling to the healthcare facility. The tolerance decay of the people who visited the healthcare facility in Scenarios 1 and 2 worked on the same principle to the tolerance decay for the benchmark, whereas the measurements were replaced by the facility attractiveness and travel time. Finally, as an improvement in the M2SFCA method, we replaced one of the decay functions $f_i(w_{ij})$ with the global decay function $f_G(w_{ij})$ that represented the tolerance level of the whole research area instead of only the catchment area. The global decay function balanced the effects of the peak values for some catchment areas, because it was a fixed curve of all catchment areas [17]. In this study, the selection of the global tolerance function was based on the entire area of Shenzhen.

6. Limitations of the Study

The limitations of this study must be mentioned as well. Although this study did not consider the variable travel time for urban and suburban areas, this simplification was still explainable for Shenzhen. First, the 2000 km^2 area was not big for a first-tier city, compared to the area of 16,410 km^2 of Beijing, 7430 km^2 of Guangzhou, and 6340 km^2 of Shanghai. Most areas in Shenzhen were accessible via a one-hour drive. Second, the CHCs in Shenzhen were accessible for most neighborhoods. Finally, the variable tolerance decay curves determined by the CDFs within the same travel time were calculated while considering the unequal distributions of healthcare facilities in the city. Thus, it is not necessary to intentionally include that the people living in rural area may be go further for visiting healthcare. However, variations in the travel time are still suggested to be considered in further studies or for other cities. The benefits include balancing the healthcare allocation in city center and suburban area, avoiding overestimate the accessibility, and being much closer to reality, which have been referred by many pieces of literature [24,39,50]. In Scenario 2, we assumed that the attractiveness and travel time had equal influences on the tolerance function, but some of the results indicated that these two factors had different effects under various situations. Further analyses are suggested to be carried out for the MT2SFCA method with different weights of travel time and attractiveness.

The maximum catchment areas of CHCs and hospitals used in this study were 30 min of walking and 30 min of driving. These values are decided according to the policy and studies focusing on the planning of healthcare facilities in China [22,33]. We also conducted a survey among local people in Shenzhen about 'the farthest distance you can tolerate to visit CHCs/hospitals'. However, they were simplified values that do not consider the discrepancies among various population groups. Several studies found that the health equity usually varies among different groups, especially for the vulnerable groups [51,52]. Exploring the health equity of the multi-tiered medical system focusing on different population groups are recommended in further works.

In this study, we considered two travel modes that aimed at two different healthcare types. The effects of travel modes on accessibility have been proposed by several studies and are debatable. In some studies, the demand or supply locations were scattered, and the different travel modes significantly affected the accessibility of the healthcare facility [53,54]. For some developed areas, the accessibility calculated for multi-travel modes resulted in similar results of those obtained for single travel mode [55]. However, various travel modes are still encouraged to be considered in further studies.

It is also important to mention that the healthcare facilities used in this study were the facilities under the multi-tiered medical system, which included the private and public hospitals/CHCs. Private clinics were not considered. The reasons are that the private clinics cannot offer referral services, and the medical insurance is not available for most of them. As a result, the patients choosing the private clinics are mainly the floating population who are different from the long-term residents discussed in this study. However, the private clinics still help improve the accessibility and equity. Further work can focus on the effects of private clinics on current medical system and health equity.

There are other aspects that can be investigated in further works. Using the geographic center of administrative region to present population location is a traditional way when calculating accessibility and equity [20,23], whereas some studies proposed the effects of commute on routes when people visiting facilities [56,57]. It is recommended to consider the commuter-based locations in further work. The empirical validation of a certain function for a certain setting are regarded as an effective way to determine the appropriate distance decay function in traditional methods. Although the MT2SFCA method adapted the variety of the value distributions within the catchment area, the validation of the logistic cumulative distribution function used in MT2SFCA is still suggested by more empirical data.

7. Conclusions

In this study, we evaluated the accessibility and spatial equity of the multi-tiered medical system in China after the referral reform was introduced. Our study area was Shenzhen, China, and we proposed the MT2SFCA method, which was an improvement of the traditional M2SFCA method by replacing the distance decay function by the tolerance decay function using the formula of the logistic CDF. The CDF reshaped the function curve to adapt the distribution of tolerance values within the catchment area for the CHCs and hospitals in the multi-tiered medical system. When calculating the accessibility, we also considered the numbers of real outpatient visits and proposed two scenarios of tolerance to determine the effects of travel time and attractiveness when people select healthcare facilities, and then compared to the benchmark value. Travel time was set as the independent variable of decay function, which was referred to as the 'benchmark'. In Scenario 1, we assumed that the tolerance was only affected by the attractiveness of facilities, and in Scenario 2, we assumed that the tolerance was influenced by both attractiveness and travel time. The outpatient visits normalized by the facility capacity represented the attractiveness of the facility.

By comparing the accessibility and spatial equity of the CHCs, hospitals, and the entire multi-tiered medical system, we deduced that the multi-tiered medical system could gain the advantages of both the CHCs and hospitals. The CHCs offset the lower accessibility of hospitals in suburban areas, and simultaneously, improved the accessibility to healthcare facilities. The hospitals balanced the inequity of accessibility caused by the CHCs. Thus, the selection of CHCs by patients relied more on travel time, whereas the facility features were more important when choosing hospitals. It was difficult to determine which factor affected the multi-tiered medical system more than the other. However, compared to the benchmark, both the scenarios portrayed lower accessibility in the central areas of the city, which indicated that the actual supply–demand relations of healthcare resources were not as optimistic as the results calculated using only the effects of travel time in the city center (via convenient transportation). Similarly, people in rural areas experienced slightly better accessibility to healthcare services, even though they had to travel longer distances.

The MT2SFCA method indicated remarkable results in evaluating the accessibility of the medical system. Under this two-way patient referral multi-tiered medical system, both the CHCs and hospitals were found to be crucial for the whole system. Only one type of healthcare facility could not reflect the real distribution of healthcare resources. Thus, when evaluating the accessibility and spatial equity of medical systems, various types of healthcare facilities must be considered. In further studies, factors other than travel time are recommended to be considered in the evaluation of healthcare equity and accessibility. Furthermore, commuter-based locations, various catchment sizes, different modes, population groups, and weights of contributing factors can be used to improve the MT2SFCA method. Further studies could move toward improving spatial accessibility and equity of healthcare services by building new facilities and pathways.

Author Contributions: Conceptualization, methodology, formal analysis, validation, visualization, writing, M.T.; Conceptualization, writing, supervision, data curation, funding acquisition, L.Y.; Conceptualization, writing, supervision, project administration, R.G.; Data curation, validation, supervision, resources, Y.W.; Data curation, formal analysis, validation, resources, X.L. All authors have read and agreed to the published version of the manuscript.

Funding: This research was funded by the Science and Technology Planning Project of Shenzhen Municipality (CN), grant number JCYJ20180305125219726 and the National and provincial supporting projects of Shenzhen collaborative innovation technology plan, grant number 2019175353.

Institutional Review Board Statement: Not applicable.

Informed Consent Statement: Not applicable.

Data Availability Statement: Not applicable.

Acknowledgments: All the authors gratefully thank the reviewers and editor for their insightful and constructive comments. We also thank all contributors to the OpenStreetMap (OSM) initiative and their updates on the crowd-sourced geodata.

Conflicts of Interest: The authors declare no conflict of interest.

References

1. Taleai, M.; Sliuzas, R.; Flacke, J. An integrated framework to evaluate the equity of urban public facilities using spatial multi-criteria analysis. *Cities* **2014**, *40*, 56–69. [CrossRef]
2. Siegel, M.; Koller, D.; Vogt, V.; Sundmacher, L. Developing a composite index of spatial accessibility across different health care sectors: A German example. *Health Policy* **2016**, *120*, 205–212. [CrossRef] [PubMed]
3. Omer, I. Evaluating accessibility using house-level data: A spatial equity perspective. *Comput. Environ. Urban Syst.* **2006**, *30*, 254–274. [CrossRef]
4. Tian, M.; Yuan, L.; Guo, R.; Wu, Y.; Liu, X. Sustainable development: Investigating the correlations between park equality and mortality by multilevel model in Shenzhen, China. *Sustain. Cities Soc.* **2021**, *75*, 103385. [CrossRef]
5. WHO. Sustainable Health Financing, Universal Coverage and Social Health Insurance. 2005. Available online: http://apps.who.int/iris/bitstream/10665/20383/1/WHA58_33-en.pdf (accessed on 5 May 2021).
6. Chinadaily. China's Development Targets for 14th Five-Year Plan Period. 2020. Available online: https://www.chinadaily.com.cn/a/202011/02/WS5f9f3940a31024ad0ba82610_1.html (accessed on 5 May 2021).
7. Zheng, Z.; Shen, W.; Li, Y.; Qin, Y.; Wang, L. Spatial equity of park green space using KD2SFCA and web map API: A case study of Zhengzhou, China. *Appl. Geogr.* **2020**, *123*, 102310. [CrossRef]
8. Aman, J.J.C.; Smith-Colin, J. Transit deserts: Equity analysis of public transit accessibility. *J. Transp. Geogr.* **2020**, *89*, 102869. [CrossRef]
9. Radke, J.; Mu, L. Spatial decompositions, modeling, and mapping service regions to predict access to social programs. *Geogr. Inf. Sci.* **2000**, *6*, 105–112. [CrossRef]
10. Joseph, A.E.; Bantock, P.R. Measuring potential physical accessibility to general practitioners in rural areas: A method and case study. *Soc. Sci. Med.* **1982**, *16*, 85–90. [CrossRef]
11. Luo, W.; Qi, Y. An enhanced two-step floating catchment area (E2SFCA) method for measuring spatial accessibility to primary care physicians. *Health Place* **2009**, *15*, 1100–1107. [CrossRef]
12. Dai, D. Racial/ethnic and socioeconomic disparities in urban green space accessibility: Where to intervene? *Landsc. Urban Plan.* **2011**, *102*, 234–244. [CrossRef]
13. Dai, D.J.; Wang, F.H. Geographic disparities in accessibility to food stores in southwest Mississippi. *Environ. Plan. B Plan. Des.* **2011**, *38*, 659–677. [CrossRef]
14. Wan, N.; Zou, B.; Sternberg, T. A three-step floating catchment area method for analyzing spatial access to health services. *Int. J. Geogr. Inf. Sci.* **2012**, *26*, 1073–1089. [CrossRef]
15. Delamater, P.L. Spatial accessibility in suboptimally configured health care systems: A modified two-step floating catchment area (M2SFCA) metric. *Health Place* **2013**, *24*, 3–43. [CrossRef]
16. Luo, W.; Whippo, T. Variable catchment sizes for the two-step floating catchment area (2SFCA) method. *Health Place* **2012**, *18*, 789–795. [CrossRef]

17. Bauer, J.; Groneberg, D.A. Measuring spatial accessibility of health care providers—Introduction of a variable distance decay function within the floating catchment area (fca) method. *PLoS ONE* **2016**, *11*, e0159148. [CrossRef]
18. Penchansky, R.; Thomas, J.W. The concept of access: Definition and relationship to consumer satisfaction. *Med. Care* **1981**, *19*, 127–140. [CrossRef]
19. Luo, J. Integrating the huff model and floating catchment area methods to analyze spatial access to healthcare services. *Trans. GIS* **2014**, *18*, 436–448. [CrossRef]
20. Shin, K.; Lee, T. Improving the measurement of the Korean emergency medical system's spatial accessibility. *Appl. Geogr.* **2018**, *100*, 30–38. [CrossRef]
21. Rong, P.; Zheng, Z.; Kwan, M.P.; Qin, Y. Evaluation of the spatial equity of medical facilities based on improved potential model and map service API: A case study in Zhengzhou, China. *Appl. Geogr.* **2020**, *119*, 102192. [CrossRef]
22. Lu, C.; Zhang, Z.; Lan, X. Impact of China's referral reform on the equity and spatial accessibility of healthcare resources: A case study of Beijing. *Soc. Sci. Med.* **2019**, *235*, 112386. [CrossRef]
23. Wang, X.; Yang, H.; Duan, Z.; Pan, J. Spatial accessibility of primary health care in China: A case study in Sichuan Province. *Soc. Sci. Med.* **2018**, *209*, 14–24. [CrossRef] [PubMed]
24. Chen, B.Y.; Cheng, X.P.; Kwan, M.P.; Schwanen, T. Evaluating spatial accessibility to healthcare services under travel time uncertainty: A reliability-based floating catchment area approach. *J. Transp. Geogr.* **2020**, *87*, 102794. [CrossRef]
25. Jiang, S.; Gu, Y.; Yang, F.; Wu, T.; Wang, H.; Cutler, H.; Zhang, L. Tertiary hospitals or community clinics? An enquiry into the factors affecting patients' choice for healthcare facilities in urban China. *China Econ. Rev.* **2020**, *63*, 101538. [CrossRef]
26. Wang, Y.; Castelli, A.; Cao, Q.; Liu, D. Assessing the design of China's complex health system—Concerns on equity and efficiency. *Health Policy OPEN* **2020**, *1*, 100021. [CrossRef]
27. Su, S.; Li, Z.; Xu, M.; Cai, Z.; Weng, M. A geo-big data approach to intra-urban food deserts: Transit-varying accessibility, social inequalities, and implications for urban planning. *Habitat Int.* **2017**, *64*, 22–40. [CrossRef]
28. SZMHC. 2018 Health Statistics of Shenzhen Municipality. Shenzhen Municipal Health Commission. 2019. Available online: http://wjw.sz.gov.cn/xxgk/ylfwxxgk/ylfwxxgk/content/post_3122213.html (accessed on 1 March 2021).
29. SZMHC. Shenzhen Municipal Planning Development of Healthcare Facilities 2016–2020. Shenzhen Municipal Health Commission. 2017. Available online: http://www.szpsq.gov.cn/xxgk/ghjh/fzgh/content/post_4181946.html (accessed on 1 March 2021).
30. SZMHC. Shenzhen Municipal Health and Family Planning Development Statistics Bulletin 2018. Shenzhen Municipal Health Commission. 2019. Available online: http://wjw.sz.gov.cn/ztzl/2018gzyd/ (accessed on 1 March 2021).
31. World Population Review. World Population Review: Shenzhen Population 2020. Available online: https://worldpopulationreview.com/world-cities/shenzhen-population (accessed on 17 December 2020).
32. Baidu Inc. Baidu Map Open Platform. 2020. Available online: http://lbsyun.baidu.com/ (accessed on 17 December 2020).
33. Cheng, L.; Yang, M.; De Vos, J.; Witlox, F. Examining geographical accessibility to multi-tier hospital care services for the elderly: A focus on spatial equity. *J. Transp. Health* **2020**, *19*, 100926. [CrossRef]
34. TBSZM. Shenzhen Traffic Performance Index System Transport Bureau of Shenzhen Municipality. Available online: http://tocc.jtys.sz.gov.cn/#/rt/road (accessed on 10 November 2021).
35. OSM. OpenStreetMap. Available online: https://www.openstreetmap.org/ (accessed on 17 December 2020).
36. Lianjia. Lianjia Real Estate Agency. Lianjia Real Estate Agency Co. Ltd. Available online: http://www.lianjia.com (accessed on 10 November 2020).
37. Esri., ArcGIS 10.7. Redlands, California: Environmental Systems Research Institute Inc. Available online: https://support.esri.com/en/Products/Desktop/arcgis-desktop/arcmap/10-8-1 (accessed on 10 November 2020).
38. Huff, D.L. Defining and estimating a trading area. *J. Mark.* **1964**, *28*, 34–38. [CrossRef]
39. Dony, C.C.; Delmelle, E.M.; Delmelle, E.C. Re-conceptualizing accessibility to parks in multi-modal cities: A variable-width floating catchment area (VFCA) method. *Landsc. Urban Plan.* **2015**, *143*, 90–99. [CrossRef]
40. Bowles, S.; Carlin, W. Inequality as experienced difference: A reformulation of the Gini coefficient. *Econ. Lett.* **2020**, *186*, 108789. [CrossRef]
41. Sinha, A.; Chakrabarti, B.K. Inequality in death from social conflicts: A Gini & Kolkata indices-based study. *Phys. A Stat. Mech. Appl.* **2019**, *527*, 121185.
42. RStudio Team. *Rstudio: Integrated Development for R*; Rstudio, PBC: Boston, MA, USA, 2015; Available online: http://www.rstudio.com/ (accessed on 17 May 2021).
43. Pan, J.; Zhao, H.; Wang, X.; Shi, X. Assessing spatial access to public and private hospitals in Sichuan, China: The influence of the private sector on the healthcare geography in China. *Soc. Sci. Med.* **2016**, *170*, 35–45. [CrossRef]
44. Dahlgren, C.; Dackehag, M.; Wändell, P.; Rehnberg, C. Simply the best? The impact of quality on choice of primary healthcare provider in Sweden. *Health Policy* **2021**, *125*, 1448–1454. [CrossRef]
45. Chen, Q.; Xu, D.; Fu, H.; Yip, W. Distance effects and home bias in patient choice on the Internet: Evidence from an online healthcare platform in China. *China Econ. Rev.* **2022**, *72*, 101757. [CrossRef]
46. Palm, M.; Sturrock, S.L.; Howell, N.A.; Farber, S.; Widener, M.J. The uneven impacts of avoiding public transit on riders' access to healthcare during COVID-19. *J. Transp. Health* **2021**, *22*, 101112. [CrossRef]
47. Lippi Bruni, M.; Ugolini, C.; Verzulli, R. Should I wait or should I go? Travelling versus waiting for better healthcare. *Reg. Sci. Urban Econ.* **2021**, *89*, 103697. [CrossRef]

48. Varkevisser, M.; van der Geest, S.A.; Schut, F.T. Do patients choose hospitals with high quality ratings? Empirical evidence from the market for angioplasty in the Netherlands. *J. Health Econ.* **2012**, *31*, 371–378. [CrossRef]
49. Yan, X.; Shan, L.; He, S.; Zhang, J. Cross-city patient mobility and healthcare equity and efficiency: Evidence from Hefei, China. *Travel Behav. Soc.* **2022**, *28*, 1–12. [CrossRef]
50. Mcgrail, M.R.; Humphreys, J.S.; Ward, B. Accessing doctors at times of need-measuring the distance tolerance of rural residents for health-related travel. *BMC Health Serv. Res.* **2015**, *15*, 212. [CrossRef]
51. Santinha, G.; Wolf, J.; Costa, C. Aging and the built environment: Is mobility constrained for institutionalized older adults? *J. Urban. Int. Res. Placemak. Urban Sustain.* **2020**, *13*, 431–447. [CrossRef]
52. Zhang, F.; Li, D.; Ahrentzen, S.; Zhang, J. Assessing spatial disparities of accessibility to community-based service resources for Chinese older adults based on travel behavior: A city-wide study of Nanjing, China. *Habitat Int.* **2019**, *88*, 101984. [CrossRef]
53. Cheng, J.; Yan, R.; Gao, Y. Exploring spatial heterogeneity in accessibility and transit mode choice. *Transp. Res. Part D Transp. Environ.* **2020**, *87*, 102521. [CrossRef]
54. Kim, C.; Tappis, H.; Mcdaniel, P.; Soroush, M.S.; Fried, B.; Weinberger, M.; Trogdon, J.G.; Kristen, H.L.; Delamater, P.L. National and subnational estimates of coverage and travel time to emergency obstetric care in Afghanistan: Modeling of spatial accessibility. *Health Place* **2020**, *66*, 102452. [CrossRef] [PubMed]
55. Mao, L.; Nekorchuk, D. Measuring spatial accessibility to healthcare for populations with multiple transportation modes. *Health Place* **2013**, *24*, 115–122. [CrossRef] [PubMed]
56. Fransen, K.; Neutens, T.; De Maeyer, P.; Deruyter, G. A commuter-based two-step floating catchment area method for measuring spatial accessibility of daycare centers. *Health Place* **2015**, *32*, 65–73. [CrossRef]
57. Niedzielski, M.A.; Kucharski, R. Impact of commuting, time budgets, and activity durations on modal disparity in accessibility to supermarkets. *Transp. Res. Part D Transp. Environ.* **2019**, *75*, 106–120. [CrossRef]

International Journal of
Environmental Research and Public Health

MDPI

Article

Spatiotemporal Evolution and Driving Mechanism of "Production-Living-Ecology" Functions in China: A Case of Both Sides of Hu Line

Yu Chen [1] and Mengke Zhu [2,*]

[1] School of Economics and Management, Zhengzhou University of Light Industry, Science Avenue 136, Zhengzhou 450000, China; 2012030@zzuli.edu.cn
[2] School of Public Administration, Huazhong Agricultural University, Wuhan 430070, China
* Correspondence: 13939045355@163.com

Abstract: In order to explore the spatiotemporal evolution of land use function and its driving factors in China, taking both sides of the Hu Line as an example, we used Exploratory Spatial Data Analysis and Geographically Weighted Regression methods to reveal dynamic evolution law, spatial characteristics and influencing factors of the "Production-Living-Ecology" functions of 288 prefecture-level cities on both sides of the Hu Line. The results show that: (1) In the temporal dimension, the coordination of "Production-Living-Ecology" functions of land use in China has been improved, and the Hu Line can be roughly used as the boundary of China's territorial space use. (2) In the spatial dimension, there is a significant positive spatial correlation between "Production-Living-Ecology" functions of land use in China, and the coordination gap between "Production-Living-Ecology" functions of land use on both sides of the Hu Line is gradually narrowing. (3) In terms of influencing mechanism, the coordination of "Production-Living-Ecology" functions is mainly driven by internal factors and is supplemented by external ones. The influence pattern of most driving factors is consistent with the layout characteristics of "strong east and weak west" of the Hu Line.

Keywords: Hu Line of land; "production-living-ecology" coordination; spatial heterogeneity; ESDA-GWR; China

Citation: Chen, Y.; Zhu, M. Spatiotemporal Evolution and Driving Mechanism of "Production-Living-Ecology" Functions in China: A Case of Both Sides of Hu Line. *IJERPH* **2022**, *19*, 3488. https://doi.org/10.3390/ijerph19063488

Academic Editor: Paul B. Tchounwou

Received: 15 January 2022
Accepted: 4 March 2022
Published: 15 March 2022

1. Introduction

In 1935, Hu Huanyong initiated the baseline—"Hu Line" [1]—or revealing the differences in China's population distribution. In essence, the Hu Line reflects the high spatial coupling between Chinese population and physical geography. It also highlights the problem of uncoordinated regional development in China's large-scale territorial space. Hu Huanyong believes that differences in natural geographical environment, social and historical conditions, and levels of economic development are the main reasons for the disparity in development between the two sides of the baseline, which coincides with the multi-functionality of land use. Based on diversified regional development goals and development needs at different levels, and under the guidance of natural, social, economic and other conditions, human beings reconstruct the original ecological space on the earth's surface, so that land use presents multi-functional characteristics such as life, production and ecology [2,3]. However, due to the inherent scarcity of land resources and the equality of opportunities for each function, conflicts between different functional spaces occur frequently, which further aggravates the confusion of the spatial development pattern of the country [4,5]. The main manifestation is that the development intensity of land space with the Hu Line as the boundary has obvious development characteristics of "strength in the east and weak in the west" [6]. As an important ecological function area, the northwest half of the wall has extremely limited space for gathering people and industries. Compared with the southeast half of the wall, the coordination degree of multi-functional land use is lower. Based on this, this paper proposes the following hypothesis:

Hypothesis 1. *The functional coordination of the land on both sides of the Hu Line has the characteristics of "high in the east and low in the west".*

In 2014, Chinese Premier Li Keqiang put forward the issue of "how to crack the Hu Line" [7], reflecting the urgency to clarify the specific factors causing the large gap between the two sides of the Hu Line and eliminate the actual development behind it. As a complete system, land is based on the background of land resources, with human beings as the main body and implementers; it has the characteristics of diversification of internal elements, diversity of utilization processes, and complexity of interaction with society, economy, and ecosystems. The internal subsystems also have synergistic and coherent effects [8]. Therefore, when researching the specific influencing factors of the functional coordination of "Production-Living-Ecology" functions, not only should it be based on the perspective of the whole system, but also the importance of the coordinated development of various subsystems within the system should be considered. Therefore, this paper proposes the following hypothesis:

Hypothesis 2. *The functional coordination of land "Production-Living-Ecology" Functions is not only affected by external factors, but also by the coordinated development of various subsystems.*

Based on this, this paper scientifically measures the functional coordination and spatial evolution law of the "Production-Living-Ecology" functions on both sides of the Hu Line, deeply explores the driving factors that cause the difference in coordination, and proposes targeted solutions, which will help alleviate the contradiction between the needs of utilization of the current land, helps to break the "Hu Line" in the national land space. The structure of this paper is as follows: Section 2 is a review of the relevant literature, covering the specific content of the Hu Line and the "Production-Living-Ecology" functions of land use; the third section introduces the research methods and the evaluation indicators of the coordination of the "Production-Living-Ecology" functions on both sides of the Hu Line. The fourth section analyzes the overall characteristics of the coordination of China's "Production-Living-Ecology" functions and the local characteristics of the southeastern half and the northwestern half bounded by the Hu Line from the perspective of space and time, focusing on the research on the two sides from the internal driving and external driving. Finally, the reason for the spatial heterogeneity of the coordination of "Production-Living-Ecology" functions is drawn, and based on this, countermeasures and suggestions are put forward for breaking through the "Hu Line of Land".

2. Literature Review

2.1. Hu Line

At this stage, the research on the Hu line mainly focuses on the extension of its connotation and the exploration of breakthrough paths.

2.1.1. Proposed Hu Line

In 1935, Hu Huanyong first quantitatively described the uneven distribution of China's population and proposed the famous Aigun Heilongjiang–Tengchong Yunnan population geographic dividing line [9], also known as the "Hu line" [10]. As a geographical boundary of population, the comprehensive geographical basis behind the Hu Line is the suitability and limitation of China's human settlement environment [11]. Furthermore, China's ecological carrying capacity has a trend of increasing gradient along the vertical direction of the Hu Line. It can be seen that the Hu Line symbolizes the transformation of China's ecological environment. As a "virtual boundary", Hu line is not actually "land". It is a high-level summary of various geographical boundaries and a deep integration of various geographical mutations, so it is also regarded as a natural geographical boundary in China [12]. In addition, the GDP, which reflects the economic development level of each geographic region, is also highly coupled with the Hu Line. Therefore, the Hu Line is also considered to be the economic geographic boundary of China [13].

2.1.2. Breaking through the Hu Line

The academic circle has come to two main viewpoints around "how to break through the Hu Line": First, there is the theory that the Hu Line cannot be broken through. From the perspective of natural environment, due to the profound geographical background on both sides of the Hu Line, it is difficult to get rid of the shackles of the environment even if measures such as technological reform and industrial upgrading are implemented. From the perspective of economic development, the difference in transportation costs caused by geographical factors is difficult to eliminate. Therefore, the competitiveness of commodity markets on both sides of the Hu Line is quite different, and this regional economic distribution law is unbreakable [14]. From the perspective of social development, China's population distribution is highly stubborn, and the gap between the two sides in basic public services, cultural and educational levels will also lead to the long-term existence of the Hu Line. Second, the Hu Line can break through. According to Krugman's point of view, the second geographic nature is the driving force to overcome the first geographic nature [15], and the development of transportation makes the population and industry agglomerate, making the west open up. In addition, informatization is the third geographic nature, which can promote trade development, knowledge spillovers, and promote preferential development in certain regions [16,17]. The construction of the "One Belt, One Road" has driven the development of the East-West linkage of the Eurasian continent, so that the northwestern half of the country has been transformed from the end of the previous opening to the east to the bridgehead opening to the west.

2.2. *"Production-Living-Ecology" Function*

At present, the research on the "production-living-ecology" function of land use mainly focuses on three aspects: concept definition, classification system and evaluation research.

2.2.1. Origin and Definition of "Production-Living-Ecology" Function

The function of "production-living-ecology" is the extension and development of the multi-functional concept of land use [18]. The multi-functional research on land use originated from the European Union's agricultural multi-functional research at the end of the 20th century [19], In 1994, the concept of Agricultural Multifunctionality was first used in Uruguay Round Agreement on Agriculture (URAA), and later, OECD defines it as "besides the functionality of food production, agriculture also has the functions of environmental protection, landscape functionality, rural employment, and food safety" [20,21]. Although academia has further expanded agricultural versatility into multi-functional land use [22–24], with the formation and promotion of the concept of sustainable development, the concept of land use multi-function emerges at the right moment. Sustainability Impact Assessment: Tools for Environmental Social and Economic Effects of Multifunctional Land Use in European Regions (SENSOR) project defines its concept as "human products and services in the process of land use in a certain region" [25], thus deriving three functional systems of society, economy and environment [26,27]. The "production-living-ecology" function is the product of the coordination and coupling of the three major systems. It further complements the multi-functional characteristics of land use and is regarded as a comprehensive system composed of production, living and ecological functions [28,29].

2.2.2. Classification System of "Production-Living-Ecology" Function

Functional classification of "production-living-ecology" is a process of discovering, representing, naming and classifying land functions [30]. It roughly includes three perspectives: ecosystem function, landscape function and land use [31,32]. Specifically, ecosystem functions derive from the ecological framework [33], but a comprehensive ecosystem service classification system has not been formed [34], and most scholars agree with the 17 ecosystem functions proposed by Costanza based on the summary of ecosystem [35]. Landscape functions evolve on the basis of landscape ecology and spatial planning [36,37]. The classification of landscape functions is very similar to that of ecosystem functions, and de Groot forms the landscape functional classification framework after adding the carrying function according to the original ecosystem functional classification system [38]. In addition, landscape functions are subdivided into three functions: production, ecology and culture [39]. The functional division of the perspective of land use is mainly economic-oriented, which is the product of the combination of land background elements with a certain natural physical and chemical structure and the form of human utilization [40]. According to the mapping relationship between land use structure and function, land use types are classified as "production, living (society) and ecology" [41]. However, this classification method can only reflect the main function of land use and fails to fully show the multi-functional characteristics of each piece of land.

2.2.3. Evaluation Research on "Production-Living-Ecology" Function

The research on the functional evaluation generally includes three parts: analysis framework, evaluation method and influencing factors. From the perspective of analysis framework, the conceptual framework of land use function developed by SENSOR project for analyzing land sustainability incorporates key indicators such as economy, culture and environment at the regional level [42], which greatly develops the multi-functional evaluation method system of land use. Due to the consideration of regional differences, a variety of evaluation frameworks emerge at the historic moment. The integrated analysis framework and participatory framework [43] that integrate various models are gradually becoming a trend. As the basis of evaluation research, the index system mainly covers functional classification and hierarchical design. In terms of specific methods, the comprehensive index method is the most widely used evaluation method. In addition, spatial analysis techniques or mathematical models are usually used to characterize the evolution of land functions [44–46]. In terms of influencing factors, the transformation of land use versatility is closely related to natural resource endowment, social and economic conditions and policy factors, but regional policy is the key cause [47]. At the same time, the influencing factors are also dynamic, which is manifested by the factors of environmental resources becoming increasingly prominent [48].

2.3. Summarize

To sum up, the Hu line has greatly enriched its connotation, but its role in dividing the spatial pattern of land use has been ignored. Moreover, most of the existing studies have not emphasized the rational layout and long-term development of land use function of land space. In terms of "Production-Living-Ecology" functions, the classification system experienced a trend from simple to complex, from one to multiple, but did not form a "universal" classification system. In terms of evaluation research, the trend of interdisciplinary analysis framework has emerged. Although the selection of indicators is relatively comprehensive, there is a lack of multi-scale research. Most of the influencing factors are qualitative explanations, and lack of analysis of regional differences. Compared with the existing literature, the innovations and contributions of this paper are as follows: (1) At the research scale, the spatial law of the coordination of "Production-Living-Ecology" functions of cities on both sides of the Hu Line is explored from the prefecture-city level, which not only extends the connotation of the Hu Line, but also breaks through the limitations of previous studies on "Production-Living-Ecology" functions focusing on large-scale studies. (2) In terms of research methods, the GWR model was adopted to seek ways to improve and optimize the land use structure on both sides of the Hu Line, which to some extent made up for the lack of discussion on the internal differences of different regions in previous studies. (3) In terms of influencing factors, on the one hand, influencing factors are set on the basis of fully considering the difference between the two sides of the Hu Line. On the other hand, the territorial space system is regarded as a complex dynamic giant system with multiple factors interacting with each other, and internal and external influencing factors are selected comprehensively. (4) Path exploration: Starting from territorial space utilization and starting from "Production-Living-Ecology" functions, it provides a new idea for the study of "how to break through Hu Line".

3. Materials and Methods

3.1. Study Area

China has a vast territory, due to the huge difference in resource endowment between the east and the west, resulting in a "strong east and weak west" distribution pattern in population, economy and other aspects with the Hu Line as the boundary. As shown in Figure 1, the population and economy west of the Hu Line only accounted for 7% of the southeast half in 2010. Although the proportion rose to 7.3% and 7.6%, respectively, in 2020, this pattern still had no substantial change in 2020. In recent years, with the continuous promotion of the main function zoning and new urbanization development strategy, the pattern of land use production, living and ecological function between urban and rural areas has changed dramatically, the strengths and weaknesses of the "Production-Living-Ecology" functions and the interlocking situations also have obvious regional colors, showing different development states on both sides of the Hu Line. There are few studies in the literature on the Hu Line in delineating the coordination characteristics of the "Production-Living-Ecology" functions of land use. Based on the availability of data, this paper selects a total of 288 prefecture-level cities on both sides of the Hu line as the study sample, involving a total of 30 provinces and autonomous regions except Tibet and three municipalities directly under the central government, Beijing, Shanghai and Tianjin, which account for 88% of China's total population and 91% of China's GDP; therefore, the results obtained using these cities have a wide range of practicality and play a role in supporting the scientific exploration of the theory of the spatial layout of China's land from the perspective of Hu line.

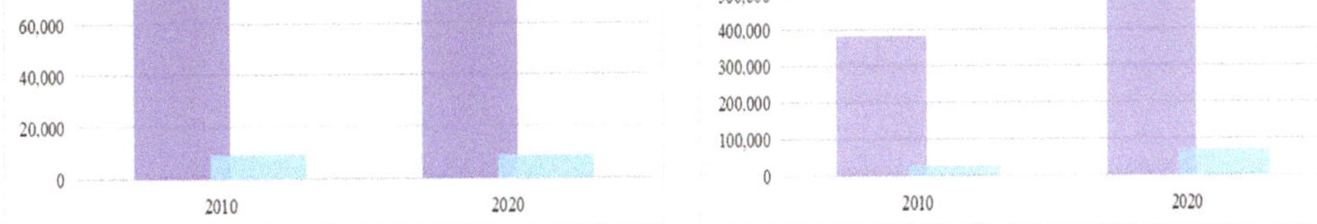

Figure 1. Population size and economic level on both sides of the Hu Line.

3.2. Research Method

3.2.1. Coupling Coordination Analysis

Coupling coordination degree can comprehensively reflect the overall function of environment and economy or the coordinated development level of comprehensive environment and economy. Referring to the existing research [49,50], this paper constructs the coupling and coordination model of production, living and ecological functions of land use to quantitatively identify the coordinated development level of "production-living-ecology" function and realize multi-scale integrated evaluation and analysis. See Equations (1)–(3) for calculation method:

$$C = \left\{ \frac{f_1 \times f_2 \times f_3}{(f_1 + f_2) \times (f_1 + f_3) \times (f_2 + f_3)} \right\}^{1/3} \quad (1)$$

$$T = \alpha f_1 + \beta f_2 + \gamma f_3 \quad (2)$$

$$D = \sqrt{C \times T} \quad (3)$$

In the formula, C is the coupling degree; f_i is the comprehensive evaluation function of each function; T is the comprehensive evaluation value of "production-living-ecology" function, reflecting the overall coordination effect; α, β, γ are undetermined weights. In this paper, since the "production-living-ecology" function of land is equally important, $\alpha = \beta = \gamma = 1/3$; D is the coupling coordination degree, the greater the D value, the better the coupling coordination. Among them, coupling degree refers to the degree of mutual influence of land "production-living-ecology" functions; coupling coordination degree reflects the level of harmony between the "production-living-ecology" functions in the land use function system in the development process.

3.2.2. Spatial Pattern Analysis

Exploratory spatial data analysis (ESDA) is an ideal data-driven analysis method. The essence of the model is to use a series of spatial data analysis methods and technologies, with spatial relevance as the core, through the description and visualization of the spatial phenomena, to find spatial agglomeration and spatial anomalies, thus revealing the spatial interaction mechanism between research objects. ESDA is divided into global spatial autocorrelation and local spatial autocorrelation. The global Moran's I index is used to describe the overall spatial characteristics of efficiency, so as to judge the spatial correlation and difference characteristics; the local Gi^* index is used to describe the local spatial heterogeneity characteristics of efficiency, so as to judge the local spatial differentiation laws. In this paper, global Moran's I and local Gi^* indexes are used to measure the spatial pattern characteristics of "production-living-ecology" function coordination degree at the city level in China.

Global Spatial Autocorrelation

The global Moran's I index measures the general trend of spatial correlation of the unit attribute values of adjacent or similar regions in the whole study area.

$$I = \frac{\sum_{i=1}^{n} \sum_{j=1}^{n} W_{ij}(X_i - \overline{X})(X_j - \overline{X})}{S^2 \sum_{i=1}^{n} \sum_{j=1}^{n} W_{ij}} \quad (4)$$

where: n is the number of research objects; X_i and X_j represent the observation values of i and j regions, respectively; W_{ij} is the spatial weight matrix (1 for spatial adjacency and 0 for non-adjacency); S^2 is the variance of observation values; and is the average of observation values. At a given significance level, a positive Moran's I value means that the overall coordination degree of urban "production-living-ecology" function coupling shows significant spatial agglomeration characteristics; if Moran's I value is negative, it means that the overall coordination degree of urban "production-living-ecology" function coupling shows significant spatial differentiation.

Hot Spot Analysis

It is used to analyze the hot and cold regions in different spatial regions, so as to measure the autocorrelation characteristics of local space.

$$G_i^* = \sum_{j=1}^{n} W_{ij} \frac{X_i}{\sum_{j=1}^{n} X_j} \quad (5)$$

where: W_{ij} is the spatial weight matrix, the spatial adjacency is 1, and the non-adjacency is 0. If it is significantly positive, it indicates that the value around i is relatively high, which belongs to the hot spot area; otherwise, the value around i is relatively low, which belongs to the cold spot area.

Driving Factor Analysis

Compared with the traditional OLS regression model, geographic weighted regression (GWR) uses spatial relations to reflect the non-stationary characteristics of parameters in different spatial locations, so that the relationship between research variables changes with the change of spatial location. Therefore, it can be used to reflect the spatial heterogeneity of the impact of different factors on the coordination of "production-living-ecology" function of land use. The model structure is as follows:

$$y_i = \beta_0(u_i, v_i) + \sum_k \beta_k(u_i, v_i) x_{ik} + \varepsilon_i \quad (6)$$

In Equation (6), y_i is the dependent variable value at the geographic location (u_i, v_i), (u_i, v_{i}) is the geocentric coordinate of the sample space unit, $\beta_0(u_i, v_i)$ is the constant value at the geographic location (u_i, v_i), $\beta_{\mathrm{k}}(u_i, v_i)$ is the value of function $\beta_{\mathrm{k}}(u, v)$ at the location of I, ε_i is the spatial random residual.

3.3. Index System Construction and Data Sources

The huge difference in natural geographical environment on both sides of the Hu Line and the inherent multi-dimensional, complex and scarce attributes of land space directly lead to the diversity of land functions on both sides. The 18th National Congress of the Communist Party of China proposed that the development and utilization of land space should be in line with "intensive and efficient production space, moderate livable space and picturesque ecological space". Therefore, on the basis of integrating the huge differences in production, life and ecology on both sides of the Hu Line, this paper constructed a three-dimensional index system (Table 1) of "production-living-ecology" from top to bottom according to the "system-element-function" theory and the "production-living-ecology" spatial optimal group theory [51]. First of all, the spatial distribution of population represented by the Hu Line is highly consistent with the spatial distribution of productive land resources, and the basic goal of production function is to achieve spatial concentration of production and guarantee social and economic development. Based on the mode of production and the level of economic development, agricultural production and non-agricultural production represent the mode of production. The former relies on agricultural land to obtain material products, while the latter relies on construction land to obtain commodities and services, therefore, the corresponding indexes are selected. From the perspective of the internal and external environment of economic development, indicators such as per capita GDP and amount of foreign capital used are selected to represent. Secondly, the Hu Line is also the demarcation line of human livability, and the basic goal of life function is to promote the concentration of living space and improve the livability level of cities. The improvement of living function cannot be separated from the people-oriented development concept. Based on Maslow's hierarchy of needs theory, the living standard, material life and spiritual life respectively represent the physiological, safety and self-actualization needs that people need to meet for survival. Living standards are reflected in the security of life, such as the need to ensure housing and travel. Material life is embodied in material wealth, such as the level of employment and consumption. Spiritual life is reflected in the provision of spiritual services, such as scientific and educational investment and cultural service provision. Therefore, the corresponding indicators are selected. Finally, the Hu Line symbolizes the transformation of China's ecological environment, and the basic goal of ecological function is to promote the integration of ecological space and maintain human living conditions. Ecological function is the prerequisite for the realization of production and living function and the natural base of land use [52]. The corresponding indicators are selected based on ecological foundation, carrying capacity and governance capacity. Based on the above analysis, this paper constructs an evaluation system of 27 basic indicators with 9 criteria levels.

Table 1. Functional coordination evaluation index system of "production-living-ecology".

Criteria Layer	Elements Layer	Basic Indicators
Production function	Agricultural production	Proportion of agricultural land
		Proportion of agricultural output value
		Per unit area yield of grain
	Non-agricultural production	Proportion of construction land
		Average gross industrial output value of land
		Average industrial output value
		Freight volume
	Economic development	Per capita GDP
		Amount of foreign capital used
		Fixed asset investment per land
		The industrial structure
Living function	Living standard	Proportion of residential land area
		Density of road network
	Material life	The employment rate
		Per capita savings balance
	Spiritual life	Proportion of science and education expenditure
		Number of books in public libraries per 10,000 people
		Number of college students per 10,000 persons
Ecological function	Ecological foundation	Green coverage rate of built-up area
		Per capita green garden area
	Ecological carrying	Average industrial wastewater discharge
		Average industrial sulfur dioxide emissions
		Average industrial smoke and dust emission
	Ecological governance	Comprehensive utilization rate general solid waste
		Sewage treatment rate
		Harmless treatment rate of domestic garbage

4. Results

4.1. Analysis on the Coordinated Space-Time Pattern of "Production-Living-Ecology" Function from the Perspective of Hu Line

This section includes two parts: characteristics of spatio-temporal changes of "production-living-ecology" function coordination and spatial differentiation of driving factors.

4.1.1. Characteristics of Spatio-Temporal Changes of "Production-Living-Ecology" Functional Coordination

According to Equations (1)–(3), calculate the coordination degree of "Production-Living-Ecology" function of 288 prefecture-level cities on both sides of the Hu Line from 2008 to 2017 (Table 2), and analyze the time variation trend of coordination degree of "Production-Living-Ecology" function on both sides. Overall, the coordination of "Production-Living-Ecology" function in China has improved as a whole, rising from 0.1207 in 2008 to 0.1364 in 2017, an increase of 13% in 10 years, but the growth rate is relatively slow. From the point of view of the Hu line, the temporal variation characteristics of the coordination of "Production-Living-Ecology" function on both sides are basically synchronous. According to the data, the coordination of "Production-Living-Ecology" function on both sides of the Hu Line is characterized by "high in the east and low in the west". Although the coordination difference between the two sides fluctuated, decreasing from 0.0154 in 2008 to 0.026 in 2017, in general, the coordination of "Production-Living-Ecology" function in the southeast half of the wall has a certain advantage compared with the northwest half. This is consistent with the basic situation of regional economic development. As the southeast half of China, which is economically developed, the first round of industrialization oriented by market economy has come to an end, while the new round of industrialization based on the principle of "industrial agglomeration, centralized layout and intensive land use" is booming. In contrast, the northwest half of China is in a transitional stage from the early stage of industrialization to the middle stage and needs to rely on a large amount of land input to promote the rapid development of industrialization, resulting in a relatively weak coordination of land use functions.

Table 2. Functional coordination of "production-living-ecology" in China from 2008 to 2017.

	2008	2011	2014	2017
Total	0.1223	0.1732	0.1320	0.1366
The Southeastern	0.1069	0.1701	0.1385	0.1341
The Northwest	0.1207	0.1729	0.1327	0.1364

ArcGIS10.0 software (Enveronmental Systems Research Institute (ESRI), RedLands, CA, USA) was used to generate the spatial distribution pattern map (Figure 2) to analyze the spatial changes of the coordination of Production-living-Ecology function of land use in China. The results are as follows:

(1) Low-level coordination area. In 2017, this type of area accounted for 44.8%, an increase of 10.8% compared with 2008, showing a significant change. Most of them appear in the west of the Hu Line and the three major forest areas, mostly in a continuous situation. Except for a few provincial capitals and municipalities, they are all at a low level. Among them, the western region accounted for 60.2% in 2008 and decreased to 48.1% in 2017. In contrast, in the east, a large number of cities have seen a significant deterioration in the functional coordination of "production-living-ecology", and the proportion of low-level coordination areas has increased from 11.2% to 23.2%. The central region has not changed much.

(2) Primary coordination area. From 2008 to 2017, there was no significant change in the primary coordination area, and the proportion declined slightly. Among them, the proportion in 2008 and 2017 was 38.5% and 35.8%, respectively. They were distributed on both sides of the Hu Line and mainly concentrated in the central and eastern regions of China, accounting for about 40%. In these areas, the "core-periphery" change pattern mostly appears, that is, the trend of decreasing outward around the advanced or intermediate coordination area, and the most obvious is in the middle and lower reaches of the Yangtze River and the Bohai Rim region.

(3) Intermediate coordination area. Contrary to the low-level coordination areas, the intermediate coordination areas are mainly distributed east of the Hu Line, and the

proportion of cities in the intermediate coordination areas decreased significantly from 2008 to 2017, from 65% to 43%, Although the change in the proportion of each area is not significant, the cities included have decreased to varying degrees, especially in the central and eastern regions, which decreased from 21 and 35 in 2008 to 13 and 23 in 2017, respectively. Among them, the Loess Plateau and the middle and lower reaches of the Yangtze River have the most significant changes from agglomerates to sporadic distribution.

(4) Advanced coordination area. From 2008 to 2017, the proportion of advanced coordination has not changed significantly, all of which are below 5%. East of the Hu Line is the most important distribution area, and most of these cities are located within the urban agglomeration. Most regions also occupy the position of central cities in the urban agglomeration. For example, Beijing, Shanghai, and Zhengzhou belong to the core cities of Beijing-Tianjin-Hebei, the Yangtze River Delta, and the Central Plains urban agglomeration. In addition, compared with 2008, the advanced coordination area has changed from a simple division in the central and eastern regions to the western and middle eastern regions, and the advanced coordination area in the west is also located within the urban agglomeration on the northern slope of Tianshan Mountain.

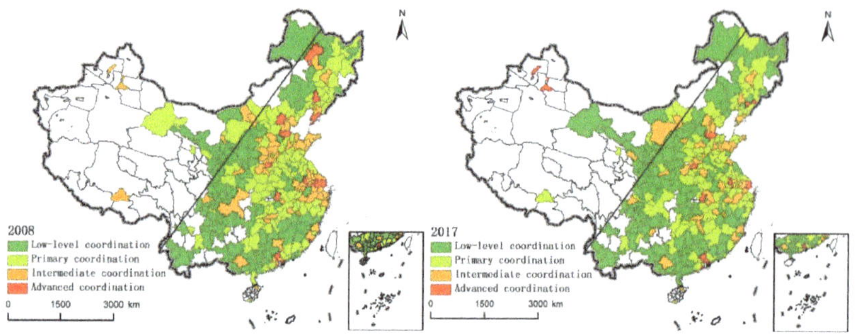

Figure 2. Distribution of "production-living-ecology" functional coordination in China from 2008 to 2017.

The above analysis shows that: First of all, the Hu Line can be interpreted to some extent as the boundary of China's territorial space utilization. With this line as the boundary, the west is mostly the low-level coordination area of land use "production-living-ecology" function, while the east is mostly the intermediate and advanced coordination area. The main reason is that the Hu Line can be used as the boundary of China's ecological environment, and the northwest is the main ecological spatial distribution area in China. Industrialization and urbanization, as the basic driving force for the transformation of "production-living-ecology" functions, are subject to their special landforms, resulting in a large gap among production, living and ecological functions. However, the southeast has significant advantages in public services and industrial development, and its land use is more reasonable due to the increasingly intensified ecological protection policies in recent years. Secondly, from the perspective of the three major regions in China, the proportion of the low-level coordination areas in the west has decreased significantly. The main reason may be that the implementation of the western development policy on the one hand promoted regional economic growth and paid more attention to ecological restoration and environmental protection, thus promoting the gradual rise of production and living functions. The proportion of intermediate coordination areas in the central and eastern regions decreased significantly. This is mainly because with the development of industry, some low-end industries have infiltrated into and threatened the development of ecological environment. Although policies such as "ecological civilization construction" and "main function zoning" have effectively restricted the development path at the expense of the environment, they have also led to the continuous compression of production and life functions. The advanced coordination area is mostly located in the central city of the eastern urban agglomeration and shows the attenuation trend that the advanced coordination area as the center gradually weakens to the outer layer. By forming a central city with strong radiation power, urban agglomerations promote the development of surrounding and peripheral cities, and form an urban agglomeration system with reasonable layout, division of labor and cooperation, and complementary functions. It is increasingly becoming the main spatial form of various development factors and the key area for industrialization and urbanization development. With many advantages, its function coordination of "production-living-ecology" can achieve rapid development.

Therefore, the above analysis can verify hypothesis 1: the coordination of land Production-Living-Ecology function on both sides of the Hu Line is characterized by "high in the east and low in the west".

4.1.2. Evolution of Spatial Pattern of "Production-Living-Ecology" Functional Coordination

In order to quantitatively study the evolution of the spatial pattern of Production-Living-Ecology function coordination, this paper established Queen's adjacency matrix and used the data of prefecture-level cities from 2008 to 2017 to calculate the Global Moran's I of the study area over the years. It was found that the Moran's I index passed the test at the significance level of 0.01 in all years, indicating that the coordination level of Production-Living-Ecology function of prefecture-level cities in China had a positive spatial autocorrelation. In addition, the global Moran's I indices in 2008 and 2017 were 0.1287 and 0.1034, respectively, indicating that the spatial distribution pattern of the coordination level of Production-Living-Ecology function in China was relatively stable in general.

To eliminate global autocorrelation to local instability of defects, and further detect the local spatial agglomeration pattern evolution characteristics, ArcGIS10.0 software (Enveronmental Systems Research Institute (ESRI), RedLands, CA, USA) was used to calculate the 2008 and 2017 in the local Gi^* index of each city. The natural breakpoint method is used to divide the values into hot spot area, second hot spot area, second cold spot area and cold spot area, and draw the clustering and evolution chart of the "production-living-ecology" functional coordination degree pattern of cities in China from 2008 to 2017 (Figure 3).

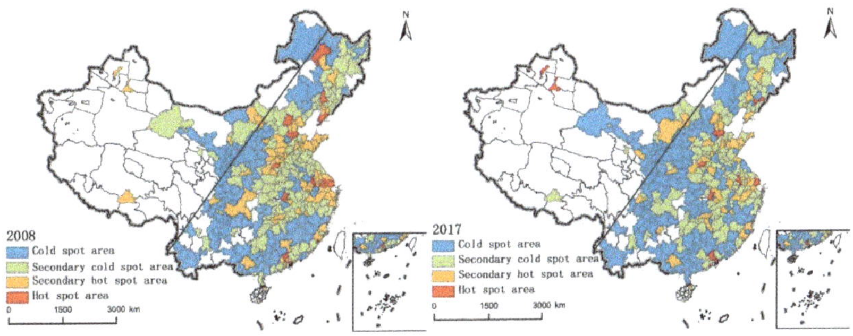

Figure 3. Spatial pattern of "production-living-ecology" functional coordination in China from 2008 to 2017.

On the whole, there has been no substantial change in the pattern of cold and hot spots in the coordination degree of "production-living-ecology" in China's cities, and the situation of "high in east and low in west" is still maintained on both sides of the boundary of the Hu Line. Among them, hot spots did not form an obvious global high-value concentration center. Most of the hot spots in 2008 were located on the east side of the Hu Line (Qiqihar, Shenyang, Dalian, Beijing, Cangzhou, Zhengzhou, Wuhan, Nanjing, Wuxi, Suzhou, Shanghai, Xiamen, Guangzhou and Shenzhen). Most of them are provincial capitals. In 2017, although cities in the southeast (Benxi, Cangzhou, Zhengzhou, Wuhan,

Nanjing, Shanghai, Guangzhou, Dongguan and Shenzhen) are still dominant, they moved westward and spread to Urumqi and Karamay on the west side of Hu Line, and some regions were reduced from hot spots to second hot spots or cold spots. At the same time, there is also a certain degree of spatial polarization in some regions, such as the Central Plains urban agglomeration and the Yangtze River Delta city group, whose agglomeration trend shows an attenuation trend from east to west. The cold spot area gradually moves to the east and spreads, and presents an obvious global agglomeration state, especially in areas such as the Loess Plateau and Sichuan Basin, accompanied by the transformation of many second cold spot areas into cold spot areas. From the overall change of the coordination degree pattern of "production-living-ecology" function from 2008 to 2017, the differences between the two sides of the Hu Line are still significant. An overall high-value concentrated central area has not been formed, which indicates that there is a lack of "leading" cities in China to promote the regional coordination of "production-living-ecology". In addition, the expansion of cold spots and second cold spots, as well as the compression of hot spots and second hot spots, indicating that the "production-living-ecology" functional coordination gap on both sides of the Hu Line in territorial space planning is gradually narrowing.

4.2. *Research on Spatial Differentiation of Driving Factors*

On the basis of determining the driving factors, an analysis of the spatial heterogeneity of driving factors is carried out.

4.2.1. Driving Factor Analysis Framework

As a complex dynamic giant system interacting with multiple elements [53], the land space system is not only strongly restricted by the relationship between subsystems within the system, but also constrained by many natural, social and economic elements outside the system. Therefore, this paper starts from the perspective of system theory, especially selects the production-living function, production-ecology function and living-ecology function to study the influence of each subsystem (Table 3). At the same time, considering the differences of human and natural environments on both sides of the Hu Line, population density, financial density, economic density and water resource density are selected as external environmental factors to study their influence on the coordination of "production-living-ecology" functions. From the perspective of an internal driving force, the coordination between two subsystems will directly affect the development of the overall coordination of "production-living-ecology" function. Among them, the coordination of production-living function means that the stronger production function is not only the economic development, but also meets the needs of infrastructure construction and social security improvement, thus strengthening the living function. The coordination of production-ecological function means that the development of industrial parks and new technologies enhances the intensity of industrial agglomeration and provides greater development space for ecological function. The coordination of living-ecological function means that the living function and ecological function can be improved synchronously by relying on powerful resources such as culture and infrastructure. From the perspective of external driving forces, the Hu Line has long been known as the dividing line of China's demographic geography, economic geography and physical geography due to huge differences in population distribution, economic development and natural environment. First of all, as the boundary of population geography, the Hu Line divides China into densely populated areas and sparse areas, so population density is chosen to represent the population driving effect. The increase in population will directly aggravate the scarcity resources in the system, and then cause obvious effect on the change of production, living and ecological function structure. Secondly, China's fiscal expenditure layout is coupled to the Hu Line to a certain extent, so the financial density is chosen to represent the investment-driven effect. As a factor of production, fiscal density directly enters into the economic production sector to improve the output level of various industries, as a financial support for developing infrastructure and ensuring people's livelihood, and indirectly increases output by improving ecological environment and production conditions. Thirdly, as the economic geographical dividing line, the economic development level of both sides of the Hu Line is always high in the east and low in the west. Therefore, economic density is chosen to represent economic driving effect. Areas with a high level of economic development tend to have a high level of intensive land use, which will promote the coordinated development of the "production-living-ecology" function. The area with a low level of economic development may also rely on "backwardness advantage" to obtain tremendous development. Finally, the Hu Line, as the boundary of abrupt ecological changes, divides China's semi-humid region and semi-arid region, and basically coincides with the 400mm annual rainfall line. Therefore, water resource density is chosen to represent water driving action. This factor restricts the development of "production-living-ecology" function through ecological water, production water and domestic water, and makes the three interact and combine organically with different water resource benefits. Therefore, this paper analyzes the driving mechanism of the "production-living-ecology" function of the national space system through two driving factors, internal and external.

Table 3. Selection of driving factors for "production-living-ecology" functional coordination.

Driving Factors	Variables	Definition
Internal driving force	Production-Living function	/
	Production-Ecological function	/
	Living-Ecological function	/
External driving force	Population density	population/total area
	Financial density	general budget expenditure/total area of local finance
	Economic density	regional GDP/ total area
	Water resource density	total water resources/total area of the region

4.2.2. Spatial Heterogeneity of Driving Factors

Unlike ordinary linear regression models, GWR considers the influence of different spatial positions on the regression results, which can be used to explore the non-stationarity of spatial relations. Geographically weighted regression model was used to set ADAPTIVE and AICc as bandwidth, and R2 was 0.7939, indicating that the model had a good overall fitting effect and could well simulate the influence of variables on the coordination of "Production-Living-Ecology" functions. The results show that each variable has different estimation results for different cities, indicating that there are spatial differences in the impact on the coordination of "Production-Living-Ecology" Functions in different regions (Table 4). This kind of influence is mainly driven by internal, and auxiliary by external. This also verifies hypothesis 2 of this paper, that the coordination of land "Production-Living-Ecology" Functions is not only affected by external factors, but also by the coordinated development of subsystems, as follows:

Production-Living function (Figure 4a) coordination has a two-way effect on "Production-Living-Ecology" Functions coordination, but it is mainly positive, 98.6% of prefecture-level cities have a positive correlation with "Production-Living-Ecology" Functions coordination. There is a certain spatial coupling with the Hu Line. The mean value of the regression coefficient of the southeast half wall is 0.1864, which is significantly higher than that of the northwest half wall, and most of the high value areas are located in the areas east of the Hu Line, with a bipolar distribution, respectively, in the northeast and some southern areas. In recent years, under the guidance of the revitalization of the Northeast policy, three northeastern provinces region have continued to optimize the production space by promoting the modernization of agriculture and industry, providing the necessary support to improve the functions of the social system and increasing the coordination of Production-life functions. In contrast, the southern high-value areas are mostly poverty-stricken zones. With the support of industrial poverty alleviation policies, a large number of abandoned home bases after relocation to alleviate poverty have been reclaimed, transforming the original construction land into arable land and land for infrastructure construction, and increasing the diversity and coordination of land use functions.

Table 4. Calculation results of the GWR model.

	Minimum	Lower Quartile	Mean	Upper Quartile	Maximum
P-L	−0.3195	0.1447	0.1765	0.2098	0.3271
P-E	−0.1798	0.0722	0.0703	0.1111	0.1214
L-E	0.3190	0.3864	0.4041	0.4033	1.3531
ED	−0.1690	0.0563	0.0565	0.0584	0.0889
FD	0.0484	0.0494	0.0537	0.0530	0.3024
PD	0.0028	0.0261	0.0345	0.0433	0.0815
WD	−0.0782	−0.0041	−0.0026	0.0014	0.0026

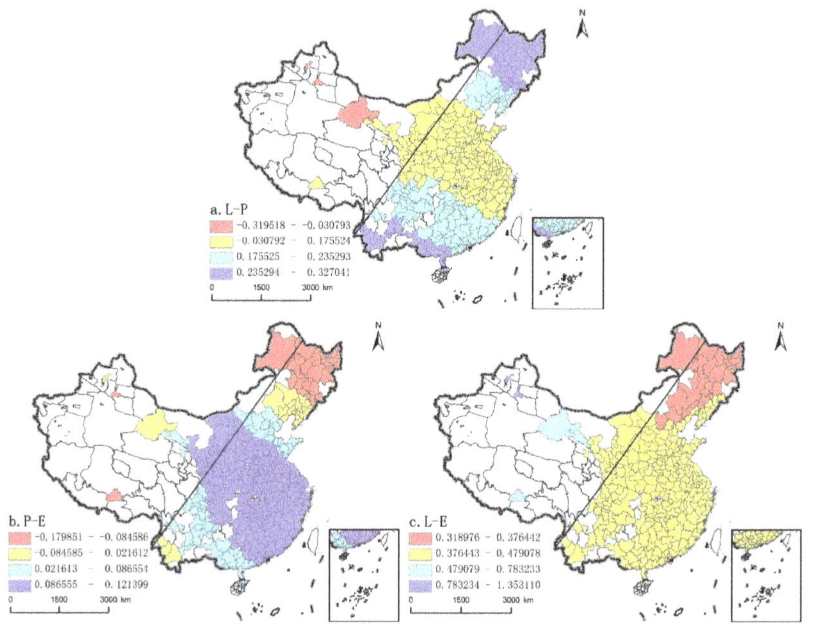

Figure 4. The spatial coefficient distribution of internal driving force (**a**) production-living function, (**b**)production-ecological function, (**c**) living-ecological function.

The degree of coordination of production-ecological functions (Figure 4b) also has a two-way influence on the coordination of the "three living" functions, but it is also mainly positive, in which 86.8% of the prefecture-level cities are positively correlated with the coordination of "Production-Living-Ecology" Functions, the spatial distribution of "Production-Living-Ecology" Functions is stepped from the central high value area to the northeast and southwest. The mean values of the regression coefficients on both sides of the Hu Line are 0.0711 and 0.0628, respectively, and most of the high value areas are located on the east side of the Hu Line, especially concentrated in some cities in the central and western parts and the eastern coast. Among them, thanks to the support of the western development strategy and ecological protection project, the ecological construction and economic development in the central and western regions can be synchronized, which is conducive to improving the coordination degree of land use function. In addition, the low concentration in northeastern China, basic negative regression coefficient, while the strategy of rejuvenating northeast to some extent inhibited the economic downturn, but as the old industrial base, its ills, mainly manifested in and out of the land quantity reduction and poor resources and environment development, etc., and the economic growth of locking problems such as path dependence or path is very prominent [54].

The coordination degree of Life-Ecology functions (Figure 4c) has a significant positive impact on the coordination degree of "Production-Living-Ecology" Functions, presenting a decreasing spatial distribution of lumpiness from west to east. Different from the distribution of "high in the east and low in the west" on both sides of the Hu Line, the mean regression coefficient of the southeast half is 0.3924, significantly lower than the 0.5133 in the northwest half. The high value area is also mainly distributed in the west of the Hu Line, among which the cities in Xinjiang are the most prominent. The western development strategy, and beautiful rural construction allows to give priority to the western region of Xinjiang improving infrastructure, combined with recent years dedicated to incorporating the ecological concept in the urbanization construction in Xinjiang, always in a good ecological resources capitalization of opportunity at the same time, the rural residential environment renovation of full swing action, to push the synchronizing lifting of life and ecological function. Low in the area mainly gathered on the Hu Line east of northeast China, the reason may lie in the traditional sense of the urbanization development of negative effects on the ecosystem is easy, but at this stage of construction land continue to increase, unreasonable land use planning problems such as the northeast to continue in a state of ecological deficit, so hindered the coordinated development of "Production-Living-Ecology" Functions.

Economy density (Figure 5a) also has a two-way impact on the "Production-Living-Ecology" Functions, but the regression coefficients of all cities except Xinjiang are positive. In space, it is similar to the pattern of "strong east and weak west" on both sides of the Hu Line, and the mean value of regression coefficient in the east is larger than that in the west. However, the high value area shows an obvious polarization trend, not only concentrated in the Pearl River Delta east of the Hu Line, but also concentrated in the northwest west of the Hu Line. Among them, as the second largest economic zone in China, the Pearl River Delta has become more mature in its economic development. Compared with its response to urbanization, land use change responds more strongly to regional timeliness policies and pays more attention to the coordinated development of land use functions. Unlike the Pearl River Delta, after China's economy enters the new normal, the rapidly developing urbanization in western China has brought about a continuous increase in the demand for construction land. However, all western regions represented by Gansu province have greatly alleviated the contradiction in land demand at this stage by vigorously developing ecological tourism industry and modern agriculture.

Finance density (Figure 5b) has a significant positive impact on the coordination of "Production-Living-Ecology" Functions, and gradually decreases from the center of the low-value area to the periphery. Unlike the distribution of the Hu Line, the distribution of regression coefficient of fiscal density shows the characteristics of "strong in the west and weak in the east", and the high value area is distributed on both sides, mainly concentrated in western China and some parts of northeast China, among which the western region dominated by Xinjiang is the most prominent. As a typical area of government-led urbanization, this top-down development mode enables Xinjiang to obtain a great financial tilt, which makes Xinjiang "build a city first, then establish a city" under the government planning, and gradually rationalize the functional structure of land use. On the contrary, fiscal density plays a small role in promoting the coordination of "production-production-production" functions in the central and eastern cities east of the Hu Line, which may be due to the inefficiency and corruption of government financial expenditure in these areas, or the excessively high level of expenditure distorts the function of market resource allocation [55], resulting in low land use efficiency, and further affecting the development and coordination of various functions.

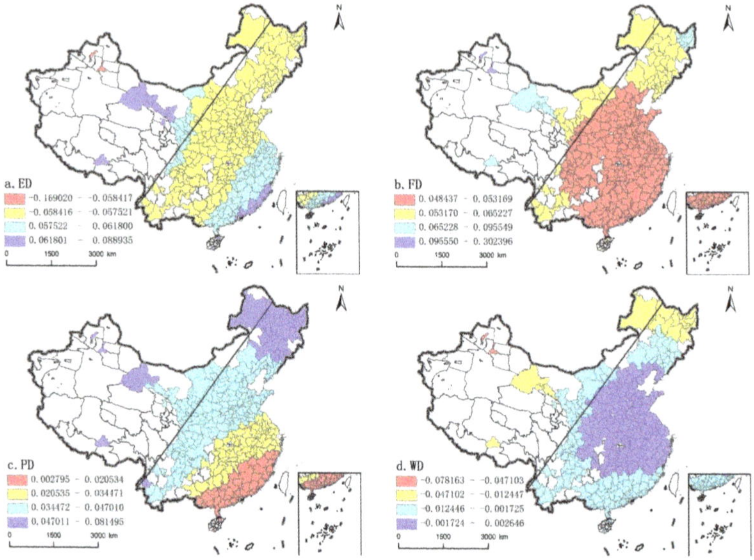

Figure 5. The spatial coefficient distribution of external driving force (**a**) economic density, (**b**) financial density, (**c**) population density, (**d**) water resource density.

Population density (Figure 5c) also has a positive impact on the coordination of "Production-Living-Ecology" Functions, presenting a stepwise spatial distribution from southeast to northwest. The mean values of regression coefficients on both sides of The Hu Line are 0.0331 and 0.0474, respectively, showing the distribution characteristics of "strong in the west and weak in the east". The high values are distributed in the northwest region west of the Hu Line and the northeast region east of the Hu Line. Among them, the new population policy and the northeast revitalization plan greatly change the stagnation of population development in the northeast, and direct effects on regional population growth and the migration process, and thus indirectly affect the transformation of land use function, in essence, it is a continuous reconstruction process from conflict to coordination of different land use functions or types in space [56]. The low value area is located in the Pearl River Delta and its surrounding areas on the east side of the Hu Line, where the population and land use show a positive allometric relationship [57], rapid economic growth continues to strengthen the "siphon effect" of population. In order to improve the living standard of urban residents, a large number of high-class residential buildings have been built in many areas, which not only failed to improve the living standard of residents, but also aggravated the disorder of urban sprawl, thus damaging the coordinated development of "Production-Living-Ecology" Functions.

Water resource density (Figure 5d) has a positive and negative bidirectional influence on the coordination of "Production-Living-Ecology" Functions. The east of the Hu Line is mostly positive, while the west of the Hu Line is mainly negative. Xinjiang region is the high value center of negative impact. The special geographical location determines that most of the cities in Xinjiang are typical oasis cities in arid areas. Urumqi and Karamay are the economic development centers at the northern foot of Xinjiang. The rapid development of industrialization leads to the continuous displacement of agricultural water by production and living water, which restricts the development of cultivated land, and the continuous encroachment of production and construction land on the basic ecological land at the outer edge of the city, resulting in the imbalance of spatial distribution of urban land use functions. The positive impact areas are almost all located in the east of the Hu Line, mainly in the Yangtze River, with abundant water resources compared with Xinjiang and other places. Especially, in recent years, the development concept of "joint efforts to protect and not to develop" has not only reversed the situation of ecological environment deterioration in the Yangtze River Basin, but also accelerated the change of industrial structure and strengthened the coordination of regional land multi-functional utilization.

5. Conclusions and Discussion

5.1. Conclusions

Based on the discussion on the coordination of Production-Living-Ecology function of land use in 288 prefecture-level cities on both sides of the Hu Line from 2008 to 2017, this study mainly verified the two hypotheses proposed in this paper.

Firstly, from the perspective of time dimension, it can be seen that the function coordination degree of "Production-living-Ecology" on the east side of the Hu Line is higher than that on the west side. From the spatial dimension, it is found that the west of the Hu Line is mostly a low-level coordination area, while the east is mostly a middle and high-level coordination area, which verifies hypothesis 1: the coordination of land Production-Living-Ecological function on both sides of the Hu Line is characterized by "high in the east and low in the west".

Secondly, GWR was used to analyze the driving mechanism that affected the coordination of Production-Living-Ecology function of land use. It was found that there were significant regional differences in the impact of each driving factor on the coordination of Production-Living-Ecology function. The order of influence degree is Life-Ecology function > Production-Living function > Production-Ecology function > Economic density > Finance density > Population density > Water resource density. It shows that the coordination of Production-Ecology function is mainly driven by internal factors and is supplemented by external factors. That is, hypothesis 2 of this paper is verified: the coordination of land Production-Living-Ecology function is not only affected by external factors, but also by the coordinated development of subsystems.

5.2. Discussion

According to the research conclusion of this paper, there are three major characteristics of the coordination of the "Production-Living-Ecology" Functions of China's land use: non-equilibrium on both sides of the Hu line, mainly internally driven and externally driven. Therefore, in order to balance the coordinated use of China's land space, countermeasures should be suggested from these three characteristics.

5.2.1. Firmly Grasp the Main Line of Coordinated Regional Development and Accelerate the Breaking of the "Land Hu Line"

The concept of "main functional area" was first proposed in 2004 and then incorporated into the regional coordinated development strategy [58]. Therefore, we can learn from its core idea and plan the utilization of the national land on both sides of the Hu Line through the spatial governance model of the main functional area and ensure the coordination and sustainable development of "Production-Life-Ecology" Functions through three levels of action mechanism of "planning, control and evaluation".

First, delineate the main functional area to ensure the balance of "Production-Living-Ecology" Functions. Through the above research, it can be found that most of the areas west of the Hu Line, mainly Xinjiang and Tibet, are ecologically fragile areas, and the contradiction between economic and social development and ecological protection is more prominent. Therefore, the balanced development of different functions can be achieved by delimiting main functional areas. The land space west of the Hu Line is divided into spatial units with cities and counties as units, and each unit is given a unique main function, thus forming a "one blueprint" for the main functional zoning at the city and county level nationwide; delineate three red lines of urban development boundary, permanent basic farmland and ecological protection, and effectively restrict the production, living and ecological protection behavior of each space by clarifying the spatial boundary of the main functional area. Second, refine the management and control development, and realize the coordinated development of "Production-Living-Ecology" Functions from the process. In the development, the development direction of each area should be clearly defined. In the key development urbanization areas, due to their strong resource and environmental carrying capacity, it is necessary to strengthen the construction of urban functions, guide the orderly clustering of industries, and strengthen the production and living functions of land use; for the main agricultural production areas with restricted development, this type of area is mainly used for the supply of agricultural products, so we should focus on the agricultural production function of land use, and appropriately strengthen its living and ecological functions; for key ecological function areas that are restricted from development, this type of area mainly provides ecological products to ensure national ecological security, and should focus on grasping the ecological function of land use. Third, the assessment of the development performance of each, from the system to ensure that the concept of "Production-Living-Ecology" accurate implementation. The supporting policies of functional areas can be implemented in accordance with the positioning of the main functional areas and categorized and managed. To provide policy support for investment, industry and population in areas with large urbanization needs, especially for industrial development west of the "Hu Line"; for the main agricultural production areas east of the Hu line can improve the living standards of farmers through the agricultural price compensation mechanism, while increasing the investment and construction of industries and public services; for the key ecological function areas west of the Hu line, on the one hand, financial transfer payments should be increased, and on the other hand, industrial access thresholds should be strictly enforced as a way to strengthen ecological functions and appropriately improve production and living functions.

5.2.2. Enhance the Internal Driving Force Coordination and Promote the Coordinated Development of "Production-Living-Ecology" Function

We should further promote the coordination degree of production, living and ecological functions, strengthen the integrated layout of "Production-Living-Ecology" Space, realize the symbiosis and co-prosperity of "Production-Living-Ecology" Function, and ensure the coordinated development of land use functions.

First, we will adopt classified policies to ease the contradiction between the use of land for production and living purposes [59]. Distinguish different industrial types and adopt corresponding layout patterns. For the first-class industrial land, the Production-Life compound layout mode is adopted, while for the second- and third-class industrial land, the independent production space mode can be adopted. The compactness of production space should be strengthened to make production space intensive and efficient based on the layout of industrial chain relations. According to the needs of different groups, improve the layout of infrastructure, strengthen the connection between production and living space, realize the co-construction and sharing of infrastructure, and achieve the overall coordination of production and living functions. Second, upgrade and restructure to promote synchronous development of production and ecological functions. For the Production-Ecology function, the key lies in the upgrading of industrial structure. By increasing industrial investment, enterprises should be guided to develop circular economies to achieve sustainable development, so as to make up for the deficiency of natural ecology with high-quality production. Reconstruct urban structure, strictly delimit land use boundary, maintain cultivated land area by urban growth boundary and cultivated land protection boundary, and restrict the disorderly expansion of urban construction land. To protect green space to isolate industrial areas, so as to reduce urban pollution and improve ecological quality, and ensure that the ecological function of land use can be brought into play. Third, we need to take multiple measures to promote the coordinated development of living and ecological functions. The living environment should be improved, the population size and distribution should be considered comprehensively, and the community life circle should be formed by improving the construction and coverage of public service facilities. Vigorously develop livable cities, build a network ecological landscape pattern of "corridors around the city, green wedge introduction, park Mosaic, multi-corridor connection", form a complete and homogeneous ecosystem, improve public service facilities and infrastructure on this basis, to create a green livable city. Deployment of pilot city double repair work actively, carry out urban repair and ecological restoration, from is closely related to the residents of "environment" of improving infrastructure, increase investment in environmental governance at the same time, the ecological red line within the scope of the houses or buildings moved or renovation, to carry out ecological restoration systemic reshape city temperament.

5.2.3. Optimize the Influence of External Drivers to Facilitate the Continuous Coordination of "Production-Living-Ecology" Function

On the basis of considering regional heterogeneity, the external impact factors should be optimized according to local conditions to help different regions realize the sustainable development of land use "Production-Living-Ecology" functions.

First, differentiated development strategies should be adopted according to different stages of economic development. The response of land use change to urbanization and economic development level is no longer obvious in some areas east of the Hu Line where economic development has become mature. Therefore, it is necessary to constantly strengthen the government's function of policy guidance and control of the bottom line, and strictly delimit the ecological red line to give consideration to economic development and ecological protection [35]. For the region west of Hu Line, which is in the stage of economic transformation and development, special attention should be paid to the coupling development of urbanization and industrialization [50], the intensity of development should be controlled in strict accordance with the red line for ecological protection, and a negative list of industrial access should be drawn up to prevent "pollution shelter effect" in key ecological function zones, so as to ensure the ecological function of land use. Second, reform the existing fiscal system to facilitate spatially balanced development. It is necessary to gradually establish a financial system that matches the balanced development of space to support the coordinated symbiosis of various functions of land use. A three-dimensional model of spatially balanced development can be constructed, which roughly includes three levels: the production layer, the secondary distribution layer and the actual consumption layer of residents, in order to meet the inevitable requirements of economic development, we adhere to an unbalanced development strategy at the production layer, and at the same time, we must establish a strong redistribution system at the secondary distribution layer, but this requires the support of a scientific transfer payment mechanism. In addition, it must have a sound legal system and establish a comprehensive spatial planning system to ensure its operation. Third, do a good job in human resource development and reserve, and start the "open source and reduce expenditure" of urban land. For the economically developed areas east of the Hu Line with a large population, we should consciously formulate policies to control population, "open source" on the basis of "reducing expenditure", strictly control the expansion of urban construction land, and avoid the deterioration of man-land relationship. While the population control policies in some eastern megacities will be effective, they will be accompanied by the local migration of the population in the central and western regions. Therefore, cities to the west of the Hu Line should do a good job in the reserve, development and utilization of various human resources. Fourthly, rational use of water resources to improve the ecological environment. For the areas west of the Hu Line, where water resources are scarce, water resources should be allocated and managed based on the overall interests of the whole basin in accordance with the general idea of "reducing agricultural water, saving domestic water, increasing ecological water and ensuring industrial water". For water source region of the east of the relatively rich Hu Line, first priority is to insist on protection priority, constantly optimize the ecological environment, in returning farmland to forest and grass measures such as to give full play to the ecosystem on the basis of self-healing, adherence to the "three line", in the reasonable range of environmental carrying capacity of the development and utilization of water resources. The effective ecological compensation mechanism should be established as soon as possible, so as to achieve long-term comprehensive management of the whole basin, so as to continuously optimize the structure and function of land use.

Author Contributions: Conceptualization, Y.C.; data curation, M.Z.; formal analysis, Y.C. and M.Z.; funding acquisition, Y.C.; methodology, M.Z. and Y.C.; software, M.Z.; supervision, Y.C.; writing—original draft, M.Z. and Y.C.; writing—review and editing, M.Z. and Y.C. All authors have read and agreed to the published version of the manuscript.

Funding: This work was supported by grants from Support Plan for Scientific and Technological Innovation Talents in Henan Institutions of Higher Learning (humanities and social sciences) (2018-cx-012); Training Plan for Key Young Teachers in Henan Institutions of Higher Learning (2018GGJS094); Good Scholar in Philosophy and Social Sciences in Henan Institutions of Higher Learning (2019-YXXZ-20); and Philosophy and Social Science Innovation Team Building Program of Henan Universities (2021-CXTD-12,2022-CXTD-05). Philosophy and Social Science planning project of Henan Province (2021BJJ112); and The Major Projects of Philosophy and Social Science Research of Hubei Province (19ZD044).

Institutional Review Board Statement: Not applicable.

Informed Consent Statement: Not applicable.

Data Availability Statement: The data presented in this study are openly available in National Bureau of Statistics, reference number 978-7-5037-9120-8, 978-7-5037-8770-6, 978-7-5037-8432-3, 978-7-5037-8082-0, 978-7-5037-7706-6, 978-7-5037-7350-1, 978-7-5037-7019-7, 978-7-5037-6754-8.

Conflicts of Interest: The authors declare no conflict of interest. The funders had no role in the design of the study; in the collection, analyses, or interpretation of data; in the writing of the manuscript, or in the decision to publish the results.

References

1. Hu, H.Y. Essays on China's population distribution. *Acta Geogr. Sin.* **1935**, *2*, 33–74.
2. OECD. *Multifunctionality: Towards an Analytical Framework*; Organization for Economic Cooperation and Development: Paris, France, 2001.
3. Steffen, W.; Crutzen, P.J.; McNeill, J.R. The anthropocene: Are humans now overwhelming the great forces of nature. *AMBIO J. Hum. Environ.* **2007**, *36*, 614–621. [CrossRef]
4. Mander, Ü.; Wiggering, H.; Helming, K. *Multifunctional Land Use: Meeting Future Demands or Landscape Goods and Services*; Springer: Berlin/Heidelberg, Germany, 2007.
5. Pagliarin, S. Linking processes and patterns: Spatial planning, governance and urban sprawl in the Barcelona and Milan metropolitan regions. *Urban Stud.* **2018**, *55*, 3650–3668. [CrossRef]
6. Yang, Y.Y.; Bao, W.K.; Liu, Y.S. Coupling coordination analysis of rural production-living-ecological space in the Beijing-Tianjin-Hebei region. *Ecol. Indic.* **2020**, *117*, 106512. [CrossRef]
7. Chen, M.X.; Gong, Y.H.; Li, Y.; Lu, D.; Zhang, H. Population distribution and urbanization on both sides of the Hu Huanyong Line: Answering the Premier's question. *J. Geogr. Sci.* **2016**, *26*, 1593–1610. [CrossRef]
8. Shi, Z.Q.; Deng, W.; Zhang, S.R. Spatial pattern and spatiotemporal change of territory space in Hengduan Mountains region in recent 25 years. *Geogr. Res.* **2018**, *37*, 607–621.
9. Balz, V.; Zonneveld, W. Transformations of planning rationales: Changing spaces for governance in recent dutch national planning. *Reg. Des.* **2018**, *19*, 363–384. [CrossRef]
10. Tien, H.Y. Demography in China: From zero to now. *Popul. Index* **1981**, *47*, 683–710. [CrossRef]
11. Lu, D.D.; Wang, Z.; Feng, Z.M.; Zeng, G.; Fang, C.; Dong, X.; Liu, S.; Jia, S.; Fang, Y.; Meng, G. Academic debates on Hu Huanyong population line. *Geogr. Res.* **2016**, *35*, 805–824.
12. Fang, C.L. New Structure and New Trend of Formation and Development of Urban Agglomerations in China. *Sci. Geogr. Sin.* **2011**, *31*, 1025–1034.
13. Fan, J.; Liang, B.; Guo, R. Strategic Emphasis of Regional Coordinated Growth Pattern Optimization in the New Era of Socialism with Chinese Characteristics. *Econ. Geogr.* **2018**, *38*, 1–10.
14. Zhang, J.Z.; Liang, J.S.; Zhu, Y.X.; Zhou, X. Land and GDP's Function on Population Distribution in China. *Sci. Geogr. Sin.* **2017**, *37*, 1006–1013.
15. Krugman, P. First nature, second nature and metropolitan location. *J. Reg. Sci.* **1993**, *33*, 129–144. [CrossRef]
16. Deng, X.; Bai, X. Sustainable urbanization in western China. *Environ. Sci. Policy Sustain. Dev.* **2014**, *56*, 12–24. [CrossRef]
17. Dewan, S.; Kraemer, K.L. Information Technology and Productivity: Evidence from Country-level Data. *Manag. Sci.* **2000**, *46*, 548–562. [CrossRef]

18. Liu, J.L.; Liu, Y.S.; Li, Y.R. Classification evaluation and spatial-temporal analysis of "production-living-ecological" spaces in China. *Acta Geogr. Sin.* **2017**, *72*, 1290–1304.
19. European Commission. *Safeguarding the Multifunctional Role of Agriculture: Which Instruments?* DG Agriculture-European Commission: Brussels, Belgium, 1999.
20. Barthelemy, D.; Nieddu, M. Non-trade concerns in agricultural and environmental economics: How J.R. Commons and Karl Polanyi can help us. *J. Econ. Issues* **2007**, *41*, 519–527. [CrossRef]
21. Wiggering, H.; Dalchow, C.; Glemnitz, M.; Helming, K.; Müller, K.; Schultz, A.; Stachow, U.; Zander, P. Indicators for multifunctional land use—Linking socio-economic requirements with landscape potentials. *Ecol. Indic.* **2006**, *6*, 238–249. [CrossRef]
22. Gadjiev, A.D.; Aral, A.; Aliev, I.A. On behaviour of the Riesz and generalized Riesz potentials as order tends to zero. *Math. Inequal. Appl.* **2007**, *10*, 875–888. [CrossRef]
23. Hediger, W. Weak and strong sustainability, environmental conservation and economic growth. *Nat. Resour. Model.* **2006**, *19*, 359–394. [CrossRef]
24. Vereijken, P.H. *Multifunctionality: Applying the OECD Framework, a Review of Literature in the Netherlands*; OECD: Paris, France, 2001.
25. Paracchini, M.L.; Pacini, C.; Jones, M.L.M.; Pérez-Soba, M. An aggregation framework to link indicators associated with multifunctional land use to the stakeholder evaluation of policy options. *Ecol. Indic.* **2011**, *11*, 71–80. [CrossRef]
26. Kienast, F.; Bolliger, J.; Potschin, M.; De Groot, R.S.; Verburg, P.H.; Heller, I.; Wascher, D.; Haines-Young, R. Assessing Landscape Functions with Broad-Scale Environmental Data: Insights Gained from a Prototype Development for Europe. *Environ. Manag.* **2009**, *44*, 1099–1120. [CrossRef] [PubMed]
27. Pérez-Soba, M.; Petit, S.; Jones, L.; Bertrand, N.; Briquel, V.; Omodei-Zorini, L.; Contini, C.; Helming, K.; Farrington, J.H.; Mossello, M.T.; et al. Land use functions—A multifunctionality approach to assess the impact of land use changes on land use sustainability. In *Sustainability Impact Assessment of Land Use Changes*; Springer: Berlin/Heidelberg, Germany, 2008.
28. Chen, J.; Shi, P.J. Discussion on functional land use classification system. *J. Beijing Norm. Univ. Nat. Sci.* **2005**, *41*, 536–540.
29. Verburg, P.H.; van de Steeg, J.; Veldkamp, A.; Willemen, L. From land cover change to land function dynamics: A major challenge to improve land characterization. *J. Environ. Manag.* **2009**, *90*, 1327–1335. [CrossRef] [PubMed]
30. Huang, J.C.; Lin, H.X.; Qi, X.X. A literature review on optimization of spatial development pattern based on ecological-production-living space. *Prog. Geogr.* **2017**, *36*, 378–391.
31. Reidsma, P.; Koenig, H.J.; Feng, S.; Bezlepkina, I.; Nesheim, I.; Bonin, M.; Sghaier, M.; Purushothaman, S.; Sieber, S.; Van Ittersum, M.K.; et al. Methods and tools for integrated assessment of land use policies on sustainable development in developing countries. *Land Use Policy* **2011**, *28*, 604–617. [CrossRef]
32. Xie, G.D.; Zhen, L.; Zhang, C.X.; Xiangzheng, D.; Koenig, H.J.; Tscherning, K.; Helming, K. Assessing the multifunctionalities of land use in China. *J. Resour. Ecol.* **2010**, *1*, 311–318.
33. Millennium Ecosystem Assessment. *Ecosystems and Human Well-Being Synthesis*; Island Press: Washington, DC, USA, 2005.
34. De Groot, R.S.; Wilson, M.A.; Boumans, R.M.J. A typology for the classification, description and valuation of ecosystem functions, goods and services. *Ecol. Econ.* **2002**, *41*, 393–408. [CrossRef]
35. Costanza, R.; d'Arge, R.; de Groot, R.; Farber, S.; Grasso, M.; Hannon, B.; Limburg, K.; Naeem, S.; O'neill, R.V.; Paruelo, J.; et al. The value of the world's ecosystem services and natural capital. *Nature* **1997**, *387*, 253–260. [CrossRef]
36. Maco, S.E.; McPherson, E.G. A practical approach to assessing structure, function, and value of street tree populations in small communities. *J. Arboric.* **2003**, *29*, 84–97. [CrossRef]
37. McPherson, E. Accounting for benefits and costs of urban greens-pace. *Landsc. Urban Plan.* **1992**, *22*, 41–45. [CrossRef]
38. De Groot, R.S. Function-analysis and valuation as a tool to assess land use conflicts in planning for sustainable, multifunctional landscapes. *Landsc. Urban Plan.* **2006**, *75*, 175–186. [CrossRef]
39. Lovell, S.T.; DeSantis, S.R.; Nathan, C.A.; Olson, M.B.; Mendez, V.E.; Kominami, H.C.; Erickson, D.L.; Morris, K.S.; Morris, W.B. Integrating agroecology and landscape multifunctionality in Vermont: An evolving framework to evaluate the design of agroecosystems. *Agric. Syst.* **2010**, *103*, 327–341. [CrossRef]
40. Foley, J.A.; DeFries, R.; Asner, G.P.; Barford, C.; Bonan, G.; Carpenter, S.R.; Chapin, F.S.; Coe, M.T.; Daily, G.C.; Gibbs, H.K.; et al. Global consequences of land use. *Science* **2005**, *309*, 570–574. [CrossRef]
41. Liang, X.Y.; Gu, Z.M.; Lei, M. The Differences Between Land Use Function and Land Use to Reflecting the Change of Land Use System and Their Impacts on Landscape Pattern: A Case Study of Lantian County in Shaanxi Province, China. *J. Nat. Resour.* **2014**, *29*, 1127–1135.
42. Schößer, B.; Helming, K.; Wiggering, H. Assessing land use change impacts–a comparison of the SENSOR land use function approach with other frameworks. *J. Land Use Sci.* **2010**, *5*, 159–178. [CrossRef]
43. Callo-Concha, D.; Denich, M. A participatory framework to assess multifunctional land-use systems with multicriteria and multivariate analyses: A case study on agrobiodiversity of agroforestry systems in Tomé Açú, Brazil. *Change Adapt. Socio-Ecol. Syst.* **2014**, *1*, 40–50. [CrossRef]
44. Fleskens, L.; Duarte, F.; Eicher, I. A conceptual framework for the assessment of multiple functions of agro-ecosystems: A case study of Trás-os-Montes olive groves. *J. Rural Stud.* **2009**, *25*, 141–155. [CrossRef]
45. Helming, K.; Pérez-Soba, M. Landscape scenarios and multifunctionality: Making land use impact assessment operational. *Ecol. Soc.* **2011**, *16*, 50. [CrossRef]

46. Wang, F.; Dong, Y.X. Spatial differences and influencing factors of land use function in Guangzhou. *Resour. Sci.* **2015**, *37*, 2179–2192.
47. Kopeva, D.; Peneva, M.; Madjarova, S. Multifunctional land use: Is it a key factor for rural development. In Proceedings of the 118th EAAE Seminar: Rural Development: Governance, Policy Design and Delivery, Ljubljana, Slovenia, 25–27 August 2010; EAAE: Ljubljana, Slovenia, 2010.
48. Wang, F.; Dong, Y.X. Dynamic evaluation of land use functions based on grey relation projection method and diagnosis of its obstacle indicators: A case study of Guangzhou City. *J. Nat. Resour.* **2015**, *30*, 1698–1713.
49. Chen, Y.; Ma, Z.H.; Gu, J.L.; Weiteng, T. Environmental cost research: Cooperation, evolution, hotspot and prospect. *J. Arid Land Resour. Environ.* **2019**, *33*, 11–22.
50. Chen, Y.; Zhu, M.K.; Su, X.Y. Study on the improvement of land use efficiency in industrial new city under the background of high-quality development. *J. Zhengzhou Univ. Light Ind. Soc. Sci. Ed.* **2019**, *20*, 97–103.
51. Fang, C.L.; Mao, H.Y.; Ye, D.N. *Theory and Method of Spatial Pattern Optimization of Urban Development in China*; Science Press: Beijing, China, 2016.
52. Kates, R.W.; Clark, W.C.; Corell, R.W.; Hall, J.M.; Jaeger, C.C.; Lowe, I.; McCarthy, J.J.; Schellnhuber, H.J.; Bolin, B.; Dickson, N.M.; et al. Sustainability Science. *Science* **2001**, *292*, 641–642. [CrossRef] [PubMed]
53. Lin, J.; Song, G.; Zhang, Y. Synergistic evolution mechanism of "production-living-ecology" functions in spatial planning system: A case study of fuxin city. *China Land Sci.* **2019**, *33*, 9–17.
54. Fan, J.; Liu, H.C.; Wang, Y.F.; Zhao, Y.; Chen, D. "The northeast china phenomenon" and prejudgment on economic revitalization in northeast China:A primary research on stable factors to impact national spatial development and protection pattern. *Sci. Geogr. Sin.* **2016**, *36*, 1445–1456.
55. Robert, J.; Growth, B.J.J.o.E. Inequality and growth in a panel of countries. *J. Econ. Growth* **2000**, *5*, 87–120.
56. Long, H.L.; Qu, Y. Land use transitions and land management: A mutual feedback perspective. *Land Use Policy* **2018**, *74*, 111–120. [CrossRef]
57. Naroll, R.S.; von Bertalanffy, L. The Principle of Allometry in Biology and the Social Sciences. *Gen. Syst. Yearb.* **1956**, *10*, 76–89.
58. Bai, S.Q.; Chen, Z.M.; Huo, Y.R. Optimization of Strategy and Policy of Main Functional Area. *China Land* **2020**, *11*, 20–23.
59. Von der Dunk, A.; Gret-Regamey, A.; Dalang, T.; Hersperger, A.M. Defining a typology of peri-urban land-use conflicts—A case study from Switzerland. *Landsc. Urban Plan.* **2011**, *101*, 149–156. [CrossRef]

International Journal of
Environmental Research and Public Health

MDPI

Article

Determinants and Willingness to Pay for Purchasing Mask against COVID-19: A Protection Motivation Theory Perspective

Qiying Ding [1], Shoufu Lin [2,*] and Shanyong Wang [3]

[1] School of Economics and Management, Dongguan University of Technology, Dongguan 523808, China; dingqy@dgut.edu.cn
[2] School of Economics, Fujian Normal University, Fuzhou 350007, China
[3] School of Public Affairs, University of Science and Technology of China, Hefei 230026, China; wsy1988@ustc.edu.cn
* Correspondence: linshf2003@126.com; Tel.: +86-591-8346-5205

Abstract: Currently, coronavirus disease 2019 (COVID-19) is spreading globally, which poses great challenges to the whole world and human beings. The aim of this research is to understand the determinants and residents' willingness to pay (WTP) for purchasing masks against COVID-19 in China. On the basis of protection motivation theory and contingent value method, this research shows that most residents are willing to purchase masks against COVID-19. COVID-19 knowledge, perceived severity, perceived vulnerability, and response efficacy are positively and significantly associated with residents' WTP and the WTP value. However, self-efficacy is only significantly associated with residents' WTP while not with WTP value. Furthermore, compared with other residents, residents in Hubei province have a higher level of COVID-19 knowledge, perceived severity, perceived vulnerability, self-efficacy and response efficacy, and the WTP value is higher. The average value of residents' WTP value for purchasing masks against COVID-19 in Hubei province is ¥120.92 ($18.73) per month during the epidemic, while it is ¥100.16 ($15.50) for other residents. In addition, the effects of demographic factors such as age, gender, income, etc., on residents' WTP and WTP value have also been examined.

Keywords: COVID-19; mask; willingness to pay; protection motivation theory; contingent value method

Citation: Ding, Q.; Lin, S.; Wang, S. Determinants and Willingness to Pay for Purchasing Mask against COVID-19: A Protection Motivation Theory Perspective. *IJERPH* **2022**, *19*, 4268. https://doi.org/10.3390/ijerph19074268

Academic Editors: Jie Chen, Qian Zhou and Ting Zhang

Received: 11 February 2022
Accepted: 30 March 2022
Published: 2 April 2022

1. Introduction

At the end of 2019, a new coronavirus disease 2019 (COVID-19) suddenly broke out and pose unique challenges for everyone around the globe. Currently, COVID-19 has become a global public health event. On 11 March 2020, Dr. Tedros Adhanom Ghebreyesus, the Director General of the World Health Organization (WHO), announced that on the basis of scientific assessment, WHO believes that COVID-19 can be called a global pandemic. Almost all countries in the world have reported confirmed cases of COVID-19. By now, COVID-19 is still spreading around the world and showing no signs of improvement.

COVID-19 has caused a serious negative impact on the global economy and resident's daily life. There is no doubt that the global economy will definitely decline. Furthermore, due to the infectivity of COVID-19 and its high fatality rate, COVID-19 also exerts a negative impact on resident's physiological health, especially psychological health [1]. During the COVID-19 epidemic, residents more easily feel panic, anxious, scared, uneasy and worried that they can be infected [2]. To reduce its negative impact, several protective actions against COVID-19 can be taken by residents. For example, going out less and staying at home more, enhancing physical exercise and ensuring adequate sleep to enhance immunity, wearing masks, washing hands with medical alcohol, etc. It is noteworthy that these preventive measures can only prevent but cannot completely guarantee residents from the virus intrusion. At present, the injection of COVID-19 vaccine is the most direct and effective preventive way to prevent viral infections [3]. Currently, governments, medical institutions and scientific research companies of various countries have worked tirelessly to develop vaccines to control the spread of COVID-19 [4].

In fact, as claimed by WHO, before the COVID-19 vaccine is launched on a large scale, among the protective measures, wearing masks, especially N95 masks, is an effective way to reduce COVID-19 spread and infection rate. It is estimated that wearing masks can reduce the spread of COVID-19 by more than 70% [5]. Given the significance of wearing masks, it is important to encourage residents to purchase and wear masks against COVID-19. However, residents need to pay a certain cost to purchase masks, and then a financial burden will be placed on them. As a result, before encouraging residents to purchase and wear masks, it is necessary to understand whether residents are willing to pay for purchasing masks against COVID-19, the value of willingness to pay (WTP) and the related determinants. Because COVID-19 is an emergency in public health, limited research attention has been focused on residents' WTP for purchasing mask against COVID-19. To close the research gap and provide recommendations to government agencies, this research aims to use survey data collected in China to analyze residents' WTP for purchasing mask against COVID-19 by using contingent valuation method.

In the public health research domain, protection motivation theory is a commonly used theory to understand individual's self-protective behavior and protective behavior decision making, and its effectiveness has been validated [6]. In this research, purchasing masks against COVID-19 is a self-protective behavior and whether and how much willing to pay for purchasing mask against COVID-19 is protective behavior decision making. Hence, protection motivation theory can be regarded as the theoretical basis in the current research, and WTP can be incorporated into the protection motivation theory conceptual framework. Meanwhile, as a new virus, residents' knowledge about COVID-19 can have an effect on residents' risk perception and subsequent behavioral responses. Lack of knowledge about COVID-19 may provide space for rumors to breed and spread, and induce residents to take incorrect protective measures. Hence, residents' knowledge about COVID-19 has been considered and added into the research framework. The main contribution of this research is that we systematically explored whether residents are willing to pay for purchasing mask against COVID-19, the value of WTP and the related determinants. To the best of our knowledge, this is the first attempts to understand residents' WTP for purchasing mask against COVID-19, which can further enrich the research on COVID-19 and provide implications for government agencies to make intervention strategies.

2. Literature Review

2.1. Protection Motivation Theory

In behavioral research context, several theoretical models and theories are well developed to explore individual's behavioral reaction, such as theory of planned behavior, cognitive dissonance theory, value-belief-norm theory, norm activation model, protection motivation theory, etc. Among them, protection motivation theory (PMT), which was originally developed by [6], has been frequently adopted to explore why individuals take protective actions. PMT has been widely used in various crisis and health risk situations (e.g., natural disasters, climate change, epidemics) and its explanatory power has been validated [6–9].

According to PMT, the aim of an individual to take protective actions is to avoid or reduce the negative influences of potential risks [6,7]. The decision to take protective actions is influenced by two factors: threat appraisal and coping appraisal [7]. Threat appraisal refers to individuals tending to assess the negative outcomes of the potential risks and the threats on themselves such as whether they are easily affected by potential risks and whether the negative effects of potential risks are severe [6]. In general, threat appraisal can be divided into two sub-variables: perceived severity and perceived vulnerability. The more severity and vulnerability individuals perceived, the more likely they are willing to take protective actions to prevent risks. Coping appraisal refers to individuals tending to assess whether they have ability and capability to take protective actions and whether the protective actions can help them avoid or lower the adverse outcome of risks [6]. Coping appraisal can be divided into two sub-variables: self-efficacy and response efficacy. PMT assumes that the higher the self-efficacy and response efficacy, the more likely individuals are prepared to take protective actions to prevent risks.

In the COVID-19 research domain, research has been done to explore residents' risk perceptions of COVID-19 and protective behaviors. Based on PMT, Ref. [10] assessed public risk perception of COVID-19 and its impact on taking protective actions, and further examined the predictors of risk perception. They found that the level of public risk perception is relatively high, and risk perception is positively correlated with the adoption of protective actions. Personal experience with the virus, trust in government, prosocial value, personal knowledge and personal efficacy are all significant predictors of risk perception. Ref. [11] investigated the perception of risk and the worries about COVID-19 infection in both healthcare workers and the general population in Italy. They found that healthcare workers report higher risk perception and more eager to take protective measures. Ref. [12] used PMT to explore the immediate risk perceptions and psychological effects of the COVID-19 pandemic among Italian participants. They noted that perceived control, perceived efficacy of containment measures and affective states affect risk perception, which further promote residents to take protective behaviors. Ref. [13] adopted PMT to analyze the motivations of residents to take protective measures and behaviors during the early phase of COVID-19. They found that risk perception can drive the adoption of protective behaviors. Ref. [14] investigated the effect of risk perception on self-reported engagement in protective behaviors based on the research samples from United States. They noted that the samples demonstrate growing awareness of risk and report engaging in protective behaviors with increasing frequency. Their research findings highlighted the importance of risk perception and further confirmed the positive relationship between risk perception and protective behavior. Ref. [15] examined the effect of the components of PMT on taking protective health behaviors related to the COVID-19 virus. They found that the components of PMT are positively and significantly associated with the adoption of protective health behaviors. Other studies such as [16–18] also explored residents' risk perceptions of COVID-19 and protective behaviors, and proposed measures to encourage residents to take protective behaviors to impede the spread of COVID-19.

Though prior research has explored the issues about residents' risk perceptions of COVID-19 and protective behaviors, limited research has been performed to explore residents' WTP for taking protection actions such as purchasing mask against COVID-19 and examined the related determinants. Thus, to enrich the research on COVID-19, the current research aims to explore the determinants and WTP for purchasing masks against COVID-19. Meanwhile, given the popularity and explanatory power, PMT has been selected as the theoretical basis of this research.

2.2. Willingness to Pay and Contingent Valuation Method

In essence, the aim of residents to purchase and wear masks against COVID-19 is to avoid infection by COVID-19 and keep the virus at bay. Health is a non-market product and cannot be traded in the market. Hence, its value cannot be decided by demand and supply functions. According to microeconomic theory, the value formation of non-market products is largely decided by how much residents are willing to pay. In this research, residents' WTP refers to how much they intend to spend on purchasing masks against COVID-19.

In practice, there are two methods to obtain information about WTP and calculate the WTP value: choice experiment method and contingent valuation method. Compared with choice experiment method, contingent valuation method is more robust and easy to understand and implement. Contingent valuation method is a typical stated preference evaluation method based on the utility maximization theory to assess the economic value of non-market products by asking the respondents' WTP directly [19,20]. The respondents' answer is based on their own ideas rather than on their previous purchase behavior. The implicit assumption of this method is that the respondents can clearly understand their preferences and express them truthfully during the inquiry process [21]. Currently, contingent valuation method is the most widely used and effective method to analyze WTP and calculate the WTP value [21]. For this consideration, contingent valuation method has been adopted to analyze residents' WTP for purchasing mask against COVID-19.

For contingent valuation method, there are four elicitation techniques to inquire the respondents' WTP information: bidding game, open-ended, payment card and dichotomous choice [22]. Bidding game elicitation technique refers to setting an initial bid value first and then continuously increase or decrease the price level to detect respondents' WTP [23]. This elicitation technique is greatly affected by the initial bid value, and the entire game process requires constant communication with the respondents, which consumes a lot of time and effort. Hence, in practice, bidding game elicitation technique is rarely adopted. Open-ended elicitation technique refers to let respondents state their WTP directly [24]. Though this elicitation technique is simple and easy to conduct, it will also cause respondents to not know how to answer or even not to answer, which in turn affects the reliability of the results [24]. Payment card elicitation technique refers to setting different WTP interval first and then ask respondents to state their WTP based on these intervals [25]. Compared with open-ended elicitation technique, this elicitation technique is convenient for respondents to state their WTP. It should be cautioned that the credibility of the results depends largely on the rationality of the interval settings. Dichotomous choice elicitation technique refers to setting an initial bid value first and then inquire respondents whether they are willing to pay the initial bid value [26]. This elicitation technique simulates the real market behavior, but it requires a very complex probability statistical model to estimate the WTP value.

3. Data and Method

3.1. Questionnaire Design

Given that N95 masks are more effective to curb COVID-19 spread than cloth masks and surgical masks, the survey aims to explore residents' WTP for buying N95 masks. The masks mentioned in the following are all refer to N95 masks. Questionnaire survey was performed to collect residents' WTP information. The questionnaire included 4 parts. The first part briefly introduced the research background and research purpose, and ensured security of the primary data [27]. The second part aimed to obtain the information related to respondents' knowledge about COVID-19 and the four variables of PMT.

Multiple measurement items were employed to measure 5 variables mentioned above. All the items were assessed on a five-point Likert scale ranging from 1 (completely disagree) to 5 (completely agree), and respondents were asked to evaluate the items based on their own feelings and perceptions. To ensure the validity of the measurement items, all of them were adapted from prior research and slightly modified to make them applicable for the current research context. Specifically, the measurement items of the four variables of PMT were adapted from [16,17,19], and each variable was measured using three items. Four items adapted from [10,24,28] were employed to measure knowledge about COVID-19. To ensure the accuracy of these items, 7 academic scholars whose research interests focus on health behavior and risk communication were invited to help us to refine these items. Based on their comments, minor revisions such as typos and phrasing were made [29]. The final items of the research variables were presented in Appendix A.

The third part of the questionnaire was used to obtain information about residents' WTP. We first inquired the respondents whether they are willing to pay for purchasing masks against COVID-19. If not, we asked the respondents to choose from five statements the one that most closely resembled their reason for not being willing to pay. If yes, we then asked them how much they are willing to pay for purchasing masks against COVID-19 per month during the epidemic. To facilitate respondents to express their WTP value, payment card elicitation technique was adopted. In total, we set 8 intervals of WTP value: (1) ¥1–30 ($0.15–4.65); (2) ¥31–60 ($4.80–9.29); (3) ¥61–90 ($9.45–13.94); (4) ¥91–120 ($14.10–18.59); (5) ¥121–150 ($18.74–23.24); (6) ¥151–180 ($23.39–27.88); (7) ¥181–210 ($28.04–32.53) and (8) ¥211–240 ($32.68–37.18). The fourth part was used to collect respondents' demographic information such as age, gender, family size, health status, etc. [13,30,31].

3.2. Data Collection

In general, there are three commonly used methods to perform questionnaire surveys: online survey method, face to face survey method, and telephone and e-mail survey method [32–35]. In this research, online survey method was adopted to perform the survey. The reasons can be stated as follows. First, the current survey was performed during the COVID-19 outbreak period. Hence, face to face survey method should not be considered. Second, the response rate of telephone and e-mail survey method was low and time-consuming. Thus, telephone and e-mail survey methods were not considered.

With the help of Questionnaire Star (www.wjx.cn (accessed on 1 January 2020)), a popular and professional online survey website in China, the questionnaire survey was performed during 1–24 February 2020 in Hubei, Anhui, Jiangsu, Zhejiang, Shandong, Guangdong and Fujian Provinces and the Municipality of Shanghai. Participants were recruited from a large sample pool maintained by the Questionnaire Star. We totally received 3471 questionnaires. After abandoning the invalid questionnaires, 3148 valid questionnaires were obtained and used to perform data analysis.

4. Data Analysis and Results

In the following data analysis, we first conducted the reliability and validity analysis [36]. Then, we introduced the demographic information of respondents and conducted descriptive analysis to describe the research data. At last, we used the relevant estimation method to identify the determinants of WTP and WTP value. Furthermore, Hubei is the province most affected by the COVID-19 in China, respondents' perception and attitude toward COVID-19 in Hubei Province may be different from respondents in other provinces. Hence, to better and fully understand the determinants and the value of WTP for purchasing mask against COVID-19, the total valid samples ($N = 3148$) have been divided into 2 sub-samples: Hubei Sample ($N = 1103$) and Non-Hubei (e.g., Anhui, Jiangsu, Zhejiang, Shandong, Guangdong and Fujian Provinces and the Municipality of Shanghai) Sample ($N = 2045$).

4.1. Reliability and Validity Analysis

The results of reliability and validity analysis were presented in Table 1. According to Table 1, it can be concluded that the values of Cronbach's alpha and composite reliability (CR) were all greater than the threshold value of 0.70 [37]. Thus, the reliability of the survey was acceptable. Furthermore, the factor loadings of the items were all larger than 0.70 and significant ($p < 0.001$), and AVE values also exceeded 0.50 (See Table 1). Thus, the convergent validity of the survey was satisfactory [37]. In addition, as shown in Table 2, the square root of AVE for each variable was greater than its correlation coefficients with the other variables, revealing good discriminant validity [37]. Meanwhile, the Heterotrait–Monotrait (HTMT) Ratio for each of the variables was smaller than 0.85, which further suggested that the discriminant validity of the survey was acceptable [38].

4.2. Demographic Information

The demographic information of the respondents was illustrated in Table 3. In the total sample, compared with males, females accounted for the largest proportion, suggesting that females are more concerned about COVID-19 and willing to engage in the survey. The respondents were young and middle-aged. More than half of the respondents were aged between 26 and 50. Nearly 80% of the respondents had more than 10 years of education. Most respondents were middle class. Nearly 70% of the respondents earned a monthly income between ¥5000–15,000 ($774–2322). More than 80% of the respondents had 2–5 family members. Nearly half of the respondents acknowledged that their health status is acceptable. Table 3 also presented the demographic information of the respondents in Hubei Sample and Non-Hubei Sample.

Table 1. Reliability and validity analysis.

Variables	Item	Loading	Cronbach's Alpha	CR	AVE
Knowledge	KN1	0.85 ***	0.80	0.89	0.68
	KN2	0.77 ***			
	KN3	0.84 ***			
	KN4	0.83 ***			
Perceived severity	PS1	0.88 ***	0.82	0.88	0.71
	PS2	0.83 ***			
	PS3	0.81 ***			
Perceived vulnerability	PV1	0.79 ***	0.77	0.84	0.64
	PV2	0.82 ***			
	PV3	0.79 ***			
Self-efficacy	SE1	0.79 ***	0.83	0.89	0.72
	SE2	0.89 ***			
	SE3	0.87 ***			
Response efficacy	RE1	0.81 ***	0.79	0.86	0.67
	RE2	0.79 ***			
	RE3	0.86 ***			

Note: *** indicates significant at 0.1% significance level.

Table 2. Discriminant validity analysis.

Variables	KN	PS	PV	SE	RE
KN	**0.82**	0.42	0.63	0.57	0.49
PS	0.53	**0.84**	0.37	0.53	0.38
PV	0.48	0.35	**0.80**	0.49	0.51
SE	0.55	0.43	0.43	**0.85**	0.50
RE	0.41	0.45	0.38	0.33	**0.82**

Note: The bold values (diagonal elements) are the square root of AVE values; the values below the diagonal are the correlation coefficients among variables; the values above the diagonal are the Heterotrait–Monotrait (HTMT) Ratio of each variable.

4.3. Descriptive Analysis

There were five main variables in this research: knowledge about COVID-19, perceived severity, perceived vulnerability, self-efficacy and response efficacy. Table 4 introduced the descriptive analysis results of variables. It indicated that the mean values of these five variables are all larger than the average value of 3. Compared with the mean values of four variables in PMT, the mean value of COVID-19 knowledge is relatively lower. Table 4 also presented the mean values of these five variables in Hubei Sample and Non-Hubei Sample. To compare whether there are differences between the mean values of these five variables in Hubei Sample and Non-Hubei Sample, ANOVA analysis was conducted. The results indicated that there are significant differences between the mean values of knowledge about COVID-19 ($T = 2.81$, $p < 0.05$), perceived severity ($T = 3.01$, $p < 0.05$), perceived vulnerability ($T = 3.11$, $p < 0.05$), self-efficacy ($T = 2.89$, $p < 0.05$) and response efficacy ($T = 4.31$, $p < 0.01$) in Hubei Sample and Non-Hubei Sample, and the mean values of these five variables in Hubei Sample were significantly higher than that in Non-Hubei Sample. Indeed, compared with respondents in Non-Hubei Sample, respondents in Hubei Sample will definitely pay more attention to COVID-19. Thus, it is understandable that the respondents in Hubei Sample have a higher level of COVID-19 knowledge, and perceive a higher level of severity, vulnerability, self-efficacy, and response efficacy than respondents in Non-Hubei Sample.

Table 3. Samples' demographic information.

Category		Total Sample		Non-Hubei Sample		Hubei Sample	
		N	%	*N*	%	*N*	%
Gender	Female	1701	54.03%	1093	53.45%	582	52.77%
	Male	1447	45.97%	952	46.55%	521	47.23%
Age	18–25	564	17.92%	350	17.11%	190	17.23%
	26–40	723	22.97%	481	23.52%	250	22.67%
	41–50	941	29.89%	623	30.46%	330	29.92%
	51–60	503	15.98%	318	15.55%	173	15.68%
	>60	417	13.25%	273	13.35%	160	14.51%
Years of education	≤6	314	9.97%	218	10.66%	121	10.97%
	7–9	316	10.04%	181	8.85%	120	10.88%
	10–12	789	25.06%	519	25.38%	271	24.57%
	13–16	1045	33.20%	691	33.79%	369	33.45%
	≥17	684	21.73%	436	21.32%	222	20.13%
Monthly Income	<¥5000 ($774)	409	12.99%	251	12.27%	162	14.69%
	¥5000–10,000 ($1548)	1101	34.97%	731	35.75%	381	34.54%
	¥10,001–15,000 ($2322)	1070	33.99%	701	34.28%	362	32.82%
	>¥15,000	568	18.04%	362	17.70%	198	17.95%
Family size	1	220	6.99%	139	6.80%	75	6.80%
	2–3	1448	46.00%	921	45.04%	516	46.78%
	4–5	1196	37.99%	775	37.90%	408	36.99%
	>5	284	9.02%	210	10.27%	104	9.43%
Health status	Not well	1045	33.20%	690	33.74%	370	33.54%
	Acceptable	1479	46.98%	952	46.55%	501	45.42%
	Very well	624	19.82%	403	19.71%	232	21.03%
Observations		3148		2045		1103	

Table 4. Descriptive analysis result of research variable.

Variables	Total Sample		Non-Hubei Sample		Hubei Sample	
	Mean	SD	Mean	SD	Mean	SD
Knowledge (KN)	3.639	0.518	3.501	0.683	3.973	0.732
Perceived severity (PS)	4.219	0.457	4.093	0.683	4.472	0.702
Perceived vulnerability (PV)	4.313	0.537	4.101	0.781	4.598	0.692
Self-efficacy (SE)	4.411	0.531	4.278	0.602	4.693	0.573
Response efficacy (RE)	4.298	0.633	4.128	0.821	4.601	0.721

Note: SD = Standard Deviation.

4.4. Determinants of Residents' WTP

To identify the determinants of residents' WTP for purchasing masks against COVID-19, we should first analyze whether residents are willing to pay or not. As shown in Table 5, among the 3148 valid samples, 2581 observations are willing to pay for purchasing masks against COVID-19, accounting for 81.99% of the total valid samples. In addition, 567 observations are unwilling to pay for purchasing masks against COVID-19, accounting for 18.01% of the total valid samples. This finding suggested that most residents are willing to pay for purchasing masks against COVID-19. Furthermore, Table 5 also presented residents' WTP for purchasing masks against COVID-19 in Hubei Sample and Non-Hubei Sample. It can be found that the ratio of willing to pay (90.03%) in Hubei Sample is much higher than that in Non-Hubei Sample (79.95%).

Table 5. Residents' WTP.

Response	Total Sample		Non-Hubei Sample		Hubei Sample	
	Frequency	Ratio	Frequency	Ratio	Frequency	Ratio
Willing to pay	2581	81.99%	1635	79.95%	993	90.03%
Unwilling to pay	567	18.01%	410	20.05%	110	9.97%
Observations	3148		2045		1103	

Moreover, the reasons why residents were unwilling to pay for purchasing masks against COVID-19 were explored as well. We summarized five reasons: (1) I am healthy and have strong immunity, so I am unwilling to spend money to purchase and wear masks; (2) I always stay at home, so I am unwilling to spend money to purchase and wear masks; (3) COVID-19 will end soon, so I am unwilling to spend money to purchase and wear masks; (4) I have no money to purchase masks and (5) the cost of purchasing masks should be paid by the government. The frequency and ratio of each reason was shown in Table 6. Table 6 suggested that the reasons why respondents are unwilling to pay for purchasing masks against COVID-19 mainly focus on two aspects: good health and strong immunity, and always stay at home. This finding was also applicable for respondents in Hubei Sample and Non-Hubei Sample.

Table 6. Reasons of unwilling to pay.

Reason	Total Sample		Non-Hubei Sample		Hubei Sample	
	Frequency	Ratio	Frequency	Ratio	Frequency	Ratio
I am healthy and have strong immunity	210	37.04%	140	34.15%	52	47.27%
I always stay at home	165	29.10%	120	29.27%	31	28.18%
COVID-19 will end soon	80	14.11%	50	12.20%	20	18.18%
I have no money	32	5.64%	25	6.10%	1	0.91%
The cost should be paid by the government	80	14.11%	75	18.29%	6	5.45%
Observations	567		410		110	

To identify the determinants of residents' WTP, we should select the appropriate estimation model and method. The dependent variable, namely residents' WTP, was a discrete variable or "0–1" variable. Traditional linear regression estimation method such as ordinary least squares (OLS) estimation method cannot accurately predict the effects of independent variables on dependent variable [39]. Following the suggestion of [40], binary logistic regression method was used. Furthermore, given that residents' WTP varies with the respondents' demographic factors such as age, gender, education, income, family size and health status, we introduced these factors as the control variables into the regression analysis. Specifically, *gender* is a dummy variable, which is equal to 1 if the respondent is male and 0 if the respondent is female. *Age* is a continuous variable, which refers to the actual age of the respondent. *Education* is a continuous variable, which refers to the number of years the respondent has received education in school. *Income* is a continuous variable, which refers to the respondent's household monthly income. *Family size* is a continuous variable, which refers to the number of family members of the respondent. Health status is a dummy variable, which is equal to 1 if the health status is acceptable and very well, and 0 if the health status is not well.

The results of logistic regression analysis were presented in Table 7. Model 1 showed the regression results of the total sample. For control variables, gender is negatively and significantly associated with residents' WTP. Family size is positively and significantly associated with residents' WTP. Other control variables such as age, education, income and health status have no significant effect on residents' WTP. Residents' knowledge about COVID-19 ($\beta = 0.345$, $p < 0.05$), perceived severity ($\beta = 0.465$, $p < 0.001$), perceived vulnerability ($\beta = 0.321$, $p < 0.05$), self-efficacy ($\beta = 0.238$, $p < 0.01$) and response efficacy ($\beta = 0.317$, $p < 0.05$) are all positively and significantly associated with residents' WTP. Among the standardized coefficients, the standardized coefficient of perceived severity is the largest.

To further evaluate the proportional contribution of each variable to the explained variance, we used the method proposed by [41,42] to perform a relative importance analysis. Table 8 presented the results of the relative weight of the importance analysis of the determinants of residents' WTP. As shown in Table 8, perceived severity explains a larger percentage of the variance (20.49%) towards residents' WTP than any other variables. Thus, by comparing the relative contribution of each variable towards the predictive criterion of residents' WTP, it can be concluded that perceived severity has the largest effect on residents' WTP.

Table 7. Determinants of residents' WTP.

Variables	Logistic Regression		
	Total Sample	Non-Hubei Sample	Hubei Sample
	Model 1	Model 2	Model 3
Knowledge	0.345 *	0.281 **	0.389 **
Perceived severity	0.465 ***	0.412 *	0.507 ***
Perceived vulnerability	0.321 *	0.318 **	0.397 *
Self-efficacy	0.238 **	0.221 *	0.313 *
Response efficacy	0.317 *	0.291 ***	0.403 ***
Gender	−0.131 **	−0.187 **	0.149
Age	0.131	0.123	0.199
Education	0.204	0.253	0.101
Income	0.181	0.153	0.271
Family size	0.208 *	0.196 **	0.314
Health status	0.217	0.253	0.318
Observations	3148	2045	1103
LR χ^2	130.218	123.679	141.783
Prob > χ^2	0.000	0.000	0.001
Pseudo R^2	0.554	0.511	0.589
Log Likelihood	−269.341	−291.327	−245.827

Notes: * <0.05, ** <0.01 and *** <0.001.

Table 8. Relative importance weights of the determinants of residents' WTP.

Variables	Raw Relative Weight	Rescaled Relative Weight
Knowledge	0.091	16.49%
Perceived severity	0.113	20.49%
Perceived vulnerability	0.081	14.77%
Self-efficacy	0.061	11.02%
Response efficacy	0.054	9.56%
Gender	0.018	3.18%
Age	0.026	4.74%
Education	0.028	5.11%
Income	0.024	4.18%
Family size	0.025	4.46%
Health status	0.033	6.01%
Pseudo R^2	0.554	100%

Models 2 and 3 in Table 7 showed the regression results of Non-Hubei Sample and Hubei Sample. Overall, the findings in Non-Hubei Sample (Model 2) and Hubei Sample (Model 3) were in line with the findings in total sample (Model 1). Compared with Non-Hubei Sample (Model 2), the standardized coefficients of knowledge about COVID-19, perceived severity, perceived vulnerability, self-efficacy and response efficacy in Hubei Sample (Model 3) are relatively larger. Meanwhile, it is worth noting that all the control variables in Hubei Sample (Model 3) are insignificant.

4.5. Determinants of Residents' WTP Value

To identify the determinants of residents' WTP value, we should analyze the distribution of residents' WTP value. The distribution of residents' WTP value was presented in Table 9. Prior research such as [43–45] noted that WTP value can be decided based on the median value of each interval. Hence, the median value of each interval can also be regarded as a reasonable representation level of residents' WTP value in this research. On the basis of residents' WTP value, we calculated the average value of residents' WTP value. By referring to the work of [45,46], the average value of residents' WTP value can be expressed as follows:

$$\text{WTP} = \sum_{i=1}^{n} \text{WTP}_i \frac{N_i}{N} \quad (1)$$

Table 9. Distribution of residents' WTP value.

Interval	Total Sample		Non-Hubei Sample		Hubei Sample	
	Frequency	Ratio	Frequency	Ratio	Frequency	Ratio
¥1–30	288	11.16%	225	13.76%	70	7.05%
¥31–60	422	16.35%	345	21.10%	70	7.05%
¥61–90	255	9.88%	195	11.93%	55	5.54%
¥91–120	481	18.64%	245	14.98%	260	26.18%
¥121–150	592	22.94%	299	18.29%	300	30.21%
¥151–180	241	9.34%	91	5.57%	130	13.09%
¥181–210	187	7.25%	125	7.65%	60	6.04%
¥211–240	115	4.46%	110	6.73%	48	4.83%
Observations	2581		1635		993	

In Equation (1), WTP means average value of residents' WTP value, WTP_i means the WTP value of respondents who select ith interval, N_i means the number of respondents who select ith interval and N means the total number of respondents who are willing to pay. According to Equation (1) and Table 9, the average value of residents' WTP value for purchasing masks against COVID-19 is ¥120.92 ($18.73) per month during the epidemic in Hubei province and it is ¥100.16 ($15.50) per month during the epidemic in non-Hubei province. Overall, the average value of residents' WTP value for purchasing masks against COVID-19 is ¥106.53 ($16.51) per month during the epidemic nationally.

In this research, the dependent variable, namely residents' WTP value, was measured by a payment card elicitation technique. Residents' WTP value was an interval value. To improve the prediction accuracy of the estimation model, the interval regression estimation model was employed [39,47]. The estimation results were presented in Table 10.

Table 10. Determinants of residents' WTP value.

Variables	Total Sample	Non-Hubei Sample	Hubei Sample
	Model 4	Model 5	Model 6
Knowledge	0.221 *	0.309 ***	0.268 **
Perceived severity	0.263 *	0.197 **	0.331 ***
Perceived vulnerability	0.280 **	0.251 **	0.342 *
Self-efficacy	0.347	0.202	0.307
Response efficacy	0.401 ***	0.344 **	0.413 ***
Gender	−0.181 **	−0.197 *	−0.287
Age	−0.207	−0.183	−0.257
Education	0.231	0.253	0.186
Income	0.136	0.187	0.256
Family size	−0.260	−0.183	0.259
Health status	−0.237 *	−0.209 **	−0.289
Observations	2581	1635	993
Wald χ^2	97.359	92.257	89.183
Prob > χ^2	0.000	0.000	0.000
Log Likelihood	−1123.387	−1242.207	−1037.342

Notes: * <0.05, ** <0.01 and *** <0.001.

As shown in Table 10, in the total sample (Model 4), residents' COVID-19 knowledge ($\beta = 0.221$, $p < 0.05$), perceived severity ($\beta = 0.263$, $p < 0.05$), perceived vulnerability ($\beta = 0.280$, $p < 0.01$) and response efficacy ($\beta = 0.401$, $p < 0.001$) are positively and significantly associated with residents' WTP value, while self-efficacy has no significant effect on residents' WTP value ($\beta = 0.347$, $p > 0.05$). As for control variables, gender ($\beta = -0.181$, $p < 0.01$) and health status ($\beta = -0.237$, $p < 0.05$) are negatively and significantly associated with residents' WTP value. Other control variables such as age, education, income and family size have no significant effect on residents' WTP value. In Non-Hubei Sample (Model 5) and Hubei Sample (Model 6), the research results are almost consistent with findings in total sample (Model 4). However, in Hubei Sample (Model 6), all control variables have no significant effect on residents' WTP value.

5. Discussion

We undertook the current research with the purpose to explore the determinants of residents' willingness to pay (WTP) for purchasing masks against COVID-19 and the value of WTP. Based on protection motivation theory, we demonstrated that perceived severity, perceived vulnerability, self-efficacy and response efficacy are the positive antecedents of residents' WTP. These findings revealed that when residents perceive a higher level of severity and vulnerability, and have a higher level of self-efficacy and response efficacy, they will be likely to pay for purchasing masks against COVID-19. The current research findings were consistent with prior research on COVID-19 such as [10,12,15], which further highlighted the importance of protection motivation theory in explaining residents' protective behaviors during the COVID-19 pandemic. Meanwhile, this research also identified the positive impact of residents' knowledge about COVID-19 on residents' WTP, indicating that the more residents are knowledgeable about COVID-19, the more likely they are to pay for purchasing masks against COVID-19. This finding mirrored prior research findings [48] and further accented the significance of public COVID-19 knowledge in COVID-19 research.

By comparing the standardized coefficients of these five variables, it can be found that the standardized coefficient of perceived severity is the largest, revealing that perceived severity has the largest effect on residents' WTP. Indeed, the primary reason why residents are willing to pay for purchasing masks against COVID-19 is that they perceive the severity of COVID-19 and wish to purchase and wear masks to reduce the negative impact of COVID-19 on them. For control variables, gender negatively impacts residents' WTP, suggesting that females are more willing to pay for purchasing masks against COVID-19 than males. While family size positively impacts residents' WTP, uncovering that the more family members, the more likely they are to pay for purchasing masks against COVID-19. Other control variables such as age, education, income and health status have no significant effect on residents' WTP. This may be due to the fact that COVID-19 has spread rapidly throughout the world and its negative outcome on human society has been known to the public [49]. Thus, anyone, regardless of age, education, income and health status, is all willing to pay for purchasing masks against COVID-19.

Furthermore, the determinants of the value of WTP for purchasing masks against COVID-19 were also explored. Findings showed that residents' COVID-19 knowledge, perceived severity, perceived vulnerability and response efficacy are the positive antecedents of WTP value. These findings indicated that when residents are knowledgeable about COVID-19, perceive a higher level of severity and vulnerability, and have a higher level of response efficacy, they are likely to pay more for purchasing masks against COVID-19. However, contrary to our expectation, this research indicated that self-efficacy has no significant effect on WTP value. This may be because that the cost paid on purchasing masks against COVID-19 is not too much and nearly all residents can afford it. That is, residents have ability and capacity to purchase masks against COVID-19 and thus the effect of self-efficacy is insignificant. Given that prior COVID-19 literature rarely discussed residents' WTP for taking protective behaviors especially purchasing and wearing mask, this research contributed to existing body of knowledge on COVID-19 and residents' protective behaviors literature, thus advancing the science in this research domain for other scholars to explore.

As for control variables, gender and health status negatively affect residents' WTP value, suggesting that female and residents in poor health are more likely to pay more for purchasing masks against COVID-19. Other control variables such as age, education, income and family size have no significant effect on residents' WTP value, revealing that anyone, regardless of age, education, income and family size, is willing to pay for purchasing masks against COVID-19.

6. Conclusions and Limitations

COVID-19 has shown a pandemic trend globally. To curb its spread and reduce its negative effect on the global economy, especially on public health, all circles in the world should take measures to against COVID-19 [49]. From an individual perspective, this research focused on residents' self-protective behaviors and aimed to examine the determinants and willingness to pay for purchasing mask against COVID-19.

This research found that most residents are willing to pay for purchasing masks against COVID-19. Residents' COVID-19 knowledge, perceived severity, perceived vulnerability, self-efficacy and response efficacy are positively and significantly associated with residents' WTP, and perceived severity has the largest effect. For control variables, only gender and family size are significantly associated with residents' WTP. Other control variables such as age, income, education and health status have no significant effect on residents' WTP. Furthermore, we also examined the determinants of residents' WTP value. The results indicated that residents' COVID-19 knowledge, perceived severity, perceived vulnerability and response efficacy are positively and significantly associated with residents' WTP value. However, self-efficacy has no significant effect on residents' WTP value. Gender and health status are significantly associated with residents' WTP value. Other control variables such as age, education, income and family size have no significant effect on residents' WTP value.

In addition, we also calculated the average value of residents' WTP value for purchasing mask against COVID-19. The average value of residents' WTP value for purchasing mask against COVID-19 is ¥106.53 ($16.51) per month during the epidemic nationally. Meanwhile, this research further noted that residents in Hubei province tending to pay more than residents in non-Hubei province. The average value of residents' WTP value for purchasing mask against COVID-19 is ¥120.92 ($18.73) per month during the epidemic in Hubei province, and it is ¥100.16 ($15.50) per month during the epidemic in non-Hubei province.

There are several limitations in this research. First, an online survey method was adopted to collect research data. In general, face to face survey method is more applicable for using contingent value method. In the following research, face to face survey methods can be used. Second, payment card elicitation technique was used in this research. The WTP value largely depends on the interval value we set. Hence, it needs caution to generalize the residents' WTP value. Third, the research sample of this study was still limited, which may affect the research findings. In future research, more data can be gathered to replicate the current research findings. Finally, we did not consider the data from 2021. In future research, the data from 2021 should be collected and analyzed.

Author Contributions: Q.D.: Writing—original draft; methodology; S.L.: Review and editing; conceptualization and formal analysis; S.W.: Review and editing. All authors have read and agreed to the published version of the manuscript.

Funding: This work was supported by the Basic and Applied Basic Research Foundation of Guangdong Province, Youth Fund Project of Regional Joint Fund (2020A1515110133), Social Science Foundation (Major Program) of Fujian Province (FJ2021Z007) and Natural Science Foundation of Fujian Province (2021J01175).

Institutional Review Board Statement: Not applicable.

Informed Consent Statement: Not applicable.

Data Availability Statement: The datasets used and/or analyzed during the current study are available from the corresponding author on reasonable request.

Conflicts of Interest: The authors declare no conflict of interest.

Appendix A. Variable and Measurement Item

Variables	Measurement Item
Knowledge (KN)	KN1: COVID-19 is a respiratory infection caused by a new species of coronavirus family KN2: COVID-19 can be transmitted through respiratory droplets such as cough and sneeze KN3: COVID-19 can be prevented through wearing mask and personal hygiene KN4: The common symptoms of COVID-19 are fever, cough and shortness of breath
Perceived severity (PS)	PS1: COVID-19 is a serious social issue PS2: COVID-19 will have negative consequences PS3: The negative effect of COVID-19 is severe
Perceived vulnerability (PV)	PV1: COVID-19 can negatively impact me PV2: I am vulnerable to the negative effects of COVID-19 PV3: My chances of being infected by COVID-19 is high
Self-efficacy (SE)	SE1: It is easy for me to purchase and wear mask SE2: If I wanted to, I could easily purchase and wear mask SE3: It is mostly up to me whether I purchase and wear mask
Response efficacy (RE)	RE1: Wearing mask can impede the spread of COVID-19 RE2: Wearing mask can lower the chances of being infected by COVID-19 RE3: Wearing mask can defeat COVID-19 as soon as possible

References

1. Cao, W.; Fang, Z.; Hou, G.; Han, M.; Xu, X.; Dong, J.; Zheng, J. The psychological impact of the COVID-19 epidemic on college students in China. *Psychiatry Res.* **2020**, *287*, 112934. [CrossRef] [PubMed]
2. Liu, S.; Yang, L.; Zhang, C.; Xiang, Y.-T.; Liu, Z.; Hu, S.; Zhang, B. Online mental health services in China during the COVID-19 outbreak. *Lancet Psychiatry* **2020**, *7*, 17–18. [CrossRef]
3. Peeples, L. News Feature: Avoiding pitfalls in the pursuit of a COVID-19 vaccine. *Proc. Natl. Acad. Sci. USA* **2020**, *117*, 8218–8221. [CrossRef] [PubMed]
4. Prem, K.; Liu, Y.; Russell, T.W.; Kucharski, A.J.; Eggo, R.M.; Davies, N.; Jit, M.; Klepac, P.; Flasche, S.; Clifford, S.; et al. The Effect of Control Strategies to Reduce Social Mixing on Outcomes of the COVID-19 Epidemic in Wuhan, China: A Modelling Study. *Lancet Public Health* **2020**, *5*, 261–270. [CrossRef]
5. MacIntyre, C.R.; Wang, Q. Physical distancing, face masks, and eye protection for prevention of COVID-19. *Lancet* **2020**, *395*, 1950–1951. [CrossRef]
6. Rogers, R.W. A Protection Motivation Theory of Fear Appeals and Attitude Change. *J. Psychol.* **1975**, *91*, 93–114. [CrossRef]
7. Maddux, J.E.; Rogers, R.W. Protection motivation and self-efficacy: A revised theory of fear appeals and attitude change. *J. Exp. Soc. Psychol.* **1983**, *19*, 469–479. [CrossRef]
8. Rainear, A.M.; Christensen, J.L. Protection motivation theory as an explanatory framework for pro-environmental be-havioral intentions. *Commun. Res. Rep.* **2017**, *34*, 239–248. [CrossRef]
9. Wang, S.; Wang, J.; Yang, F. From willingness to action: Do push-pull-mooring factors matter for shifting to green transportation? *Transp. Res. Part D Transp. Environ.* **2020**, *79*, 102242. [CrossRef]
10. Dryhurst, S.; Schneider, C.R.; Kerr, J.; Freeman, A.L.; Recchia, G.; Van Der Bles, A.M.; Spiegelhalter, D.; van der Linden, S. Risk per-ceptions of COVID-19 around the world. *J. Risk Res.* **2020**, *23*, 994–1006. [CrossRef]
11. Simione, L.; Gnagnarella, C. Differences Between Health Workers and General Population in Risk Perception, Behaviors, and Psychological Distress Related to COVID-19 Spread in Italy. *Front. Psychol.* **2020**, *11*, 2166. [CrossRef] [PubMed]

12. Lanciano, T.; Graziano, G.; Curci, A.; Costadura, S.; Monaco, A. Risk Perceptions and Psychological Effects during the Italian COVID-19 Emergency. *Front. Psychol.* **2020**, *11*, 2434. [CrossRef] [PubMed]
13. Vai, B.; Cazzetta, S.; Ghiglino, D.; Parenti, L.; Saibene, G.; Toti, M.; Verga, C.; Wykowska, A.; Benedetti, F. Risk Perception and Media in Shaping Protective Behaviors: Insights from the Early Phase of COVID-19 Italian Outbreak. *Front. Psychol.* **2020**, *11*, 563426. [CrossRef] [PubMed]
14. Wise, T.; Zbozinek, T.D.; Michelini, G.; Hagan, C.C.; Mobbs, D. Changes in risk perception and self-reported protective behaviour during the first week of the COVID-19 pandemic in the United States. *R. Soc. Open Sci.* **2020**, *7*, 200742. [CrossRef] [PubMed]
15. Kowalski, R.M.; Black, K.J. Protection Motivation and the COVID-19 Virus. *Health Commun.* **2021**, *36*, 15–22. [CrossRef] [PubMed]
16. Bhati, A.S.; Mohammadi, Z.; Agarwal, M.; Kamble, Z.; Donough-Tan, G. Motivating or manipulating: The influence of health-protective behaviour and media engagement on post-COVID-19 travel. *Curr. Issues Tour.* **2021**, *24*, 2088–2092. [CrossRef]
17. Collins, A.; Florin, M.-V.; Renn, O. COVID-19 risk governance: Drivers, responses and lessons to be learned. *J. Risk Res.* **2020**, *23*, 1073–1082. [CrossRef]
18. Tomczyk, S.; Rahn, M.; Schmidt, S. Social distancing and stigma: Association between compliance with behavioral recommendations, risk perception, and stigmatizing attitudes during the COVID-19 outbreak. *Front. Psychol.* **2020**, *11*, 1821. [CrossRef]
19. Duffield, J.W.; Patterson, D.A. Inference and Optimal Design for a Welfare Measure in Dichotomous Choice Contingent Valuation. *Land Econ.* **1991**, *67*, 225. [CrossRef]
20. Neumann, P.J.; Johannesson, M. The willingness to pay for in vitro fertilization: A pilot study using contingent valuation. *Med. Care* **1994**, *32*, 686–699. [CrossRef]
21. Sun, C.; Zhu, X. Evaluating the public perceptions of nuclear power in China: Evidence from a contingent valuation survey. *Energy Policy* **2014**, *69*, 397–405. [CrossRef]
22. Ryan, M.; Scott, D.A.; Donaldson, C. Valuing health care using willingness to pay: A comparison of the payment card and dichotomous choice methods. *J. Health Econ.* **2004**, *23*, 237–258. [CrossRef] [PubMed]
23. Ezebilo, E.E.; Mattsson, L.; Afolami, C.A. Economic value of ecotourism to local communities in the Nigerian rainforest zone. *J. Sustain. Dev.* **2010**, *3*, 51. [CrossRef]
24. Romano, K.R.; Finco, F.D.B.A.; Rosenthal, A.; Finco, M.V.A.; Deliza, R. Willingness to pay more for value-added pomegranate juice (*Punica granatum* L.): An open-ended contingent valuation. *Food Res. Int.* **2016**, *89*, 359–364. [CrossRef] [PubMed]
25. Mataria, A.; Luchini, S.; Daoud, Y.; Moatti, J.-P. Demand assessment and price-elasticity estimation of quality-improved primary health care in palestine: A contribution from the contingent valuation method. *Health Econ.* **2007**, *16*, 1051–1068. [CrossRef]
26. Bateman, I.J.; Day, B.H.; Dupont, D.P.; Georgiou, S. Procedural invariance testing of the one-and-one-half-bound di-chotomous choice elicitation method. *Rev. Econ. Stat.* **2009**, *91*, 806–820. [CrossRef]
27. Wang, Y.; Wang, S.; Wang, J.; Wei, J.; Wang, C. An empirical study of consumers' intention to use ride-sharing services: Using an extended technology acceptance model. *Transportation* **2020**, *47*, 397–415. [CrossRef]
28. Taghrir, M.H.; Borazjani, R.; Shiraly, R. COVID-19 and Iranian Medical Students; A Survey on Their Related-Knowledge, Preventive Behaviors and Risk Perception. *Arch. Iran. Med.* **2020**, *23*, 249–254. [CrossRef]
29. Wang, S.; Wang, J.; Li, J.; Yang, F. Do motivations contribute to local residents' engagement in pro-environmental behaviors? Resident-destination relationship and pro-environmental climate perspective. *J. Sustain. Tour.* **2019**, *28*, 834–852. [CrossRef]
30. Gao, L.; Wang, S.; Li, J.; Li, H. Application of the extended theory of planned behavior to understand individual's energy saving behavior in workplaces. *Resour. Conserv. Recycl.* **2017**, *127*, 107–113. [CrossRef]
31. Shi, H.; Wang, S.; Zhao, D. Exploring urban resident's vehicular PM2.5 reduction behavior intention: An application of the extended theory of planned behavior. *J. Clean. Prod.* **2017**, *147*, 603–613. [CrossRef]
32. Wang, S.; Fan, J.; Zhao, D.; Yang, S.; Fu, Y. Predicting consumers' intention to adopt hybrid electric vehicles: Using an extended version of the theory of planned behavior model. *Transportation* **2016**, *43*, 123–143. [CrossRef]
33. Ru, X.; Wang, S.; Yan, S. Exploring the effects of normative factors and perceived behavioral control on individual's en-ergy-saving intention: An empirical study in eastern China. *Resour. Conserv. Recycl.* **2018**, *134*, 91–99. [CrossRef]
34. Ru, X.; Qin, H.; Wang, S. Young people's behavior intentions towards reducing PM2. 5 in China: Extending the theory of planned behavior. *Resour. Conserv. Recycl.* **2018**, *141*, 99–108. [CrossRef]
35. Wang, Y.; Liang, J.; Yang, J.; Ma, X.; Li, X.; Wu, J.; Yang, G.; Ren, G.; Feng, Y. Analysis of the environmental behavior of farmers for non-point source pollution control and management: An integration of the theory of planned behavior and the protection motivation theory. *J. Environ. Manag.* **2019**, *237*, 15–23. [CrossRef]
36. Wang, S.; Wang, J.; Lin, S.; Li, J. Public perceptions and acceptance of nuclear energy in China: The role of public knowledge, perceived benefit, perceived risk and public engagement. *Energy Policy* **2019**, *126*, 352–360. [CrossRef]
37. Fornell, C.; Larcker, D.F. Evaluating structural equation models with unobservable variables and measurement error. *J. Mark. Res.* **1981**, *18*, 39–50. [CrossRef]
38. Henseler, J.; Ringle, C.M.; Sarstedt, M. A new criterion for assessing discriminant validity in variance-based structural equation modeling. *J. Acad. Mark. Sci.* **2015**, *43*, 115–135. [CrossRef]
39. He, K.; Zhang, J.; Zeng, Y. Households' willingness to pay for energy utilization of crop straw in rural China: Based on an improved UTAUT model. *Energy Policy* **2020**, *140*, 111373. [CrossRef]
40. Brock, W.A.; Durlauf, S.N. Discrete Choice with Social Interactions. *Rev. Econ. Stud.* **2001**, *68*, 235–260. [CrossRef]

41. Tonidandel, S.; Lebreton, J.M. Determining the Relative Importance of Predictors in Logistic Regression: An Extension of Relative Weight Analysis. *Organ. Res. Methods* **2009**, *13*, 767–781. [CrossRef]
42. Kantakumar, L.N.; Kumar, S.; Schneider, K. What drives urban growth in pune? A logistic regression and relative im-portance analysis perspective. *Sustain. Cities Soc.* **2010**, *60*, 102269. [CrossRef]
43. Armbrecht, J. Use value of cultural experiences: A comparison of contingent valuation and travel cost. *Tour. Manag.* **2014**, *42*, 141–148. [CrossRef]
44. Chen, J.M.; Zhang, J.; Nijkamp, P. A regional analysis of willingness-to-pay in Asian cruise markets. *Tour. Econ.* **2016**, *22*, 809–824. [CrossRef]
45. Seetaram, N.; Song, H.; Ye, S.; Page, S. Estimating willingness to pay air passenger duty. *Ann. Tour. Res.* **2018**, *72*, 85–97. [CrossRef]
46. Gupta, M. Willingness to pay for carbon tax: A study of Indian road passenger transport. *Transp. Policy* **2016**, *45*, 46–54. [CrossRef]
47. Stewart, M.B. On Least Squares Estimation when the Dependent Variable is Grouped. *Rev. Econ. Stud.* **1983**, *50*, 737–753. [CrossRef]
48. Li, J.-B.; Yang, A.; Dou, K.; Wang, L.-X.; Zhang, M.-C.; Lin, X.-Q. Chinese public's knowledge, perceived severity, and perceived controllability of COVID-19 and their associations with emotional and behavioural reactions, social participation, and precautionary behaviour: A national survey. *BMC Public Health* **2020**, *20*, 1589. [CrossRef]
49. Gilbert, M.; Pullano, G.; Pinotti, F.; Valdano, E.; Poletto, C.; Boëlle, P.-Y.; D'Ortenzio, E.; Yazdanpanah, Y.; Eholie, S.P.; Altmann, M.; et al. Preparedness and vulnerability of African countries against importations of COVID-19: A modelling study. *Lancet* **2020**, *395*, 871–877. [CrossRef]

International Journal of
Environmental Research and Public Health

MDPI

Review

Trends, Issues and Future Directions of Urban Health Impact Assessment Research: A Systematic Review and Bibliometric Analysis

Wenbing Luo [1,2], Zhongping Deng [1], Shihu Zhong [3,*] and Mingjun Deng [4]

1 School of Business, Hunan University of Science and Technology, Xiangtan 411201, China; wbluo@hnust.edu.cn (W.L.); 21021502041@mail.hnust.edu.cn (Z.D.)
2 School of Accounting, Hunan University of Technology and Business, Changsha 410205, China
3 Shanghai National Accounting Institute, Shanghai 201702, China
4 Big Data and Intelligent Decision Research Center, Hunan University of Science and Technology, Xiangtan 411201, China; mjdeng@hnust.edu.cn
* Correspondence: zhongshihu@163.sufe.edu.cn

Abstract: Health impact assessment (HIA) has been regarded as an important means and tool for urban planning to promote public health and further promote the integration of health concept. This paper aimed to help scientifically to understand the current situation of urban HIA research, analyze its discipline co-occurrence, publication characteristics, partnership, influence, keyword co-occurrence, co-citation, and structural variation. Based on the ISI Web database, this paper used a bibliometric method to analyze 2215 articles related to urban HIA published from 2012 to 2021. We found that the main research directions in the field were Environmental Sciences and Public Environmental Occupational Health; China contributed most articles, the Tehran University of Medical Sciences was the most influential institution, Science of the Total Environment was the most influential journal, Yousefi M was the most influential author. The main hotspots include health risk assessment, source appointment, contamination, exposure, particulate matter, heavy metals and urban soils in 2012–2021; road dust, source apposition, polycyclic aromatic hydrocarbons, air pollution, urban topsoil and the north China plain were always hot research topics in 2012–2021, drinking water and water quality became research topics of great concern in 2017–2021. There were 25 articles with strong transformation potential during 2020–2021, but most papers carried out research on the health risk assessment of toxic elements in soil and dust. Finally, we also discussed the limitations of this paper and the direction of bibliometric analysis of urban HIA in the future.

Keywords: urban; health impact assessment; bibliometric analysis; CiteSpace; knowledge mapping

Citation: Luo, W.; Deng, Z.; Zhong, S.; Deng, M. Trends, Issues and Future Directions of Urban Health Impact Assessment Research: A Systematic Review and Bibliometric Analysis. *IJERPH* **2022**, *19*, 5957. https://doi.org/10.3390/ijerph19105957

Academic Editor: Paul B. Tchounwou

Received: 18 March 2022
Accepted: 12 May 2022
Published: 13 May 2022

1. Introduction

The European Union Environmental Impact Assessment (EIA) Directive (2011/92/EU as amended by 2014/52/EU) requires EIAs to consider the effects that a project might have on human health [1]. Over the past two decades, health impact assessment (HIA) practice has expanded across the world [2], HIA has been regarded as an important means and tool for urban planning to promote public health and further promote the integration of health concept. More and more professionals in the fields of spatial planning, transportation planning and public health all over the world are beginning to pay attention to and use HIA tools [3–7]. Many cities around the world set "improving public health" as an important development goal to promote the construction of healthy cities by expanding their understanding and continuously carrying out healthy city planning practice, constructing an HIA theoretical model and carrying out evaluation practice [8–12].

Over the past decade, scholars have increasingly focused on urban HIA research and have issued an increasing number of papers; this makes it difficult for us to grasp the focus of research from thousands of papers, resulting in a major risk of ignoring basic problems and research improvement fields. It will provide an important theoretical basis for researchers, practitioners, decision makers and stakeholders from different backgrounds to carry out urban HIA research and management practice more effectively by presenting the structure, law, and distribution of scientific knowledge in the field of urban HIA. Who have been the famous scholars in urban HIA related research fields? Which countries and institutions have close exchanges in urban HIA related research fields? What are the research topics and development trends in urban HIA related research fields? These problems need to be further analyzed. In order to solve this problem, it is necessary to use a bibliometric analysis method, as this method can better find knowledge status and development trends in a given field [13,14]; additionally use of scientometric software (such as VOSviewer, CoPalRed, Bibexcel, Sci2, VantagePoint, CiteSpace and Online Analysis Platform for Bibliometrics) to realize the visual analysis of citations, so as to reveal how the research field has evolved, the obvious knowledge turning points on the critical path and which topics have attracted people's attention [15]. However, to the best of our knowledge, there is no bibliometric analysis on urban HIA at a global scale. Therefore, we intuitively displayed the knowledge structure and development trends of urban HIA related research fields through bibliometric analysis, in order to guide scholars and practitioners to determine the research interests and emerging themes of urban HIA, so as to enhance their understanding and evaluation of urban HIA.

This paper is organized as follows. After this introduction, Section 2 provides the primary research materials and methods. Section 3 presents the research findings and analyses. Section 4 presents research-related conclusions.

2. Materials and Methods

2.1. Data Acquisition

According to the data resources required by CiteSpace, we took the Web of Science Core Collection as the data collection platform. As people are paying increasing attention to the impact of contaminated sites on the environment and public health, health risk assessment methods were used to describe and quantify the health impact on neighbouring people and guide public health interventions [16]. At the same time, we found that if only "health impact assessment" was used as the search term, the total number of literature studies was less than 400 under the same search conditions. Therefore, this paper juxtaposes "health risk assessment" as a search term. Figure 1 shows the number of papers published each year from 1992 to 2021 according to the retrieval strategy used in this paper. We found that the number of papers published in the early stages was small. CiteSpace software (Version 5.8.R3, Chaomei Chen, Drexel University, Philadelphia, PA, USA) developers pointed out that the longer the literature time span, the poorer the knowledge map. Therefore, this paper focuses on the bibliometric analysis of urban health impact assessment research over the last ten years.

Finally, the search strategy of bibliometric analysis was as follows: This study regards the Web of Science Core Collection as a data-collection platform according to data resources required in CiteSpace; The bibliometric search strategy can be described as the following: TS = (urban OR city OR cities) AND TS = ("health risk assessment" OR "health impact assessment"), Publication years = (1 January 2012 to 14 November 2021), Indexes = (SCI-EXPANDED, SSCI, ESCI), Document types = "Articles". A total of 2215 publications were selected on 14 November 2021.

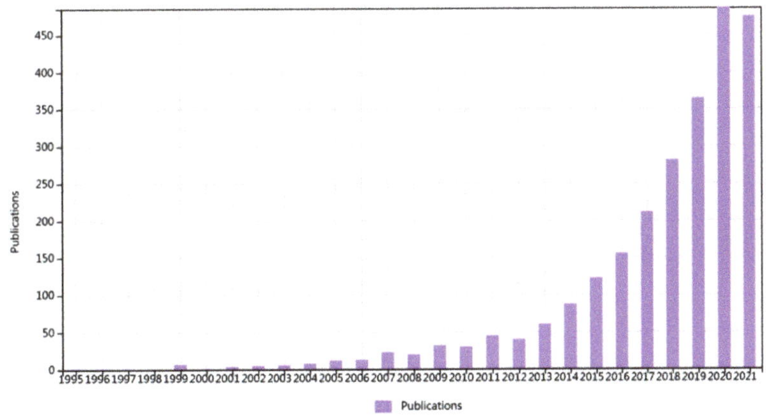

Figure 1. Number of publications over the years.

2.2. *Bibliometric Analysis Methods*

Bibliometrics is an interdisciplinary study that utilizes mathematics, statistics, and bibliography to quantitatively analyze academic literature [17]. The common methods of bibliometrics include statistical analysis, citation analysis, sharing analysis, etc. In addition, mapping knowledge can show the relationship between the development process and structure of scientific knowledge, focus on the evolution process of a certain knowledge field, and help scholars understand the hot spots, frontiers, and trends of research in this field [18].

Generally, the knowledge of the development status on a research subject is carried out using reviews as systematic or integrative approaches. However, the statistical analysis of journals, authors, countries, institutions and influence can help us quickly grasp the basic information and development status of literature in a certain field [19]. We used the Online Analysis Platform for Bibliometrics (https://bibliometric.com/ (accessed on 16 November 2021)) to conduct publication year, journal, countries and influence analysis, so as to quickly obtain the information of influential institutions, authoritative publications and experts in relevant fields.

Partnership analysis mainly analyzes the relationship between countries, the relationship between institutions and the relationship between authors. We used Online Analysis Platform for Bibliometrics and VOSviewer to analyze the cooperation network among countries, institutions, and authors.

Keyword co-occurrence analysis is an effective method, which can find hot topics and develop research frontiers in specific research fields. In this paper, we made a keyword co-occurrence network map by VOSviewer and monitored hot topics in urban HIA research through keyword co-occurrence network analysis.

Co-citation analysis can map the knowledge structure of a research field, detect the trends in the research field (by the authors engaged in these topics and their interrelationships) and highlight the findings with significant impact [20]. Understanding trends and emerging topics in a research area is important for future and current researchers, policymakers, funding agencies and other stakeholders [21]. CiteSpace enables us to understand a certain field quickly and systematically. CiteSpace can label co-citation clusters and use time-sliced snapshots to form timeliness and pivotal points [14]. In this study, we used CiteSpace (Version 5.8.R3) to find major research areas in the knowledge domain and journal overlay maps. In order to better understand the development of urban HIA research in different periods, we carried out co-citation analysis in two periods: (1) Set a time span from 2012 to 2016, set "years per slice = 1", "node types = reference", "Selection Criteria: Select top = 100" and "Pruning = Pathfinder and Pruning sliced networks" in CiteSpace to analyze their intellectual structure and the dynamics of co-citation clusters; (2) Set a time span from 2017 to 2021, set "years per slice = 1", "node types = reference", "Selection Criteria: g-index, k = 50" and "Pruning = Pathfinder and Pruning sliced networks" in CiteSpace to analyze their intellectual structure and the dynamics of co-citation clusters.

3. Results and Analyses

3.1. Discipline Co-Occurrence Analysis

Via the "dual-map overlay" function of CiteSpace, we can construct the discipline co-occurrence network, as shown in Figure 2. The original map shows more than 10,000 journals indexed in Web of Science, which are divided into different disciplines in different colors and are located in different locations of the source (or left) region and the reference (or right) region. Among them, "source" refers to the relevant papers in a certain field for a certain period of time and "reference" refers to all references of the above papers. For example, the discipline "ECONOMICS, ECONOMIC, POLITICAL" is in lake-blue and it ranks the 10th in the source region and the 12th in the reference region [22]. Then we added a layer containing the 2215 bibliographic records on urban HIA, which became the colorful links between the source region and the reference region.

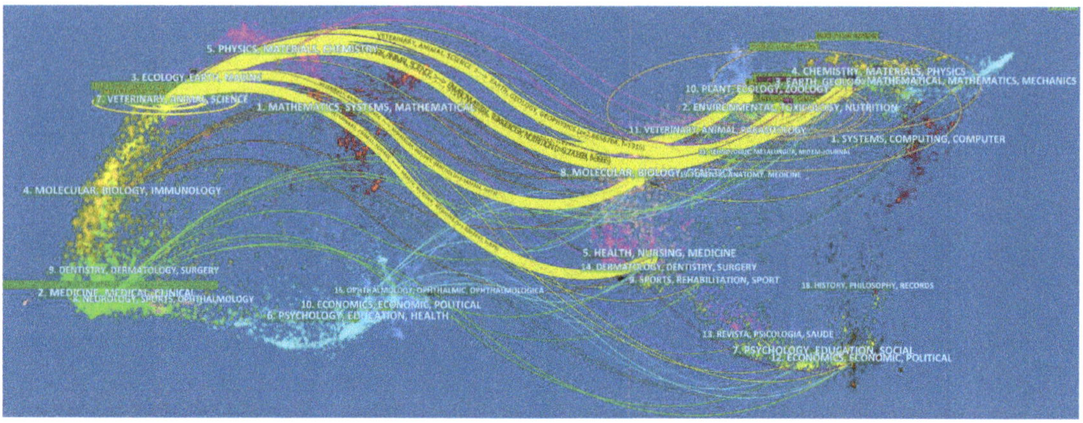

Figure 2. A dual map overlay of literature on urban HIA research.

From Figure 2, the impact of the city and health "7. VETERINARY, ANIMAL, SCIENCE". As for the distribution of the reference journals, "7. VETERINARY, ANIMAL, SCIENCE" links going to "2. ENVIRONMENTAL, TOXICOLOGY, NUTRITION", "3. EARTH, GEOLOGY, GEOPHYSICS", "10. PLANT, ECOLOGY, ZOOLOGY", "8. MOLECULAR, BIOLOGY, GENETICS" and "5. HEALTH, NURSING, MEDICINE" account for higher percentage. This just reflects that the research on urban HIA is a typical interdisciplinary research field.

3.2. Publication Characteristics Analysis

The top 10 countries in the number of annual publications are shown in Figure 3. Since the Online Analysis Platform for Bibliometrics can only automatically generate the top ten countries, the situation of annual publications in other countries cannot be seen in this figure. The number of articles issued in China, Iran and India has shown a rapid growth trend from 2012 to 2021.

As shown in Table 1: (1) Among the top 10 WOS of categories in the total number of papers published; (2) Among the top 10 publication titles in terms of publication volume; (3) Among the top 10 authors in the number of papers published.

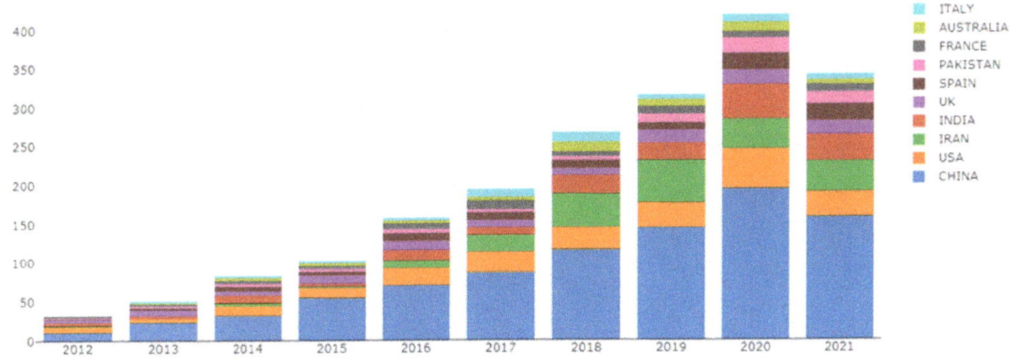

Figure 3. Number of papers published by countries each year.

Table 1. Top 10 WOS of categories, publication titles and authors.

WOS Categories	Record Count	Publication Titles	Record Count	Authors	Record Count
Environmental Sciences	1640	Environmental Science and Pollution Research	161	Li J	27
Public Environmental Occupational Health	408	Science of the Total Environment	146	Wang Q	27
Engineering Environmental	233	International Journal of Environmental Research and Public Health	106	Radfard M	25
Water Resources	217	Environmental Geochemistry and Health	101	Rojas-rueda D	24
Toxicology	178	Human and Ecological Risk Assessment	93	Latif MT	21
Meteorology Atmospheric Sciences	115	Ecotoxicology and Environmental Safety	88	Mohammadi MJ	21
Biodiversity Conservation	99	Environmental Pollution	81	Lu XW	20
Multidisciplinary Sciences	76	Chemosphere	80	Zhang H	19
Geosciences Multidisciplinary	58	Atmospheric Environment	43	Zhang JQ	18
Chemistry Analytical	49	Environmental Research	43	Li F	17

3.3. Partnership Analysis

The cooperative relationship between countries is shown in Figure 4. Among them, authors from CHINA, IRAN, USA, and SPAIN have more cooperation with authors from other countries.

The cooperation between institutions is shown in Figure 5. Institutions include universities, research institutes and national research institutions; According to the statistics of the number of articles jointly published by institutions, the organization represented by the red node has a cooperative relationship with the node where the mouse is located. The core of institutional cooperation network mainly includes Chinese Academy of Sciences, Tehran University of Medical Sciences, Beijing Normal University, Indian Institute of Technology, etc.

The cooperation between authors is shown in Figure 6. In the main author cooperation network, the authors who play a key role include Mohammadi M J, Radfard M, Rojas-rueda D, Lu XW, Liu G, Wang Q, Li J, etc.

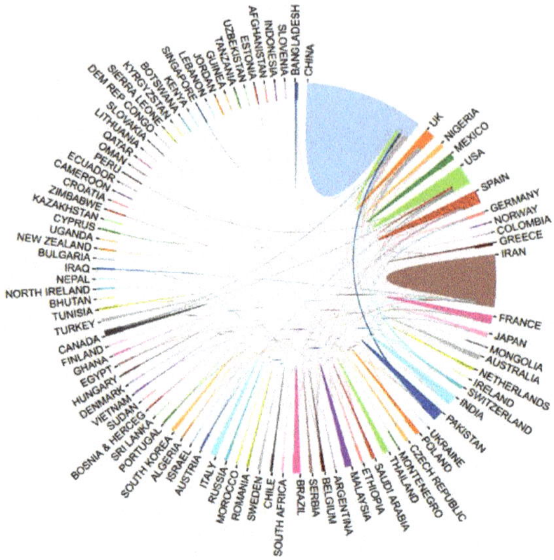

Figure 4. Cooperation between countries.

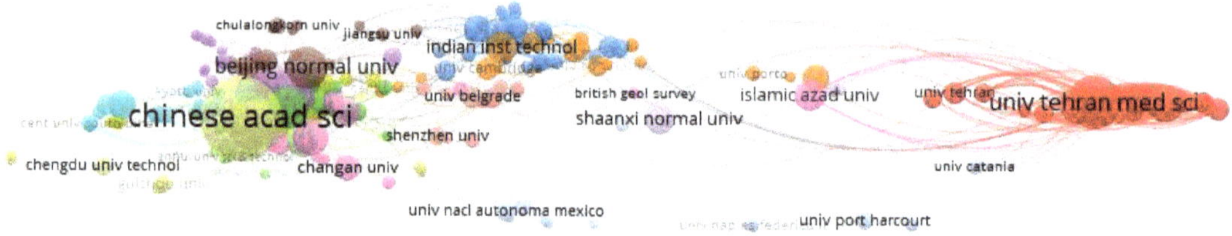

Figure 5. Cooperation between institutions.

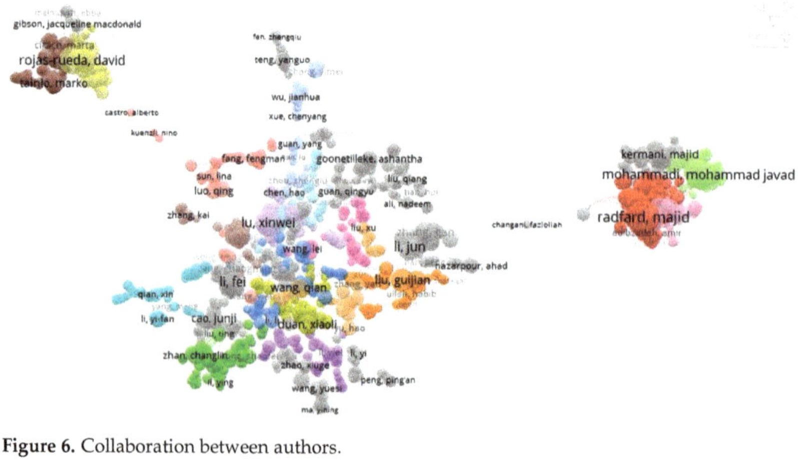

Figure 6. Collaboration between authors.

3.4. Influence Analysis

The top 10 institutions with influence are shown in Table 2. Univ Tehran Med Sci, Beijing Normal Univ and Chinese Acad Sci ranked the top three in the total number of references.

Table 2. Top 10 institutions with influence.

Institution Name	Total Number of Articles	Total References	Average Cited Times	Total Number of First Authors	Number of Citations of the First Author	Average Citation of the First Author
Univ Tehran Med Sci	107	801	7.49	30	276	9.20
Beijing Normal Univ	56	617	11.02	35	301	8.60
Chinese Acad Sci	215	539	2.51	84	217	2.58
Ahvaz Jundishapur Univ Med Sci	106	437	4.12	20	109	5.45
Univ Kebangsaan Malaysia	64	356	5.56	19	112	5.89
Chinese Res Inst Environm Sci	53	260	4.91	19	171	9.00
Shiraz Univ	25	256	10.24	15	154	10.27
China Univ Geosci	54	211	3.91	26	90	3.46
Zhejiang Univ	30	200	6.67	12	157	13.08
Shahid Beheshti Univ Med Sci	50	184	3.68	3	6	2.00

The top 10 publication titles with influence are shown in Table 3. "Science of the Total Environment", "Ecotoxicology and Environmental Safety", and "Environmental Science and Pollution Research" ranked the top three in the total number of references.

Table 3. Top 10 publication titles with influence.

Publication Titles	Total Number of Articles	Total References	Average Cited Times
Science of the Total Environment	146	742	5.08
Ecotoxicology and Environmental Safety	88	565	6.42
Environmental Science and Pollution Research	147	429	2.92
Chemosphere	80	421	5.26
Human and Ecological Risk Assessment	93	257	2.76
Environmental Geochemistry and Health	90	242	2.69
Atmospheric Environment	43	241	5.60
Environmental Pollution	81	195	2.41
Environment International	41	187	4.56
International Journal of Environmental Research and Public Health	106	179	1.69

The top 10 authors with influence are shown in Table 4. Yousefi M, Mahvi AH and Lu XW ranked the top three in the total number of references.

Table 4. Top 10 authors with influence.

Author	Total Number of Articles	Total References	Average Cited Times	Total Number of First Authors	Number of Citations of the First Author
Yousefi M	15	207	13.8	5	79
Mahvi AH	14	186	13.29	0	0
Lu XW	20	157	7.85	3	31
Keshavarzi B	13	148	11.38	3	71
Nabizadeh R	10	141	14.1	0	0
Radfard M	19	139	7.32	5	37
Teng YG	6	134	22.33	0	0
Rojas-Rueda D	24	127	5.29	3	34
Chen HY	5	127	25.4	2	124
Wang YY	9	125	13.89	1	0

3.5. Keyword Co-Occurrence Analysis

The knowledge map of keyword co-occurrence can suggest hot topics [5]. We made the keyword co-occurrence network from 2012 to 2021, as shown in Figure 7. Hot keywords include "health risk assessment", "source appointment", "contamination", "exposure", "particulate matter", "heavy metals", "urban soils", "spatial-distribution", "pm2.5", "health impact assessment", "polycyclic aromatic-hydrocarbons", "air-pollution", etc.

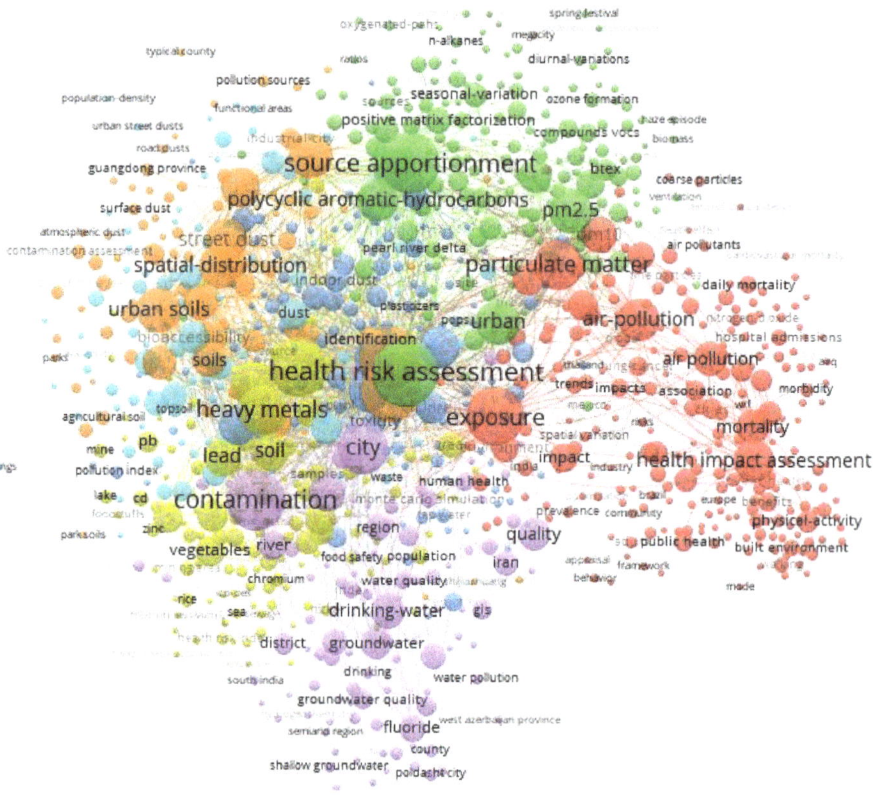

Figure 7. The keyword co-occurrence network.

3.6. Co-Citation Analysis

The co-citation map of references estimated the scientific relevance of publications [23]. Co-citation cluster analysis was used to explore the research patterns, new trends and their relationships in urban HIA research. Timeline visualization in CiteSpace described clusters through a horizontal timeline. Each cluster was displayed in left-to-right order. The largest cluster was shown at the top of the view. Large nodes or nodes with a red tree structure are particularly interesting because they are either highly referenced, have referenced bursts, or both. Below each timeline, the top three references cited in a particular year are displayed [14].

3.6.1. Timeline View (2012–2016)

Based on the literature records from 2012 to 2016, we generated a cited reference map with 458 nodes and 984 links (Figure 8). The results show, the mean silhouette (S = 0.9113) and the modularity (Q = 0.7918), that the modular Q value was greater than 0.7, which indicated that it was reasonable for the network to be divided into loosely coupled clusters.

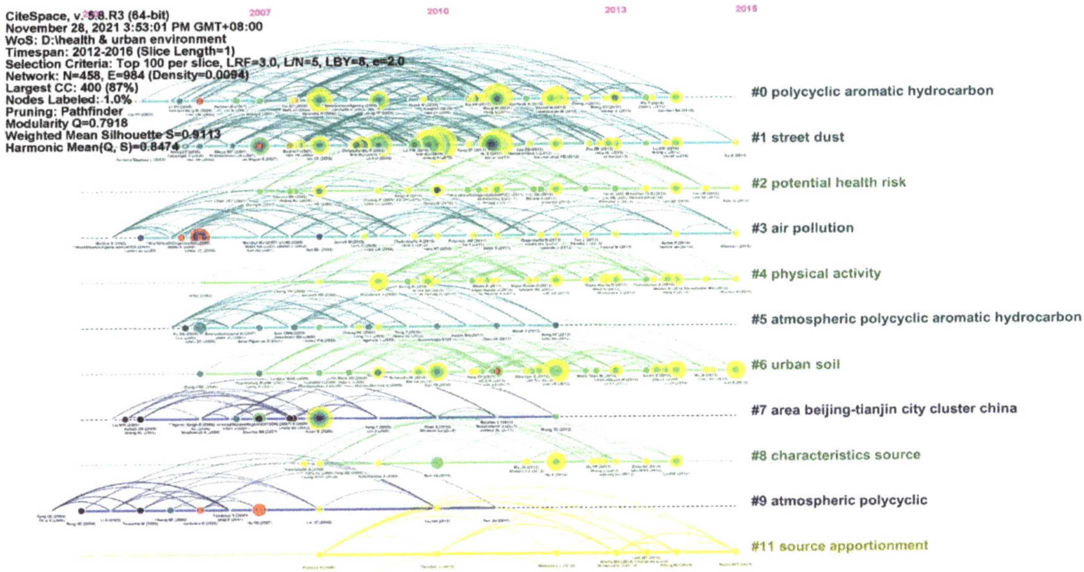

Figure 8. A timeline visualization of clusters on urban HIA research in 2012–2016.

The five salient clusters were sorted by size (Table 5). The literature with high co-citation frequency became a representative publication in the cluster, which affected the annotation of the cluster and revealed the research frontier.

Cluster #0 was the largest cluster and represented "polycyclic aromatic hydrocarbons" with 64 members. In the representative publications, Yu et al. (2014) identified the potential sources of polycyclic aromatic hydrocarbons (PAHs) in 87 urban street dust samples from Tianjin as a Chinese megacity and evaluated the risk of PAHs to urban residents using the incremental lifetime cancer risk model [24].

Cluster #1 represented "street dust" with 58 members. In the representative publications, Lu et al. (2014) applied the potential ecological risk index to assess the risk of heavy metals in street dust of cities in China on urban ecosystems and applied the human exposure model to assess the risk of heavy metals to human health. The authors emphasized that further research on street dust exposure parameters and transportation factors was needed to reduce the uncertainty related to risk calculation [25].

Cluster #2 represented "potential health risk" with 45 members. In the representative publications, Fu et al. (2015) estimated the rice's potential health risk to inhabitants in Fuzhou, China by target hazard quotient (THQ), hazard index (HI) and target cancer risk (TR) [26].

Cluster #3 represented "air pollution" with 42 members. In the representative publications, Lai et al. (2013) systematically evaluated and analyzed the mortality and incidence rate of four typical air pollutants (PM_{10}, NO_2, SO_2, and O_3) in the Chinese population. The authors emphasized that the short-term impact of air pollution could be used for health impact assessment, but the evidence of long-term impact was still insufficient [27].

Cluster #4 represented "physical activity" with 40 members. In the representative publications, Gerike et al. (2016) investigated the determinants of active mobility and the evaluation of measures to increase it through a large-scale longitudinal survey conducted in seven Physical Activity through Sustainable Transport Approaches (PASTA) case study cities. The results would provide data on the health benefits of cycling and/or walking to the WHO's online health economic assessment tool [28].

Table 5. Summary of the largest five clusters in 2012–2016.

Cluster ID	Size	Silhouette	Cluster Label (LLR)	Representative Publication
#0	64	0.894	polycyclic aromatic hydrocarbons	Yu et al. (2014) [24], Jiang et al. (2014) [29], Tuyen et al. (2014) [30], Hoseini et al. (2016) [31], Bulejko et al. (2016) [32], Yue et al. (2015) [33]
#1	58	0.895	street dust	Lu et al. (2014) [25], Han et al. (2016) [34], Sun et al. (2015) [35], Keshavarzi et al. (2015) [36], Han et al. (2016) [37]
#2	45	0.783	potential health risk	Fu et al. (2015) [26], Varol & Davraz (2015) [38], Islam et al. (2015) [39]
#3	42	0.969	air pollution	Lai et al. (2013) [27], Morelli et al. (2016) [40], Arranz et al. (2014) [41], Baccini et al. (2013) [42], Izhar et al. (2016) [43]
#4	40	0.985	physical activity	Gerike et al. (2016) [28], Mansfield & Jacqueline (2015) [44], Gibson et al. (2015) [45], Zapata-Diomedi et al. (2016) [46]

Table 6 lists the detailed information of the top 13 references with strongest citation bursts in 2012–2016. The Sigma metric measures are both citation burstness and structural centrality of a cited reference. Most references were published in top journals.

Table 6. Top 13 references with strongest citation bursts in 2012–2016. The black line represents the year of citation burstness of the paper.

Title	Strength	Begin	End	2012–2016
Use of health impact assessment in the United States: 27 case studies, 1999–2007 (Dannenberg, 2008)	3.87	2012	2013	
Health effects of fine particulate air pollution: Lines that connect (Chow et al., 2006)	3.22	2012	2014	
Seasonal and site-specific variation in vapour and aerosol phase PAHs over Flanders (Belgium) and their relation with anthropogenic activities (Ravindra et al., 2006)	2.25	2012	2014	
Use of health impact assessment in incorporating health considerations in decision making (Davenport et al., 2006)	2.21	2012	2013	
The 2005 world health organization reevaluation of human and mammalian toxic equivalency factors for dioxins and dioxin-like compounds (den Berg et al., 2006)	2.21	2012	2013	
Geochemistry and risk assessment of street dust in Luanda, Angola: A tropical urban environment (Ferreira-Baptista & Migu et al., 2005)	2.21	2012	2013	
Risk-based evaluation of the exposure of children to trace elements in playgrounds in Madrid (Spain) (De Miguel et al., 2007)	2.84	2013	2016	
Health risk assessment for traffic policemen exposed to polycyclic aromatic hydrocarbons (PAHs) in Tianjin, China (Hu et al., 2007)	2.33	2013	2014	
Apheis: Health Impact Assessment of Long-term Exposure to $PM_{2.5}$ in 23 European Cities (Boldo et al., 2006)	1.94	2013	2014	
The status of soil contamination by semivolatile organic chemicals (SVOCs) in China: A review (Cai et al., 2008)	1.94	2013	2014	
Emission of polycyclic aromatic hydrocarbons in China (Xu et al., 2006)	1.94	2013	2014	
Probabilistic risk assessment for personal exposure to carcinogenic polycyclic aromatic hydrocarbons in Taiwanese temples (Liao et al., 2006)	1.94	2013	2014	
Distribution, availability and sources of trace metals in different particle size fractions of urban soils in Hong Kong: Implications for assessing the risk to human health (Luo et al., 2011)	1.95	2014	2016	

3.6.2. Timeline View (2017–2021)

Based on the literature records from 2017 to 2021, we generated a cited reference map with 888 nodes and 1470 links (Figure 9). The results show that with the mean silhouette (S = 0.9258) and the modularity (Q = 0.7937), the modular Q value was greater than 0.7, which indicated that it was reasonable for the network to be divided into loosely coupled clusters.

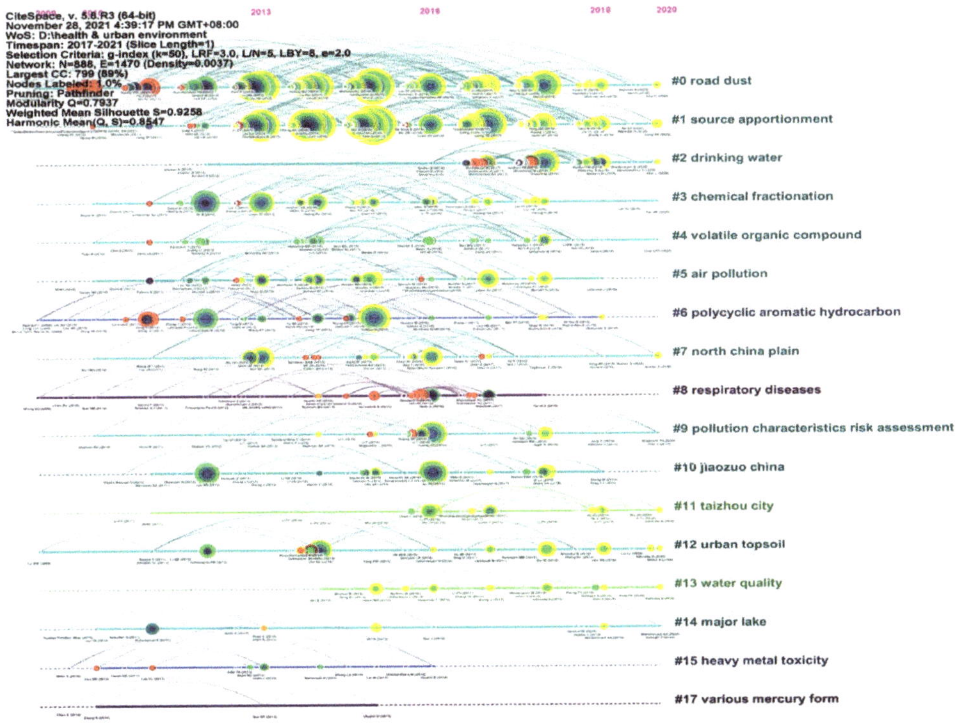

Figure 9. A timeline visualization of clusters on urban HIA research in 2017–2021.

The nine salient clusters were sorted by size (Table 7). The literature with high co-citation frequency became a representative publication in the cluster, which affected the annotation of the cluster and revealed the research frontier.

Cluster #0 represented "road dust" with 121 members. In the representative publications, Moryani et al. (2020) evaluated the pollution level of heavy metals (Cu, Pb, Zn, CD, Ni, Sb, Cr) in five parts of road dust in four different regions of Karachi and Shikarpur by calculating the pollution index enrichment factor and Igeo; the health risk assessment was carried out according to the carcinogenic risk methods and hazard index [47].

Cluster #1 represented "source apportionment" with 119 members. In the representative publications, Cai et al. (2019) studied the levels, distribution, and source apportionment of metals in soils from a typical rapidly developing county, Southern China [48].

Cluster #2 represented "drinking water" with 68 members. In the representative publications, Hamed et al. (2018) assessed the nitrate concentration and also the microbial quality of bottled water in a number of brands produced in the Torbat-e Heydarieh city in 2017 [49].

Cluster #3 represented "chemical fractionation" with 63 members. In the representative publications, Sah et al. (2019) identified the migration potential of metals (As, Cd, Co, Cr, Ni, and Pb) in urban fine particulate matter and assessed the health risks of these metals to infants, young children, children, males, and females. The research conclusions showed that urban aerosols have potential risks to humans [50].

Cluster #4 represented "volatile organic compounds" with 61 members. In the representative publications, Gu et al. (2020) analyzed the chemical characteristics and sources of volatile organic compounds (VOCs) in Tianjin, China, using 1-h resolution VOC-species data between 1 November 2018 and 15 March 2019 [51].

Cluster #5 represented "air pollution" with 52 members. In the representative publications, Lehtomaki et al. (2020) quantified the number of deaths caused by ambient air pollution in Nordic countries using selected assessment tools, identified the main differences and stressed that high spatial resolution should be used to avoid underestimating the health effects of ambient air pollution [52].

Cluster #6 represented "polycyclic aromatic hydrocarbons" with 46 members. In the representative publications, Najmeddin and Keshavarzi (2019) used toxic equivalency factors and increased lifetime cancer risk to assess the health risk of PAHs in PM_{10} and road dust samples [53].

Cluster #7 represented "north China plain" with 45 members. In the representative publications, Zhang et al. (2019) evaluated the potential health risks of PAHs (including gas and particle phases) by combining methods of benzo[a]pyrene equivalent concentration and incremental lifetime cancer risk and identified the potential source regions of $PM_{2.5}$-bound PAHs in Jinan by the Concentration Weighted Trajectory model [54].

Cluster #8 represented "respiratory diseases" with 37 members. In the representative publications, Geravandi et al. (2017) studied the relationship between the number of hospitalized respiratory diseases (including asthma attacks, acute bronchitis, and chronic obstructive pulmonary disease) caused by PM_{10} and normal/dust event days in Ahvaz, Iran, from 2010 to 2012 [55].

Table 7. Summary of the largest nine clusters in 2017–2021.

Cluster ID	Size	Silhouette	Cluster Label (LLR)	Representative Publication
#0	121	0.847	road dust	Moryani et al. (2020) [47], Faisal et al. (2021) [56], Chen et al. (2019) [57], Ahamad et al. (2021) [58], Shabanda et al. (2019) [59], Mondal & Singh (2021) [60], Jiang et al. (2018) [61], Othman & Latif (2020) [62], Heidari et al. (2021) [63], Shahab et al. (2020) [64], Wang et al. (2021) [65]
#1	119	0.874	source apportionment	Cai et al. (2019) [48], Duan et al. (2020) [66], Zhang et al. (2021) [67], Li et al. (2021) [68], Sun et al. (2020) [69], Tang et al. (2020) [70]
#2	68	0.982	drinking water	Hamed et al. (2018) [49], Qasemi et al. (2019) [71], Badeenezhad et al. (2021) [72], Radfard et al. (2019) [73], Mirzabeygi et al. (2018) [74]
#3	63	0.962	chemical fractionation	Sah et al. (2019) [50], Long et al. (2021) [75], Jan et al. (2018) [76], Guo et al. (2021) [77], Jiang et al. (2020) [78]
#4	61	0.971	volatile organic compounds	Gu et al. (2020) [51], Li et al. (2020) [79], Ding et al. (2020) [80], Tohid et al. (2019) [81], Xiong et al. (2020) [82], Wang et al. (2020) [83], Li et al. (2020) [84]
#5	52	0.967	air pollution	Lehtomaki et al. (2020) [52], Izquierdo et al. (2020) [85], Luo et al. (2020) [86], Giallouros et al. (2020) [87], Sacks et al. (2018) [88], Sohrabi et al. (2020) [89], Khomenko et al. (2021) [90], Gamarra et al. (2021) [91]
#6	46	0.970	polycyclic aromatic hydrocarbons	Najmeddin et al. (2019) [53], Abbasnejad et al. (2019) [92], Najmeddin et al. (2018) [93], Qishlaqi & Beiramali (2019) [94], Liang et al. (2019) [95]
#7	45	0.904	north China plain	Zhang et al. (2019) [54], Shen et al. (2019) [96], Zhang et al. (2019) [97], Luo et al. (2021) [98], Gao et al. (2019) [99]
#8	37	0.969	respiratory diseases	Geravandi et al. (2017) [55], Khaniabadi et al. (2017) [100]

Table 8 lists the detailed information of the top 30 references with strongest citation bursts in 2017–2021. There are 85 references with the strongest citation bursts in 2017–2021, we chose 30 representative references. The citation burstness and structural centrality of the cited references can be measured by Sigma metric. The early foundational documents and these 85 highly cited documents together constitute the intellectual base of urban HIA research in 2017–2021.

Table 8. Top 30 references with strongest citation bursts in 2017–2021. The black line represents the year of citation burstness of the paper.

Title	Strength	Begin	End	2012–2021
Health risk assessment of heavy metal exposure to street dust in the zinc smelting district, Northeast of China (Zheng et al., 2010)	16.11	2017	2018	
A review of heavy metal contaminations in urban soils, urban road dusts and agricultural soils from China (Wei et al., 2010)	12.64	2017	2018	
Multivariate statistical analysis of heavy metals in street dust of Baoji, NW China (Lu et al., 2010)	9.56	2017	2018	
Study of ground-level ozone and its health risk assessment in residents in Ahvaz City, Iran during 2013 (Yari et al., 2016)	6.88	2017	2018	
Health risk assessment of abandoned agricultural soils based on heavy metal contents in Hong Kong, the world's most populated city (Luo et al., 2011)	6.49	2017	2018	
A comparative study of health risk of potentially toxic metals in urban and suburban road dust in the most populated city of China (Shi et al., 2011)	5.97	2017	2019	
Polycyclic aromatic hydrocarbons (PAHs) in urban surface dust of Guangzhou, China: Status, sources and human health risk assessment (Wang et al., 2011)	5.46	2017	2019	
Bioaccessibility and health risk of arsenic, mercury and other metals in urban street dusts from a mega-city, Nanjing, China (Hu et al., 2011)	5.46	2017	2019	
Integrating hierarchical bioavailability and population distribution into potential eco-risk assessment of heavy metals in road dust: A case study in Xiandao District, Changsha city, China (Huang et al., 2016)	5.35	2017	2018	
An evaluation of hospital admission respiratory disease attributed to sulfur dioxide ambient concentration in Ahvaz from 2011 through 2013 (Goudarzi et al., 2016)	4.96	2017	2018	
Heavy metals exposure of children from stairway and sidewalk dust in the smelting district, northeast of China (Zheng et al., 2010)	4.96	2017	2018	
Polycyclic aromatic hydrocarbons in urban soils of Beijing: Status, sources, distribution and potential risk (Peng et al., 2011)	4.94	2017	2019	
Multivariate and geostatistical analyses of the spatial distribution and sources of heavy metals in agricultural soil in Dehui, Northeast China (Sun et al., 2013)	4.58	2017	2018	
Exposure to PM_{10}, NO_2 and O_3 and impacts on human health (Khaniabadi et al., 2017)	4.2	2017	2018	
Cardiovascular and respiratory mortality attributed to ground-level ozone in Ahvaz, Iran (Goudarzi et al., 2015)	4.2	2017	2018	
Impact of Middle Eastern Dust storms on human health (Khaniabadi et al., 2017)	4.2	2017	2018	
Heavy metal contamination and health risk assessment in drinking water of Sistan and Baluchistan, Southeastern Iran (Mirzabeygi et al., 2017)	5.18	2018	2019	
The concentration data of fluoride and health risk assessment in drinking water in the Ardakan city of Yazd province, Iran (Mirzabeygi et al., 2018)	4.75	2018	2019	
Drinking water quality and human health risk in Charsadda district, Pakistan (Khan et al., 2013)	3.16	2018	2019	
Risk assessment and implication of human exposure to road dust heavy metals in Jeddah, Saudi Arabia (Shabbaj et al., 2018)	3.16	2018	2019	
Association of Hypertension, Body Mass Index and Waist Circumference with Fluoride Intake; Water Drinking in Residents of Fluoride Endemic Areas, Iran (Yousefi et al., 2018)	3.16	2018	2019	

Table 8. *Cont.*

Title	Strength	Begin	End	2012–2021
Source apportionment of atmospheric $PM_{2.5}$-bound polycyclic aromatic hydrocarbons by a PMF receptor model. Assessment of potential risk for human health (Callen et al., 2014)	2.87	2018	2019	
Sources identification of heavy metals in urban topsoil from inside the Xi'an Second Ringroad, NW China using multivariate statistical methods (Chen et al., 2012)	2.87	2018	2019	
Levels, sources and health risks of carbonyls and BTEX in the ambient air of Beijing, China (Zhango et al., 2012)	3.53	2019	2021	
Spatial variation and probabilistic risk assessment of exposure to fluoride in drinking water (Fallahzadeh et al., 2018)	3.31	2019	2021	
Probabilistic risk assessment of Chinese residents' exposure to fluoride in improved drinking water in endemic fluorosis areas (Zhang et al., 2017)	3.09	2019	2021	
Investigation of outdoor BTEX: Concentration, variations, sources, spatial distribution and risk assessment (Miri et al., 2016)	3.09	2019	2021	
Inhalation exposure and related health risks of BTEX in ambient air at different microenvironments of a terai zone in north India (Masih et al., 2016)	2.87	2019	2021	
Pollution, ecological-health risks and sources of heavy metals in soil of the northeastern Qinghai-Tibet Plateau (Wu et al., 2018)	2.65	2019	2021	
Trends of BTEX in the central urban area of Iran: A preliminary study of photochemical ozone pollution and health risk assessment (Hajizadeh et al., 2018)	2.2	2019	2021	

3.7. Structural Variation Analysis (SVA)

3.7.1. Articles with Transformative Potentials

The main limitation of citation-based indicators is that they may ignore newly published articles. SVA is a method to focus on the impact of newly published papers on the conceptual structure of related knowledge fields [101]. The SVA program looks for new connections that may change the global structure [102]. The purpose of applying SVA is to evaluate the potential of an article to establish abnormal or unexpected connections between different clusters. From the perspective of scientific discovery theory, many significant contributions come from the idea of crossing borders [14]. To assess the recent papers' transformative potentials, we used the SVA of CiteSpace—we used 3-year span sliding windows. Table 9 shows a list of articles with a high transformative potential based on the ΔModularity and ΔCluster Linkage.

Table 9. Some of the articles with the strongest transformative potentials, M is ΔModularity, C-L is for ΔCluster Linkage, C-D is for ΔCentrality Divergence.

Year	M	C-L	C-D	Title
2020	98.94	21.2	0.31	The effects of urban vehicle traffic on heavy metal contamination in road sweeping waste and bottom sediments of retention tanks (Nawrot et al., 2020)
2020	98.87	33.48	0.06	Contamination characteristics of heavy metals in particle size fractions from street dust from an industrial city, Central China (Zhong et al., 2020)
2020	98.27	75.03	0.06	Pollution, sources and human health risk assessment of potentially toxic elements in different land use types under the background of industrial cities (Xia et al., 2020)
2020	97.99	19.56	0.06	Characteristics and health risk assessment of heavy metals in street dust for children in Jinhua, China (Bartholomew et al., 2020)
2020	97.87	59.56	0.06	Pollution characteristics and toxicity of potentially toxic elements in road dust of a tourist city, Guilin, China: Ecological and health risk assessment (Shahab et al., 2020)

Table 9. *Cont.*

Year	M	C-L	C-D	Title
2020	97.46	15.64	0.08	Geostatistical mapping and quantitative source apportionment of potentially toxic elements in top- and sub-soils: A case of suburban area in Beijing, China (Duan et al., 2020)
2020	97.4	9.11	0.08	Spatial distribution of pollution characteristics and human health risk assessment of exposure to heavy elements in road dust from different functional areas of Zhengzhou, China (Wang et al., 2020)
2020	97.16	10.86	0.07	Hazard, ecological and human health risk assessment of heavy metals in street dust in Dezful, Iran (Sadeghdoust et al., 2020)
2021	97.13	−14.03	0.10	Potentially toxic elements in soil and road dust around Sonbhadra industrial region, Uttar Pradesh, India: Source apportionment and health risk assessment (Ahamad et al., 2021)
2020	97.11	12.5	0.06	Pollution status and human health risk assessment of potentially toxic elements and polycyclic aromatic hydrocarbons in urban street dust of Tyumen city, Russia (Konstantinova et al., 2020)
2021	96.88	−17.27	0.03	Contamination and health risk assessment of potentially harmful elements associated with roadside dust in Dhanbad India (Patel and Jain, 2021)
2021	96.75	−18.19	0.02	Heavy metals in indoor dust across China: Occurrence, sources and health risk assessment (Liu et al., 2021)
2021	96.62	−20.82	0.04	A comprehensive exploration of risk assessment and source quantification of potentially toxic elements in road dust: A case study from a large Cu smelter in central China (Wang et al., 2021)
2021	96.62	−17.14	0.01	Risk and sources of heavy metals and metalloids in dust from university campuses: A case study of Xi'an, China (Fan et al., 2021)
2020	96.57	25.28	0.08	Pollution characteristics, sources and health risk assessments of urban road dust in Kuala Lumpur City (Othman and Latif, 2020)
2021	96.49	−14.5	0.01	Pollution effect assessment of industrial activities on potentially toxic metal distribution in windowsill dust and surface soil in central China (Han et al., 2021)
2021	96.41	−25.84	0	Heavy metal pollution of road dust in a city and its highly polluted suburb; quantitative source apportionment and source-specific ecological and health risk assessment (Heidari et al., 2021)
2021	96.33	−14.85	0.04	Spatio-temporal distribution and source identification of heavy metals in particle size fractions of road dust from a typical industrial district (Zhu et al., 2021)
2021	95.71	−17.24	0.01	Contamination, distribution and health risk assessment of risk elements in topsoil for amusement parks in Xi'an, China (Guo et al., 2021)
2021	95.58	−9.36	0.04	Urban street dust in the Middle East oldest oil refinery zone: Oxidative potential, source apportionment and health risk assessment of potentially toxic elements (Naraki et al., 2021)
2021	94.97	−13.77	0.06	Water quality and health risk assessment based on hydrochemical characteristics of tap and large-size bottled water from the main cities and towns in Guanzhong Basin, China (Deng et al., 2021)
2021	94.77	−28.26	0.01	Human health risk assessment of heavy metals in the urban road dust of Zhengzhou metropolis, China (Faisal et al., 2021)
2021	94.75	−14.34	0.08	Pollution evaluation, human health effect and tracing source of trace elements on road dust of Dhanbad, a highly polluted industrial coal belt of India (Mondal and Singh, 2021)
2021	92.61	−30.86	0.08	Status, spatial distribution and health risk assessment of potentially harmful element from road dust in steel industry city, China (Wang et al., 2021)
2021	91.84	−17.22	0.01	Pollution, human health risk assessment and spatial distribution of toxic metals in urban soil of Yazd City, Iran (Soltani-Gerdefaramarzi et al., 2021)

3.7.2. Trajectories of Citations across Cluster Boundaries

There were six examples of articles with high modularity change rates, as shown in Figure 10. The visualization reveals the distribution of the references cited by these articles across different clusters.

(1) Zhong et al. (2020) analyzed two particle size distributions of heavy metals in street dust from an industrial city, explored their possible sources and assessed their health

risks [103]. The papers cited in this paper are mainly distributed in clusters #0, #1, #9, #10, and #12.

(2) Xia et al. (2020) explored the source of six potentially toxic elements (PTEs) in topsoil of three different land use types (residential land, industrial land, and farmland) in Tonghua City and evaluated the ecological risk and human health risk of PTEs in different types of soil [104]. The papers cited in this paper are mainly distributed in clusters #0, #1, #10, and #12.

(3) Shahab et al. (2020) evaluated the pollution level and health risk from heavy metals in road dust collected in three functional areas in the tourist city Guilin using the geoaccumulation index (Igeo), ecological risk index, spatial interpolation, and array-based risk assessment model [64]. The papers cited in this paper are mainly distributed in clusters #0, #1, #12 and #15.

(4) Ahamad et al. (2021) identified the sources of potentially toxic elements (As, Cd, Cr, Cu, Fe, Hg, Mn, Ni, Pb, Zn) of 48 samples of soil and road dust from industrial clusters in the Sonbhadra region of Uttar Pradesh (India) and assessed their human health risks [58]. The papers cited in this paper are mainly distributed in clusters #0, #1, #9 and #14.

(5) Wang et al. (2021) evaluated the pollution characteristics and spatial distribution characteristics of 12 PTEs (Mn, Ni, Cu, Zn, Hg, Cd, As, Cr, Pb, Tl, Co, and Sb) in a large copper smelter in Central China and evaluated the potential ecological and health risks of PTEs by combining with positive matrix decomposition [105]. The papers cited in this paper are mainly distributed in clusters #0, #1, #2, #6, #9, and #12.

(6) Heidari et al. (2021) assessed the related specific source-ecological and health risks of heavy metals (As, Cd, Co, Cr, Cu, Mn, Ni, Pb, and Zn) in road dust in Bandar Abbas (Iran) and its western suburb [63]. The papers cited in this paper are mainly distributed in clusters #0, #1, #3, #5, and #6.

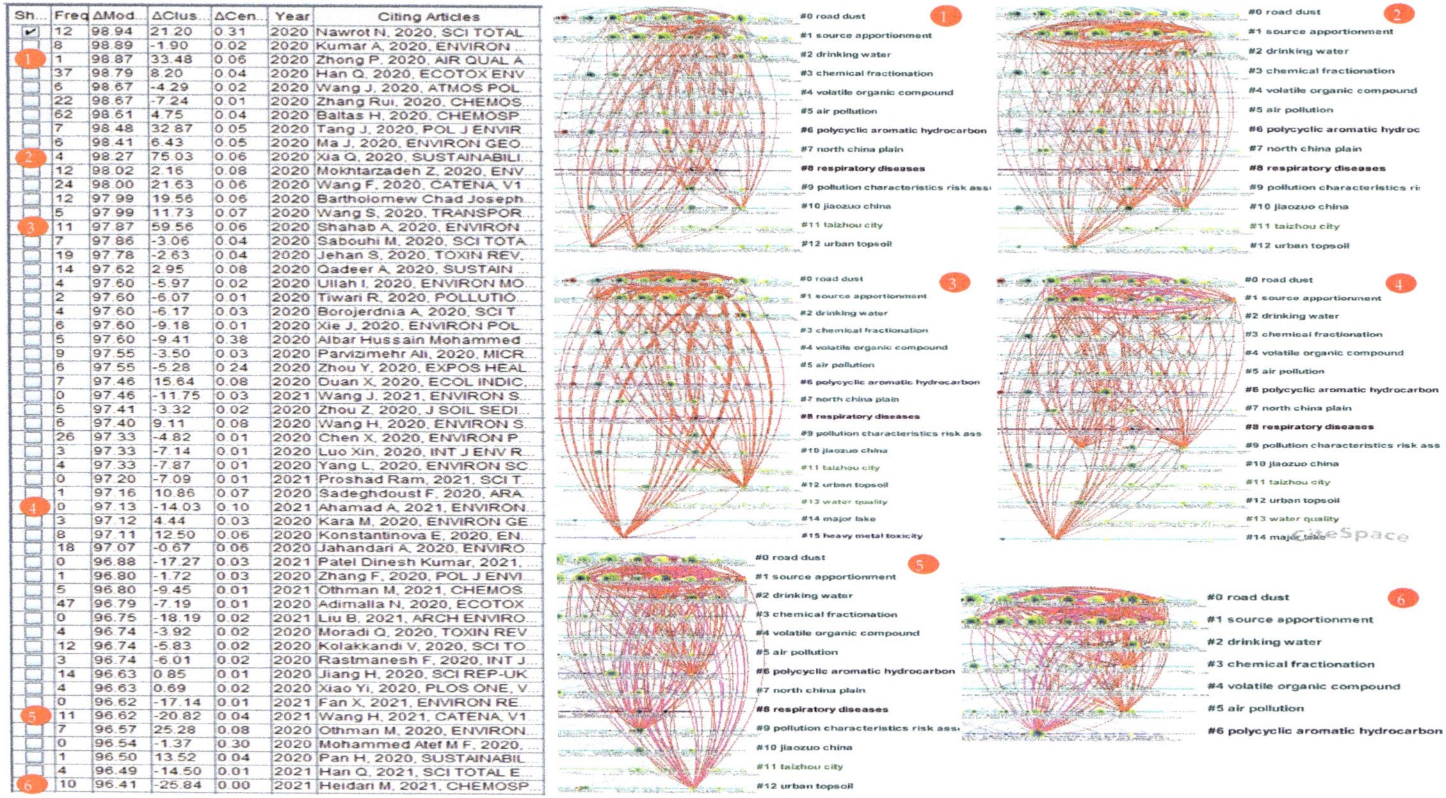

Sh...	Freq	ΔMod...	ΔClus...	ΔCen...	Year	Citing Articles
✓	12	98.94	21.20	0.31	2020	Nawrot N, 2020, SCI TOTAL ...
	8	98.89	-1.90	0.02	2020	Kumar A, 2020, ENVIRON ...
1	1	98.87	33.48	0.06	2020	Zhong P, 2020, AIR QUAL A...
	37	98.79	8.20	0.04	2020	Han Q, 2020, ECOTOX ENV...
	6	98.67	-4.29	0.02	2020	Wang J, 2020, ATMOS POL...
	22	98.67	-7.24	0.01	2020	Zhang Rui, 2020, CHEMOS...
	62	98.61	4.75	0.04	2020	Baltas H, 2020, CHEMOSP...
	7	98.48	32.87	0.05	2020	Tang J, 2020, POL J ENVIR...
	6	98.41	6.43	0.05	2020	Ma J, 2020, ENVIRON GEO...
2	4	98.27	75.03	0.06	2020	Xia Q, 2020, SUSTAINABILI...
	12	98.02	2.16	0.08	2020	Mokhtarzadeh Z, 2020, ENV...
	24	98.00	21.63	0.06	2020	Wang F, 2020, CATENA, V1...
	12	97.99	19.56	0.06	2020	Bartholomew Chad Joseph...
	5	97.99	11.73	0.07	2020	Wang S, 2020, TRANSPOR...
3	11	97.87	59.56	0.06	2020	Shahab A, 2020, ENVIRON ...
	7	97.86	-3.06	0.04	2020	Sabouhi M, 2020, SCI TOTA...
	19	97.78	-2.63	0.04	2020	Jehan S, 2020, TOXIN REV,...
	14	97.62	2.95	0.08	2020	Qadeer A, 2020, SUSTAIN ...
	4	97.60	-5.97	0.02	2020	Ullah I, 2020, ENVIRON MO...
	2	97.60	-6.07	0.01	2020	Tiwari R, 2020, POLLUTIO...
	4	97.60	-6.17	0.03	2020	Borojerdnia A, 2020, SCI T...
	6	97.60	-9.18	0.01	2020	Xie J, 2020, ENVIRON POL...
	5	97.60	-9.41	0.38	2020	Albar Hussain Mohammed ...
	9	97.55	-3.50	0.03	2020	Parvizimehr Ali, 2020, MICR...
	6	97.55	-5.28	0.24	2020	Zhou Y, 2020, EXPOS HEAL...
	7	97.46	15.64	0.08	2020	Duan X, 2020, ECOL INDIC,...
	0	97.46	-11.75	0.03	2021	Wang J, 2021, ENVIRON S...
	5	97.41	-3.32	0.02	2020	Zhou Z, 2020, J SOIL SEDI...
	6	97.40	9.11	0.08	2020	Wang H, 2020, ENVIRON S...
	26	97.33	-4.82	0.01	2020	Chen X, 2020, ENVIRON P...
	3	97.33	-7.14	0.01	2020	Luo Xin, 2020, INT J ENV R...
	4	97.33	-7.87	0.01	2020	Yang L, 2020, ENVIRON SC...
	0	97.20	-7.09	0.01	2021	Proshad Ram, 2021, SCI T...
	1	97.16	10.86	0.07	2020	Sadeghdoust F, 2020, ARA...
4	0	97.13	-14.03	0.10	2021	Ahamad A, 2021, ENVIRON...
	3	97.12	4.44	0.03	2020	Kara M, 2020, ENVIRON GE...
	8	97.11	12.50	0.06	2020	Konstantinova E, 2020, EN...
	18	97.07	-0.67	0.06	2020	Jahandari A, 2020, ENVIRO...
	0	96.88	-17.27	0.03	2021	Patel Dinesh Kumar, 2021, ...
	1	96.80	-1.72	0.03	2020	Zhang F, 2020, POL J ENVI...
	5	96.80	-9.45	0.01	2021	Othman M, 2021, CHEMOS...
	47	96.79	-7.19	0.01	2020	Adimalla N, 2020, ECOTOX ...
	0	96.75	-18.19	0.02	2021	Liu B, 2021, ARCH ENVIRO...
	4	96.74	-3.92	0.02	2020	Moradi Q, 2020, TOXIN REV...
	12	96.74	-5.83	0.02	2020	Kolakkandi V, 2020, SCI TO...
	3	96.74	-6.01	0.02	2020	Rastmanesh F, 2020, INT J...
	14	96.63	0.85	0.01	2020	Jiang H, 2020, SCI REP-UK...
	4	96.63	0.69	0.02	2020	Xiao Yi, 2020, PLOS ONE, V...
	0	96.62	-17.14	0.01	2021	Fan X, 2021, ENVIRON RE...
5	11	96.62	-20.82	0.04	2021	Wang H, 2021, CATENA, V1...
	7	96.57	25.28	0.08	2020	Othman M, 2020, ENVIRON...
	0	96.54	-1.37	0.30	2020	Mohammed Atef M F, 2020, ...
	1	96.50	13.52	0.04	2020	Pan H, 2020, SUSTAINABIL...
	4	96.49	-14.50	0.01	2021	Han Q, 2021, SCI TOTAL E...
6	10	96.41	-25.84	0.00	2021	Heidari M, 2021, CHEMOSP...

Figure 10. Six examples of articles with high modularity change rates.

4. Discussions

The limitations of this study are shown as follows:

First, the data only comes from English papers in the WoS Core Collection, resulting in the exclusion of a large number of English documents in Scopus, PubMed/Medline and other databases, as well as a large number of documents in other language countries [106]. It is necessary to conduct bibliometric analysis of urban HIA related literature in other databases and urban HIA related literature in other languages [107], so as to grasp the global research progress more comprehensively on urban HIA.

Second, as urban HIA is a global topic, the situation of each country is different, so the research content may also be different. In the future, we can select country samples for comparative research, so as to understand the research progress of various countries in the field of urban HIA.

Finally, due to the limitation of the software itself, in the co-citation analysis, some important research topics in the field of urban HIA might have been omitted, for example, the urban HIA practice issues [1,2,108–110] and HIA in urban planning [111–113]. These important research topics should be employed in a bibliometric analysis in the future.

5. Conclusions

This paper used the bibliometric method to analyze the trends, issues and future directions of urban HIA research. We advance the following main conclusions:

First, the main research directions in the field were Environmental Sciences and Public Environmental Occupational Health.

Second, China contributed most articles; the Univ Tehran Med Sci was the most influential institution; Science of the Total Environment was the most influential journal; Yousefi M was the most influential author.

Third, the main hotspots included health risk assessment, source appointment, contamination, exposure, particulate matter, heavy metals and urban soils in 2012–2021.

Fourth, the road dust, source apposition, PAHs, air pollution, urban topsoil and north China plain were always hot research topics in 2012–2021. Drinking water and water quality became research topics of great concern in 2017–2021.

Finally, there were 25 articles with strong transformation potential during 2020–2021, but most papers carried out research on health risk assessment of toxic elements in soil and dust.

Author Contributions: Conceptualization, W.L. and Z.D.; methodology, M.D. and S.Z.; formal analysis, S.Z.; data curation, Z.D. and M.D.; writing—original draft preparation, M.D., S.Z. and W.L.; writing—review and editing, W.L. and S.Z.; funding acquisition, W.L. All authors have read and agreed to the published version of the manuscript.

Funding: This study was supported by the National Social Science Foundation of China (20BGL201) and Hunan Provincial Natural Science Foundation of China (2021JJ30281).

Institutional Review Board Statement: Not applicable.

Informed Consent Statement: Not applicable.

Data Availability Statement: Not applicable.

Conflicts of Interest: The authors declare no conflict of interest.

References

1. Cave, B.; Pyper, R.; Fischerbonde, B.; Humboldtdachroeden, S.; Martinolmedo, P. Lessons from an international initiative to set and share good practice on human health in environmental impact assessment. *Int. J. Environ. Res. Public Health* **2021**, *18*, 1392. [CrossRef] [PubMed]
2. Winkler, M.S.; Furu, P.; Viliani, F.; Cave, B.; Divall, M.; Ramesh, G.; Harris-Roxas, B.; Knoblauch, A.M. Current global health impact assessment practice. *Int. J. Environ. Res. Public Health* **2020**, *17*, 2988. [CrossRef] [PubMed]
3. Simos, J.; Arrizabalaga, P. Using the synergies between strategic environmental evaluation and hia to advance the integration of environmental and health issues in public decision-making processes. *Soz.-Und Prav.* **2006**, *51*, 133. [CrossRef] [PubMed]

4. Yoo, W.S.; Kim, K.Y.; Koh, K.W. Introduction of health impact assessment and healthy cities as a tool for tackling health inequality. *J. Prev. Med. Public Health* **2007**, *40*, 439. [CrossRef]
5. Harris, P.; Harris-Roxas, B.; Wise, M.; Harris, L. Health impact assessment for urban and land-use planning and policy development: Lessons from practice. *Socioecol. Pract. Res.* **2010**, *25*, 531–541. [CrossRef]
6. Hoshiko, M.; Hara, K.; Ishitake, T. Assessing the validity of health impact assessment predictions regarding a Japanese city's transition to core city status: A monitoring review. *Public Health* **2012**, *126*, 168–176. [CrossRef]
7. Forsyth, A.; Slotterback, C.S.; Krizek, K. Health impact assessment (hia) for planners: What tools are useful? *Urb. Plan. Int.* **2016**, *24*, 231–245. [CrossRef]
8. Boldo, E.; Medina, S.; Tertre, A.L.; Hurley, F.; Mücke, H.G.; Ballester, F.; Aguilera, I. Apheis: Health impact assessment of long-term exposure to $PM_{2.5}$ in 23 European cities. *Eur. J. Epidemiol.* **2006**, *21*, 449–458. [CrossRef]
9. Bacigalupe, A.; Esnaola, S.; Calderon, C.; Zuazagoitia, J.; Aldasoro, E. Health impact assessment of an urban regeneration project: Opportunities and challenges in the context of a southern European city. *J. Epidemiol. Commun. Health* **2010**, *64*, 950–955. [CrossRef]
10. Keuken, M.; Zandveld, P.; Elshout, S.; Janssen, N.; Hoek, G. Air quality and health impact of PM_{10} and EC in the city of Rotterdam, the Netherlands in 1985–2008. *Atmos. Environ.* **2011**, *45*, 5294–5301. [CrossRef]
11. Kheirbek, I.; Wheeler, K.; Walters, S.; Kass, D.; Matte, T. $PM_{2.5}$ and ozone health impacts and disparities in New York city: Sensitivity to spatial and temporal resolution. *Air Qual. Atmos. Health* **2013**, *6*, 473–486. [CrossRef] [PubMed]
12. Fatima, B.; Nichole, M.C.; Rezak, A.; Isabella, A.M. Short-term health impact assessment of urban PM_{10} in Bejaia city (Algeria). *Can. Respir. J.* **2016**, *2016*, 8209485.
13. Aleixandre-Benavent, R.; Aleixandre-Tudó, J.L.; Castelló-Cogollos, L.; Aleixandre, J.L. Trends in scientific research on climate change in agriculture and forestry subject areas (2005–2014). *J. Clean. Prod.* **2017**, *147*, 406–418. [CrossRef]
14. Chen, C. Science mapping: A systematic review of the literature. *J. Data Inf. Sci.* **2017**, *2*, 1–40. [CrossRef]
15. Shi, Y.; Liu, X. Research on the literature of green building based on the web of science: A scientometric analysis in CiteSpace (2002–2018). *Sustainability* **2019**, *11*, 3716. [CrossRef]
16. Xiong, K.; Kukec, A.; Rumrich, I.K.; Rejc, T.; Hnninen, O. Methods of health risk and impact assessment at industrially contaminated sites: A systematic review. *Epidemiol. Prev.* **2018**, *42*, 49–58.
17. Hood, W.W.; Wilson, C.S. The literature of bibliometrics, scientometrics, and informetrics. *Scientometrics* **2001**, *52*, 291–314. [CrossRef]
18. Ellegaard, O.; Wallin, J.A. The bibliometric analysis of scholarly production: How great is the impact? *Scientometrics* **2015**, *105*, 1809–1831. [CrossRef]
19. Liu, W.; Wang, J.; Li, C.; Chen, B.; Sun, Y. Using bibliometric analysis to understand the recent progress in agroecosystem services research. *Ecol. Econ.* **2019**, *156*, 293–305. [CrossRef]
20. Zhao, D.; Strotmann, A. Analysis and visualization of citation networks. *Synth. Lect. Inf. Concepts Retr. Serv.* **2015**, *7*, 207. [CrossRef]
21. Uddin, S.; Khan, A.; Baur, L.A. A Framework to Explore the Knowledge Structure of Multidisciplinary Research Fields. *PLoS ONE* **2015**, *10*, e0123537. [CrossRef] [PubMed]
22. Yi, Y.; Luo, J.; Wübbenhorst, M. Research on political instability, uncertainty and risk during 1953–2019: A scientometric review. *Scientometrics* **2020**, *123*, 1051–1076. [CrossRef]
23. Ma, X.; Zhang, L.; Wang, J.; Luo, Y. Knowledge domain and emerging trends on echinococcosis research: A scientometric analysis. *Int. J. Environ. Res. Public Health* **2019**, *16*, 842. [CrossRef] [PubMed]
24. Yu, B.; Xie, X.; Ma, L.; Kan, H.; Zhou, Q. Source, distribution, and health risk assessment of polycyclic aromatic hydrocarbons in urban street dust from Tianjin, China. *Environ. Sci. Pollut. Res. Int.* **2014**, *21*, 2817–2825. [CrossRef]
25. Lu, X.; Xing, W.; Wang, Y.; Hao, C.; Gao, P.; Yi, F. Risk assessment of toxic metals in street dust from a medium-sized industrial city of China. *Ecotoxicol. Environ. Saf.* **2014**, *106*, 154–163. [CrossRef]
26. Fu, Q.; Li, L.; Achal, V.; Jiao, A.; Liu, Y. Concentrations of heavy metals and arsenic in market rice grain and their potential health risks to the population of Fuzhou, China. *Hum. Ecol. Risk Assess. Int. J.* **2015**, *21*, 117–128. [CrossRef]
27. Lai, H.K.; Tsang, H.; Wong, M. Meta-analysis of adverse health effects due to air pollution in Chinese populations. *BMC Public Health* **2013**, *13*, 360. [CrossRef]
28. Gerike, R.; Nazelle, A.D.; Nieuwenhuijsen, M.; Panis, L.I.; Götschi, T.; Anaya, E.; Avila-Palencia, I.; Boschetti, F.; Brand, C.; Dons, E. Tom Cole-HunterPhysical activity through sustainable transport approaches (Pasta): A study protocol for a multicentre project. *BMJ Open* **2016**, *6*, e009924. [CrossRef]
29. Jiang, Y.; Hu, X.; Yves, U.J.; Zhan, H.; Wu, Y. Status, source and health risk assessment of polycyclic aromatic hydrocarbons in street dust of an industrial city, NW China. *Ecotoxicol. Environ. Saf.* **2014**, *106*, 11–18. [CrossRef]
30. Tuyen, L.H.; Tue, N.M.; Takahashi, S.; Suzuki, G.; Viet, P.H.; Subramanian, A.; Bulbule, K.A.; Parthasarathy, P.; Ramanathan, A.; Tanabe, S.; et al. Methylated and unsubstituted polycyclic aromatic hydrocarbons in street dust from Vietnam and India: Occurrence, distribution and in vitro toxicity evaluation. *Environ. Pollut.* **2014**, *194*, 272–280. [CrossRef]
31. Hoseini, M.; Yunesian, M.; Nabizadeh, R.; Yaghmaeian, K.; Ahmadkhaniha, R.; Rastkari, N.; Parmy, S.; Faridi, S.; Rafiee, A.; Naddafi, K. Characterization and risk assessment of polycyclic aromatic hydrocarbons (PAHs) in urban atmospheric particulate of Tehran, Iran. *Environ. Sci. Pollut. Res.* **2016**, *23*, 1820–1832. [CrossRef] [PubMed]

32. Bulejko, P.; Adamec, V.; Schüllerová, B.; Skeřil, R. Levels, sources, and health risk assessment of polycyclic aromatic hydrocarbons in Brno, Czech Republic: A 5-year study. *Environ. Sci. Pollut. Res.* **2016**, *23*, 20462–20473. [CrossRef] [PubMed]
33. Yue, H.; Yun, Y.; Gao, R.; Li, G.; Sang, N. Winter polycyclic aromatic hydrocarbon-bound particulate matter from peri-urban north china promotes lung cancer cell metastasis. *Environ. Sci. Technol.* **2015**, *49*, 14484. [CrossRef] [PubMed]
34. Han, X.; Lu, X.; Zhang, Q.; Wuyuntana; Hai, Q.; Pan, H. Grain-size distribution and contamination characteristics of heavy metal in street dust of Baotou, China. *Environ. Earth Sci.* **2016**, *75*, 468. [CrossRef]
35. Zhou, Q.; Zheng, N.; Liu, J.; Wang, Y.; Sun, C.; Liu, Q.; Wang, H.; Zhang, J. Residents health risk of Pb, Cd and Cu exposure to street dust based on different particle sizes around zinc smelting plant, Northeast of China. *Environ. Geochem. Health* **2015**, *37*, 207–220. [CrossRef]
36. Keshavarzi, B.; Tazarvi, Z.; Rajabzadeh, M.A.; Najmeddin, A. Chemical speciation, human health risk assessment and pollution level of selected heavy metals in urban street dust of Shiraz, Iran. *Atmos. Environ.* **2015**, *119*, 1–10. [CrossRef]
37. Han, L.; Gao, B.; Wei, X.; Xu, D.; Gao, L. Spatial distribution, health risk assessment, and isotopic composition of lead contamination of street dusts in different functional areas of Beijing, China. *Environ. Sci. Pollut. Res.* **2016**, *23*, 3247–3255. [CrossRef]
38. Varol, S.; Davraz, A. Evaluation of potential human health risk and investigation of drinking water quality in Isparta city center (Turkey). *J. Water Health* **2015**, *14*, 471–488. [CrossRef]
39. Islam, M.S.; Ahmed, M.K.; Habibullah-Al-Mamun, M.; Raknuzzaman, M. The concentration, source and potential human health risk of heavy metals in the commonly consumed foods in Bangladesh. *Ecotoxicol. Environ. Saf.* **2015**, *122*, 462–469. [CrossRef]
40. Morelli, X.; Rieux, C.; Cyrys, J.; Forsberg, B.; Slama, R. Air pollution, health and social deprivation: A fine-scale risk assessment. *Environ. Res.* **2016**, *147*, 59–70. [CrossRef]
41. Arranz, M.C.; Moreno, M.F.M.; Medina, A.A.; Capitán, M.A.; Vaquer, F.C.; Gómez, A.A. Health impact assessment of air pollution in Valladolid, Spain. *BMJ Open* **2014**, *4*, e005999. [CrossRef] [PubMed]
42. Baccini, M.; Biggeri, A.; Accetta, G.; Alessandrini, E.R.; Zero, F. Short-term impact of air pollution among Italian cities covered by the EpiAir2 project. *Epidemiol. Prev.* **2013**, *37*, 252. [PubMed]
43. Izhar, S.; Goel, A.; Chakraborty, A.; Gupta, T. Annual trends in occurrence of submicron particles in ambient air and health risk posed by particle bound metals. *Chemosphere* **2016**, *146*, 582–590. [CrossRef] [PubMed]
44. Mansfield, T.J.; Jacqueline, M. Health impacts of increased physical activity from changes in transportation infrastructure: Quantitative estimates for three communities. *BioMed Res. Int.* **2015**, *2015*, 812325. [CrossRef] [PubMed]
45. Gibson, J.M.; Rodriguez, D.; Dennerlein, T.; Mead, J.; Hasc, T.; Meacci, G.; Levin, S. Predicting urban design effects on physical activity and public health: A case study. *Health Place* **2015**, *35*, 79–84. [CrossRef] [PubMed]
46. Zapata-Diomedi, B.; Herrera, A.; Veerman, J.L. The effects of built environment attributes on physical activity-related health and health care costs outcomes in Australia. *Health Place* **2016**, *42*, 19–29. [CrossRef]
47. Moryani, H.T.; Kong, S.; Du, J.; Bao, J. Health risk assessment of heavy metals accumulated on $PM_{2.5}$ fractioned road dust from two cities of Pakistan. *Int. J. Environ. Res. Public Health* **2020**, *17*, 7124. [CrossRef]
48. Cai, L.M.; Jiang, H.H.; Luo, J. Metals in soils from a typical rapidly developing county, Southern China: Levels, distribution, and source apportionment. *Environ. Sci. Pollut. Res.* **2019**, *26*, 19282–19293. [CrossRef]
49. Hamed, A.; Hamed, S.; Majid, R.; Abbas, A.; Bayram, H.; Hesam, A.; Adibzadeh, A. Data on investigating the nitrate concentration levels and quality of bottled water in Torbat-e Heydarieh, Khorasan Razavi province, Iran. *Data Brief* **2018**, *20*, 463–467.
50. Sah, D.; Verma, P.K.; Kumari, K.M.; Lakhani, A. Chemical fractionation of heavy metals in fine particulate matter and their health risk assessment through inhalation exposure pathway. *Environ. Geochem. Health* **2019**, *41*, 1445–1458. [CrossRef]
51. Gu, Y.; Liu, B.; Li, Y.; Zhang, Y.; Feng, Y. Multi-scale volatile organic compound (voc) source apportionment in Tianjin, China, using a receptor model coupled with 1-hr resolution data. *Environ. Pollut.* **2020**, *265*, 115023. [CrossRef] [PubMed]
52. Lehtomki, H.; Geels, C.; Brandt, J.; Rao, S.; Hnninen, O. Deaths attributable to air pollution in Nordic countries: Disparities in the estimates. *Atmosphere* **2020**, *11*, 467. [CrossRef]
53. Najmeddin, A.; Keshavarzi, B. Health risk assessment and source apportionment of polycyclic aromatic hydrocarbons associated with PM_{10} and road deposited dust in Ahvaz Metropolis of Iran. *Environ. Geochem. Health* **2019**, *41*, 1267–1290. [CrossRef] [PubMed]
54. Zhang, Y.; Yang, L.; Zhang, X.; Li, J.; Wang, W. Characteristics of $PM_{2.5}$-bound PAHs at an urban site and a suburban site in Jinan in north China plain. *Aerosol Air Qual. Res.* **2019**, *19*, 871–884. [CrossRef]
55. Geravandi, S.; Sicard, P.; Khaniabadi, Y.O.; Marco, A.D.; Sadeghi, S. A comparative study of hospital admissions for respiratory diseases during normal and dusty days in Iran. *Environ. Sci. Pollut. Res.* **2017**, *24*, 18152–18159. [CrossRef]
56. Faisal, M.; Wu, Z.; Wang, H.; Hussain, Z.; Azam, M.I. Human health risk assessment of heavy metals in the urban road dust of Zhengzhou metropolis, China. *Atmosphere* **2021**, *12*, 1213. [CrossRef]
57. Chen, X.; Guo, M.; Feng, J.; Liang, S.; Han, D.; Cheng, J. Characterization and risk assessment of heavy metals in road dust from a developing city with good air quality and from Shanghai, China. *Environ. Sci. Pollut. Res. Int.* **2019**, *26*, 11387–11398. [CrossRef]
58. Ahamad, A.; Raju, N.J.; Madhav, S.; Gossel, W.; Ram, P.; Wycisk, P. Potentially toxic elements in soil and road dust around Sonbhadra industrial region, Uttar Pradesh, India: Source apportionment and health risk assessment. *Environ. Res.* **2021**, *202*, 111685. [CrossRef]

59. Shabanda, I.S.; Koki, I.B.; Low, K.H.; Zain, S.M.; Bakar, N. Daily exposure to toxic metals through urban road dust from industrial, commercial, heavy traffic, and residential areas in Petaling Jaya, Malaysia: A health risk assessment. *Environ. Sci. Pollut. Res.* **2019**, *26*, 37193–37211. [CrossRef]
60. Mondal, S.; Singh, G. Pollution evaluation, human health effect and tracing source of trace elements on road dust of Dhanbad, a highly polluted industrial coal belt of India. *Environ. Geochem. Health* **2021**, *43*, 2081–2103. [CrossRef]
61. Jiang, Y.; Shi, L.; Guang, A.; Mu, Z.; Zhan, H.; Wu, Y. Contamination levels and human health risk assessment of toxic heavy metals in street dust in an industrial city in Northwest China. *Environ. Geochem. Health* **2018**, *40*, 2007–2020. [CrossRef] [PubMed]
62. Othman, M.; Latif, M.T. Pollution characteristics, sources, and health risk assessments of urban road dust in Kuala Lumpur city. *Environ. Sci. Pollut. Res.* **2020**, *27*, 11227–11245. [CrossRef] [PubMed]
63. Heidari, M.; Darijani, T.; Alipour, A. Heavy metal pollution of road dust in a city and its highly polluted suburb; quantitative source apportionment and source-specific ecological and health risk assessment. *Chemosphere* **2021**, *273*, 129656. [CrossRef] [PubMed]
64. Shahab, A.; Zhang, H.; Ullah, H.; Rashid, A.; Xiao, H. Pollution characteristics and toxicity of potentially toxic elements in road dust of a tourist city, Guilin, China: Ecological and health risk assessment. *Environ. Pollut.* **2020**, *266*, 115419. [CrossRef] [PubMed]
65. Wang, J.; Huang, Y.; Cheng, X. Status, spatial distribution, and health risk assessment of potentially harmful element from road dust in steel industry city, China. *Arab. J. Geosci.* **2021**, *14*, 318. [CrossRef]
66. Duan, X.C.; Yu, H.H.; Ye, T.R.; Huang, Y.; Albanese, S. Geostatistical mapping and quantitative source apportionment of potentially toxic elements in top- and sub-soils: A case of suburban area in Beijing, China. *Ecol. Indic.* **2020**, *112*, 106085. [CrossRef]
67. Zhang, H.; Cai, A.; Wang, X.; Wang, L.; Wang, Q.; Wu, X.; Ma, Y. Risk assessment and source apportionment of heavy metals in soils from Handan city. *Appl. Sci* **2021**, *11*, 9615. [CrossRef]
68. Li, P.; Wu, T.; Jiang, G.; Pu, L.; Li, Y.; Zhang, J.; Xu, F.; Xie, X. An integrated approach for source apportionment and health risk assessment of heavy metals in subtropical agricultural soils, Eastern China. *Land* **2021**, *10*, 1016. [CrossRef]
69. Sun, T.; Huang, J.; Wu, Y.; Yuan, Y.; Xie, Y.; Fan, Z.; Zheng, Z. Risk assessment and source apportionment of soil heavy metals under different land use in a typical estuary alluvial island. *Int. J. Environ. Res. Public Health* **2020**, *17*, 4841. [CrossRef]
70. Tang, J.; He, M.; Luo, Q.; Adeel, M.; Jiao, F. Heavy metals in agricultural soils from a typical mining city in China: Spatial distribution, source apportionment, and health risk assessment. *Pol. J. Environ. Stud.* **2020**, *29*, 1379–1390. [CrossRef]
71. Qasemi, M.; Afsharnia, M.; Farhang, M.; Ghaderpoori, M.; Zarei, A. Spatial distribution of fluoride and nitrate in groundwater and its associated human health risk assessment in residents living in western Khorasan Razavi, Iran. *Desalin. Water Treat.* **2019**, *170*, 176–186. [CrossRef]
72. Badeenezhad, A.; Darabi, K.; Heydari, M.; Amrane, A.; Ghelichi-Ghojogh, M.; Parseh, I.; Darvishmotevalli, M.; Azadbakht, O.; Javanmardi, P. Temporal distribution and zoning of nitrate and fluoride concentrations in Behbahan drinking water distribution network and health risk assessment by using sensitivity analysis and Monte Carlo simulation. *Int. J. Environ. Anal. Chem.* **2021**, *101*, 1903455. [CrossRef]
73. Radfard, M.M.; Yunesian, M.; Nodehi, R.N.; Biglari, H.; Nazmara, S.; Hadi, M.; Yousefi, N.; Yousefi, M.; Abbasnia, A.; Mahvi, A.H. Drinking water quality and arsenic health risk assessment in Sistan and Baluchestan, southeastern province, Iran. *Human Ecol. Risk Assess.* **2018**, *25*, 949–965. [CrossRef]
74. Mirzabeygi, M.; Yousefi, M.; Soleimani, H.; Mohammadi, A.A.; Mahvi, A.H.; Abbasnia, A. The concentration data of fluoride and health risk assessment in drinking water in the Ardakan city of Yazd province, Iran. *Data Brief* **2018**, *18*, 40–46. [CrossRef] [PubMed]
75. Long, L.; He, J.; Yang, X. Characteristics, emission sources and health risk assessment of trace elements in size-segregated aerosols during haze and non-haze periods at Ningbo, China. *Environ. Geochem. Health* **2021**, *43*, 2945–2963. [CrossRef]
76. Jan, R.; Roy, R.; Yadav, S.; Satsangi, P.G. Chemical fractionation and health risk assessment of particulate matter-bound metals in Pune, India. *Environ. Geochem. Health* **2016**, *40*, 1–16. [CrossRef]
77. Guo, Q.; Li, L.; Zhao, X.; Yin, B.; Liu, Y.; Wang, X.; Yang, W.; Geng, C.; Wang, X.; Bai, Z. Source Apportionment and Health Risk Assessment of Metal Elements in $PM_{2.5}$ in Central Liaoning's Urban Agglomeration. *Atmosphere* **2021**, *12*, 667. [CrossRef]
78. Jiang, H.; Xiao, H.; Song, H.; Liu, J.; Wang, Z. A long-lasting winter haze episode in Xiangyang, central China: Pollution characteristics, chemical composition, and health risk assessment. *Aerosol Air Qual. Res.* **2020**, *20*, 2859–2873. [CrossRef]
79. Li, Y.; Yin, S.; Yu, S.; Yuan, M.; Zhang, R. Characteristics, source apportionment and health risks of ambient VOCs during high ozone period at an urban site in central plain, China. *Chemosphere* **2020**, *250*, 126283. [CrossRef]
80. Ding, Y.; Lu, J.; Liu, Z.; Li, W.; Chen, J. Volatile organic compounds in Shihezi, China, during the heating season: Pollution characteristics, source apportionment, and health risk assessment. *Environ. Sci. Pollut. Res.* **2020**, *27*, 16439–16450. [CrossRef]
81. Tohid, L.; Sabeti, Z.; Sarbakhsh, P.; Benis, K.Z.; Shakerkhatibi, M.; Rasoulzadeh, Y.; Rahimian, R.; Darvishali, S. Spatiotemporal variation, ozone formation potential and health risk assessment of ambient air VOCs in an industrialized city in Iran. *Atmos. Pollut. Res.* **2018**, *10*, 556–563. [CrossRef]
82. Xiong, Y.; Bari, M.A.; Xing, Z.; Du, K. Ambient volatile organic compounds (VOCs) in two coastal cities in western canada: Spatiotemporal variation, source apportionment, and health risk assessment. *Sci. Total Environ.* **2020**, *706*, 135970. [CrossRef] [PubMed]
83. Wang, X.; Liu, G.; Hu, R.; Zhang, H.; Zhang, F. Distribution, sources, and health risk assessment of volatile organic compounds in Hefei city. *Arch. Environ. Contam. Toxicol.* **2020**, *78*, 392–400. [CrossRef] [PubMed]

84. Li, C.; Li, Q.; Tong, D.; Wang, Q.; Tan, L. Environmental impact and health risk assessment of volatile organic compound emissions during different seasons in Beijing. *J. Environ. Sci.* **2019**, *93*, 1–12. [CrossRef]
85. Izquierdo, R.; Dos Santos, S.G.; Borge, R.; de la Paz, D.; Sarigiannis, D.; Gotti, A.; Boldo, E. Health impact assessment by the implementation of Madrid city air-quality plan in 2020. *Environ. Res.* **2020**, *183*, 109021. [CrossRef]
86. Luo, H.; Guan, Q.; Lin, J.; Wang, Q.; Wang, N. Air pollution characteristics and human health risks in key cities of Northwest China. *J. Environ. Manag.* **2020**, *269*, 110791. [CrossRef]
87. Giallouros, G.; Kouis, P.; Papatheodorou, S.I.; Woodcock, J.; Tainio, M. The long-term impact of restricting cycling and walking during high air pollution days on all-cause mortality: Health impact assessment study. *Environ. Int.* **2020**, *140*, 105679. [CrossRef]
88. Sacks, J.D.; Lloyd, J.M.; Zhu, Y.; Anderton, J.; Jang, C.J.; Hubbell, B.; Fann, N. The environmental benefits mapping and analysis program—community edition (BenMAP-CE): A tool to estimate the health and economic benefits of reducing air pollution. *Environ. Model. Softw.* **2018**, *104*, 118–129. [CrossRef]
89. Sohrabi, S.; Zietsman, J.; Khreis, H. Burden of disease assessment of ambient air pollution and premature mortality in urban areas: The role of socioeconomic status and transportation. *Int. J. Environ. Res. Public Health* **2020**, *17*, 1166. [CrossRef]
90. Khomenko, S.; Cirach, M.; Pereira-Barboza, E.; Mueller, N.; Nieuwenhuijsen, M. Premature mortality due to air pollution in European cities: A health impact assessment. *Lancet Planet. Health* **2021**, *5*, 121–134. [CrossRef]
91. Gamarra, A.R.; Lechón, Y.; Vivanco, M.G.; Garrido, J.L.; Martín, F.; Martín, F.; Theobald, M.R.; Gil, V.; Santiago, J.L. Benefit analysis of the 1st Spanish air pollution control programme on health impacts and associated externalities. *Atmosphere* **2020**, *12*, 32. [CrossRef]
92. Abbasnejad, B.; Keshavarzi, B.; Mohammadi, Z.; Moore, F.; Abbasnejad, A. Characteristics, distribution, source apportionment, and potential health risk assessment of polycyclic aromatic hydrocarbons in urban street dust of Kerman Metropolis, Iran. *Int. J. Environ. Res. Public Health* **2019**, *29*, 668–685. [CrossRef] [PubMed]
93. Najmeddin, A.; Moore, F.; Keshavarzi, B.; Sadegh, Z. Pollution, source apportionment and health risk of potentially toxic elements (ptes) and polycyclic aromatic hydrocarbons (PAHs) in urban street dust of Mashhad, the second largest city of Iran. *J. Geochem. Explor.* **2018**, *190*, 154–169. [CrossRef]
94. Qishlaqi, A.; Beiramali, F. Potential sources and health risk assessment of polycyclic aromatic hydrocarbons in street dusts of Karaj urban area, Northern Iran. *J. Environ. Health Sci. Eng.* **2019**, *17*, 1029–1044. [CrossRef] [PubMed]
95. Liang, M.; Liang, H.; Rao, Z.; Hong, X. Characterization of polycyclic aromatic hydrocarbons in urban-rural integration area soil, north china: Spatial distribution, sources and potential human health risk assessment. *Chemosphere* **2019**, *234*, 875–884. [CrossRef] [PubMed]
96. Shen, R.; Liu, Z.; Chen, X.; Wang, Y.; Wang, L.; Liu, Y.; Li, X. Atmospheric levels, variations, sources and health risk of pm2.5-bound polycyclic aromatic hydrocarbons during winter over the north China plain. *Sci. Total Environ.* **2019**, *655*, 581–590. [CrossRef]
97. Zhang, Y.; Yang, L.; Gao, Y.; Chen, J.; Wang, W. Comparative study of PAHs in PM_1 and $PM_{2.5}$ at a background site in the north China plain. *Aerosol Air Qual. Res.* **2019**, *19*, 2281–2293. [CrossRef]
98. Luo, M.; Ji, Y.; Ren, Y.; Gao, F.; Zhang, H.; Zhang, L.; Yu, Y.; Li, H. Characteristics and health risk assessment of $PM_{2.5}$-bound PAHs during heavy air pollution episodes in winter in urban area of Beijing, China. *Atmosphere* **2021**, *12*, 323. [CrossRef]
99. Gao, P.; Hu, J.; Song, J.; Chen, X.; Xing, B. Inhalation bioaccessibility of polycyclic aromatic hydrocarbons in heavy $PM_{2.5}$ pollution days: Implications for public health risk assessment in northern China. *Environ. Pollut.* **2019**, *255*, 113296. [CrossRef]
100. Khaniabadi, Y.O.; Fanelli, R.; De Marco, A.; Daryanoosh, S.M.; Kloog, I.; Hopke, P.K.; Conti, G.O.; Ferrante, M.; Mohammadi, M.J.; Babaei, A.A.; et al. Hospital admissions in Iran for cardiovascular and respiratory diseases attributed to the middle eastern dust storms. *Environ. Sci. Pollut. R.* **2017**, *24*, 16860–16868. [CrossRef]
101. Chen, C. Predictive effects of structural variation on citation counts. *J. Am. Soc. Inf. Sci. Technol.* **2012**, *63*, 431–449. [CrossRef]
102. Chen, W.; Geng, Y.; Zhong, S.; Zhuang, M.; Pan, H. A bibliometric analysis of ecosystem services evaluation from 1997 to 2016. *Environ. Sci. Pollut. Res.* **2020**, *27*, 23503–23513. [CrossRef] [PubMed]
103. Zhong, P.; Zhang, J.Q.; Xu, D.M.; Tian, Q.; Qi, S.H. Contamination characteristics of heavy metals in particle size fractions from street dust from an industrial city, central China. *Air Qual. Atmos. Health* **2020**, *13*, 871–883. [CrossRef]
104. Xia, Q.; Zhang, J.; Chen, Y.; Ma, Q.; Peng, J.; Rong, G. Pollution, sources and human health risk assessment of potentially toxic elements in different land use types under the background of industrial cities. *Sustainability* **2020**, *12*, 2121. [CrossRef]
105. Wang, H.; Cai, L.; Wang, Q.; Hu, G.; Chen, L. A comprehensive exploration of risk assessment and source quantification of potentially toxic elements in road dust: A case study from a large Cu smelter in central China. *Catena* **2021**, *196*, 104930. [CrossRef]
106. Zhou, Y.; Chen, L. Twenty-year span of global coronavirus research trends: A bibliometric analysis. *Int. J. Environ. Res. Public Health* **2020**, *17*, 3082. [CrossRef]
107. Pereira, C.; Perisse, A.R.S.; Knoblauch, A.M.; Utzinger, J.; Hacon, S.D.S.; Winkler, M.S. Health impact assessment in Latin American countries: Current practice and prospects. *Environ. Impact Asses. Rev.* **2017**, *65*, 175–185. [CrossRef]
108. Green, L.; Gray, B.J.; Ashton, K. Using health impact assessments to implement the sustainable development goals in practice: A case study in Wales. *Impact Assess. Proj. Apprais.* **2020**, *38*, 214–224. [CrossRef]
109. Claudio, F.; Rijke, K.D.; Page, A. The csg arena: A critical review of unconventional gas developments and best-practice health impact assessment in Queensland, Australia. *Impact Assess. Proj. Apprais.* **2018**, *36*, 105–114. [CrossRef]
110. Roué-Le Gall, A.; Jabot, F. Health impact assessment on urban development projects in france: Finding pathways to fit practice to context. *Glob. Health Promot.* **2017**, *24*, 25–34. [CrossRef]

111. Iungman, T.; Khomenko, S.; Nieuwenhuijsen, M.; Barboza, E.P.; Mueller, N. The impact of urban and transport planning on health: Assessment of the attributable mortality burden in Madrid and Barcelona and its distribution by socioeconomic status. *Environ. Res.* **2021**, *196*, 110988. [CrossRef] [PubMed]
112. Thondoo, M.; Mueller, N.; Rojas-Rueda, D.; Vries, D.D.; Nieuwenhuijsen, M.J. Participatory quantitative health impact assessment of urban transport planning: A case study from eastern Africa. *Environ. Int.* **2020**, *144*, 106027. [CrossRef] [PubMed]
113. Gamache, S.; Diallo, T.A.; Shankardass, K.; Lebel, A. The elaboration of an intersectoral partnership to perform health impact assessment in urban planning: The experience of Quebec city (Canada). *Int. J. Environ. Res. Public Health* **2020**, *17*, 7556. [CrossRef] [PubMed]

International Journal of
Environmental Research and Public Health

MDPI

Article

Social Stability Risk Assessment of Disaster-Preventive Migration in Ethnic Minority Areas of Southwest China

Linyi Zhou [1], Demi Zhu [1] and Wei Shen [2,*]

1 School of International and Public Affairs, Shanghai Jiao Tong University, Shanghai 200030, China; zhoulinyi1017@sjtu.edu.cn (L.Z.); zhudemi@sjtu.edu.cn (D.Z.)
2 School of Economics and Management, Tongji University, Shanghai 200092, China
* Correspondence: semleorain@tongji.edu.cn

Abstract: Disaster-preventive migration (DPM) is an important method for disaster risk management, but migration itself entails a potential social stability risk. This study took County D in Yunnan Province, one of the counties most severely threatened by geological disasters in China, as an example to construct an indicator system of social stability risk factors for disaster-preventive migration based on a literature survey and in-depth interviews. The system consists of 5 first-level risk factors and 14 s-level risk factors. The social stability risk of DPM in County D was assessed using a fuzzy comprehensive evaluation method based on experts' weights. The results showed that the overall social stability risk level of disaster-preventive migration in County D is 'high'. In terms of importance, the five first-level risk factors were ranked as follows: public opinion risk > compensation risk > livelihood recovery risk > cultural risk > geological disaster risk. Among the risk factors, the level of public opinion risk and compensation risk appeared to be high, whereas that of livelihood recovery risk, cultural risk and geological disaster risk resulted to be medium. To our knowledge, this paper is the first research to evaluate the social stability risk of DPM; it not only enriches the theories of social stability risk assessment, but also has important guiding significance for people relocation and resettlement in Chinese ethnic minority areas.

Keywords: disaster-preventive migration (DPM); social stability risk; fuzzy comprehensive evaluation (FCE); ethnic minority area; China

Citation: Zhou, L.; Zhu, D.; Shen, W. Social Stability Risk Assessment of Disaster-Preventive Migration in Ethnic Minority Areas of Southwest China. *IJERPH* **2022**, *19*, 6192. https://doi.org/10.3390/ijerph19106192

Academic Editors: Jie Chen, Qian Zhou, Ting Zhang and Paul B. Tchounwou

Received: 26 April 2022
Accepted: 18 May 2022
Published: 19 May 2022

1. Introduction

According to the Global Risks Report 2020, natural disasters rank third in terms of likelihood and seventh in terms of impact, among all potential global risks [1]. From 1975 to 2015, the number of people exposed to risks associated with all types of natural disasters has doubled globally as a result of urbanization, population growth, and socioeconomic development [2]. Natural disasters pose a greater risk to and have a more devastating impact on less developed countries or regions, and poor people are the most vulnerable to their effects [3]. China is particularly prone to natural disasters [4]. In 2020, 138 million people were affected by various natural disasters in China; furthermore, 591 people died or went missing due to such disasters, while the direct economic losses are estimated to be 370.15 billion yuan [5]. Geological disasters are natural disasters caused by a geological process and include earthquakes, volcanic eruptions, landslide, mud-rock flow, etc. [6]. Compared with the eastern and central regions, western China is ecologically sensitive and more susceptible to natural disasters; these areas also have a lower capacity to avert the risk of natural disasters, which means that a natural disaster has severe consequences in these regions. For example, a magnitude-6.4 quake hit Yunnan province in southwest China at 9.48 p.m. on Friday 21 May 2021 local time, and just hours later, a magnitude 7.4 earthquake hit the Qinghai Province in northwest China. The two massive earthquakes killed at least three people and injured dozens of others.

Migration is one of the most effective methods by which human beings respond to recurrent natural disasters [7]. When people are unable to adapt to or mitigate the impact of natural disasters in an area prone to such disasters, there is no alternative to migration [8]. To minimize the risk of natural disasters, the Chinese central government formulated the Decisions on Strengthening the Prevention and Control of Geological Disasters, which emphasized accelerating the relocation and evacuation of people living within areas particularly vulnerable to geological disasters. The document suggested that this process should be accelerated through a series of planned steps, and that priority must be given to the relocation of people living around potential spots of geological disasters that were highly hazardous or difficult to manage [9]. After more than a decade of development, the Chinese government recently implemented a relocation and resettlement plan in parallel with the risk identification and management of natural disasters [10].

However, there are several potential risks associated with disaster-preventive migration. Downing identified nine major risks of resettlement, namely, joblessness, homelessness, marginalization, food insecurity, loss of common land and resources, increased health risks, social disarticulation, disruption of formal educational activities, and loss of civil rights [11]. Migration may also lead to a decline in the productivity and standard of living of people compared with their lifestyle in their place of origin, disrupt their customs and the living environment, as well as create ongoing conflicts between the affected population and the local authorities when government compensation falls short of expectations [12–15]. In some cases, this situation may give rise to violent resistance and bloody conflicts, thereby posing a threat to the harmony and stability of the society [16].

In this context, relocation in County D of Yunnan Province, China, is a much more complicated issue compared with regular relocation—the county is multi-ethnic, is located at a high altitude, and is prone to natural disasters. Disaster-preventive migration in this county has threatened social stability and therefore has faced significant resistance. This leads to a research question: how to identify and evaluate the social stability risk of DPM in County D? A solution to this problem would not only promote the development of social stability risk assessment but may also serve as an important guide for the relocation and resettlement of DPM populations belonging to minority groups.

Concretely speaking, this paper attempts to answer the following two fundamental issues:

(1) What are the core risk factors for social stability associated with disaster-preventive migration in county D?
(2) How to use scientific methods to assess the social stability risk?

2. Literature Review

Natural disasters are closely associated with property damage and migration [17,18]. Disaster-preventive migration is a risk management strategy for relocating and resettling people exposed to the risks of natural hazards [19]. Disaster-preventive migration, which is different from migration for specific projects, ecological restoration, and natural resource conservation, aims to protect the property and lives of populations exposed to natural disasters and may cause negative impacts on the resettled population [20,21]. While resettlement may result in better housing quality for people, their economic well-being may be negatively affected [22]. In addition, some people who relocate may not be able to adapt to the new environment, leading to a deterioration in their mental health status [23] and a decrease in subjective well-being [24]. As a result, disaster-preventive migration is often used as the last option for the prevention of risks linked to natural disasters [25].

Disaster-induced migration is divided into post-disaster migration and disaster-preventive migration. Post-disaster migration takes place when it is not possible for residents to return to the original settlement after a disaster [19]. Disaster-preventive migration is considered a possible strategy to cope with disaster risks linked with the increased possibility of natural disasters [26,27]. Some countries have begun to include disaster-preventive migration as an important component of their national disaster management strategies [28]. However, even when people's means of living are threatened by natural disasters, sentimental attachment to the local residence is an important reason for their reluctance to relocate [29,30]. Therefore, distant and permanent resettlement as part of disaster-preventive migration is an important cause of social instability [31,32].

To prevent projects' failure, international organizations and the national migration planning authorities of numerous countries require an ex ante assessment of the potential harmful consequences of migration projects [33]. Social impact assessment (SIA) is a method commonly adopted internationally for managing the social issues related to projects [34]. SIA originated from the environmental impact assessment (EIA) [35] framework in the United States and has now become a complete assessment system over the course of 50 years [33,36,37]. The application of SIA around the world has contributed significantly to the success of many projects. However, due to policy and institutional issues, SIA has faced many obstacles during the implementation stage in developing countries [38] such as China [39]. Social stability risk assessment is a nascent system that respects Chinese particularities and was developed based on SIA. Although the institutional framework for SSRA in China has been refined thereafter, current studies have focused on the construction of large engineering projects [40–42], meteorological disasters [43], land acquisition [33], and migration engineering [44], among other issues. There is a lack of research on the SSRA of preventive migration in areas at high risk of experiencing geological disasters.

It is undeniable that social stability risk assessment is a tool for planning better resettlement [34]. The social stability risk linked to DPM comes from various sources including livelihood recovery, land compensation, cultural factors, and so on [45,46]. The immigrant livelihood issue is a topic of common concern for scientific research and policy debates [47]. As livelihood recovery is the key to sustainable development in disaster-affected areas [48], current research has focused on livelihood asset assessment [49–51], livelihood vulnerability assessment [52,53], and livelihood risk mitigation strategies [54,55]. Land compensation policies are directly related to the livelihood of immigration, especially of farmers, and have a major influence on disaster-related migration aspirations [56]. Cultural factors play both positive and negative roles in natural disaster risk management. Religion is considered to be a part of culture and communities and plays an important role in natural disaster management because it has access to resources that are vital to emergency rescue in a disaster [57]. However, some believers misinterpret natural disasters, for example, earthquake and tsunami in Japan are regarded as God's warning, and this has a negative impact on natural disaster management [58].

Involuntary migration disrupts people's routine life and causes them to become uncomfortable. Studies have shown that involuntary migration can be extremely detrimental to the social stability of the relocated communities [59]. Most residents, living in areas identified as particularly prone to natural disasters, are reluctant to leave their homes [60] because of place attachment [61,62], loverhood, and religion [63–65]. Improving the risk perception of natural disasters is an important measure to promote relocation decisions [66]. Risk perception is a subjective judgment that people make about the characteristics and severity of a risk [67]. A high natural disaster risk perception is reflected in the purchasing of a natural disaster insurance [68], the enhancement of DPM willingness, and the adoption of a natural disaster risk reduction strategy [69,70].

The possible marginal contributions of this paper include: (1) risk perceptions was incorporated into the index system of SSRA, thus improving the SSRA framework; (2) this study focuses on the SSRA of geological disaster migrants, which may broaden the research field of SSRA; (3) in terms of evaluation method, we established a fuzzy comprehensive evaluation method considering multi-experts' weights to assess the social stability risk of DPM; the method not only considers the ambiguity of the evaluation problem, but also solves the inconsistent problem of experts' views.

3. Materials and Methods

3.1. Study Area

County D, in Diqing Tibetan Autonomous Prefecture in Yunnan Province, is located between 98°35′6″–99°32′20″ E and 27°33′44″–29°15′2″ N in the Hengduan mountain range in the northwestern part of Yunnan Province. There are two towns and six townships in County D, with a total area of 7291 square kilometers and a population density of eight people per square kilometer. S Town, the county capital, is located at 3400 m above sea level; it is 182 km from Shangri-La, the state capital, and 889 km from Kunming, the provincial capital. Since ancient times, S town has presented an intersection of Chinese and Tibetan cultures, served as the 'foreign market center' along the southwestern Tea Horse Road, and operated as the Tibetan-Chinese trade and cultural distribution center. It is known locally as the 'snow mountain foreign market'. S town is an important transportation hub from Yunnan to Sichuan and Tibet and occupies a special strategic location for political, economic, and cultural communication between Yunnan, Sichuan, and Tibet. It is also the political, economic, and cultural center of County D. S town is one of the main settlements of ethnic minorities. Major ethnic groups include the Tibetan, Han, Hui, and Naxi. It is also a typical multi-religious area, including Tibetan Buddhism, Catholicism, and Islam, among others. Due to a complex geological structure, this area is prone to geological disasters such as landslides and mudslides and it is one of the key target areas for geological disaster prevention and control [71]. The disaster-preventive migration in focus involved two communities and one village in S town of County D, comprising more than 1700 households and approximately 6000 people (Figure 1).

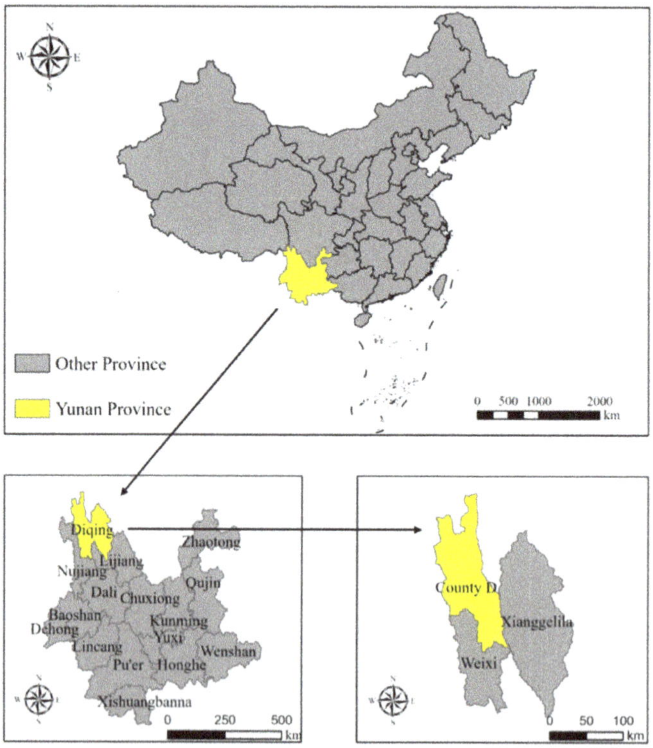

Figure 1. Study area.

3.2. Data Sources

The data in this study were derived from on-site expert surveys, symposiums, and face-to-face interviews. In July 2020, a survey team was selected by the People's Government of County D and was divided into five groups to investigate the social stability risks from disaster-preventive migration in County D. First, symposiums for experts were held for government departments and scholars in the field of migration in County D. Questionnaires were distributed to the experts who took part in the symposiums, to collect data. These experts belonged to the People's Government office of County D, the Development and Reform Commission, the Planning and Land Bureau, the Housing and Urban-Rural Development Bureau, the Agriculture and Rural Affairs Bureau, the Forestry and Grassland Bureau, the Emergency Management Bureau, the Public Complaints and Proposals Administration, the Natural Resources Bureau, the Ecological and Environmental Bureau, the Audit Office, the Finance Bureau, consulting agencies, universities, and other institutions. A total of 30 experts were invited to the symposium, with 15 experts from government departments (50%), 7 from consulting agencies (23.33%), and 8 from universities (26.67%). We obtained 30 completed expert questionnaires in the symposiums, the response rate was 100%.

Second, a typical survey was used to select 72 representative residents for face-to-face interviews according to the degree of impact, to listen to their specific views on DPM and demands for related interests. Specifically, firstly, a list of groups affected by DPM was obtained from government departments and categorized by occupation. Secondly, these residents were ranked according to their occupation and degree of disaster impact, with priority given to those who were most affected. Finally, the sample size of different occupational residents was determined according to the population proportion in each occupation and rounded up. The 72 representative residents included 25 farmers, 18 enterprise employees, 6 representatives of individual businesses, 4 representatives of local enterprises, 12 grassroot government officials, 5 retired workers, and 2 imams.

3.3. Identification of Social Stability Risks

Risk identification is a prerequisite for conducting social stability risk analysis. The main risk identification techniques included a literature review, brainstorming, flowcharting, discussions, and interviews [72]. The information from face-to-face interviews, which were conducted in July 2020, County D with 72 residents, and related literature [33,47] was combined to identify social stability risk factors for disaster-preventive migration in County D, which included 5 first-level risk factors and 14 s-level risk factors (Table 1).

Table 1. Social stability risk factors for disaster-preventive migration.

Target Layer	First-Level Risk Factors	Second-Level Risk Factors
Social stability risk factors of DPM	Compensation risks	Housing compensation Compensation for land acquisition Settlement allowance
	Cultural risks	Inability to adapt to the lifestyle Integration of ethnicities Changes in social networks
	Livelihood recovery risks	Loss of forest and land resources Job opportunities and income issues Inability to meet expectations of living environment
	Risk of geological hazards	Possibility of geological hazards Magnitude of damage caused by geological hazards
	Risks linked to public opinion	Level of openness and transparency of information Level of public participation Government response to public opinion

3.4. Fuzzy Comprehensive Evaluation Model

Fuzzy comprehensive evaluation (FCE) is a method for comprehensive evaluation in a multi-criteria fuzzy decision environment using fuzzy sets [73]. The basic idea was to obtain the overall risk assessment results by constructing a mathematical model that comprehensively considered the level of influence of all risk factors. The method combined qualitative and quantitative approaches and enhanced the scientific validity of the SSRA. The FCE was divided into six steps, as follows.

In the first step, a set of influencing factors for the evaluation object was created. The influence factor set consisted of factors that affected the evaluation object. The influence factor set was denoted as:

$$U = \{u_1, u_2, \cdots, u_i, \cdots, u_n\} \tag{1}$$

$$u_i = \{u_{i1}, u_{i2}, \cdots, u_{ij}, \cdots, u_{ik}\} \tag{2}$$

where U is the set of influencing factors, n is the number of first-level risk factors included in U, u_i $(i = 1, 2, \cdots, n)$ is the ith first-level risk factor in U, u_{ij} $(j = 1, 2, \cdots, n)$ is the jth second-level factor in u_i, and k is the number of second-level risk factors.

The second step was to construct an evaluation set. The evaluation set included the evaluation values assigned to a certain evaluation indicator of the object. The evaluation set was expressed as:

$$V = \{v_1, v_2, \cdots, v_m\} = \{1, 2, \cdots, m\} \tag{3}$$

Here, V is the risk assessment set, v_1, v_2, $\cdots$, v_m represent the risk level, and its corresponding rating values are $1, 2, \cdots, m$.

The third step was to determine the weight assignment set. This information is often missing in comprehensive multi-indicator evaluations; the weight of each indicator should be determined based on expert opinions and knowledge. In this study, the frequency count [32] was used to determine the weights of first-level and second-level risk factors. Take the first-level risk factor set as an example:

(1) A weighting scheme was proposed by T $(T > 30)$ experts for each of the factors u_i $(i = 1, 2, \cdots, n)$ in the influencing factor set U.
(2) For the weights a_{it} $(t = 1, 2, \cdots, T)$ for factor u_i provided by T experts, the maximum weight G_i and the minimum weight g_i were identified.
(3) An appropriate positive integer p was chosen such that $d = \frac{G_i - g_i}{p}$. The weights a_{it} $(t = 1, 2, \cdots, T)$ were divided into p groups, from the largest to the smallest, according to the group distance d.
(4) The frequencies or rates of the weights that fell within each group were calculated, and the group median $\bar{a}_i$ of the group with the maximum number of frequencies or rates was taken as the weight of factor u_i. Then, $\bar{a}_i$ was normalized to obtain the weight vector:

$$A = \{A_1, A_2, \cdots, A_n\} = \left\{ \frac{\bar{a}_1}{\sum_{i=1}^{n} \bar{a}_i}, \frac{\bar{a}_2}{\sum_{i=1}^{n} \bar{a}_i}, \cdots, \frac{\bar{a}_n}{\sum_{i=1}^{n} \bar{a}_i} \right\} \tag{4}$$

Similarly, for the weights a_{ijt} $(t = 1, 2, \cdots, T)$ provided by T experts for the influencing factors of $u_{ij} (j = 1, 2, \cdots, k)$ in u_i, the group median $\bar{a}_{ij}$ of the group with the maximum frequencies or rates, as obtained in the preceding steps, was regarded as the weight for factor u_{ij}. The weight vector of second-level risk factors was obtained after the normalization of $\bar{a}_{ij}$.

$$A'_i = \{A'_{i1}, A'_{i2}, \cdots, A'_{ik}\} = \left\{ \frac{\bar{a}_{i1}}{\sum_{j=1}^{k} \bar{a}_{ij}}, \frac{\bar{a}_{i1}}{\sum_{j=1}^{k} \bar{a}_{ij}}, \cdots, \frac{\bar{a}_{i1}}{\sum_{j=1}^{k} \bar{a}_{ij}} \right\} \tag{5}$$

In the fourth step, the fuzzy judgement matrices R and R_i of U and u_i, respectively, were determined. In this study, the fuzzy judgement matrices were determined using fuzzy assessment methods based on the experts' weights [74] by considering differences in the education level, cultural background, and familiarity with the assessment items of the experts. For the second-level risk factors, the weights of T experts were assumed to be $w_1, w_2, \cdots, w_T$ and $w_1 + w_2 + \cdots + w_T = 1$. The weight of one expert evaluating factor u_{ij} as v_h was denoted as $w_t^{(ijh)}$; then, the weight of the factor u_{ij} being evaluated as v_h $(h = 1, 2, \cdots, m)$ was: $\sum_{t=1}^{T} w_t^{(ijh)}$. The membership of the evaluation factors u_{ij} to the evaluation result v_h in the evaluation set V was $r_{ijh} = \sum_{t=1}^{T} w_t^{(ijh)} / \sum_{t=1}^{T} w_t$, where $\sum_{t=1}^{T} w_t$ was the sum of all expert weights. After calculating the memberships of all factors of u_{ij} using the aforementioned method, the fuzzy judgement array R_i of the second-level risk factors was obtained, as follows:

$$R_i = \left(r_{ijh}\right)_{k \times m} = \begin{bmatrix} r_{i11} & r_{i12} & \cdots & r_{i1m} \\ r_{i21} & r_{i22} & \cdots & r_{i2m} \\ \cdots & \cdots & \cdots & \cdots \\ r_{ik1} & r_{ik2} & \cdots & r_{ikm} \end{bmatrix} \tag{6}$$

R was obtained through calculating R_i, namely, let $B_i = A_i' \cdot R_i$, then $R = [B_1, B_2, \cdots, B_n]^T$.

In the fifth step, FCE was performed. The first level of FCE was performed among the lowest layer of factors, while the second level of FCE was performed among the higher layers. The FCE vector of the first level was denoted as B_i, and that of the second level was denoted as B. The specific calculation process is shown in Equations (7) and (8).

$$B_i = A_i' \cdot R_i \tag{7}$$

$$B = A \cdot R \tag{8}$$

The fuzzy comprehensive matrices of different levels of evaluation factors were calculated according to Equations (7) and (8), and the risk levels were determined based on the maximum membership values [75].

The sixth step was to calculate the specific risk values. The second-level risk values were denoted as Z, and the first-level risk values were denoted as Z_i'. The specific calculation process is shown in Equations (9) and (10).

$$Z = B \times V^T \tag{9}$$

$$Z_i' = B_i \times V^T \tag{10}$$

The first- and second-level risk values were obtained through Equations (9) and (10) to provide the basis for risk management decisions. Social stability risks level and reference standard are shown in Table 2.

Table 2. Social stability risks' level and reference standard.

Social Stability Risks	Very Low	Low	Medium	High Risk	Very High
Risk value (Z)	(0, 1]	(1, 2]	(2, 3]	(3, 4]	(4, 5]
Grade	1	2	3	4	5

4. Results

The social stability risks of disaster-preventive migration were assessed according to the FCE steps described earlier.

(1) The influencing factor set of the evaluation object was established. The influencing factor set of an evaluation object was $U'' = ''\{social\ stability\ risk\ of\ DPM\}'' = \{''u\_1'', ''u\_2'', ''u\_3'', ''u\_4'', ''u\_5''\} =$ $\{''compensation\ risk,\ cultural\ risk,\ livelihood\ recovery\ risk,\ geological\ disaster\ risk,\ public\ opinion\ risk''\}''$, $u_i = \{u_{i1}, u_{i2}, \ldots, u_{ik}\} i = 1, 2, \ldots, 5$.

(2) The evaluation set was $V = \{v_1, v_2, v_3, v_4, v_5,\} = \{1,2,3,4,5\}$. These five levels represented the five possible evaluation results, defined as follows: very low risk level, low risk level, medium risk level, high risk level, and very high-risk level.

(3) Taking $p = 6$, the weight vectors of second-level risk factors and first-level risk factors were obtained:

$$A'_1 = \{A'_{11}, A'_{12}, A'_{13}\} = \{0.308, 0.333, 0.359\}$$

$$A'_2 = \{A'_{21}, A'_{22}, A'_{23}\} = \{0.363, 0.392, 0.245\} Z'_i = B_i \times V^T$$

$$A'_3 = \{A'_{31}, A'_{32}, A'_{33}\} = \{0.449, 0.187, 0.364\}$$

$$A'_4 = \{A'_{41}, A'_{42}\} = \{0.530, 0.470\}$$

$$A'_5 = \{A'_{51}, A'_{52}, A'_{53}\} = \{0.508, 0.209, 0.283\}$$

$$A = \{A_1, A_2, A_3, A_4, A_5\} = \{0.407, 0.116, 0.233, 0.093, 0.151\}$$

(4) The expert weights were determined through the questionnaires administered to the experts, based on which the fuzzy judgement matrices R_i and R of the first- and second-level indicators were established using an FCE method:

$$R_1 = \begin{Bmatrix} 0.119 & 0.151 & 0.175 & 0.325 & 0.230 \\ 0.095 & 0.127 & 0.278 & 0.294 & 0.206 \\ 0.159 & 0.175 & 0.206 & 0.214 & 0.246 \end{Bmatrix}$$

$$R_2 = \begin{Bmatrix} 0.135 & 0.167 & 0.357 & 0.167 & 0.175 \\ 0.294 & 0.349 & 0.151 & 0.095 & 0.111 \\ 0.151 & 0.119 & 0.373 & 0.159 & 0.198 \end{Bmatrix}$$

$$R_3 = \begin{Bmatrix} 0.056 & 0.127 & 0.087 & 0.468 & 0.262 \\ 0.278 & 0.317 & 0.159 & 0.111 & 0.135 \\ 0.317 & 0.341 & 0.135 & 0.143 & 0.063 \end{Bmatrix}$$

$$R_4 = \begin{Bmatrix} 0.278 & 0.214 & 0.262 & 0.183 & 0.063 \\ 0.127 & 0.540 & 0.127 & 0.135 & 0.071 \end{Bmatrix}$$

$$R_5 = \begin{Bmatrix} 0.056 & 0.111 & 0.183 & 0.397 & 0.254 \\ 0.032 & 0.119 & 0.278 & 0.365 & 0.206 \\ 0.063 & 0.151 & 0.294 & 0.270 & 0.222 \end{Bmatrix}$$

$$R = \begin{Bmatrix} 0.125 & 0.151 & 0.220 & 0.275 & 0.228 \\ 0.201 & 0.227 & 0.280 & 0.137 & 0.156 \\ 0.193 & 0.241 & 0.118 & 0.283 & 0.166 \\ 0.207 & 0.367 & 0.198 & 0.160 & 0.067 \\ 0.053 & 0.124 & 0.234 & 0.354 & 0.235 \end{Bmatrix}$$

(5) The indicator system of the social stability risks of disaster-preventive migration was divided into two levels. FCE was performed first for second-level indicators and then for first-level indicators.

The FCE results of social stability risks of disaster-preventive migration were obtained as follows:

$$B_1 = A'_1 \cdot R_1 = [0.308, 0.333, 0.359] \cdot \begin{bmatrix} 0.119 & 0.151 & 0.175 & 0.325 & 0.230 \\ 0.095 & 0.127 & 0.278 & 0.294 & 0.206 \\ 0.159 & 0.175 & 0.206 & 0.214 & 0.246 \end{bmatrix} = [0.125, 0.151, 0.220, 0.275, 0.228]$$

$$B_2 = A_2'\cdot R_2 = [0.363, 0.392, 0.245]\cdot\begin{bmatrix} 0.135 & 0.167 & 0.357 & 0.167 & 0.175 \\ 0.294 & 0.349 & 0.151 & 0.095 & 0.111 \\ 0.151 & 0.119 & 0.373 & 0.159 & 0.198 \end{bmatrix} = [0.201, 0.227, 0.280, 0.137, 0.156]$$

$$B_3 = A_3'\cdot R_3 = [0.449, 0.187, 0.364]\cdot\begin{bmatrix} 0.056 & 0.127 & 0.087 & 0.468 & 0.262 \\ 0.278 & 0.317 & 0.159 & 0.111 & 0.135 \\ 0.317 & 0.341 & 0.135 & 0.143 & 0.063 \end{bmatrix} = [0.193, 0.241, 0.118, 0.283, 0.166]$$

$$B_4 = A_4'\cdot R_4 = [0.530, 0.470]\cdot\begin{bmatrix} 0.278 & 0.214 & 0.262 & 0.183 & 0.063 \\ 0.127 & 0.540 & 0.127 & 0.135 & 0.071 \end{bmatrix} = [0.207, 0.367, 0.198, 0.160, 0.067]$$

$$B_5 = A_5'\cdot R_5 = [0.508,\ 0.209,\ 0.283]\cdot\begin{bmatrix} 0.056 & 0.111 & 0.183 & 0.397 & 0.254 \\ 0.032 & 0.119 & 0.278 & 0.365 & 0.206 \\ 0.063 & 0.151 & 0.294 & 0.270 & 0.222 \end{bmatrix} = [0.053, 0.124, 0.234, 0.354, 0.235]$$

where B_1 indicated compensation risks, B_2 cultural risks, B_3 livelihood restoration risks, B_4 geohazard risks, and B_5 public opinion risks.

The following was obtained based on the results of the preceding evaluation:

$$R = [B_1, B_2, \cdots, B_n]^T = \begin{bmatrix} 0.125 & 0.151 & 0.220 & 0.275 & 0.228 \\ 0.201 & 0.227 & 0.280 & 0.137 & 0.156 \\ 0.193 & 0.241 & 0.118 & 0.283 & 0.166 \\ 0.207 & 0.367 & 0.198 & 0.160 & 0.067 \\ 0.053 & 0.124 & 0.234 & 0.354 & 0.235 \end{bmatrix}$$

A comprehensive evaluation based on Equation (8) yielded the following comprehensive evaluation vector:

$$B = A\cdot R = [0.407, 0.116, 0.233, 0.093, 0.151]\cdot\begin{bmatrix} 0.125 & 0.151 & 0.220 & 0.275 & 0.228 \\ 0.201 & 0.227 & 0.280 & 0.137 & 0.156 \\ 0.193 & 0.241 & 0.118 & 0.283 & 0.166 \\ 0.207 & 0.367 & 0.198 & 0.160 & 0.067 \\ 0.053 & 0.124 & 0.234 & 0.354 & 0.235 \end{bmatrix} = [0.146, 0.197, 0.204, 0.262, 0.191]$$

(6) The SSRA value for disaster-preventive migration and the first-level risk factor values for social stability Z_i' in disaster-preventive migration were calculated based on Equations (9) and (10):

$$Z = B \times V^T = [0.146, 0.197, 0.204, 0.262, 0.191] \times [1, 2, 3, 4, 5] = 3.155$$

$$Z_1' = B_1 \times V^T = [0.125, 0.151, 0.220, 0.275, 0.228] \times [1, 2, 3, 4, 5] = 3.327$$

$$Z_2' = B_2 \times V^T = [0.201, 0.227, 0.280, 0.137, 0.156] \times [1, 2, 3, 4, 5] = 2.819$$

$$Z_3' = B_3 \times V^T = [0.193, 0.241, 0.118, 0.283, 0.166] \times [1, 2, 3, 4, 5] = 2.989$$

$$Z_4' = B_4 \times V^T = [0.207, 0.367, 0.198, 0.160, 0.067] \times [1, 2, 3, 4, 5] = 2.514$$

$$Z_5' = B_5 \times V^T = [0.053, 0.124, 0.234, 0.354, 0.235] \times [1, 2, 3, 4, 5] = 3.595$$

where Z_1' is the assessment value of compensation risks, Z_2' is the assessment value of cultural risks, Z_3' is the assessment value of livelihood recovery risks, Z_4' is the assessment value of geological hazard risks, and Z_5' is the assessment value of public opinion risks.

The results of the comprehensive SSRA showed that the overall social stability risk of disaster-preventive migration in County D is 'high'. Specifically, compensation risks and public opinion risks were classified as 'high', while cultural risks, livelihood restoration risks, and geological hazard risks were classified as 'medium'. Figure 2 shows the scores of first-level risk factors for social stability in the risk assessment of disaster-preventive migration in County D, ranked in descending order: Public opinion risks (u_5) > compensation risks (u_1) > livelihood recovery risks (u_3) > cultural risks (u_2) > geological hazard risks (u_4).

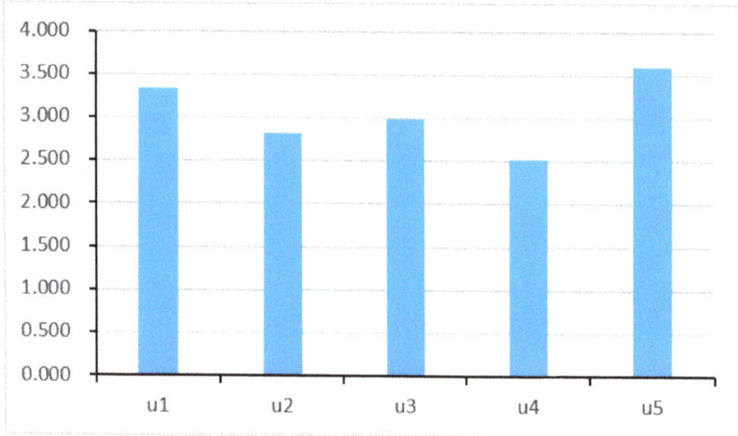

Figure 2. Social stability risk level of first-level risk factors.

5. Discussion

The results showed a 'high' overall social stability risk of disaster-preventive migration in County D, which may lead to social instability if risk prevention measures are not taken. The risk values of public opinion risks and compensation risks were the highest among the first-level risk factors, and geological disaster risks have a major influence on the willingness of DPM. Thus, to control the social stability risks of DPM in County D, decision-makers should primarily consider these three major risk factors.

(1) Public opinion risks: This risk showed three aspects, namely, the level of openness and transparency of information on disaster-preventive migration, the level of public participation, and the government's response to public opinions. Information plays an important role in risk management and is fundamental to risk communication [76]. The open and transparent flow of public information on disaster-preventive migration between the government and the society has become one of the important factors affecting the validity of risk governance [77]. Transparent information on disaster-preventive migration can help reduce public fears and avoid misunderstandings among affected people and can enable them to trust disaster-preventive resettlement projects [78,79]. Public opinion risks stemmed from a lack of information transparency. Moreover, the government's suppression, minimization, non-response, or inappropriate response to public opinion would aggravate public opinion and may have significant impacts.

Voluntariness and prior informed consent are important principles in the relocation and resettlement of disaster-affected migrants, and public participation is key for the implementation of these principles [80]. The central government, local governments, as well as several stakeholders and actors were involved in disaster-preventive migration in County D, with different stakeholders and actors having different interests and motivations in the project [81]. The World Bank has pointed out the importance of timely consultation with stakeholders on resettlement programs and of providing them with opportunities to participate in the planning, implementation, and monitoring of resettlement [82]. Furthermore, studies have shown that inadequate public participation in disaster-preventive migration may lead to conflicts among the stakeholders [83].

In fact, the government of County D had proposed a plan for relocation as early as 2003 and had conducted preliminary research on several proposed relocation sites. However, the county relocation plan was placed on hold. For a decade or so, the government failed to disclose information on the rationale for the relocation and the mode of relocation, which resulted in a widespread negative public opinion. Moreover, the government's evasive responses to such public opinion resulted in inadvertent harm to the residents. For example, some residents wanted to build new houses to improve their living conditions, but the overwhelming negative public opinion on county relocation prevented them from doing so. In 2019, the Ministry of Natural Resources dispatched a 'Letter of Recommendations on the Prevention and Control of Geological Disasters in County D, Diqing Prefecture, Yunnan Province' to the General Office of the Yunnan Provincial People's Government; this letter clearly stated that 'County D has become one of the counties most seriously threatened by geological disasters in Yunnan province and even in the country. The current development of the county exceeds its urban environmental capacity, posing severe potential risk from geological disasters to people's lives and properties', thereby bringing the relocation of County D back on the agenda. However, relevant information has remained 'confidential', and there was a lack of public participation in the formulation of the county's relocation plan, which led to the risks of public opinion being ranked first among all first-level risk factors. It is recommended that the People's Government of County D should seek instructions from the relevant departments at higher levels as soon as possible to clarify the policies and measures involved in relocation and to disclose the information to the public in a timely manner.

(2) Compensation risks: This risk was reflected in the compensation for houses and attached buildings, land and its appurtenances, and disaster-preventive resettlement of migrants. Studies have shown that the relocation compensation program is a core factor influencing the willingness of people to relocate and is also a key factor in reducing social stability risks [33,84,85]. County D is a multi-ethnic area where Tibetans are the main ethnic group; the residents' houses consist of wooden houses, brick houses, and cement houses. With the development of the tourism economy in County D, housing rental income has become an important source of income for the residents in the area. Therefore, residents had high expectations from relocation housing subsidies. Residents hoped to receive additional compensation for relocation in ethnic minority areas on top of the national compensation standard.

County D is rich in forestry resources, and the main forestry products are cordyceps and pine mushrooms. Therefore, farmers in Town S of County D currently have higher income levels than farmers in other parts of the county. Compensation for the forest land and its associated above-ground appurtenances in the relocation was one of the main concerns of farmers. Although the government promised that the mountain and forestry rights of S town would remain after the relocation and that residents could still return to S town to collect matsutake, cordyceps, and other forest products, the residents said that they basically would not come back to collect the forest products because the planned relocation site is too far from S town, and the cost of coming back to collect the forest products is too high. In addition, they stated that if they do not live there, the forest products, such as matsutake and cordyceps in the contracted forest land, would be collected by other people, and new conflicts and disputes would arise. These factors have led the residents to increase their compensation expectations.

In the implementation of resettlement, the provided compensation included cash, land, and employment [31]. Cash compensation is the simplest form of compensation and is used often in resettlement. However, cash compensation is not always effective. Some relocatees were not good at managing cash, and some used resettlement subsidies for weddings or gambling, which prevented them from relocating [86]. S town is a Tibetan settlement. Tibetan residents have the tradition of living in compact family communities, with several generations living together and building a single Tibetan house with front and back yards and livestock sheds, among other things. They are unable to accept apartments. The demand for resettlement homesteads became a priority during relocation, surpassing the demand for cash and employment compensation. Therefore, the relocation compensation scheme should fully consider the demands of different types of people, respect the customs of ethnic minorities, and meet the specified cultural requirements of ethnic minorities.

(3) Geological disaster risks: This risk is measured in terms of the "likelihood of occurrence" and the "magnitude of damage caused by geological hazards", which correspond to the "likelihood" and "threat" dimensions of risk perception, respectively [87–89]. Therefore, the geological disaster risks in this paper is, in fact, geological disaster risk perception. Some studies have found that disaster risk perception has a significant impact on DPM willingness [90]. Different measures of risk perception have inconsistent effects on migration decisions [91]. People's willingness to relocate will increase when the potential of a disaster is higher and the threat is greater [92]. The willingness of DPM has a direct impact on the social stability risk. Forced migration is more likely to cause social instability than voluntary migration [93,94]. The geological disaster risk is an inverse indicator, and its risk value is the lowest among the five primary risk factors, which suggests that experts had a higher risks perception of geological disaster in County D. However, during interviews with residents, we found that most residents' risk perception of geological disaster in County D was opposite to that of the experts. They believe that although minor geological disasters were once very common there, there had never been a serious geological disaster. They appeared very sure that disasters would not happen in the future, because the local government has already invested a lot of manpower and resources in the prevention and control of geological disasters.

Expert versus nonexpert (local resident) differences in geological disaster risk perception will cause great obstacles to the implementation of DPM. To make the DPM project in County D proceed smoothly, the People's Government of County D should resolve the potential differences in geological disaster risk perception between experts and nonexperts (aboriginal) as quickly as possible by highlighting the potential severity of geological disasters, their effects on people's lives and safety, and the restricted future development of the county, among other points.

6. Conclusions

Southwestern China is an area prone to geological disasters. To reduce the risk of disasters, many disaster-preventive relocation and resettlement programs have been implemented. Although disaster-preventive migration is an important method for disaster risk management, migration itself entails potential social stability risks, which would affect the harmony and stability of the society if not implemented properly [95]. How to identify and evaluate the social stability risk of DPM in County D is the core issue of this paper. In order to make the conclusions scientific and reasonable, this study identified the social stability risk of DPM in County D based on feedback from symposiums, in-depth interviews, and literature and assessed it by a fuzzy comprehensive evaluation method considering multiple experts' weights. The following conclusions were obtained from the research:

(1) The social stability risk of DPM in County D includes five first-level risk factors, which are public opinion risks, compensation risks, livelihood recovery risks, cultural risks, geological disaster risks.

(2) The overall social stability risk level of DPM in County D is 'high'. In terms of importance, the five first-level risk factors were ranked as follows: public opinion risks > compensation risks > livelihood recovery risks > cultural risks > geological disaster risks. Expert versus nonexpert differences in geological disaster risk perception will cause great obstacles to the implementation of DPM.

Author Contributions: Conceptualization, L.Z. and W.S.; methodology, L.Z.; formal analysis, L.Z.; investigation, D.Z.; supervision, D.Z.; validation, D.Z.; writing—original draft preparation, W.S.;

writing—review and editing, W.S. All authors have read and agreed to the published version of the manuscript.

Funding: This research was funded by the National Social Science Foundation of China (No. 13ZD176), the Shenzhen Philosophy and Social Science Planning Project (SZ2021A003).

Institutional Review Board Statement: The study was conducted according to the guidelines of the Declaration of Helsinki, and approved by the National Social Science Foundation of China.

Informed Consent Statement: Informed consent was obtained from all subjects involved in the study.

Data Availability Statement: Data sharing not applicable.

Conflicts of Interest: The authors declare no conflict of interest.

References

1. World Economic Forum Global Risks 2020 Report. Available online: https://www.weforum.org/reports/the-global-risks-report-2020 (accessed on 5 March 2022).
2. Corban, C.; Florczyk, A.; Freire, S.; Kemper, T.; Ehrlich, D.; Siragusa, A.; Pesaresi, M. *Atlas of the Human Planet 2017: Global Exposure to Natural Hazards*; EUR 28556 EN; European Commision Joint Research Centre (JRC): Ispra, Italy, 2017. [CrossRef]
3. Deraniyagala, S. Economic Recovery after Natural Disasters. *UN Chron.* **2016**, *53*, 31–34. [CrossRef]
4. Shi, P. (Ed.) *Natural Disasters in China*; Springer: Berlin/Heidelberg, Germany, 2016.
5. Ministry of Emergency Management of the People's Republic of China. National Natural Disaster Fundamentals for 2020. 8 January 2021. Available online: https://www.mem.gov.cn/xw/yjglbgzdt/202101/t20210108376745.shtml (accessed on 6 March 2022).
6. Ashar, F.; Amaratunga, D.; Sridarran, P.; Haigh, R. Practices of Tsunami Evacuation Planning in Padang, Indonesia. In *Coastal Management*; Academic Press: Cambridge, MA, USA, 2019; pp. 399–433.
7. Drabo, A.; Mbaye, L.M. Natural disasters, migration and education: An empirical analysis in developing countries. *Environ. Dev. Econ.* **2015**, *20*, 767–796. [CrossRef]
8. Field, C.B.; Barros, V.R. (Eds.) *Climate Change 2014–Impacts, Adaptation and Vulnerability: Regional Aspects*; Cambridge University Press: Cambridge, UK, 2014.
9. State Council of the People's Republic of China. Decision of the State Council on Strengthening the Prevention and Control of Geological Disasters. 17 June 2011. Available online: https://www.gov.cn/zwgk/2011-06/17/content_1886569.htm (accessed on 6 March 2022).
10. Lu, X.; Han, Z. Emergency management in China: Towards a comprehensive model? *J. Risk Res.* **2019**, *22*, 1425–1442. [CrossRef]
11. Downing, T.E. *Avoiding New Poverty: Mining-Induced Displacement and Resettlement*; International Institute for Environment and Development: London, UK, 2002.
12. Webber, M.; McDonald, B. Involuntary resettlement, production and income: Evidence from Xiaolangdi, PRC. *World Dev.* **2004**, *32*, 673–690. [CrossRef]
13. Cernea, M.M. For a new economics of resettlement: A sociological critique of the compensation principle. *Int. Soc. Sci. J.* **2003**, *55*, 37–45. [CrossRef]
14. Bui, T.M.H.; Schreinemachers, P.; Berger, T. Hydropower development in Vietnam: Involuntary resettlement and factors enabling rehabilitation. *Land Use Policy* **2013**, *31*, 536–544. [CrossRef]
15. Liu, Z.Z.; Zhu, Z.W.; Wang, H.J.; Huang, J. Handling social risks in government-driven mega project: An empirical case study from West China. *Int. J. Proj. Manag.* **2016**, *34*, 202–218. [CrossRef]
16. González-Parra, C.; Simon, J. All that glitters is not gold: Resettlement, vulnerability, and social exclusion in the Pehuenche community Ayin Mapu, Chile. *Am. Behav. Sci.* **2008**, *51*, 1774–1789. [CrossRef]
17. Hikichi, H.; Aida, J.; Kondo, K.; Tsuboya, T.; Kawachi, I. Residential relocation and obesity after a natural disaster: A natural experiment from the 2011 Japan Earthquake and Tsunami. *Sci. Rep.* **2019**, *9*, 374. [CrossRef]
18. Fernando, N.; Warner, K.; Birkmann, J. Migration and natural hazards: Is relocation a secondary disaster or an opportunity for vulnerability reduction? In *Environment, Forced Migration and Social Vulnerability*; Springer: Berlin/Heidelberg, Germany, 2010; pp. 145–156.
19. Correa, E. *Populations at Risk of Disaster: A Resettlement Guide*; Ramirez, F., Sanahuja, H., Eds.; World Bank and GFDRR: Washington, DC, USA, 2011.
20. Wilmsen, B.; Webber, M.; Yuefang, D. Development for whom? Rural to urban resettlement at the Three Gorges Dam, China. *Asian Stud. Rev.* **2011**, *35*, 21–42. [CrossRef]
21. Xue, L.; Wang, M.Y.; Xue, T. 'Voluntary'poverty alleviation resettlement in China. *Dev. Chang.* **2013**, *44*, 1159–1180. [CrossRef]
22. Hwang, S.S.; Cao, Y.; Xi, J. The short-term impact of involuntary migration in China's Three Gorges: A prospective study. *Soc. Indic. Res.* **2011**, *101*, 73–92. [CrossRef]

23. Snodgrass, J.G.; Upadhyay, C.; Debnath, D.; Lacy, M.G. The mental health costs of human displacement: A natural experiment involving indigenous Indian conservation refugees. *World Dev. Perspect.* **2016**, *2*, 25–33. [CrossRef]
24. Li, C.; Li, M. The Policy Information Gap and Resettlers' Well-Being: Evidence from the Anti-Poverty Relocation and Resettlement Program in China. *Int. J. Environ. Res. Public Health* **2020**, *17*, 2957. [CrossRef]
25. Barnett, J.; Webber, M. *Accommodating Migration to Promote Adaptation to Climate Change*; Policy Research Working Paper 5270; World Bank: Washington, DC, USA, 2010.
26. Artur, L.; Hilhorst, D. Floods, resettlement and land access and use in the lower Zambezi, Mozambique. *Land Use Policy* **2014**, *36*, 361–368. [CrossRef]
27. Vlaeminck, P.; Maertens, M.; Isabirye, M.; Vanderhoydonks, F.; Poesen, J.; Deckers, S.; Vranken, L. Coping with landslide risk through preventive resettlement. Designing optimal strategies through choice experiments for the Mount Elgon region, Uganda. *Land Use Policy* **2016**, *51*, 301–311. [CrossRef]
28. Claudianos, P. Out of Harm's Way; Preventive Resettlement of at Risk Informal Settlers in Highly Disaster Prone Areas. *Procedia Econ. Financ.* **2014**, *18*, 312–319. [CrossRef]
29. Lübken, U. Chasing a ghost? Environmental change and migration in history. *Glob. Environ.* **2012**, *5*, 4–24. [CrossRef]
30. Berg, T.M.V. "We are not compensating rocks": Resettlement and traditional religious systems. *World Dev.* **1999**, *27*, 271–283. [CrossRef]
31. Tadgell, A.; Doberstein, B.; Mortsch, L. Principles for climate-related resettlement of informal settlements in less developed nations: A review of resettlement literature and institutional guidelines. *Clim. Dev.* **2018**, *10*, 102–115. [CrossRef]
32. Peng, S.; Shi, G.; Zhang, R. Social stability risk assessment: Status, trends and prospects—A case of land acquisition and resettlement in the hydropower sector. *Impact Assess. Proj. Apprais.* **2021**, *39*, 379–395. [CrossRef]
33. Mathur, H.M. Social impact assessment: A tool for planning better resettlement. *Soc. Chang.* **2011**, *41*, 97–120. [CrossRef]
34. Esteves, A.M.; Franks, D.; Vanclay, F. Social impact assessment: The state of the art. *Impact Assess. Proj. Apprais.* **2012**, *30*, 34–42. [CrossRef]
35. Freudenburg, W.R. Social impact assessment. *Annu. Rev. Sociol.* **1986**, *12*, 451–478. [CrossRef]
36. International Association for Impact Assessment (IAIA). *International Principles and Guidelines for Social Impact Assessment*; International Association for Impact Assessment (IAIA): Fargo, ND, USA, 2003.
37. Vanclay, F. International principles for social impact assessment. *Impact Assess. Proj. Apprais.* **2003**, *21*, 5–12. [CrossRef]
38. Tang, B.S.; Wong, S.W.; Lau, M.C.H. Social impact assessment and public participation in China: A case study of land requisition in Guangzhou. *Environ. Impact Assess. Rev.* **2008**, *28*, 57–72. [CrossRef]
39. Ip, D.F.-K. Difficulties in implementing social impact assessment in China: Methodological considerations. *Environ. Impact Assess. Rev.* **1990**, *10*, 113–122.
40. He, Z.; Huang, D.; Zhang, C.; Fang, J. Toward a stakeholder perspective on social stability risk of large hydraulic engineering projects in China: A social network analysis. *Sustainability* **2018**, *10*, 1223. [CrossRef]
41. Guo, X.; Kapucu, N. Examining stakeholder participation in social stability risk assessment for mega projects using network analysis. *Int. J. Disaster Risk Manag.* **2019**, *1*, 1–31. [CrossRef]
42. Jiang, T.; Shi, G.; Pu, Y. How does a single community grant multiple social licences for a problematic metro project? Reflections from a dynamic perspective. *Impact Assess. Proj. Apprais.* **2021**, *39*, 96–109. [CrossRef]
43. Li, C.; Xi, Z. Social stability risk assessment of land expropriation: Lessons from the Chinese case. *Int. J. Environ. Res. Public Health* **2019**, *16*, 3952. [CrossRef]
44. Xu, X.H.; Wang, C.H.; Cai, C.G.; Xue, M. Evolution and coping research for flood disaster social stability risk based on the complex network. *Nat. Hazards* **2015**, *77*, 1491–1500. [CrossRef]
45. Vanclay, F. Reflections on Social Impact Assessment in the 21st century. *Impact Assess. Proj. Apprais.* **2020**, *38*, 126–131. [CrossRef]
46. Guadagno, L. Human mobility in the Sendai framework for disaster risk reduction. *Int. J. Disaster Risk Sci.* **2016**, *7*, 30–40. [CrossRef]
47. Jaquet, S.; Shrestha, G.; Kohler, T.; Schwilch, G. The effects of migration on livelihoods, land management, and vulnerability to natural disasters in the Harpan watershed in western Nepal. *Mt. Res. Dev.* **2016**, *36*, 494–505. [CrossRef]
48. Sina, D.; Chang-Richards, A.Y.; Wilkinson, S.; Potangaroa, R. What does the future hold for relocated communities post-disaster? Factors affecting livelihood resilience. *Int. J. Disaster Risk Reduct.* **2019**, *34*, 173–183. [CrossRef]
49. Xu, Y.; Qiu, X.; Yang, X.; Lu, X.; Chen, G. Disaster risk management models for rural relocation communities of mountainous southwestern China under the stress of geological disasters. *Int. J. Disaster Risk Reduct.* **2020**, *50*, 101697. [CrossRef]
50. Chen, Y.; He, L.; Zhou, D. Consequences of post-disaster policies and relocation approaches: Two communities from rural China. *Disaster Prev. Manag. Int. J.* **2020**, *30*, 340–353. [CrossRef]
51. Li, C.; Li, S.; Feldman, M.W.; Li, J.; Zheng, H.; Daily, G.C. The impact on rural livelihoods and ecosystem services of a major relocation and settlement program: A case in Shaanxi, China. *Ambio* **2018**, *47*, 245–259. [CrossRef]
52. Zhao, F.; Yang, Y.Y. Vulnerability of immigrants' livelihood in reservoir resettlement caused by external force and its solution: A case study of the reservoir zone of the south-to-north water diversion. *Popul. Econ.* **2009**, *175*, 1–7.
53. Huong, N.T.L.; Yao, S.; Fahad, S. Assessing household livelihood vulnerability to climate change: The case of Northwest Vietnam. *Hum. Ecol. Risk Assess. Int. J.* **2019**, *25*, 1157–1175. [CrossRef]

54. Paul, M., Jr.; Boakye, J.A.; Muliro, M. Mitigating the impacts of floods using adaptive and resilient coping strategies: The role of the emergency Livelihood Empowerment Against Poverty program (LEAP) in Ghana. *J. Environ. Manag.* **2020**, *270*, 110809.
55. Xiao, Q.; Liu, H.; Feldman, M. Assessing livelihood reconstruction in resettlement program for disaster prevention at Baihe county of China: Extension of the impoverishment risks and reconstruction (IRR) model. *Sustainability* **2018**, *10*, 2913. [CrossRef]
56. Randell, H. Structure and agency in development-induced forced migration: The case of Brazil's Belo Monte Dam. *Popul. Environ.* **2016**, *37*, 265–287. [CrossRef]
57. Sheikhi, R.A.; Seyedin, H.; Qanizadeh, G.; Jahangiri, K. Role of religious institutions in disaster risk management: A systematic review. *Disaster Med. Public Health Prep.* **2021**, *15*, 239–254. [CrossRef]
58. Ha, K.M. The role of religious beliefs and institutions in disaster management: A case study. *Religions* **2015**, *6*, 1314–1329. [CrossRef]
59. Colson, E. Forced migration and the anthropological response. *J. Refug. Stud.* **2003**, *16*, 1–18. [CrossRef]
60. UNDRR. Disaster Risk Reduction in Sri Lanka: Status Report 2019. Available online: https://www.unisdr.org/files/68230_10srilankadrmstatusreport.pdf (accessed on 10 March 2022).
61. Xu, Y.; Wu, D.; Chen, N.C. Here I belong!: Understanding immigrant descendants' place attachment and its impact on their community citizenship behaviors in China. *J. Environ. Psychol.* **2022**, *79*, 101743. [CrossRef]
62. Qing, C.; Guo, S.; Deng, X.; Wang, W.; Song, J.; Xu, D. Stay in Risk Area: Place Attachment, Efficacy Beliefs and Risk Coping. *Int. J. Environ. Res. Public Health* **2022**, *19*, 2375. [CrossRef]
63. McDowell, C. (Ed.) *Understanding Impoverishment: The Consequences of Development-Induced Displacement*; Berghahn Books: New York, NY, USA, 1996; Volume 2.
64. Swapan, M.S.H.; Sadeque, S. Place attachment in natural hazard-prone areas and decision to relocate: Research review and agenda for developing countries. *Int. J. Disaster Risk Reduct.* **2021**, *52*, 101937. [CrossRef]
65. Askman, J.; Nilsson, O.; Becker, P. Why people live in flood-prone areas in Akuressa, Sri Lanka. *Int. J. Disaster Risk Sci.* **2018**, *9*, 143–156. [CrossRef]
66. Xu, D.; Qing, C.; Deng, X.; Yong, Z.; Zhou, W.; Ma, Z. Disaster risk perception, sense of pace, evacuation willingness, and relocation willingness of rural households in earthquake-stricken areas: Evidence from Sichuan Province, China. *Int. J. Environ. Res. Public Health* **2020**, *17*, 602. [CrossRef]
67. Slovic, P. Perception of risk. *Science* **1987**, *236*, 280–285. [CrossRef]
68. Xu, D.; Liu, E.; Wang, X.; Tang, H.; Liu, S. Rural households' livelihood capital, risk perception, and willingness to purchase earthquake disaster insurance: Evidence from southwestern China. *Int. J. Environ. Res. Public Health* **2018**, *15*, 1319. [CrossRef]
69. Shah, A.A.; Ye, J.; Abid, M.; Ullah, R. Determinants of flood risk mitigation strategies at household level: A case of Khyber Pakhtunkhwa (KP) province, Pakistan. *Nat. Hazards* **2017**, *88*, 415–430. [CrossRef]
70. Xu, D.; Zhou, W.; Deng, X.; Ma, Z.; Yong, Z.; Qin, C. Information credibility, disaster risk perception and evacuation willingness of rural households in China. *Nat. Hazards* **2020**, *103*, 2865–2882. [CrossRef]
71. Wang, J.; Guan, J.; Wei, Y.; Gao, P.; Mei, A.; Zhang, D. A study of the disaster model and movement process simulation of debris flow in the Zhixi River of Deqin County. *Hydrogeol. Eng. Geol.* **2021**, *48*, 187–195.
72. Samaras, G.D.; Gkanas, N.I.; Vitsa, K.C. Assessing risk in dam projects using AHP and ELECTRE I. *Int. J. Constr. Manag.* **2014**, *14*, 255–266. [CrossRef]
73. Du, Y.W.; Wang, S.S.; Wang, Y.M. Group fuzzy comprehensive evaluation method under ignorance. *Expert Syst. Appl.* **2019**, *126*, 92–111. [CrossRef]
74. Li, W.; Liang, W.; Zhang, L.; Tang, Q. Performance assessment system of health, safety and environment based on experts' weights and fuzzy comprehensive evaluation. *J. Loss Prev. Process Ind.* **2015**, *35*, 95–103. [CrossRef]
75. Liu, W.; Hui, L.; Lu, Y.; Tang, J. Developing an evaluation method for SCADA-Controlled urban gas infrastructure hierarchical design using multi-level fuzzy comprehensive evaluation. *Int. J. Crit. Infrastruct. Prot.* **2020**, *30*, 100375. [CrossRef]
76. Shi, J.; Hu, X.; Guo, X.; Lian, C. Risk information seeking behavior in disaster resettlement: A case study of ankang city, China. *Int. J. Environ. Res. Public Health* **2020**, *17*, 7352. [CrossRef] [PubMed]
77. Zheng, S.; Meng, T. Government Information Disclosure and Governance Effectiveness in Public Crisis Governance-Based on a Survey Experiment. *Public Manag. Policy Rev.* **2022**, *11*, 88–103.
78. Zhang, W.; Wang, M.; Zhu, Y.C. Does government information release really matter in regulating contagion-evolution of negative emotion during public emergencies? From the perspective of cognitive big data analytics. *Int. J. Inf. Manag.* **2020**, *50*, 498–514. [CrossRef]
79. Asiama, K.; Lengoiboni, M.; Van der Molen, P. In the land of the dammed: Assessing governance in resettlement of Ghana's Bui Dam Project. *Land* **2017**, *6*, 80. [CrossRef]
80. Ty, P.H.; Van Westen, A.C.M.; Zoomers, A. Compensation and resettlement policies after compulsory land acquisition for hydropower development in Vietnam: Policy and practice. *Land* **2013**, *2*, 678–704. [CrossRef]
81. Singer, J.; Pham, H.T.; Hoang, H. Broadening stakeholder participation to improve outcomes for dam-forced resettlement in Vietnam. *Water Resour. Rural Dev.* **2014**, *4*, 85–103. [CrossRef]
82. World Bank. *Involuntary Resettlement Sourcebook: Planning and Implemention in Development Projects*; The World Bank: Washington, DC, USA, 2004.

83. Chung, J. Conflicts and natural disaster management: A comparative study of flood control in the Republic of Korea and the United States. *Disasters* **2016**, *40*, 554–572. [CrossRef]
84. Bukvic, A.; Smith, A.; Zhang, A. Evaluating drivers of coastal relocation in Hurricane Sandy affected communities. *Int. J. Disaster Risk Reduct.* **2015**, *13*, 215–228. [CrossRef]
85. Seebauer, S.; Winkler, C. Should I stay or should I go? Factors in household decisions for or against relocation from a flood risk area. *Glob. Environ. Chang.* **2020**, *60*, 102018. [CrossRef]
86. Al Atahar, S. Development-driven forced displacement and compensation-based resettlement: Experiences from the Jamuna multi-purpose bridge project. *Dev. Pract.* **2014**, *24*, 258–271. [CrossRef]
87. Xu, D.; Peng, L.; Su, C.; Liu, S.; Wang, X.; Chen, T. Influences of mass monitoring and mass prevention systems on peasant households' disaster risk perception in the landslide-threatened Three Gorges Reservoir area, China. *Habitat Int.* **2016**, *58*, 23–33. [CrossRef]
88. Lazo, J.K.; Bostrom, A.; Morss, R.E.; Demuth, J.L.; Lazrus, H. Factors affecting hurricane evacuation intentions. *Risk Anal.* **2015**, *35*, 1837–1857. [CrossRef] [PubMed]
89. Xue, K.; Guo, S.; Liu, Y.; Liu, S.; Xu, D. Social networks, trust, and disaster-risk perceptions of rural residents in a multi-disaster environment: Evidence from Sichuan, China. *Int. J. Environ. Res. Public Health* **2021**, *18*, 2106. [CrossRef] [PubMed]
90. Stein, R.M.; Dueñas-Osorio, L.; Subramanian, D. Who evacuates when hurricanes approach? The role of risk, information, and location. *Soc. Sci. Q.* **2010**, *91*, 816–834. [CrossRef]
91. Wang, H.; Shi, G.; Zhang, R.; Xu, J.; Shangguan, Z. Risk perceptions and mining-induced displacement and resettlement: A case study from Anhui Province, China. *Impact Assess. Proj. Apprais.* **2021**, *39*, 366–378. [CrossRef]
92. Xu, D.; Peng, L.; Liu, S.; Su, C.; Wang, X.; Chen, T. Influences of sense of place on farming households' relocation willingness in areas threatened by geological disasters: Evidence from China. *Int. J. Disaster Risk Sci.* **2017**, *8*, 16–32. [CrossRef]
93. Martins-Borges, L. Involuntary migration as a risk factor for mental health. *REMHU Rev. Interdiscip. Mobilidade Hum.* **2013**, *21*, 151–162. [CrossRef]
94. Shaojun, C. A study of poverty risks based on involuntary migration of Chinese village dwellers. *Chin. Sociol. Anthropol.* **2006**, *38*, 19–39. [CrossRef]
95. Chen, Y.; Li, Q.; He, L.; Xu, Y.; Xue, N. Factors Influencing People's Perception of Dual Risks in Population Resettlement: A Case Study of Resettlement in Mountain Areas of Western China. *J. Southwest Pet. Univ. Soc. Sci. Ed.* **2021**, *23*, 24–33.

International Journal of
Environmental Research and Public Health

MDPI

Article

The Spatiotemporal Evolutionary Trend and Driving Factors of the Coupling Coordinated Development between Regional Green Finance and Ecological Environment

Tao Shi

Economics Institute, Henan Academy of Social Science, Fengchan Road 21, Zhengzhou 450002, China; taoshi_ccp@163.com

Abstract: Based on the 30 inland provincial samples of China from 2003 to 2019, this article analyzes the evolutionary characteristics of the coupling coordination between green finance and the ecological environment (CCFE) using ArcGIS 10.5 software and employs the spatial Durbin model to analyze the driving factors of the CCFE. The results can be concluded as follows: (1) the CCFE of China is at a moderately low level, with a fluctuating upward trend. Spatially, it presents a spatial distribution pattern—higher in the east and lower in other regions. In terms of types, the regions of the CCFE are more in primary coordination and basic un-coordination and less in moderate un-coordination and moderate coordination. There are more regions of the green finance lagged type, and relatively few regions have achieved the financial ecological synchronization type. (2) The CCFE hotspots are concentrated in the Pearl River Delta, with a spatial "increase–decrease" development trend. Additionally, the CCFE cold spots are concentrated in the upper Yellow River Basin, with a relatively stable spatial scope. (3) The CCFE shows a positive spillover effect and accumulative delivery effect in the economic geospatial space. The population urbanization rate and the number of granted patent applications have a significant positive impact on the CCFE, and the percentage of secondary industries to GDP has a negative impact accordingly. Spatially, the percentage of secondary industries to GDP and the number of granted patent applications of nearby provinces in the economic geospatial space have a negative impact on the local CCFE. (4) The impact and spatial effect of different factors on the CCFE are obviously different. Finally, policy implications on the coordinated development of green finance and the ecological environment are also made.

Keywords: green finance; ecological environment; coupling coordination rate; spatiotemporal evolution; driving factor

Citation: Shi, T. The Spatiotemporal Evolutionary Trend and Driving Factors of the Coupling Coordinated Development between Regional Green Finance and Ecological Environment. *IJERPH* **2022**, *19*, 6211. https://doi.org/10.3390/ijerph19106211

Academic Editors: Jie Chen, Qian Zhou and Ting Zhang

Received: 6 April 2022
Accepted: 17 May 2022
Published: 20 May 2022

1. Introduction

The ecological environment is the foundation of human survival and development; promoting the high-quality development of the ecological environment has received great attention. In the past 10 years, China has been committed to ecological environment construction and protection and has achieved remarkable results. According to the ecological environment bulletin in China (2020) and the annual report of the electricity industry in China (2021), in the "13th-Five-Year-Plan" period, China's coal-fired power generation units meted the ultra-low emission limit and reached a total of 950 million kilowatts, the proportion of good days in the prefecture-level cities and above increased to 87.0% (target 84.5%), the average concentration ratio of PM2.5 in the prefecture-level cities that have not reached the standard decreased to 28.8% compared to that in 2015 (target 18%), the proportion of surface water with excellent quality increased to 83.74% (target 70%), and the safe utilization rate of polluted land reached 90%. Nowadays, green finance development in China has reached the international first-class level, and the effective development of the ecological environment cannot be separated from China's earlier implementation of green finance policy [1]. Since China launched green loan products in 2012, China has gradually established an integrated green finance system, covering green credit, green bonds, green insurance, green security, and so forth. According to the annual report on green finance development in China (2021), up to June 2021, the accumulative issuance of green bonds in domestic China and abroad exceeded RMB 1.73 trillion, and the transaction value of the carbon emission rights trading market reached RMB 100 billion; this has strengthened the promotion of ecological environment protection and construction. However, there is a spatial unbalance in the development of green finance and the ecological environment in China [2]. China's financial resources are mainly concentrated in the economically developed eastern regions, the carbon emission rights trading pilot regions. Except for Chongqing city and Hubei province, which are located in the central and western regions, Beijing, Shanghai, Guangdong, and Shenzhen are located in the eastern regions. Meanwhile, China's ecological fragile regions are mainly located in the central and western regions, such as the northwestern arid region and the upper Yellow River Basin. In 2020, China announced that it would promote "3060" targets in the future and that green finance and ecological development would play important roles in the "3060" development process. Therefore, it is obviously significant to explore the coupling coordination development between green finance and the ecological environment (CCFE) and the driving forces.

The issues about green finance and the ecological environment have also attracted scholars' attention. Based on 30 inland city samples in China, adopting the GMM model, H. Zhou & Xu (2022) [3] concluded that green finance has a negative impact on ecological development in China; there is an invert U-shaped relationship between green finance and the regions' ecological development, and the inverted U-shaped relationship is more obvious in the central and western regions. Furthermore, R. Wang et al. (2022) [4] confirmed the conclusions above and considered that there is a nonlinear U-shaped relationship between green finance and regional ecological efficiency, especially in the central and western regions. In addition, some scholars have studied green finance and high-quality development [5] and green finance and economic growth [6]. The scholars have discussed the causal relationship between green finance and the ecological environment but have not explored the dependence and degree of dependence between the green finance system and the ecological environmental system. Based on the views above, this article will focus on the coupling coordinated relationship between green finance and the ecological environment and analyze the overall characteristics, spatiotemporal distributed patterns, spatial aggregation evolution characteristics, and driving forces of the CCFE. Additionally, the potential contributions are as follows: (1) Adopting the coupling coordination model, this article calculates the CCFE index of 30 inland sample provinces in China from 2003 to 2020 and, using ArcGIS 10.5, analyzes the spatiotemporal evolution of the overall characteristics and regional pattern characteristics of CCFE, showing the systematic development of CCFE in China. (2) Appling the spatial hot–cold model, this article analyzes the spatiotemporal evolution of different regions with a high or low value of CCFE. (3) Using the spatial Durbin model with a two-order lag period, this article analyzes the driving force affecting the CCFE and explores the spatial heterogeneity and spatial spillover effects of different factors.

The rest part of this article is structured as follows. Section 1.1 provides a brief literature review on green finance and the ecological environment. Section 2 presents the calculated index of green finance and the ecological environment, the coupling coordination model, and the spatial Durbin model and describes the panel data used in this article. Section 3 reports the empirical estimation results, and we discuss the results in Section 4. Section 5 concludes the results and provides policy implications.

1.1. Literature Review

1.1.1. The Appraisal of the Ecological Environment

Recently, scholars have had a consensus on the definition of ecological environment, and ecological environment appraisals have become a research hotspot. From the view of an evaluation system, most scholars have evaluated the ecological environment from the perspectives of comprehensive index evaluation and efficiency evaluation [7], and most related factors can be divided into the two aspects of natural factors and human factors. Among them, the natural factors include the forest cover rate, atmosphere variation, and nature protection region, and the human factors include urbanization and land use. A typical comprehensive evaluation system is similar to systems created by Yibo et al. (2021) [8], who constructed an ecological environment quality index system that includes natural ecology and social indicators, and Xiao et al. (2021) [9], who constructed an ecological environment evaluation index system that includes 13 aspects, such as per capita green area, per capita water resources, and energy consumption per unit of GDP. Meanwhile, a typical ecological environment efficiency evaluation system, such as the one studied by Zhang et al. (2022) [10], analyzes China's environmental development efficiency; the input index includes the employed population, capital investment, and water use and the output index includes GDP, CO_2 emissions, SO_2 emissions, and soot emissions. Zhang et al. believe that environmental development in China shows a spatial distribution that is high in the east and low in other regions. Therefore, a comprehensive index evaluation system can better show the development of the ecological environment from more detailed perspectives, and we adopt this in this article.

Accordingly, scholars have used the principal component analysis method, the entropy method, the fuzzy Delphi analytic hierarchy process, and multiple normalization methods combined with pixel-phenology to evaluate the ecological environment [11]. Additionally, the typical method, such as Chang et al.'s method (2019) [12], uses spatial principal component analysis to analyze the ecological index in the upper Hanjiang river regions. Shi et al. (2020) [13] adopted the entropy method to calculate the regional ecological environment index in the tropical and subtropical regions in China from 2003 to 2016, and Y. Liu et al. (2022) [14] applied the DEA-SBM model to analyze ecological security. In addition, some scholars have used artificial intelligence and complex numerical optimization to analyze the ecological environment management problem [15].

1.1.2. The Definition and Appraisal of Green Finance

Focusing on the improvement of the ecological environment, scholars have earlier studied green finance. Salazar (1998) [16] believed that financial innovation must base on environmental protection to improve social progress, achieving a dynamic balance between environmental protection and economic development. This is the first conception of green finance, and it emphasizes that the development target of green finance is environmental protection and social progress. Along with the more complex ecological environment development, environmental risk has begun to be more obvious, and the conception of green finance brings more detail and focus to environmental risk. Labatt and White (2002) [17] believed that green finance is a kind of financial innovation required to prevent environmental risk in financial instruments and product innovation. In 2016, China integrated the green development concept into the G20 agenda and reached a global consensus on the development of green finance; the target of green finance has been raised to emphasize the human survival situation, strengthening the ecological balance through financial services and product innovation [18]. Recently, the most recognized concept of green finance is to provide financial services for environmental protection, energy savings, clean energy, and green transportation, to support environmental improvement, resource savings, and efficient use, and to combat climate change [19,20], and we follow this definition in this article.

Based on the concept of green finance, few scholars have analyzed the evaluation of green finance from a quantitative perspective. Scholars have calculated the development of green finance using green bonds, green securities, and green insurance as the replacement variables of green finance [21]. Additionally, a single index cannot efficiently reflect the development level of green finance; some scholars have tried to construct a comprehensive evaluation system, including bonds and securities. [22]. In addition, some scholars have appraised green finance development efficiency from the input and output perspectives [23].

1.1.3. The Relationship between Green Finance and the Ecological Environment

Scholars believe that green finance has efficiently promoted ecological environment development [24]. In one aspect, the government guides the development direction of the market to clean technology, such as carbon capture, tidal energy, and nuclear energy [25]. Meanwhile, using environmental regulation tools such as an environmental tax, the government can dispose of environmentally destructive actions to promote the high-quality development of the ecological environment. In another aspect, sustainable energy investment can be promoted to advance industrial decarbonization [26] using green financial tools, such as green bonds [27]. Additionally, it can also guide the green low-carbon transformation of energy consumption structures and industry structures [28] to promote the green low-carbon development of the economy, reducing the environmental pollution caused by economic and social development. Especially in the COVID-19 pandemic period, green financial policies such as carbon pricing and tradable green certificates can efficiently reduce the financial cost and counteract the negative shock of the pandemic [29]. In addition, green finance is a key factor for high technology to drive green growth, keeping resource prices and economic development stable [30].

However, some scholars believe that green finance does not bring clean energy but that green financial investments are only impelled by the demand for clean energy [31], and environmental regulations will constrain the role of green finance [32]. Therefore, combined with the modern concept of green finance, we can see that green finance emphasizes the coordinated development of financial activities, environmental protection, and ecological balance to realize the continuous development of economies and society [33], and green finance and the ecological environment show a merged and interactive developmental relationship. Indeed, from 1998 to 2018, the ecological environment of only one-third of China has improved [34] with the rapid development of green finance development. Therefore, according to the study above, we propose hypotheses H1 and H2:

Hypothesis 1 (H1). *The mutual and interactive developmental relationship between green finance and the ecological environment in China is at a low level with spatial heterogeneity.*

Hypothesis 2 (H2). *There are some factors that constrict the mutual and interactive developmental relationship between green finance and the ecological environment in China.*

1.1.4. Summary

As discussed above, scholars have analyzed the related issues on green finance and the ecological environment from different perspectives, with more study on the concept, impact, and appraisal and less on the relationship between green finance and the ecological environment. Few scholars have explored green finance and green development, economic growth, and ecological development efficiency, and we lacked a study on the CCFE. Therefore, based on the 30 inland provincial samples from 2003 to 2020 in China, this article will systematically analyze the overall characteristics, spatiotemporal evolution, and driving factors of the CCFE to promote green finance and the ecological environmental development of China in the "14th-Five-Year-Plan" period. Figure 1 shows the technological path of this article.

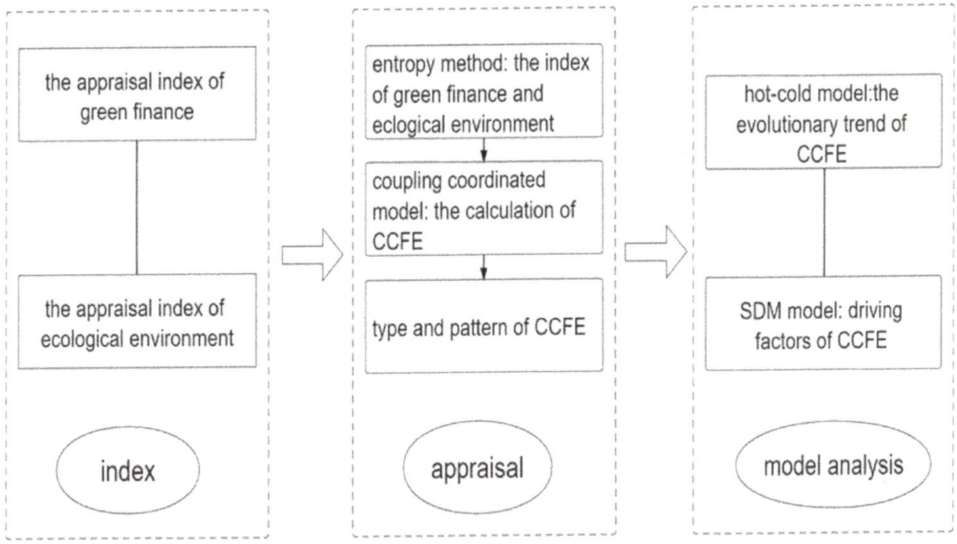

Figure 1. The technological path of this article.

2. Materials and Methods

2.1. The Calculation of Green Finance and the Ecological Environment

Referring to the current research [35,36], adhering to the principle of systematicness, scientificity, comprehensiveness, and accessibility, combined with the reality of China's green finance and ecological development, we constructed a comprehensive evaluation index system of green finance and the ecological environment. Table 1 shows the index and statistical descriptions; the values presented in Table 1 are for regions in China.

Table 1. Comprehensive appraisal index system and statistical descriptions.

Description	Unit	Mean	Std. Dev.	Min	Max
The market value proportion of environmental protection enterprises to total enterprises	%	1.479	2.485	0.000	22.427
The proportion of fixed asset investments in water conservancy, environment, and the public facilities management industry to total social fixed asset investment	%	10.269	5.234	3.484	45.650
The proportion of interest expenses in the output of six high-energy-consumption industries to the total industry	%	58.616	18.655	16.451	116.258
The proportion of completed investment in industrial pollution to GDP	%	0.147	0.131	0.001	0.992
Total industrial wastewater discharge	10,000 tons	71,570.25	59,639.56	3453.0	296,318.0
Total industrial waste air emission discharge	100 million standard m^3	18,079.460	15,778.840	533.000	87,297.970
Total industrial solid waste production	10,000 tons	12,512.900	21,066.850	91.000	265,481.500
The number of environmental pollution incidents	times	22.248	41.412	0.000	406.000

Table 1. *Cont.*

Description	Unit	Mean	Std. Dev.	Min	Max
The percentage of fiscal expenditure on environmental pollution to GDP	%	0.709	0.511	0.019	3.614
The percentage of environmental pollution governance investment to GDP	%	1.319	0.683	0.121	4.240
The harmless treatment rate of domestic waste	%	78.761	23.270	11.800	100.393
Total industrial wastewater treatment	10,000 tons	214,968.900	273,059.700	4213.491	2,125,782.000
The city sewage treatment rate	%	76.298	21.515	0.210	100.000
Treatment capacity of industrial waste gas treatment facilities	10,000 m^3/h	118,491.00	301,661.10	449.361	3,190,759.0
Comprehensive utilization rate of industrial solid waste	%	66.100	20.374	15.903	99.600
The area of natural protection	10,000 hectares	356.988	560.576	9.038	2183.698
Public green area per capita	m^2	11.033	3.457	3.100	21.795
Green space rate of built-up area	%	33.082	5.543	15.640	47.305
Forest coverage	%	30.768	17.791	2.940	66.971
Electricity consumption	100 million kwh	1556.901	1291.464	56.620	6940.000
Energy consumption	10,000 tons of standard coal	12,832.900	8441.495	684.000	42,441.410
Energy consumption per unit GDP	ton of standard coal/10,000 yuan	1.066	0.673	0.207	4.524
Total apparent CO_2 emissions	mt	94.206	132.486	0.200	879.816
Carbon intensity	ton/10,000 Yuan	1.363	2.079	0.001	12.085

Note: (1) Data shown in Table 1 range from 2003 to 2020 in China; (2) the data source mentioned in Section 2.3.

Green finance aims to support economic activities, such as environmental improvement and tackling climate change [37], by using comprehensive tools. Therefore, we chose green securities, green industries, green credit, and green investments to comprehensively calculate the development level of green finance, calculating the index of the market value proportion of environmental protection enterprises to total enterprises; the proportion of fixed asset investments in water conservancy, environment, and the public facilities management industry to total social fixed asset investment; the proportion of interest expenses in the output of six high-energy-consumption industries to the total industry; and the proportion of completed investments in industrial pollution to GDP correspondingly. Among them, according to the industrial category in the software of Tonghuasun, we chose the environmental protection pattern of the enterprise as air governance, water governance, solid waste governance, comprehensive environment governance, and environmental protection equipment.

The ecological environment is a complex ecosystem related to the sustainable development of society and the economy, and it is a comprehensive reflection of environmental pollution and environmental governance [38]. Therefore, we chose the pollution intensity of the ecological environment, the governance intensity of the ecological environment, the construction level of the ecological environment, and energy intensity to calculate ecological environmental development. Among them, the pollution intensity of the ecological environmental represents the ecological polluted level caused by different types of pollution, such as air and solid waste; an index of total industrial wastewater discharge, total industrial waste air emission discharge, total industrial solid waste production, and the number of environmental pollution incidents was chosen. Ecological environment governance intensity reflects the governance performance of the different roles of government, enterprises, and individuals [39,40]; an index of the percentage of fiscal expenditure on environmental pollution to GDP, the percentage of environmental pollution governance investment to GDP, the harmless treatment rate of domestic waste, total industrial wastewater treatment, the city sewage treatment rate, the treatment capacity of industrial waste gas treatment facilities, and the comprehensive utilization rate of industrial solid waste was chosen. The construction level of the ecological environment is the realistic manifestation of ecological environment condition improvements, such as regional forest cover, and an important foundation promoting ecological environment development [41]; an index of the area of natural protection, public green area per capita, green space rate of built-up area, and forest coverage was chosen. Traditional resources such as oil are an important source that leads to ecological environment pollution, while clean energy, such as electricity, can efficiently improve the ecological environment. Different production modes also play an important role in changes in the ecological environment [42]; an index of electricity consumption, energy consumption, energy consumption per unit GDP, total apparent CO_2 emissions, and carbon intensity was chosen.

2.2. The Analysis of CCFE and Driving Force

2.2.1. The Calculated Method of CCFE

Compared to comprehensive calculated methods, such as the analytic hierarchy process, the entropy method can avoid subjective factors impacting the results and more objectively evaluate the index [43,44]. Therefore, based on the entropy method, we calculate the ecological environmental development level $iecolg_i$ in year i as follows:

$$iecolg_i = \sum_{j=1}^{m} w_j \times x_i' \tag{1}$$

In Formula (1), w_j represents the weight of different samples; x_i' refers to the standardized index and is calculated as follows:

$$\begin{cases} x_i' = \frac{x_i - \min\{x_1,\ldots,x_n\}}{\max\{x_1,\ldots,x_n\} - \min\{x_1,\ldots,x_n\}} \\ p_i = (1 + x_i') / \sum_{i=1}^{n} (1 + x_i') \\ e_j = -k \sum_{i=1}^{n} p_i \times \ln(p_i), k = 1/\ln(n) \\ w_j = d_j / \sum_{j}^{m} d_j, d_j = 1 - e_j \end{cases} \tag{2}$$

In Formula (2), x_i refers to the index value correspondently. A change in the numerator of x_i' to ($\max\{x_1, \ldots, x_n\}$-x_i) will negatively standardize the value of x_i. Additionally, p_i represents the weight of the sample index, e_j refers to the information entropy in index j, d_j is the utility of index j, and n is the sample number; lastly, we calculate the weight of different indices, w_j. Similarly, we calculate the green finance development index $igreen_i$ using the same method above.

2.2.2. The Calculation of Coupling Coordination

Referring to the definition of capacity coupling and the coefficient model in physics [45,46] and setting the couple value between green finance and the ecological environment, we obtained the coupling appraisal model between green finance and the ecological environment; the couple value C_j in region j is calculated as follows:

$$C_j = \left\{ \frac{S_{iecolg} \times S_{igreen}}{\left(\frac{S_{iecolg} + S_{igreen}}{2}\right)^2} \right\}^k, (k \geq 2) \tag{3}$$

In Formula (3), k represents the number of coupling indices, and setting $k = 2$. However, the couple level cannot efficiently reflect the high and low levels of the coordinated development between green finance and the ecological environment, especially since it is difficult to represent the "overall efficacy" and "coordination effect" of regional green finance and the ecological environment [47]. Additionally, we need to calculate the CCFE of $iccdn_j$, as follows:

$$iccdn_j = \sqrt{c_j \times t_j},\ t_j = \alpha S_{iecolg} + \beta S_{igreen} \tag{4}$$

In Formula (4), α and β are the important indicators of green finance and the ecological environment, respectively. In the current global economic development condition, green finance is as important as the ecological environment, setting $\alpha = \beta = 0.5$. Referring to the current research, we divided the CCFE types, as shown in Table 2.

Table 2. The CCFE type.

CCFE Level	Type	Efficacy	Pattern
$0.8 < iccdn_j \le 0.1$	Quality coordination (TCC)	$S_{iecolg} < S_{igreen}$	Ecological environment lagged
		$S_{iecolg} \approx S_{igreen}$	Green finance and ecological environment synchronization
		$S_{iecolg} > S_{igreen}$	Green finance lagged
$0.6 < iccdn_j \le 0.8$	High coordination (HCC)	$S_{iecolg} < S_{igreen}$	Ecological environment lagged
		$S_{iecolg} \approx S_{igreen}$	Green finance and ecological environment synchronization
		$S_{iecolg} > S_{igreen}$	Green finance lagged
$0.5 < iccdn_j \le 0.6$	Middle coordination (MCC)	$S_{iecolg} < S_{igreen}$	Ecological environment lagged
		$S_{iecolg} \approx S_{igreen}$	Green finance and ecological environment synchronization
		$S_{iecolg} > S_{igreen}$	Green finance lagged
$0.4 < iccdn_j \le 0.5$	Primary coordination (UCC)	$S_{iecolg} < S_{igreen}$	Ecological environment lagged
		$S_{iecolg} \approx S_{igreen}$	Green finance and ecological environment synchronization
		$S_{iecolg} > S_{igreen}$	Green finance lagged
$0.3 < iccdn_j \le 0.4$	Basic un-coordination (EUCC)	$S_{iecolg} < S_{igreen}$	Ecological environment lagged
		$S_{iecolg} \approx S_{igreen}$	Green finance and ecological environment synchronization
		$S_{iecolg} > S_{igreen}$	Green finance lagged
$0.2 < iccdn_j \le 0.3$	Middle un-coordination (MUCC)	$S_{iecolg} < S_{igreen}$	Ecological environment lagged
		$S_{iecolg} \approx S_{igreen}$	Green finance and ecological environment synchronization
		$S_{iecolg} > S_{igreen}$	Green finance lagged
$0 < iccdn_j \le 0.2$	Extreme un-coordination (DUCC)	$S_{iecolg} < S_{igreen}$	Ecological environment lagged
		$S_{iecolg} \approx S_{igreen}$	Green finance and ecological environment synchronization
		$S_{iecolg} > S_{igreen}$	Green finance lagged

Note: $S_{iecolg} \approx S_{igreen}$ refers to $|S_{iecolg} - S_{igreen}| \le 0.1$.

2.2.3. The Spatial Analysis Method

Firstly, using the hot–cold model, we analyze the spatiotemporal evolution of the CCFE. The hot-cold model can efficiently reflect the variation of variables with high or low values [48,49] and remedy the shortcoming of the global or local Moran I index. Therefore, we adopt the Getis-Ord Gi^* index to depict the spatiotemporal evolutionary characteristics of the CCFE, as follows:

$$Gi* = \frac{\sum_{i=1}^{n}\sum_{j=1}^{n} w_{ij}x_i x_j}{\sum_{i=1}^{n}\sum_{j\neq 1}^{n} x_i x_j} \tag{5}$$

In Formula (5), $x_i > 0$, $x_j > 0$, and w_{ij} refers to the spatial weight matrix reflecting the relationship between spatial units, calculated by the particle distance between provincial capital cities as: $w_{ij} = 1/d_{ij}$. Meanwhile, it is the hot regions of the CCFE when $Gi^* > 1.96$, and it is the cold regions of the CCFE when $Gi^* < 1.96$. In addition, we observe the hot–cold characteristics of spatial unit i using the local Getis-Ord Gi^* index, as follows:

$$Gi* = \frac{\sum_{j\neq i}^{n} w_{ij}x_j}{\sum_{j\neq i}^{n} x_j} \tag{6}$$

Using the spatial hot–cold model, we can explore the evolutionary trend of the CCFE, but we do not know why the evolutionary trend of the CCFE in different regions is different, and we need to further analyze the driving forces of the CCFE. In fact, under the national strategy of strengthening and promoting the financial services supporting ecological environmental protection, the spatial correlation of the CCFE is more closed than before [50]. Additionally, the spatial Durbin model (SDM) can better reflect the impacted factor from spatial and temporal perspectives [51]. Therefore, we establish an SDM model using the eco-geographical distance matrix (W), as follows:

$$ln(iccdn_{it}) = \alpha + \beta lnX_{it} + \rho W_{ij} ln(iccdn_{it}) + \mu_i + v_i + \varepsilon_{it} \tag{7}$$

$$\varepsilon_{it} = \lambda W_{ij}\varepsilon_{it} + \eta_{it} \tag{8}$$

In Formulas (7) and (8), μ_i refers to the regional effect, v_i refers to the time effect, ε_{it} represents the random error item, and ρ is the spatially lagged item coefficient. W_{ij} refers to the spatial weight matrix in line i and column j, and it is defined as the product of the economic weight matrix and the geographical weight matrix; the economic weight matrix is calculated by the reciprocal difference in absolute values of GDP per capita. X refers to the serial impacted factors; η refers to the random item. According to the current reference, we analyze the driving factor of the CCFE from the perspectives of economic development, industrial structure, population, and investment. Among them, the industrial structure is calculated by the proportion of secondary industries to GDP (rsecd). Compared to the other variables reflecting the technological innovation level, the number of granted patent applications can realistically reflect the regional technological innovation level [52]; hence, the number of granted patent applications was chosen to reflect the regional technological innovation level (rpatent). The high-education resource is the human resource of a region's green finance and ecological environment development [53], and the average number of students in high school was chosen to reflect regional human resources (nedu). Investment is an important driving force promoting regional economic development, and it is an important support for improving regional ecological environment development [54]; the proportion of fixed investments to GDP (rfixed) was chosen to reflect the regional investment level. Population is a key variable in changing the ecological environment. The overloaded ecological pressure of population will restrict ecological environment development, while a higher population will also promote regional economic development [55]; the population urbanization rate (rurban) was chosen to reflect regional economic development and population concentration intensity.

2.3. *The Sources of Materials*

Without special statements, the data used in this article are from the China Statistics Yearbook, the China Financial Statistics Yearbook, the China Fiscal Statistics Yearbook, and the China Ecological Statistics Yearbook. Meanwhile, excluding the sample available in hard copy from Tibet, we constructed panel data with 30 inland samples from 2003 to 2020 in China. Additionally, for the vacancy value in the samples, the five-year moving average value was used to supplement the information. The logarithmic method in all variables was used to reduce the impact of variation, and Table 3 shows the statistic descriptions.

Table 3. Urban resilience evaluation index system.

Variable	Mean	Std. Dev.	Min	Max	Obs.
lniccdn	−0.996	0.183	−1.644	−0.544	540
lnrurban	3.953	0.269	3.215	4.495	540
lnrsecd	3.789	0.225	2.760	4.119	540
lnrpatent	9.277	1.716	4.248	13.473	540
lnnedu	7.682	0.416	6.547	8.839	540
lnrfixed	4.158	0.432	2.359	5.250	540

Note: (1) ln refers to the logarithm of variables. (2) Std.Dev represents the standard deviation of the variable. (3) Obs. is the total number of samples.

3. Results

3.1. *The Spatiotemporal Evolution of the Regional CCFE*

3.1.1. The Spatiotemporal Development Trend of the Regional CCFE

Using the Jackknife nature breakpoint method, Figure 2 shows the spatiotemporal distribution of the green financial index, the ecological environmental development index, the coupling index, and the regional CCFE in China. Among them, the circle size represents the high or low level of the index, and the number of circles indicates the variation of the CCFE.

Figure 2a shows the spatiotemporal evolution of the green finance index. Generally, the average value of the green finance index ranges between 0.13 and 0.93, indicating that green finance development in China is at a middle and low level, with a fluctuating upward trend. Recently, China's economy has entered a new stage of high-quality development, strengthening the financial support for the green low-carbon transformation of industry and life, and green finance development has improved steadily. Spatially, there are fewer regions with low green finance indices; these are mainly concentrated in the eastern economic development regions and the green development pilot zones in the central and western regions. The eastern region has higher economic development to promote the high-quality development of green finance, with more green financial institutions and stronger financial innovation ability. The green financial pilot zones, such as Hubei province and Chongqing city, had earlier explored the development of green finance and accumulated development experiences to promote green finance development. Notably, the development level of green finance in most regions has obviously changed, while Hubei province and Chongqing city are stably developed, with a high development level. In 2011, Hubei province became a trading pilot zone of carbon emission rights, and it has vigorously explored the trading model of carbon emission rights, the Clean Development Model, and promoted regional green finance development. Similar to Hubei province, Chongqing has also been a trading pilot zone of carbon emission rights in China since 2011, and, in 2017, Chongqing issued a "13th-Five-Year-Plan" to build a national functional financial center and was the first to take the lead in launching a pilot project of green finance development at the provincial level, especially protecting the ecological environment of the Yangtze River; accordingly, Chongqing's green finance development level is higher than in other regions.

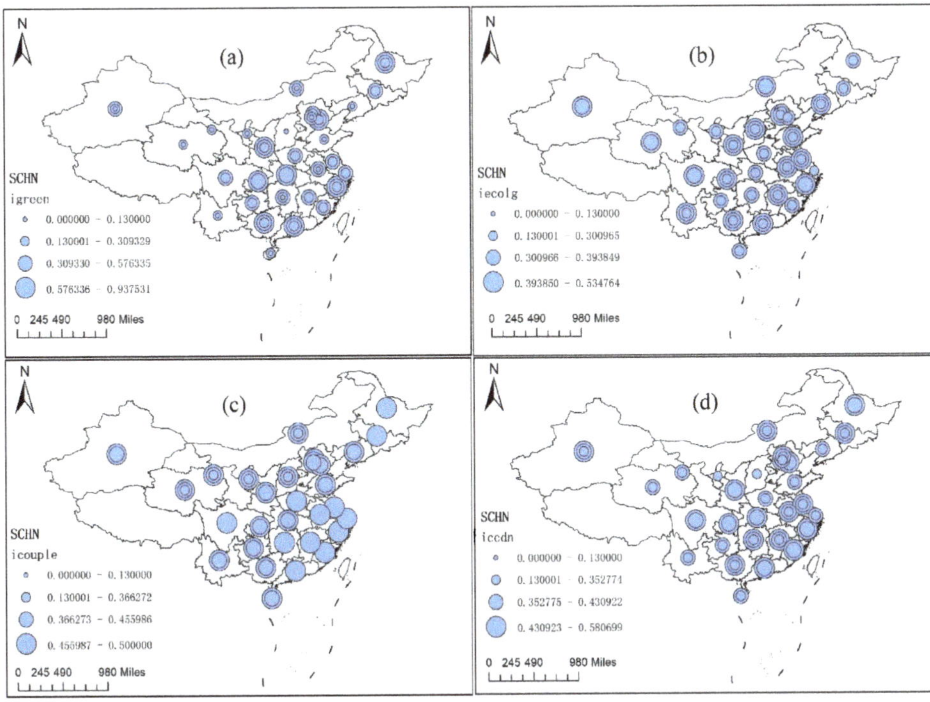

Figure 2. The evolutionary trend of related indices from 2003 to 2020. Note: (1) The symbol (**a–d**) refers to the green finance index, the ecological environment index, the coupling index between green finance and the ecological environment, and CCFE respectively.

Figure 2b shows the spatiotemporal evolution of the ecological environment index. Generally, the average value of the ecological environment index ranges from 0.19 to 0.53, indicating that ecological environment development in China is also at a middle and low level, with a steady upward trend. Recently, China has vigorously promoted environmental protection and successively issued many environmental protection laws and regulations to strengthen the governance of air pollution and carbon emissions; China has also implemented the construction of shelter forest systems in key regions such as the Yangtze River and coastal areas, construction projects of natural forest protection, sandstorm governance in "Beijing-Tianjin-Hebei", and fast-growing forests, which have obviously improved the ecological environment. Spatially, there are more regions with relatively higher ecological environment indices, and these regions are mainly concentrated in the southeastern and northeastern regions. Additionally, there are fewer regions with relatively lower ecological environment indices; these are mainly concentrated in the central regions. In recent years, China has strengthened the ecological environmental governance in the regions such as the Pearl River, enhanced the supervision of ecological environment protection, promoted the green production transformation of core carbon reduction, and improved the ecological development in related regions. At the same time, the central regions with more natural resources, such as Shanxi province and Henan province, have had more pressure on their ecological environments, such as air pollution and wastewater governance, which have restricted the development of their ecological environments.

Figure 2c shows the spatiotemporal evolution of the coupling index between green finance and the ecological environment. Generally, the average value of the coupling index between green finance and the ecological environment ranges from 0.13 to 0.51, indicating that the coupling index between green finance and the ecological environment in China is at a middle and low level, with a steady upward trend. Recently, in order to improve the ecological environment, China has successively issued many policies, such as green bond guidelines, and continuously constructed the green finance system, including green credits, green stocks, green development funds, and green insurance. Additionally, the objective reality faced by the ecological environment also provided a basis for green finance innovation, deepening the mutual relationship between green finance and the ecological environment. Spatially, the number of regions with higher coupling indices is large, with small changes, and they are mainly located in the eastern developed regions, owing to the developed finance development level and low-carbon industrial structure. The number of regions with lower coupling indices is small, with obvious changes, and they are mainly located in the northwestern regions and depend on less-green finance resources.

Figure 2d shows the spatiotemporal evolution of the CCFE. Generally, the average value of the CCFE ranges from 0.10 to 0.60, indicating that the CCFE level in China is at a middle and low level and in a primary coordinated stage, with a steady upward trend; Hypothesis 1 is verified. Additionally, the results indicate that the interactive effect between green finance and ecological development is more obvious. In fact, depending on the development of the ecological environment, the innovation development of green finance in China has been at the forefront of the world. Up to 2020, green loans in China reached RMB 12 trillion, with a proportion of 6.9% of total loans, and green bond stocks also reached RMB 813.2 billion, with zero default cases. Additionally, due to green finance innovations, such as the carbon emission rights quota trading rule (CEA) and the securitization of environmental rights and interests, the ecological environment has obviously improved, especially in carbon reduction. As of 2020, the trade of CEA reached 76.92 million tons. Moreover, the production methods of China are more obviously green. In 2021, the new grid-connected capacity of photovoltaic power generation in China reached 54.88 million kilowatts, and the proportion of clean energy in total energy consumption reached 25.5%, increasing by 1.2% compared to 2020. Among them, the percentage of coal consumption declined to 56.0%, decreasing by 0.95% compared to 2020. Spatially, the number of regions with higher CCFE indices is small, and the regions with stable CCFE indices are mainly located in the eastern developed regions and western green finance pilot zones, owing to the related high development of financial and low-carbon industrial structures. The regions with more fluctuating CCFE indices are mainly located in the central regions, restricted by the high-carbon industry, similar to the above. The number of regions with lower CCFE indices is large, with obvious changes, and they are mainly located in the central and western regions. Similar to the above, the green finance resources in the central and western regions cannot efficiently match the industrial green transformation development as they are limited by the higher proportion of high-carbon industries and relatively fewer financial resources.

3.1.2. The Spatiotemporal Evolution of Regional CCFE Type

Figure 3 shows the evolutionary trend of CCFE types in the years 2003, 2009, 2015, and 2020, respectively. Generally, the CCFE level has steadily increased, showing a relatively concentrated distribution. In 2003, there were fewer regions with the primary type of CCFE, such as Zhejiang and Sichuan, with a relatively spatially concentrated distribution, and more regions with the basic un-coordination type of CCFE, such as Qinghai and Yunnan. There is also a middle un-coordination type of CCFE, such as Gansu and Shanxi, with a spatially concentrated contiguous distribution. In 2009, the regions with the middle un-coordination type and the primary coordination type continuously narrowed, while the regions with the basic un-coordination type and the middle coordination type gradually expanded; accordingly, the spatial distribution is similar to 2005. Among them, the number of regions with the basic un-coordination type expanded the most, and the number of regions with the middle un-coordination type narrowed the least. In 2015, the regions with primary coordination continuously expanded, while the regions with the middle coordination type and the basic un-coordination type obviously narrowed. Among them, the number of regions with the primary coordination type expanded the most, showing a more spatially concentrated contiguous distribution. In 2020, the number of regions, such as Chongqing, with the middle coordination type and Guangxi and Jiangxi with the primary coordination type, expanded to 1 and 18, respectively, and the number of regions, such as Sichuan and Liaoning, with the basic un-coordination type and Shanxi with the middle un-coordination type narrowed to 10 and 1 respectively. Among them, the number of regions with the primary coordination type expanded the most, and the number of regions with the middle un-coordination type narrowed the least. Spatially, the regions with the middle coordination type are scattered and located in the western developed provinces. The regions with the primary coordination type are contiguously concentrated and distributed in the eastern coastal provinces. The regions with the basic un-coordination type are concentrated and distributed in the southwestern and northeastern provinces, and the regions with the middle un-coordination type are scattered and located in the central provinces.

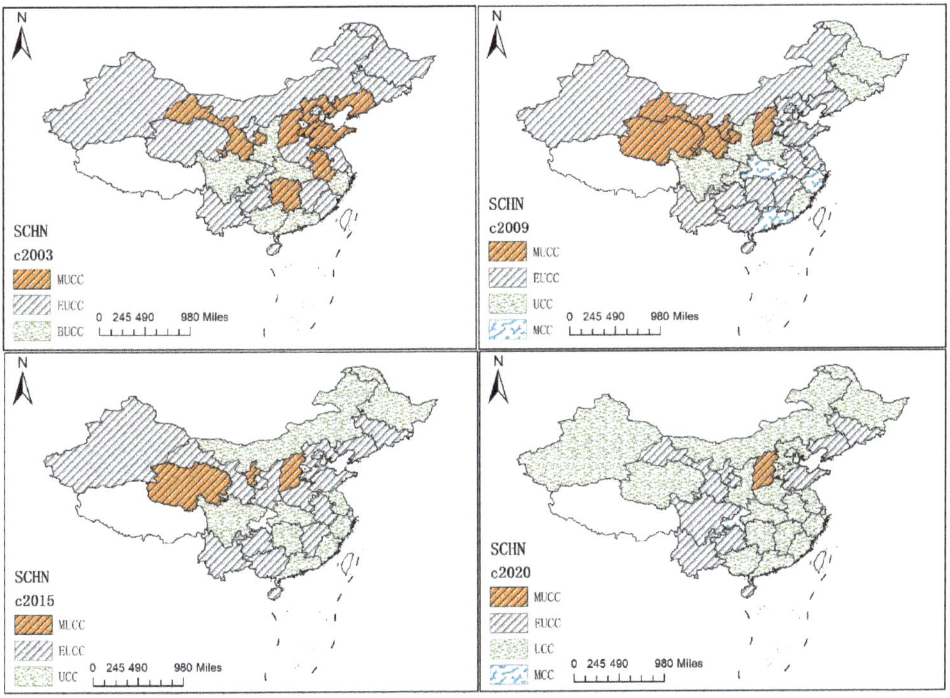

Figure 3. The evolutionary trend of CCFE type in years 2003, 2009, 2015, and 2020. Note: (1) The abbreviations of MUCC, EUCC, UCC, and MCC are the CCFE types mentioned above.

Further, according to Table 3, Table 4 shows the CCFE pattern in 2003, 2009, 2015, and 2020. In Table 4, the spatial distributions of the four different CCFE patterns are quite different in the samples. The ecological lagged regions are located in the eastern economically developed areas, the green finance development lagged regions are located in the central and western areas, and the green finance and ecological environment synchronized regions are mainly located in the western areas. Additionally, the green financial lagged pattern is the main pattern of the CCFE; the number of regions in the green finance lagged pattern, the ecological environment lagged pattern, and the green finance and ecological environment synchronized pattern are 15 (more than), 14 (less than), and 8 (less than), respectively. Meanwhile, regions with the ecological environmental development lagged pattern and the green finance and ecological environment synchronized pattern are mainly with the primary coordination type, and regions with the green finance lagged pattern are mainly in the basic un-coordination pattern. Therefore, the green finance lagged pattern is the main pattern of the CCFE in the samples and less in the synchronized pattern, indicating that there are more regions in the un-coordination relationship between green finance and the ecological environment.

Table 4. The pattern of CCFE in the years 2003, 2009, 2015, and 2020, respectively.

Pattern	2003	2009	2015	2020
Ecological environment lagged	Jiangsu, Guangdong, Zhejiang, Heilongjiang, Hubei, Chongqing, Guizhou, Tianjin, Shaanxi	Shaanxi, Guizhou, Jilin, Zhejiang, Guangdong, Hubei, Tianjin	Guizhou, Hubei, Tianjin, Chongqing	Heilongjiang, Anhui, Guangdong, Jiangxi, Zhejiang, Hubei, Hunan, Tianjin, Fujian, Shanghai, Shaanxi, Chongqing
Green finance and ecological environment synchronization	Jilin, Jiangxi, Sichuan, Ningxia, Henan	Chongqing, Henan	Shanghai, Shaanxi, Fujian, Zhejiang, Hunan, Guangdong, Sichuan, Heilongjiang	Sichuan, Beijing
Green finance lagged	Gansu, Liaoning, Shanxi, Shandong, Qinghai, Hebei, Guangxi, Anhui, Xinjiang, Inner Mongolia, Hainan, Hunan, Yunnan, Beijing, Shanghai, Fujian	Gansu, Qinghai, Shanxi, Inner Mongolia, Ningxia, Hebei, Shandong, Yunnan, Guangxi, Liaoning, Hainan, Xinjiang, Beijing, Hunan, Anhui, Jiangsu, Sichuan, Heilongjiang, Shanghai, Jiangxi, Fujian	Qinghai, Ningxia, Xinjiang, Shanxi, Yunnan, Shandong, Inner Mongolia, Hebei, Liaoning, Guangxi, Anhui, Hainan, Henan, Jiangsu, Jiangxi, Beijing, Jilin	Shanxi, Ningxia, Hainan, Qinghai, Yunnan, Shandong, Gansu, Xinjiang, Jiangsu, Hebei, Guizhou, Jilin, Liaoning, Henan, Inner Mongolia

3.1.3. The Spatial Agglomerated Evolutionary Trend of the CCFE

Furthermore, Figure 4 shows the spatial agglomerated evolutionary trend of hot–cold spot regions of the CCFE in 2003, 2009, 2015, and 2020. In 2003, Guizhou province in the western region was in the high-value cluster of the CCFE, forming a hotspot region for the coordinated development of green finance and the ecological environment. Guangxi province in the western region was in the low-value cluster of the CCFE, forming a cold spot region for the coordinated development of green finance and the ecological environment. In 2009, the spatial distribution of the hot–cold spot regions of the CCFE changed in an obvious manner. Zhejiang province, Fujian province, and Guangdong province in the southeastern economically developed regions; Hubei province, Anhui province, and Jiangxi province in the central region; and Guizhou province in the western region were in the high-value cluster of the CCFE, forming a hotspot region for the coordinated development of green finance and the ecological environment. Gansu province and Qinghai province in the western region were in the low-value cluster of CCFE, forming a cold spot region for the coordinated development of green finance and the ecological environment. In 2015, the spatial distribution of the hot–cold spot regions of the CCFE also changed in an obvious manner. Fujian province and Guangdong province in the southeastern economically developed regions; Anhui province, Hubei province, and Jiangxi province in the central region; and Guangxi province and Guizhou province in the western region were in the high-value cluster of the CCFE, forming a hotspot region for the coordinated development of green finance and the ecological environment, with no cold spot regions. In 2020, the spatial distribution of the hot–cold spot regions of the CCFE changed greatly. Fujian province and Guangdong province in the southeastern economically developed regions and Jiangxi province in the central region were in the high-value cluster of the CCFE, forming a hotspot region for the coordinated development of green finance and the ecological environment. The Inner Mongolia Autonomous Region in the western region was in the low-value cluster of the CCFE, forming a cold spot region for the coordinated development of green finance and the ecological environment.

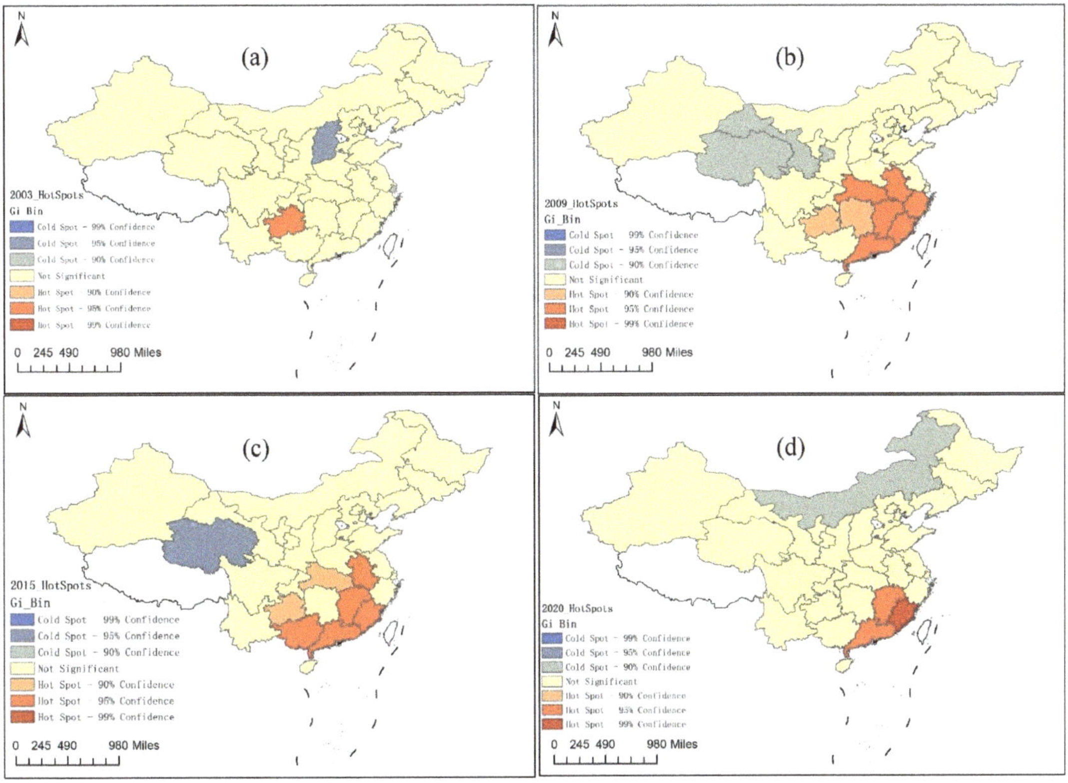

Figure 4. The spatial agglomerated evolutionary trend of hot–cold spot regions of the CCFE in the years 2003, 2009, 2015, and 2020, respectively. Note: (1) The symbol (**a–d**) refers to the green finance index, the ecological environment index, the coupling index between green finance and the ecological environment, and CCFE re-spectively.

Therefore, the hot spot regions of the CCFE are mainly located in the eastern region, while cold spots are mainly distributed in the western region; the results are basically consistent with the spatial distribution of the three patterns of the CCFE in Figure 2. Compared to other regions, the eastern coastal region is an area with a high economic development level, especially with more green financial resources and lower carbon industrial structures; most cities there are hot spots of the CCFE.

3.2. The Driving Force Analysis of CCFE

3.2.1. The Analysis of the Benchmark Model

According to the result of the Hausman test, reducing the impact of the endogenous problem, this study controlled the time effect and spatial effect of the samples and adopted the fixed-effect SDM model with a two-order lag and eco-geographical matrix to estimate the results of the benchmark model. Meanwhile, in order to test the stability of the estimation results, the stepwise regression model was used; Table 5 shows the estimation results of the benchmark model. In Table 5, the spatial correlation coefficients of spatial rho are significantly positive at the 1% confidence level, indicating that the coordinated development of green finance and the ecological environment in the eco-geographical adjacent province is conducive to promoting the coordinated development of green finance and the ecological environment at the local level, showing a significantly positive spatial spillover effect.

Table 5. The estimation results of the benchmark model.

Variable	(1)	(2)	(3)	(4)	(5)
L.Wlniccdn	1.474 ***	1.585 ***	1.356 ***	1.018 **	0.859 *
	(3.78)	(4.09)	(3.33)	(2.30)	(1.94)
lnrurban	0.143 **	0.234 ***	0.183 **	0.228 **	0.274 ***
	(2.21)	(3.26)	(2.39)	(2.19)	(2.58)
lnrsecd		−0.166 ***	−0.172 ***	−0.159 ***	−0.162 ***
		(−3.29)	(−3.40)	(−3.05)	(−3.13)
lnrpatent			0.0217	0.0246	0.0281 *
			(1.35)	(1.50)	(1.72)
lnnedu				−0.0423	−0.0791
				(−0.84)	(−1.49)
lnrfixed					0.00875
					(0.48)
W×lnrurban	−1.582 ***	−1.198 *	−0.0603	−0.846	−0.120
	(−2.60)	(−1.77)	(−0.07)	(−0.81)	(−0.11)
W×lnrsecd		−1.203 *	−1.751 **	−2.108 ***	−2.185 ***
		(−1.80)	(−2.53)	(−2.92)	(−3.03)
W×lnrpatent			−0.384 **	−0.403 **	−0.373 **
			(−2.23)	(−2.29)	(−2.12)
W×lnnedu				0.932	1.059 *
				(1.52)	(1.66)
W×lnrfixed					−0.611 ***
					(−2.84)
Spatial rho	0.716 ***	0.694 ***	0.693 ***	0.753 ***	0.781 ***
	(2.68)	(2.61)	(2.62)	(2.79)	(2.88)
R2	0.004	0.053	0.022	0.067	0.072
N	510	510	510	510	510

Note: (1) *, **, *** represent significance at the 10%, 5%, 1% confidence levels. (2) The number in parentheses is the t-value. (3) L. refers to the first-order lag. (4) W is the spatial weight matrix. (5) N refers to the number of samples. (6) R2 refers to the coefficient of determination. (7) The chi2(5) value of the LR test in column (5) is 29.48, with a p-value equal to 0.0000, indicating that the SDM model chosen is more suitable than the others; in the other columns, this conclusion is still valid.

The lag term of the CCFE is significantly positive at the 1% confidence level, indicating that the CCFE in previous periods had a significant positive impact on the development of the period and the coordinated development of green finance and the ecological environment has a positive cumulative transfer effect. As mentioned above, the CCFE in China showed a steady upward trend and objectively confirmed the positive cumulative transfer effect. The coordinated development model of green finance and the ecological environment in previous periods can provide an improvement and innovation basis in the future by processing the "improving–optimizing–improving- … " process to continuously promote the coordinated development of green finance and the ecological environment.

The population urbanization rate is significantly positive at the 1% confidence level, indicating that the increase in urbanization rate is conducive to promoting the CCFE. Currently, China is continuously developing new urbanization without sacrificing the development of agriculture, ecology, and the environment and promoting infrastructure integration and public services equalization between urban and rural spaces. Additionally, ecological environment development will enter into a healthy track and improve accordingly when the increase in the population urbanization rate matches the corresponding social resources, such as the economy, medical care, education, and material resources such as water and energy. Therefore, the development of new human-centered urbanization will improve the development of the ecological environment and be beneficial to promoting the coordinated development of green finance and the ecological environment.

The percentage of secondary industries to GDP is significantly negative at the 1% confidence level, indicating that the increase in the proportion of secondary industries is not conducive to the development of the CCFE. The proportion increase of secondary industries will continuously enhance ecological pollution pressures such as carbon emissions if it ignores the structure optimization of raising the percentage of newly strategized industries, such as the manufacturing service industry, and green low-carbon transformation, such as the production of clean energy. Additionally, the customized secondary industries with high carbon emissions and high waste energy will increase the compliance risk and operation risk of market actors such as enterprises, reducing the green credit motion of financial institutions such as banks, and this will not favor the coordinated development of green finance and ecological development. Meanwhile, the spatially lagged coefficients W×lnrsecd are significantly negative at the 10% (at least) confidence level, indicating that the proportion increase of secondary industries in eco-geographical adjacent provinces will siphon local provincial resources such as green finance, ecological talents, and technology and be detrimental to the local development of the CCFE.

The number of granted patent applications is significantly positive at the 10% confidence level, indicating that the development of the regions' technological innovation will promote the development of the CCFE. Improving regional technological innovation, on one hand, can enhance the development quality of the ecological environment, using clean energy and green buildings such as tidal energy, nuclear energy, carbon capture, clean buildings, and incineration flue gas purification technology. On the other hand, embedding advanced technology such as blockchain, cloud computing, artificial intelligence, and big data in the innovation of financial products and services can efficiently improve the efficiency of green finance by servicing ecological environment development and realizing the efficient and coordinated development of green finance and the ecological environment. The spatially lagged coefficients W×lnrpatent are significantly negative at the 5% confidence level, indicating that the improvement of technological innovation in eco-geographical adjacent provinces will siphon local, provincial resources such as talents and technology and be detrimental to the local development of the CCFE. Therefore, Hypothesis 2 is verified.

3.2.2. The Heterogeneity Analysis

Furthermore, we analyzed the heterogeneity of driving forces on the CCFE. Time-wise, we set the year 2014 as the time split point, considering the environment protection law of China was formally implemented in 2015, and explored the impact difference of this driving force before or after the implementation of the law. Spatially, we divided the samples into four regions—east, center, west, and northeast—according to the National Development and Reform Commission of China and analyzed the impact of the heterogeneity of different factors on different regions. Table 6 shows the estimation results.

Table 6. The heterogeneity estimation results of influence factors.

Variable	(6)	(7)	(8)	(9)	(10)	(11)
	≤2014	>2014	East	Center	West	Northeast
L.lniccdn	0.566 ***	0.361 ***	0.436 ***	0.507 ***	0.464 ***	0.115
	(13.25)	(4.82)	(8.37)	(7.17)	(7.69)	(1.01)
lnrurban	0.00583	0.0472	0.424 *	−1.655 ***	−0.907 ***	1.869 *
	(0.04)	(0.17)	(1.77)	(−2.62)	(−2.67)	(1.70)
lnrsecd	−0.0715	−0.319 ***	0.0326	0.137	−0.191	0.351
	(−1.16)	(−3.18)	(0.28)	(0.82)	(−1.36)	(1.44)
lnrpatent	−0.00470	0.0194	−0.0124	0.0358	0.129 ***	−0.0288
	(−0.28)	(0.67)	(−0.49)	(0.80)	(2.76)	(−0.30)
lnnedu	−0.0178	0.0736	−0.312 ***	0.502 **	0.266 **	−0.400
	(−0.30)	(0.59)	(−2.84)	(2.39)	(2.09)	(−0.59)

Table 6. *Cont.*

Variable	(6)	(7)	(8)	(9)	(10)	(11)
	≤2014	>2014	East	Center	West	Northeast
lnrfixed	0.0346	−0.0833 ***	−0.155 ***	−0.0830	−0.137 *	−0.0758 **
	(1.05)	(−3.22)	(−2.82)	(−1.57)	(−1.66)	(−2.00)
W × lnrurban	−1.145 **	6.191 **	−0.325	1.516 *	1.044 *	−2.882 *
	(−2.15)	(2.41)	(−0.73)	(1.75)	(1.88)	(−1.69)
W × lnrsecd	−1.027 ***	−3.170 ***	−0.103	−0.412 *	−0.00163	−0.813 *
	(−4.46)	(−2.87)	(−0.66)	(−1.69)	(−0.01)	(−1.80)
W × lnrpatent	0.102	0.370	−0.0307	−0.0684	−0.183 **	0.0474
	(1.62)	(1.16)	(−0.90)	(−0.81)	(−2.18)	(0.35)
W × lnnedu	0.234 *	−0.754	0.361 **	−0.395	−0.327	0.429
	(1.81)	(−0.53)	(2.33)	(−1.52)	(−1.57)	(0.59)
W × lnrfixed	−0.107	−0.321	0.299 ***	0.196 *	0.332 **	0.225 **
	(−0.93)	(−1.09)	(2.67)	(1.91)	(2.07)	(2.08)
Spatial rho	0.535 ***	1.168 **	0.496 ***	0.397 ***	0.321 **	0.331 *
	(4.65)	(2.36)	(5.26)	(2.59)	(2.15)	(1.72)
R2	0.689	0.044	0.387	0.799	0.609	0.002
N	330	180	170	102	187	51

Note: (1) *, **, *** represents significance at the 10%, 5%, 1% confidence levels. (2) The number in parentheses is the t-value. (3) L., R2, W, N are similar to the above.

From the perspective of time heterogeneity, in the years after 2015, the percentage of secondary industries and the percentage of fixed investments are significantly negative at the 1% confidence level, indicating that the increase in the proportions of secondary industries and fixed investments is not conducive to the development of the CCFE after 2015. After 2015, the implementation of the national environment protection law obviously increased the trade cost of illegal environmental activities such as environmental disruption and ecological pollution. Currently, the industry proportion of high energy consumption, high pollution, and wastewater in secondary industries is also high in China; increasing traditional secondary industries will raise the operational cost of enterprises and enhance the risk pressure of green financial institutions such as commercial banks, decoupling the development of the CCFE. In addition, the spatially lagged coefficients W×lnrsecd are still significantly negative at the 1% confidence level and are not affected by the time changes.

From the perspective of regional heterogeneity, the population urbanization rate is significantly positive at the 10% confidence level in the eastern region and the northeastern region and significantly negative in the western region. The result indicates that the increase in the population urbanization rate in the new urbanization is conducive to the development of the CCFE in the eastern and northeastern regions and not in the western region. As mentioned above, the eastern region in China is an economically developed area, and the development of new urbanization can promote the high-quality development of the CCFE, while the northeastern region has incremental development at a low level. Meanwhile, the western and central regions face serious constraints of ecological protection issues, especially the low-carbon transformation pressure of green industries, ecological fragility such as soil erosion, and an overly high proportion of heavy industries in the upper Yellow River Basin; the slowing construction of new urbanization has restricted the development of CCFE correspondingly. Additionally, the spatially lagged coefficients W×lnrurban in the central and western regions are still significantly negative at the 10% confidence level and significantly negative at the 10% confidence level, indicating that the increase in the population urbanization rate in eco-geographically adjacent provinces has a spatial positive spillover effect on local provinces in the central and western regions and a negative spatial spillover effect on the northeastern region.

The number of granted patent applications is significantly positive at the 1% confidence level in the western region, indicating that the development of technological innovation is conducive to the development of the CCFE in the western region. Additionally, the spatially lagged coefficients W×lnrpatent in the western region is significantly negative at the 5% confidence level, indicating that the development of technological innovation in eco-geographically adjacent provinces has a spatial negative spillover effect on the local provinces; the siphon effect is more obvious in the western region.

The number of students of high education per 100,000 inhabitants in the population in the eastern region is significantly negative at the 1% confidence level and significantly positive at the 5% confidence level in the central and western regions, indicating that there should be more emphasis on the structure and not the scale of talents in the eastern region; strengthening the scale of talents in the central and western regions is conducive to promote the development of the CCFE correspondingly. Additionally, the spatially lagged coefficients W×lnnedu in the eastern region are significantly negative at the 1% confidence level, indicating that the expansion of high education resources in the eastern region has a spatial positive spillover effect, promoting the development of the CCFE in local provinces. Similar to the results above, the proportion of fixed investments is significantly negative at the 10% confidence level in the eastern region, western region, and northeast region, and the spatially lagged coefficients W×lnrfixed are significantly negative at less than the 10% confidence level.

3.2.3. The Analysis of the Spatial Spillover Effect

In addition, according to Formula (7) and the results in Table 5, Table 7 shows the total spatial effect, direct effect, and indirect effect of the CCFE.

Table 7. The estimation result of the spatial spillover effect.

Variable	(12)	(13)	(14)	(15)	(16)	(17)
	SR_Direct	SR_Indirect	SR_Total	LR_Direct	LR_Indirect	LR_Total
lnrurban	0.268 ***	−0.188	0.080	0.266 **	−0.115	0.151
	(2.56)	(−0.28)	(0.11)	(2.09)	(−0.07)	(0.08)
lnrsecd	−0.167 ***	−1.183 ***	−1.350 ***	−0.233 ***	−2.664 *	−2.897 *
	(−3.29)	(−2.78)	(−3.06)	(−2.98)	(−1.6)	(−1.68)
lnrpatent	0.026 **	−0.218 **	−0.192 **	0.016	−0.428	−0.412
	(1.62)	(−2.1)	(−1.77)	(0.79)	(−1.39)	(−1.28)
lnnedu	−0.073	0.640	0.567	−0.043	1.261	1.218
	(−1.5)	(1.54)	(1.39)	(−0.71)	(0.98)	(0.92)
lnrfixed	0.006	−0.359 ***	−0.353 **	−0.012	−0.749	−0.761
	(0.34)	(−2.57)	(−2.46)	(−0.47)	(−1.53)	(−1.5)
lnrurban	0.268 ***	−0.188	0.080	0.266 **	−0.115	0.151
	(2.56)	(−0.28)	(0.11)	(2.09)	(−0.07)	(0.08)

Note: (1) *, **, *** represents significance at the 10%, 5%, 1% confidence levels. (2) The number in parentheses is the t-value. (3) SR and LR refer to the short-term and long-term periods, respectively.

The direct effects of the population urbanization rate in the short and long term are significantly positive at the 1% confidence level, indicating that the increase in the population urbanization rate can promote the development of the CCFE in the inner regions. The total effect, direct effect, and indirect effect of the proportion of secondary industries in the long and short term are significantly negative at less than the 10% confidence level, indicating that the enhancement of the proportion of secondary industries is not conducive to CCFE development in the overall, local, and eco-geographically adjacent regions. Accordingly, the direct effect of the proportion of secondary industries is larger than the indirect effect, showing that the restricted effect is obvious in external regions. The direct effect of the number of granted patent applications in the short term is significantly positive at the 5% confidence level, and the total effect and indirect effect in the short term are significantly negative at the 5% confidence level, indicating that the improvement of technological innovation is not conducive to the development of the CCFE in the short term. Particularly, the inhibitory effect of technological innovation is especially obvious in the local region, while the promoted effect is significant in the eco-geographically adjacent region. The total effect and indirect effect of the proportion of fixed investments in the short term are significantly negative at the 5% confidence level, indicating that increasing the proportion of fixed investments will restrict the development of the CCFE in the overall sample and eco-geographically adjacent provinces.

4. Discussion

This article analyzes the evolutionary trend of the CCFE from 2003 to 2020 in China, and the results show that the CCFE in China is at a primary stage, with a fluctuating upward trend. Spatially, the CCFE shows spatiotemporal evolutionary characteristics, such as higher values with fewer changes in the eastern region and lower values with more changes in other regions. Most regions are dominated by the primary coordination type, followed by the basic un-coordination type, and there are fewer regions with the middle un-coordination type and the middle coordination type. Correspondingly, the green finance lagged pattern is the main type in all samples, and few regions have reached the economic-ecological synchronized pattern. Consistent with Zhang et al. (2022) [56], it is believed that green finance and environmental performance in China are in the primary coordinated stage, with a spatial distribution pattern of orderly decrease from east to west. Using the Getis Ord Gi* index, we analyzed the hot–cold spot evolutionary trend of the CCFE, and the result showed that the hot spots of CCFE are concentrated in the eastern region, such as the Pearl River, with an "increase–decrease" development trend in the spatial space, while the cold spots are located in the western region, such as the upper Yellow River Basin, with a stable spatial space. Similar to the results of Lv et al. (2021) [57], it is believed that there is a development gap in green finance, especially in the eastern region, with a polarization phenomenon.

The spatial Durbin model was used to analyze the driving force of the CCFE. The development of the CCFE in eco-geographically adjacent provinces shows a significantly positive spatial spillover effect and a cumulative transfer effect. Enhancing the population urbanization rate is conducive to the development of the CCFE, and the promoted effect is obviously significant in the eastern and northeastern regions, while it is negative in the western region. Actually, the development of the ecological environment and urbanization in the western regions is relatively lower than in other regions [58]; this has restricted CCFE development accordingly. The overly high proportion of secondary industries is not conducive to the development of the CCFE [59], especially after 2015. The improvement in regional technological innovation is conducive to CCFE development [60,61]. However, technological innovation shows a competitive effect that is especially obvious in the western region. Additionally, the high education resources in the eastern region are not conducive to the development of the CCFE, and the positive spatial spillover effect is significantly obvious in the eco-geographically adjacent province. In contrast, the high education resources in the central and western regions are conducive to the development of the CCFE. In addition, the proportion of fixed investments is not conducive to the development of the CCFE in the eastern region, western region, and northeastern region, showing a positive spillover effect in eco-geographically adjacent spaces.

Finally, according to the spatial Durbin model, we found the spatial spillover effects of different driving forces. The increase in the population urbanization rate promotes the development of the CCFE in the sample, significantly reducing ecology and natural resource pressures such as water for humans, similar to the findings of Kassouri (2021) [62]. The increase in the proportion of secondary industries is not conducive to the development of the CCFE, and the direct effect of the proportion of secondary industries is more obvious than the indirect effect. In contrast, the restricted effect of the proportion of secondary industries in the development of the CCFE is stronger in the external regions [63]. The improvement of technological innovation in the short term has a negative impact on the development of the CCFE, and the restricted effect on the local level is more obvious, promoting the development of the CCFE in eco-geographically adjacent provinces. In addition, the increase in the proportion of fixed investments is not conducive to the development of the CCFE in the overall sample and the eco-geographically adjacent provinces.

However, our study has several limitations. Firstly, the study period was from 2003 to 2020. For data limitation, we did not extend the data to 2021 or before 2003, and statistical bias may underestimate the development of the CCFE. Second, limiting data accessibility, green finance was not calculated by more micro-related indicators in the green finance field, such as provincial green investments and loans. This might have resulted in the underestimation of the green finance impact. Third, this article analyzed the macro driving force of the CCFE directly but did not emphasize the factors and mechanism of any aspect deeply. Therefore, we may have to empirically analyze the driving force of one or more micro aspects in the future.

5. Conclusions

This article analyzes the overall characteristics, spatiotemporal distribution patterns, and evolutionary characteristics of the spatial clustering and driving force of the CCFE, and the results can be concluded as follows:

(1) The CCFE in China is at the primary stage, with a fluctuating upward trend, showing spatial distribution characteristics, such as being higher in the eastern region and lower in other regions. Additionally, there are more regions with the types of primary coordination and basic un-coordination and fewer regions with the middle un-coordination and middle coordination types. Moreover, most regions dominated with the green finance lagged pattern, and fewer regions reached the finance-ecology synchronized pattern.

(2) The hot spots of the CCFE are located in the eastern region, such as the Pearl River, showing an "increase–decrease" development trend in the spatial space. Additionally, the cold spots of the CCFE are concentrated in the central and western regions, such as the Yellow River Basin, with a stably spatial space.

(3) There is a positive spatial spillover effect in the eco-geographically adjacent space in the development of the CCFE, with a significant cumulative transfer effect. The population urbanization and the number of granted patent applications have a significant positive impact on the CCFE, and the proportion of secondary industries has a significant negative impact. Spatially, the proportion of secondary industries and the number of granted patent applications have a negative impact on the development of CCFE in the eco-geographically adjacent space. Meanwhile, the influence and spatial effect of different factors on the development of the CCFE have an obvious heterogeneity in the different time and spatial ranges.

6. Policy Implications

Realizing the synchronized development of green finance and the ecological environment is an important direction of China's green finance development and ecological environment protection in the "14th-Five-Year-Plan" period. Combined with the conclusions above, some policy implications are as follows:

(1) Continuously promote the coordinated development of green finance and the ecological environment. On one hand, in top-level rule design, it is necessary to take improvements in ecological environment quality as the fundamental goal and promote the quality development of green finance [64]. Green development should be closely integrated with the development targets of China in the 14th-Five-Year-Plan period. The production and service innovation of green finance should be combined with goals such as energy conservation, emission reduction, and clean production at each stage to place green finance into the micro construction circle of the ecological environment. On the other hand, it is necessary to accelerate green finance innovation to promote the high-quality construction of the ecological environment. In the national and provincial green finance reform and innovation demonstration zones, innovative experience as a model, production, service, and technology of green finance should

be continuously explored to create a replicable and popularized model of coordinated development of green finance and the ecological environment, playing on positive cumulative transfer effects of CCFE.

(2) Classify and orderly complement the developmental shortcomings of green finance and the ecological environment. In one aspect, under the premise of continuously enhancing innovations such as green bonds and green securities, the eastern developed region should focus on the construction of the ecological environment, emphasize environmental issue governance such as soil erosion, soil salinization, water pollution, haze, and carbon emission, and supplement the infrastructure construction of rural environmental protection. Meanwhile, the eastern region should raise their regulatory standards and accelerate the transmission velocity of low-carbon industries. In other aspects, under the premise of reinforcing the construction of the ecological environment, the central and western regions should comprehensively use green financial tools such as green standards, environmental risk management [65], and fiscal discounts to improve the high-quality development of green finance. Especially in the key fields of current green technology, such as carbon capture and storage, they should strengthen the support of green finance.

(3) Strengthen the cooperation and the regional demonstration effect of coordinated development. China should take full advantage of the coordinated development of green finance and ecological environment development in different regions and deeply embed the coordination relationship between green finance and the ecological environment to create a healthy interactive development [66]. On one hand, it should continuously take advantage of the demonstration and leading effects of national green finance reform and innovation zones such as Guangzhou and Zhejiang, promote the green finance model, green credit resources, and green technological talent spillovers into the periphery region, and improve the high-quality development of green finance in adjacent regions. On the other hand, it should continuously take advantage of the demonstration and leading effects of national ecological environment zones such as Fujian, Jiangxi, Guizhou, and Hainan, replicate and promote the demonstration experience, such as water resource and environmental governance, rural living environment governance, ecological protection and restoration, ecological poverty alleviation, and ecological compensation, and improve the high-quality development of the ecological environment in adjacent regions.

(4) Fully release the element dividends, such as population, green industry, and technological innovation. Authorities in the eastern region, such as the Zhejiang and Guangdong authorities, should optimize the talent structure in green finance and the ecological environment and introduce high-level talent to the field of technological innovation and green corporation governance. The government in central and western regions should expand the talent scale in the coordinated development of green finance and the ecological environment and encourage and support the innovation and entrepreneurship of talent from eastern economically developed regions. Additionally, on the premise of adhering to the high-quality development of the real economy, the decision-makers should enhance the percentage of green industries, such as clean energy, green transportation, and green buildings, accelerate the green and low-carbon transformation of industrial structures [67], reduce emissions such as carbon emissions, and build a carrier for the coordinated development of green finance and the ecological environment. In addition, policymakers should strengthen innovation in technology, such as big data and cloud computing, promote the innovation of green service models and products, and improve the service efficiency of green finance. Moreover, it should enhance the basic research on applications such as the large-scale utilization of renewable energy, energy conservation, power batteries, and new power systems; accelerate technological innovation in electrical safety, high-efficiency photovoltaics, low-cost carbon dioxide capture, utilization and

storage, and large-capacity energy storage; and improve the efficiency of different technology services for ecological environment construction.

Funding: This work was supported by grants from the National Social Science Foundation of China (20CJY064) and the annual innovation project of the Henan Academy of Social Science (22A06).

Institutional Review Board Statement: The study was conducted according to the guidelines of the Declaration of Helsinki, and approved by the Institutional Review Board.

Informed Consent Statement: Not applicable for studies not involving humans.

Data Availability Statement: The data presented in this study are openly available from the China Statistical Yearbook, available at the website: http://www.stats.gov.cn/tjsj/ndsj, (accessed on 5 January 2022); the China Financial Statistics Yearbook, available at the website: https://data.cnki.net/yearbook/Single/N2022010064, (accessed on 3 January 2022); and the China Environmental Statistical Yearbook, available at the website: https://data.cnki.net/yearbook/Single/N2021070128, (accessed on 3 January 2022).

Conflicts of Interest: The authors declare no conflict of interest.

References

1. Song, M.; Xie, Q.; Shen, Z. Impact of green credit on high-efficiency utilization of energy in China considering environmental constraints. *Energy Policy* **2021**, *153*, 112267. [CrossRef]
2. Yu, C.-H.; Wu, X.; Zhang, D.; Chen, S.; Zhao, J. Demand for green finance: Resolving financing constraints on green innovation in China. *Energy Policy* **2021**, *153*, 112255. [CrossRef]
3. Zhou, H.; Xu, G. Research on the impact of green finance on China's regional ecological development based on system GMM model. *Resour. Policy* **2022**, *75*, 102454. [CrossRef]
4. Wang, R.; Zhao, X.; Zhang, L. Research on the impact of green finance and abundance of natural resources on China's regional eco-efficiency. *Resour. Policy* **2022**, *76*, 102579. [CrossRef]
5. Yang, Y.; Su, X.; Yao, S. Nexus between green finance, fintech, and high-quality economic development: Empirical evidence from China. *Resour. Policy* **2021**, *74*, 102445. [CrossRef]
6. Sinha, A.; Mishra, S.; Sharif, A.; Yarovaya, L. Does green financing help to improve environmental & social responsibility? Designing SDG framework through advanced quantile modelling. *J. Environ. Manag.* **2021**, *292*, 112751.
7. Liu, D. Value evaluation system of ecological environment damage compensation caused by air pollution. *Environ. Technol. Innov.* **2021**, *22*, 101473. [CrossRef]
8. Yan, Y.; Chai, Z.; Yang, X.; Simayi, Z.; Yang, S. The temporal and spatial changes of the ecological environment quality of the urban agglomeration on the northern slope of Tianshan Mountain and the influencing factors. *Ecol. Indic.* **2021**, *133*, 108380.
9. Xiao, Y.; Tian, K.; Huang, H.; Wang, J.; Zhou, T. Coupling and coordination of socioeconomic and ecological environment in Wenchuan earthquake disaster areas: Case study of severely affected counties in southwestern China. *Sustain. Cities Soc.* **2021**, *71*, 102958. [CrossRef]
10. Zhang, S.; Wu, Z.; Wang, Y.; Hao, Y. Fostering green development with green finance: An empirical study on the environmental effect of green credit policy in China. *J. Environ. Manag.* **2021**, *296*, 113159. [CrossRef]
11. Zhang, D.; Wu, L.; Huang, S.; Zhang, Z.; Ahmad, F.; Zhang, G.; Shi, N.; Xu, H. Ecology and environment of the Belt and Road under global climate change: A systematic review of spatial patterns, cost efficiency, and ecological footprints. *Ecol. Indic.* **2021**, *131*, 108237. [CrossRef]
12. Chang, Y.; Hou, K.; Wu, Y.; Li, X.; Zhang, J. A conceptual framework for establishing the index system of ecological environment evaluation—A case study of the upper Hanjiang River, China. *Ecol. Indic.* **2019**, *107*, 105568. [CrossRef]
13. Shi, T.; Yang, S.; Zhang, W.; Zhou, Q. Coupling coordination degree measurement and spatiotemporal heterogeneity between economic development and ecological environment—Empirical evidence from tropical and subtropical regions of China. *J. Clean. Prod.* **2020**, *244*, 118739. [CrossRef]
14. Niu, L.; Xiao, L. Ecological environment management system based on artificial intelligence and complex numerical optimization. *Microprocess. Microsyst.* **2021**, *80*, 103627. [CrossRef]
15. Liu, Y.; Qu, Y.; Cang, Y.; Ding, X. Ecological security assessment for megacities in the Yangtze River basin: Applying improved emergy-ecological footprint and DEA-SBM model. *Ecol. Indic.* **2022**, *134*, 108481. [CrossRef]
16. Salazar, J. Environmental finance: Linking two worlds. In *A Workshop on Financial Innovations for Biodiversity*; Salazar, J.: Bratislava, Slovakia, 1998; Volume 1, pp. 2–18.
17. Labatt, S.; White, R.R. *Environmental Finance: A Guide to Environmental Risk Assessment and Financial Products*; John Wiley & Sons Ltd.: Chichester, UK, 2002.
18. Chen, Y.; Zhao, Z.J. The rise of green bonds for sustainable finance: Global standards and issues with the expanding Chinese market. *Curr. Opin. Environ. Sustain.* **2021**, *52*, 54–57. [CrossRef]

19. Li, M.; Hamawandy, N.M.; Wahid, F.; Rjoub, H.; Bao, Z. Renewable energy resources investment and green finance: Evidence from China. *Resour. Policy* **2021**, *74*, 102402. [CrossRef]
20. Xiang, X.; Liu, C.; Yang, M. Who is financing corporate green innovation? *Int. Rev. Econ. Finance* **2022**, *78*, 321–337. [CrossRef]
21. Feng, H.; Liu, Z.; Wu, J.; Iqbal, W.; Ahmad, W.; Marie, M. Nexus between Government spending's and Green Economic performance: Role of green finance and structure effect. *Environ. Technol. Innov.* **2022**, *27*, 102461. [CrossRef]
22. Yin, X.; Xu, Z. An empirical analysis of the coupling and coordinative development of China's green finance and economic growth. *Resour. Policy* **2022**, *75*, 102476. [CrossRef]
23. Lee, C.-C.; Lee, C.-C. How does green finance affect green total factor productivity? Evidence from China. *Energy Econ.* **2022**, *107*, 105863. [CrossRef]
24. Arif, A.; Vu, H.M.; Cong, M.; Wei, L.H.; Islam, M.M.; Niedbała, G. Natural resources commodity prices volatility and economic performance: Evaluating the role of green finance. *Resour. Policy* **2022**, *76*, 102557. [CrossRef]
25. Wang, X.; Wang, Q. Research on the impact of green finance on the upgrading of China's regional industrial structure from the perspective of sustainable development. *Resour. Policy* **2021**, *74*, 102436. [CrossRef]
26. Al Mamun, M.; Boubaker, S.; Nguyen, D.K. Green Finance and Decarbonization: Evidence from around the World. *Finance Res. Lett.* **2022**, *46*, 102807. [CrossRef]
27. Li, Z.; Kuo, T.-H.; Siao-Yun, W.; The Vinh, L. Role of green finance, volatility and risk in promoting the investments in Renewable Energy Resources in the post-COVID-19. *Resour. Policy* **2022**, *76*, 102563. [CrossRef]
28. Sun, H.; Chen, F. The impact of green finance on China's regional energy consumption structure based on system GMM. *Resour. Policy* **2022**, *76*, 102588. [CrossRef]
29. Tu, Q.; Mo, J.; Liu, Z.; Gong, C.; Fan, Y. Using green finance to counteract the adverse effects of COVID-19 pandemic on renewable energy investment—The case of offshore wind power in China. *Energy Policy* **2021**, *158*, 112542. [CrossRef]
30. Zhou, G.; Zhu, J.; Luo, S. The impact of fintech innovation on green growth in China: Mediating effect of green finance. *Ecol. Econ.* **2022**, *193*, 107308. [CrossRef]
31. Madaleno, M.; Dogan, E.; Taskin, D. A step forward on sustainability: The nexus of environmental responsibility, green technology, clean energy and green finance. *Energy Econ.* **2022**, *109*, 105945. [CrossRef]
32. Xu, Y.; Li, S.; Zhou, X.; Shahzad, U.; Zhao, X. How environmental regulations affect the development of green finance: Recent evidence from polluting firms in China. *Renew. Energy* **2022**, *189*, 917–926. [CrossRef]
33. Scholtens, B. Why Finance Should Care about Ecology. *Trends Ecol. Evol.* **2017**, *32*, 500–505. [CrossRef] [PubMed]
34. Jiang, L.; Liu, Y.; Wu, S.; Yang, C. Analyzing ecological environment change and associated driving factors in China based on NDVI time series data. *Ecol. Indic.* **2021**, *129*, 107933. [CrossRef]
35. Yusheng, K.; Ntarmah, A.H. Developing a rural ecological assessment index for Jiangsu Province, China. *J. Nat. Conserv.* **2021**, *64*, 126093. [CrossRef]
36. Cojoianu, T.F.; Clark, G.L.; Hoepner, A.G.F.; Veneri, P.; Wójcik, D. Entrepreneurs for a low carbon world: How environmental knowledge and policy shape the creation and financing of green start-ups. *Res. Policy* **2020**, *49*, 103988. [CrossRef]
37. Dikau, S.; Volz, U. Central bank mandates, sustainability objectives and the promotion of green finance. *Ecol. Econ.* **2021**, *184*, 107022. [CrossRef]
38. Cheng, K.; He, K.; Fu, Q.; Tagawa, K.; Guo, X. Assessing the coordination of regional water and soil resources and ecological-environment system based on speed characteristics. *J. Clean. Prod.* **2022**, *339*, 130718. [CrossRef]
39. Jun, L.; Jundong, H.; Yang, L. Analysis of Rural Ecological Environment Governance in the Two-Oriented Society Construction: A Case Study of Xiantao City in Hubei Province. *Procedia Environ. Sci.* **2011**, *11*, 1278–1284. [CrossRef]
40. Stanford, H.R.; Garrard, G.E.; Kirk, H.; Hurley, J. A social-ecological framework for identifying and governing informal greenspaces in cities. *Landsc. Urb. Plan.* **2022**, *221*, 104378. [CrossRef]
41. Yang, Y.; Wang, L.; Yang, F.; Hu, N.; Liang, L. Evaluation of the coordination between eco-environment and socioeconomy under the "Ecological County Strategy" in western China: A case study of Meixian. *Ecol. Indic.* **2021**, *125*, 107585. [CrossRef]
42. Li, C.; Wu, X.; Wang, X.; Yin, J.; Zheng, A.; Yang, X. Ecological environment and socioeconomic factors drive long-term transmission and extreme outbreak of dengue fever in epidemic region of China. *J. Clean. Prod.* **2021**, *279*, 123870. [CrossRef]
43. Wang, Z.; Xie, B.; Xia, X.; Yang, H.; Zuo, Q.; Liu, Z. Energy loss of radial inflow turbine for organic Rankine cycle using mixture based on entropy production method. *Energy* **2022**, *245*, 123312. [CrossRef]
44. Li, G.; Wang, Y.X.; Zeng, Y.; He, W.H. A new maximum entropy method for estimation of multimodal probability density function. *Appl. Math. Model.* **2021**, *102*, 137–152. [CrossRef]
45. Chen, Q.; Lu, S.; Xiong, K.; Zhao, R. Coupling analysis on ecological environment fragility and poverty in South China Karst. *Environ. Res.* **2021**, *201*, 111650. [CrossRef] [PubMed]
46. Chen, P.; Shi, X. Dynamic evaluation of China's ecological civilization construction based on target correlation degree and coupling coordination degree. *Environ. Impact Assess. Rev.* **2022**, *93*, 106734. [CrossRef]
47. Zhang, D.; Chen, Y. Evaluation on urban environmental sustainability and coupling coordination among its dimensions: A case study of Shandong Province, China. *Sustain. Cities Soc.* **2021**, *75*, 103351. [CrossRef]
48. Ma, Q.; Li, Y.; Xu, L. Identification of green infrastructure networks based on ecosystem services in a rapidly urbanizing area. *J. Clean. Prod.* **2021**, *300*, 126945. [CrossRef]

49. Moonga, G.; Chisola, M.N.; Berger, U.; Nowak, D.; Yabe, J.; Nakata, H.; Nakayama, S.; Ishizuka, M.; Bose-O'Reilly, S. Geospatial approach to investigate spatial clustering and hotspots of blood lead levels in children within Kabwe, Zambia. *Environ. Res.* **2022**, *207*, 112646. [CrossRef]
50. Ahmad, M.; Wu, Y. Combined role of green productivity growth, economic globalization, and eco-innovation in achieving ecological sustainability for OECD economies. *J. Environ. Manag.* **2022**, *302*, 113980. [CrossRef]
51. Wang, F.; Wang, R.; He, Z. The impact of environmental pollution and green finance on the high-quality development of energy based on spatial Durbin model. *Resour. Policy* **2021**, *74*, 102451. [CrossRef]
52. Yang, C.; Zeng, W.; Yang, X. Coupling coordination evaluation and sustainable development pattern of geo-ecological environment and urbanization in Chongqing municipality, China. *Sustain. Cities Soc.* **2020**, *61*, 102271. [CrossRef]
53. Chen, Y.; Tian, W.; Zhou, Q.; Shi, T. Spatiotemporal and driving forces of Ecological Carrying Capacity for high-quality development of 286 cities in China. *J. Clean. Prod.* **2021**, *293*, 126186. [CrossRef]
54. Yu, D.; Cao, Y.; Cao, M.; Xu, H. Enhancing China's ecological sustainability through more optimized investment. *Glob. Ecol. Conserv.* **2022**, *34*, e02049. [CrossRef]
55. Chen, Y.; Zhu, M.; Lu, J.; Zhou, Q.; Ma, W. Evaluation of ecological city and analysis of obstacle factors under the background of high-quality development: Taking cities in the Yellow River Basin as examples. *Ecol. Indic.* **2020**, *118*, 106771. [CrossRef]
56. Zhang, H.; Geng, C.; Wei, J. Coordinated development between green finance and environmental performance in China: The spatial-temporal difference and driving factors. *J. Clean. Prod.* **2022**, *346*, 131150. [CrossRef]
57. Lv, C.; Bian, B.; Lee, C.-C.; He, Z. Regional gap and the trend of green finance development in China. *Energy Econ.* **2021**, *102*, 105476. [CrossRef]
58. Ding, M.; Liu, W.; Xiao, L.; Zhong, F.; Lu, N.; Zhang, J.; Zhang, Z.; Xu, X.; Wang, K. Construction and optimization strategy of ecological security pattern in a rapidly urbanizing region: A case study in central-south China. *Ecol. Indic.* **2022**, *136*, 108604. [CrossRef]
59. Yang, X.; Liu, S.; Jia, C.; Liu, Y.; Yu, C. Vulnerability assessment and management planning for the ecological environment in urban wetlands. *J. Environ. Manag.* **2021**, *298*, 113540. [CrossRef]
60. Morgan, T. The techno-finance fix: A critical analysis of international and regional environmental policy documents and their implications for planning. *Prog. Plan.* **2018**, *119*, 1–29. [CrossRef]
61. Xue, X.; Wang, Z. Impact of finance pressure on energy intensity: Evidence from China's manufacturing sectors. *Energy* **2021**, *226*, 120220. [CrossRef]
62. Kassouri, Y. Monitoring the spatial spillover effects of urbanization on water, built-up land and ecological footprints in sub-Saharan Africa. *J. Environ. Manag.* **2021**, *300*, 113690. [CrossRef]
63. Wang, A.; Liao, X.; Tong, Z.; Du, W.; Zhang, J.; Liu, X.; Liu, M. Spatial-temporal dynamic evaluation of the ecosystem service value from the perspective of "production-living-ecological" spaces: A case study in Dongliao River Basin, China. *J. Clean. Prod.* **2022**, *333*, 130218. [CrossRef]
64. Wang, M.; Li, X.; Wang, S. Discovering research trends and opportunities of green finance and energy policy: A data-driven scientometric analysis. *Energy Policy* **2021**, *154*, 112295. [CrossRef]
65. Debrah, C.; Chan, A.P.C.; Darko, A. Green finance gap in green buildings: A scoping review and future research needs. *Build. Environ.* **2022**, *207*, 108443. [CrossRef]
66. Hafner, S.; Jones, A.; Anger-Kraavi, A.; Monasterolo, I. Modelling the macroeconomics of a 'closing the green finance gap' scenario for an energy transition. *Environ. Innov. Soc. Transit.* **2021**, *40*, 536–568. [CrossRef]
67. Liu, T.; Song, Y.; Xing, X.; Zhu, Y.; Qu, Z. Bridging production factors allocation and environmental performance of China's heavy-polluting energy firms: The moderation effect of financing and internationalization. *Energy* **2021**, *222*, 119943. [CrossRef]

International Journal of
Environmental Research and Public Health

MDPI

Article

The Sharing of Costs and Benefits of Rural Environmental Pollution Governance in China: A Qualitative Analysis through Guanxi Networks Perspective

Yanqiang Du [1], Pingyang Liu [2], Shipeng Su [3] and Linyi Zhou [4,*]

1 College of Public Administration, Nanjing Agricultural University, Nanjing 210095, China; dyqiang2088@njau.edu.cn
2 Department of Environmental Science and Engineering, Fudan University, Shanghai 200433, China; pyliu@fudan.edu.cn
3 School of Public Management, Fujian Agriculture and Forestry University, Fuzhou 350002, China; ssp@fafu.edu.cn
4 School of International and Public Affairs, Shanghai Jiao Tong University, Shanghai 200030, China
* Correspondence: zhoulinyi1017@sjtu.edu.cn

Abstract: Concern has been expressed in many parts of the world that community relations in rural areas are breaking down, making issues such as rural environmental degradation harder to resolve without external regulation. Guanxi is a specific Chinese idiom for characterizing social networks, as a broad term to represent existing relations among people, which can be loosely translated as "relationship". Based on a case study of an underdeveloped mountainous area of Southern China, this paper examined the problem from the perspective of guanxi, and explored the impacts of internal group differentiation catalyzed by pig farming pollution and the subsequent influences on the distribution of costs and benefits of different shareholders. It was found that the guanxi in the village were changed from blood relationship centered to economic interest centered. This disparity exerts a significant influence on the distribution of costs and benefits of pollution control and exacerbates environmental inequalities. This means that pig farmers dominated the narrative of pig farming pollution, while the ordinary villagers chose to suffer without protesting, which hinders the advancement of pollution control, and pig farmers took the benefits of weak pollution control and managed to transfer the external cost to others, while others became direct victims. The paper concludes that the rich become richer and the poor become poorer in both economic and environmental perspectives. It is strongly suggested that guanxi should be integrated into the consideration and decision-making process of rural environmental governance in order to guarantee the efficiency and efficacy of its implementation.

Keywords: environmental equality; guanxi network; pig farming pollution; cost and benefit sharing; China

Citation: Du, Y.; Liu, P.; Su, S.; Zhou, L. The Sharing of Costs and Benefits of Rural Environmental Pollution Governance in China: A Qualitative Analysis through Guanxi Networks Perspective. *IJERPH* **2022**, *19*, 6587. https://doi.org/10.3390/ijerph19116587

Academic Editors: Jie Chen, Qian Zhou and Ting Zhang

Received: 16 April 2022
Accepted: 26 May 2022
Published: 28 May 2022

1. Introduction

Environmental problems in rural or farming areas have become a major obstacle for creating a "beautiful countryside" and implementing the Rural Revitalization Strategy in China [1,2]. Increasing rural environmental pollution has been shown to threaten the physical and mental health of farmers, as well as regional ecological safety; this poses a serious challenge for state-led rural environmental governance, which has, thus far, failed to address the complex challenge of balancing economic development and environmental pollution control in rural areas [3]. Pig farming pollution is a big challenge for rural environmental protection and sustainable development in rural China. For example, in 2017, 689 million pigs were sold, and the chemical oxygen demand of the livestock and poultry industry reached 100.55 million tons, accounting for 93.8% of the total emissions from agricultural sources. Even though national policies for the control of livestock and poultry pollution were introduced and related public investments increased, many problems remain unsolved, while new problems and conflicts emerge [4–7].

One easily observable—yet often neglected—factor here is rural guanxi networks. Many scholars note that "guanxi" are extremely important in underdeveloped rural areas of developing countries, particularly when they serve as a mechanism for addressing problems in the transformation of rural society, in the absence of official laws and regulations [8,9]. According to Grootaert's study on rural Indonesia [10], guanxi networks assist the poor more, because for them, returns on guanxi are higher than they are for the rich. Meanwhile, some scholars find that in rural areas, the rich or the elite have much stronger guanxi networks than the poor, and that the benefits they obtain from them are much greater than those obtained by the poor [11]. In the field of rural environmental governance, studies find that difficulties in implementing rural environmental policies can be attributed to rural guanxi networks, and that these are also closely related to rural social inequities [12]. The traditional guanxi is a very important factor in driving rural environmental improvement in China [13].

Guanxi networks are embedded in every aspect of rural society [9,13–15]. As a localized society in nature, rural China's development and governance mechanisms have been profoundly shaped by guanxi networks [16–18]. In the context of rapid urbanization and dramatic rural transformation in China, traditional mechanisms are disintegrating, while market mechanisms have not yet taken shape; therefore, guanxi networks still play an important role [13,19]. Specifically, the influence of guanxi networks on the governance of public rural affairs is highly likely to trigger new social inequalities, thereby further affecting governance efficiency and even social stability. However, these problems have not received adequate attention—practically or theoretically.

Thus, this study attempted to answer the following two issues based on a case study of an underdeveloped mountainous area of Southern China:

(1) how do the guanxi networks among the villagers change by livestock farming?
(2) how do guanxi networks shape the way in which the costs and benefits of pig farming are distributed?

2. Literature Review

Guanxi is frequently mentioned in Chinese society, and is also an indispensable analysis perspective [20]. After comparing the social system of China and that of the West, Studies found that Chinese society is neither individual-based nor society-based, but guanxi-based [21]. A large part of the literature suggests that guanxi networks appear particularly important to understand the economy, politics, and culture of Chinese rural society [21–23] Literally, it is similar to "relationship", but with more emphasis on connection and interaction. It is regarded as both "social networks" and "social capital" [16,22], especially in Western literature. In a Chinese context, guanxi also refers to "private contacts". Studies summarize its fundamental characteristics: (1) as constituted by relations among different actors and may be deemed a series of social contacts of actors; (2) these contacts are of a relatively long duration; and (3) its main function is to offer mutual assistance in need [24].

The controversy surrounding the definition of guanxi remains, and more studies are starting to apply the concept of guanxi inter-disciplinarily because of its strong explanatory power [20,25]. Thus, the purpose of this study was not to provide an accurate understanding of guanxi or relationships, but to use its common understanding with special emphasis on its function and subsequent impacts on rural environmental governance. Based on existing research, our starting point was that guanxi networks comprise interpersonal relationships between individuals and their peers on the basis of ethics, emotions, and interests; it also represents social contacts produced and reproduced in a constant exchange process.

It has been widely discussed that guanxi contributes significantly to rural societies. For example, studies find that guanxi can significantly promote the development of rural enterprises [26]. During the process of urbanization and industrialization, guanxi networks also boost rural labor mobility [27]. In addition, guanxi is critical for the implementation of top-down policies [28] and improves the efficiency and efficacy of rural public goods supply [15].

However, the influence of guanxi networks on rural environmental governance has not attracted much attention [13,29,30]. Unlike relationship networks in Western cultures, guanxi networks in China are not official organizational ones, even though they play a crucial role in rural governance, such as by organizing environmental movements and promoting their success [23]. It has been widely recognized that Chinese top-down environmental governance is faced with serious challenges in rural areas. For example, environmental governance may lead to conflicts between local demands and those prioritized by the central government [31,32]. Furthermore, there are other factors that weaken the government's policy enforcement capability in rural areas, such as the dispersed, non-point sources of environmental pollution, difficulties in identifying and monitoring pollution sources, the high costs of information access, and the excessive number of actors involved [33,34]. Consequently, more attention should be paid to the rural community itself. Hodge (2001) recommended that agricultural environmental policy should establish a broader institutional framework between different organizations and individuals, including considering rural informal institutions [35]. North (1990) demonstrated that guanxi networks exist as a form of informal rural institution [36]. Therefore, it appears particularly important to explore environmental governance within rural communities from the perspective of guanxi networks [37,38]. Considering the cultural "fertile soil" for the development of guanxi in rural China, it is particularly important to understand the economy, politics, and culture of Chinese rural society from the perspective of guanxi [39].

Rural environmental management is a typical regional public good, and many studies center on its efficiency and efficacy [2,40,41]. Yet, existing studies have not conducted in-depth analyses on the distribution of cost and benefit related to rural environmental treatment among different stakeholders, even though some might be beneficiaries, while others are victims [42]. Hanson argued that an overall high efficiency does not guarantee equality [43]; instead, in the overwhelming majority of cases, unbalanced distribution results in environmental inequalities [44]. For example, considering products/services that are harmful to the environment, the poor often take greater environmental risks to achieve cost-effectiveness, and are unable to enjoy the benefits of environment-friendly products/services [45]. This indicates that the costs of environmental policies disproportionately fall upon low-income groups, while the benefits of environmental policies are often largely reaped by high-income groups [46].

At present, Chinese rural society has become seriously stratified, meaning that the disparity between villagers in income, occupation, and social capital, among other factors, has brought about unequal access to resources, services, and social status. Moreover, it differentially affects villagers' benefits from the supply of rural public goods (i.e., roads and environmental governance) [31]. It is therefore imperative to systematically investigate the influence of guanxi networks among different groups in Chinese rural society and its effects on the costs and benefits of industry growth and pollution from pig farming, and their distribution.

While not related specifically to China, solving the rural environmental pollution through various ways in many developing countries, such as top-down ways and bottom-up ways, is important. This paper offers a new perspective for better understanding the interaction of guanxi networks and rural environmental governance in China. This may help others to better understand why policy fails in rural pollution prevention. A lack of understanding of guanxi results in an ineffective control of animal waste and the failure of environmental regulations. Instead, improving trust-based networks is a better option to control pig farming pollution and promote environmental justice in China, as well as in similar societies in other countries.

3. Materials and Methods

3.1. Study Area

The target village for our case study was S village, located in the undeveloped mountainous area in northern Fujian Province, China. The village comprises 248 households, which are divided into 6 villager groups, with a total of 998 villagers. In 2015, its per capita annual income was around 5900 RMB. In 2020, S village had 890 villagers, and its per capita annual income was around 8100 RMB. The village has hardly any collective fiscal revenue, and the situation was exacerbated by the rapid urbanization process. The large scale of population hollowing out led to the collapse of this traditional community, significantly weakening the influence and appeal of the village collective.

In the early 1990s, the pig farming industry was first introduced to S village, and developed rapidly. At the time, many rural migrant workers, who had been working in cities, returned to farm pigs in the village area because of its relatively high profits. Later, the village saw the constant expansion of the scale of pig farming; however, no pollution treatment facilities were built, and pig excrement and urine were discharged directly into local rivers. The local government adopted a series of measures to control this pollution, for example, ordering unqualified households to demolish their farms and subsidizing other households to construct biogas digesters. However, these measures did not work well; on the contrary, as soon as the restrictive government policies were relaxed, the industry rebounded. Many demolished pigpens reappeared, becoming larger and more numerous, causing increasingly serious environmental pollution. The nearby river was sometimes reported to be black and smelly. The village's drinking water sources were contaminated by waste water several times (subsequently, villagers used mountain spring water instead), which adversely affected the health of villagers.

3.2. Data Collection

The data in this study were collected mainly through long-term observations at the village, in-depth interviews, and questionnaire surveys. First, since 2013, a research team of at least four researchers stayed in the village for about two weeks every quarter to observe it. By living together with the villagers, we were able to understand the production, lifestyles, and interpersonal relationships within the community. While observing the principles of understanding and recognizing our respondents' rights to confidentiality and privacy, we generated data in the form of photos, videos, and village field survey reports, among other data.

Second, a questionnaire survey involving the entire village was conducted from March 2013 to July 2014. All the households (except those unavailable at that time, such as migration workers) were visited and questionnaires were completed face to face, considering the literacy issues among villagers. A total of 110 questionnaires were collected, of which 64 were from farmers (refers to ordinary villagers who do not have pigs), and 46 from pig farmers.

Third, based on the information gained from observation and the questionnaire survey, semi-structured interviews were carried out with key figures in the village using a snowball sampling method. In S village, the main stakeholders included pig farmers, farmers, village committee cadres, and officials of the township government. We conducted 55 interviews, including the village cadres and reputable clan figures. All the interviews were transcribed when finished and translated into English. Deep reading of transcripts was applied for coding and analyzing.

Finally, data from official reports and supplementary interviews by telephone calls were also analyzed. To clarify any ambiguities and double check quantitative data, the lead researcher called the village cadres, reputable clan figures, and some villagers on occasion, from April to December 2016, January 2019, and July 2021.

Based on all the data above, we conducted qualitative research based on a case study. This paper illustrates the role of guanxi in mobilizing resources in rural environmental struggles in China following the bidirectional mechanism framework of guanxi—socioeconomic impacts–environmental behaviors. The extent to which village-level guanxi networks have survived the increasingly narrow market-focused interests of specific villager groups, such as the differentiation between pig farmers and farmers, was analyzed and the subsequent economic, environmental, and social costs and benefits of pig farming were estimated. Finally, the environmental behavior and governance of the villagers were analyzed. While qualitative methods were used, they were mainly used to show the functions of guanxi networks.

4. Results

4.1. Changing of Guanxi Networks and the Differentiation of Households

4.1.1. The Changing of Guanxi Networks

S village used to be clan-dominated, with characteristics typical of traditional communities. Clan relations played significant roles in traditional rural society to provide many common goods, like roads and education, especially in the Fujian province where clan relations were strong. For example, when a family in difficulty seeks help, it mainly resorts to neighbors, relatives, and friends. Public commodities at a village level, such as the construction of bridges and roads, were also supplied mainly through collective action, which is described by the Chinese saying "those with money contribute money and those with strength give strength." Addressing changes in rural society, the director of the Women's Federation in this village said:

> *Nowadays, community relations and village regulations are generally unimportant, because people are just judged on their fortune rather than their moral character. (Female, 46, village director of the Women's Federation)*

However, traditional community governance has been seriously challenged by rapid urbanization and industrialization since the 1980s. As an undeveloped mountainous village, S village used to depend heavily on rice planting, a labor-intensive but low-output crop. The population hollowing out continued among the younger generation and able-bodied men, and households became atomized, driven by maximization of private interests, which led to the collapse of the community. Due to its rapid growth, the pig farming industry became the pillar industry and a major income source for many farmers; this turned out to reshape the community with its economic power. Driven by profits, people joined the industry eagerly. However, not every household had the same opportunities. According to the data from our interviews, there are underlying requirements for pig farming: economically, a large initial capital should be available for investment in building pigsties and buying piglets; socially, information sources on markets, technology, and the availability of types of services are necessary. For farmers with no industry experience and who depend heavily on the community, these prerequisites are beyond their capabilities; therefore, they have to seek help from their guanxi network. In fact, the growth of pig farming in S village can be attributed to relatives or friends "passing on experience, helping, and guiding newcomers." As farmer (non-pig farmer) C stated in the survey,

> *Pig farming in the village depends completely on relatives or friends... because people who have good relationships often discuss the situation with the price of pigs, farming techniques and government policies together. The main reason why most ordinary agricultural households do not raise pigs is that they do not have start-up funds or people to give them technical guidance...These things require help from nearby pig farmers. (Male, 52, farmer)*

Catalyzed by the pig farming industry, the traditional blood relation-based guanxi was gradually replaced by economic interest-centered guanxi. As a result, interpersonal contacts, social morality, and the supply of village-level public commodities were changed significantly. Villagers were always busy making money rather than bonding with each other. When they were short of something, such as labor, they did not seek help from their neighbors or relatives, but rather paid to hire workers. As the compiler of the clan pedigree in the village put it:

"Over these years, people have just done their own thing . . . They just maintain so-so relationships with other villagers in this village, and only greet each other, and their relationships with each other are not so close as before. For example, if a family happened to be eating and another person came by, then the host would invite the visitor to dine and drink together. But now the visitor will refuse to dine even if the host adds a pair of chopsticks." (Male, 56, compiler of the clan pedigree)

We further discovered that the main reason why villagers are unwilling to eat in other people's homes is because they are afraid of owing favors (i.e., "I will invite you next time"). This reflects a more pecuniary interest-based relationship, and almost everyone just associates with people they get along with. There are many kinds of guanxi networks in rural China caused by different factors, and this research focused on the guanxi network caused by pig breeding.

4.1.2. The Characteristics of Guanxi Networks in Different Groups

The village was divided by two guanxi groups: pig farmers and farmers. As our survey shows, in S village, there are 46 pig farmers, including 22 large-scale ones, 22 scattered ("san yang") households, and four households that gave up raising pigs by demolishing their pig farms in July 2014, as they wanted to move to the city. With high incomes, these groups are better able to attract capable people, including young people, to join them. The average age of the pig farming group is 48 years old, and they are mostly men (74% of pig farmers are men). Farmers, who were "excluded" from the sector in the village are the group that do not raise pigs. The traditional industry of S village was crop production, which was highly labor intensive in this mountainous area and brought in little income. Our survey indicated that farmers are 51 years old on average. Our findings indicated that pig farmers are younger, which means that the pig farming industry has a certain attractiveness (Table 1).

Table 1. The scale of each group.

Item	Sample Class	Farmers		Pig farmers	
		Percentage (%)	Mean Value	Percentage (%)	Mean Value
Family scale	Not less than 4	42.2	5.3	45.7	5.2
	5 to 8	51.5		47.8	
	Over 8	6.3		6.5	
Educational level	Primary school and lower	68.8	/	67.4	/
	Junior middle school and above	31.2		32.6	
	Junior college and above	0.0		0.0	
Gender	Man	62.5	/	73.9	/
	Woman	37.5		26.1	
Age	Not less than 40	20.3	51.2	21.7	48.4
	41 to 50	34.4		41.3	
	Over 50	45.3		40.0	

Meanwhile, different groups have different kinds of guanxi networks. Pig farmers have stronger guanxi networks and are more capable than farmers who access external resources. As Table 2 indicates, each pig farmer has an average of 1.9 relatives, who are similarly engaged in the industry and earning an average annual household income of 76,349 RMB. The survey indicated that the villager cadres in S village are hardly separable from the pig farming group (17% of pig farmers are or were village cadres). Moreover, all the village cadres in S village are pig farmers, and as "capable people" in the village, pig farmers who successfully make money are more likely to be elected as village cadres. The village cadres were therefore categorized in the "pig farmers" group. In contrast, the number of relatives of farmers is 1.6, and their average annual household income is 54,840 RMB. There is a positive correlation between the scales of the resources. As the pig farming sector has grown, the difference in the return for crop production and animal husbandry has further widened the economic gap between pig farmers and non-farmers.

Table 2. The capability of each group.

Item	Sample Class	Farmers		Pig Farmers	
		Percentage (%)	Mean Value	Percentage (%)	Mean Value
Gross income	Not Less than 10,000	12.5	54,840.6	7.6	76,349.1
	10,001 to 50,000	64.1		59.1	
	50,001 to 100,000	20.3		24.1	
	Over 100,000	3.1		8.2	
Pig breeding by relatives	None	45.3	1.6	30.4	1.9
	1 to 5	46.9		59.1	
	Over 5	7.8		10.5	
Village cadres or not	No	87.5	/	82.6	/
	Were	10.9		4.3	
	The proportion of Christianity	1.6		13.1	

We also found that pig farming shaped the nature of guanxi in different groups. For the pig farmers, the guanxi network is growing, driven by the economic benefits—this means that they are self-enforcing, being perpetrators; the farmers' guanxi networks are shrinking, turning them into victims. Through the industry chain, pig farmers are more able to extend their relationships vertically and associate with people outside their family. As a result, they were able to acquire more information and take advantage of resources. Farmers mostly engage in traditional agriculture and associate with a limited group of older people on the basis of blood and geographical relationships; this constrains their access to information and resources. Our interview material indicated this clearly:

> *The scope of our associations is limited to our village or some relatives and friends...But pig farmers have much greater interpersonal relationships than us. We often see them inviting their friends to dine and drink at home. Some large pig farming households, in particular, have extremely good relationships with the town government, village cadres, pig dealers and so on. (Male, 49, farmer)*

These different guanxi networks have an impact on the effectiveness of pollution control in the following ways.

(1) Pig farmers gradually expand the scope of their external associations and take advantage of their powerful guanxi to get close to government officials. Through these strong guanxi networks, they are able to obtain information and resources relating to governance policies—for example, biogas digester subsidies or the planned scope of demolition—or the timing of inspections. Some government officials can use their power over pollution control to make a profit. In this way, environmental governance is transformed into a power-for-money deal, and for this reason many top-down pollution control measures are not really implemented. For example, in an interview, a pig farmer indicated:

> *Whenever the Spring Festival and other festivals come, I always give some cigarettes and wine to village cadres, and some precious tea to the town leader in charge of this village. My son is the driver for a leader of this town. So other pig farmers also seek connections with my son. (Male, 50, pig farmer)*

(2) Some pig farmers work with each other to resist pollution control. Given their shared economic interests and close relationships within the group, pig farmers have a greater incentive to seek the maximization of group interests. For example, during surprise inspections launched by the government, these households are often informed in advance, and some backyard pig farmers drive their pigs to the pigpens of farmers with larger facilities that they have good relationships with, to thereby bypass the requirements to construct pollution control facilities or biogas digesters.

(3) Farmers have weak guanxi networks and are gradually marginalized in terms of rural public affairs. They are not able to raise pigs themselves or to escape the impact of the pollution caused by other villagers, who do. Facing the strong pig farming group, they can only choose to "keep silent" for the following reasons. First, they must have at least some social contact with pig farmers; they prefer to become a "silent majority", rather than cause offense, so as to maintain these relationships and put a good face on things. Second, because they are still based on kinship relations, the guanxi networks of farmers are looser and they are marginalized in terms of their ability to speak out on village affairs, especially in contrast to pig farmers. Third, pig farmers have a lot economic power, and farmers must often rely on them for job opportunities or to borrow money, or in other ways. For example, pig farmers may give the dissatisfied victims of pollution some pork, or pay them to work on their farms. As this village is not rich, most farmers who do not raise pigs have accepted pollution, instead of choosing to resist it, as long as they can get some benefits from their pig farming neighbors.

It follows that these different guanxi networks place various groups in the position of being "perpetrators" or "victims", in terms of their relationship to pollution control. Although pig farmers are the perpetrators of pollution, they can rely on the benefits from pig farming to further strengthen their guanxi networks; farmers, however, end up as "victims" of environmental pollution. Meanwhile, government-led top-down policies persist, even though they are not really implemented, due to the powerful influence of the pig farmers. The vast majority of pig farmers have not even constructed the most basic facilities (such as biogas digesters), and the disadvantaged position and silence of farmers that are excluded from the sector means that government policy is not supported from below.

4.2. *Influence of Different Guanxi Networks on the Distribution of Costs and Benefits of Pollution Control*

The "perpetrator–victim" situation described in the preceding section is just an external characterization of the unsatisfactory effects of pollution control. The different guanxi networks among these two groups also create a situation of "prosperity and poverty", mainly through their influence on the way that the costs and benefits of pollution control are shared. Although all the members of S village are victims of pig farming pollution, some groups are more capable of evading the consequences of environmental pollution and environmental risks, while others bear a disproportionate share of the costs.

4.2.1. Costs and Benefits to Pig Farmers

The benefits gained by pig farmers come mainly from selling pigs. Although the labor opportunity cost of raising pigs is low, the returns are quite high; this is why many villagers are willing to raise pigs instead of leaving the village for work. We performed telephonic follow-up interviews with some villagers in January 2019 and July 2021, and analyzed the returns on pig farming for 2015 and 2016; the results are shown in Table 3. In terms of pig cost, the gross cost per head of pig on average was 1300 RMB (feed cost 1100 RMB, disease prevention 150 RMB, water and electricity costs 20 RMB, and loss due to pigs that died of disease 30 RMB), the labor input and environmental cost was not calculated. We found that every pig brought a profit of 950 RMB in peak season. Moreover, small-scale farmers could make a net annual profit of 30,000 RMB, and large-scale farmers a net annual profit of 50,000 RMB.

These economic benefits are realized on the basis that environmental costs and social costs are not considered, even though these are considerable. Pig farmers in S village mostly have sties with cement floors, on which excrement and urine accumulate, causing a strong odor. Pig farmers wash the excrement and urine away with clean water twice a day, usually at 8:00–9:00 a.m. and 4:00–5:00 p.m. The waste water is discharged directly into nearby rivers. In this way, they gain an economic advantage by exploiting the ecological environment of the village without paying any cost. The wealth of this group ultimately originates from the loss of natural and social resources.

Table 3. Costs and benefits of pig farmers.

Costs/Benefits	Contents	Data Standard	Remarks
Breeding cost	Feed cost	The cost of young pigs 200 RMB, the cost of medium pig 500 RMB, pig rearing large cost 1000 RMB.	The average weight of a piglet is 15–30 kg, a medium pig is 50–60 kg, and a large pig is 100–130 kg.
	Labor cost	one labor wage is 1500–2000 RMB/month; 8 pigs or more require 1 laborer to be responsible for feeding and management.	/
Environmental cost	Cost of treatment facilities (biogas digesters etc.)	The average cost of a biogas digester is 900 RMB/square meter; it costs about 10,000 to 20,000 RMB to build a biogas digester.	Only talk about the construction cost, ignore the manual processing and post-maintenance.
	External cost	Loss of neighborhood relations in the community.	/
Other costs	Depreciation cost of pig house	The cost of building a pig house is 70–90 RMB/square meter, and it will run for about 10 years.	The land belongs to the individual contracted land of pig farmers.
	Other	Disease prevention is 150 RMB, charges for water and electricity are 20 RMB, and loss due to pigs that died of disease is the equivalent of 30 RMB.	/
Benefits	Peak season	The price of a pig is 14–16 RMB/kg, a small part is 18–20 RMB/kg.	/
	Off-season	The price of a pig is 8–12 RMB/kg.	/
Government subsidies	Environment subsidies	The government will provide a subsidy of 1200 RMB when the biogas digester is checked and accepted.	/

When faced with breeding pollution control, pig farmers' income was unchanged, but they experienced a substantial increase in the cost. If governance is required in terms of discharge standards, the pig farmers must bear the costs of aquaculture waste water treatment. For example, it costs approximately 10,000–20,000 RMB to build a biogas digester (the government gives a subsidy of 1200 RMB for every biogas digester), and this is equivalent to the profit that can be made from 40–80 heads of pigs. Because of the lack of supervision and penalties, as well as the mismatch between the costs and benefits, most pig farmers do not construct biogas digesters, but choose to directly—and illegally—discharge waste water into rivers and streams.

4.2.2. Costs and Benefits of Farmers

Farmers bear the brunt of the costs of pollution related to pig farming. The direct losses include a decrease in agricultural production due to pollution, and the pollution of water sources used for drinking and household activities, which means higher costs to buy water. The indirect losses include a drop in the value of their property, as well as the negative social impact. Pollution from pig farming has made S village virtually uninhabitable, and the disappearance of development opportunities has led to a sharp decline in the value of real estate. Moreover, the worsening relationships and conflicts over pig farming are also an invisible burden on villagers, as we discuss further below.

In the early years of the development of pig farming, farmers derived some benefits from it; for example, they could acquire pig manure and urine to use as fertilizer. However, after the scale of the industry expanded, only few farmers got the chance to work as wage laborers on large-scale farms, which paid approximately 1500–2000 RMB/month, while most farmers suffered various direct and indirect losses. Because most pig farmers in S village "save" the cost of treating waste water and directly discharge nearly all pig excrement and urine into rivers, the bodies of water approximate to pig farms have suffered severe eutrophication. The water is not fit for drinking and cannot even be used to irrigate farmland. In our survey, many farmers reported that "our crops die from excessive pig farming waste water", "rice seedlings grow well but bear no fruit", and other problems. One farmer complained that crop losses were a heavy burden, because he did not have any other source of income:

> *My crops are affected by waste sludge and water from nearby pig farming households, and my rice is all damaged by the excessive phosphorus and nitrogen content in the irrigation water, which is over the standard. I got no harvest this year! (Male, 48, farmer)*

Water sources for household use are also polluted, and water costs are higher. Waste water from pig farming not only affects irrigation water, it also contaminates water in deep wells and rivers through surface and underground penetration. S village therefore has to draw on drinking water from sources higher up the mountain, which has significantly increased the cost of the water supply. The use of polluted surface water and underground water by people or animals is still very difficult to avoid, which might cause potential health problems. A female farmer we interviewed said:

> *Nearly all the wells, from which we used to fetch water, could no longer be used. Our current drinking water comes from a mountain (where there are no farms) very far from the village. We laid pipes from that mountain to our homes. The costs were equally shared by our villagers, including pig farmers and other farmers. (Female, 42, farmer)*

Farmers' indirect losses are mainly of three types: (1) Property loss. Pollution from pig farming has made S village almost uninhabitable. Heavy pollution accelerated the hollowing out of the rural population, especially those with knowledge and wealth. Even the pig farmers themselves have moved to cities with the money they earned, leaving hired workers in the village. Although the market value of rural housing is not available as these transactions are forbidden according to China's laws, it usually takes more than 100 thousand RMB to build a modest house in the village; however, it is highly possible that houses in S village have become negative assets due to the serious pollution. (2) Collapse of community. The irregular development of the pig farming sector has fostered a money-oriented attitude in S village, undermining traditional clan rules and community virtues. There have been many conflicts over pig farming in the community and relationships among different groups have deteriorated. For example, the pig farm of resident R is located near the home of farmer T. T has been complaining to R about the pollution for a long time.

> *"You are too unconscionable. Your conscience has been eaten by dogs. If your farm had been there for a year or two, I would not complain to you. But you have been raising pigs for so long here and your farm has always been making that smell. How are we supposed to live here? Do you want me to die in your pigpen?"*

Pig farmer R countered farmer T by saying:

> *"This plot of land is mine. I constructed the farm on my own land. If you are dissatisfied with the farm, will you give me another plot of land to build a farm? Moreover, it's hard for us to make money, like a gamble! You complain this way every day. So no wonder that our pigs do not grow well. You envy my good luck. If you have the ability, you can raise pigs. I would let you to build a similar farm next to our home!"*

(3) Loss of development opportunities. As General Secretary Xi Jinping of China puts it, "Clear waters and lush mountains are invaluable assets." When serious pollution from

pig farming destroys the ecological environment, villagers are deprived of their future, and later generations of the right to development. Unfortunately, however, short-term interests still play the leading role in decision-making in the consciousness of most villagers.

4.2.3. Influence of Guanxi Networks on the Cost and Benefit Sharing of Different Groups

As can been seen in the above analysis, pig farmers do not bear the costs of environmental governance caused by pollution, but often cause innocent farmers to bear more of these costs. The crux of the matter lies in that the pig farmers and farmers are very different in terms of the guanxi networks they can draw on to pursue their interests. As a result, the rich have become richer and the poor have become poorer, and for village S, inequalities in rural environmental governance have worsened.

Specifically, pig farmers transfer the costs of pollution by taking advantage of their relatively strong guanxi networks; in this way, they minimize their direct losses from pollution. If the waste water was to be discharged according to the official standard, they would have to pay for the treatment costs, and their net profits would be greatly reduced. In the case of a sudden decrease in pork prices, they might suffer a loss. Pig farmers, therefore, do everything they can to avoid bearing increased environmental costs (for example, giving township government officials gifts, and performing small favors for the victim group at the Spring Festival and other festivals), and even ingeniously transfer the costs of pollution control to the public. These actions have led to serious negative externalities. Moreover, pig farmers also avoid indirect losses, such as exposure to environmental pollution, by migrating elsewhere in the region. In S village, large-scale pig farmers often damage the environment more seriously, but they have more economic strength, and therefore greater ability to cope with supervision. They have not engaged in raising pigs themselves for a long time and they no longer live in the village. For example, in recent years, some pig farmers have purchased housing in cities in the district or prefecture that have a better environment, thereby avoiding the impact of pollution on their daily lives; this behavior has contributed to a rapid rise in house prices in the local prefecture and district. Pig farmers are therefore not exposed to the negative effects of pollution on their health.

Farmers bear more pollution costs because of their weak guanxi networks. On the one hand, this discourages them to protest or fight back, as they feel nobody would listen to them or support them. They take it for granted that those rich pig farmers have the power to monopolize the right to speak and suppress others. Further, farmers sometimes seek help from pig farmers, such as borrowing money for emergencies or receiving occasional petty favors; these victims can be seen as the "silent majority". On the other hand, due to their poor financial conditions and weak guanxi network, farmers are rarely able to move to cities to avoid the environmental risks. Thus, they have to stay in the village and bear the costs of environmental governance, hoping that ecological remediation may eventually be possible.

In conclusion, different groups in S village share the costs and benefits of pollution related to pig farming in very unequal ways, and this result is mainly due to different groups' guanxi networks. The wealth of pig farmers ultimately originates from the conversion of natural and social resources. Compared with farmers, pig farmers have stronger guanxi networks, receive more environmental benefits, and generate greater environmental pressure. In the face of pollution control, pig farmers transfer the costs of pollution by taking advantage of their relatively strong guanxi networks, who have mastered the community's right to control the relationship between individuals. These strong guanxi networks serve the maximum demand of the interests of pig farmers, but play a negative role in rural environmental governance. A study by Du et al. [2,10] agreed that the guanxi network is the third resource allocation method in rural China, in addition to government and market allocation.

Under the influence of this warped guanxi network, rural environmental governance suffers a double loss: the environment is not governed, and the economic growth is not sustainable. For pig farmers and farmers, both have suffered losses: the environment continues to deteriorate, leading to stricter government supervision and governance measures; finally, more stringent cultured control measures will be adopted to shut down pig farms. In March 2017, the pig farms were forcibly demolished by the local government. The case of rural environmental governance in S village, our results show that the guanxi network-led bottom-up governance and government-led top-down governance still need to find a valid combination path to further promote efficient and sustainable rural environmental governance.

5. Discussion

Previous studies found that Guanxi has a significant influence on environmental governance, but the conclusions are different [47]. Some researchers believe that high level social capital have a significant and negative impact on environmental pollution [48–50], while other studies draw opposite conclusions [13,51,52]. Specifically, the social capital plays a role through the impact on environmental behavior [53]. In the present study, we found that pig breeding enhanced the guanxi network of pig farmers, which directly led to the gradual deterioration of rural environmental pollution. This finding supports the conclusion that guanxi is not conducive to promote rural environmental protection. The polluter-pays principle is difficult to implement in rural pig breeding China because of pig farmer guanxi networks [54].

Different guanxi networks affect the way in which the costs and benefits of pollution control are shared. As a result, the rich have become richer and the poor have become poorer, and environmental inequalities have worsened [55,56]. The relevant literature showed that stronger social relation networks may lead to stronger willingness to protect the environment [57]. However, it has actually a precondition that the social norms are strong [53,58,59]. Because of the lack of social norms, pig farmers accrue economic advantage by massively transferring environmental costs and become "wealthy perpetrators" while farmers that are forced to bear serious pollution and costs becoming "poor victims".

This study reflects on the nature and strength of the dyadic personal relationships and networks that are at the heart of Chinese rural culture, and the extent to which they could offer a new way of thinking about rural policy more generally. As this suggests, the role of guanxi and other informal institutions must not be ignored in rural environmental governance. In the changes and differentiation of guanxi in the current rural areas, we should pay more attention on local characteristics and even adopt uniform, institutionalized measures to address the rural environment, such as environmental regulation and ecological remediation policies, which have been proposed to address these issues. Besides, guanxi networks lead to costs and benefits being shared among different groups, which, in turn, leads to environmental inequities. Farmers, as the environmentally vulnerable groups, should be should be targeted by government policies.

In concluding, therefore, this paper offers new insights to an extant literature on global rural change. At its core, the issue is that not only is traditional class habitus and place identity declining in rural areas, but that it is being replaced by new, plural forms of network and association that challenge not only local cultures, but also the institutions that have provided stable governance. This is a significant finding given the governance of pollution from pig farming and others, in China and elsewhere, that often drive rural environmental issues through top-down governance and control regulations. At a time when rural society in China is being transformed, we should recognize the influence of guanxi networks on the sharing of costs and benefits of control of pollution from pig farming, and which have some effect on rural environmental equalities. As rural society develops, along with improvements in institutional frameworks, guanxi networks should come to play a weaker role in rural environmental governance. In this situation, institutions will need to play a role in reducing the environmental inequalities induced by different guanxi networks.

In present study, we wanted to discover the changing of guanxi networks and the impact on the sharing of costs and benefits through a long period of observation, and the rural environmental inequality by pig farming pollution. The qualitative method enabled extensive insights into these issues—why the guanxi networks have changed, why the government treatment did not take effect, and why the farmers did organize and collectively do something.

However, the study has some limitations. First, the long-term observations at the village, in-depth interviews, and questionnaire surveys in this study were only conducted in S village, and thus the transferability of the results to other areas may be limited due to complex guanxi networks. Second, the study only considered the guanxi network of pig farmers and farmers, and other guanxi networks were ignored. Third, due to environmental cost, depreciation costs of pig houses are difficult to measure precisely, and we did not pay much attention to the precise measurement of cost benefits. Additional research is necessary and should use quantitative or experimental research methods to assess the cost and benefit of rural environment pollution governance through the perspective of guanxi networks.

6. Conclusions

In the quick transformation period in rural China, pollution from livestock and poultry breeding is not a simple environmental or economic problem. Guanxi plays an important role in the rural environmental pollution governance. Pig farming shaped the nature of guanxi in different groups. For the pig farmers, their guanxi networks are growing, while the farmers' guanxi networks are shrinking. The different guanxi networks have an impact on the effectiveness of rural environmental pollution governance, and affect the way in which the costs and benefits of pollution control are shared; the rich have become richer and the poor have become poorer, and environmental inequalities have worsened. At a time when rural society in China is being transformed, we should recognize the influence of guanxi networks on the sharing of costs and benefits of controlling pollution related to pig farming, which and have some effect on rural environmental inequalities.

Author Contributions: Conceptualization, P.L.; data curation, L.Z.; investigation, S.S.; methodology, L.Z.; writing—original draft, Y.D.; writing—review & editing, L.Z. All authors have read and agreed to the published version of the manuscript.

Funding: This research was funded by the Shenzhen Philosophy and Social Science Planning Project (SZ2021A003).

Institutional Review Board Statement: All interviewees agreed with and understood the main idea of this study, the data were recorded and collected under anonymity or provided willingly, and the interviewees all agreed to cooperate in the provision of relevant data. Therefore, the research design and data collection process complied with ethical standards, and there was no need to apply for ethical certification.

Informed Consent Statement: Informed consent was obtained from all subjects involved in the study.

Data Availability Statement: Data sharing is not applicable.

Conflicts of Interest: The authors declare no conflict of interest.

References

1. Jin, S.; Bluemling, B.; Mol, A.P. Mitigating land pollution through pesticide packages—The case of a collection scheme in Rural China. *Sci. Total Environ.* **2018**, *622*, 502–509. [CrossRef] [PubMed]
2. Liu, P.; Qi, S.; Li, D.; Rayenscroft, N. Promoting agricultural innovation as a means of improving China's rural environment. *J. Environ. Manag.* **2021**, *280*, 1–9. [CrossRef] [PubMed]
3. Xie, L.; Flynn, A.; Tan-Mullins, M.; Cheshmehzangi, A. Water and land: Environmental governance and Chinese eco-development. *J. Clean. Prod.* **2019**, *221*, 839–853. [CrossRef]
4. He, C.; Chen, T.; Mao, X.; Zhou, Y. Economic transition, urbanization and population redistribution in China. *Habitat Int.* **2016**, *51*, 39–47. [CrossRef]
5. Gatto, A.; Polselli, N.; Bloom, G. Empowering gender equality through rural development: Rural markets and micro-finance in Kyrgyzstan. *L'Europa Comunità Internazionale Difronte Alle Sfide Dello Svilupp.* **2016**, 65–89.

6. Morrow, N.; Mock, N.B.; Gatto, A.; LeMense, J.; Hudson, M. Protective Pathways: Connecting Environmental and Human Security at Local and Landscape Level with NLP and Geospatial Analysis of a Novel Database of 1500 Project Evaluations. *Land* **2022**, *11*, 123. [CrossRef]
7. Agovino, M.; Cerciello, M.; Gatto, A. Policy efficiency in the field of food sustainability. The adjusted food agriculture and nutrition index. *J. Environ. Manag.* **2018**, *218*, 220–233. [CrossRef]
8. Wang, C.; Woods, M. The role of guanxi in rural social movements: Two case studies from Taiwan. *J. Agrar. Change* **2013**, *13*, 197–212. [CrossRef]
9. King, B.; Fielke, S.; Bayne, K.; Klerkx, L.; Nettle, R. Navigating shades of social capital and trust to leverage opportunities for rural innovation. *J. Rural Stud.* **2019**, *68*, 123–134. [CrossRef]
10. Grootaert, C. Social capital, household welfare and poverty in Indonesia. *Policy Res. Work. Pap. Ser.* **1999**, *11*, 4–38.
11. Morduch, J.; Sicular, T. Politics, growth and inequality in rural China: Does it pay to join the party? *Harv. Inst. Econ. Res. Work. Pap.* **1998**, *77*, 331–356. [CrossRef]
12. Swanson, K.E.; Kuhn, R.G.; Xu, W. Environmental Policy Implementation in Rural China: A Case Study of Yuhang, Zhejiang. *Environ. Manag.* **2001**, *27*, 481–491. [CrossRef] [PubMed]
13. Du, Y.; Liu, P.; Ravenscroft, N.; Su, S. Changing community relations in southeast China: The role of Guanxi in rural environmental governance. *Agric. Hum. Values* **2020**, *37*, 833–847. [CrossRef]
14. Zhang, N. The impact of guanxi networks on the employment relations of rural migrant women in contemporary China. *Ind. Relat. J.* **2011**, *42*, 580–595. [CrossRef]
15. Cecchi, C. Public Goods and Public Services—The Process of Building Social Capital in Rural Areas. 2003. Available online: SSRN:https://ssrn.com/abstract=941196 (accessed on 10 January 2021).
16. Fan, Y. Questioning guanxi: Definition, classification and implications. *Int. Bus. Rev.* **2002**, *11*, 543–561. [CrossRef]
17. Xin, K.R.; Pearce, J.L. Guanxi: Connections as substitutes for formal institutional support. *Acad. Manag. J.* **1996**, *39*, 1641–1658.
18. Chen, X. A phenomenological explication of guanxi in rural tourism management: A case study of a village in China. *Tour. Manag.* **2017**, *63*, 383–394. [CrossRef]
19. Peng, Y. Kinship Networks and Entrepreneurs in China's Transitional Economy. *Am. J. Sociol.* **2004**, *109*, 1045–1074. [CrossRef]
20. Tsang, E.W.K. Can guanxi be a source of sustained competitive advantage for doing business in China? *Acad. Manag. Exec.* **1998**, *12*, 64–74. [CrossRef]
21. Taormina, R.J.; Gao, J.H. A research model for Guanxi behavior: Antecedents, measures, and outcomes of Chinese social networking. *Soc. Sci. Res.* **2010**, *39*, 1195–1212. [CrossRef]
22. Arias, J.T.G. A relationship marketing approach to guanxi. *Eur. J. Mark.* **1998**, *32*, 145–156. [CrossRef]
23. Xie, L.; Mol, A.P.J. The role of guanxi in the emerging environmental movement in China. *Community Ecol. Dyn. Place Sustain. Politics* **2006**, *10*, 269–292.
24. Yang, Z.; Cheng, L.W. Guanxi as a governance mechanism in business markets: Its characteristics, relevant theories, and future research directions. *Ind. Mark. Manag.* **2011**, *40*, 492–495. [CrossRef]
25. Gezelius, S.S. Exchange and Social Structure in Norwegian Agricultural Communities: How Farmers Acquire Labour and Capital. *Sociol. Rural.* **2014**, *54*, 206–226. [CrossRef]
26. Bian, Y. Bringing Strong Ties Back in: Indirect Ties, Network Bridges, and Job Searches in China. *Am. Sociol. Rev.* **1997**, *62*, 366. [CrossRef]
27. Knight, J.; Yueh, L. The role of social capital in the labour market in China. *Econ. Transit.* **2010**, *16*, 389–414. [CrossRef]
28. LaPalombara, J.; Putnam, R.D. Making Democracy Work: Civic Traditions in Modern Italy. *Contemp. Sociol.* **1994**, *26*, 306–308. [CrossRef]
29. Bhandari, P.B. Rural livelihood change? Household capital, community resources and livelihood transition. *J. Rural Stud.* **2013**, *32*, 126–136. [CrossRef]
30. Yu, H.; Deng, Y.; Lu, Z.N.; Hao, C. Is environmental regulation effective in China? Evidence from city-level panel data. *J. Clean. Prod.* **2018**, *188*, 966–976.
31. Tang, S.Y.; Lo, W.H.; Fryxell, G.E. Governance reform, external support, and environmental regulation enforcement in rural China: The case of Guangdong province. *J. Environ. Manag.* **2010**, *91*, 2008–2018. [CrossRef]
32. Liu, P.; Zhao, Y.; Ravenscroft, N.; Harder, M.K. Responsibility-driven collective action in the context of rapid rural depopulation. *J. Rural Stud.* **2020**, *75*, 48–56. [CrossRef]
33. Lo, K. How authoritarian is the environmental governance of China? *Environ. Sci. Policy* **2015**, *54*, 152–159. [CrossRef]
34. Zhang, X. Implementation of Pollution Control Targets in China: Has a Centralized Enforcement Approach Worked? *China Q.* **2017**, *231*, 749–774. [CrossRef]
35. Hodge, I. Beyond agri-environmental policy: Towards an alternative model of rural environmental governance. *Land Use Policy* **2001**, *18*, 99–111. [CrossRef]
36. North, D.C. *Institutions, Institutional Change and Economic Performance*; Cambridge University Press: Cambridge, UK, 1990.
37. Prager, K.; Nienaber, B.; Neumann, B.; Phillips, A. How should rural policy be evaluated if it aims to foster community involvement in environmental management? *J. Rural. Stud.* **2015**, *37*, 120–131. [CrossRef]
38. Liu, P.; Rayenscroft, N. Collective action in implementing top-down land policy: The case of Chengdu, China. *Land Use Policy* **2017**, *65*, 45–52. [CrossRef]

39. Zhang, X.; Li, G. Does guanxi matter to nonfarm employment? *J. Comp. Econ.* **2003**, *31*, 315–331. [CrossRef]
40. Clarkson, P.M.; Li, Y.; Richardson, G.D.; Vasvari, F.P. Revisiting the relation between environmental performance and environmental disclosure: An empirical analysis. *Account. Organ. Soc.* **2008**, *33*, 303–327. [CrossRef]
41. Xu, Y.; Huang, X.; Bao, H.X.H.; Ju, X.; Zhong, T.; Chen, Z.; Zhou, Y. Rural land rights reform and agro-environmental sustainability: Empirical evidence from China. *Land Use Policy* **2018**, *74*, 73–87. [CrossRef]
42. Pellow, D.N. Environmental justice and rural studies: A critical conversation and invitation to collaboration. *J. Rural Stud.* **2016**, *47*, 381–386. [CrossRef]
43. Hanson, L.L. Environmental Justice across the Rural Canadian Prairies: Agricultural Restructuring, Seed Production and the Farm Crisis. *Local Environ.* **2007**, *12*, 599–611. [CrossRef]
44. Mullin, K.; Mitchell, G.; Nawaz, N.R.; Waters, R.D. Natural capital and the poor in England: Towards an environmental justice analysis of ecosystem services in a high income country. *Landsc. Urban Plan.* **2018**, *176*, 10–21. [CrossRef]
45. Brulle, R.J.; Pellow, D.N. ENVIRONMENTAL JUSTICE: Human Health and Environmental Inequalities. *Annu. Rev. Public Health* **2006**, *27*, 103–124. [CrossRef] [PubMed]
46. Bento, A.; Freedman, M.; Lang, C. Who Benefits from Environmental Regulation? Evidence from the Clean Air Act Amendments. *Rev. Econ. Stat.* **2015**, *97*, 610–622. [CrossRef]
47. Wang, Y.; Xiong, J.; Li, W.; Na, M.; Yao, M. The Effect of Social Capital on Environmental Pollution in China—Suppression or Promotion? *Int. J. Environ. Res. Public Health* **2020**, *17*, 9459. [CrossRef]
48. Ibrahim, M.; Law, S.H. Social capital and CO2 emission—output relations: A panel analysis. *Renew. Sustain. Energy Rev.* **2014**, *29*, 528–534. [CrossRef]
49. Marbuah, G.; Gren, I.-M.; Tirkaso, W.T. Social capital, economic development and carbon emissions: Empirical evidence from counties in Sweden. *Renew. Sustain. Energy Rev.* **2021**, *152*, 111691. [CrossRef]
50. Zhou, D.; Liu, T.; Wang, Q. How Social Capital Affects Environmental Performance in China. *Front. Energy Res.* **2020**, *7*. [CrossRef]
51. Du, Y.Q.; Liu, P.Y.; Bao, C.K.; Su, S.P. A Study on the rural environmental governance through the lens of social capital—A case of livestock farming pollution in the undeveloped region. *J. Public Manag.* **2016**, *13*, 101–112.
52. Jianxiang, W.; Shanshan, W. Can Social Capital Promote the Growth of Environmental Total Factor Productivity in China? *Manag. Rev.* **2019**, *31*, 15.
53. Farrow, K.; Grolleau, G.; Ibanez, L. Social Norms and Pro-environmental Behavior: A Review of the Evidence. *Ecol. Econ.* **2017**, *140*, 1–13. [CrossRef]
54. Zheng, H.; Chen, S.; Sun, X.; Su, S. Why polluter-pays principle is difficult to implement in rural areas?—A case study of pig-farmer paying behavior under the third party governance of pig-farming pollution in Nanping. *Zhongguo Shengtai Nongye Xuebao/Chin. J. Eco-Agric.* **2017**, *25*, 1081–1089.
55. Himley, M. Geographies of Environmental Governance: The Nexus of Nature and Neoliberalism. *Geogr. Compass* **2008**, *2*, 433–451. [CrossRef]
56. Pulido, L. Rethinking Environmental Racism: White Privilege and Urban Development in Southern California. *Ann. Assoc. Am. Geogr.* **2000**, *90*, 12–40. [CrossRef]
57. Jones, N. Investigating the influence of social costs and benefits of environmental policies through social capital theory. *Policy Sci.* **2010**, *43*, 229–244. [CrossRef]
58. Polyzou, E.; Jones, N.; Evangelinos, K.; Halvadakis, C. Willingness to pay for drinking water quality improvement and the influence of social capital. *J. Socio-Econ.* **2011**, *40*, 74–80. [CrossRef]
59. Nyborg, K.; Anderies, J.M.; Dannenberg, A.; Lindahl, T.; Schill, C.; Schluter, M.; Adger, W.N.; Arrow, K.J.; Barrett, S.; Carpenter, S.; et al. Social norms as solutions. *Science* **2016**, *354*, 42–43. [CrossRef]

International Journal of
Environmental Research and Public Health

MDPI

Article

The Impact of Coordinated Development of Ecological Environment and Technological Innovation on Green Economy: Evidence from China

Lining Su

School of Management, Anhui University, Hefei 230601, China; sulining@vip.163.com; Tel.: +86-138-6678-6803

Abstract: Promoting the coordinated development of ecological environment and technological innovation is significant to the development of a green economy. In this study, we construct an index system of ecological environment, technological innovation, and green economy based on the panel data of 30 provinces and cities in China from 2005 to 2016, using the entropy weight method, the coupling coordination model, and the panel vector autoregressive model (PVAR) to calculate the comprehensive development levels of ecological environment, technological innovation, and green economy and the coordination degree between ecological environment and technological innovation, and then further explore the impact of the coordinated development level of ecological environment and technological innovation on the development of a green economy. The research results include: First, from 2005 to 2016, the comprehensive development levels of ecological environment, technological innovation, and green economy in China's 30 provinces and cities achieved different degrees of improvement as a whole. Among them, the comprehensive development level of green economy was the highest, followed by the development level of technological innovation, and the comprehensive development level of ecological environment was the lowest. Second, from 2005 to 2016, the coordination degree between ecological environment and technological innovation in China's provinces and cities increased year by year, but on the whole, the coordination degree between ecological environment and technological innovation in various regions was in a state of imbalance. Third, there was a long-term equilibrium relationship among the coordinated development levels of ecological environment, technological innovation, and green economy. Fourth, through pulse analysis and Monte Carlo simulation, we found that the coordinated development level of ecological environment and technological innovation had a lagging positive impact on green economy. Finally, we provide a summary of the results of this study.

Keywords: ecological environment; technological innovation; coupling coordination; green economy

Citation: Su, L. The Impact of Coordinated Development of Ecological Environment and Technological Innovation on Green Economy: Evidence from China. *IJERPH* **2022**, *19*, 6994. https://doi.org/10.3390/ijerph19126994

Academic Editors: Jie Chen, Qian Zhou and Ting Zhang

Received: 27 April 2022
Accepted: 1 June 2022
Published: 7 June 2022

1. Introduction

Since the reform and opening up in 1978, China's economy has grown rapidly with China becoming the largest developing country; China's GDP exceeded 100 trillion yuan in 2020, second only to the United States in overall economic strength [1]. However, during the process of economic development, a serious environmental crisis has appeared in China in recent years; according to statistics, economic losses caused by environmental pollution account for 2–3% of the gross domestic product (GDP) every year. In addition, China's economic growth rate is facing increasing downward pressure. In order to cope with the environmental crisis and enhance the power of economic development, China proposes to vigorously develop green economy (GE) and technological innovation (TI), in order to achieve sustainable economic and social development through vigorously developing a green economy and scientific and technological innovations. Technological innovation is the driving force for high-quality development of a green economy [2], and an ecological environment (EE) is an important guarantee for high-quality development of a green economy [3]. Protecting an ecological environment and promoting technological innovation play important driving roles in developing a green economy. However, it is still unclear how the coordination degree between ecological environment and technological innovation affect a green economy. Analyzing the impact of the coordination level between ecological environment and technological innovation on green economy is of practical significance for China's high-quality development. In this study, we evaluate the comprehensive development levels of ecological environment, technology innovation, and green economy, and then evaluate the coordination degree between ecological environment and technological innovation and analysis the impact of coordination level between ecological environment and technological innovation on green economy. Finally, based on the research findings, we provide some policy suggestions.

The arrangement of this paper is as follows: First, we identify and describe the related research by searched and reading the literature related to the relationships among ecological environment, technological innovation, and green economy from the Web of Science database. Then, we introduce the research methods and data sources; explain the entropy method, the coupling coordination model, and the PVAR model; and design an index system of environmental, technology innovation, and green economy. Next, we display and discuss the results, which include assessing thecomprehensive development levels of environment, technological innovation and green economy; assessing the coordination degree between environment and technological innovation; and analyzing the impact of the coordination level between environment and technological innovation on green economy. Finally, we summarize the research findings.

2. Literature Review

At present, there are many studies on the relationship between ecological environment and economic development. Among them, Shi et al. (2019) measured and analyzed the coupling coordination and spatio-temporal heterogeneity of economic development and ecological environment in 17 tropical and subtropical regions from 2003 to 2016 by using a geographical and time weighted regression (GTWR) method, and found that there was significant spatio-temporal heterogeneity between economic development and ecological environment with most regions belonging to the economic lag type [4]. Zhu et al. (2021) took Guangdong Province of China as an example, and established a model of the coordination degree between ecological environment and economic development, then analyzed the coordination degree between ecological environment and economic development in Guangdong Province. They found that the coordination degree showed an increasingly high trend, which indicated that with the rapid economic development of Guangdong Province, more and more attention had been paid to environmental protection [5]. In addition, some scholars have used an improved entropy weight method to calculate the coupling and coordinated development of high-quality economic development and ecological environment in the Yellow River Basin of China from 2008 to 2018, and found that high-quality economic development, ecological environment quality, and their coupling and coordination level in the Yellow River Basin showed different degrees of improvement [6].

Regarding the relationship between technological innovation and economy, as early as the last century, some scholars had proven the role of technological innovation in promoting economic growth through research [7]. Later, scholars studied the specific impact of technological innovation on economic development. Among them, Liu, C. (2016) suggested that technological innovation was an important driving force for a country's sustainable economic development and social progress, and technological innovation could be achieved through R&D investment, thereby achieving sustainable economic growth [8]. Wang et al. (2020) found that technological innovation could drive the transformation of the economic development mode, and economic development provided financial support for technological innovation, which showed coordination [9]. Some scholars have proposed to use technological innovation to promote the development of agricultural economy, and have pointed out that it was necessary to promote the role of technological innovation in the transformation of agricultural economic development from various aspects such as policy, investment, organizational construction, and the creation of an entrepreneurial environment [10].

Regarding the relationship between ecological environment and technological innovation, research on the relationship between them is also relatively early. For example, Frank (1997) and others proved that technology research was helpful to protect the ecological environment and put forward the concept of "ecological innovation" [11]. Chen (2010) and others explored the impact of technological innovation efficiency on the ecological environment by constructing a technological innovation index system and using data envelopment analysis (DEA) [12]. From the perspective of input and output, other scholars have used collected panel data to evaluate the green technology level and environmental governance performance of provincial enterprises in Anhui Province from multiple dimensions [13]. In addition, regarding the relationships among ecological environment, technological innovation, and green economy, most studies have focused on measuring the relationship between two of the three [14,15], while there are few studies on the relationships among the three. Among them, Zhao et al. (2021) used an entropy weight method, coupling coordination model, and gravity model to study the spatio-temporal coupling coordination relationship and spatio-temporal characteristics of the economy, energy, and ecological environment in the Yellow River Basin of China [16].

After reviewing the literature, we found that existing studies have mainly focused on analyzing the relationships between ecological environment and technological innovation, between ecological environment and economic development, as well as between technological innovation and economic development. Few studies in the literature have analyzed the relationships among ecological environment, technological innovation, and economic development together. Therefore, based on the panel data of 30 provinces and cities in China from 2005 to 2016, in this study, we construct an index system of ecological environment, technological innovation, and green economy by using the entropy weight method, a coupling coordination model, and a PVAR model to explore the impact of the coordinated development level of ecological environment and technological innovation on green economy, and finally put forward policy suggestions according to the research findings.

3. Research Methods and Data Sources

The purpose of this study is to analyze the impact of coordinated development of ecological environment and technological innovation on green economy. The research design mainly consisted of two parts. In the first part, we measure the level of coordinated development between ecological environment and technological innovation. In the second part, based on the calculation results of the coordination level of ecological environment and technological innovation, we analyze the impact of their coordination level on green economy. However, before the above analysis, it is necessary to evaluate the comprehensive development levels of ecological environment, technological innovation, and green economy separately. Therefore, the specific research design included three parts: First, it is necessary to evaluate the comprehensive development levels of ecological environment, technological innovation, and green economy. Then, the coordination level of ecological environment and technological innovation needs to be calculated. Finally, the impact of the coordination level between ecological environment and technological innovation on green economy is analyzed.

3.1. Index System for Ecological Environment, Technological Innovation, and Green Economy

Comprehensive development level is a description of the development state of a thing. At present, to evaluate the comprehensive development levels of ecological environment, technological innovation, and green economy, scholars have either used a single index to measure, or they have designed an index system, and then used factor analysis, the analytic hierarchy process, and other methods to calculate the data in the index system, and finally, evaluated the development levels of ecological environment, technological innovation, and green economy. In this study, an index system is designed to evaluate the comprehensive development levels of ecological environment, technological innovation, and green economy. This is mainly because an index system can comprehensively investigate the state of ecological environment, technological innovation, and green economy.

In terms of ecological environment, referring to the existing studies [17,18], in this study, we decompose the ecological environment into three first-level indicators: environmental pollution generation, environmental pollution control, and natural environment foundation. We build eleven secondary-level indicators, which include industrial solid waste generation (ten thousand tons), total wastewater discharge (ten thousand tons), total sulfur dioxide discharge (ten thousand tons), industrial solid waste investment (100 million yuan), industrial wastewater treatment investment (100 million yuan), wetland area (ten thousand hm^2), and forest coverage (%), etc. (see Table 2). In terms of technological innovation, based on the existing research [19–21], we divide technological innovation into three first-level indicators, which include investment in scientific and technological innovation, the output of technological innovation, and technological innovation effectiveness, and secondary-level indicators which include the proportion of enterprises that include Research and Experimental Development (R&D) institutions (%), the full-time equivalent of ten thousand R&D personnel, the number of scientific papers (article), the number of patent authorizations (items), the sales revenue of new products (ten thousand yuan) and the export value of high-tech products (100 million yuan), etc. (see Table 2). In terms of green economy, based on existing studies [22,23], we divide economic growth into three first-level indicators, which include economic growth scale, economic growth structure, and economic growth benefits [22,23]. Based on first-level indicators, we build thirteen secondary-level indicators, including GDP (100 million yuan), industrial production value (100 million yuan), tertiary industry added value as a percentage of GDP (%), retail sales of consumer goods per capita (yuan), income gap (yuan), urbanization rate (%), etc. (see Table 1).

Table 1. Index system for EE, TI, and GE.

Total System	First Indicator	Secondary Indicator
Ecological environment	Environmental pollution generation	Industrial solid waste generation (ten thousand tons), total wastewater discharge (ten thousand tons), total sulfur dioxide discharge (ten thousand tons)
	Environmental pollution control	Completion of investment in forestry fixed assets (100 million yuan), investment in industrial waste gas treatment (100 million yuan), industrial solid waste investment (100 million yuan), industrial wastewater treatment investment (100 million yuan)
	Natural environment foundation	Wetland area (ten thousand hm^2), area of nature reserve (thousand hm^2), total groundwater resources (a hundred million m^3), forest coverage (%)
Technological innovation	Technological innovation investment	The full-time equivalent of R&D personnel per 10,000 people, the proportion of R&D expenditure in GDP (%), the proportion of enterprises with R&D institutions (%), the proportion of R&D expenditure in main business income (%)
	Scientific and technological innovation output	Number of scientific papers (article), number of patents (items), technology market turnover (100 million yuan)
	Scientific and technological innovation effectiveness	Sales revenue of new products (ten thousand yuan), export value of high-tech products (100 million yuan), energy consumption per unit GDP (ton of standard coal/ten thousand yuan), labor productivity (ten thousand yuan/person)

Table 1. *Cont.*

Total System	First Indicator	Secondary Indicator
Economic growth	Economic growth scale	GDP (100 million yuan), industrial production value (100 million yuan), social fixed asset investment (100 million yuan), financial development level, fiscal revenue (ten thousand yuan)
	Economic growth structure	The proportion of the added value of the tertiary industry in GDP (%), the proportion of the added value of the secondary industry in GDP (%), and the retail sales of consumer goods per capita (yuan)
	Economic growth benefits	Per capita GDP (yuan), income gap (Yuan), urbanization rate (%), kilometer density (km/10,000 square meters), total savings of urban and rural residents (100 million yuan),per capita GDP (yuan), income gap (Yuan), urbanization rate (%), kilometer density (km/10,000 square meters), total savings of urban and rural residents (100 million yuan)

3.2. Comprehensive Evaluation of Ecological Environment, Technological Innovation, and Green Economy

In this study, it is necessary to comprehensively evaluate the comprehensive development levels of ecological environment, technological innovation, and green economy. We chose the entropy method to evaluate the comprehensive development levels of environment, technological innovation, and green economy. The purpose of the entropy method is to objectively determine the weight of indicators through the dispersion degree of indicators in the samples. Generally speaking, the smaller the information entropy of an indicator is, the higher the degree of aggregation of the indicator, and the greater the role of the indicator on behalf of the whole indicator system. Therefore, the weight of the indicator is also higher. The specific process is as follows:

First, the original data need to be standardized to eliminate the impact of different measurement units and dimensions on the indicators. The calculation formulas are as follows:

$$\text{Positive indicator}: \ y_{kij} = \frac{x_{ij} - \min(x_{ij})}{\max(x_{ij}) - \min(x_{ij})} \tag{1}$$

$$\text{Negative indicator}: \ y_{kij} = \frac{\max(x_{ij}) - x_{ij}}{\max(x_{ij}) - \min(x_{ij})} \tag{2}$$

where x_{ij} represents sample value; max $(_{kij})$ and min (x_{ij}), respectively, represent maximum and minimum values in the sample data.

Second, the entropy method in the objective weighting method is used to calculate the weight of each index as follows:

$$p_{kij} = \frac{y_{ij}}{\sum_{i=1}^{m} y_{ij}} \ ; \ e_{kj} = \left[-\frac{1}{ln(m)}\right] \sum_{i=1}^{m} p_{ij} ln p_{ij} \tag{3}$$

$$w_j = (1 - e_i) / \sum_{i=1}^{m} (1 - e_i) \tag{4}$$

Finally, the comprehensive development levels of ecological environment (U_E), technological innovation (U_T), and green economy (U_G) are calculated. The specific calculation formulas are as follows:

$$U = \sum_{i=1}^{m} w_{ij} y_{ij} \ ; \ \sum_{i=1}^{m} w_{ij} = 1 \tag{5}$$

3.3. *Coupling Coordination Model*

Coupling originally comes from physics and refers to the interaction between two or more objects. At present, the coupling coordination degree model is widely used to analyze the coordination development level between different systems [24]. In this research, we analyze the coordinated development correlation between ecological environment and technological innovation through the coupling coordination model. The specific calculation formulas are as follows:

$$C = 2\sqrt{\frac{U_E \times U_T}{(U_E + U_T)^2}}, C \in [0,\ 1] \tag{6}$$

$$T = \alpha U_E + \beta U_T, \alpha + \beta = 1 \tag{7}$$

$$D = \sqrt{C \times T}, D \in [0,\ 1] \tag{8}$$

In Equation (6), U_E is ecological environment, U_T is technological innovation, and C is system coupling degree which can reflect consistent development between ecological environment and technological innovation. The larger C is, the higher the coupling and the better the synergy effect between ecological environment and technological innovation. When $C = 0$, the coupling degree between ecological environment and technological innovation reaches its lowest, indicating that the two systems are independent. When $C = 1$, the coupling degree between ecological environment and technological innovation reaches its peak, which shows that the two systems are in an orderly development state. However, a higher coupling degree can also be obtained when ecological environment and technological innovation are at a low level. Therefore, the coordination degree model is established based on the coupling degree model to explore the coordinated development level between ecological environment and technological innovation, as shown in Equations (7) and (8).

In Equations (7) and (8), T denotes a comprehensive evaluation index that can reflect the overall synergistic effect of ecological environment and technological innovation. It also reflects the impact of comprehensive development level on cooperative dispatching, which are undetermined coefficients. In this study, we assumed $\alpha = \beta = 0.5$; D is coordination degree. The greater the value of D, the higher the degree of coordination between ecological environment and technological innovation, and the better coordinated development level of the two systems.

In this study, we divide the coordinated development level of ecological environment and technological innovation by referring to the research of previous scholars [25,26] (see Table 2).

Table 2. Classification of coordination degree.

Stage	Antagonistic Stage				Run-In Stage				Coordination Stage	
Coordination degree	$0 \le D < 0.4$				$0.4 \le D < 0.8$				$0.8 \le D < 1.0$	
D	$0 \le D < 0.1$	$0 \le D < 0.2$	$0.2 \le D < 0.3$	$0.3 \le D < 0.4$	$0.4 \le D < 0.5$	$0.5 \le D < 0.6$	$0.6 \le D < 0.7$	$0.7 \le D < 0.8$	$0.8 \le D < 0.9$	$0.9 \le D \le 1.0$
Classification	Extreme imbalance	Serious disorder	Moderate Disorder	Mild disorder	On the verge of maladjustment	Barely coordinated	Primary coordination	Intermediate-coordination	Good coordination	Quality coordination

3.4. *Panel Vector Autoregressive Model*

Sims (1980) established a single dimensional vector autoregressive model (VAR) to describe the impact of variables on a specific variable [27]. A characteristic of this model is that all variables are regarded as endogenous variables, that is, each endogenous variable is taken as a function of the lag value of all endogenous variables in the system to construct the model, and therefore, truly reflects the interaction between each variable. However, the VAR model does not support panel data. Therefore, later, Holtz Eakin, Newey, and Rosen (1988) extended it to panel data structure (PVAR) [28]. PVAR considers the individual and time fixed effects, increases the precision of estimation, and any and no presuppositions are made about the relationship among variables. In particular, no assumptions are made about the direction of mutual causation among variables. Therefore, in this study, we used the PAVR model to analyze the impact of the coordination level between ecological environment and technological innovation on green economy [29]. The PVAR model is as follow:

$$Y_{it} = \beta_0 + \alpha_i + \sum_{j=1}^{p} \beta_j Y_{t-j} + \varepsilon_{it} \ (i = 1, 2, 3, \ldots\ldots, 30\ ,\ t = 1, 2, 3 \ldots\ldots, 12) \quad (9)$$

where i represents province; t represents year; Y_{it} includes two column vectors, namely coordinated development level (*CO*) between ecological environment and technological innovation and green economy (*EC*); β_0 represents intercept term; p represents lag order, β_j represents parameter matrix of lag j order; α_i represents variable of individual fixed effects; and ε_{it} represents random disturbance term.

3.5. Data Sources

The data used in this study were derived from the China Statistical Yearbook (2006–2017) [30], the China Science and Technology Statistical Yearbook (2006–2017) [31], the China High Technology Statistical Yearbook (2006–2017) [32], the China Demographic and Employment Statistical Yearbook (2006–2017), and the China Economic and Social Data Research Platform [33,34]. Some data also came from the website of the National Bureau of Statistics and local statistical bulletins [35].

4. Results

4.1. The Comprehensive Development Levels of Ecological Environment, Technological Innovation, and Green Economy

The comprehensive calculation model is used to calculate the comprehensive development levels of ecological environment, technological innovation, and green economy in 30 provinces and cities. The results are shown in Tables 3–5 and Figure 1.

Table 3. The comprehensive development levels of ecological environment.

Province	2005	2006	2007	2008	2009	2010	2011	2012	2013	2014	2015	2016
Beijing	0.04	0.06	0.06	0.05	0.03	0.02	0.03	0.03	0.07	0.04	0.07	0.07
Tianjin	0.04	0.03	0.03	0.03	0.03	0.02	0.05	0.01	0.04	0.05	0.06	0.03
Hebei	0.14	0.05	0.05	0.06	0.1	0.04	0.05	0.03	0.04	0.05	0.05	0.04
Shanxi	0.08	0.15	0.15	0.18	0.13	0.11	0.08	0.06	0.08	0.04	0.06	0.04
Inner Mongolia	0.09	0.12	0.13	0.13	0.14	0.09	0.11	0.08	0.28	0.18	0.2	0.2
Liaoning	0.06	0.06	0.07	0.06	0.05	0.04	0.03	0.02	0.07	0.05	0.13	0.07
Jilin	0.09	0.07	0.08	0.08	0.08	0.08	0.05	0.03	0.04	0.04	0.06	0.06
Heilongjiang	0.07	0.08	0.11	0.09	0.15	0.11	0.08	0.04	0.14	0.11	0.18	0.17
Shanghai	0.01	0.05	0.01	0.02	0.02	0.01	0.01	0.01	0.02	0.04	0.05	0.1
Jiangsu	0.09	0.08	0.12	0.09	0.08	0.03	0.06	0.04	0.13	0.06	0.14	0.15
Zhejiang	0.04	0.06	0.06	0.05	0.06	0.03	0.03	0.03	0.09	0.1	0.19	0.18
Anhui	0.03	0.04	0.05	0.04	0.04	0.03	0.02	0.02	0.05	0.04	0.07	0.17
Fujian	0.19	0.1	0.05	0.05	0.04	0.04	0.03	0.03	0.08	0.07	0.2	0.19
Jiangxi	0.09	0.08	0.08	0.08	0.13	0.08	0.06	0.03	0.06	0.05	0.11	0.11
Shandong	0.2	0.13	0.14	0.23	0.12	0.1	0.16	0.09	0.06	0.07	0.19	0.16
Henan	0.13	0.09	0.12	0.12	0.05	0.05	0.03	0.01	0.07	0.04	0.07	0.07
Hubei	0.05	0.05	0.06	0.05	0.08	0.06	0.02	0.02	0.06	0.06	0.09	0.32
Hunan	0.11	0.13	0.1	0.1	0.12	0.12	0.08	0.19	0.08	0.07	0.11	0.11
Guangdong	0.15	0.13	0.12	0.08	0.07	0.06	0.05	0.06	0.08	0.07	0.19	0.13
Guangxi	0.08	0.06	0.12	0.1	0.11	0.18	0.14	0.12	0.3	0.32	0.33	0.18
Hainan	0.05	0.06	0.05	0.05	0.07	0.03	0.05	0.02	0.05	0.06	0.06	0.07
Chongqing	0.05	0.04	0.07	0.08	0.06	0.03	0.04	0.01	0.05	0.04	0.08	0.06
Sichuan	0.16	0.15	0.19	0.18	0.2	0.06	0.09	0.05	0.12	0.12	0.17	0.16
Guizhou	0.05	0.09	0.07	0.09	0.07	0.05	0.08	0.02	0.05	0.05	0.07	0.06
Yunnan	0.1	0.11	0.12	0.11	0.07	0.07	0.04	0.03	0.08	0.11	0.14	0.09
Shaanxi	0.04	0.03	0.06	0.04	0.09	0.07	0.07	0.04	0.07	0.05	0.08	0.07
Gansu	0.08	0.11	0.12	0.07	0.13	0.08	0.05	0.07	0.07	0.07	0.07	0.1
Qinghai	0.12	0.14	0.14	0.15	0.2	0.17	0.15	0.08	0.18	0.21	0.3	0.21
Ningxia	0.03	0.05	0.05	0.05	0.05	0.02	0.02	0.02	0.03	0.06	0.04	0.05
Xinjiang	0.12	0.15	0.15	0.15	0.16	0.11	0.09	0.06	0.16	0.12	0.18	0.17
Average	0.09	0.09	0.09	0.09	0.09	0.07	0.06	0.05	0.09	0.08	0.12	0.12

Table 4. The comprehensive development levels of technological innovation.

Province	2005	2006	2007	2008	2009	2010	2011	2012	2013	2014	2015	2016
Beijing	0.08	0.11	0.18	0.23	0.31	0.42	0.42	0.46	0.47	0.52	0.59	0.58
Tianjin	0.06	0.07	0.1	0.14	0.14	0.23	0.23	0.21	0.26	0.29	0.33	0.34
Hebei	0.01	0.02	0.03	0.04	0.05	0.09	0.09	0.08	0.09	0.1	0.11	0.11
Shanxi	0.01	0.02	0.03	0.04	0.04	0.09	0.08	0.07	0.08	0.09	0.1	0.1
Inner Mongolia	0.02	0.02	0.03	0.03	0.03	0.08	0.07	0.05	0.06	0.06	0.07	0.08
Liaoning	0.02	0.03	0.06	0.07	0.09	0.12	0.12	0.12	0.13	0.15	0.17	0.18
Jilin	0.01	0.02	0.03	0.03	0.04	0.06	0.06	0.06	0.06	0.07	0.07	0.08
Heilongjiang	0.01	0.02	0.03	0.03	0.05	0.07	0.07	0.07	0.07	0.08	0.09	0.09
Shanghai	0.05	0.06	0.11	0.16	0.21	0.32	0.32	0.31	0.34	0.37	0.41	0.42
Jiangsu	0.09	0.11	0.15	0.22	0.27	0.37	0.37	0.35	0.4	0.44	0.49	0.49
Zhejiang	0.07	0.08	0.12	0.16	0.17	0.29	0.29	0.25	0.28	0.31	0.35	0.36
Anhui	0.03	0.04	0.05	0.07	0.08	0.16	0.16	0.13	0.14	0.15	0.17	0.17
Fujian	0.02	0.03	0.06	0.07	0.09	0.16	0.15	0.13	0.17	0.18	0.21	0.22
Jiangxi	0.01	0.02	0.03	0.04	0.04	0.07	0.06	0.06	0.07	0.08	0.09	0.09
Shandong	0.03	0.04	0.07	0.1	0.11	0.17	0.17	0.16	0.18	0.2	0.22	0.23
Henan	0.01	0.02	0.03	0.04	0.05	0.09	0.08	0.07	0.07	0.08	0.09	0.09
Hubei	0.04	0.05	0.06	0.08	0.08	0.12	0.12	0.13	0.13	0.14	0.16	0.16
Hunan	0.02	0.03	0.04	0.06	0.07	0.12	0.11	0.1	0.1	0.11	0.12	0.13
Guangdong	0.06	0.08	0.12	0.17	0.22	0.3	0.3	0.28	0.36	0.4	0.43	0.44
Guangxi	0.01	0.01	0.01	0.02	0.02	0.03	0.03	0.03	0.03	0.04	0.04	0.04
Hainan	0.01	0.01	0.02	0.02	0.03	0.05	0.05	0.04	0.06	0.06	0.07	0.07
Chongqing	0.02	0.03	0.05	0.07	0.07	0.14	0.13	0.11	0.12	0.13	0.16	0.16
Sichuan	0.01	0.02	0.03	0.03	0.04	0.11	0.11	0.08	0.05	0.06	0.07	0.07
Guizhou	0.01	0.01	0.01	0.01	0.01	0.04	0.04	0.03	0.03	0.03	0.03	0.03
Yunnan	0.01	0.02	0.02	0.03	0.03	0.06	0.06	0.05	0.06	0.06	0.07	0.07
Shaanxi	0.02	0.03	0.05	0.06	0.07	0.15	0.14	0.13	0.1	0.11	0.13	0.13
Gansu	0.01	0.01	0.02	0.03	0.03	0.06	0.06	0.05	0.04	0.05	0.06	0.06
Qinghai	0.01	0.01	0.02	0.02	0.02	0.06	0.05	0.03	0.04	0.05	0.05	0.05
Ningxia	0.01	0.02	0.03	0.04	0.04	0.1	0.09	0.06	0.07	0.08	0.09	0.1
Xinjiang	0.01	0.01	0.02	0.02	0.02	0.07	0.06	0.04	0.05	0.05	0.06	0.06
Average	0.026	0.04	0.05	0.07	0.08	0.14	0.14	0.12	0.14	0.15	0.17	0.17

Table 5. The comprehensive development levels of green economy.

Province	2005	2006	2007	2008	2009	2010	2011	2012	2013	2014	2015	2016
Beijing	0.3	0.26	0.28	0.34	0.48	0.52	0.47	0.52	0.56	0.62	0.71	0.84
Tianjin	0.2	0.24	0.32	0.36	0.41	0.49	0.49	0.54	0.59	0.63	0.76	0.84
Hebei	0.14	0.19	0.23	0.29	0.38	0.45	0.49	0.55	0.6	0.6	0.74	0.85
Shanxi	0.17	0.21	0.23	0.28	0.4	0.45	0.47	0.55	0.51	0.65	0.75	0.83
Inner Mongolia	0.16	0.2	0.23	0.3	0.41	0.48	0.53	0.59	0.66	0.66	0.72	0.79
Liaoning	0.18	0.22	0.25	0.33	0.41	0.48	0.51	0.58	0.64	0.66	0.66	0.67
Jilin	0.17	0.23	0.25	0.28	0.38	0.43	0.42	0.56	0.56	0.64	0.75	0.86
Heilongjiang	0.18	0.21	0.21	0.28	0.37	0.44	0.47	0.54	0.59	0.66	0.73	0.84
Shanghai	0.17	0.23	0.3	0.37	0.44	0.51	0.49	0.51	0.52	0.56	0.64	0.84
Jiangsu	0.17	0.22	0.25	0.31	0.41	0.48	0.48	0.53	0.59	0.66	0.72	0.78
Zhejiang	0.16	0.22	0.27	0.37	0.45	0.53	0.53	0.56	0.66	0.68	0.69	0.79
Anhui	0.16	0.21	0.23	0.3	0.39	0.45	0.44	0.5	0.55	0.65	0.76	0.89
Fujian	0.12	0.17	0.19	0.28	0.4	0.43	0.46	0.52	0.59	0.69	0.76	0.82
Jiangxi	0.13	0.16	0.18	0.23	0.31	0.39	0.41	0.46	0.52	0.59	0.68	0.86
Shandong	0.18	0.22	0.24	0.29	0.38	0.45	0.47	0.54	0.58	0.65	0.73	0.84
Henan	0.19	0.23	0.26	0.29	0.37	0.42	0.4	0.51	0.58	0.65	0.73	0.84
Hubei	0.14	0.18	0.19	0.27	0.39	0.45	0.45	0.5	0.57	0.65	0.75	0.87
Hunan	0.13	0.16	0.2	0.28	0.38	0.44	0.45	0.49	0.56	0.64	0.75	0.88
Guangdong	0.17	0.22	0.27	0.33	0.4	0.44	0.47	0.53	0.58	0.65	0.7	0.84
Guangxi	0.18	0.2	0.21	0.26	0.35	0.42	0.44	0.51	0.59	0.67	0.78	0.89
Hainan	0.13	0.18	0.22	0.27	0.33	0.44	0.49	0.56	0.61	0.69	0.78	0.84
Chongqing	0.13	0.19	0.22	0.31	0.39	0.46	0.48	0.54	0.59	0.68	0.76	0.84
Sichuan	0.13	0.16	0.18	0.26	0.36	0.44	0.49	0.54	0.62	0.68	0.75	0.77
Guizhou	0.14	0.17	0.17	0.21	0.34	0.43	0.36	0.58	0.46	0.51	0.56	0.65
Yunnan	0.11	0.22	0.17	0.21	0.31	0.4	0.53	0.43	0.47	0.55	0.63	0.76
Shaanxi	0.19	0.21	0.24	0.31	0.38	0.45	0.5	0.55	0.62	0.69	0.78	0.74
Gansu	0.15	0.19	0.21	0.27	0.42	0.5	0.47	0.55	0.63	0.69	0.76	0.7
Qinghai	0.15	0.18	0.2	0.23	0.39	0.47	0.44	0.51	0.57	0.64	0.71	0.81
Ningxia	0.14	0.18	0.2	0.22	0.32	0.38	0.41	0.47	0.54	0.59	0.64	0.86
Xinjiang	0.18	0.22	0.26	0.34	0.36	0.41	0.4	0.59	0.67	0.74	0.78	0.84
Average	0.16	0.20	0.23	0.29	0.38	0.45	0.46	0.53	0.58	0.64	0.72	0.82

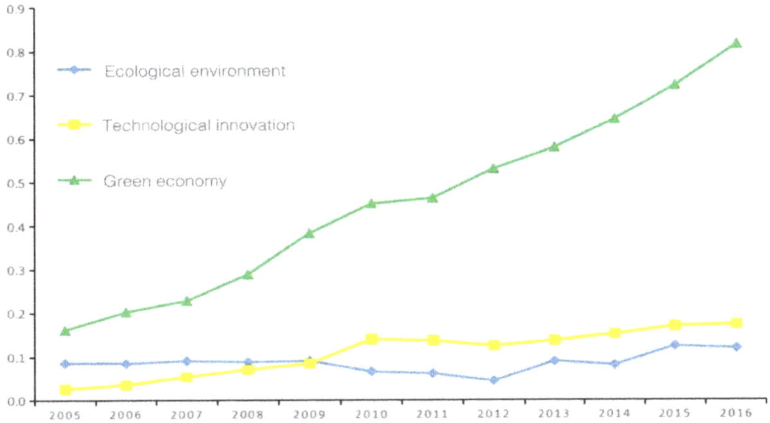

Figure 1. Comprehensive development levels of EE, TI, and GE (2005–2016).

Combining Tables 3–5, it can be seen that from 2005 to 2016, the comprehensive development levels of ecological environment, technological innovation, and green economy in China achieved various degrees of improvement as a whole. The average annual comprehensive development level of ecological environment increased from 0.09 to 0.12, increasing by 133.3%. The development level of technological innovation increased from 0.03 to 0.17, with a huge growth rate of 566.7%. The average annual comprehensive development level of green economy increased from 0.16 to 0.82, and the growth rate also reached an alarming 512.5%. It can be seen that from 2005 to 2016, the comprehensive development level of the green economy improved the most, the development level of and technological innovation was second, and the comprehensive development level of the ecological environment improved the least. This shows that China has indeed achieved great success in transforming its development model and moving towards high-quality development. China's green economy development trend has achieved good results. China has always paid attention to the country's technological innovation capabilities, and has achieved good results by continuously supporting the development of high-tech industries. Although the development of the ecological environment has also been improved, it has not achieved the obvious effect, China still needs to invest more in ecological and environmental protection.

As can be seen from Figure 1, the comprehensive development levels of China's ecological environment, technological innovation, and green economy generally shows a continuous development trend from 2005 to 2016. The development curve of green economy shows a steady upward trend year by year, the comprehensive curve of technological innovation shows a slow rise at first, then a slight decline, and then a slow upward trend, showing a slow rise as a whole. Specifically, it gradually increased slightly from 2005 to 2010, began to decline after reaching a small peak in 2010, and gradually increased two years later from 2012 to 2016. The ecological environment curve shows a trend of first falling and then rising, and generally shows a slow development trend. Specifically, it continued to decline from 2009 to 2012, and the lowest point in 2012 was 0.05, and then slowly fluctuated until 2016, with the annual average rising from 0.09 to 0.12. It can be found that the fluctuation trends of the technological innovation curve and the ecological environment curve are relatively close, and the two intersected once in 2009. The two are quite different from the green economic curve, which shows a rapid upward trend. This shows that, as compared with the rapid development of China's green economy, the development trend of technological innovation and ecological environment is not satisfactory. Although China's technological innovation has made progress in recent years, there are still "bottlenecks" in high-tech industries, and many cutting-edge technologies have not been broken through. With the rapid development of China's economy, all types of environmental pollution have also followed, resulting in significant harm to the ecological environment. Even if the

Chinese government advocates vigorously developing green economy and environmental protection, the actual results are not good.

4.2. Coordination Degree between Ecological Environment and Technological Innovation

By using the coupling coordination model, the coordination degree between ecological environment and technological innovation is calculated as described below (see Table 6).

Table 6. Coordination degree between ecological environment and technological innovation.

Province	2005	2006	2007	2008	2009	2010	2011	2012	2013	2014	2015	2016
Beijing	0.16	0.2	0.22	0.23	0.22	0.22	0.24	0.24	0.3	0.27	0.32	0.32
Tianjin	0.16	0.16	0.17	0.19	0.17	0.18	0.23	0.14	0.23	0.24	0.26	0.21
Hebei	0.15	0.13	0.14	0.16	0.19	0.17	0.18	0.15	0.17	0.18	0.19	0.18
Shanxi	0.13	0.16	0.19	0.2	0.19	0.22	0.2	0.18	0.2	0.17	0.2	0.18
Inner Mongolia	0.14	0.15	0.17	0.18	0.17	0.2	0.21	0.18	0.25	0.23	0.25	0.25
Liaoning	0.14	0.14	0.18	0.17	0.18	0.19	0.18	0.15	0.22	0.21	0.27	0.23
Jilin	0.13	0.13	0.15	0.15	0.16	0.18	0.16	0.14	0.16	0.16	0.18	0.19
Heilongjiang	0.12	0.13	0.17	0.17	0.21	0.21	0.19	0.16	0.22	0.22	0.25	0.25
Shanghai	0.11	0.17	0.14	0.17	0.18	0.16	0.17	0.16	0.19	0.25	0.27	0.32
Jiangsu	0.21	0.22	0.26	0.27	0.27	0.24	0.28	0.25	0.34	0.28	0.36	0.37
Zhejiang	0.17	0.19	0.2	0.21	0.23	0.22	0.21	0.2	0.28	0.3	0.36	0.36
Anhui	0.12	0.14	0.16	0.17	0.17	0.19	0.18	0.16	0.2	0.2	0.24	0.29
Fujian	0.18	0.17	0.16	0.17	0.17	0.2	0.19	0.17	0.24	0.24	0.32	0.32
Jiangxi	0.13	0.14	0.16	0.16	0.19	0.19	0.18	0.14	0.18	0.18	0.23	0.22
Shandong	0.2	0.19	0.22	0.27	0.24	0.26	0.29	0.24	0.23	0.24	0.32	0.31
Henan	0.14	0.14	0.17	0.18	0.15	0.18	0.16	0.12	0.19	0.16	0.2	0.2
Hubei	0.15	0.16	0.17	0.18	0.2	0.21	0.17	0.15	0.21	0.21	0.24	0.34
Hunan	0.16	0.18	0.18	0.2	0.21	0.24	0.22	0.27	0.21	0.2	0.24	0.24
Guangdong	0.21	0.22	0.24	0.24	0.25	0.26	0.24	0.25	0.29	0.29	0.38	0.34
Guangxi	0.11	0.11	0.14	0.14	0.15	0.19	0.18	0.17	0.22	0.23	0.24	0.21
Hainan	0.1	0.11	0.12	0.13	0.15	0.14	0.15	0.12	0.17	0.18	0.18	0.19
Chongqing	0.13	0.13	0.17	0.19	0.18	0.18	0.19	0.13	0.2	0.19	0.24	0.22
Sichuan	0.15	0.15	0.19	0.2	0.21	0.2	0.22	0.18	0.2	0.21	0.23	0.23
Guizhou	0.09	0.11	0.12	0.13	0.13	0.15	0.17	0.1	0.13	0.14	0.16	0.15
Yunnan	0.12	0.15	0.16	0.18	0.16	0.18	0.15	0.14	0.19	0.21	0.22	0.2
Shaanxi	0.13	0.12	0.16	0.15	0.2	0.22	0.22	0.19	0.21	0.2	0.22	0.22
Gansu	0.12	0.14	0.15	0.15	0.18	0.18	0.17	0.17	0.17	0.17	0.18	0.2
Qinghai	0.12	0.13	0.16	0.16	0.17	0.22	0.21	0.16	0.21	0.22	0.25	0.23
Ningxia	0.1	0.12	0.14	0.14	0.14	0.16	0.14	0.12	0.16	0.19	0.17	0.19
Xinjiang	0.12	0.13	0.16	0.16	0.17	0.21	0.19	0.16	0.21	0.2	0.23	0.23

It can be seen from Table 6 that coordination degrees between ecological environment and technological innovation increase year by year from 2005 to 2016, but on the whole, the coordination degrees between ecological environment and technological innovation in various regions were in a state of imbalance. Taking 2005, 2010, and 2016 as examples, in 2005,coordination degrees between ecological environment and technological innovation in China's provinces and cities ranged from 0.09 to 0.21, and most were in a seriously unbalanced state. By 2010, as compared with 2005, the coordination degrees between ecological environment and technological innovation in China's provinces cities had slightly improved, ranging from 0.14 to 0.22, and were still in a serious state of imbalance. By 2016, the coordination degrees between ecological environment and technological innovation in China's provinces and cities further improved, ranging from 0.19 to 0.36, and were in a state of moderate imbalance. It can be seen that although the coordination degrees between ecological environment and technological innovation in China's provinces and cities show an upward trend year by year, coordination levels have always been in a state of serious imbalance.

4.3. Analysis of the Impact of Coordination Degree between Ecological Environment and Technological Innovation on Green Economy

4.3.1. Unit Root Test

First, a unit root is used to test stationary; it examines whether a variable is in the same order and a single integer or not, to avoid deviation of estimation results from the existence of pseudo regression. It can be seen from Table 7 that the original data of the coordinated development level (CO) is not stable. In order to achieve a single integration of the same order, we performed first-order difference processing on the coordinated development level (EC) data. The results show that the green economy data of all regions are stable after the first-order difference, and the co-integration test can be carried out. Similarly, the unit root test of green economy data shows that the original data and the first-order difference data are stable. It can be seen that the coordinated development degree and green economy are stable after the first-order difference.

Table 7. Unit root test results.

Variable	LLC Inspection	IPS Inspection	ADF Inspection	PP Inspection	Conclusion
CO	−2.85 ***	0.48	−5.04	−5.17	unstable
ΔCO	−4.81 ***	−4.81 ***	6.83 ***	8.89 ***	smooth
GE	−5.83 ***	−3.94 ***	3.74 ***	1.52	smooth
ΔGE	−7.17 ***	−8.17 **	5.88 **	36.64 ***	smooth

Note: *** means $p < 0.001$; ** means $p < 0.01$.

4.3.2. Co-Integration Test

According to the unit root test, there is a single integration of the same order between the coordinated development level and green economy. Therefore, a co-integration test can be performed to test whether or not a long-term equilibrium relationship exists between the two. According to the co-integration test method of Pedroni, we tested two variables. The results are shown in Table 8. According to the results of the Pedroni co-integration test, the results are not significant, based on the statistics of Panel v, Panel rho, and Group PP, while they are significant at the 1% level in the Group ADF statistics. and they are significant at the 0.1% level in the statistics of Panel ADF, Panel PP, and Group rho. According to the results of the Johansen co-integration test, there is at least one co-integration relationship. In conclusion, there is a long-term equilibrium relationship between the level of coordinated development and the green economy.

Table 8. Co-integration test results.

Test Method	Test Statistics	Test Result	Conclusion
Pedroni	Panelv-Statistic	−2.42	Co-integration correlation
	Panelrho-Statistic	0.56	
	PanelPP-Statistic	−6.31 ***	
	PanelADF-Statistic	−2.58 ***	
	Grouprho-Statistic	1.72 ***	
	GroupPP-Statistic	−7.28	
	GroupADF-Statistic	−2.02 **	
Johansen	None	177.7 ***	Co-integration correlation
	Atmost1	276.4 ***	

Note: *** means $p < 0.001$; ** means $p < 0.01$.

4.3.3. Optimal Lag Order Test

It is necessary to discover optimal lag order to test the panel vector autoregressive model. The test results of the maximum lag order of the PVAR model are shown in Table 9. Among them, AIC, BIC, and HQIC show that the PVAR model with a lag order of two should be constructed.

Table 9. Test results of optimal lag order.

Lag	AIC	BIC	HQIC
1	−4.83	−4.04	4.51
2	−5.13 *	−4.23 *	−4.77 *

Note: * means $p < 0.05$.

4.3.4. Granger Causality Test

After the co-integration relationship test, it is found that there is a long-term equilibrium relationship between coordinated development level (CO) and green economy (GE). Therefore, the Granger causality test can be performed to explore a causal relationship [30,31]. The specific test results are shown in Table 10. According to the test results, the original hypothesis that green economy is not the cause of an increase in coordinated development level is rejected at the significance level of 0.1% between coordinated development level (CO) and green economy (GE), and the original hypothesis that coordinated development level is not the cause of green economy is rejected at the significance level of 0.1%. This shows that there is a Granger causality relationship between coordinated development level (CO) and green economy (GE) after the first-order difference at the significance level of 0.1%.

Table 10. Granger causality test results.

Null Hypothesis	Observations	df	chi2 Statistics	Conclusion
GE is not the cause of L_CO	270	2	7.21 ***	Reject the null hypothesis
CO is not the cause of L_GE	270	2	32.33 ***	Reject the null hypothesis

Note: *** means $p < 0.001$.

4.3.5. Pulse Response Analysis

In this study, we used the impulse response function and the Monte Carlo simulation method to study the impact of the coordination of ecological environment and technological innovation on green economy. In the simulation process, the number of periods set by the model is 15 and the number of repetitions of data simulation is 500; the impulse response function results are shown in Figure 2. The abscissa represents the number of lag periods; the ordinate represents the corresponding degree; the two curves at the top and bottom represent the upper and lower bounds of 95% confidence interval, respectively; and the middle curve represents the point estimation value of impulse response function.

Figure 2 represents the impulse response results of the coordinated development level and green economy. Figure 2a,d, respectively, show the response of coordinated development level and green economy to the impact of one standard deviation unit; both reach their peak in the current period and show a maximum positive response. Then, the impact gradually weakens and approaches zero response in Phase 1. Then, the green economy has a negative impact on the coordinated development level, and the negative impact gradually increases and reaches the maximum in Phase 2. Since then, the negative impact gradually weakens and approaches zero. Figure 2b shows the dynamic impact of green economy on the level of coordinated development. It can be seen from the Figure 2 that the coordinated development level has a significant negative response to green economy in the current period and reaches the maximum negative response, but then the negative impact of green economy on the coordinated development level gradually weakens. In phase 2, the impact of green economy on the coordinated development level is close to zero, then, presents a positive impact and reaches the maximum positive impact in phase 3, and then, the impact gradually weakens, close to zero. Figure 2c shows the dynamic relationship between the level of coordinated development and the impact of green economy. After the impact of a standard deviation of the current green economy, the initial response of the level of coordinated development is zero, but then there is a positive response, which gradually increases, reaches a peak in phase 2, and then gradually approaches zero, indicating that the level of coordinated development has a lagging positive impact on green economy.

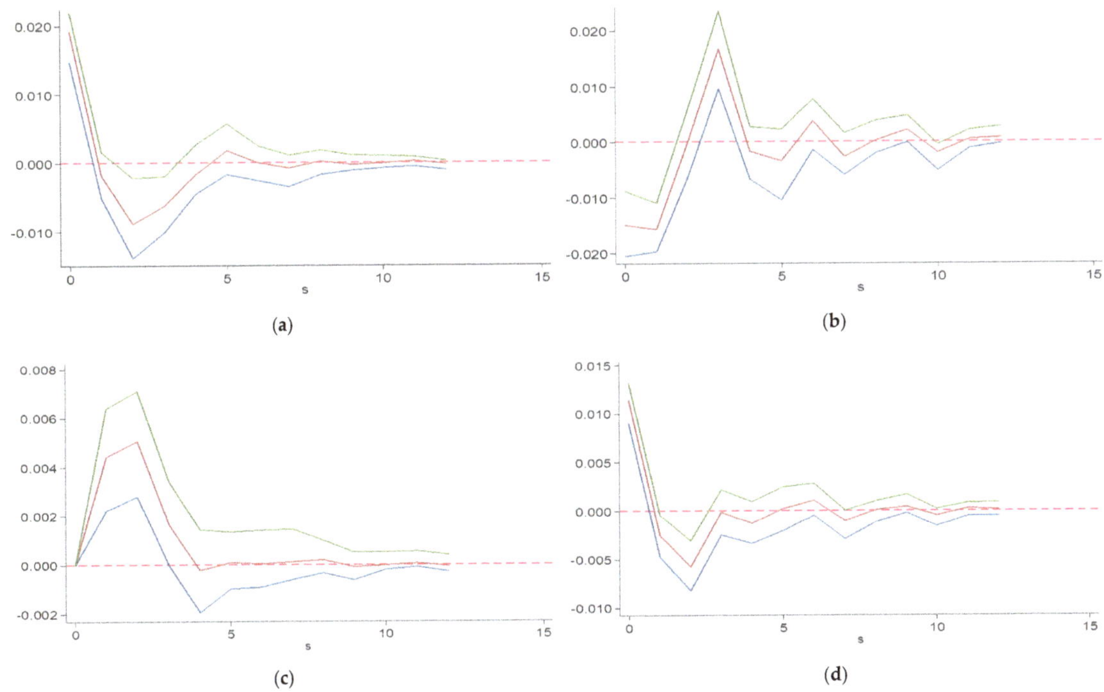

Figure 2. Corresponding results of pulses: (**a**) GE response to GE shock; (**b**) GE response to CO shock; (**c**) CO response to GE shock; (**d**) CO response to CO shock.

5. Conclusions and Prospect

5.1. Conclusions

Based on the panel data of 30 provinces and cities in China from 2005 to 2016, in this study, we adopt the entropy weight method, coupling coordination model, and PAVR model to analyze the impact of coordinated development of ecological environment and technological innovation on green economy. The research finding include: First, from 2005 to 2016, the level of ecological environment, technological innovation, and green economy in 30 provinces and cities in China has achieved varying degrees of improvement. Among them, the level of green economy is the highest, followed by technological innovation, and the level of ecological environment is the lowest. This is mainly because China has increased economic stimulus and investment in technological innovation and the Chinese government attaches more importance to the economy and technology than to environmental protection. Second, the levels of coordination degree between ecological environment and technological innovation increased year by year from 2005 to 2016, but on the whole, the degree of coordination between ecological environment and technological innovation in different regions was unbalanced. Thirdly, the coordination degree between ecological environment and technological innovation has a backward positive impact on green economy, that is, coordinated development between ecological environment and technological innovation has a positive impact on the development of green economy, but the coordination level of the two is low, and therefore, it plays a small role in promoting the development of a green economy. This shows that China needs to promote the development of a green economy by promoting technological innovation and environmental protection. Based on the above results, it can be found that improving the coordination level of technology and ecological environment can promote the development of green economy, but China's work on ecological environment is still insufficient as compared with technological innovation and the development of green economy.

5.2. Research Limitation and Prospect

Based on China's provincial panel data, we conducted an empirical analysis by using the coupling coordination model and panel vector autoregressive model. Our results show that the coordinated development level of China's ecological environment and technological innovation is increasingly important to the development of green economy, which provides theoretical support for the sustainable and healthy development of a green economy. However, there are still some shortcomings. First, in this study, we did not analyze various regions in China, and the research time was only ten years. In the future, if conditions permit, China could be divided into specific regions, and research could be carried out according to different regional characteristics to explore the impact of the coordinated development level of ecological environment and technological innovation in different regions on the development of green economy. At the same time, the research period could be appropriately increased. Second, econometric models are diverse and complex. In this study, we only used the coupling coordination model and panel vector autoregressive model. Therefore, using other models to study this topic should become a research direction in the future.

Funding: This research received no external funding.

Institutional Review Board Statement: Not applicable.

Informed Consent Statement: Not applicable.

Data Availability Statement: Data available in a publicly accessible repository that does not issue DOIs. Publicly available datasets were analyzed in this study.This data can be found here: https://navi.cnki.net/knavi/yearbooks/YINFN/detail?uniplatform=NZKPT (accessed on 4 April 2022).

Conflicts of Interest: The author declares no conflict of interest.

References

1. Wu, J.; Zhang, K. How to Evaluate the Coordination of Green Economy, Education Development, and Technological Innovation? Take China as Example. *Discret. Dyn. Nat. Soc.* **2022**, *2022*, 2027636. [CrossRef]
2. Li, Q. Regional technological innovation and green economic efficiency based on DEA model and fuzzy evaluation. *J. Intell. Fuzzy Syst.* **2019**, *37*, 6415–6425. [CrossRef]
3. Junhan, L. Green Transformation of Circular Economy from The Perspective of Ecological Environment Protection. *J. Environ. Prot. Ecol.* **2020**, *21*, 1517–1525.
4. Shi, T.; Yang, S.; Zhang, W.; Zhou, Q. Coupling coordination degree measurement and spatiotemporal heterogeneity between economic development and ecological environment—Empirical evidence from tropical and subtropical regions of China. *J. Clean. Prod.* **2020**, *244*, 118739. [CrossRef]
5. Zhu, W.; Liu, S. Evaluation and analysis of coordinated development of ecological environment and economy. *Fresenius Environ. Bull.* **2021**, *30*, 4798–4803.
6. Liu, K.; Qiao, Y.; Shi, T.; Zhou, Q. Study on coupling coordination and spatiotemporal heterogeneity between economic development and ecological environment of cities along the Yellow River Basin. *Environ. Sci. Pollut. Res.* **2021**, *28*, 1–15. [CrossRef] [PubMed]
7. Harrod, R. Why Growth Rates Differ: Postwar Experience in Nine Western Countriesby Edward, F. Denison. *Economica* **1969**, *36*, 323–325. [CrossRef]
8. Liu, C.; Xia, G. Research on the Dynamic Interrelationship among R&D Investment, Technological Innovation, and Economic Growth in China. *Sustainability* **2018**, *10*, 4260.
9. Wang, Y.; Deng, Q.; Zhang, Y. Research on the Coupling and Coordinated Development of Marine Technological Innovation and Marine Ecological Economic Development. *J. Coast. Res.* **2020**, *99*, 419–427. [CrossRef]
10. Qi-Qi, C.; Jun-Biao, Z.; Yu, H. A study on research hot-spots and frontiers of agricultural science and technology innovation-visualization analysis based on the Citespace III. *Agric. Econ.* **2016**, *62*, 429–445. [CrossRef]
11. Hond, F.D. Book review: Driving eco-innovation; A Brcakthrough disciplinge for innovation and sustainability by Claude Fussler with Peter James, 1996. Pitman Publishing, xx + 364 pp, 45.00 (hbk), ISBN 0 273 62207 2. *Bus. Strategy Environ.* **1997**, *6*, 297. [CrossRef]

12. Chen, H.M.; Wu, Z.Y.; Jin, W. Evaluation of Regional Technological Innovation Efficiency Based on Principal Component Analysis and DEA. *Appl. Mech. Mater.* **2010**, *33*, 378–382. [CrossRef]
13. Zhang, K.; Jiang, W.; Xu, Y.; Hou, Y.; Zhang, S.; Liu, W. Assessing the corporate green technology progress and environmental governance performance based on the panel data on industrial enterprises above designated size in Anhui Province, China. *Environ. Sci. Pollut. Res.* **2021**, *28*, 1151–1169. [CrossRef] [PubMed]
14. Yang, B.; Jahanger, A.; Ali, M. Remittance inflows affect the ecological footprint in BICS countries: Do technological innovation and financial development matter? *Environ. Sci. Pollut. Res.* **2021**, *8*, 23482–23500. [CrossRef] [PubMed]
15. Ahmad, M.; Jiang, P.; Majeed, A.; Umar, M.; Khan, Z.; Muhammad, S. The dynamic impact of natural resources, technological innovations and economic growth on ecological footprint: An advanced panel data estimation. *Resour. Policy* **2020**, *69*, 101817. [CrossRef]
16. Zhao, J.; Tian, L.; Ding, L.; Sun, H.; Li, P. Research on Energy-Environment-Economy-Ecology Coupling Development in the Yellow River Basin. *E3S Web Conf.* **2021**, *267*, 1003. [CrossRef]
17. Li, M.; Liang, X.; Xiao, C.; Zhang, X.; Li, G.; Li, H.; Jang, W. Evaluation of Reservoir-Induced Hydrological Alterations and Ecological Flow Based on Multi-Indicators. *Water* **2020**, *12*, 2069. [CrossRef]
18. Zhang, Y.; Fan, J.; Wang, S. Assessment of Ecological Carrying Capacity and Ecological Security in China's Typical Eco-Engineering Areas. *Sustainability* **2020**, *12*, 3923. [CrossRef]
19. Shang, J.; Wang, Z.; Li, L.; Chen, Y.; Li, P. A study on the correlation between technology innovation and the new-type urbanization in Shaanxi province. *Technol. Forecast. Soc. Chang.* **2018**, *135*, 266–273. [CrossRef]
20. Jiang, B.; Ding, L.; Fang, X. Sustainable Development of New Urbanization from the Perspective of Coordination: A New Complex System of UrbanizationTechnology Innovation and the Atmospheric Environment. *Atmosphere* **2019**, *10*, 652. [CrossRef]
21. Yi-Qiong, H.U. Indicators and application for corporate's capacity of independent innovation on evaluation. *Technol. Dev. Enterp.* **2006**, *11*, 37–40.
22. Wang, D.; Zhou, T.; Lan, F.; Wang, M. ICT and socio-economic development: Evidence from a spatial panel data analysis in China. *Telecommun. Policy* **2021**, *45*, 102173. [CrossRef]
23. McGranahan, D.V. Analysis of socio-economic development through a system of indicators. *Ann. Am. Acad. Political Soc. Sci.* **1971**, *393*, 65–81. [CrossRef]
24. Liao, K.C.; Yue, M.Y.; Sun, S.W.; Xue, H.B.; Liu, W.; Tsai, S.B.; Wang, J.T. An evaluation of coupling coordination between tourism and finance. *Sustainability* **2018**, *10*, 2320. [CrossRef]
25. Zi, T. An integrated approach to evaluating the coupling coordination between tourism and the environment. *Tour. Manag.* **2015**, *46*, 11–19.
26. Liao, K.; Dai, S.; Duan, X. Research on the Coordination Effect Evaluation and Dynamic Relationship of Technological Innovation and Green Governance. *Sci. Technol. Prog. Policy* **2019**, *36*, 34–43.
27. Sims, C.A. Macroeconomics and reality. *Econometrica* **1980**, *48*, 1–48. [CrossRef]
28. Holtz-Eakin, D.; Newey, W.; Rosen, H.S. Estimating Vector Autoregressions with Panel Data. *Econometrica* **1988**, *56*, 1371–1395. [CrossRef]
29. Jawadi, F.; Mallick, S.K.; Sousa, R.M. Fiscal and monetary policies in the BRICS: A panel VAR approach. *Econ. Model.* **2016**, *58*, 535–542. [CrossRef]
30. China Statistical Yearbook. Available online: https://navi.cnki.net/knavi/yearbooks/YINFN/detail?uniplatform=NZKPT (accessed on 4 April 2022).
31. China Science and Technology Statistical Yearbook. Available online: https://navi.cnki.net/knavi/yearbooks/YBVCX/detail?uniplatform=NZKPT (accessed on 4 April 2022).
32. China High-Tech Industry Statistical Yearbook. Available online: https://navi.cnki.net/knavi/yearbooks/YZGGJ/detail?uniplatform=NZKPT (accessed on 3 April 2022).
33. China Population & Employment Statistical Yearbook. Available online: https://navi.cnki.net/knavi/yearbooks/YZGRL/detail?uniplatform=NZKPT (accessed on 5 April 2022).
34. Available online: https://data.cnki.net/ (accessed on 4 April 2022).
35. National Bureau od Statistics. Available online: http://www.stats.gov.cn/ (accessed on 8 April 2022).

International Journal of
Environmental Research and Public Health

MDPI

Article

The Role of Housing Tenure Opportunities in the Social Integration of the Aging Pre-1970 Migrants in Beijing

Ye Zhu, Weiyu Cao, Xin Li and Ran Liu *

College of Resource Environment and Tourism, Capital Normal University, No. 105 West 3rd Ring Road North, Beijing 100048, China; 1190902032@cnu.edu.cn (Y.Z.); 1190902002@cnu.edu.cn (W.C.); 1190902010@cnu.edu.cn (X.L.)
* Correspondence: liu.ran.space@hotmail.com

Abstract: This study focuses on the social integration of the pre-1970 first-generation migrants in reformist China, who were born before the year 1970 while getting old in the destination cities. The pre-1970 first-generation migrants are not a homogeneous group but are composed of: (a) those over 45 years old and still working but facing age discrimination; and (b) the elderly granny as nanny assuming the domestic and child-care work for their sons or daughters in the destination cities. We conceptualized and re-defined the aging migrants' social integration into three dimensions (i.e., participation practices, communication contacts, and subjective perceptions), and used the 2017 Migrant Dynamics Monitoring Survey (MDMS) data from Beijing to measure and explain the varied integration levels among a total of 1267 aging migrant samples in the Beijing metropolis. It is proven that housing tenure matters and housing tenure entitlement would be conductive to beefing up aging migrants' integration. However, informal housing should not be "stigmatized" as a segregated world, since those dwelling in the informal housing have reported a higher probability of perceiving a fully integrated status (namely subjective well-being, SWB) than those living in the dormitory-like housing. Additionally, an employment-income paradox is found, which shows that higher economic achievement is NOT equivalent to a higher social integration status for the aging migrants.

Keywords: aging migration; housing tenure; social integration; Beijing

Citation: Zhu, Y.; Cao, W.; Li, X.; Liu, R. The Role of Housing Tenure Opportunities in the Social Integration of the Aging Pre-1970 Migrants in Beijing. *IJERPH* **2022**, *19*, 7093. https://doi.org/10.3390/ijerph19127093

Academic Editors: Jie Chen, Qian Zhou and Ting Zhang

Received: 23 April 2022
Accepted: 6 June 2022
Published: 9 June 2022

1. Introduction

The integration and health of the aging migrants have become a global issue in recent years and attracted much attention in both the OECD countries and the developing world [1,2]. The aging migrants are easier exposed to integration and health risks owing to their floating and therefore disadvantaged socioeconomic status, and a series of cultural, institutional, and language barriers have associations with their social integration and health-seeking behaviors. Existing studies have revealed such disadvantages, vulnerability, and discrimination facing the aging migrants in different contexts. The healthy aging schemes, however, have not expanded the health and quality of life-related benefit packages to cover the entire spectrum of migrant populations (especially aging migrants) in many countries. For instance, the World Health Organization (WHO) and its members had created a Global Strategy and Action Plan for Ageing and Health (2016–2020), stressing that everyone can live a long and healthy life [3]. However, this Global Strategy mentioned little about the disadvantageous aging migrants and their integration and health benefits. In recent years, the European Healthy Cities Network began to target the aging migrants (for instance, migrant women of Moroccan origin aged 55 years and over in the specific context of Rotterdam) at risk of loneliness [4]. Other case studies from Italy, Finland, Sweden, and Ireland of the European Healthy Cities Network had proposed a whole-of-society approach to target the vulnerable groups and their related networks (e.g., families and migrant communities) to catalyze their integration across society [4].

Similar to the process of population aging and increased migration that have close associations with the demographics of Europe, the aging migrants have been an important part of China's urban population, too. Massive migration in China began after market-oriented reforms at the end of the 1970s when China relaxed its *hukou*-based household registration system and allowed its populations to move freely between different cities or from rural to urban areas. This great transformation marked a historical turning point in the 1970s. The pre-1970 generation (who were born before 1970) has been regarded as the first-generation migrants in reformist China. Migrants who were born during the 1980s, 1990s, and 2000s are termed the "New Generation Migrants" in China, namely the post-1980, post-1990, and post-2000 generations [5]. The existing studies noticed a sea-change in the industrial and labor relations and societal structures faced by the new generation of migrants [6]. Little attention, however, was given to the social integration of the "aging first-generation migrants" (the pre-1970 generation born before the year 1970) in China.

The pre-1970 migrants have a wide range of age cohorts in urban China: (a) those over 45 years old and still working; and (b) de facto elderly migrants already retired. Such an aging process deserves attention, as it would incur more risk factors for exclusion and disease. For instance, some recent research began to stress the unemployment and exclusion risks exposed to people over 45 years old (as a specific vulnerable group in the employment market) in times of crisis and restructuring in both the OECD and developing countries. A study on Spanish unemployment revealed the socio-professional context that rejects and excludes people over 45 years old from the job market [7]. The empirical studies in the UK confirmed this conclusion [8]. Another research on the age limit in recruitment advertisements in China also pointed out the age discrimination against job seekers: the upper age limit of selected four types of jobs (handyman, technician, engineer, and manager) has a trend of convergence towards 45 years old [9]. The de facto elderly migrants who are already retired also face difficulties adapting to the living environments, because they assume the domestic and child-care work (namely granny as a nanny) for their sons or daughters but have few chances for out-of-home leisure or local communication contact. The above continuity but heterogeneity of the aging process (ranging from the migrant labor over 45 years to the retired granny) deserves further investigation.

In this paper, we tentatively re-define the social integration dimensions of the aging pre-1970 migrants in Beijing. The aging- and migrant-specific integration-seeking behaviors and perceptions matter, involving (a) aging migrants' participation in local affairs (rather than engagement with their own clan/lineage), (b) extensiveness of communication contacts (migrant-local ties, rather than within migrant networks), and (c) self-identification and perceptions of their social integration status. The specific measures of participation, communication contact, and perception are clarified. We then outline the key demographic, migratory, and contextual factors that shape the differentiated social integration profiles of the aging migrants in the transitional Beijing metropolis. Recent studies have proved that better housing opportunities are accompanied by a higher level of social integration [10]. However, relevant studies focused only on the physical context (e.g., physical quality, characteristics, arrangement, and environment) of housing [11], and did not mention the housing tenure context. We innovatively list the housing tenure (as an outcome of migrants' self-selection and socio-spatial stratification) as the contextual factor, which has associations with the social interaction behaviors and perceptions of the aging pre-1970 migrants. This research uses the Migrant Dynamics Monitoring Survey (MDMS) data in 2017 in the Beijing metropolis and employs logistic regression analysis to attest to whether the housing opportunities (owning, renting, employer- or government-provided, informality) have significant associations with the social integration of the aging pre-1970 migrants in Beijing. In conclusion, there is a need for more attention given to the healthy aging scheme providing the aging migrants better housing opportunities, creating a positive sense of self, and more chances for participation, communication, and empowerment. This is important to accommodate the needs of the growing number of aging migrants in China.

2. Social Integration of Aging Migrants in China: Review and Conceptualization

2.1. Migration, Aging, and the Role of the Housing Regime in the Social Stratification and Inclusion

In contrast to the Western countries, the household registration system (namely *hukou*) is a particular institution that links people's place of origin to their daily life, social services, and welfare in China, and it has exerted an impact on the social stratification between local vs. nonlocal *hukou* holders and between talented vs. less-skilled migrant workers [12,13]. The New-Styled Urbanization Plan and *hukou* reforms have been implemented during the 13th Five-Year Plan period (2015–2020) to integrate migrants in terms of employment opportunities, housing acquisition, and social services delivery [14]. The recent *hukou* reform ensured that the migrants can get urban *hukou* in medium-sized cities (with three million residents and below), but *hukou* restrictions remain strong in first-tier cities and megacities such as Beijing. Megacities began to open their *hukou* doors to talented youth, although policy makers still stress the importance of the *hukou* system to avoid urban ills and population over-crowding [15].

Migrants' integration and willingness to settle in the destination cities have become the focus of current research on migration in China. The existing studies revealed the positive impact of human capital and social networks on the migrants' socioeconomic and psychological integration [16,17]. More recent research began to compare migrants' integration in the different neighborhood types in urban China [18–20] since neighbor networks and socioeconomic and physical environments of neighborhoods are vital components of integration [21–23].

China has the largest elderly population in the world and its pace of aging (i.e., fast-growing number and proportion of the elderly people in cities) has become rapid in recent years. However, relatively little attention has been given to the pre-1970 generation migrants (born before 1970), who were the first-generation migrants in reformist China who are aging now. In recent years, researchers began to discuss the pre-1970 migrants' social integration issues. For instance, Lin and Huang used the 2015 national scale data issued by the China Household Financial Survey (CHFS) to analyze the cohort differences among migrants, concerning the community environmental satisfaction and their impact on migrants' subjective well-being (SWB) [24]. It was found that the satisfying social environment (rather than the physical environment) exhibited the positive associations with happiness among the pre-1970 migrants, and at the same time, the positive associations of a satisfying social life with SWB were more observable in the pre-1970 migrants than their younger cohorts. It was found that the social integration (including social environment and social life as revealed in Lin and Huang's studies) exerts a prominent impact on the health and quality of life of the pre-1970 first-generation migrants. However, little is known regarding the "localized" participation and communication behaviors and perceptions of social integration among the pre-1970 migrants, who are getting old.

The pre-1970 migrants straddle a wide range of life courses. They are facing quite different situations under China's retirement policy, if they are under 60 years old (mostly still working) or over 60 years old (mostly retired). More attention needs to be put on the sizeable aging migrants in China, including (a) de facto elderly migrants (mostly retired, living with their sons or daughters and caring for grand-children in the destination city), and (b) aging-but-still working migrant workers (still employed but relatively disadvantaged compared with the post-1980 and post-1990 new generations in terms of their adaptation to the new economies in megacities). The aging migrants are called "*laopiao*", having left the familiar environment and social networks in their hometown and floating in a destination city, either as aging migrant workers or granny as a nanny. Such aging migration in transitional China is not for recreation or retirement purposes but is an economic or family-unification driven migration. The aging migrants face difficulties adapting to the living environments in megacities (such as Beijing), regardless of whether co-residing with their children or not. If they assume the domestic and child-care work for their sons or daughters, they have fewer chances for out-of-home leisure and local communication contacts [25]. As revealed, the language barrier can reduce the elderly migrants' abilities to build up a social network in the destination city and result in poorer health conditions [26]. The older migrants face mobile vulnerability in big cities such as Beijing, but they can develop coping strategies to improve their socio-cultural mobility in the destination [27]. It is also found that social environment and social activities can contribute to old adults' health in the megacities such as Shanghai [28]. Scholars have examined the impact of different neighborhood types on the quality of life among elderly people in Nanjing and Beijing megacities [29,30]. These aging and healthy living studies, however, have not been extended to the aging migrants who are more disadvantaged than the local elderly people.

Less attention has been paid to the role of housing types in integration. Housing provides housing security, public services, and upward mobility opportunities (such as school provisions organized around the catchment areas) for the migrants [31]. In China, *hukou* imposes limits on the social integration of migrants, but recent studies have indicated that the migrants tend to achieve permanent settlement through more flexible channels such as purchasing urban housing in the destination city, even though the migrants have limited housing opportunities than residents since that house prices are particularly high in big cities [32,33]. Moreover, housing is a symbol of the living quality of the migrants and an important indicator and a result of social stratification in the destination city in China [34,35]. As early as the 1960s, the new Weber School represented by Rex put forward the concept of housing class and emphasized that individual possession of housing tenure is one of the criteria for dividing the social classes [36]. Housing type or housing choice is the primary factor directly related to the migrants' social stratification and inclusion, especially in transitional economies such as China with a profound housing commodification reform since the 1990s. Interestingly, the concept of "housing type" and "community type" is seemingly exchangeable in the previous studies on the so-called community-level integration studies. For instance, it is proved that migrants living in the government-sponsored "affordable housing" community exhibited a much higher level of social integration than those living in other "rental" communities [37]. It is also found that migrants who live in "commodity housing" neighborhoods achieve a higher level of integration, but those living in "urban villages" cannot find a path to integrate into the mainstream city [20,38,39]. What is more important, housing tenure itself would stimulate interaction and integration [40]. The recent studies on neighborhood-level integration also stressed the significance of housing tenure type. A recent empirical study on migrants in peri-urban neighborhoods in Beijing pointed out that a low sense of belonging among migrants is not necessarily a result of homogenous tenure, but of living with uncertainty and exclusion from the formal urban economy, and scholars have revealed the role of tenure heterogeneity in providing a sense of privilege and privacy [19]. It is uncertain whether this conclusion can be held in other contexts, but housing type indeed matters in the integration process. In addition, housing unaffordability is found negatively correlated with migrants' mental health, and compared with migrants who are home-occupiers, the tenant migrants are more easily excluded from the psychological integration in the face of high rental costs [41,42]. However, we know little about the role of housing stratification in inclusion/exclusion processes, especially among the aging migrant populations.

2.2. Conceptualization, Framework, and Hypotheses

The existing studies on the migrants' social integration under China's *hukou* regime have measured the willingness to settle down or not, and the willingness to make *hukou* conversion or not, as a representation of the migrants' sense of belonging and identity to the city [43,44]. However, for older migrants, having or lacking strong ties/networks with locals, and engaging in local affairs are profoundly important predictors of well-being and health status. As pointed out by the Sociologist Louis Wirth, "If men of diverse experiences and interests are to have ideas and ideals in common, they must have the ability to communicate". The integration process requires the extensiveness of contact among migrant populations and local society [45,46]. Existing studies, however, tended to define integration to be a small network within the neighborhoods. The social integration interpretation (as well as integration into local society in general) should build up and maintain the larger networks (such as the city-wide housing tenure system, the urban-bound participation activities, and perceptions) rather than neighborhood-bound within some specific mosaic-like enclaves or the recommended socio-ethnically mixed neighborhoods. The previous studies had tried to prove that the overall best direct predictor of social integration was community or neighborhood [47,48]. The Western experience focused on the associations of the mixed neighborhood with integration and believed that physical mixing can promote interclass interaction [49]. However, Musterd, Ostendorf, and Galster pointed out it is unclear whether a neighborhood mixing between different people does indeed result in a higher level of integration [50,51]. The community-level mechanism of integration is still opaque, and the analysis results vary with the specific contexts.

Ager and Strang proposed a conceptual framework for understanding integration in 2008, and they listed the key domains of integration: (a) achievement and access across the sectors of employment, housing, education, and health; (b) practices regarding citizenship and rights; (c) processes of social connection within and between groups; and (d) structural barriers to such connection related to language, culture and the local environments [52]. Among them, housing is stressed as one of the most researched areas of integration, and as important as employment and education. They paid attention to the associations that housing has with the physical and emotional well-being, the financial security of tenancies and ownership, their ability to feel at home, settled (as well as the continuity of relationships associated with being settled), safe, secure and stable, and other social and cultural impact of housing. Ager and Strang's conceptualizations are likely to remain controversial [53], but they can embrace the significant questions regarding the specific processes that can facilitate integration (for instance, concerning targeted housing policies that can make opportunities for social connection or a sense of safety) [52]. Chen and Wang adopted Ager and Strang's conceptual framework on what is integration and developed the three-dimensional measurement of the Chinese new generation migrants' social integration process: (a) participation in community activities; (b) connection with the community, and (c) accustomed to social norms [54]. They then used the relevant factors and processes that facilitate integration to explain the younger migrants' integration in Shanghai.

It is important to see the aging migrants' integration as a practical and relational process and multiple measurements, not a purely perceptual outcome concerning satisfaction, happiness, or willingness to settle down or make *hukou* conversion to a destination city. Here, as elaborated by Robert Brown (2010: 2), the social integration refers to the range of a person's communication contacts (regardless of individual-level, small group, or mass communication) rather than to their frequency of communication, as the integration process requires some extensiveness of communication contacts [46]. We can assume that integration is itself dependent on extensive communication with the local population and that migrants who report a variety of communication contacts with the locals differ from those who report few or no such contacts.

Because housing choice and housing type are vital components of social stratification statuses and city/neighbor networks, we examine the housing stratification-related integration perspectives to explain the impact of "housing tenure type" on the aging pre-1970 migrants' "integration" in the Chinese metropolises such as Beijing. The aging migrants' social integration is defined from three dimensions (i.e., participation practices, communication contacts, and subjective perceptions, similar to Ager and Strang's conceptualization and Chen and Wang's adoption of it in the Chinese megacity contexts [52,54]):

(a) Their actual participation in local affairs (regardless of a small group-like community/neighborhood or the mass society of a city);
(b) Communication contacts with the locals, beyond their own patriarchal family- and clan-relationship (namely "*laoxiang*" as people from similar originating areas); and
(c) Migrants' relevant perceptions of subjective well-being (SWB).

Can a housing tenure regime be better designed to promote the aging migrants' social integration with their local social capital and environments? Next, we will use the survey evidence from the 2017 Migrant Dynamics Monitoring Survey (MDMS) data in Beijing and the logistic regression to examine this possibility by testing the relationships between varying types of housing tenure and the strength of integration: (a) whether housing tenure opportunities can predict the aging migrants' social integration; and (b) which kind of housing tenure attainment/arrangement is more conducive to (or can best support) the integration of aging migrants in the metropolises such as Beijing?

The typical housing tenure opportunities available to the migrants in Beijing are composed of: (a) self-owned commercial housing; (b) dormitory-like housing provided by governments or employer units; (c) rental commercial housing; and (d) informal housing involving "urban village" housing, small property housing and other types of informalities [55,56]. Figure 1 displays the main housing types accessible to the migrants in Beijing, and Figure 2 demonstrates the conceptual framework that constructs and interprets the aging pre-1970 migrants' integration into Beijing's local society. As shown in Figure 2, we construct a three-tiered measurement of integration (practical, relational, and perceptual), and examine the main determinants of integration (from perspectives of household, migratory, and housing-related) to interpret the variance of aging migrants' integration levels. The housing-related explanatory factors involve housing tenure types and housing expenditure stress. The definitions and measurements of dependent and explanatory factors will be elaborated in Section 3, based on the data availability of the 2017 MDMS.

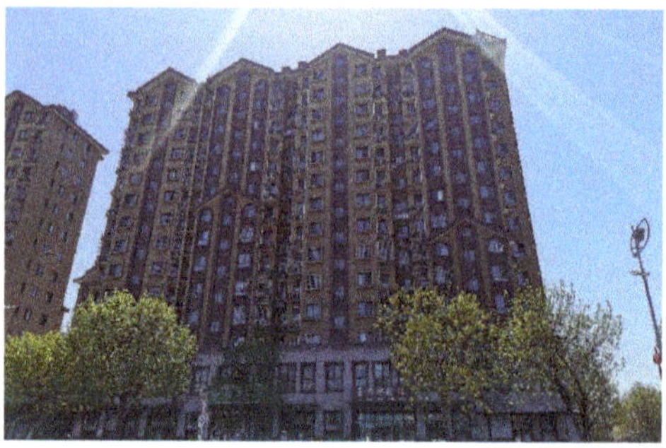

(a)

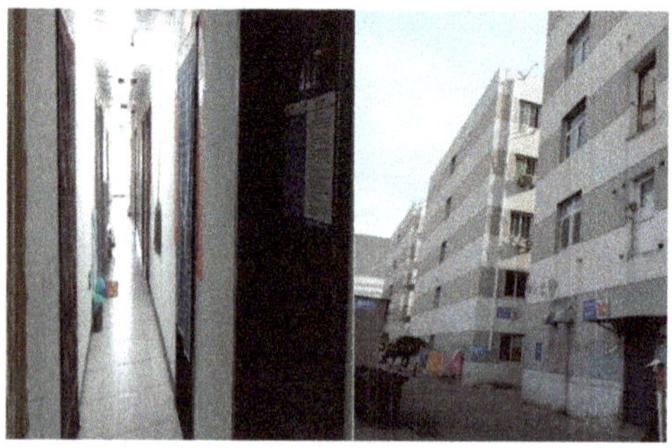

(b)

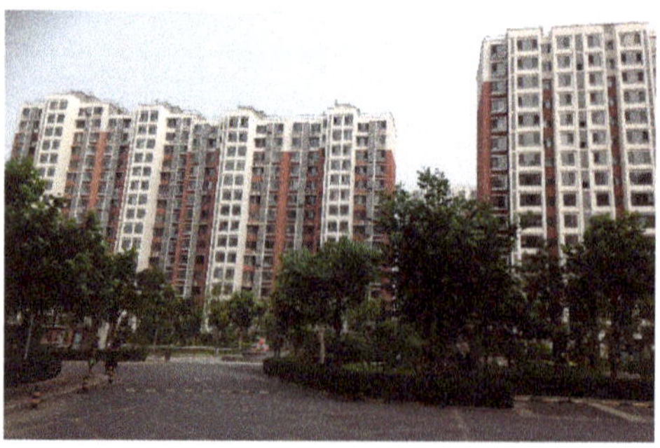

(c)

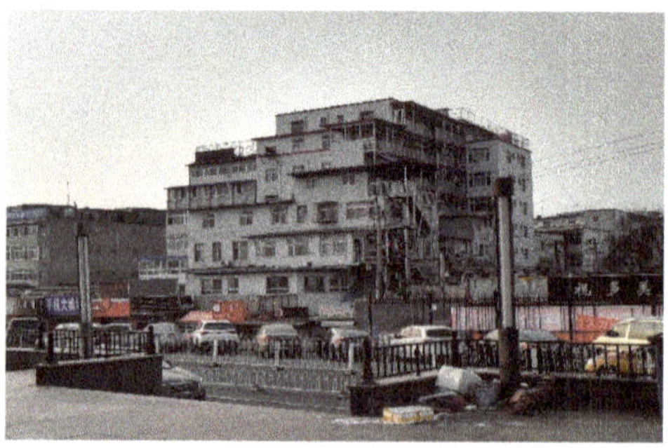

(d)

Figure 1. Housing tenure types accessible for migrants in the Beijing metropolis in China (**a**) commercial housing for self-owning or renting; (**b**) dormitory provided by employers in the industrial park; (**c**) public rented housing prepared for talented migrant workers; (**d**) "urban village" housing. Photos were taken by authors.

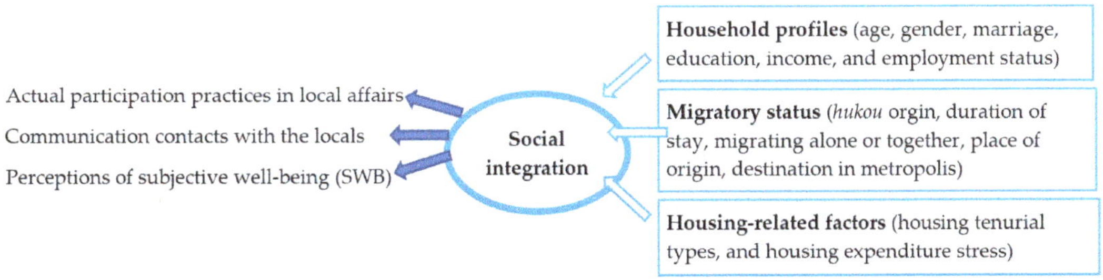

Figure 2. The three-tiered measurement of social integration (practical, relational, and perceptual), and its determinants (household, migratory, and housing-related). Originated and adapted from Ager and Strang's conceptualization and Chen and Wang's empirical studies in the Chinese megacity contexts [52,54].

Considering that the pre-1970 migrants straddle a wide range of life courses, we try to separate the whole pre-1970 migrants into two age cohort groups according to China's retirement policy: (a) ≥60 years old (mostly retired), and (b) pre-1970 and <60 years old (mostly still working). They are facing quite different situations, and the housing impact on their respective social integration would be quite different, too.

We hypothesize that:

Hypothesis 1: *The insecurities of housing tenure can lower the aging migrants' integration, and home-owning can beef up their integration; and*

Hypothesis 2: *Those in a paid employment status (<60 years old) vs. those in a retired status (≥60 years old) would indicate the differentiated integration processes faced by the aging migrants.*

3. Data and Method

3.1. Research Area and Data Source

The data is derived from the 2017 Migrant Dynamics Monitoring Survey (MDMS) collected and issued by the National Health Commission in China. This survey adopted a stratified three-stage probability proportion to size (PPS) random sampling method and involved the investigation questions on the migrants' social integration in the destination city. We selected the migrant samples collected in the Beijing metropolis. In total valid 6999 samples in Beijing, we select 1267 samples of pre-1970 generation migrants (aged between 48 and 84 years old), who were born before 1970 and became the first-generation migrants in reformist China but getting aging now. The migrants had lived in Beijing for one month or more but did not get local *hukou* in Beijing.

We choose Beijing as the case study. First, Beijing is the most important destination city of the Chinese domestic migration in the north, accommodating migrants with different economic-cultural backgrounds in a diversity of housing types. Migrants' housing choice in Beijing was repetitively investigated in previous studies [57,58], and the Beijing metropolis is deemed an ideal case to study the integration of diverse migrant populations including the aging migrants. Second, Beijing itself has a large elderly population, and it is believed that the inflow of younger migrants can slow down the process of population aging. Policy makers paid more attention to how to serve the aging local population and attract educated young migrants while ignoring the integration and health issues of the aging migrant populations. For instance, recent studies investigated the role of changing the urban environment in the everyday aging experiences in Beijing, and the surveys were conducted on the older people living at home in Beijing [59]. It was found that the growing housing inequality in post-reform urban China reflects how older people assess their built environment change in the Beijing metropolis, but such studies did not focus on the aging migrant populations. More research is needed to fill in this research gap.

The purpose of this study is to understand the role of different housing tenure types (i.e., self-owned housing; dormitory-like housing provided by governments or employers; rental housing; and informal housing, see Figure 1) in the integration of the aging migrants into the Chinese metropolises such as Beijing. The statistical analysis will be conducted in the next section. The self-owned commercial housing is the most "secure" housing type and a place more like a "home" for migrants. The surveyed aging migrants displayed a higher home-owing ratio (30.1%) than an average level in the total migrant samples (19.8%) in Beijing, due to their higher capacity to acquire an owned home after years of adaptation and success, or due to their kids' home-owning status in Beijing. Interestingly, there is little variance between the proportion of aging migrants living in informal housing (29.80%) and the average level of total migrant populations (33.6%). It is thus indicated that the associations between housing inequality and stratification would be greater with the aging migrants than it is in the total migrant populations. Informal housing in Beijing is highly concentrated in Chaoyang, Haidian, and Fengtai districts in the Urban Function Extended Districts. The map for Beijing Municipality is shown in Figure 3. Additionally, the dormitory-like housing proportion of the aging migrants (14.7%) keeps the same as the total migrant population (12.6%), too. However, living in the dormitories often means sharing a room with other workers, and for this reason, dormitories would not be the first choice for many migrant households.

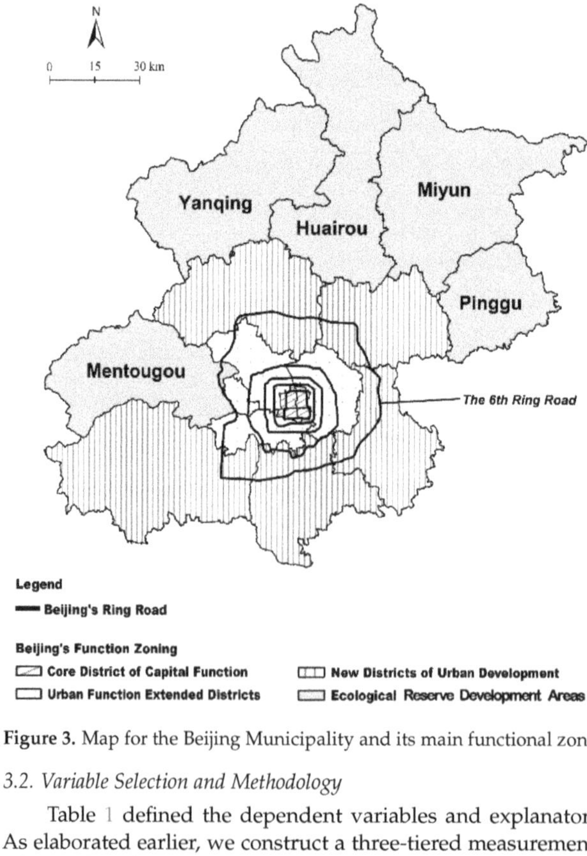

Figure 3. Map for the Beijing Municipality and its main functional zones.

3.2. Variable Selection and Methodology

Table 1 defined the dependent variables and explanatory variables in this study. As elaborated earlier, we construct a three-tiered measurement of integration (practical, relational, and perceptual). The aging migrants' social integration is defined as listed in Table 1. The relevant questions were listed in the questionnaire of the 2017 MDMS, which contains the specific "social integration" section.

Table 1. Indicators.

		Indicators	Descriptions	Mean	Standard Deviation
Dependent variables					
	1	Local affairs participation	No = 0, Yes = 1	0.44	0.49
	2	Communication with the locals as the most frequent daily contact	No = 0, Yes = 1	0.26	0.44
	3	A full integration status perceived (subjective well-being)	No = 0, Yes = 1	0.19	0.39
Explanatory variables					
• Household profiles		Age (years old)	Continuous variable	57.74	8.25
		Gender	Male = 1, Female = 2	1.43	0.50
		Marital status	Married = 1, Unmarried = 2	1.10	0.30
		Educational attainment	Primary and below = 1, Junior secondary = 2, Senior/technical secondary = 3, College and above = 4	2.22	0.96
		Household monthly income (logged, unit: yuan)	Continuous variable	3.85	0.33
		Employment status	Employed = 1, Unemployed or retired = 2	1.41	0.49
• Migratory status		Hukou origin	Rural hukou = 1, Urban hukou = 2	1.42	0.49
		Duration of stay in Beijing (years)	Continuous variable	9.73	7.73
		Migrate alone or together	Yes (migrate alone) = 1, No (migrate together with family) = 2	1.96	0.21
		Place of origin	Eastern Region = 1, North Region = 2, Central Region = 3, South-Western Region = 4, North-Western Region = 5, North-Eastern Region = 6	3.18	2.22
		Destination in Beijing metropolis	Core District of Capital Function = 1, Urban Function Extended Districts = 2, New Districts of Urban Development = 3, Ecological Reserve Development Areas = 4	2.24	0.77
• Housing-related factors		Housing tenure types	Self-owned commercial housing = 1, Dormitory-like housing provided by governments or employer units = 2, Rental commercial housing = 3, Informal housing = 4	2.55	1.20
		Housing stress (housing expenditure-to-income ratio)	Continuous variable	0.14	0.39

Note: 1. The rare samples from the South-Eastern Region (N = 4) are detected as outliers and are deleted for this reason. 2. In the Beijing metropolis, (a) Core District of Capital Function (Inner Cities) includes Dongcheng and Xicheng Districts; (b) Urban Function Extended Districts (Inner Suburbs) include Chaoyang, Fengtai, Shijingshan, and Haidian Districts; (c) New Districts of Urban Development (Outer Suburbs) includes Fangshan, Tongzhou, Shunyi, Changping and Daxing Districts; and (d) Ecological Reserve Development Areas (Mountainous Areas) includes Mentougou, Huairou, Pinggu, Miyun and Yanqing Districts. Data source: MDMS, 2017.

First, from a practical dimension, we assign the value of 1 to the "local affair participation" variable, if the aging migrants had participated in the local affairs in Beijing (e.g., the labor union, volunteers' association, supervising or offering advice for the management of their workplace and community, reporting to governments and giving policy making suggestions, online comments and discussions on the national affairs and social news, donating, blood donation, volunteer activities, and participating in the Party's branch meetings and activities). Otherwise, we give the value of 0 to the 1st tier of the dependent variable.

Second, from a relational perspective, we assign the value of 1 to the 2nd tier of the dependent variable "communication with the locals as the most frequent daily contacts", if the aging migrants have chosen the local Beijingese as the primary communication contacts instead of their own family- and clan-relationship or other populations. Otherwise, we give the value of 0 to this tier of the dependent variable.

Third, from a subjective and perceptual definition, we assign the value of 1 to the 3rd tier of the dependent variable "a full integration status perceived", if the aging migrants give full marks in the questionnaire questions concerning migrants' perceptions of subjective well-being (SWB). The five positive and inclusive settings of subjective well-being (SWB) are inquired about in the five questions of the 2017 MDMS: (a) I like the city I am living in now; (b) I pay attention to the change of this city; (c) I am willing to integrate into the local society and become a member; (d) I think the locals are willing to accept me as one of them, and (e) I think I am already a "local" resident. Each of the five questions is assigned 1 to 4 points to the four choices (i.e., complete disagreement, disagreement, basic agreement, and complete agreement, respectively). If the aging migrants gave a full score of 20 for the five questions, we consider them able to integrate fully into the local city and assign the value of 1 to this dependent variable. Otherwise, we give the value of 0 to the 3rd tier of the dependent variable.

Next, we examine the main determinants of integration and select three types of attributes including household profiles, migratory status, and housing-related factors to interpret the variance of the aging migrants' integration level. Table 1 lists a total of 13 exploratory variables in the above three attribute groups. The focus would be put on the impact of the different housing tenure on the social integration of the aging migrants in Beijing. The housing tenure categories and related landscapes were mentioned earlier in Figure 1.

3.3. Regression Model Selection

This paper uses a binary logistic regression model to study the associations of social integration among the aging migrants with differential housing tenures. The calculation formula is listed as follows:

$$\log\left[\frac{p}{1-p}\right] = a + b_1X_1 + b_2X_2 + b_3X_3 + \ldots + b_kX_k \quad (1)$$

where X_1, X_2, X_3 ... X_K are independent variables, a is a constant term, b_1, b_2, b_3 ... b_K represent the regression coefficients of the respective explanatory variables.

The dependent variables are participation, communication contact, and subjective identity, as listed in Table 1. P is the probability of being willing to integrate, and 1-P is the probability of not planning to integrate.

Logistic regression is widely used when the dependent variables are categorical (e.g., No = 0, Yes = 1 as listed in Table 1). Regression results are reported in the results section.

4. Results

4.1. Descriptive Statistical Analysis

The descriptive statistics are summarized in Table 2. Most of the aging pre-1970 migrants were living in self-owned commercial housing (30.1%) and informal housing such as "urban villages" (29.8%). Such a tenurial divide often displays a large socioeconomic difference and a contrasting integration status.

Table 2. Descriptive statistics of the aging pre-1970 migrants across the different housing tenure types in Beijing.

		Self-Owned Commercial Housing		Dormitory-Like Housing Provided by Governments or Employer Units		Rental Commercial Housing		Informal Housing		Total	
Sampling		382	30.1%	186	14.7%	321	25.3%	378	29.8%	1267	100%
Dependent variables											
1 Local affairs participation	Yes	208	54.5%	88	47.3%	145	45.2%	122	32.3%	563	44.4%
	No	174	45.5%	98	52.7%	176	54.8%	256	67.7%	704	55.6%
2 Communication with locals as the most frequent daily contact	Yes	155	40.6%	34	18.3%	67	20.9%	70	18.5%	326	25.7%
	No	227	59.4%	152	81.7%	254	79.1%	308	81.5%	941	74.3%
3 Full integration perceived (SWB)	Yes	116	30.4%	20	10.8%	49	15.3%	57	15.1%	242	19.1%
	No	266	69.6%	166	89.2%	272	84.7%	321	84.9%	1025	80.9%
Explanatory variables											
• **Household profiles**											
Gender	Male	181	47.4%	124	66.7%	179	55.8%	237	62.7%	721	56.9%
	Female	201	52.6%	62	33.3%	142	44.2%	141	37.3%	546	43.1%
Marital Status	Single	39	10.2%	27	14.5%	23	7.2%	36	9.5%	125	9.9%
	Married	343	89.8%	159	85.5%	298	92.8%	342	90.5%	1142	90.1%
Education	Primary and below	54	14.1%	51	27.4%	85	26.5%	132	34.9%	322	25.4%
	Junior secondary	103	27.0%	82	44.1%	139	43.3%	166	43.9%	490	38.7%
	Senior/technical secondary	127	33.2%	48	25.8%	67	20.9%	65	17.2%	307	24.2%
	College and above	98	25.7%	5	2.7%	30	9.3%	15	4.0%	148	11.7%
Employment status	Employed	61	16.0%	164	88.2%	237	73.8%	283	74.9%	745	58.8%
	Unemployed or retired	321	84.0%	22	11.8%	84	26.2%	95	25.1%	522	41.2%
• **Migratory status**											
Hukou origin	Rural *hukou*	82	21.5%	144	77.4%	217	67.6%	294	77.8%	737	58.2%
	Urban *hukou*	300	78.5%	42	22.6%	104	32.4%	84	22.2%	530	41.8%
Migrate alone or not	Migrate alone	10	2.6%	19	10.2%	13	4.0%	15	4.0%	57	4.5%
	Migrate together with family	372	97.4%	167	89.8%	308	96.0%	363	96.0%	1210	95.5%
Place of origin	Eastern Region	77	20.2%	41	22.0%	80	24.9%	85	22.5%	283	22.3%
	North Region	121	31.7%	66	35.5%	84	26.2%	120	31.7%	391	30.9%
	Central Region	53	13.9%	36	19.4%	82	25.5%	73	19.3%	244	19.3%
	South-Western Region	19	5.0%	10	5.4%	23	7.2%	29	7.7%	81	6.4%
	North-Western Region	26	6.8%	8	4.3%	13	4.0%	4	1.1%	51	4.0%
	North-Eastern Region	86	22.4%	25	13.4%	39	12.2%	67	17.7%	217	17.1%
Destination in Beijing metropolis	Core District of Capital Function	38	9.9%	34	18.3%	58	18.1%	34	9.0%	164	12.9%
	Urban Function Extended Districts	256	67.0%	112	60.2%	220	68.5%	143	37.8%	731	57.7%
	New Districts of Urban Development	57	14.9%	29	15.6%	28	8.7%	166	43.9%	280	22.1%
	Ecological Reserve Development Areas	31	8.1%	11	5.9%	15	4.7%	35	9.3%	92	7.3%

Note: The rare samples from the South-Eastern Region (N = 4) are detected as outliers and are deleted for this reason. Data source: MDMS, 2017.

The aging migrants living in owned housing have probably the family members (e.g., spouse, kids, son/daughter-in-law), who have already acquired Beijing *hukou*. Compared with the other three types of housing, these aging occupiers demonstrate the obvious advantages in all the practical, relational, and perceptual dimensions of integration, reportedly, 54.5% participate in the local affairs, 40.6% list communication with the locals as a prominent daily contact means, and 30.4% regarding themselves fully integrated into local society. This more inclusive status can be evidenced by the fact that 84.0% of these aging home-occupiers have got retired or are unemployed, and 78.5% of them have an urban origin (instead of a rural origin), as listed in Table 2.

A comparative study on the integration level is quite illuminating, between the aging migrants living in (a) dormitory-like housing provided by the governments or employers, (b) rental commercial housing, and (c) informal housing. It is believed that those in informal housing are more disadvantaged and segregated. However, the relational and perceptual measurements of integration (communication contacts index and SWB index in Table 2) in the informal housing are reported at the same level or even higher than that in the dormitory-like housing provided by the governments or employers. The values of SWB are also the same between those living in rental commercial housing and informal housing.

It is impressive that those living in the formal housing are congregated in the Urban Function Extended Districts in Beijing, while those in informal housing are present mostly in the New Districts of Urban Development in Beijing (see Table 2). A massive demolition of urban villages in Haidian, Fengtai, and Chaoyang Districts since 2009 can explain such a geographical disparity between the formal and informal housing in Beijing [60].

4.2. Regression on the Pre-1970 Migrants' Integration Status

We have tested how to partition the whole pre-1970 migrants into two cohorts (majority still working vs. majority being retired), who are at two very distinct life stages. In sum, 48–59 years old are more likely in a still working status (labor force ratio as high as 78.2%), and this situation is consistent with China's retirement policy that men retire at 60 and women retire at 55. We thus select 60 years old as a threshold to stratify the whole pre-1970 migrants into (a) 48–59 years old cohort and (b) ≥60 years old for further comparative studies. The majority (78.2%) of the 48–59 years old age cohort are still working. According to the 2017 MDMS, it is reported that among the still working 48–59 years old age cohort, 59.7% of them are factory workers in the secondary industry assuming hard physical labor jobs. 8.3% of them came to Beijing to continue their agricultural activities. Only 7.4% of them are white-collars with more decent jobs in the governments, enterprises, and institutions. Few (0.6%) are engaged in the service work. The remaining 2.2% of them engage in flexible work.

Table 3 summarizes the main findings from the regression analysis. We will elaborate on the analysis results in the three models on the three-tiered measurement of social integration (practical, relational, and perceptual), respectively.

4.2.1. Explaining the Practical Dimension of Aging Migrants' Integration

Participation in local affairs (a binary variable: yes or no) is an indicator of aging migrants' integration measured by their actual participation practices (regardless of a small group-like community/neighborhood or the mass society of a city).

First, in the whole pre-1970 migrant population, the regression results in Table 3 display that a younger age ($p < 0.05$, OR = 0.976), higher educational level (significant, OR < 0.7), an employed status ($p < 0.1$, OR = 1.390), a longer stay in Beijing ($p < 0.001$, OR = 1.043) would be the significant indicators for those more active in local participation. Among all the indicators, human capital is the strongest to predict the aging migrants' probability of participation in local affairs. Well-educated aging migrants are more active in local affairs participation. The probability of local affairs participation in poorly educated populations (primary and below) is merely 0.251 times ($p < 0.001$), compared with those with a college degree and higher. It is thus proved that a lower educational background presents a significantly negative correlation to participation. Housing tenure type is proved the second strongest indicator to explain the variance of aging migrants' local affairs participation. Homeowners are more likely to participate in the local affairs in Beijing than those living in informal housing ($p < 0.001$, OR = 2.641).

Second, the regression analysis on the two age cohorts (48–59 years old and ≥60 years old) has reported the similar findings that younger age ($p < 0.001$, OR = 0.908; $p < 0.05$, OR = 0.942), higher educational level (significant, OR < 0.6), and a longer stay in Beijing (significant, OR = 1.041, OR = 1.061) are the significant indicators for those more active in local participation. The employed status is an insignificant factor when modeling the two age cohorts. There has been a decisive divide in employment status between the two age cohorts, and for this reason, the within-group variance of employment status in each age cohort becomes minor. Moreover, the housing tenure factor displays different associations with the participation in local affairs in Beijing. For instance, for the 48–59 age cohorts who are still working, living in the dormitory-like housing indicates a significantly higher odds of local affairs participation than living in the owned homes.

Table 3. Logistic regress on the pre-1970 migrants' integration: (a) all pre-1970; (b) ≥ 60 years old; and (c) < 60 years old & pre-1970.

	All Pre-1970 Migrants in Beijing						≥60 Years Old						<60 Years Old & Pre-1970					
	1. Local Affairs Participation		*2. Communication with Locals as the Most Frequent Contacts*		*3. Full Integration Perceived (SWB)*		*1. Local Affairs Participation*		*2. Communication with Locals as the Most Frequent Contacts*		*3. Full Integration Perceived (SWB)*		*1. Local Affairs Participation*		*2. Communication with Locals as the Most Frequent Contacts*		*3. Full Integration Perceived (SWB)*	
Predictors	*B*	*Exp(β)*	*B*	*Exp(β)*	*B*	*Exp(β)*	*B*	*Exp(β)*	*B*	*Exp(β)*	*B*	*Exp(β)*	*B*	*Exp(β)*	*B*	*Exp(β)*	*B*	*Exp(β)*
Household profile																		
Age (years old)	−0.024 **	0.976	−0.001	0.999	0.008	1.008	−0.060 **	0.942	−0.018	0.982	0.029	1.030	−0.096 ***	0.908	−0.081 **	0.923	0.042	1.043
Gender (ref = female)	0.016	1.016	−0.276 *	0.759	−0.048	0.953	0.051	1.052	−0.308	0.735	−0.511 **	0.600	0.101	1.106	−0.290	0.748	0.173	1.189
Marriage (ref = unmarried)	−0.276	0.759	−0.035	0.966	0.092	1.096	−0.303	0.739	0.254	1.277	0.731	2.078	−0.398	0.672	−0.821 *	0.440	−0.667	0.513
Education level (ref = college and higher)																		
Primary and below	−1.382 ***	0.251	−0.714 **	0.490	−0.338	0.713	−1.441 ***	0.237	−0.654	0.524	0.111	1.117	−1.089 **	0.337	−0.995 **	0.370	−0.978 *	0.376
Junior secondary	−1.002 ***	0.367	−0.326	0.722	−0.218	0.804	−1.182***	0.307	0.188	1.207	0.113	1.119	−0.649 *	0.523	−0.770 *	0.463	−0.868 *	0.420
Senior/technical secondary	−0.42 *	0.657	−0.172	0.842	0.300	1.349	−0.691**	0.501	−0.096	0.908	0.368	1.445	0.102	1.107	−0.224	0.799	−0.137	0.872
Logged familial income (annual, unit: yuan)	−0.494 **	0.610	−0.190	0.827	−0.228	0.796	−0.653 **	0.520	−0.246	0.782	0.100	1.105	−0.084	0.919	0.095	1.100	−0.753 *	0.471
Employment status (ref = retired/ unemployed)	0.329 *	1.390	−0.228	0.796	−0.555 **	0.574	0.227	1.255	0.073	1.076	−1.864 **	0.155	−0.087	0.917	−0.054	0.947	0.123	1.131
Migratory status																		
Hukou origin (ref = urban *hukou*)	−0.227	0.797	−0.512 **	0.599	0.118	1.125	−0.265	0.767	−0.476	0.621	0.012	1.012	−0.212	0.809	−0.523**	0.588	0.324	1.383
Duration of stay in Beijing (years)	0.042 ***	1.043	0.039 ***	1.040	0.043 ***	1.044	0.059 **	1.061	0.037 **	1.037	0.056 **	1.058	0.040 ***	1.041	0.043 ***	1.044	0.036 **	1.037
Migrate alone or together (ref = with family)	0.131	1.140	−0.361	0.697	0.383	1.467	0.390	1.477	−0.751	0.472	1.113	3.044	0.045	1.046	−0.699	0.497	−0.565	0.568
Place of origin (ref = North–Eastern China)																		
Eastern Region	−0.079	0.924	−0.066	0.936	−0.165	0.848	−0.316	0.729	−0.042	0.959	−0.679 *	0.507	0.101	1.106	0.058	1.060	0.147	1.158
North China	−0.013	0.987	0.215	1.240	−0.251	0.778	−0.039	0.962	0.038	1.038	−0.377	0.686	−0.021	0.979	0.375	1.455	−0.201	0.818
Central China	−0.001	0.999	0.002	0.995	−0.040	0.961	−0.311	0.733	−0.066	0.936	−0.063	0.939	0.129	1.137	0.183	1.210	0.150	1.162
South−Western Region	−0.130	0.874	−0.917 **	0.400	−0.051	0.951	−0.502	0.605	−0.150	0.860	−0.821	0.440	−0.026	0.974	−1.751 **	0.174	0.389	1.475
North−Western Region	−0.032	0.969	0.660 *	1.936	0.523	1.687	0.201	1.222	0.903 *	2.468	0.740	2.095	−0.241	0.786	−0.020	0.981	−0.056	0.946
Destination in Beijing metropolis (ref = Ecological Reserve Development Areas)																		
Core District of Capital Function	0.328	1.388	−0.891 **	0.410	−0.377	0.686	0.349	1.417	−2.109 ***	0.121	0.163	1.177	0.431	1.539	−0.520	0.595	−0.615	0.541
Urban Function Extended Districts	0.406	1.501	−1.112 ***	0.329	−0.487 *	0.614	0.796 *	2.216	−2.320 ***	0.098	−0.078	0.925	0.238	1.268	−0.659 *	0.517	−0.434	0.648
New Districts of Urban Development	0.304	1.355	−0.709 **	0.492	0.106	1.112	0.792	2.208	−1.844 **	0.158	0.895	2.448	0.079	1.082	−0.248	0.780	−0.043	0.958

Table 3. *Cont.*

	All Pre-1970 Migrants in Beijing						≥60 Years Old						<60 Years Old & Pre-1970					
	1. Local Affairs Participation		*2. Communication with Locals as the Most Frequent Contacts*		*3. Full Integration Perceived (SWB)*		*1. Local Affairs Participation*		*2. Communication with Locals as the Most Frequent Contacts*		*3. Full Integration Perceived (SWB)*		*1. Local Affairs Participation*		*2. Communication with Locals as the Most Frequent Contacts*		*3. Full Integration Perceived (SWB)*	
Housing−related factors																		
Housing tenure types (ref = Informal housing)																		
Self−owned commercial housing	0.971 ***	2.641	0.647 **	1.909	0.654 **	1.923	1.204 **	2.784	0.504	1.656	0.393	1.482	0.387	1.472	0.574 *	1.776	1.056 **	2.876
Dormitory−like from gov or employer units	0.475 **	1.607	0.142	1.153	−0.191	0.826	−0.002	0.998	0.797 *	2.219	0.146	1.158	0.697 **	2.008	−0.175	0.839	−0.428	0.652
Rental commercial housing	0.498 **	1.645	0.117	1.125	0.126	1.134	0.477	1.611	−0.145	0.865	0.083	1.086	0.401 *	1.493	0.121	1.128	0.183	1.201
Housing stress (expenditure−to−income ratio)	−0.214	0.807	0.212	1.237	0.219	1.244	−0.373	0.689	0.148	1.159	0.401	1.493	0.331	1.392	0.398	1.490	−0.479	0.619
Constant	2.857 **	17.415	0.800	2.226	−1.154	0.316	5.856 **	349.257	3.059	22.095	−4.642 **	0.010	5.088 **	162.008	4.089 *	59.675	−0.409	0.664
N	1267		1259		1267		495		495		495		772		772		772	
df	23		23		23		23		23		23		23		23		23	
λ^2	152.633		141.969		95.174		83.028		65.398		68.257		96.555		92.361		45.571	
−2 Log−Likelihood	1577.344		1285.410		1131.423		590.522		564.252		476.144		959.008		670.304		621.15	
Nagelkerke R^2	0.153		0.157		0.117		0.209		0.173		0.194		0.158		0.180		0.099	
Percent correctly classified	66.2%		76.2%		81.7%		67.2%		71.3%		75.4%		67.4%		81.1%		84.7%	

Note: Significant at * 0.1; ** 0.05; *** 0.001 level. The rare samples from the South-Eastern Region (N = 4) are detected as outliers and are deleted for this reason. Data source: MDMS, 2017.

4.2.2. Explaining the Relational Dimension of Aging Migrants' Integration

From a relational perspective, we use the "whether communication with the locals as the most frequent daily contacts" (the binary variable: yes or no) as the second dependent variable in this study. Daily communication contact is an important means for the aging migrants to integrate into mainstream society.

First, in the whole pre-1970 migrant population, regression results in Table 3 show that the female aging migrants ($p < 0.1$, OR = 0.759), those better educated ($p < 0.05$, OR = 0.490), an urban *hukou* origin ($p < 0.05$, OR = 0.599), and the longer stay in Beijing ($p < 0.001$, OR = 1.040) are more likely to list the local *Beijingese* as the primary communication contacts (instead of their own family- and clan-relationship or other populations). It is also found that geographical and locational-related factors matter. It is reported in Table 3 that the aging migrants whose place of origin shares similarities (in terms of customs, cultures, and languages) with Beijing are more easily inclusive in this contact dimension. Those from the South-Western Region in China ($p < 0.05$, OR = 0.400) face more barriers to integration. Beijing as a destination city is more inclusive for those migrating from vast North China. Moreover, those choosing a residential location in Beijing's more peripheral Ecological Reserve Development Areas (significant, OR < 0.5) are more probably interactive with the local *Beijingese*. Aging migrants living in the urban centers are more easily excluded from the local people's network. However, these peripheral areas are more inclusive, as native people in peripheries hold an "outsider identity" in the capital-city culture which is urban-center-dominated. In addition, Ecological Reserve Development Areas are located in the nature-human interface, creating a better contact and recreation atmosphere for the aging migrants. More research can be conducted to explore the inter-variance of integration between different locations within a metropolis.

The impact of housing tenure type on the aging migrants' daily communication contacts is significant ($p < 0.05$, OR = 1.909), but not as prominent as those when modeling the associations with local affairs participation. Compared with those in informal housing, homeowners are significantly more interactive and communicative with the local *Beijingese* ($p < 0.05$, OR = 1.909). However, such a contact difference is insignificant between those living in the dormitory-like housing (provided by governments or employer units), rental commercial housing, and informal housing.

Second, the regression analysis on the two age cohorts (48–59 years old and ≥60 years old) has reported that the gender is insignificant. The education level and *hukou* origin are insignificant for older age cohorts (≥60 years old), but remain significant for younger still working age cohorts (48–59 years old); higher educational level (significant, OR < 0.5), and urban *hukou* origin ($p < 0.05$, OR = 0.588) are the significant indicators for still working groups' daily communication contacts. The longer stays in Beijing (significant, OR = 1.044, OR = 1.037) are a significant indicator for both age cohorts' daily communication contacts. The similarity or disparity between the place of origin and Beijing also plays a significant role in the older or younger age cohorts' local communications. A similar inter-variance of integration between different locations within a metropolis is reported, too, in the modeling of the two age cohorts (48–59 years old and ≥60 years old). However, housing is found to have different associations with the younger or older cohorts' daily communication contacts. For instance, when younger still working age cohorts (48–59 years old) are living in the owned homes, they have significantly higher odds of local communications than those living in informal housing. However, when older age cohorts (≥60 years old) are living in the dormitory-like housing, they would report the highest odds of local communications. The complicated two- or three-generation co-living status can explain such a difference for the retired migrant populations.

4.2.3. Explaining the Perceptual Dimension of Aging Migrants' Integration

Subjective well-being (SWB) is a widely used integration indicator in previous studies. Interestingly, human capital did not report significant associations of educational levels with the aging migrants' integration.

First, in the whole pre-1970 migrant population, the subjective identity of retired or unemployed aging migrants is significantly stronger than that of their still working peers ($p < 0.05$, OR = 0.574)—that is, the probability of a full integration status perceived (SWB) among bread earners is only 57.4% of that for the retired or unemployed aging migrants. Age discrimination against job seekers has a trend of convergence towards 45 years old [9]. Disadvantaged aging migrants face more difficulties adapting to the age limit in the employment markets. However, those who have retired may have more pride than the migrant workers, as they dwell with kids who have probably already acquired Beijing *hukou*. In addition, a longer stay in Beijing ($p < 0.001$, OR = 1.044) predicts a higher probability of full integration status perceived (SWB) by the aging migrants. Those living in the "Urban Function Extended Districts" report the lowest probability (61.4%) to perceive a fully integrated status (SWB), compared with those in the Ecological Reserve Development Areas ($p < 0.1$, OR = 0.614). A rampant migrant enclave demolition in the Urban Function Extended Districts can explain this result [60].

The homeowners report the highest probability of perceiving a fully integrated status (SWB), compared with those living in informal housing ($p < 0.05$, OR = 1.923). Interestingly, those dwelling in the dormitory-like housing (from governments or employers) report a lower ratio of perceiving a fully integrated status (SWB) than those living in informal housing, despite that the regression coefficient is insignificant. More case studies are needed to explore the specific reasons behind it.

Second, the regression analysis on the two age cohorts (48–59 years old and ≥60 years old) has reported that a longer stay in Beijing can predict a higher probability of full integration status perceived (SWB) in both the two age cohorts. The employment status is still significant for older age cohorts (≥60 years old), but insignificant for younger still working age cohorts (48–59 years old)—that is, the odds of the full integration status perceived (SWB) among the bread earners in the older age cohorts (≥60 years old) is merely 15.5% of that for the retired or unemployed peers. It is also reported that the education level is significant for younger still working age cohorts (48–59 years old); a higher educational level can predict a higher odds of full integration status perceived (SWB) for still working groups. Interestingly, housing tenure is insignificant for the older age cohorts' (≥60 years old) full integration status perceived (SWB), but home-owning plays a significant role to predict the higher odds of the full integration status perceived (SWB) among the younger still working age cohorts (48–59 years old). Among the older age cohorts who have retried, homeowners in Beijing are probably their sons or daughters. The household-level tenure- and *hukou* structure within the two- and three-generation relationships can shed light on this nuance.

5. Discussion

5.1. Reinterpreting Social Integration in the Chinese Urbanizing Regime

One of the most classic theories concerning social integration is assimilationism, which was originally put forward by the Chicago School during the prosperous Western industrialization and immigrant flow-in periods before World War II [61]. Social integration has been defined as a process of fusion, in which immigrants and locals adopt the memories, sentiments, and attitudes of one another, and through such incorporation form a common cultural life. Interestingly, the Chicago School drew on Emile Durkheim and Herbert Spencer's thoughts to understand the complex processes of socio-spatial differentiation that involve both social fragmentation and social integration (namely the secondary institutions performing the crucial social integration functions) and at the same time can achieve relative stability and equilibrium.

In the post-World War II studies in the OECD countries, social integration refers to a person's sense of belonging or attachment. As defined by Keyes (1998: 122), integration is "the extent to which people feel they have something in common with others who constitute their social reality, as well as the degree to which they feel that they belong to their communities and society" [62]. As revealed by Fischer in his review of the social integration literature, the older adults, homeowners, the better educated, the wealthy, women, whites, longtime residents, and people with children were found to be more socially integrated than their younger, renting, less-educated, poorer, male, nonwhite, short-term residents, and childless counterparts [63]. In addition to those social status characteristics, urbanism has close associations with social interaction, too, though no clear consensus exists. For instance, Fischer suggested that people in urban centers are just as socially integrated and satisfied with their lives as suburban residents if analysis controls for socioeconomic and demographic factors [63]. Community and investments in it have associations with social integration, too. Long-term residents and homeowners are found more likely to participate in local events and have friends, and for this reason, home ownership and length of residence are treated as indicators of social ties and integration [64–66].

However, new waves of immigration in the post-World War II had transformed American cities into spaces of ethnic diversity and reproduced a highly differentiated social landscape in contemporary metropolises such as Los Angeles. One of the central interests of urban studies has been the quest to understand the extent of social isolation or social segregation, which is the opposite of social integration. The Los Angeles School drew from Marxist, poststructuralist, and postmodern theories to interpret the city as a highly differentiated, conflictual, and divided space. Social isolation or social segregation represents a breakdown of social integration that otherwise can provide social support or a sense of belonging. The social and spatial dimensions of integration (or lack of it) are considered interchangeable in the emerging "divided cities" in the USA, but Musterd, Ostendorf, and Galster pointed out it is still unclear whether more social contact or neighborhood mixing between different people does indeed result in a higher level of integration [50,51,67]. The UK attracted most immigrants from former colonies in the post-World War II period but triggered some serious conflicts, too. The focus is on how to establish social unity and welfare equality in a culturally diverse society. Adachi defined social integration as a situation in which social unity co-exists with cultural diversity, and people with different backgrounds can share the same concept of society [68].

Under the profound impact of the *hukou* system, the definition and demonstration of social integration in China are different from that in the Western contexts. For instance, the existing studies on the massive internal migration in China paid much attention to the integration, permanent settlement, and *hukou* transfer initiatives. However, little attention is given to the integration of the pre-1970 first-generation migrants, who were born before the year 1970 and getting old in the destination cities. The pre-1970 migrants have a wide range of age cohorts in urban China: (a) those over 45 years old and still working but facing the age discrimination challenges in employment markets; and (b) de facto elderly migrants who are already retired but also facing the difficulties adapting to living environments in the destination city, because they assume the domestic and child-care work for their sons or daughters but have few chances for out-of-home leisure or local communication contact.

In this study, we have adopted and improved Ager and Strang's conceptualization of social integration, as well as Chen and Wang's migrant integration analysis framework in the Chinese megacity contexts [52,54], and then re-defined aging migrants' social integration in an innovated triple dimension (i.e., participation practices, communication contacts, and subjective perceptions). We use the social integration data from Beijing's aging migrant samples, which were collected from the 2017 Migrant Dynamics Monitoring Survey (MDMS), to measure and explain the varied integration levels among a total of 1267 aging migrant samples. The three dimensions of social integration in the Chinese urbanizing context can fill the practical, relational, and perceptual/psychological aspects in conventional social integration studies.

5.2. Main Findings

First, the housing tenure security has proven to be a strong indicator to explain the variance of aging migrants' local affairs participation (Hypothesis 1). When explaining the local affairs participation of all the pre-1970 migrants, the practical-dimensional integration stays almost the same when living in a dormitory-like housing (provided by local governments or employer units) or a rental commercial housing acquired from markets (OR = 1.607, OR = 1.645, respectively). It thus indicates that the formality/informality is an important indicator of aging migrants' local affairs participation. However, the variance of suppliers (governments, employers, markets) is not a convincing indicator of integration levels. Home occupation matters in integration. The associations between tenure and local affairs participations vary with the different age cohorts. For instance, in all pre-1970 migrant populations, homeowners are more likely to participate in local affairs than those living in informal housing. A similar conclusion stands when it refers to the older age cohorts who are above 60 years old and mostly retired. Interestingly, the analysis did not detect a significant variance of tenure-participation nexus between home-owning and informal housing dwelling for the 48–59 age cohorts who are still working. For the 48–59 age cohorts, living in the dormitory-like housing indicates the significantly higher odds of local affairs participation than living in the owned homes. A relatively low proportion of the 48–59 age cohorts in well-paid occupations can explain the homeowning-participation paradox in the still working groups.

Second, the analysis results also show that the life cycle matters (Hypothesis 2), and the analysis reveals the employment-income paradox in explaining aging migrants' social integration in Beijing. In the whole pre-1970 migrants in Beijing, a higher income level predicts a lower probability of local affairs participation ($p < 0.05$, OR = 0.610), which was in contradiction with previous research findings. The bread earners report a higher ratio for local affairs participation ($p < 0.1$, OR = 1.390) than those retired or unemployed, while the income level has an opposite association with local affairs participation ($p < 0.05$, OR = 0.610). Such an employment-income paradox is interpretative when there exists a large group of retired migrants, living with their sons or daughters and caring for grandchildren in the destination city. Their aggregated household income is reported high, but "granny as a nanny" has little time for out-of-home leisure and local communication contacts, when assuming domestic and child-care work for sons or daughters. This reported high-income status is accompanied by the specific segregation status, as "granny as a nanny" has left their familiar environment and social networks in their hometown while floating in the destination city. This demonstrates that higher economic achievement is NOT equivalent to a higher social integration status for the aging migrants in a great metropolis such as Beijing.

Third, we can also detect a complex interplay between housing tenure heterogeneity and life cycle heterogeneity (Hypothesis 1 × Hypothesis 2). For instance, for the whole pre-1970 migrant population, the homeowners are significantly more interactive and communicative with the local *Beijingese* ($p < 0.05$, OR = 1.909) than those in informal housing. However, housing is found to have different associations with the different cohorts' communication contacts. Homeownership is still a significant indicator for the younger still working age cohorts' (48–59 years old) local communication contacts. Yet when it comes to the older age cohorts ($\geq$60 years old), those living in the dormitory-like housing have reported the highest odds of the local communications. Further research is needed to explore the two- or three-generation co-living structure. More detailed household-level data analysis can explain this nuance. It is also found that housing tenure is insignificant for the older age cohorts' ($\geq$60 years old) full integration status perceived (SWB), but home-owning plays a significant role to predict higher odds of the full integration status perceived (SWB) among the younger still working age cohorts (48–59 years old). Among the older age cohorts who have retried, homeowners in Beijing are probably their sons or daughters. The household-level tenure- and *hukou* structure within the two- and three-generation relationships can shed light on this nuance.

6. Conclusions

The data analysis findings are illuminating to guide follow-up studies. First, housing tenure matters. The securities of migrants' housing tenure (i.e., migrants as home-occupiers in the destination cities) can significantly beef up their integration, while the insecurities of housing tenure (e.g., informal housing) can lower their integration. Housing tenure entitlement is therefore conducive to beefing up the aging migrants' integration. This research result can fulfill the findings from previous studies. For instance, Lin et al. divided housing into different types, and then put them into three models to measure the migrants' urban attachment [69]. Yang et al. also used different types of urban villages in Shenzhen as an independent variable to analyze their impact on the migrants' social integration [70]. Our empirical study contributed to another case study on Beijing's pre-1970 migrants, and further supported the conclusion that the housing tenure security and entitlement are conducive to the aging migrants' social integration process.

Second, different indicators exert a differentiated impact on the three-tiered measurement of social integration (practical, relational, and perceptual). For instance, the associations of human capital with integration are significant in the practical and relational dimensions, but insignificant in the perceptual dimension. The contrast between the paid employment status vs. those in a retired status (see the indicator of "employment status") has indeed reported the differentiated impact on integration processes, and this differentiation is significant in the practical and perceptual dimensions, but insignificant in a relational dimension. This research also pointed out an employment-income paradox, which shows that higher economic achievement is NOT equivalent to a higher social integration status for the aging migrants. Their aggregated household income is reported high, but the "granny as a nanny" faces segregation problems in terms of local affair participation. More detailed surveys on representative migrant households would be helpful to figure out the specific mechanism behind such an employment-income paradox on integration. It is also reported that the still working migrants have less satisfaction or pride than their retired peers in the perceptual dimension of integration. The retired groups may dwell with their kids who have probably already acquired the Beijing *hukou*, and probably, for this reason, a retirement status indicates a higher probability of full integration status perceived (SWB). The family data of the 2017 MDMS shows that: (a) among all the pre-1970 samples, 224 households are co-living between the granny/grandpa and the grandson/granddaughter (approaching 20% in all the targeted pre-1970 samples); and (b) interestingly, among them, 115 grandsons/granddaughters hold the local Beijing *hukou*. Such a unified three-generation family structure can support the saying of "granny as a nanny", which is a popular *"laopiao"* phenomenon in Beijing. Further research is needed to probe into the complicated *hukou* arrangement within a family and its impact on the aging people's social integration.

Finally, is informal housing a sign of segregation? The answer is uncertain and varies with specific case studies. As reported in Table 2 concerning with communication contacts index and SWB index, those dwelling in informal housing have reported the same or even higher level of integration, compared with those living in the dormitory-like housing provided by the local governments or employers. The regression results also report that the contact variance is insignificant between those living in informal housing, dormitory-like housing, and rental commercial housing. It is also reported that those dwelling in the dormitory-like housing have a lower ratio of perceiving a fully integrated status (SWB) than those living in informal housing, despite that its regression coefficient is insignificant. Is it reasonable to justify the dispossession by stigmatizing informal housing as a segregated world [71]? More empirical studies are needed to reveal the relational and functional nature of the so-called "informal" property rights in transitional China.

This research contributed another empirical study on Beijing's aging migrants to social integration studies. First, the aging of the global population is the most important medical and social demographic problem worldwide. The World Health Organization (WHO) has defined healthy aging as a process of maintaining the functional ability to enable well-being in older age. This article focuses on social integration as crucial to measuring the healthy aging of migrants, filling for the practical, relational, and perceptual/psychological aspects (see Figure 2) of healthy aging studies. The second contribution is the findings on the housing tenure impact on the social integration of the pre-1970 first-generation migrants in reformist China. Hypothesis 1 on housing tenure heterogeneity is proved in our study. However, it is found that those living in the informal housing have a higher probability of perceiving a fully integrated status (subjective well-being, SWB) than those living in the formalized dormitory-like housing. These findings shed light on the housing formalization policies in megacities in China: the physical demolition of migrant enclaves would also cut down their active social bonding and positive subjective well-being, which deserves more attention in policy making. More comparative studies on the social impact of informal migrant enclaves in the fast-urbanizing countries (i.e., China, India, and Latin America) can shed light on the global debates on "ageism and urbanization" [72]. For instance, is the destination city age-friendly, and how can we promote the urbanization pattern through the lens of old age? Third, our research reveals the geographies of aging among migrants, and different situations between younger (48–59 years old) and older (≥60 years old) of the pre-1970 cohorts. Hypothesis 2 on the life cycle heterogeneity is proved, too. This nuance of aging migrants deserves more attention in further studies.

As elaborated above, the strengths of this research are manifested: (a) a more comprehensive definition of aging migrants' social integration, filling for the practical, relational, and perceptual/psychological aspects (see Figure 2) of healthy aging studies; (b) critical thinking on the role of informal housing and migrant enclaves in the migrants' integration that can shed more light on the global debates on "ageism and urbanization"; and (c) the nuance of aging migrants in terms of "housing tenure heterogeneity" (Hypothesis 1) and "life cycle heterogeneity" (Hypothesis 2) in their social integration processes. The weakness of this study is that we have started to pay attention to the complicated life cycle and the family-based *hukou* package that have exerted profound impact on the aging migrants' integration into Beijing. However, we did not investigate and reveal their mechanism at a more detailed household scale. Further research can depict the specific impact of life cycle and household-level strategies (such as the *hukou* package within a family and three-generation relations) on the aging migrants' social integration. Policy makers should take some conservative interventions in the informal housing management, including providing more age-friendly environments, facilities, and services in the migrant enclaves. The age-friendly *hukou* reforms are needed, too, to entitle more benefits for the two- or three-generation migrant households.

Author Contributions: Writing—original draft preparation, Y.Z., W.C., X.L.; supervision, R.L. All authors have read and agreed to the published version of the manuscript.

Funding: This research was funded by a grant from the National Natural Science Foundation of China (NSFC project number: 42071201), and a grant from the Beijing Philosophy and Social Science Planning Program and Social Science Research Key Program of Beijing Municipal Commission of Education (project number: SZ202010028016).

Institutional Review Board Statement: Not applicable.

Informed Consent Statement: Not applicable.

Data Availability Statement: Data use of the 2017 Migrant Dynamics Monitoring Survey (MDMS) is supported and approved by the Migrant Population Service Center, the National Health Commission of China. https://www.chinaldrk.org.cn/wjw/#/home (accessed on 11 April 2022).

Conflicts of Interest: The authors declare no conflict of interest.

References

1. Montes de Oca, V.; García, T.R.; Sáenz, R.; Guillén, J. The Linkage of Life Course, Migration, Health, and Aging: Health in Adults and Elderly Mexican Migrants. *J. Aging Health* **2011**, *23*, 1116–1140. [CrossRef]
2. Kristiansen, M.; Razum, O.; Tezcan-Güntekin, H.; Krasnik, A. Aging and health among migrants in a European perspective. *Public Health Rev.* **2016**, *37*, 1–14. [CrossRef]
3. World Health Organization. Global strategy and action plan on ageing and health 2016–2020: Towards a world in which everyone can live a long and healthy life. In Proceedings of the Sixty-Ninth World Health Assembly, Geneva, Switzerland, 23–29 May 2016.
4. The WHO Regional Office for Europe. Building healthy cities: Inclusive, safe, resilient and sustainable. In Proceedings of the WHO European Healthy Cities Network Annual Business and Technical Conference, Pécs, Hungary, 1–3 March 2017.
5. Warner, M.; Zhu, Y. The challenges of managing "new generation" employees in contemporary China: Setting the scene. *Asia Pac. Bus. Rev.* **2018**, *24*, 429–436. [CrossRef]
6. He, S.; Wang, K. China's New Generation Migrant Workers' Urban Experience and Well-Being. In *Mobility, Sociability and Well-being of Urban Living*; Wang, D., He, S., Eds.; Springer: Berlin/Heidelberg, Germany, 2016; pp. 67–91.
7. Amber, D.; Domingo, J. The Discourse on the Unemployment of People over 45 Years Old in Times of Crisis. A Study of Spanish Blogs. *J. Aging Soc. Policy* **2016**, *7*, 63–78.
8. Drydakis, N.; MacDonald, P.; Chiotis, V.; Somers, L. Age Discrimination in the UK Labour Market. Does Race Moderate Ageism? An Experimental Investigation. *Appl. Econ. Lett.* **2018**, *25*, 1–4. [CrossRef]
9. Wu, K.; Sun, C.L. Research on Age Discrimination against Job Seekers Based on Recruitment Advertisements. *Open Access Libr. J.* **2021**, *8*, 1–11. [CrossRef]
10. Liu, Z.; Wang, Y.; Tao, R. Social capital and migrant housing experiences in urban China: A structural equation modeling analysis. *Hous. Stud.* **2013**, *28*, 1155–1174. [CrossRef]
11. King, K. Jane Jacobs and "the need for aged buildings": Neighbourhood historical development pace and community social relations. *Urban Stud.* **2013**, *50*, 2407–2424. [CrossRef] [PubMed]
12. Chan, K.W. China's *Hukou* System at 60: Continuity and Reform. In *Handbook on Urban Development in China*; Yep, R., Wang, J., Johnson, T., Eds.; Edward Elgar: Cheltenham, UK, 2019; pp. 59–79.
13. Gu, H. Understanding the migration of highly and less-educated labourers in post-reform China. *Appl. Geogr.* **2021**, *137*, 102605. [CrossRef]
14. State Council. Opinion on Further Reform of the Hukou System. Beijing; 30 July 2014. Available online: http://www.gov.cn/zhengce/content/2014-07/30/content_8944.htm (accessed on 12 April 2022). (In Chinese)
15. NDRC (National Development and Reform Commission). Memo on Promoting Experiences Based on the Third Group of Comprehensive Pilot Cities in New-Type of Urbanization. 26 August 2021. Available online: http://www.gov.cn/zhengce/zhengceku/2021-08/31/content_5634330.htm (accessed on 12 April 2022). (In Chinese)
16. Li, Y.; Xiong, C.; Zhu, Z.; Lin, Q. Family Migration and Social Integration of Migrants: Evidence from Wuhan Metropolitan Area, China. *Int. J. Environ. Res. Public Health* **2021**, *18*, 12983. [CrossRef]
17. Yue, Z.; Li, S.; Jin, X.; Feldman, M. The Role of Social Networks in the Integration of Chinese Rural-Urban Migrants: A Migrant-Resident Tie Perspective. *Urban Stud.* **2013**, *50*, 1704–1723. [CrossRef]
18. Zou, J.; Chen, Y.; Chen, J. The complex relationship between neighbourhood types and migrants' socio-economic integration: The case of urban China. *J. Hous. Built Environ.* **2020**, *35*, 65–92. [CrossRef]
19. Lin, S.; Zhang, F.; Wu, F. Contrasting migrants' sense of belonging to the city in selected peri-urban neighbourhoods in Beijing. *Cities* **2022**, *120*, 103499.
20. Lin, S.; Wu, F.; Li, Z. Social integration of migrants across Chinese neighbourhoods. *Geoforum* **2020**, *112*, 118–128. [CrossRef]
21. Logan, J.R.; Spitze, G.D. Family Neighbors. *Am. J. Sociol.* **2002**, *100*, 453–476. [CrossRef]
22. Campbell, K.E.; Lee, B.A. Sources of Personal Neighbor Networks: Social Integration, Need, or Time? *Soc. Forces* **1992**, *70*, 1077–1100. [CrossRef]
23. Kweon, B.S.; Sullivan, W.C.; Wiley, A.R. Green Common Spaces and the Social Integration of Inner-City Older Adults. *Environ. Behav.* **1998**, *30*, 832–858. [CrossRef]
24. Lin, S.; Huang, Y. Community environmental satisfaction: Its forms and impact on migrants' happiness in urban China. *Health Qual. Life Outcomes* **2018**, *16*, 236. [CrossRef]
25. Tang, S.; Lee, H.; Feng, J. Social capital, built environment and mental health: A comparison between the local elderly people and the "*laopiao*" in urban China. *Ageing Soc.* **2020**, *42*, 179–203. [CrossRef]
26. Lu, S.; Chen, S.; Wang, P. Language barriers and health status of elderly migrants: Micro-evidence from China. *China Econ. Rev.* **2019**, *54*, 94–112. [CrossRef]
27. Cheng, Y.; Rosenberg, M.; Winterton, R.; Blackberry, I.; Gao, S. Mobilities of Older Chinese Rural-Urban Migrants: A Case Study in Beijing. *Int. J. Environ. Res. Public Health* **2019**, *16*, 488. [CrossRef]
28. Liu, Y.; Dijst, M.; Faber, J.; Geertman, S.; Cui, C. Healthy urban living: Residential environment and health of older adults in Shanghai. *Health Place* **2017**, *47*, 80–89. [CrossRef]
29. Feng, J.; Tang, S.; Chuai, X. The impact of neighbourhood environments on quality of life of elderly people: Evidence from Nanjing, China. *Urban Stud.* **2018**, *55*, 2020–2039. [CrossRef]

30. Yan, B.; Gao, X.; Lyon, M. Modeling satisfaction amongst the elderly in different Chinese urban neighborhoods. *Soc. Sci. Med.* **2014**, *118*, 127–134. [CrossRef] [PubMed]
31. Wang, Y.; Wang, Z.; Zhou, C.; Liu, Y.; Liu, S. On the Settlement of the Floating Population in the Pearl River Delta: Understanding the Factors of Permanent Settlement Intention versus Housing Purchase Actions. *Nat. Sustain.* **2020**, *12*, 9771. [CrossRef]
32. Yang, S.; Guo, F. Breaking the barriers: How urban housing ownership has changed migrants' settlement intentions in China. *Urban Stud.* **2018**, *55*, 3689–3707. [CrossRef]
33. Song, Y.; Zhang, C. City size and housing purchase intention: Evidence from rural–urban migrants in China. *Urban Stud.* **2020**, *57*, 1866–1886. [CrossRef]
34. Wang, M.; Ning, Y. The Social Integration of Migrants in Shanghai's Urban Villages. *China Rev.* **2016**, *16*, 93–120.
35. Wu, Y.; Chen, J.; Bian, Z.; Wang, H.; Wang, Z. Housing, Housing Stratification, and Chinese Urban Residents' Social Satisfaction: Evidence from a National Household Survey. *Soc. Indic. Res.* **2020**, *152*, 653–671. [CrossRef]
36. Rex, J. The Concept of Housing Class and the Sociology of Race Relations. *Race Cl.* **1971**, *12*, 293–301. [CrossRef]
37. Zheng, S.; Song, Z.; Sun, W. Do affordable housing programs facilitate migrants' social integration in Chinese cities? *Cities* **2020**, *96*, 102449. [CrossRef]
38. Zeng, H.; Yu, X.; Zhang, J. Urban village demolition, migrant workers' rental costs and housing choices: Evidence from Hangzhou, China. *Cities* **2019**, *94*, 70–79. [CrossRef]
39. Xie, S.; Chen, J. Beyond homeownership: Housing conditions, housing support and rural migrant urban settlement intentions in China. *Cities* **2018**, *78*, 76–86. [CrossRef]
40. Manturuk, K.; Lindblad, M.; Quercia, R. Friends and Neighbors: Homeownership and Social Capital among Low- To Moderate-Income Families. *J. Urban Aff.* **2010**, *32*, 471–488. [CrossRef]
41. Joshi, N.K. Local house prices and mental health. *Int. J. Health Econ. Manag.* **2016**, *16*, 89–102. [CrossRef]
42. Park, G.R.; Jung, Y. Housing insecurity and health among people in South Korea: Focusing on tenure and affordability. *Public Health* **2019**, *171*, 116–122. [CrossRef]
43. Chen, C.; Fan, C. China's *Hukou* puzzle: Why don't rural migrants want urban *Hukou*? *China Rev.* **2016**, *16*, 9–39.
44. Chen, J.; Wang, W. Economic incentives and settlement intentions of rural migrants: Evidence from China. *J. Urban Aff.* **2019**, *41*, 372–389. [CrossRef]
45. Fanelli, A. Extensiveness of Communication Contacts and Perceptions of the Community. *Am. Sociol. Rev.* **1956**, *21*, 439–445. [CrossRef]
46. Brown, R. *Explanation in Social Science*; Routledge: New York, NY, USA, 2010.
47. Gracia, E.; Herrero, J. Determinants of social integration in the community: An exploratory analysis of personal, interpersonal and situational variables. *J. Community Appl. Soc.* **2004**, *14*, 1–15. [CrossRef]
48. Lewicka, M. What makes neighborhood different from home and city? Effects of place scale on place attachment. *J. Environ. Psychol.* **2010**, *30*, 35–51. [CrossRef]
49. Kleinhans, R. Social implications of housing diversification in urban renewal: A review of recent literature. *J. Hous. Built Environ.* **2004**, *19*, 367–390. [CrossRef]
50. Vaughan, L.; Arbaci, S. The Challenges of Understanding Urban Segregation. *J. Hous. Built Environ.* **2011**, *37*, 128–138. [CrossRef]
51. Galster, G.; Andersson, R.; Musterd, S. Who is affected by neighbourhood income mix? Gender, age, family, employment and income differences. *Urban Stud.* **2010**, *47*, 2915–2944. [CrossRef]
52. Ager, A.; Strang, A. Understanding Integration: A Conceptual Framework. *J. Refug. Stud.* **2008**, *21*, 166–191. [CrossRef]
53. Castles, S.; Korac, M.; Vasta, E.; Vertovec, S. *Integration: Mapping the Field*; Report of a project carried out by the Centre for Migration and Policy Research and Refugee Studies Centre for the Home Office; University of Oxford: Oxford, UK, 2001.
54. Chen, Y.; Wang, J. Social integration of new-generation migrants in Shanghai China. *Habitat Int.* **2015**, *49*, 419–425. [CrossRef]
55. Huang, Y.; Tao, R. Housing migrants in Chinese cities: Current status and policy design. *Environ. Plan. C* **2015**, *33*, 640–660. [CrossRef]
56. Liu, R.; Wong, T.C.; Liu, S. Peasants' counterplots against the state monopoly of the rural urbanization process: Urban villages and "small property housing" in Beijing, China. *Environ. Plan. A* **2012**, *44*, 1219–1240. [CrossRef]
57. Wu, W. Sources of Migrant Housing Disadvantage in Urban China. *Environ. Plan. A* **2004**, *36*, 1285–1304. [CrossRef]
58. Huang, Y.; Yi, C. Invisible migrant enclaves in Chinese cities: Underground living in Beijing, China. *Urban Stud.* **2015**, *52*, 2948–2973. [CrossRef]
59. Yu, J.; Rosenberg, M.W. Aging and the changing urban environment: The relationship between older people and the living environment in post-reform Beijing, China. *Urban Geogr.* **2019**, *41*, 162–181. [CrossRef]
60. Liu, R.; Wong, T.C. Urban village redevelopment in Beijing: The state-dominated formalization of informal housing. *Cities* **2018**, *72*, 160–172. [CrossRef]
61. Park, R.E.; Burgess, E.W. *Introduction to the Science of Sociology*; University of Chicago Press: Chicago, IL, USA, 1921.
62. Keyes, C. Social Well-Being. *Soc. Psychol. Q.* **1998**, *61*, 121–140. [CrossRef]
63. Fischer, C. *To Dwell among Friends*; University of Chicago Press: Chicago, IL, USA, 1982.
64. Dorvil, H.; Morin, P.; Beaulieu, A.; Robert, D. Housing as a social integration factor for people classified as mentally ill. *Hous. Stud.* **2005**, *20*, 497–519. [CrossRef]

65. Keene, D.; Bader, M.; Ailshire, J. Length of residence and social integration: The contingent effects of neighborhood poverty. *Health Place* **2013**, *21*, 171–178. [CrossRef]
66. Adams, R.E.; Serpe, R.T. Social Integration, Fear of Crime, and Life Satisfaction. *Sociol. Perspect.* **2000**, *43*, 605–629. [CrossRef]
67. Musterd, S.; Ostendorf, W. Residential segregation and integration in the Netherlands. *J. Ethn. Migr. Stud.* **2009**, *35*, 1515–1532. [CrossRef]
68. Adachi, S. Social Integration in Post-Multiculturalism: An Analysis of Social Integration Policy in Post-war Britain. *Int. J. Jpn. Sociol.* **2011**, *20*, 107–120. [CrossRef]
69. Lin, S.; Wu, F.; Li, Z. Beyond neighbouring: Migrants' place attachment to their host cities in China. *Popul. Space Place* **2021**, *27*, e2374. [CrossRef]
70. Yang, G.; Zhou, C.; Jin, W. Integration of migrant workers: Differentiation among three rural migrant enclaves in Shenzhen. *Cities* **2020**, *96*, 102453. [CrossRef]
71. Zhang, M.; He, S. Informal Property Rights as Relational and Functional: Unravelling the Relational Contract in China's Informal Housing Market. *Int. J. Urban Reg. Res.* **2020**, *44*, 967–988. [CrossRef]
72. Finlay, J.M.; Finn, B.M. Geography's blind spot: The age-old urban question. *Urban Geogr.* **2021**, *42*, 1061–1078. [CrossRef]

International Journal of
Environmental Research and Public Health

MDPI

Article

How to Evaluate Investment Efficiency of Environmental Pollution Control: Evidence from China

Xiaochun Zhao [1], Laichun Long [1], Qun Sun [1] and Wei Zhang [2,*]

[1] School of Management, Anhui University, Hefei 230601, China; 14006@ahu.edu.cn (X.Z.); l21201027@stu.ahu.edu.cn (L.L.); sunqun320@126.com (Q.S.)
[2] School of Public Administration, Sichuan University, Chengdu 610065, China
* Correspondence: hbue_wb@163.com; Tel.: +86-180-6200-9973

Abstract: Clarifying the efficiency of investment in environmental pollution control is conducive to better control of environmental pollution. Based on panel data of 30 provinces and cities in China from 2008 to 2017, this study combines the three-stage super-efficient SBM-DEA model and the Global-Malmquist-Luenberger index to measure the efficiency of investment in environmental pollution control in China and analyze regional differences. The results show that: First, the investment efficiency of environmental pollution control in China shows a rising trend year by year, but there are significant differences among provinces and regions; the presence of random factors and environmental variables makes the control efficiency underestimated. Second, excluding the effects of both, the national investment efficiency of environmental pollution control has improved significantly, but still has not reached the optimal effect; the gap between provinces and regions has narrowed while the investment efficiency of environmental pollution control has improved, and there is still an unbalanced situation. Third, the main driver of the year-on-year improvement in China's environmental pollution control efficiency is technological progress; compared with northeastern China, technological progress has a more significant role in promoting eastern, central, and western China. Finally, based on the results, this paper focuses on making suggestions to promote environmental pollution control in China in terms of making regional cooperation, making good environmental protection investment and strengthening environmental protection technology research and development.

Keywords: environmental pollution control investment efficiency; three-stage DEA; super-efficient SBM; Global-Malmquist-Luenberger index; regional differences

Citation: Zhao, X.; Long, L.; Sun, Q.; Zhang, W. How to Evaluate Investment Efficiency of Environmental Pollution Control: Evidence from China. *IJERPH* **2022**, *19*, 7252. https://doi.org/10.3390/ijerph19127252

Academic Editors: Jie Chen, Qian Zhou and Ting Zhang

Received: 25 April 2022
Accepted: 9 June 2022
Published: 13 June 2022

1. Introduction

Since the reform and opening up in 1978, China has experienced rapid economic growth. From a poor and backward developing country to become the second largest economy in the world and has the largest foreign exchange reserves in the world. However, the process of industrialization and urbanization has also brought serious environmental pollution problems [1], which is becoming increasingly serious and directly affects the daily lives of residents as well as the long-term development. Nearly half of China's water sources cannot be used for drinking water, and the water quality of large reservoirs and lakes is generally poor [2]. The annual generation of industrial solid waste is among the highest in the world, and white pollution caused by plastic packaging and agricultural films can be seen everywhere [3,4]. While the economy is developing rapidly, it is urgent to seek a harmonious relationship between humans and the environment. It is noteworthy that the Chinese government has long been aware of the destruction of the environment due to various types of pollution, and a large amount of funds and various policies have gradually tilted toward the field of environmental pollution management. From 1981 to 2017, the investment in environmental protection increased from 2.5 billion yuan to

953.89 billion yuan. The increasing scale of environmental protection investment amount has failed to address the root cause of environmental pollution problems, and the effect of environmental pollution management in China is still not optimistic, with different degrees of environmental pollution problems in various provinces. However, the actual situation of the efficiency of investment in environmental pollution management in China's regions and provinces is currently unclear. There are differences in environmental protection investment efforts, environmental protection awareness, and environmental protection policies among regions, and how to accurately evaluate the efficiency of their investment in environmental pollution control while taking into account these external differences is of great relevance to the Chinese government in formulating environmental protection policies.

With the rapid development of China's economy, environmental pollution has become increasingly serious. The Chinese government also recognized this early and attached great importance to the treatment of environmental pollution, and continuously increased the investment in environmental pollution treatment [5]. Is China's environmental pollution control investment efficiency gradually improving? China is a vast country with differences in economic volume and resource endowment in different regions, and environmental policies are supported differently in each region [6]. Are there regional differences in the efficiency of investment in environmental pollution control in China? Economically developed provinces have more investment in environmental protection, more research and development in environmental protection technology, higher education level and higher awareness of environmental protection, while economically backward provinces have relatively less investment in environmental protection [7]. Are there regional differences in the efficiency of investment in environmental pollution control in China? This paper takes 30 provinces and cities in China from 2008–2017 as the research object (due to the problem of missing data in Tibet, Hong Kong, Macao and Taiwan, they are excluded from the research object), selects input and output indicators by referring to scholars' studies, and uses the super-efficient SBM model and the Global-Malmquist-Luenberger index to analyze the current situation of investment efficiency in environmental pollution control in China. The main research objectives of this study include the following: First, to evaluate the efficiency of investment in environmental pollution control in China; second, to clarify the changing trend of investment efficiency of environmental pollution control in China; then, comparing the differences in environmental pollution control efficiency among different regions; finally, identifying the main factors that affect the efficiency of environmental pollution control. Based on the research findings, relevant suggestions are made for environmental pollution control in China.

The arrangement of this paper is as follows: It first sorts out the related research about the efficiency of environmental pollution control. Afterwards, it introduces the research methods and data sources of this paper. Next, it displays and discusses the specific research results. Finally, it puts forward the research findings and corresponding policy recommendations and summarizes the shortcomings of this paper.

2. Literature Review

The research about the efficiency of environmental pollution control can be traced back to the end of the last century. Scholars used different methods to study the efficiency of environmental pollution control from various perspectives. In terms of research methods, they can be divided into two main categories. The first category is Data Envelopment Analysis (DEA) based on inputs and outputs. Reinhard (2000) was one of the first scholars to apply environmental variables to DEA input-output analysis, and they used the DEA method to measure environmental efficiency on dairy farms in the Netherlands and explained that the DEA method is capable of calculating any form of environmental efficiency score [8]. Mandal, S.K et al. (2010) used DEA analysis to estimate the environmental efficiency of the Indian cement industry by using the combustion of coal for cement production to produce a large amount of carbon dioxide as an undesired output [9]. Cecchini et al. (2018) used the DEA model and combined the results of life-cycle analysis to estimate the environmental efficiency and CO_2 reduction potential of 10 dairy farms in Umbria, Italy, proposing that the marginal emission reduction costs showed a positive correlation with the measured environmental efficiency scores [10]. Other scholars constructed a system of input-output indicators based on provincial panel data in China and used DEA to evaluate the efficiency of eco-environmental management in rural China [11]. The second category is Stochastic Frontier Analysis (SFA) for regression equation analysis. For example, some scholars estimated the input efficiency of industrial environmental management in China using SFA models based on data from three types of industrial wastes and explored the overall characteristics of input efficiency [12]. Other scholars used stochastic frontier analysis (SFA) models to analyze the effects of energy consumption and environmental pollution on the efficiency of technological innovation in industrial enterprises [13]. Moreover, some scholars have used the improved DEA method to measure the efficiency of environmental governance. Goto et al. (2014) used three modified data envelopment analysis (DEA) models to assess the operational and environmental efficiency of regional industries in Japan [14]. Xiao S et al. (2019) conducted a study on environmental efficiency using three-stage DEA [15]. There is also Zou et al. who proposed to measure the regional environmental efficiency in China using non-desired outputs through the SBM model [16]. Among the methods to evaluate the efficiency of environmental pollution control, besides the two mainstream methods of DEA and SFA, other scholars have used methods to assess the economic efficiency of investments. For example, Akoto et al. (2020) used the net present value (NPV) and financial benefit-cost ratio (FBCR) methods to evaluate the environmental impact and economic profitability of several bioenergy sources [17]. Zhao et al. (2021) used the internal rate of return index (IRR) to study the waste treatment system in Beijing and made effective recommendations to improve the energy recovery efficiency of the waste treatment system [18].

The research results of these studies are beneficial to environmental pollution management, but they still have shortcomings. From the literature, it can be seen that the traditional DEA method and SFA method are the main choices of the pollution control efficiency evaluation method in the existing studies. First, these research methods adopted by scholars are either subject to large random errors and environmental factors, or they can only be scaled down equivalently in terms of input-output adjustment, which cannot guarantee the objectivity of efficiency evaluation results, or they only focus on analyzing investment efficiency of environmental pollution control at the static level. Second, there is a lack of research on the efficiency of environmental pollution control investment in different regions of China by combining the three-stage super-efficiency SBM-DEA model with the Malmquist index method. Therefore, in order to fill the above research gaps, this paper tries to combine these two approaches and conduct empirical analysis based on panel data of 30 provinces in China from 2008 to 2017, analyze the level of pollution control investment efficiency and its change characteristics in China from the overall level, and compare regional differences. Eastern China has a large population and the highest level of economic development. Central China is not as economically developed as Eastern China and has the second largest population, but has great development potential. Western China has a vast territory, the smallest population density, and the third highest level of economic development. In contrast, northeastern China has the smallest population and a smaller economy, but has a developed heavy industrial sector. In 2018, eastern China accounted for 51.75% of the national share of GDP and had 11 large cities (with a resident population of more than 5 million people); northeastern China, with 5.03% of the national GDP, had 4 large cities; central China, with 25.76% of the national GDP, had 3 large cities; and western China, with 17.10% of the national GDP, had 4 large cities [19,20]. Comparing the efficiency difference of environmental pollution control investment among different regions can provide policy recommendations for environmental pollution control in China.

3. Materials and Methods

3.1. Research Methods

3.1.1. First Stage Super-Efficient SBM Model

The global super-efficient SBM (Slacks-based model) model with variable scale payoffs was proposed by Tone (2001) [21]. This model avoids the absence of feasible solutions and "technical regression" in the case of variable payoffs of scale; it ensures accurate efficiency results without the need for uniformity of scales. The equation is shown in (1).

$$\rho = \min \frac{\frac{1}{m}\sum_{i=1}^{1}\frac{\overline{x}}{x_{ik}}}{\frac{1}{s_1+s_2}\left(\sum_{t=1}^{s_1}\frac{\overline{y}_l^d}{y_{l0}^d}+\sum_{k=1}^{s_2}\frac{\overline{y}_k^u}{\overline{y}_{k0}^u}\right)} \tag{1}$$

$$s.t.\begin{cases} \overline{x} \geq \sum\limits_{j\neq 1,j\neq j_0}^{n} x_{ij}\lambda_j; \overline{y}^d \leq \sum\limits_{j=1,j\neq j_0}^{n} y_{l_j}^d\lambda; \overline{y}^u \geq \sum\limits_{j=1,j\neq j_0}^{n} y_{k_j}^d\lambda_j \\ \overline{y}^d \leq y_{l_j}^d; \overline{y}^u \geq y_{k_j}^d \\ \lambda_j \geq 0, i = 1,2,\ldots,m; j = 1,2,\ldots,s_1; k = 1,2,\ldots,s_2 \end{cases}$$

where, n denotes the number of decision-making units (DMU), i.e., y^u represents the number of provinces; x represents the data in the input index m; y^d represents the data in the desired output index s_1; y^u represents the data in the non-desired output index s_2; λ represents the weight of DMU; ρ denotes the efficiency value of environmental pollution control, $\rho \geq 1$, which means the efficiency is relatively effective. Larger ρ represents the higher level of environmental pollution control.

3.1.2. Second Stage Stochastic Frontier SFA Model

The stochastic frontier SFA (Stochastic Frontier Analysis) model proposed by Aigner, Lovell, and Schmidt (1977) [22] was used to quantify the errors and find the most influential stochastic factors and environmental errors. The true input and output values are calculated. With the input orientation, if there are n decision-making units (DMU), the initial slack value equation for i inputs of each DMU is shown in (2).

$$S_{in} = f_i(Z_n; \beta_i) + V_{in} + U_{in} \tag{2}$$

where i = 1, 2,..., M, n = 1, 2,..., N. represents the nth decision-making unit (DMU) observable external environmental variables; β_i represents the parameter vector of external environmental factors; $f_i(Z_n; \beta_i)$ represents the effect of external environmental variables on the input redundancy slack values, usually taken as $f_i(Z_n; \beta_i) = \beta_i Z_n$; V_{in} represents the effect of random factors, following $N(0, {\sigma_{un}}^2)$; U_{in} represents the effect of internal management status and input size, following $N(0, {\sigma_{un}}^2)$; V_{in} and U_{in} are independent of each other. The regression results obtained from the calculation are used to adjust the input values of other relatively inefficient DMU, and Equation (3) is as follows:

$$(X_{in})^* = X_{in} + [\max_n(\beta_i Z_n) - \beta_i Z_n] + [\max_n(V_{in}) - V_{in}] \tag{3}$$

where, X_{in} represents the actual input value; $(X_{in})^*$ denotes the adjusted input value; $[\max_n(\beta_i Z_n) - \beta_i Z_n]$ represents that all decision-making units (DMU) are in a homogeneous environment; $[\max_n(V_{in}) - V_{in}]$ represents the random error term that will be adjusted to the same condition for all DMU.

3.1.3. The Third Stage after Adjustment Is again Substituted into the Super-Efficient SBM Model

It is brought into the global super-efficient scale payoff variable SBM model, i.e., Equation (1), for calculation to obtain more objective and accurate efficiency values and for empirical analysis.

3.1.4. GML (Global-Malmquist-Luenberger) Index

The efficiency values measured by the super-efficient SBM are only static descriptions, while the GML index is a good complement to the SBM model and can dynamically analyze the changes in efficiency values between two years before and after. Therefore, the GML index proposed by Oh (2010) is introduced to measure the changes and influencing factors of governance efficiency in different periods and to conduct dynamic comparative analysis among regions [23]. The GML index can be further decomposed into the technical efficiency change index (EC index) and the technical progress change index (TC index), which respectively represent the contribution of technical efficiency improvement and technical improvement to the improvement of environmental pollution control efficiency in the period from t to $t + 1$ of the evaluation decision-making unit (DMU). The formula is shown in (4).

$$\begin{aligned} GML(x^{t+1}, y^{t+1}, b^{t+1}, x^t, y^t, b^t) &= \frac{E(x^{t+1}, y^{t+1}, b^{t+1})}{E(x^t, y^t, b^t)} \\ &= \frac{E^{t+1}(x^{t+1}, y^{t+1}, b^{t+1})}{E^t(x^t, y^t, b^t)} \times \left[\frac{E(x^{t+1}, y^{t+1}, b^{t+1})}{E^{t+1}(x^{t+1}, y^{t+1}, b^{t+1})} \times \frac{E^t(x^t, y^t, b^t)}{E(x^t, y^t, b^t)} \right] \\ &= EC \times TC \end{aligned} \quad (4)$$

3.2. *Variables Selection*

At present, many studies have been carried out on the efficiency of environmental pollution management in academia, and on the basis of the excellent results of related scholars [24–29], considering the typicality, accessibility, and feasibility of relevant variable indicators, environmental pollution management is divided into three first-level indicators of input variables, output variables, and external environmental variables, and finally constructed into an indicator system containing 11 three-level indicators(See Table 1 for details).

Table 1. Investment efficiency indicators of environmental governance.

Tier 1 Indicators	Tier 2 Indicators	Tier 3 Indicators
Input variables	Financial input	Industrial pollution control investment (billion yuan)
		Urban environmental pollution management infrastructure investment amount (billion yuan)
	Material input	Household garbage harmless treatment plants (seat)
		Urban sewage treatment plants (seat)
Output variables	Industrial emissions treatment	general solid waste comprehensive utilization (million tons)
		The number of industrial waste gas pollution treatment facilities (sets)
	Living pollution treatment	Household garbage harmless treatment rate (%)
		Urban sewage treatment rate (%)
Environmental variables	Government environmental support efforts	The proportion of environmental pollution treatment investment in GDP (%)
	Local economic development level	GDP (billion yuan)
	Socialization level	Urbanization rate (%)

3.3. Data Sources

This paper selects the data of 30 provinces and cities in China from 2008 to 2017 for the analysis (see Table 1 for detailed indicators). All data are from the official information released by the National Bureau of Statistics, mainly including the China Statistical Yearbook (2009–2018), China Environmental Statistical Yearbook (2009–2018) and the official information data of various provinces. Based on the exist studies and the situation of China's economic and social development, the provinces covered in this study can be divided into four regions, the eastern region (Beijing, Tianjin, Hebei, Shanghai, Jiangsu, Zhejiang, Fujian, Shandong, Guangdong, Hainan), the northeastern region (Liaoning, Jilin, Heilongjiang,), the central region (Shanxi, Anhui, Jiangxi, Henan, Hubei, Hunan), and the western region (Inner Mongolia, Guangxi, Chongqing, Sichuan, Guizhou, Yunnan, Shaanxi, Gansu, Qinghai, Ningxia, Xinjiang) [30–32].

4. Results

4.1. First Stage Initial Super-Efficient SBM Analysis

The initial efficiency of environmental pollution control investments in 30 provinces and cities from 2008–2017 was measured by using the global super-efficient payoffs of scale variable SBM model, and the results are shown in columns 3, 4 of Table 2, and Figure 1.

Table 2. Efficiency averages and rankings by province from 2008 to 2017.

Region	Province	Stage 1		Stage 3	
		Average Efficiency	Ranking	Average Efficiency	Ranking
Eastern China	Beijing	0.443	25	0.534	30
	Tianjin	0.852	8	0.904	7
	Hebei	0.977	3	0.986	5
	Shanghai	0.727	11	0.792	15
	Jiangsu	0.490	22	0.719	21
	Zhejiang	0.665	13	0.760	18
	Fujian	0.549	19	0.739	19
	Shandong	0.640	16	0.817	14
	Guangdong	0.655	15	0.736	20
	Hainan	0.956	5	1.004	2
Northeastern China	Liaoning	0.684	12	0.894	8
	Jilin	0.388	28	0.582	28
	Heilongjiang	0.301	30	0.562	29
Central China	Shanxi	0.956	4	0.991	4
	Anhui	0.768	10	0.885	9
	Jiangxi	0.658	14	0.803	14
	Henan	0.575	18	0.767	16
	Hubei	0.389	27	0.658	25
	Hunan	0.474	23	0.677	24
Western China	Nei Monggol	0.533	20	0.842	11
	Guangxi	0.581	17	0.769	17
	Chongqing	0.833	9	0.869	10
	Sichuan	0.495	21	0.694	22
	Guizhou	0.866	7	0.822	12
	Yunnan	0.946	6	0.941	6
	Shaanxi	0.436	26	0.692	23
	Gansu	0.449	24	0.600	27
	Qinghai	1.009	1	0.998	3
	Ningxia	0.993	2	1.018	1
	Xinjiang	0.341	28	0.626	26

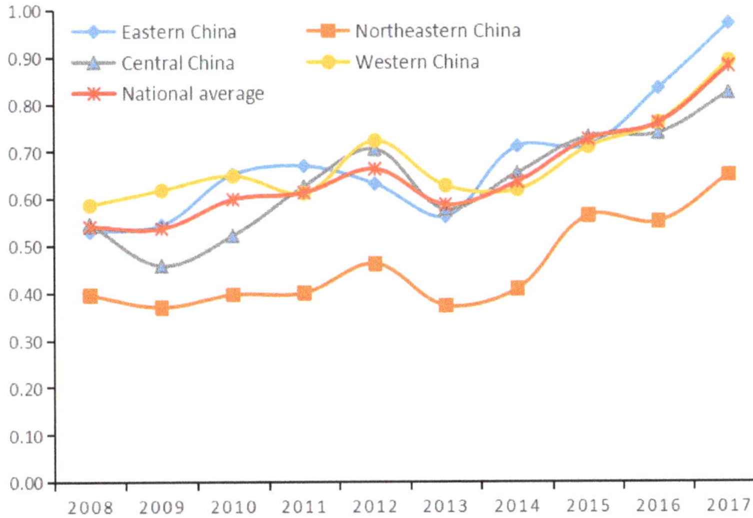

Figure 1. Change in the average value of efficiency in the first stage from 2008 to 2017.

From the inter-provincial comparison in Table 2, there are obvious inter-provincial differences in the efficiency of investment in environmental pollution control in China. Qinghai Province has the highest level of investment efficiency of environmental pollution control, ranking first with an efficiency value of 1.009; Heilongjiang Province has the lowest level of efficiency, ranking last with an efficiency value of 0.301. The investment efficiency of environmental pollution control of economically developed provinces does not rank as high as one might expect, such as Shanghai ranking eleventh and Guangdong Province ranking fifteenth. On the contrary, some of the less developed provinces ranked more highly in investment efficiency of environmental pollution control, such as Qinghai Province and Ningxia Hui Autonomous Region ranked first and second, and Yunnan and Guizhou ranked sixth and seventh, respectively. This indicates that there are various factors affecting the investment efficiency of environmental pollution treatment in each province. From an overall perspective, there are also obvious regional differences in the efficiency of governance investment. Among the four regions, the eastern region has the highest pollution control efficiency, with an average efficiency value of 0.682; the western region is the second, with an average efficiency value of 0.680; the central region has an average efficiency value of 0.637; and the northeastern region has the lowest level of control efficiency, with an average value of 0.458. By comparing the data, we can find that the efficiency values of the eastern region and the western region are close to each other and rank high; the difference between the efficiency values of the eastern region and the northeastern region is as high as 0.224. This may be due to the fact that the eastern region has developed earlier and has sufficient economic support for environmental pollution control [33,34]. The Chinese government, considering the balanced development between regions, has placed the development of the western region in a strategic position and focused on local environmental protection while carrying out the development of the western region, taking various measures to protect the ecological environment of the western region [35,36]. Therefore, the efficiency of governance has been improving year by year, and is approaching that of the eastern region. The industrial sector in the northeast has been developing since the early years, and is known as "China's old industrial base". These industries have caused serious environmental pollution over the years, resulting in the pollution control effect not being very obvious [37,38].

As shown in Figure 1 from the national perspective, on average, the efficiency value was always less than 1 from 2008 to 2017 without removing the influence of environmental factors and random variables, which indicates that the initial efficiency of environmental pollution control in China was always ineffective. However, with the passage of time, the overall trend shows a gradual increase. The increasing efficiency of investment in environmental pollution control is closely related to the fact that the Chinese government has been paying more and more attention to environmental pollution control over the years and actively promoting the construction and improvement of environmental protection [39,40]. The Chinese government has gradually recognized the importance of environmental protection, proposed the goal of building a beautiful China, formulated various environmental pollution control policies, and increased the scale of environmental protection investment [41–43]. However, the investment efficiency of environmental pollution control value has never reached 1, indicating that the effectiveness of China's environmental pollution control is still not optimistic and there is still much room for improvement.

4.2. Second Stage SFA Regression Analysis

The input indicator slack variables and the three external environment variables calculated in the first stage were substituted into the stochastic frontier regression equation (Stochastic Frontier Analysis, SFA), and the results are shown in Table 3.

Table 3. Results of the second stage stochastic frontier regression.

	Redundant Investment in Industrial Pollution Control		Redundant Investment in Urban Environmental Pollution Management Infrastructure	
	Coefficient	**Standard Deviation**	**Coefficient**	**Standard Deviation**
Constants	−0.406374 *	−3.848926	−194.687790 ***	47.858103
government environmental support efforts	2.302858 ***	0.925156	70.570078 ***	8.950301
local economic development level	0.000153	0.000058	0.001269 **	0.000511
socialization level	−0.091174 *	0.066246	1.091758 *	0.716531
sigma-squared	106.984520 ***	20.322746	10011.500000 ***	1.437268
gamma	0.295561 **	0.127572	0.411285 ***	0.052723
loglikelihoodfunction	−1094.0241		−1751.6127	
LR one-sided error	46.32686 ***		30.99629 ***	
	Household Garbage Harmless Treatment Plant Redundancy		**Urban Sewage Treatment Plant Redundancy**	
	Coefficient	**Standard Deviation**	**Coefficient**	**Standard Deviation**
Constants	−3.5224076 *	3.8623349	−23.451946 **	13.765248
government environmental support efforts	0.22772769 *	0.60479266	2.6279131 *	1.9546761
local economic development level	−0.00017399 **	0.000070359	−0.000456998 **	0.000256776
socialization level	0.059836647 *	0.064210501	0.36500775 *	0.2223983
sigma-squared	200.45879 ***	72.527272	1578.6747 **	632.2929
gamma	0.87481371 ***	0.048841983	0.83143444 ***	0.072676693
loglikelihoodfunction	−955.29407		−1308.6314	
LR one-sided error	144.03577 ***		168.24658 ***	

Note: "***", "**" and "*" indicate significant at the 1%, 5% and 10% levels, respectively.

According to the regression results in Table 3, the slack variable coefficient of government environmental support efforts input on the four inputs is positive, which indicates that government environmental support efforts have negative impact on the four inputs. In particular, it has the greatest negative impact on the amount of investment in urban environmental pollution control infrastructure, far exceeding the other three inputs. This shows that although China has invested heavily in environmental pollution, but it is not effective and there is great deal of redundancy. Investment redundancy refers to the fact that the investment does not produce the expected results and there is a large gap between the actual input and output levels. Investment redundancy in government environmental investments is due to inefficient management. Duplication of functions between government departments, implementation of environmental policies by local agencies are still at low level, and management and planning of environmental inputs needs to be improved [44,45].

The slack variable coefficient of the local economic development level on household garbage harmless treatment plant and urban sewage treatment plants is negative, and it is significant at the level of 5%, which indicates that it has a positive impact on these two inputs. The slack variable coefficient of this variable is positive for the amount of investment in urban environmental pollution control infrastructure and the amount of investment in industrial pollution control. It indicates that the level of local economic development has negative impact on these two inputs.

The coefficients of slack variables of socialization level on the amount of investment in urban environmental pollution management infrastructure, household garbage harmless treatment plants, and urban sewage treatment plants are positive. It shows that the increase in the level of socialization is not conducive to reducing the gap between the actual and optimal levels of these three inputs. This may be due to the fact that with the increase of urbanization, many people gather to live in towns and cities, which intensifies the production of domestic waste and sewage, adding to the burden of pollution control in these areas [46]. On the contrary, this variable has positive effect on the amount of investment in industrial pollution control. This may be due to the fact that with the increase in urbanization, the population was increasingly gathering in cities, and the government has increased its efforts to control industrial pollution for the sake of people's healthy life [47].

From the above analysis, it can be concluded that the efforts of government environmental support, the level of local economic development, and the level of socialization, have different effects on the redundancy of various inputs to environmental pollution control. In addition, in the first stage the efficiency of pollution control in economically developed provinces did not rank as high as we thought, such as Shanghai ranked eleventh and Guangdong Province ranked fifteenth. On the contrary, some less developed provinces ranked more highly in pollution control efficiency, such as Yunnan Province and Guizhou Province ranked sixth and seventh respectively. This also indicated that the calculation results of the first stage deviated from the actual situation. This may be due to the large differences in random factors in terms of area size, resources, population, industrial structure, and technological progress between different regions and provinces, which affected the accuracy of investment efficiency in environmental pollution treatment. Therefore, it is necessary to adjust the relevant data in the first stage input indicators, for example, the amount of redundancy in urban environmental pollution control infrastructure investment and industrial pollution control investment in 30 Chinese provinces and cities are adjusted, and these redundancies affect the objective evaluation of the efficiency of environmental pollution control, and, re-calculate to arrive at a more accurate value of investment efficiency in environmental pollution control.

4.3. Analysis of Governance Efficiency after the Third Stage of Adjustment

Based on the second stage Stochastic Frontier Analysis (SFA) regression equation calculations, the original input index data values were adjusted and substituted into the first stage super-efficient SBM model to produce more accurate and realistic efficiency values. The results are shown in columns 5 and 6 of Table 2 and in Figure 2. The adjusted efficiency values in the third stage show significant changes compared to the first stage.

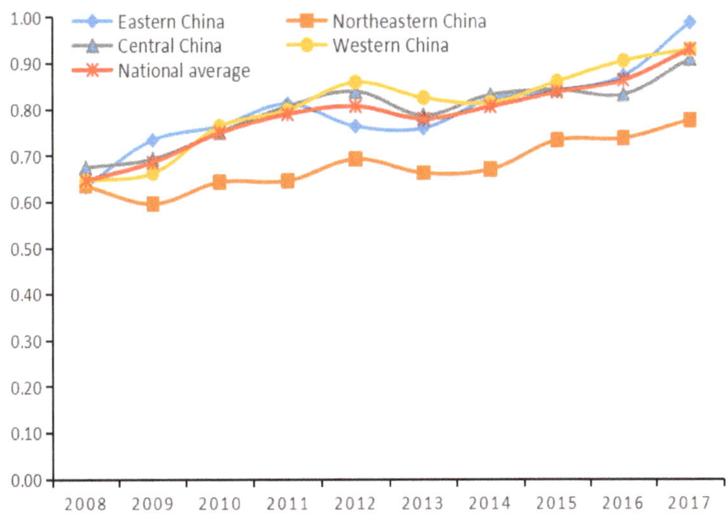

Figure 2. Change in the mean value of efficiency in the third stage from 2008 to 2017.

From the overall analysis of the country (see Figure 2), after adjustment, the investment efficiency value of China's environmental pollution control has increased significantly. The average efficiency value has increased from 0.654 in the first stage to 0.789, an increase of 20.6%. This shows that the existence of external environmental variables and random factors makes the value of investment efficiency of environmental pollution control underestimated. The average efficiency value shows a gradual upward trend in ten years, and it is gradually close to 1 compared with the first stage. This shows that China has achieved certain results in environmental pollution control in the past ten years [48]. If the growth trend continues, China's future environmental pollution control investment efficiency will gradually reach a good state. Lu, W et al. (2022) study on the efficiency of urban green development in developing countries concluded that the efficiency of environmental pollution control investment was from 0 to 1, 0 meant no efficiency, 1 meant fully effective, if it exceeded 0.75 was a relatively high level of efficiency [49]. Therefore, the efficiency value of 0.75 or even higher is the expected level. Government plays the main role in the environmental system, because in China's environmental governance system, government is in a dominant position [50]. The Chinese government has launched a series of treatment measures in the areas of air pollution control, water environmental protection, soil protection, and domestic pollution control. In 2016, the Chinese government conducted a hard-fought battle against environmental pollution and released the "13th Five-Year Plan for the Implementation of Environmental Impact Assessment Reform", which focuses on improving environmental quality and enhancing the effectiveness of environmental impact assessment in a comprehensive manner [51]. In 2017, the Chinese government issued the Opinions on the Delineation and Strict Compliance of Ecological Protection Red Line, which was expected to basically establish the ecological protection red line system within three years [52]. In 2018, China introduced regulations for the Environmental Access Conditions for Domestic Waste Incineration and Power Generation Construction Projects, which can improve the efficiency of domestic waste and wastewater treatment by regulating land use for waste treatment facilities, incineration technology, project water use, waste transportation, exhaust gas pollution control measures, and equipment [53,54].

Analysis from the perspective of provinces (see columns 5 and 6 of Table 2), the gap in investment efficiency of environmental pollution control between provinces has narrowed. Among the 30 provinces studied, 24 provinces, or 80% of all provinces, have changed their investment efficiency of environmental pollution control rankings. In the first stage, Qinghai Province ranked first in investment efficiency of environmental pollution control, and after adjustment, the efficiency value of Ningxia Hui Autonomous Region improved by 3%, surpassing the first place achieved by Qinghai Province; the efficiency of Inner Mongolia Autonomous Region improved by 9 places, with an increase of 58%; Beijing dropped from the first stage ranking 25 to 30th place, with a 20% decrease in efficiency value. This shows that the development of different provinces, environmental policies and other factors affect the efficiency of environmental pollution control in each province [55]. From a practical point of view, although there is a gap in environmental investment efficiency of environmental pollution control between provinces, it is not as large as in the first phase.

From the analysis of each region (Figure 1, Figure 2 comparison), it was different from the large fluctuation in the first stage. After the adjustment, the fluctuation range of the change level of the efficiency value in each region was small. At the same time, the gap in the investment efficiency of environmental pollution control of each region has also narrowed compared with the first stage, and the regional investment efficiency of environmental pollution control has been improved to varying degrees. This shows that the influence of random factors and environmental variables reduces the actual efficiency value. The ranking of investment efficiency of environmental pollution control across regions also changed. After the adjustment, the western region's investment efficiency of environmental pollution control ranked first, surpassing the eastern region, reaching the first place, with an average efficiency value of 0.806; the eastern region ranked second in terms of investment efficiency of environmental pollution control, with an average efficiency value of 0.799; the central region ranked third in terms of investment efficiency of environmental pollution control, with an average efficiency value of 0.797; the investment efficiency of environmental pollution control of the Ministry of Finance improved the most, with an increase of 48%, but it still ranks last, with an average efficiency value of 0.679. This may be due to the fact that although the efficiency of environmental pollution control in the eastern region was high in the past, the development speed was too fast, and the ability of environmental pollution control was far behind the speed of pollution diffusion, thus reducing the efficiency of governance in the eastern region. The western region has unique natural resources. In addition, the Chinese government attaches great importance to local environmental protection while implementing the western development policy. The introduction of large-scale funds and various supporting policies has promoted the efficiency of environmental pollution control in the western region improvement [56].

4.4. Analysis of GML Index of Environmental Pollution Control Investment Efficiency in China

4.4.1. Overall Time Series Variation Characteristics

The DEA software (MaxDEA Software Ltd, Beijing, China) was used to find out the average GML index of investment efficiency of environmental pollution control in China for each year from 2008 to 2017 and decomposed, and the results are shown in Table 4 and Figure 3.

Table 4. Average GML index and its decomposition by year in China.

Year	GML Mean Value	EC Mean Value	TC Mean Value
2008–2009	1.110	1.034	1.069
2009–2010	1.111	0.978	1.149
2010–2011	1.111	1.079	1.054
2011–2012	1.044	1.022	1.028
2012–2013	0.977	1.006	0.977
2013–2014	1.048	1.003	1.052
2014–2015	1.042	0.970	1.084
2015–2016	1.057	1.007	1.054
2016–2017	1.173	1.076	1.079

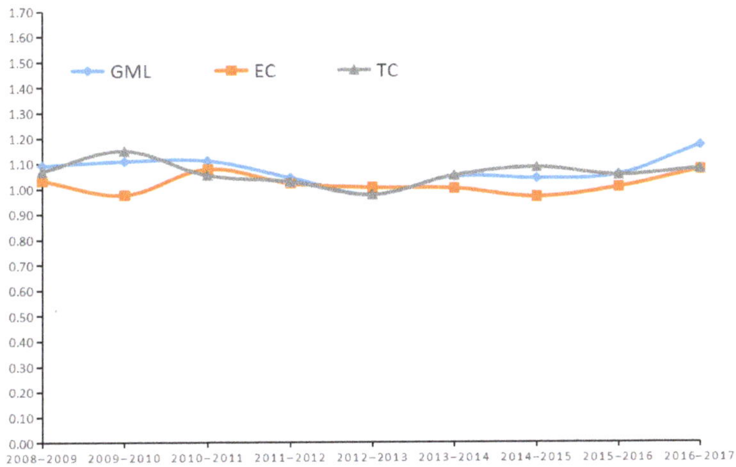

Figure 3. Average GML index and its decomposition line chart of each Year in China.

According to the average GML index for each year in China, it was greater than 1 for the remaining years except for 2012–2013, which was less than 1. This indicates that the efficiency of investment in environmental pollution control in China is gradually improving in general. This also coincides with the trend of efficiency values calculated in the third stage above.

As shown in Figure 3, China's GML index shows a general "W" pattern of falling, then oscillating up, then falling and then rising again. Since 2013, the investment efficiency of environmental pollution control has started to climb year by year. This is probably due to the fact that the Chinese government has introduced several environmental pollution control policies during this period to strengthen environmental protection in various aspects. For example, the Regulations on Urban Drainage and Sewage Treatment, the Action Plan on Prevention and Control of Air Pollution, and the Opinions on Accelerating the Development of Energy Conservation and Environmental Protection Industry [57–59]. From the decomposition of the GML index, the overall trend of the GML index is closer to the trend of the TC index, while it is more different from the trend of the EC index. This indicates that the GML index is more obviously influenced by the TC index, while it is less influenced by the EC index. That is, the improvement of investment efficiency of environmental pollution control in China is more influenced by technological progress. Fan, M et al.'s (2018) study of industrial CO_2 emission performance concluded that the more the number of TC (technological progress) index greater than 1, the better. All TC index (technological progress) greater than 1 was the best result and represented a significant contribution of technological progress. Currently, only one year

(2012–2013) of China's TC (technological progress) index was less than 1, and the rest were greater than 1. Therefore, in the future, the TC (technological progress) index all above 1 is the expected level to be reached [60]. The main investment in environmental pollution control is government investment. This is because enterprises are profit-seeking and do not have a strong willingness to take the initiative to invest in environmental pollution control. China has been increasing its investment in environmental pollution control, both financially and materially, with particular emphasis on the development of environmental protection science and technology [61,62]. The Chinese government has formulated and completed the 12th Five-Year Plan for the Development of Science and Technology for National Environmental Protection, and by the end of 2015, 675 achievements in basic theory, soft science and applied technology were registered with the National Environmental Protection Science and Technology Achievements [63]. China's rapid development in environmental protection science and technology has provided a powerful boost to environmental pollution control, the technology is mainly applied to environmental pollution monitoring and prevention. Remote sensing monitoring of haze and air pollution source emissions can be carried out efficiently using satellite platforms [64], and the application of Geographic Information System (GIS) technology has strengthened the supervision of environmental pollution management [65].

4.4.2. Inter-Provincial GML Index and Decomposition Index Analysis

The arithmetic mean of the annual average GML index and its decomposition results EC index and TC index for each province in China from 2008 to 2017 were used for the analysis, and the results are shown in Table 5.

Table 5. Average annual GML index and its decomposition by province from 2008 to 2017.

Region	Province	GML	EC	TC
Eastern China	Beijing	1.475	1.170	1.232
	Tianjin	1.130	0.999	1.130
	Hebei	1.037	1.001	1.037
	Shanghai	1.143	1.001	1.131
	Jiangsu	1.057	0.995	1.063
	Zhejiang	1.123	0.992	1.112
	Fujian	1.059	0.982	1.070
	Shandong	1.060	0.999	1.062
	Guangdong	1.098	1.080	1.105
	Hainan	0.999	0.995	1.004
Northeastern China	Liaoning	1.010	0.999	1.012
	Jilin	1.046	1.017	1.064
	Heilongjiang	1.049	0.995	1.111
Central China	Shanxi	1.002	1.009	0.994
	Anhui	1.041	0.996	1.045
	Jiangxi	1.075	1.006	1.071
	Henan	1.022	0.998	1.041
	Hubei	1.045	1.062	1.025
	Hunan	1.054	1.028	1.032
Western China	Nei Monggol	1.046	0.998	1.048
	Guangxi	1.058	0.999	1.060
	Chongqing	1.064	0.998	1.065
	Sichuan	1.021	1.010	1.020
	Guizhou	1.096	1.028	1.070
	Yunnan	1.013	1.005	1.010
	Shaanxi	1.051	1.002	1.060
	Gansu	1.177	1.083	1.103
	Qinghai	1.003	1.035	0.974
	Ningxia	1.002	0.999	1.004
	Xinjiang	1.122	1.095	1.064

Among the 30 provinces in China, the annual average GML index was greater than 1 in 29 provinces, except for Hainan Province, which was less than 1. This indicates that in general, the efficiency of investment in environmental management in Chinese provinces was improved year by year. Looking at the annual average EC index of 30 provinces, 18 provinces were greater than

1, accounting for 60%. In terms of the annual average TC index of 30 provinces, 28 provinces were greater than 1, accounting for 93%. This indicates that the improvement of investment efficiency in environmental pollution control in Chinese provinces is mainly due to the progress of self technology.

4.4.3. Regional GML Index and Decomposition Index Analysis

Based on the data analyzed above, the trend of the annual average GML index for the four regions of China from 2008 to 2017 was derived based on the GML index, as shown in Figure 4.

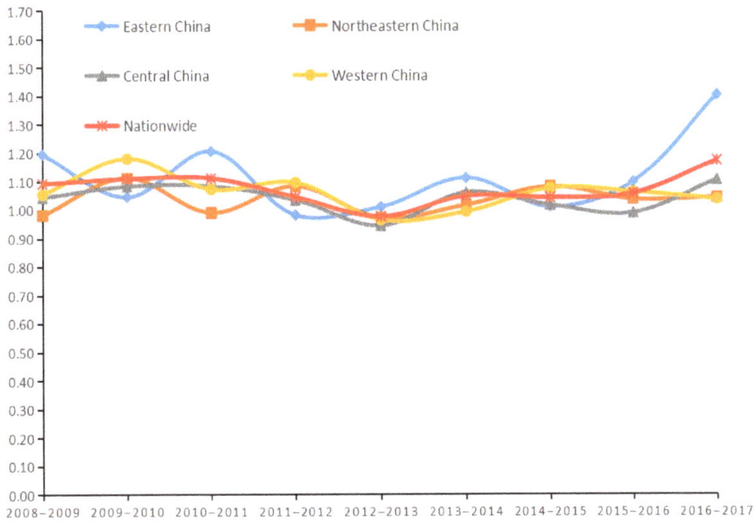

Figure 4. Trends in the annual average GML index in the four regions from 2008 to 2017.

The change trend of the annual average GML index in the four regions from 2008 to 2017 was similar, and all of them were in oscillating and fluctuating state. The trend of change in the central region was basically consistent with the national trend, with a slow rise during 2008–2011, and began to decline after 2011, reaching the lowest in 2013 with an average value of 0.945, and then a fluctuating upward trend, reaching the highest in 2017 with an average value of 1.105, and generally speaking, the efficiency of investment in environmental pollution control has improved. The western and northeastern regions fluctuate in a basically consistent state, and the overall was in an upward trend. The eastern region has the largest fluctuation. During the period of 2008–2015, it showed repeated fluctuations of falling, then rising, and then falling, and after 2015, it gradually showed an upward trend and reached the highest in 2017, with a mean value of 1.402, and the overall efficiency has improved. In order to clarify the reasons for the changes in the efficiency of environmental pollution control investment in each region, the annual average GML index of the four regions is also decomposed, and the results are shown in Table 6.

Overall, the EC index and TC index of the four regions were both higher than 1 during the decade, which indicates that both the efficiency and technology of environmental China pollution control investment have improved during this period. The TC indexes of all four regions were greater than the EC indexes, which indicates that the improvement in the efficiency of environmental pollution control investment in each region was mainly due to the progress in technology. In terms of the ten-year national average, the EC index was greater than 1 in 2009, 2011, 2012, 2013, 2014, 2016, and 2017, indicating that the improvement in technical efficiency during the period was conducive to the improvement in the efficiency of environmental pollution control investment. In contrast, the TC index was higher than 1 in all years except 2013 when it was less than 1, indicating that the improvement of technology contributes significantly to the improvement of investment efficiency in environmental pollution control in the rest of the period except 2013. The TC index was higher than 1 for the three regions of East, Central, and West except for three years in 2011, 2012, and 2013, which indicates that for these three regions, the improvement in the efficiency of investment in environmental pollution control was more obvious due to the improvement of technology.

Table 6. Decomposition results of the average GML index by year for the four regions.

Index	Region	08–09	09–10	10–11	11–12	12–13	13–14	14–15	15–16	16–17	Mean
EC	Eastern China	1.003	0.942	1.105	0.995	1.003	0.991	0.933	0.995	1.226	1.021
	Northeastern China	1.015	1.048	0.866	1.253	0.898	1.132	0.863	1.088	0.869	1.004
	Central China	1.011	0.960	1.131	0.968	1.019	1.011	1.025	0.957	1.067	1.017
	Western China	1.079	1.001	1.084	1.011	1.032	0.973	1.002	1.023	1.000	1.023
	Whole country	1.033	0.978	1.079	1.022	1.006	1.003	0.970	1.007	1.076	1.019
TC	Eastern China	1.193	1.138	1.131	0.981	1.007	1.122	1.087	1.098	1.097	1.095
	Northeastern China	0.965	1.074	1.179	0.878	1.103	0.928	1.254	0.963	1.217	1.062
	Central China	1.036	1.131	0.970	1.077	0.927	1.053	1.009	1.054	1.055	1.035
	Western China	1.003	1.190	0.995	1.084	0.941	1.022	1.076	1.039	1.039	1.043
	Whole country	1.069	1.149	1.054	1.028	0.976	1.052	1.084	1.054	1.079	1.061

5. Discussion

The conclusions drawn from the panel data of China's environmental pollution control investment from 2008–2017 can provide a reference for China's control of environmental pollution, but there are still some shortcomings that need to be further improved. First, such as the data collection is not very comprehensive. The panel data of Hong Kong, Macau, Taiwan, and Tibet Autonomous Region provinces can be complemented by software model simulations in the future, and also the research years can be extended. Second, this study analyzes the investment efficiency of environmental pollution control in China and each region from the macro level, without considering the special situation of different regions, and more in-depth analysis and research can be conducted in the future for the characteristics of different regions and explore the related influencing factors. For example, the eastern region has a developed economy and a large population, which generates more environmental pollution, but why is the environmental pollution control efficiency high [66,67]? Assuming that the possible reasons are sufficient capital, advanced technology and concentration of talents, what is the magnitude of the contribution of these factors to environmental protection? What is the root cause of the inefficiency of environmental pollution control in the northeast region compared to other regions, and how can this problem be addressed [68,69]?

6. Conclusions

This paper analyzes the investment efficiency of environmental pollution control in China from 2008 to 2019 by using the three-level super-efficiency SBM-DEA model and the GML index, and draws the following conclusions: First, the investment efficiency of environmental pollution control in China is improving, but there are obvious disparities among different regions. Affected by random factors and environmental variables, the actual efficiency value decreases. Second, excluding the effects of both, the national investment efficiency of environmental pollution control has improved significantly, but still has not reached the optimal effect. For example, after adjustment, the average efficiency of environmental pollution control in China has increased from 0.654 in the first stage to 0.789 in the third stage, with an increase of 20.6%, but the efficiency is always less than 1. At the same time, the gap between provinces and regions has narrowed while the investment efficiency of environmental pollution control has improved, and there is still an unbalanced situation. For instance, the average efficiency of the western region was far higher than that of the northeast region, which is 0.806 and 0.679 respectively. Third, overall, China's environmental pollution control efficiency has improved year by year, and the main driver is technological progress; compared with northeastern China, technological progress has a more significant role in promoting eastern, central, and western China.

Based on the above research conclusions, in order to promote the construction of environmental pollution control in China, the following suggestions are put forward:

(1) Strengthen regional cooperation to jointly control environmental pollution [70]. From the panel data of 30 Chinese provinces, it can be concluded that there is a regional development imbalance in the efficiency of investment in environmental pollution control in China. In order to achieve the improvement of overall environmental pollution treatment efficiency, the eastern region can export advanced environmental protection technology to the central and western regions, and the western region can use its abundant natural resources to cooperate with the eastern region. Other regions should lend a helping hand to the northeast region by sharing environmental governance experience, advanced environmental technologies, etc., and exporting environmental governance talents [71].

(2) Vigorously develop the rural economy. As concluded in the previous article, with the increasing level of urbanization, the concentration of residents living in towns and cities has intensified the generation of domestic waste and sewage. The development of rural economy can relieve the pressure of environmental pollution management caused by the concentration of urban population. In the process, attention should also be paid to the environmental protection of rural areas [72].
(3) Environmental protection investment should be targeted [73]. From the results of the impact analysis of the external environment, the Chinese government's annual funding for environmental pollution control is increasing, but the positive impact on various output indicators has not improved. Therefore, environmental protection investment should be targeted to prevent investment redundancy.
(4) Increase support for environmental protection technology research. According to the GML index and its decomposition, the main reason for the annual increase in the investment efficiency of China's environmental pollution control is technological progress. Therefore, it is necessary to increase support for the research and development of environmental protection technology, such as introducing policies that are conducive to the development of the environmental protection technology industry, increasing the research and development funds of environmental protection technology, and cultivating talents in the field of environmental protection [74–77].

Author Contributions: Conceptualization, X.Z.; methodology, L.L.; software, X.Z.; writing—original draft preparation, X.Z.; writing—review and editing, Q.S.; supervision, W.Z. All authors have read and agreed to the published version of the manuscript.

Funding: This work was supported by the Key research of Philosophy and Social Sciences of the 14th Five-year Plan of Sichuan University "Chengdu-chongqing Area Twin Cities Economic Circle Construction Research Project" (#SCJJ-12), The Fundamental Research Funds for the Central Universities of Sichuan University (# 2022 Self-research—School of Public Administration 05), the National Natural Science Foundation of China (#71804056), Basic scientific research business expenses in Chinese universities (#YD2110002004).

Institutional Review Board Statement: Not applicable.

Informed Consent Statement: Not applicable.

Data Availability Statement: Data available in a publicly accessible repository that does not issue DOIs. Publicly available datasets were analyzed in this study. This data can be found here: [https://navi.cnki.net/knavi/yearbooks/YINFN/detail, accessed on 4 April 2022] [https://navi.cnki.net/knavi/yearbooks/YHJSD/detail, accessed on 4 April 2022].

Conflicts of Interest: The authors declare no conflict of interest.

References

1. Li, Y.; Wu, H.; Shen, K.; Hao, Y.; Zhang, P. Is environmental pressure distributed equally in China? Empirical evidence from provincial and industrial panel data analysis. *Sci. Total Environ.* **2020**, *718*, 137363. [CrossRef] [PubMed]
2. Wang, Q.; Yang, Z. Industrial water pollution, water environment treatment, and health risks in China. *Environ. Pollut.* **2016**, *218*, 358–365. [CrossRef] [PubMed]
3. Qin, C.; Zhang, W. Green, poverty reduction and spatial spillover: An analysis from 21 provinces of China. *Environ. Dev. Sustain.* **2022**, 1–20. [CrossRef]
4. Zhang, W.; Zhang, M.; Wu, S.; Liu, F.A. complex path model for low-carbon sustainable development of enterprise based on system dynamics. *J. Clean. Prod.* **2021**, *321*, 128934. [CrossRef]
5. Feng, Q.; Sun, T. Comprehensive evaluation of benefits from environmental investment: Take China as an example. *Environ. Sci. Pollut. Res.* **2020**, *27*, 15292–15304. [CrossRef]
6. Liu, Z.; Geng, Y.; Lindner, S.; Guan, D. Uncovering China's greenhouse gas emission from regional and sectoral perspectives. *Energy* **2012**, *45*, 1059–1068. [CrossRef]
7. Ma, Y.; Ji, Q.; Fan, Y. Spatial linkage analysis of the impact of regional economic activities on PM2.5 pollution in China. *J. Clean. Prod.* **2016**, *139*, 1157–1167. [CrossRef]
8. Reinhard, S.; Lovell, C.K.; Thijssen, G.J. Environmental efficiency with multiple environmentally detrimental variables; Estimated with SFA and DEA. *Eur. J. Oper. Res.* **2000**, *121*, 287–303. [CrossRef]
9. Mandal, S.K.; Madheswaran, S. Environmental efficiency of the Indian cement industry: An interstate analysis. *Energy Policy* **2010**, *38*, 1108–1118. [CrossRef]

10. Cecchini, L.; Venanzi, S.; Pierri, A.; Chiorri, M. Environmental efficiency analysis and estimation of CO_2 abatement costs in dairy cattle farms in Umbria (Italy): A SBM-DEA model with undesirable output. *J. Clean. Prod.* **2018**, *197*, 895–907. [CrossRef]
11. Huang, Y.; Zhou, Z.; Huang, J.; Management, E.A. The management efficiency of rural ecological environment in different regions. *J. Arid. Land Resour. Environ.* **2015**, *3*, 78–83.
12. Zheng, Y.; Yang, R. Determining the efficiency of investments and evolving temporal-spatial trends in environmental governance using the stochastic frontier analysis (sfa) model. *Environ. Eng. Manag. J.* **2018**, *17*, 2767–2779.
13. Miao, C.L.; Meng, X.N.; Duan, M.M.; Wu, X.Y. Energy consumption, environmental pollution, and technological innovation efficiency: Taking industrial enterprises in China as empirical analysis object. *Environ. Sci. Pollut. Res.* **2020**, *27*, 34147–34157. [CrossRef] [PubMed]
14. Goto, M.; Otsuka, A.; Sueyoshi, T. DEA (Data Envelopment Analysis) assessment of operational and environmental efficiencies on Japanese regional industries. *Energy* **2014**, *66*, 535–549. [CrossRef]
15. Shi, X. Environmental efficiency evaluation of chinese industry systems by using Non-Cooperative Two-Stage DEA model. *Math. Probl. Eng.* **2019**, *2019*, 9208367. [CrossRef]
16. Zou, H.L.; Wang, C. Calculation of China's environmental efficiency based on the SBM model with undesirable outputs. *Eur. J. Oper. Res.* **2014**, *18*, 196–200.
17. Akoto, D.S.; Partey, S.T.; Denich, M.; Kwaku, M.; Borgemeister, C.; Schmitt, C.B. Environmental and financial assessment of producing bioenergy from *Bambusa balcooa*, *Anogeissus leiocarpa* and *Senna siamea* in Ghana. *J. Clean. Prod.* **2020**, *275*, 123147. [CrossRef]
18. Zhao, R.; Sun, L.; Zou, X.; Fujii, M.; Dong, L.; Dou, Y.; Geng, Y.; Wang, F. Towards a Zero Waste city-an analysis from the perspective of energy recovery and landfill reduction in Beijing. *Energy* **2021**, *223*, 120055. [CrossRef]
19. Liu, S.M.; Zang, M.L.; Statistics, S.O. Evaluation on the accuracy of provincial GDP growth data in China: An empirical study on revised "keqiang index" including the space light data. *J. Yunnan Univ. Financ. Econ.* **2018**, *6*, 27–37.
20. Guan-Cen, W.U.; Niu, X.; Tian, W.L. Study on new mechanism of urban regeneration in China's megalopolis: Compare and implication of three global cities. *China Soft Sci.* **2016**, *9*, 88–98.
21. Tone, K. A slacks-based measure of efficiency in data envelopment analysis. *Eur. J. Oper. Res.* **2001**, *130*, 498–509. [CrossRef]
22. Aigner, D.; Lovell, C.; Schmidt, P. Formulation and estimation of stochastic frontier production function models. *J. Econom.* **1977**, *6*, 21–37. [CrossRef]
23. Oh, D.H. A global Malmquist-Luenberger productivity index. *J. Prod. Anal.* **2010**, *34*, 183–197. [CrossRef]
24. Zhang, J.Q.; Shu-Di, B.U. Measuring allocation efficiency of regional green s&t resource based on three- stage SBM- DEA—Taking guilin city as an example. *Resour. Dev. Mark.* **2017**, *1*, 3–9.
25. Yu, H.; Lin, X. Study of environmental pollution control investment efficiency and its influence in Beijing-Tianjin-Hebei region. *J. Ind. Technol. Economics* **2018**, *5*, 138–146.
26. Yu, L.; Accounting, S.O. The Conceptual Problem and its Interpretation on Fair Value: Discussion on Reconstruction of the Objective of Financial Reporting. *J. Zhongnan Univ. Econ. Law* **2016**, *1*, 132–161.
27. Jing, L.; Ni, D.; Economics, S.O. China's industrial green production and governance efficiency research—based on two-stage SBM network model and global malmquist method. *Ind. Econ. Res.* **2015**, *3*, 46–57.
28. Yan, X. Research on Dynamic Efficiency of Industrial Pollution Control in China. *J. Ind. Technol. Econ.* **2012**, *5*, 155–162.
29. Xiang, T.D. Research on Regional Carbon Efficiency and Total Factor Productivity in China—Based on a Three-Stage DEA Model. *Econ. Surv.* **2017**, *1*, 26–31.
30. Liu, K.; Daly, K.; Varua, M.E. Determinants of regional distribution of FDI inflows across China's four regions. *Int. Bus. Res.* **2012**, *5*, 119. [CrossRef]
31. Ning, J.; Liu, J.; Kuang, W.; Xu, X.; Zhang, S.; Yan, C.; Li, R.; Wu, S.; Hu, Y.; Du, G. Spatiotemporal patterns and characteristics of land-use change in China during 2010–2015. *J. Geogr. Sci.* **2018**, *28*, 547–562. [CrossRef]
32. Kuang, B.; Lu, X.; Zhou, M.; Chen, D. Provincial cultivated land use efficiency in China: Empirical analysis based on the SBM-DEA model with carbon emissions considered. *Technol. Forecast. Soc.* **2020**, *151*, 119874. [CrossRef]
33. Li, T.; Han, Y.; Li, Y.; Lu, Z.; Zhao, P. Urgency, development stage and coordination degree analysis to support differentiation management of water pollution emission control and economic development in the eastern coastal area of China. *Ecol. Indic.* **2016**, *71*, 406–415. [CrossRef]
34. Chang, B.; Chen, L. Land economic efficiency and improvement of environmental pollution in the process of sustainable urbanization: Case of eastern China. *Land* **2021**, *10*, 845. [CrossRef]
35. Hu, X.; Zhang, H.; Hao, H.; Feng, D.; Liu, H.; Zhang, Q. Understanding the relationships between poverty alleviation and ecosystem conservation: Empirical evidence from western China. *Front. Earth Sci.* **2020**, *14*, 209–220. [CrossRef]
36. Li, W.; Zhang, L.; Guo, R. The measurement of tourism environmental pollution and tourism efficiency in western China. *J. Coastal Res.* **2020**, *104*, 660–664. [CrossRef]
37. Li, F.; Fan, Z.; Xiao, P.; Oh, K.; Ma, X.; Hou, W. Contamination, chemical speciation and vertical distribution of heavy metals in soils of an old and large industrial zone in Northeast China. *Environ. Ment. Geol.* **2009**, *57*, 1815–1823. [CrossRef]
38. Xiancheng, Z.; Zeyuan, L. Prospering revolution of resource efficiency in northeast industrial area in China. *Chin. J. Popul. Resour. Environ.* **2007**, *5*, 81–84. [CrossRef]

39. Zhang, Y.; Zheng, C. Eco-budget application oriented by environmental governance: Evidence from Beijing. *Environ. Eng. Manag. J.* **2020**, *19*, 1491–1498. [CrossRef]
40. Zhang, K.; Wen, Z. Review and challenges of policies of environmental protection and sustainable development in China. *J. Environ. Manag.* **2008**, *88*, 1249–1261. [CrossRef]
41. Chen, M.; Liang, L.; Wang, Z.; Zhang, W.; Yu, J.; Liang, Y. Geographical thoughts on the relationship between 'Beautiful China' and land spatial planning. *J. Geogr. Sci.* **2020**, *30*, 705–723. [CrossRef]
42. Marinelli, M. How to build a 'Beautiful China' in the anthropocene. The political discourse and the intellectual debate on ecological civilization. *J. Chin. Political Sci.* **2018**, *23*, 365–386. [CrossRef]
43. Wan, J. The philosophical wisdom and action implications of "beautiful China". *Soc. Sci. China* **2013**, *34*, 143–153.
44. Wang, M.; Wang, Y.; Feng, X.; Zhao, M.; Du, X.; Wang, Y.; Wang, P.; Wu, L. The effects of Intensive Supervision Mechanism on air quality improvement in China. *J. Air Waste Manag.* **2021**, *71*, 1102–1113. [CrossRef]
45. Zhang, T.; Yao, H. The improvement on the implementation level of environmental policies is demanded in China. *Environ. Sci. Pollut. Res.* **2018**, *25*, 36035–36038. [CrossRef] [PubMed]
46. Hao, Y.; Zheng, S.; Zhao, M.; Wu, H.; Guo, Y.; Li, Y. Reexamining the relationships among urbanization, industrial structure, and environmental pollution in China-New evidence using the dynamic threshold panel model. *Energy Rep.* **2020**, *6*, 28–39. [CrossRef]
47. Xie, H.; Liu, M.; Jiang, W. Balanced development and industrialization and urbanization serving as a strategy for pollution agglomeration control. *Ekoloji* **2019**, *28*, 2431–2441.
48. Zhang, B.; Cao, C.; Hughes, R.M.; Davis, W.S. China's new environmental protection regulatory regime: Effects and gaps. *J. Environ. Manag.* **2017**, *187*, 464–469. [CrossRef]
49. Lu, W.; Zhang, G. Green development efficiency of urban agglomerations in a developing country: Evidence from Beijing-Tianjin-Hebei in China. *Environ. Dev. Sustain.* **2022**, 1–24. [CrossRef]
50. Duan, X.; Dai, S.; Yang, R.; Duan, Z.; Tang, Y. Environmental collaborative governance degree of government, corporation, and public. *Sustainability* **2020**, *12*, 1138. [CrossRef]
51. Wan, J.; Qin, C.; Wang, Q.; Xiao, Y.; Niu, R.; Li, X.; Su, J. A brief overview of the 13th Five-Year plan for the protection of ecological environment. *Environ. Strategy Plan. China* **2022**, 57–85. [CrossRef]
52. Jiang, B.; Bai, Y.; Wong, C.P.; Xu, X.; Alatalo, J.M. China's ecological civilization program–Implementing ecological redline policy. *Land Use Policy* **2019**, *81*, 111–114. [CrossRef]
53. Han, Z.; Duan, Q.; Fei, Y.; Zeng, D.; Shi, G.; Li, H.; Hu, M. Factors that influence public awareness of domestic waste characteristics and management in rural areas. *Integr. Environ. Asses.* **2018**, *14*, 395–406. [CrossRef] [PubMed]
54. Wu, G.; Miao, Z.; Shao, S.; Jiang, K.; Geng, Y.; Li, D.; Liu, H. Evaluating the construction efficiencies of urban wastewater transportation and treatment capacity: Evidence from 70 megacities in China. *Resour. Conserv. Recycl.* **2018**, *128*, 373–381. [CrossRef]
55. Wei, J.; Jia, R.; Marinova, D.; Zhao, D. Modeling pollution control and performance in China's provinces. *J. Environ. Manage.* **2012**, *113*, 263–270. [CrossRef] [PubMed]
56. Hu, X.Z. The Relation between Environment Pollution and Economic Growth in Western of China—Taking Chongqing as an Example. *Appl. Mech. Mater.* **2012**, *209*, 1261–1264. [CrossRef]
57. Chang, Y.J.; Zhu, D. Urban water security of China's municipalities: Comparison, features and challenges. *J. Hydrol.* **2020**, *587*, 125023. [CrossRef]
58. Jiang, X.; Hong, C.; Zheng, Y.; Zheng, B.; Guan, D.; Gouldson, A.; Zhang, Q.; He, K. To what extent can China's near-term air pollution control policy protect air quality and human health? A case study of the Pearl River Delta region. *Environ. Res. Lett.* **2015**, *10*, 104006. [CrossRef]
59. Wang, J.; Li, L. Sustainable energy development scenario forecasting and energy saving policy analysis of China. *Renew. Sust. Energy Rev.* **2016**, *58*, 718–724. [CrossRef]
60. Fan, M.; Shao, S.; Yang, L. Combining global Malmquist–Luenberger index and generalized method of moments toinvestigate industrial total factor CO_2 emission performance: A case of Shanghai (China). *Energy Policy* **2015**, *79*, 189–201. [CrossRef]
61. Ren, S.; Hao, Y.; Wu, H. How Does Green Investment Affect Environmental Pollution? Evidence from China. *Environ. Resour. Econ.* **2022**, *81*, 25–51. [CrossRef]
62. Yi, M.; Fang, X.; Wen, L.; Guang, F.; Zhang, Y. The heterogeneous effects of different environmental policy instruments ongreen technology innovation. *Int. J. Env. Res. Public Health* **2019**, *16*, 4660. [CrossRef] [PubMed]
63. Wang, Q.; Qu, J.; Wang, B.; Wang, P.; Yang, T. Green technology innovation development in China in 1990–2015. *Sci. Total Environ.* **2019**, *696*, 134008. [CrossRef] [PubMed]
64. Zhao, S.; Wang, Q.; Li, Y.; Liu, S.; Wang, Z.; Zhu, L.; Wang, Z. An overview of satellite remote sensing technology used in China's environmental protection. *Earth Sci. Inform.* **2017**, *10*, 137–148. [CrossRef]
65. Zhang, G.Z.; Zhao, W.N.; Liu, H. A GIS-based decision support system for water trade management of river basin cities. *Procedia Environ. Sci.* **2010**, *2*, 650–655. [CrossRef]
66. Zhang, K.; Xu, D.; Li, S. The impact of environmental regulation on environmental pollution in China: An empirical study based on the synergistic effect of industrial agglomeration. *Environ. Sci. Pollut. Res.* **2019**, *26*, 25775–25788. [CrossRef]
67. Guo, Q.; Luo, K. The spatial convergence and drivers of environmental efficiency under haze constraints-Evidence from China. *Environ. Impact Asses.* **2021**, *86*, 106513. [CrossRef]

68. Niu, Z.; Sun, P.; Li, X.; He, Y.; Huang, C.; He, M.; Huang, H.; Wang, N. Spatial characteristics and geographical determinantsof mercury and arsenic in snow in northeastern China. *Atmos. Pollut. Res.* **2020**, *11*, 2068–2075. [CrossRef]
69. Du, M.; Liu, W.; Hao, Y. Spatial correlation of air pollution and its causes in Northeast China. *Int. J. Environ. Res. Public Health* **2021**, *18*, 10619. [CrossRef]
70. Shan, H.; Yang, J. Promoting the implementation of extended producer responsibility systems in China: A behavioral game perspective. *J. Clean. Prod.* **2019**, *250*, 119446. [CrossRef]
71. Hou, H.; Zhu, Y. Analysis of spillover effects of regional environmental pollution: An interprovincial study in China based on spatiotemporal lag model. *Environ. Sci. Pollut. Res.* **2022**, *29*, 836–853. [CrossRef] [PubMed]
72. Wang, J.; Liu, P. Study on environmental pollution and governance in rural development. *Fresenius Environ. Bull.* **2019**, *28*, 9218–9222.
73. Tong, C.; Ding, S.; Wang, B.; Yang, S. Assessing the target-availability of China's investments for green growth using time series prediction. *Phys. A Stat. Mech. Appl.* **2020**, *537*, 122724. [CrossRef]
74. Fujii, H.; Managi, S. Research and development strategy for environmental technology in Japan: A comparative study of the private and public sectors. *Technol. Forecast. Soc.* **2016**, *112*, 293–302. [CrossRef]
75. Zhang, W.; Zhang, M.; Zhang, W.; Zhou, Q.; Zhang, X. What influences the effectiveness of green logistics policies? A grounded theory analysis. *Sci. Total Environ.* **2020**, *714*, 136731. [CrossRef]
76. Zhang, W.; Zhang, X.; Wu, G. The network governance of urban renewal: A comparative analysis of two cities in China. *Land Use Policy* **2021**, *106*, 105448. [CrossRef]
77. Peng, B.; Sheng, X.; Wei, G. Does environmental protection promote economic development? From the perspective of coupling coordination between environmental protection and economic development. *Environ. Sci. Pollut. Res.* **2020**, *27*, 39135–39148. [CrossRef]

International Journal of
Environmental Research and Public Health

MDPI

Article

Can Digital Financial Inclusion Promote Green Innovation in Heavily Polluting Companies?

Long Xue * and Xuemang Zhang

School of Economics and Management, Zhengzhou University of Light Industry, Science Avenue 136, Zhengzhou 450000, China; xuemang_z@163.com
* Correspondence: xl2017018@sina.com

Abstract: This paper takes the China A-shares listed companies in heavy polluting industries from 2011 to 2020 as samples, combines the digital financial inclusion index to empirically examine the impacts of digital financial inclusion development on the green technology innovation of heavily polluting companies, and reveals its mechanism of action and its heterogeneity of the impacts of enterprises' green technology innovation in different development stages. The empirical research results show that the development of digital financial inclusion is able to promote the green innovation of heavy-polluting enterprises. Its main manifestation is that the development of digital financial inclusion helps the increase of green patent applications of heavy-polluting enterprises. This conclusion is validated through the endogeneity and robustness tests. The test results of the mechanism of action show that digital financial inclusion promotes green innovation of enterprises by alleviating corporate financing constraints and financial mismatch problems. Further research results show that the role of digital financial inclusion in promoting green technology innovation in heavy-polluting enterprises is more pronounced in mature enterprises. Therefore, this study provides a theoretical basis for the development of digital financial inclusion to promote heavy-polluting enterprises to achieve green transition through green technology innovation, thus achieving the "dual carbon" goal.

Keywords: digital financial inclusion; green innovation; financing constraints; life cycle

Citation: Xue, L.; Zhang, X. Can Digital Financial Inclusion Promote Green Innovation in Heavily Polluting Companies. *IJERPH* **2022**, *19*, 7323. https://doi.org/10.3390/ijerph19127323

Academic Editors: Jie Chen, Qian Zhou and Ting Zhang

Received: 22 April 2022
Accepted: 13 June 2022
Published: 15 June 2022

1. Introduction

Since the Chinese government proposed the "dual carbon" goal at the 75th United Nations General Assembly in 2020, how to achieve this goal has become a hot issue for policy-makers and academia [1,2]. High-speed economic development brought about by heavy-polluting enterprises at the expense of the environment pollution will bring serious environmental issues [3]. Therefore, whether they can achieve green transition is critical to achieving the "dual carbon" goal on schedule. Green technology innovation is a general term for new technologies, new processes, and new products that help reduce environmental pollution and save resources. Therefore, it is one of the key paths for heavy-polluting enterprises to achieve green transition. However, green technology innovation requires stable and continuous funds. There is a high degree of uncertainty, which leads to the problem of strong financing constraints for heavy-polluting enterprises to implement green technology innovation. Digital financial inclusion is an action to promote financial inclusion through the use of digital financial services [4]. In recent years, digital inclusive finance has developed rapidly, driven by modern information technologies, such as mobile payment, big data, and cloud computing. Digital inclusive finance has broken the boundaries of traditional financial services and alleviated information asymmetry in traditional financial services. The resulting high cost has broken through the limitations of time and geography and further expanded the reach and service depth of inclusive finance. Therefore, the development of digital inclusive finance provides the possibility of financial support for heavily polluting enterprises to implement green technology innovation. In the existing literature, although some scholars have paid attention to the influencing factors of corporate green technology innovation and the impact of digital financial inclusion on it [5–8], few scholars have studied whether digital financial inclusion can promote green technology innovation in heavy-polluting enterprises, and no scholar has revealed its mechanism of action and its heterogeneity. It can be seen from the above sentences that the main contributions of this paper are: First, taking heavy-polluting enterprises as the research object, it reveals the influencing mechanism of digital financial inclusion on the green innovation of heavy-polluting enterprises from the perspectives of financing constraints and financial mismatches, which not only expands the relevant literature on the impact of digital financial inclusion on enterprises, but also provides a new perspective for analyzing the influencing factors of enterprise green innovation. Second, on the basis of systematically expounding how digital financial inclusion affects the green innovation mechanism of enterprises, it further explores whether this impact will be affected by the heterogeneity of the enterprise life cycle, and clarifies the differences in the effects of digital financial inclusion on green innovation for enterprises at different development stages. This research has important theoretical and practical significance for government supports of the development of digital financial inclusion and promotion of the green technology innovation in heavy-polluting enterprises, and in turn it can promote the green transition of heavy-polluting enterprises, and help China achieve the "dual carbon" goal.

2. Literature Review and Hypothesis

2.1. Green Innovation

In the context of the "two-carbon" goal, green innovation, as an important activity to promote sustainable environmental development, has received extensive attention from scholars. A review of the existing research finds that the factors affecting the green innovation of enterprises are mainly concentrated in two aspects: environmental effects and resource supply. In terms of environmental effects, Lyubich et al. believe that when companies face higher environmental standards, they will be more inclined to develop and apply clean technologies to reduce the environmental pollution caused by their productions and operations and implement environmental regulations such as environmental taxes [9]. It is an effective way to improve environmental standards. Yu Lianchao et al. found that environmental taxes can effectively promote the green innovation of enterprises [10], which verifies the views of Lyubich et al. Furthermore, environmental regulations represented by taxes stimulate the green innovation of enterprises, and the incentive effect varies by differences in types of firms and regions [11]. The above research shows that scientific and reasonable environmental regulations and the policy mix can actively guide and motivate enterprises to carry out green technology innovation [12]. In addition to the abovementioned mandatory environmental effects, incentive-based environmental measures also have a positive impact on green innovation [11], such as government subsidies and some voluntary agreements [13,14]. In terms of resource supply, green innovation is characterized by high investments, long cycles, and high benefit uncertainty compared with other innovation activities and requires greater resource investment [15]. Green innovation resources, such as FDI, environmental investment, and foreign investment, have a positive impact on green innovation behavior and efficiency [16,17], and if the green loan interest rate provided by banks is lower than the threshold, enterprises tend to accept bank loans to implement green innovation [18]. In addition, corporate financial and governance status is also a cornerstone of green innovation resources. Good finance can provide sufficient material and human resources for green innovation [19]. The environmental protection orientation of corporate stakeholders and equity financing are also conducive to green innovation [20,21].

2.2. Digital Financial Inclusion

As an important engine for the country's high-quality development, digital inclusive finance provides new impetus and opportunities for promoting economic development [22], and its stable development has important macro and micro impacts. At the macro level, the development of digital inclusive finance has positive significance for promoting entrepreneurship, stimulating residents' consumption, accelerating inclusive growth, narrowing the urban-rural income gap, and driving the digital innovation of commercial banks [23–27]. At the microlevel, digital inclusive finance can, on the one hand, carry out an accurate risk assessment for enterprises under conditions of digital technology [28] and, on the other hand, enhance the information processing capabilities of financial institutions and investors, effectively reducing the relationship between enterprises and the market. The problem of information asymmetry between enterprises [29] increases the source channels and availability of funds for enterprises, thereby easing their financing constraints. In addition, some scholars have paid attention to the significant impact of digital financial inclusion on corporate innovation. The development of digital inclusive finance can alleviate the financing constraints and financial mismatches faced by enterprises and promote enterprise innovation through R&D investment, the accumulation of redundant expansion effects, and human capital upgrade effects [29–31].

2.3. Digital Financial Inclusion and Green Innovation

A large number of studies have shown that digital financial inclusion has a positive impact on corporate innovation activities, investment, and income [29,32]. Specifically, from the perspective of green innovation, the development of digital finance promotes urban economic agglomeration and optimizes the regional financial structure, provides a good external financial environment for the development of enterprises' green innovations, eases the financing constraints faced by enterprises [33], and then promotes enterprises' green innovations [34]. Jiang Jianxun et al. proved this conclusion from the perspective of new energy enterprises [35]. Based on the above research, we believe that the development of digital financial inclusion has a similar positive effect on the green innovation of heavy-polluting enterprises.

The Porter hypothesis proposes that innovation can offset the cost of complying with environmental requirements, and when the environmental system can be improved, it can further guide enterprises toward innovation. The mainstream view holds that both mandatory and incentive environmental effects can have a positive impact on corporate green innovation [10,14]. Currently, however, for heavily polluting enterprises mainly concentrated in the manufacturing sector, green innovation is closely related to capital market opening [36], resource acquisition and input [16], and the Green Credit System is formulated for the sustainable development of the environment and the transformation of green development of enterprises. The implementation of green credit policies, such as the "Guidelines", has changed the external credit environment, making it more difficult to obtain loans and increasing the financing constraints of such enterprises [37]. In addition, there is currently no complete green innovation mechanism in China to ensure that enterprises obtain public resources. Due to the nature of the industry, it is relatively difficult for heavily polluting enterprises to obtain public resources, such as government subsidies, which also deepens the financing constraints and weakens the incentive to engage in green innovation and, thus, is not conducive to the green innovation output of heavily polluting enterprises [38]. According to the theory of resource allocation efficiency, however, the limited financial capital in the market should flow into high-efficiency enterprises to achieve the overall effective allocation of resources and Pareto optimality, the misallocation of financial resources is a deviation from "effective allocation" [30]. The external financing that heavily polluting enterprises can obtain is limited. The main financing methods come from bond financing provided by financial institutions such as banks and equity financing in the capital market [39]. This type of financing not only pays more attention to the ability of enterprises to obtain profits and competitive advantages but also considers whether the funds can be recovered safely and whether the loan income is higher than the cost, including time value, etc., and is also affected by policy bias. Economic development allocates more financial resources to projects with quick returns and short cycles, while green innovation and development are characterized by long cycles, high costs, unclear market demands, and uncertain returns, making them vulnerable to misallocation of financial resources [30].

The financial environment is one of the main factors affecting the business activities of enterprises, and the supply of financial resources significantly affects the progress of business activities [40]. Compared with the "backward-looking" preference of the traditional credit model, the development of digital inclusive finance has effectively corrected the "stage mismatch" in the traditional financial system, making it easier for enterprises to obtain financial resources than before; that is, the development of digital inclusive finance can hedge financing. The "financial dilemma" was brought about by constraints [41]. First, the issue of information asymmetry is a leading problem that results in corporate financing constraints. Digital financial inclusion can reduce the information asymmetry between investors and companies by virtue of its digital technology [42]. Furthermore, digital inclusive finance makes up for the under covered long-tail groups in the traditional financial model and incorporates small and medium-sized enterprises, individual industrial and commercial households, and individual investors who are not able to participate in investment under the traditional financial model into the new financial system. It increases the investor group and broadens the source of funds, which effectively alleviates the problem of corporate financing constraints [29]. Second, digital inclusive finance improves the ability of information collection and integration. Through the capture and analysis of corporate behavioral data, it is possible to conduct more accurate risk assessments for enterprises and then strengthen the control of risks and credit, thus, forcing traditional transformation and upgrading of financial institutions to alleviate the misallocation of financial resources and improve the supply efficiency of financial resources [30]. Third, digital inclusive finance relies on its artificial intelligence technology, big data technology, machine learning technology, and other emerging technologies to make the production and operation of heavily polluting enterprises more scientific and efficient. It also contributes to the organizational structure becoming more rational and flexible, thereby reducing the cost of enterprises and expenses to provide more capital space for green innovation and ensure the smooth progress of green innovation of enterprises [31]. Based on the above analysis, the following hypothesis is proposed:

Hypothesis 1a (H1a). *Digital financial inclusion effectively promotes green innovation in enterprises.*

Hypothesis 1b (H1b). *Digital inclusive finance promotes the green innovation of enterprises by reducing the financing constraints and financial mismatches faced by enterprises.*

3. Variables, Data and Methods

3.1. Variable Setting

3.1.1. Explanatory Variables

Digital financial inclusion (Dindex). This paper uses the China Digital Financial Inclusion Index released by the Digital Finance Research Center of Peking University to measure the development degree of digital financial inclusion [43]. In addition, in order to ensure the accuracy of the research, we matched the prefecture-level city digital financial inclusion index with the enterprise micro-data (the selection of cities is based on those enterprises' registration places).

3.1.2. Dependent Variable

Green innovation (Patent). Due to the special nature of the industry, heavily polluting enterprises will inevitably cause some damage to the ecological environment. Their innovative output to eliminate or reduce pollution and damage caused to the ecological environment and weaken negative ecological effects is called green innovation. Referring to the practice of Wang Xin and Wang Ying [44], this paper adopts the natural logarithm method to measure the green innovation of enterprises by adding 1 to the number of green patent applications in the current year.

3.1.3. Mechanism Variables

(1) Financing constraints (Sa). In the current research on financing constraints in academia, KZ, WW, and Sa indices all measure the degree of financing constraints, but forSa, the basic data used in the calculation of the index are the scale and age of the enterprise, which has a strong exogenous and objective nature. Therefore, this paper refers to the research of Hadlock and Pierce [45], using an Sa index to measure the financing constraints faced by firms. The index calculation method is $\mathrm{Sa} = -0.737 \times \mathrm{Size} + 0.043 \times \mathrm{Size}^2 - 0.040 \times \mathrm{Age}$. (2) Financial mismatch (Fm). Limited financial capital in the market should flow into high-efficiency enterprises to achieve the effective allocation of overall resources, while the misallocation of financial resources is a deviation from the "effective allocation". This paper draws on the research of Shao Ting [46], using the cost of capital of enterprises. The financial mismatch is measured by the degree of deviation from the industry average cost of capital. The calculation method of this indicator is $[\mathrm{Interestexpense}/(\mathrm{Debt} - \mathrm{Accountspayable})]/\mathrm{Industryaveragecostofcapital}$.

3.1.4. Control Variables

This paper controls the variables at the financial and governance levels that may affect the green innovation of enterprises. The control variables at the financial level include enterprise scale (Size), which is the natural logarithm of the total assets of the enterprise; asset-liability ratio (Lev), which is the ratio of total liabilities to total assets; return on assets (Roa), which is the ratio of net profit to total assets; and fixed asset ratio (PPe), which is the ratio of net fixed assets to total assets. The control variables at the governance level include the combination of two positions (Dual); if the chairman and the general manager are the same person, the assignment is 1, otherwise, the assignment is 2; management shareholding (Msh) is the ratio of the number of shares held by management to the total number of shares; shareholding concentration ratio (Top) is the sum of the shareholding ratios of the top ten shareholders of the enterprise; and shareholding balance ratio (Balance) is the ratio of the sum of the shareholding ratios of the second-largest shareholder to the tenth largest shareholder and the shareholding ratio of the first largest shareholder. In addition, this paper also controls the industry effect (Ind) and year effect (Year) by setting dummy variables.

3.2. Data

This paper takes the China A-shares listed companies in heavy polluting industries from 2011 to 2020 as samples. The Digital Financial Inclusion Index, which is derived from the "Peking University Digital Financial Inclusion Index," compiled and released by the Peking University Financial Research Center. The green patent data used to measure green innovation is from the China Research Data Service Platform (CNRDS). The Guotai Security Database (CSMAR) provided the data on governance and financial aspects of heavy polluting industries. In addition, considering the quality of observation samples, this paper adopts the following principles to screen and process the data of listed companies: (1) The sample data of ST and ST* companies are excluded; (2) the sample data of the year with missing data were excluded to ensure the comparability of the data; (3) to eliminate the influence of outliers, this paper performs the Winsorization process on the 1% quantile of the data at the enterprise level.

3.3. Methods

3.3.1. Full Sample Regression

In order to explore how digital financial inclusion affects the green innovation of enterprises, this paper refers to the practice of Wan Jiayu et al. to construct a two-way fixed effect Model (1), and conducts an estimation test on the sample data [29].

$$Patent_{it} = \alpha_0 + \alpha_1 \times Dindex_{it} + \alpha_2 \times Controls_{it} + \Sigma Year + \Sigma Ind + \varepsilon_{it} \quad (1)$$

Model (1) Patent represents the green innovation of heavily polluting enterprises; α_0 represents the constant term of the equation; Dindex represents digital financial inclusion; Controls represents a set of corporate governance and financial control variables selected in this paper; Year and Ind represent the year dummy variable and industry dummy variable, respectively, used to control for time effects and industry effects; and ε represents a random error term. In Model (1), we focus on the preregression coefficient α_1 of digital financial inclusion. If the coefficient is significantly greater than zero, it indicates that digital financial inclusion will promote green innovation in heavily polluting enterprises; thus, H1a of this paper is verified.

3.3.2. Mechanism Effect Regression

In order to verify that financing constraints and financial mismatches are the mechanisms by which digital financial inclusion affects green innovation, this paper introduces a cross multiplication Model (2) of digital financial inclusion, financing constraints, and financial mismatches on the basis of Model (1).

$$\begin{aligned} Patent_{it} &= \lambda_0 + \lambda_1 \times Dindex_{it} \times Sa/Fm_{it} + \lambda_2 \times Dindex_{it} + \lambda_3 \times Sa/Fm_{it} \\ &+ \lambda_4 \times Controls_{it} + \Sigma Year + \Sigma Ind + \varepsilon_{it} \end{aligned} \quad (2)$$

Consistent with the meaning of Model (1), except for digital financial inclusion and financing constraints, the multiplication term of financial mismatch (Dindex × Sa/Fm) and mechanism variable financing constraints (Sa) and financial mismatch (Fm) are added. In Model (2), we mainly focus on the regression coefficient before the multiplication term λ_1. If the coefficient is significantly greater than zero, it indicates that the interactive effect of digital financial inclusion, financing constraints, and financial mismatch promotes green innovation; that is, the mechanism by which digital inclusive finance affects green innovation is through financing constraints and financial mismatch.

4. Analysis of Empirical Results

4.1. Descriptive Statistical Characteristics

Table 1 reports the descriptive statistics of the main variables. From this, it can be found that the maximum value of green innovation in the selected sample is 3.970, far exceeding the average value of 0.736. However, there are also samples with green innovation values of zero, which shows that there are large differences in the degree of green innovation between different enterprises. The standard deviation of digital inclusive finance is 0.718, indicating that digital financial inclusion is relatively concentrated near the average value, but the difference between the maximum value and the minimum value is still large. Judging from the descriptive statistical results of enterprise-level data, because the selected sample is a heavily polluting industry concentrated in manufacturing enterprises, its asset-liability ratio and fixed assets ratio are 0.426 and 0.311, respectively, which are relatively higher than those of other industries.

4.2. Collinearity and Correlation Test

To avoid the error caused by multicollinearity in the regression results, this paper conducts a VIF test among the variables. The test results are shown in the first column of Table 2, and the VIF values are all less than 10. Table 2 lists the correlation analysis results. It can be seen from the table that the correlation coefficient between digital financial inclusion

(Dindex) and green innovation (Patent) is 0.181, which is significant at the 1% level, providing preliminary validation of this paper. The main assumption is that digital financial inclusion can effectively promote green innovation in heavily polluting enterprises. On the whole, the highest correlation coefficient between digital financial inclusion and each control variable is 0.127, and the absolute value of the correlation coefficient between each control variable does not exceed 0.5, which is a low level. The above results show that the control variables selected in this paper do not have serious multicollinearity problems, and the regression results obtained are robust and reliable.

Table 1. Descriptive statistics of the main variables.

Variable	N	Mean	Std.Dev	Min	Max
Patent	6611	0.736	1.018	0	3.970
Dindex	6611	2.026	0.718	0.446	3.208
Size	6611	22.270	1.344	19.950	26.270
Lev	6611	0.426	0.209	0.051	0.950
Roa	6611	0.038	0.057	−0.193	0.204
PPe	6611	0.311	0.172	0.022	0.772
Dual	6611	1.756	0.429	1	2
Msh	6611	0.127	0.201	0	0.679
Top	6611	59.18	15.39	22.15	91.58
Balance	6611	0.874	0.766	0.035	3.772

Table 2. Correlation coefficient matrix.

Variable	VIF	Patent	Dindex	Size	Lev	Roa	PPe	Dual	Msh	Top	Balance
Patent	-	1									
Dindex	1.10	0.181 ***	1								
Size	1.81	0.487 ***	0.097 ***	1							
Lev	1.87	0.192 ***	−0.120 ***	0.486 ***	1						
Roa	1.35	0.00500	0.083 ***	−0.022 *	−0.432 ***	1					
PPe	1.30	0.124 ***	−0.112 ***	0.352 ***	0.398 ***	−0.209 ***	1				
Dual	1.10	0.117 ***	−0.108 ***	0.207 ***	0.162 ***	−0.054 ***	0.179 ***	1			
Msh	1.42	−0.125 ***	0.109 ***	−0.363 ***	−0.355 ***	0.198 ***	−0.309 ***	−0.243 ***	1		
Top	1.23	0.096 ***	0.067 ***	0.205 ***	−0.116 ***	0.247 ***	−0.041 ***	−0.045 ***	0.206 ***	1	
Balance	1.09	−0.061 ***	0.127 ***	−0.156 ***	−0.176 ***	0.080 ***	−0.150 ***	−0.050 ***	0.233 ***	0.00200	1

Note: *, **, and *** indicate significance at the 10%, 5%, and 1% levels, respectively.

4.3. Benchmark Regression

Table 3 reports the regression results of digital financial inclusion (Dindex) and green innovation (Patent) in Model (1), where column (1) is the regression result without control variables and column (2) is the regression result with control variables. The results show that the coefficients of digital financial inclusion are 0.2882 and 0.0031, respectively, both of which are significant at the 1% level, indicating that the development of digital financial inclusion can promote green innovation in heavily polluting enterprises.

Considering the endogeneity problem, this paper uses the independent variable with one lag period (Tool) as an instrumental variable to re-estimate the model by the two-stage least squares method. Column (3) is the regression result of the first stage after adding instrumental variables, tool variables and digital financial inclusion are significantly correlated at the 1% level, which fulfills the requirement of correlation of instrumental variables. Column (4) is the regression result of the second stage. Digital financial inclusion has a positive impact on the green innovation of enterprises at the 1% level. In summary, in the benchmark regression and the two-stage least squares regression, the coefficient of digital financial inclusion is significantly positive, indicating that the development of digital financial inclusion can effectively promote the green innovation of heavily polluting enterprises.

Table 3. Digital financial inclusion and green innovation.

Variable	(1)	(2)	(3)	(4)
			2SLS Regression	
	Patent	Patent	Dindex	Patent
			First	Two
Dindex	0.2882 ***	0.0031 ***		0.3310 ***
	(5.23)	(6.18)		(6.06)
Tool			1.0255 ***	
			(248.05)	
Size		0.3991 ***	0.0006	0.4128 ***
		(35.05)	(0.93)	(32.34)
Lev		−0.2052 ***	−0.0056	−0.1671 **
		(−3.11)	(−1.29)	(−2.25)
Roa		−0.2130	−0.0237 *	−0.0979
		(−1.06)	(−1.69)	(−0.44)
PPe		−0.3551 ***	−0.0104 **	−0.3956 ***
		(−4.51)	(−2.15)	(−4.57)
Dual		0.1094 ***	−0.0038 **	0.1350 ***
		(4.63)	(−2.11)	(5.14)
Msh		0.0764	0.0059	0.1128 *
		(1.38)	(1.51)	(1.78)
Top		−0.0010	−0.0001 **	−0.0012
		(−1.37)	(2.28)	(−1.42)
Balance		−0.0234 *	−0.0003	−0.0267 *
		(−1.68)	(0.31)	(−1.70)
Cons	0.5690 ***	−8.5870 ***	0.0301	−9.6591 ***
	(8.13)	(−34.52)	(1.54)	(−30.23)
Year	YES	YES	YES	YES
Ind	YES	YES	YES	YES
N	6611	6611	5516	5516
Adj-R^2	0.0976	0.3010	0.9932	0.2954

Note: Robust standard errors are in parentheses. *, **, and *** indicate significance at the 10%, 5%, and 1% levels, respectively.

4.4. Robustness Test

To ensure the reliability of the previous conclusions, the aspects that may have an impact are considered here, namely, the variable measurement problem and the dynamic problem, and the solutions are as follows. (1) Replacing the explained variables, innovation is divided into innovation input and innovation output. As a necessary condition for innovation output, innovation input can also reflect the green innovation of enterprises. Therefore, the green innovation of enterprises is remeasured from the perspective of innovation input. Drawing on the practice of Guo Ping [47], the proportion of R&D investment in the company's main business income (RD) is used as a proxy variable for corporate green innovation (Patent), and the regression results are shown in column (1) in Table 4. There was a significant positive correlation between the main variables. (2) Replacing explanatory variables, the prefecture-level city digital financial inclusion index is used to measure the explanatory variables in the previous article. Considering the problem of regional development, the provincial digital financial inclusion index (PDindex) is used here as a proxy for digital financial inclusion (Dindex) variables, the regression results are shown in column (2) in Table 4, and there is a significant positive correlation between the main variables. (3) For the explanatory variables with one lag period, considering the endogeneity caused by the dynamic problem, the explanatory variables with one lag period are brought back into the model for regression, and the regression results are shown in column (3) of Table 5. There was a significant positive correlation between them. In summary, the conclusions of this paper are robust.

Table 4. Robustness test.

Variable	(1)	(2)	(3)
	RD	**Patent**	**Patent**
Dindex	1.0832 ***		
	(10.77)		
PDindex		0.1780 ***	
		(4.29)	
L.Dindex			0.3310 ***
			(6.06)
Controls	YES	YES	YES
Cons	9.0161 ***	−8.5056 ***	−9.6591 ***
	(17.42)	(−34.33)	(−32.26)
Year	YES	YES	YES
Ind	YES	YES	YES
N	5399	6611	5516
Adj-R^2	0.2984	0.2989	0.3029

Note: Robust standard errors are in parentheses. *, **, and *** indicate significance at the 10%, 5%, and 1% levels, respectively.

4.5. Examination of the Mechanism of Action

Combined with the previous theoretical analysis, this paper believes that digital financial inclusion may promote green innovation in heavily polluting enterprises by alleviating the financing constraints at the enterprise level and financial mismatch at the market level. Therefore, this paper examines the impact mechanism of digital financial inclusion on the green innovation of heavily polluting enterprises from the perspectives of financing constraints and financial mismatch.

The impact of the interaction between digital financial inclusion and financing constraints (Dindex×Sa) and financial mismatch (Dindex×Fm) on green innovation is shown. The regression results show that the regression coefficient before the multiplication of digital financial inclusion and financing constraints is 0.1307, which is significant at the 10% level, and the regression coefficient before the multiplication of digital financial inclusion and financial mismatch is 0.0650, also at the 10% level. The above results show that financing constraints and financial mismatches are the mechanisms by which digital inclusive finance affects green innovation. In addition, this paper tests the action mechanism of the subdivision index coverage (Dcover) of digital financial inclusion to further verify the effectiveness of the action mechanism of financing constraints and financial mismatch. The test principle is the same as the above, and the results are shown in columns (3) and (4) of Table 5. It can be seen that the regression coefficients before the multiplication of digital inclusive finance coverage and financing constraints (Dcover×Sa) and financial mismatch (Dcover×Fm) are 0.1508 and 0.0601, respectively, both of which are significant at the 10% level. The above results show that digital inclusive finance alleviates financing constraints and financial mismatches through coverage, thereby promoting green innovation and verifying H1b.

4.6. Further Research

Based on the above analysis, we believe that digital financial inclusion has a greater effect on promoting green innovation in more mature enterprises. Enterprises with different life cycles have different characteristics, with obvious differences in market pressure, capital demand, financing constraints, and risk management [48]. Relatively speaking, enterprises in the growth stage have good development prospects, high growth potential, and high investment returns. They are expected to become benchmark enterprises in the industry in the future, and it is the best time for enterprises to realize the expansion of territory. During this period, companies usually implement expansion-oriented strategies, which lead to relatively high demand for capital, while the high capital demand caused by the long continuous cycle of green innovation also requires a high-quality capital supply [34,49], a crowding effect may occur. In terms of the utility of green innovation, the expected results of green innovation are highly uncertain, and it is a risky investment for growth-stage enterprises. The short-term benefits that can be achieved by using funds for green innovation investment are lower than the income that can be brought from investing capital in production and sales [50]. It may go against the company's strategic intention of increasing market share at the current stage, thus the subjective initiative of growing companies to carry out green innovation is relatively weak. For enterprises in the mature stage, their product production and sales tend to be stable. At this time, through green innovation, enterprises can not only improve the utilization efficiency and recycling rate of raw materials, and reduce resource costs and environmental costs [51,52], but can also draw consumers' attentions to the corporate environmental behavior, establish a good corporate image, and promote the growth of enterprise developable performance [53]. Compared with companies in the growth stage, companies in the mature stage are relatively complete in all aspects. With the help of the development of digital inclusive finance, they have more R&D strength and risk-taking ability to carry out green projects with high capital requirements and high-risk levels. Therefore, from the perspective of a life cycle, the high growth of enterprises may not be conducive to the promotion of digital inclusive finance for green innovation; that is, the development of digital inclusive finance may have a more significant incentive effect on the green innovation of enterprises in the mature stage of development.

Table 5. Mechanism of action test.

	(1)	(2)		(3)	(4)
Variable	**Dindex**		**Variable**	**Dcover**	
	Patent	**Patent**		**Patent**	**Patent**
Dindex × Sa	0.1307 * (1.65)		Dcover × Sa	0.1508 * (1.84)	
Sa	0.6681 *** (10.65)		Sa	0.6672 *** (10.62)	
Dindex×Fm		0.0650 * (1.83)	Dcover×Fm		0.0601 * (1.65)
Fm		−0.0472 * (−1.65)	Fm		−0.0477 * (−1.67)
Dindex	0.3185 *** (5.38)	0.3845 *** (6.19)	Dcover	0.2282 *** (5.07)	0.2791 *** (5.93)
Controls	YES	YES	Controls	YES	YES
Cons	−5.8539 *** (−14.98)	−9.2352 *** (−32.47)	Cons	−5.7958 *** (−14.85)	−9.1828 *** (−32.29)
Year	YES	YES	YES	YES	YES
Ind	YES	YES	YES	YES	YES
N	4799	4799	N	4799	4799
Adj-R^2	0.3441	0.3377	Adj-R^2	0.3437	0.3370

Note: Robust standard errors are in parentheses. *, **, and *** indicate significance at the 10%, 5%, and 1% levels, respectively.

To confirm this analysis, this paper refers to the practice of Liang Shangkun et al. [54] and ranks the growth rate of corporate sales revenue and capital expenditure rate from high to low and the retained rate of return and corporate age from low to high. The comprehensive score is calculated by assigning values, and then the comprehensive score is sorted and classified according to the industry. Companies belonging to the growth stage and mature stage are screened out, and the heterogeneous impact of digital inclusive finance on green innovation is tested in groups.

As shown in Table 6, the coefficient of digital financial inclusion in the growth stage group is 0.1802, and the coefficient of digital financial inclusion in the mature stage group is 0.4146, both of which are significant. This indicates that whether firms are in the growth stage or the mature stage, digital inclusive finance can have an incentive effect on green innovation. Furthermore, the grouping regression results obtained support the conclusion that the two are comparable through a seemingly uncorrelated test; that is, the predigital financial inclusion coefficient in the mature group is higher than the predigital financial inclusion coefficient in the growth period, which indicates that digital financial inclusion is important for green innovation. The promotion effect is stronger in mature enterprises.

Table 6. Heterogeneity test.

Variable	(1)	(2)
	Growth	Maturity
	Patent	Patent
Dindex	0.1802 *	0.4146 ***
	(1.80)	(4.66)
Controls	YES	YES
Cons	−9.0829 ***	−8.3315 ***
	(−17.28)	(−20.49)
Year	YES	YES
Ind	YES	YES
N	1618	2106
Adj-R^2	0.2910	0.3174
Suest	chi2(1) = 3.16 Prob > chi2 = 0.0754	

Note: Robust standard errors are in parentheses. *, **, and *** indicate significance at the 10%, 5%, and 1% levels, respectively.

5. Conclusions and Recommendations

5.1. Research Conclusions

Based on the green patent application data of listed companies in Shanghai and Shenzhen, A-share heavy polluting industries from 2011 to 2020 and the digital financial inclusion index compiled and released by the Financial Research Center of Peking University, this paper empirically analyzes the effect of digital financial inclusion on the green innovation of heavily polluting companies. The impact effect and its specific impact mechanism are further explored for life cycle heterogeneity. The main conclusions are as follows:

(1) Digital financial inclusion effectively stimulates the green innovation of heavily polluting enterprises, and the conclusion still holds after considering endogeneity and robustness.
(2) Digital financial inclusion alleviates corporate financing constraints, and the traditional problem of financial mismatch in financial services promotes the green innovation of heavily polluting enterprises.
(3) From the perspective of a life cycle, the effect of digital inclusive finance on the green innovation of heavily polluting enterprises in the mature stage is higher than that of those in the growth stage.

From the above conclusions, it can be seen that this study reveals the influencing mechanism of digital financial inclusion on the green innovation of heavy-polluting enterprises from the perspective of financing constraints and financial mismatch. It not only expands the relevant literature on the impact of digital financial inclusion on enterprises, but also provides a new perspective for analyzing the influencing factors of corporate green innovation. This study also clarifies the differences in the effects of digital financial inclusion on corporate green innovation at different development stages. However, this study also has certain limitations, mainly due to the availability of data. Moreover, the impact of the COVID-19 pandemic on green technology innovation in heavy-polluting enterprises was not considered in the research process. This is also an area worthy of further research in the future.

5.2. Policy Suggestions

This paper not only reveals the impact of the development of digital inclusive finance on the green innovation of heavily polluting enterprises but also clarifies its influence mechanism, which has important policy implications for promoting the green innovation of heavily polluting enterprises and the development of digital inclusive finance in China. First, the financing support system for green innovation of enterprises should be improved to promote the green transformation of heavily polluting enterprises. Green innovation in heavily polluting enterprises requires stable and continuous financial support. However, due to the nature of heavily polluting enterprises and the influence of national policies, obtaining financing is difficult because they face severe financing constraints and are easily affected by the misallocation of financial resources. Green innovation requires significant funds, thus the government should improve financing mechanisms to support the green innovation of heavily polluting enterprises. This will further encourage and support the development of digital inclusive finance through the application of information technology to support the financial needs for green innovation of heavily polluting enterprises. It will also improve the financing support mechanisms through green credit and tax incentives and the timely introduction of government subsidies to support the capital requirements for green innovation of heavily polluting enterprises. Second, for heavily polluting enterprises, it is necessary to strengthen their green business philosophy, enhance their environmental protection awareness, improve their information disclosure, reduce the degree of information asymmetry in the financing market, improve their financing capabilities, and avoid green credit. The punishment mechanism makes heavily polluting enterprises vulnerable to financing difficulties, resulting in insufficient funding sources for green innovation. Finally, for financial institutions such as banks, the channels for providing financial support to heavily polluting enterprises should be improved, including special loans to heavily polluting enterprises to support the adoption of green technology innovation.

Author Contributions: Conceptualization, L.X. and X.Z.; data curation, X.Z.; formal analysis, L.X. and X.Z.; funding acquisition, L.X. and X.Z.; methodology, X.Z. and L.X.; software, X.Z.; supervision, L.X.; writing—original draft, X.Z. and L.X.; writing—review and editing, X.Z. and L.X. All authors have read and agreed to the published version of the manuscript.

Funding: This work was supported by the Key scientific research projects of colleges and universities of Henan Province (22A790024).

Institutional Review Board Statement: Not applicable.

Informed Consent Statement: Not applicable.

Data Availability Statement: The data presented in this study are openly available in the China Research Data Service Platform and the Guotai Security Database.

Conflicts of Interest: The authors declare no conflict of interest. The funders had no role in the design of the study; in the collection, analyses, or interpretation of data; in the writing of the manuscript, or in the decision to publish the results.

References

1. Wang, S.R.; Zhu, F.E. Research on realizing the goal of "double carbon" under the overall layout of ecological civilization construction. *Theor. Discuss.* **2022**, 125–129. [CrossRef]
2. Zhu, X.K.; Gong, B.L. The risk challenge and path choice of realizing the "double carbon" goal under the background of high-quality development. *Gov. Res.* **2022**, *38*, 13–23.
3. Lun, X.B.; Liu, Y. Digital government, digital economy and green technology innovation. *J. Shanxi Univ. Financ. Econ.* **2022**, *44*, 1–13.
4. Sun, T.Q. G20 Advanced Principles for Digital Inclusive Finance: Background, framework and outlook. *Tsinghua Financ. Rev.* **2016**, 29–33. [CrossRef]
5. Yu, B. How does the green credit policy affect the technological innovation of heavily polluting enterprises? *Econ. Manag.* **2021**, *43*, 35–51.
6. Zhang, Y.M.; Xing, C.; Zhang, Y. Research on the impact of media attention on green technology innovation of heavily polluting enterprises. *J. Manag.* **2021**, *18*, 557–568.

7. Ionescu, L. Corporate Environmental Performance, Climate Change Mitigation, and Green Innovation Behavior in Sustainable Finance. *Econ. Manag. Financ. Mark.* **2021**, *16*, 94–106.
8. Qiao, B.; Zhao, G.T.; Shen, S.H. Can digital inclusive finance promote green innovation of enterprises? *South. Financ.* **2022**, *1*, 14–27.
9. Lyubich, E.; Shapiro, J.; Walker, R. Regulating mismeasured pollution: Implications of firm heterogeneity for environmental policy. *AEA Pap. Proc.* **2018**, *108*, 136–142. [CrossRef]
10. Yu, L.C.; Zhang, W.G.; Bi, Q. Will environmental tax force green innovation of enterprises? *J. Audit. Econ.* **2019**, *34*, 79–90.
11. Peng, X.; Li, B. Research on China's industrial green transformation under different types of environmental regulation. *J. Financ. Econ.* **2016**, *42*, 134–144.
12. Nie, A.Y.; He, X.G. The development of enterprise green technology innovation: Environmental regulation and policy combination. *Reform* **2012**, *218*, 102–108.
13. Stucki, T.; Woerter, M.; Arvanitis, S.; Peneder, M.; Rammer, C. How different policy instruments affect green product innovation: A differentiated perspective. *Energy Policy* **2018**, *114*, 245–261. [CrossRef]
14. Li, X.A. Environmental regulation, government subsidies, and regional green technology innovation. *Econ. Surv.* **2021**, *38*, 14–23.
15. Wang, B.; Zhang, Y.Z.; Chen, L.S.; Yao, X. Decomposition of green innovation level and influential factor contribution degree of Chinese cities. *Sci. Res. Manag.* **2020**, *41*, 123–134.
16. Bi, K.X.; Wang, Y.H.; Yang, C.J. The impact of innovation resource input on the green innovation capability of green innovation system: An empirical study based on the perspective of manufacturing FDI inflow. *China Soft Sci. Mag.* **2014**, *279*, 153–166.
17. Qian, L.; Wang, W.P.; Xiao, R.Q. A study on the differences in green innovation efficiency of Chinese regional industrial enterprises from the perspective of shared input correlation. *China Popul. Resour. Environ.* **2018**, *28*, 27–39.
18. Huang, Z.; Liao, G.; Li, Z. Loaning scale and government subsidy for promoting green innovation. *Technol. Forecast. Soc. Change* **2019**, *144*, 148–156. [CrossRef]
19. Ren, S.G.; Xiang, Q.L.; He, D.J. Will voluntary environmental regulation promote green innovation of enterprises?—Take the ISO14001 standard as an example. *Res. Dev. Manag.* **2018**, *30*, 1–11.
20. Xiao, X.H.; Tian, Q.H.; Wang, Z.J. Can stakeholders' environmental protection orientation promote green innovation?—A moderated mediating effect model. *Sci. Res. Manag.* **2021**, *42*, 159–166.
21. Wang, X.; Chu, X. Green technology innovation and financing contract selection in China's manufacturing industry. *Stud. Sci. Sci.* **2019**, *37*, 351–361.
22. Teng, L.; Ma, D.G. Can digital finance promote high-quality development? *Stat. Res.* **2020**, *37*, 80–92.
23. Xie, X.L.; Shen, Y.; Zhang, H.X.; Guo, F. Can digital finance promote entrepreneurship?—Evidence from China. *China Econ. Q.* **2018**, *17*, 1557–1580.
24. Yi, X.J.; Zhou, L. Does the development of digital inclusive finance significantly affect residents' consumption: Micro-evidence from Chinese households. *J. Financ. Res.* **2018**, *11*, 47–67.
25. Zhang, X.; Wan, G.H.; Zhang, J.J.; He, Z.Y. Digital economy, inclusive finance, and inclusive growth. *Econ. Res. J.* **2019**, *54*, 71–86.
26. Zhou, L.; Feng, D.W.; Yi, X.J. Digital inclusive finance and urban-rural income gap: "Digital dividend" or "Digital divide". *Economist* **2020**, 99–108. [CrossRef]
27. Wang, S.H.; Xie, X.L. Economic pressure or social pressure: Digital finance development and digital innovation of commercial banks. *Economist* **2021**, 100–108. [CrossRef]
28. Huang, H. Formation and challenges of digital financial ecosystem—Experience from China. *Economist* **2018**, 80–85. [CrossRef]
29. Wan, J.Y.; Zhou, Q.; Xiao, Y. Digital finance, financing constraints, and enterprise innovation. *Econ. Rev.* **2020**, *1*, 71–83.
30. Zhao, X.; Zhong, S.; Guo, X. Development of digital inclusive finance, financial mismatch mitigation, and enterprise innovation. *Sci. Res. Manag.* **2021**, *42*, 158–169.
31. Jiang, D.C.; Pan, X.W. The impact of digital economy development on corporate innovation performance: Based on empirical evidence of listed companies in China. *J. Shanxi Univ.* **2022**, *45*, 149–160.
32. Guo, P.Y.; Yin, Z.C. Driving force of independent innovation of small and micro enterprises—Evidence from the perspective of digital Inclusive. *Financ. Econ. Trends* **2022**, *732*, 85–104.
33. Wei, S.W.; Du, L.M.; Pan, S. How can digital economy promote green innovation—Empirical evidence from Chinese cities. *Financ. Econ.* **2022**, 1–14. [CrossRef]
34. Feng, S.L.; Zhang, R.; Li, G.X. Environmental decentralization, digital finance and green technology innovation. *Struct. Change Econ. Dyn.* **2022**, *61*, 70–83. [CrossRef]
35. Jiang, J.X.; Tang, Y.C.; Li, X.J. Digital finance enables green innovation of new energy enterprises in the context of dual carbon: From the perspective of financing constraints. *Contemp. Econ. Manag.* **2022**, *44*, 81–89.
36. Sha, Y.Z.; Zhang, P.; Wang, Y.R.; Xu, Y.F. Capital market opening and green innovation—Evidence from Shanghai-Hong Kong stock connect and the Shenzhen-Hong Kong stock connect. *Energy Econ.* **2021**, *111*, 106048. [CrossRef]
37. Tan, X.; Yan, Y.; Dong, Y. Peer effect in green credit induced green innovation: An empirical study from China's Green Credit Guidelines. *Resour. Policy* **2022**, *76*, 102619. [CrossRef]
38. Yang, L.Y.; Zhang, Z.Y. The impact of green credit policy on green innovation of enterprises. *Stud. Sci. Sci.* **2022**, *40*, 345–356.
39. Yang, G.Z.; Xi, Y.T. Empirical Study on financing constraints of green technology innovation activities of enterprises. *Ind. Technol. Econ.* **2019**, *38*, 70–76.

40. Hsu, P.H.; Tian, X.; Xu, Y. Financial development and innovation: Cross-country evidence. *J. Financ. Econ.* **2014**, *112*, 116–135. [CrossRef]
41. Duan, Y.Q.; He, L.Z.; Ke, X. Digital finance, technology intensive manufacturing and green development. *Shanghai Econ. Res.* **2021**, 89–105. [CrossRef]
42. Tang, S.; Wu, X.C.; Zhu, J. Digital finance and enterprise technological innovation—Structural characteristics, mechanism identification and effect differences under financial supervision. *Manag. World* **2020**, *36*, 52–66.
43. Guo, F.; Wang, J.Y.; Wang, F.; Kong, T.; Zhang, X.; Cheng, Z.Y. Measuring the development of digital financial inclusion in China: Index compilation and spatial characteristics. *China Econ. Q.* **2020**, *19*, 1401–1418.
44. Wang, X.; Wang, Y. Research on green credit policy to promote green innovation. *J. Manag. World* **2021**, *37*, 173–188.
45. Hadlock, C.J.; Pierce, J.R. New evidence on measuring financial constraints: Moving beyond the KZ index. *Rev. Financ. Stud.* **2010**, *23*, 1909–1940. [CrossRef]
46. Shao, T. Financial misallocation, ownership structure and return on capital: A study of China's industrial enterprises from 1999 to 2007. *J. Financ. Res.* **2010**, *4*, 51–68.
47. Guo, P. Policy uncertainty and corporate R&D investment: "Delay effect" or "Preemption effect"—An analysis based on the world bank Chinese enterprise survey data. *Shanxi Univ. Financ. Econ.* **2016**, *38*, 1–12.
48. Chen, H.; Zhang, Y.; Liu, D.X. Government subsidies, tax incentives and enterprise innovation performance: An empirical study at different life cycle stages. *Nankai Manag. Rev.* **2019**, *22*, 187–200.
49. Wang, Q.G.; Xu, X.Y. Value creation mechanism and empirical test of corporate social responsibility—Based on Stakeholder Theory and life cycle theory. *China Soft Sci.* **2016**, *2*, 179–192.
50. Wu, J.Z.; Fan, H.L. Research on enterprise green innovation driving mode based on configuration perspective. *Res. Dev. Manag.* **2021**, *33*, 41–53.
51. Deng, Y.P.; Wang, L.; Zhou, W.J. Does environmental regulation promote green innovation capability—Empirical evidence from China. *Stat. Res.* **2021**, *38*, 76–86.
52. Zhou, H.; Liu, J.; Jiang, W.Y.; Wan, M.Y. Product green innovation decision and green channel incentive mechanism design. *J. Syst. Sci.* **2020**, *28*, 61–66.
53. Xi, L.S.; Zhao, H. Executives' dual environmental awareness, green innovation and enterprise sustainable development performance. *Econ. Manag.* **2022**, *44*, 139–158.
54. Liang, S.K.; Zhang, Y.; Wang, Y.C. Internal remuneration gap and company value: A new exploration based on life cycle theory. *J. Financ. Res.* **2019**, *466*, 188–206.

International Journal of
Environmental Research and Public Health

MDPI

Article

Research on the Policy Effect and Mechanism of Carbon Emission Trading on the Total Factor Productivity of Agricultural Enterprises

Junguo Hua, Di Zhu and Yunfei Jia *

School of Economics and Management, Henan Agricultural University, Ping An Avenue 218, Zhengzhou 450000, China; hjghnnd168@163.com (J.H.); 18203749635@163.com (D.Z.)
* Correspondence: jiayunfei@henau.edu.cn

Abstract: Given the rural revitalization strategy in the new era, agricultural development is faced with the dual constraints of resources and the environment. Promoting the green development of agriculture is one of the important missions to solve major social issues in the new era. The implementation goal of the carbon emission trading system is to achieve a win-win situation between carbon emission reduction and green development. To evaluate the effectiveness of the carbon emission trading system on agricultural enterprises, this paper uses a double-difference model to analyze the policy effect and mechanism research path of the impact of the carbon emission trading system on the total factor productivity of agricultural enterprises. The results based on the panel data of listed agricultural companies from 2010 to 2020 show that (1) carbon emission trading rights have significantly improved the total factor productivity of agricultural enterprises; (2) green innovation in carbon emission trading rights have an impact on the total factor productivity of agricultural enterprises; and (3) heterogeneity analysis shows that the effect of carbon emission trading rights on the total factor productivity of agricultural enterprises mainly exists in large-scale, nonstate-owned, high-debt enterprises, enterprises in the eastern region, and enterprises with government subsidies. Therefore, in the future, China should continue to implement the current carbon emission trading rights system in air pollution control, and at the same time, it needs to be supplemented by government intervention and other means for long-term governance. In conclusion, the study provides a reference value for promoting the realization of the long-term goal of "low carbon" and "high quality" green development of agricultural economy and for making reasonable and effective behavioral decisions for the survival and development of enterprises.

Keywords: carbon emissions trading; total factor productivity of agricultural enterprises; green innovation; double difference

Citation: Hua, J.; Zhu, D.; Jia, Y. Research on the Policy Effect and Mechanism of Carbon Emission Trading on the Total Factor Productivity of Agricultural Enterprises. *IJERPH* **2022**, *19*, 7581. https://doi.org/10.3390/ijerph19137581

Academic Editors: Jie Chen, Qian Zhou and Ting Zhang

Received: 26 May 2022
Accepted: 19 June 2022
Published: 21 June 2022

1. Introduction

The frequent occurrence of extreme weather has made the problem of environmental pollution an important issue in countries around the world. To protect the natural environment and alleviate air pollution, the European Union Emissions Trading System (EUETS) came into being in the early 20th century and developed rapidly as an important driver for the high-quality development of enterprises. According to the research data of the World Bank, the carbon emission trading policies reduced carbon emissions by 2–5% during the period of 2005–2007, with an annual reduction of 40–100 million tons of carbon emissions. This shows that the carbon emission trading policies are of great significance in reducing emissions and promoting the development of global green technology applications. Since the implementation of the reform and opening-up policy, China's carbon emissions have continued to grow. Especially after China's entry into the WTO, with the advantages of resources and demographic dividends and the "4 trillion" plan in 2008, the scale of foreign trade has continued to increase, the manufacturing industry has expanded rapidly, and carbon dioxide emissions have increased. China's carbon dioxide emissions account for nearly 30% of global emissions. From 2002 to 2007, the average growth rate of carbon emissions reached 14%, making China gradually become the world's largest energy consumer and carbon dioxide emitter. As a responsible major country, China has realized the importance of harmonious coexistence between economic development and the natural environment, and has begun to emphasize "green development". The five development concepts of "innovation, coordination, greenness, openness, and sharing" put forward by the Fifth Plenary Session of the 18th Central Committee have elicited a top-to-bottom consensus at the national level. In response to global warming, the Chinese government has adopted a series of policy measures. In 2011, the National Development and Reform Commission issued the "Notice on Carrying out the Pilot Work of Carbon Emissions Trading", formally approving pilot work on carbon emissions trading in Beijing, Shanghai, Shenzhen, Guangdong, Tianjin, Hubei, and Chongqing. In 2012, carbon emission trading markets were established in Beijing, Shanghai, and other regions. In December 2017, the construction of the national carbon emission trading market was launched. China has entered the era of carbon emissions trading [1]. The Fifth Plenary Session of the 19th Central Committee of the Communist Party of China once again emphasized that the shift of economic growth to the mode supported by the promotion of total factor productivity of enterprises is the inevitable choice for China's economy to face the decline of capital returns and the disappearance of demographic dividends and the source of power for achieving high-quality economic development [2]. Agriculture is a barometer of the national economy; listed agricultural companies are the leaders of the agricultural industry, shouldering the important mission to drive farmers to increase production and income, promote agricultural industrial structure adjustment, and promote the process of agricultural industrialization. Their management level represents the reality of China's agricultural industry and development prospects. Therefore, it is of great significance to study the impact of the carbon trading pilot policies implemented in China on the total factor productivity of listed agricultural enterprises under the actual market environment and institutional conditions. The carbon emission trading policy mainly focuses on regulating carbon emission reduction at the enterprise level. Agricultural enterprises regulated by carbon emission trading may respond by accelerating green innovation from the perspective of compliance cost and innovation compensation [3], thereby indirectly affecting the full factor production rates of enterprises. Therefore, effectively quantifying the impact of carbon emission trading policies on agricultural enterprises' total factor productivity and its internal mechanism is helpful for the study of improving enterprises' total factor productivity against the background of "carbon peaking" and "carbon neutrality" and further promoting the quality of economic growth, the coordinated promotion of high-quality economic development in China, and the implementation of new development concepts play a pivotal role.

Taking listed agricultural companies from 2010 to 2020 as samples, this paper uses endogenous growth theory and cost and innovation compensation theory as the basis, with the help of logical reasoning and mathematical derivation, to analyze the impact of carbon emission trading rights on the total factor productivity of agricultural enterprises and explore its mechanism. On this basis, an empirical test is carried out, and the effect of heterogeneity is further analyzed. The possible marginal contributions of this paper are as follows: First, this paper makes an accurate assessment of the environmental and economic effects of the carbon emission trading pilot policy to provide direct empirical evidence for the further improvement of the carbon emission trading policy, which is a useful supplement to the empirical research field of carbon trading in China. Second, from the perspective of microagricultural enterprises, this paper examines the impact of emission trading policies on the total factor productivity of listed agricultural enterprises and the possible emission reduction mechanism and expands the research perspective in related fields to provide a reference for agricultural enterprises to meet the current "low carbon" and "high quality" economic development requirements. Third, this paper provides new evidence and explanations for the use of market-oriented environmental regulation to improve the total factor productivity of listed agricultural companies, thereby promoting the high-quality transformation of China's agricultural economy, and enriches the literature on the economic effects of carbon emission trading policies from a micro perspective. Fourth, the evidence and findings obtained from this study can provide a supportive experience and policy suggestions for China to improve the carbon trading mechanism and implement a unified national carbon trading market.

2. Literature Review

Domestic and foreign studies on the impact of environmental regulation on total factor productivity have not reached a consistent conclusion. "Follow the cost" theorists believe that the cost of environmental regulation inhibits the improvement of enterprise productivity and international competitiveness, resulting in a decline in the total factor productivity of enterprises [4–6]. In contrast, the "innovation compensation" theorists believe that the public nature of environmental protection determines the inefficiency of the market mechanism in its allocation. Enterprises will not take the initiative to carry out technological innovation, but environmental regulation can enable enterprises to internalize external costs and stimulate them. Enterprises carry out innovation and promote the improvement of the total factor productivity of enterprises [7–10]. At the same time, some scholars believe that the impact of environmental regulation on total factor productivity depends on the relative magnitude of the above two effects, so they pay more attention to the nonlinear relationship between environmental regulation and total factor productivity. The effectiveness and cross-effect of green innovation were re-examined [11,12], while others pointed out that there were regional differences in the promotion of environmental regulation and technological innovation, and there was a "U"-shaped relationship between the two [13]. Liu Siming believes that the relationship between environmental regulation and productivity growth is nonlinear or uncertain, and the relationship between the two will vary due to different industries and types of environmental regulation [14]. Although there are abundant studies on the impact of environmental regulation on total factor productivity, few scholars have explored it from the perspective of agricultural enterprises.

The types of environmental regulation in China can be roughly divided into three types: command-and-control, market-incentivized, and public participation. Previous studies have investigated the command-and-control environmental regulation represented by the "two-control zone", which increases the production cost of regulated enterprises and leads to a decrease in the total factor productivity of enterprises. Market-incentivized environmental regulation, represented by sulfur dioxide emission rights, improves the total factor productivity of enterprises by promoting enterprise innovation [15]. Public participation in environmental regulation represented by environmental information disclosure can also promote the total factor productivity of enterprises [16]. However, there are relatively few studies examining the impact of carbon emissions trading, one of China's current important carbon emission reduction policies, on total factor productivity. In addition, related studies on the impact of carbon emission rights trading have also given more attention to carbon intensity, carbon emissions [17], carbon allocation [18], enterprise value [19], enterprise innovation [20], enterprise green innovation [21], and low-carbon technology collaborative sharing against the background of carbon emissions trading [22], and less research on the impact on agricultural enterprises' total factor productivity has been conducted.

The main goal of traditional technological innovation is to bring economic benefits to enterprises, while green technological innovation, as an important part of traditional technological innovation, emphasizes the comprehensive benefits of the economy, environment and society. In recent years, with the continuous evolution of the needs of economic and social development, green technology has been frequently applied in the fields of energy conservation and environmental protection, clean energy, cleaner production, and the circular economy [23]. Due to the characteristics of the "dual externalities" of green technology innovation, in the absence of market pricing mechanism constraints and policy interventions, there will be insufficient motivation for enterprises to innovate. As an important market-based environmental policy, carbon emission trading has a reasonable price formation mechanism and government management mechanism, which can eliminate "double externalities" to a large extent and encourage enterprises to carry out green technology innovation. As the best way to solve the contradiction between the environment and development, technological innovation requires enterprises to pay more attention to ecological and environmental factors when solving the above problems [24]. Therefore, it is of great significance to explore the impact of green technology innovation on the total factor productivity of agricultural enterprises under the carbon emission mechanism.

By sorting out the relevant literature, it is not difficult to see that there are few studies evaluating the environmental and economic effects of carbon emission trading in China. From the perspective of microagricultural enterprises, this paper uses the double-difference method to study and analyze the data of listed agricultural companies from 2010 to 2020, focusing on the impact of the total factor productivity of listed agricultural companies after the implementation of the carbon emission trading system. Introducing variables of green technology innovation can better explain the impact of the carbon emission trading system on enterprise productivity and its influential mechanism. The study conclusions provide a basis for the government to establish a national carbon emission trading market for the evaluation of the economic effects of carbon emission rights and have great practical significance for making reasonable and effective behavioral decisions for the survival and development of enterprises.

3. Materials and Methods

3.1. Theoretical Mechanism of Carbon Emission Trading Rights and Total Factor Productivity of Agricultural Enterprises

Carbon emissions trading internalizes the external cost of carbon emissions of agricultural enterprises through the price mechanism to reduce the carbon dioxide emissions of enterprises [25]. The direct effect of it has two aspects. One is the cost-push effect. To achieve the emission reduction target, the Chinese government sets a strict total carbon emission amount according to social needs and then decomposes the total carbon emission target layer by layer to each lower level. In this way, carbon emission rights are commercialized. After agricultural enterprises are constrained by the carbon emission rights trading mechanism, if they want to discharge more than the quota, they need to purchase from the government or the market, which will weaken the technological innovation ability of enterprises and reduce the overall efficiency of the factor productivity of agricultural enterprises [26], otherwise it will be punished accordingly, which will undoubtedly increase the extra cost of relevant subjects, thus forcing each subject to use carbon emission allowances efficiently. The second is the income incentive effect. By designing a system that meets the environmental conditions of the Chinese market, carbon emission rights are allowed to be traded under certain rules, and relevant entities gain more choice space and can choose to buy or sell under their own cost constraints without quota. When the carbon price in the trading market is higher than the emission reduction cost, the relevant entities can have excess emission allowances through emission reduction and sell the allowances in the carbon emission rights trading market; when the carbon price in the trading market is lower than the emission reduction cost, the relevant entities can buy carbon emission allowances in the market through carbon emission trading. Carbon trading can form an effective allocation of the market so that enterprises with lower emission reduction costs can reduce carbon emissions more, and enterprises with higher emission reduction costs can reduce carbon emissions less so that the total cost of emission reduction in society can reach the lowest value. Therefore, agricultural enterprises have incentives to benefit from carbon emission trading by selling multiple carbon emission quotas and improving the competitiveness of enterprises. At the same time, higher productivity is generated by innovation incentives, efficiency improvement, and redistribution [27]. Based on this,

this paper proposes Hypothesis 1 for the emission reduction effect of carbon emission trading policies:

Hypothesis 1 (H1). *The pilot policy of carbon emission trading promotes the improvement of the total factor productivity of agricultural enterprises.*

3.2. Theoretical Mechanism of Green Innovation in Carbon Emission Trading Rights and Total Factor Productivity of Agricultural Enterprises

If China's carbon emission trading pilot policy can effectively improve the total factor productivity of agricultural enterprises, how does it achieve this effect? On the one hand, under the conditions of a given carbon quota, for enterprises in the carbon emission pilot areas, the pilot policy will increase the carbon emission cost of enterprises in the pilot areas, thereby increasing the operational burden of enterprises. Enterprises actively carry out technology research and development, which can reduce carbon emissions, thereby reducing the pressure on corporate emissions. On the other hand, companies carry out green technology innovations to reduce their carbon emissions to obtain excess carbon emission credits. These excess carbon emission credits can generate profit for companies selling them in the carbon emissions trading market. In the long run, when profit-seeking enterprises face the constraints of carbon emission limits, realizing low-carbon production through green innovation is the optimal choice for enterprises. Therefore, carbon trading policies force companies to carry out green innovation activities and reduce carbon emissions per unit of output. This approach can not only make the total carbon emissions of the enterprise meet the established carbon emission constraint target but also make a profit by selling the saved carbon emission credit in the carbon emission rights trading market. The technological innovation capability of an enterprise is an important factor affecting the total factor productivity of an enterprise. To this end, this paper selects the green innovation effect path to test the transmission mechanism. To investigate whether the pilot policy of carbon emissions trading can improve the total factor productivity of enterprises in the pilot area by improving the level of green innovation of enterprises, this paper proposes Hypothesis 2:

Hypothesis 2 (H2). *The pilot policy of carbon emissions trading improves the total factor productivity of enterprises by promoting enterprise innovation.*

4. Research Design

4.1. Sample Selection and Data Sources

To test the above assumptions, according to the CSRC industry classification standard, this paper selects all A shares listed on the Shanghai and Shenzhen Stock Exchanges and GEM belonging to agriculture; forestry; animal husbandry and fishery; agricultural and sideline food processing; food manufacturing and wine, beverage, and refined tea manufacturing enterprises as the research object. The annual data of enterprises during the sample period from 2010 to 2020 are selected, and the relationship between carbon emission trading rights, green innovation, and total factor productivity of agricultural enterprises is analyzed. Before using the data, we processed the data as follows: (1) ST and *ST-listed agricultural companies were removed; (2) listed agricultural companies with missing main financial variables and listed agricultural companies with abnormal and missing data were removed; (3) all nonvirtual variable values were processed by 1% pre- and post-tailing to eliminate the influence of extreme values. Finally, 1340 observations were obtained. The financial data of listed companies are from the China Stock Market Accounting Research (CSMAR) Database, and the patent data of green technology of enterprises are from the National Patent Database. The total factor productivity data of agricultural enterprises are from the CSMAR and Rethink Databases, assisting Tonghuashun and Sina Finance and Economics (CSMAR: http://cndata1.csmar.com/ (accessed on 1 January 2022); National Patent Database: https://www.cnpat.com.cn/ (accessed on 1 January 2022); Rethink Databases: http://www.resset.cn/db (accessed on 1 January 2022); Tonghuashun: https://www.10jqka.com.cn/ (accessed on 1 January 2022); Sina Finance and Economics: https://finance.sina.com.cn/ (accessed on 1 January 2022)).

4.2. Variable Definition and Interpretation

4.2.1. Explained Variables

This paper refers to the research of Li Dandan and Li DoudouLu [28] and Czyzewski et al. [29]. Considering the endogeneity problems in sample selection and statistical methods, this paper uses semiparametric methods (OP method and LP method, etc.) to calculate total factor productivity data at the firm level. First, the calculation results of the LP method are used for benchmark regression, and then the calculation results of the OP method are used for robustness testing. The calculation *TFP* method and index selection of this calculation method are as follows:

$$TFP_{ijt} = \alpha_{jt} + \beta_{jt}L_{ijt} + \gamma_{jt}K_{ijt} + \delta_{jt}M_{ijt} + \varepsilon_{ijt}$$

In the above formula, TFP_{ijt}, L_{ijt}, K_{ijt}, and M_{ijt} are the t logarithms of total factor productivity, labor input, capital input, and intermediate input of private enterprises in industry i, respectively; j and ε_{ijt} are random disturbance terms. The above variables are all based on 2010.

4.2.2. Mechanism Variables

Corporate green innovation. There are three types of patents in China: invention, utility model, and appearance, of which technology-related patents are mainly inventions and utility models. Referring to the research of Liu Jiamin et al., the green innovation of enterprises is measured by the number of green patent applications [30]. The data on the green innovation of listed companies come from the National Patent and Property Office. The data are cleaned and screened by using the classification of green technology patents defined by the World Intellectual Property Organization (WIPO), and the total number of green patents, the number of green invention patents, and the number of green utility model patents applied for by listed companies each year are obtained. The larger the value is, the higher the level of green innovation.

4.2.3. Control Variables

To reduce the estimation bias caused by omitted variables, this paper draws on the factors that may affect the total factor productivity of agricultural enterprises in the literature and selects the following variables as control variables: enterprise size (Size), return on assets (Roa), asset-liability ratio (Lev), agency cost (Agencost), cash flow from operating activities (Cflow), factor intensity (Capital), and the shareholding ratio of the largest shareholder (Top1). The specific definition of each variable is shown in Table 1.

Table 1. Definition of each variable.

Variable Symbol	Variable Name	Variable Description
TFP	total factor productivity of agribusiness	by CD production function method, OP method, LP method
Size	Enterprise size	Ln (total assets at the end of the period)
Roa	Return on Assets	Net profit/Total assets
Lev	Assets and liabilities	Total liabilities at the end of the period/total assets at the end of the period
Agencost	agency cost	Administrative expenses/main business income
Cflow	cash flow from operating activities	Net cash flow from operating activities/total assets at the end of the period
Capital	factor density	Ln (real net fixed assets per capita)
Top1	Shareholding ratio of the largest shareholder	Shareholding ratio of the largest shareholder
Patent	Enterprise green innovation	The total number of green patent applications
Invent	Enterprises invent green innovation	Number of green invention patent applications
Actual	Enterprise practical green innovation	Green utility model patent application

4.3. Model Establishment

The impact of carbon emission rights on the total factor productivity of agricultural enterprises in the double-difference model constructed in this paper is as follows:

$$TFP_{it} = \alpha_0 + \alpha_1 Treat_i * Time_t + \alpha_2 Controls_{it} + \varepsilon_i + \varepsilon_t + \varepsilon_{it} \quad (1)$$

To test for the existence of a mechanism effect, the following model was constructed:

$$TFP_{it} = \gamma_0 + \gamma_1 Treat_i * Time_t * Patent_{it} + \gamma_2 Treat_i * Time_t + \gamma_3 Patent_{it} + \gamma_4 \text{Controls}_{it} + \varepsilon_i + \varepsilon_t + \varepsilon_{it} \quad (2)$$

In Equations (1) and (2), TFP_{it} reflects the total factor productivity i of agricultural enterprises of sample companies α_0 during the observation period, where t is a constant term, $Treat_t$ represents a dummy variable for policy treatment (1 for provinces located in pilot areas, 0 for provinces located in nonpilot areas), and $Time_t$ represents the time dummy variable (1 after the policy, 0 before the policy), which is the $Treat_i * Time_t$ cross term of the treatment effect, that is, the core explanatory variable of this paper, and its estimated coefficient reflects the impact of carbon emission rights and the agricultural enterprises not affected by carbon emission rights. Regarding the average difference in total factor productivity, if $\alpha_1 > 0$, it shows that the total factor productivity of agricultural enterprises affected by carbon emission rights has a significant improvement compared with those not affected by carbon emission rights; that is, the carbon emission rights policy promotes the improvement in total factor productivity of agricultural enterprises. *Patent* is the mediating variable, $Controls_{it}$ is the control variable, ε_i is the individual fixed effect, ε_t is the year fixed effect, and ε_{it} is the random disturbance term.

First, Model (1) is regressed to test the impact of carbon emission rights on the total factor productivity of agricultural enterprises. If the coefficient is significantly positive, it means that carbon emission rights have significantly improved the total factor productivity of agricultural enterprises. Then, we regress Model (2). Whether the green innovation of enterprises has played a mechanistic role in the impact of carbon emission rights on the total factor productivity of agricultural enterprises is tested. If the coefficient of the interaction term is significantly positive, it means that the green innovation of enterprises has played a mechanistic role.

5. Empirical Analysis

5.1. Descriptive Statistics

Table 2 shows the descriptive statistical results of the main variables. The average value of the total factor productivity (*TFP*) of agricultural enterprises is 9.081, the minimum value is 6.733, the maximum value is 11.670, and the standard deviation is 1.016, indicating that on the whole, the total factor productivity of private enterprises fluctuates greatly, and the data have a large degree of dispersion. The average value of enterprise green innovation is 1.726, and the standard deviation is 4.519. The number of green patent applications of enterprises varies greatly.

5.2. Analysis of Regression Results

The Hausman test rejects the null hypothesis. Therefore, this paper uses a fixed-effect double-difference model to explore the impact of the carbon emission trading pilot policy on the total factor productivity of agricultural enterprises. At the same time, the reliability of the estimated results is tested by adding control variables. The regression results of Model (1) are shown in Table 3. Column (3) shows the regression result of the double-difference model, and Columns (1) and (2) show the regression results of the double-difference model after controlling for individual and year-fixed effects.

Table 2. Descriptive statistics of the main variables.

Variable	N	Mean	P50	Sd	Min	Max
TFP (OP)	1340	6.600	6.547	0.750	4.905	8.363
TFP (LP)	1340	9.081	8.985	1.016	6.733	11.670
Patent	1340	1.726	0.000	4.519	0.000	30.000
Invent	1340	1.058	0.000	3.033	0.000	20.000
Actual	1340	0.590	0.000	1.651	0.000	11.000
TreatPost	1340	0.219	0.000	0.414	0.000	1.000
Age	1340	18.880	19.000	5.042	7.000	31.000
Roa	1340	0.049	0.042	0.076	−0.243	0.258
Size	1340	7.916	7.793	1.211	5.112	11.020
Lev	1340	0.387	0.370	0.184	0.043	0.900
Agencost	1340	0.079	0.063	0.063	0.014	0.439
Cflow	1340	0.069	0.065	0.087	−0.183	0.319
Capital	1340	0.266	0.247	0.137	0.017	0.609
Subsidy	1340	11.900	15.290	6.921	0.000	19.620
Top1	1219	36.270	35.880	14.680	9.270	70.320
GDP	1340	10.920	10.890	0.470	9.889	12.010

Table 3. Basic regression results.

Variable	TFP (1)	TFP (2)	TFP (3)
Treat * Time	0.316 ***	0.149 ***	0.181 ***
	(7.09)	(4.87)	(5.47)
Size		0.325 ***	0.551 ***
		(15.80)	(41.09)
Roa		0.806 ***	2.101 ***
		(5.51)	(7.91)
Lev		0.480 ***	0.851 ***
		(6.37)	(9.74)
Agencost		−3.503 ***	−4.456 ***
		(−19.00)	(−18.66)
Cflow		0.450 ***	0.654 ***
		(4.28)	(3.19)
Capital		−1.387 ***	−1.795 ***
		(−12.98)	(−16.30)
Top1		−0.009 ***	−0.002 **
		(−6.67)	(−2.14)
Constant	9.015 ***	7.212 ***	5.114 ***
	(650.79)	(42.47)	(48.75)
Year fixed effects	control	control	not controlled
Individual fixed effects	control	control	not controlled
Observations	1330	1210	1219
R-squared	0.890	0.960	0.976
F	206.8	206.8	206.8

Note: *, **, *** indicate significance at the 10%, 5%, and 1% levels, respectively.

The regression results in Column (1) of Table 3 show that the coefficient of the interaction term is significantly positive at the 1% level; compared with the control group, the carbon emission trading pilot will increase the total factor productivity of agricultural enterprises in the treatment group, and the carbon emission trading pilot policy will increase the total factor productivity of agricultural enterprises by about 0.316% on average. In Column (2), control variables are added on the basis of Column (1), and the regression results are still significantly positive. After considering the influence of other factors, the pilot carbon emissions trading policy increased the total factor productivity of agricultural enterprises by about 0.149% on average; R2 also increased significantly, indicating that after adding control variables, the model fit was better, and the research conclusions were still robust, while Column (3) controlled the individual and time fixed effects on the basis of Column (2). R2 in Column (3) increased significantly, indicating that there are indeed differences at the individual and time levels that can affect the total factor productivity of agricultural enterprises. Therefore, it is reasonable to add individual and time-fixed effects to the benchmark regression in this paper. Regardless of which method is used for regression, the coefficient of the interaction term of the explanatory variables is significantly positive, indicating that the pilot policy of carbon emission trading can improve the total factor productivity of agricultural enterprises to a certain extent. Hypothesis 1 was preliminarily verified. To make the research conclusions more credible, this paper conducts a series of robustness tests. In addition, the R2 of the model in Table 3 is greater than 0.1, which is acceptable considering the complexity of the research phenomenon.

5.3. Robustness Test

5.3.1. Parallel Trend Test

Satisfying the parallel trend assumption of the experimental group and the control group is one of the basic prerequisites for using the double-difference method. Therefore, before the carbon trading pilot (2013), the evolution of the indicators in the experimental group and the reference group should remain basically the same and consistent; otherwise, the regression results may be biased. This paper refers to the practice of predecessors and uses the dummy variable Pre4~$After5$ to replace (1) in the formula. The $Treat * Time$ specific regression equation is as follows:

$$\begin{aligned} TFP_{it} = \alpha_1 + \alpha_{-4}\text{Pre4}_{it} + \alpha_{-3}\text{Pre3}_{it} + \alpha_{-2}\text{Pre2}_{it} + \alpha_{-1}\text{Pre1}_{it} + \alpha_0 Current_{it} + \alpha_1{}'\text{After1}_{it} \\ + \alpha_2{}'\text{After2}_{it} + \alpha_3{}'\text{After3}_{it} + \alpha_4{}'\text{After4}_{it} + \alpha_5{}'\text{After5}_{it} + \alpha_2 Controls + \varepsilon_{it} \end{aligned} \quad (3)$$

In Equation (3), Pre4_{it} means that t in the fourth year i before the enterprise is affected by the carbon trading pilot, when the enterprise is in the fourth year before being affected by it, the variable takes a value of 1; otherwise, it takes a value of 0. $After1_{it}$ means the t in the first year i after the enterprise is affected by the carbon trading pilot; when the enterprise is in the first year after being affected by it, the variable takes the value 1; otherwise, it takes a value of 0. $Current_{it}$ means that t in the current period when the enterprise is affected by the carbon trading pilot, when the enterprise is in the current period i affected by it, the variable takes a value of 1; otherwise, it takes a value of 0. The definitions of the remaining variables are the same as the regression results, and from the test results in Column (1) of Table 4, it can be seen that the regression coefficients of Pre3~$Current$ are not significant, and the regression coefficients of $After1$~$After6$ are all significant. The above results show that before the arrival of the carbon trading pilot, there was no significant difference between the experimental group and the control group, which satisfies the parallel trend hypothesis. The carbon trading pilot has a good effect in promoting the total factor productivity of agricultural enterprises, but the implementation of the policy has a certain lag. On the whole, the research design of this paper conforms to the premise of using the double-difference method.

Table 4. Robustness check.

Variable	TFP		
	(1) Parallel Trend Test	**(2) Test 2012**	**(3) Test 2011**
Pre3	−0.009		
	(−0.08)		
Pre2	0.135		
	(1.33)		
Pre1	0.060		
	(0.61)		

Table 4. *Cont.*

Variable	TFP		
	(1) Parallel Trend Test	**(2) Test 2012**	**(3) Test 2011**
Current	0.121		
	(1.23)		
After1	0.207 **		
	(2.12)		
After2	0.220 **		
	(2.37)		
After3	0.168 *		
	(1.90)		
After4	0.175 **		
	(2.05)		
After5	0.241 ***		
	(2.85)		
After6	0.209 **		
	(2.34)		
Placebox1		0.067	0.159
		(0.57)	(1.21)
Size	0.577 ***	0.262 ***	0.196 ***
	(38.45)	(9.14)	(5.98)
Roa	2.282 ***	1.061 ***	2.326 ***
	(8.71)	(3.92)	(5.21)
Lev	0.934 ***	0.325 **	1.134 ***
	(9.71)	(2.03)	(4.46)
Agencost	−1.021 ***	−4.752 ***	−6.979 ***
	(−8.63)	(−10.74)	(−9.05)
Cflow	0.599 ***	0.181	0.302
	(2.84)	(1.05)	(1.35)
Capital	−1.836 ***	−0.775 ***	−0.768 ***
	(−14.81)	(−3.72)	(−2.97)
Top1	−0.003 **	−0.001	−0.002
	(−2.37)	(−0.23)	(−0.59)
Constant	4.634 ***	7.282 ***	7.578 ***
	(41.37)	(30.00)	(27.50)
Year fixed effect	Control	Control	Control
Individual fixed effect	Control	Control	Control
Observations	1219	308	196
R-squared	0.717	0.001	0.001
F	178.6	0.982	0.982

Note: *, **, *** indicate significance at the 10%, 5%, and 1% levels, respectively.

5.3.2. Parallel Trend Test

To ensure the robustness of the experimental results, this paper draws on the practice of Topalova [31] and uses the idea of a counterfactual test to conduct a placebo test. Specifically, we set the sample data before the carbon trading pilot, assuming that the carbon trading pilot occurred in 2012 and 2011 and conducted regression analysis again. If the increase in the total factor productivity of agricultural enterprises was indeed caused by the carbon trading pilot in 2013, the coefficient of the interaction term should be insignificant in the regression results of the fictitious carbon trading pilot year. Columns (2) and (3) of Table 4 report the test results, and the coefficients of the interaction terms are 0.067 and 0.159, but not significant. This means that the fictitious policies have increased the total factor productivity of agricultural enterprises by about 0.067% and 0.159% on average, but the impact is not significant, that is, the increase in the total factor productivity of agribusiness was indeed brought about by the 2013 carbon trading pilot. It can be seen that the pilot carbon trading significantly improved the total factor productivity of agricultural enterprises.

5.3.3. Propensity Score Matching

The coefficients of the interaction term in the previous regression results only represent an "average effect", that is, the average impact of the carbon trading pilot on the total factor productivity of agricultural enterprises. It is difficult to confirm the real causal relationship between the carbon trading pilot and the total factor productivity of agricultural enterprises. At the same time, whether enterprises are affected by the carbon trading pilot is not random. The change in the total factor productivity of agricultural enterprises is related to enterprise size, R&D investment, and other factors. If the influence of these factors is not excluded, it will inevitably cause sample selection bias. Therefore, this paper adopts the propensity score-matching method to correct the sample selectivity bias to reduce the interference of the experimental results and ensure that the results are more robust. Columns (1)–(3) of Table 5 show the regression results of total factor productivity (TFP) of agribusiness and the implementation of digital finance ($Treat * Time$) after adjacent matching, radius matching, and core matching tests, respectively. The estimated coefficients of the interaction item ($Treat * Time$) are all significantly positive, the pilot policies of carbon emissions trading increased the total factor productivity of agricultural enterprises by about 0.171%, 0.149%, and 0.149% on average, which once again indicates that the carbon trading pilot significantly improves the total factor productivity of agricultural enterprises. These tables show that the coefficient signs and significance levels of the interaction terms are consistent with the results of the previous analysis. This also verifies the basic regression results; that is, the carbon trading pilot is beneficial to improve the total factor productivity of agricultural enterprises and ensures the robustness of the basic regression results.

Table 5. Robustness check.

Variable	TFP				
	(1)	**(2)**	**(3)**	**(4)**	**(5)**
Treat * Time	0.171 ***	0.149 ***	0.149 ***	0.165 ***	0.179 ***
	(3.40)	(4.87)	(4.88)	(4.57)	(5.20)
Size	0.340 ***	0.325 ***	0.323 ***	−0.054 **	0.339 ***
	(9.75)	(15.80)	(15.68)	(−2.40)	(13.60)
Roa	0.556 **	0.806 ***	0.770 ***	1.110 ***	0.961 ***
	(2.36)	(5.51)	(5.18)	(7.73)	(6.46)
Lev	0.440 ***	0.480 ***	0.470 ***	0.677 ***	0.551 ***
	(3.33)	(6.37)	(6.21)	(7.95)	(6.22)
Agencost	−3.292 ***	−3.503 ***	−3.521 ***	−0.885 ***	−0.813 ***
	(−10.84)	(−19.00)	(−19.05)	(−12.88)	(−12.08)
Cflow	0.510 ***	0.450 ***	0.472 ***	0.472 ***	0.468 ***
	(2.73)	(4.28)	(4.44)	(4.28)	(4.10)
Capital	−1.410 ***	−1.387 ***	−1.381 ***	−1.428 ***	−1.676 ***
	(−8.41)	(−12.98)	(−12.93)	(−11.50)	(−13.27)
Top1	−0.007 ***	−0.009 ***	−0.009 ***	−0.011 ***	−0.010 ***
	(−3.06)	(−6.67)	(−6.68)	(−6.74)	(−5.87)
Constant	7.022 ***	7.212 ***	7.232 ***	7.507 ***	6.964 ***
	(23.54)	(42.47)	(42.44)	(41.09)	(34.87)
Time effect	control	control	control	control	control
Individual effect	control	control	control	control	control
Observations	479	1210	1209	1210	1109
R-squared	0.972	0.960	0.960	0.900	0.950
F	205.3	205.3	205.3	84.33	30.61

Note: *, **, *** indicate significance at the 10%, 5%, and 1% levels, respectively.

5.3.4. Explained Variable Replacement

This paper changed the measurement method of the explained variable and tested it again. The results are shown in Column (4) of Table 5. The regression coefficient between the carbon trading pilot and total factor productivity of agricultural enterprises is still significantly positive, the pilot policies of carbon emissions trading increased the total factor productivity of agricultural enterprises by about 0.171%, 0.149%, and 0.165% on average, and the regression result is consistent with the above.

5.3.5. One-Period Lag Explanatory Variable

Considering that the implementation of policies may have a lag effect, this paper conducts basic regression again with the core explanatory variable lagging by one period. The results are shown in Column (5) of Table 5. The regression result is still significantly positive, the pilot policies of carbon emissions trading increased the total factor productivity of agricultural enterprises by about 0.171%, 0.149%, and 0.165% on average, which verifies Hypothesis 1 in this paper.

5.4. Mechanism Inspection

The results of the above analysis indicate that the pilot policy of carbon emission trading significantly contributes to the total factor productivity of agricultural enterprises. Then, how does the pilot policy of carbon emission trading affect the total factor productivity of agricultural enterprises? According to the literature, technological innovation affects the level of total factor productivity. Environmental regulation affects total factor productivity through R&D inputs (Wu et al., 2013) [32]. Therefore, this paper chooses green innovation as a mediating variable and uses the mediating effect model to test the mechanism of carbon emission trading rights affecting the total factor productivity of agricultural enterprises. The regression results are shown in Table 6.

Table 6. Mechanism inspection.

Variable	TFP (1)	(2)	(3)
Treat * Time * Patent/Invent/Actual	0.011 *	0.019 **	0.024
	(1.92)	(2.03)	(1.54)
Treat * Time	0.112 ***	0.114 ***	0.114 ***
	(3.19)	(3.30)	(3.20)
Size	0.543 ***	0.543 ***	0.545 ***
	(39.57)	(39.72)	(39.83)
Roa	2.181 ***	2.178 ***	2.186 ***
	(8.16)	(8.14)	(8.16)
Lev	0.889 ***	0.888 ***	0.886 ***
	(10.13)	(10.13)	(10.10)
Agencost	−4.455 ***	−4.454 ***	−4.455 ***
	(−18.55)	(−18.55)	(−18.54)
Cflow	0.613 ***	0.612 ***	0.608 ***
	(2.97)	(2.97)	(2.95)
Capital	−1.779 ***	−1.779 ***	−1.783 ***
	(−16.16)	(−16.16)	(−16.19)
Top1	−0.002 *	−0.002 *	−0.002 *
	(−1.87)	(−1.84)	(−1.93)
Constant	5.159 ***	5.156 ***	5.150 ***
	(48.47)	(48.61)	(48.42)
Year fixed effect	Control	Control	Control
Individual fixed effect	Control	Control	Control
Observations	1219	1219	1219
R-squared	0.779	0.779	0.779
F	460.3	460.5	459.6

Note: *, **, *** indicate significance at the 10%, 5%, and 1% levels, respectively.

Table 6 shows the regression results of the mechanism effect. Columns (1)–(3) list the regression results after adding enterprise green technology innovation, green practical technology innovation, and green invention technology innovation, respectively, into the basic model. The results show that after adding enterprise green technology innovation, the interaction item is significantly positive at the 10% statistical level; for every additional unit of enterprise green technology innovation, the total factor productivity of agricultural enterprises will increase by about 0.011% on average; after adding green practical technology innovation, the interaction item is significantly positive at the 5% statistical level; for each additional unit of green practical technology innovation, the total factor productivity of agricultural enterprises will increase by about 0.019% on average. After adding green invention technology innovation, the coefficients of the interaction terms are all positive but insignificant; for each additional unit of green invention technology innovation, the total factor productivity of agricultural enterprises increases by about 0.024% on average, but the improvement effect is not obvious, indicating that under the pilot policy of carbon emission trading, enterprise green technology innovation significantly promotes the improvement in the total factor productivity of agricultural enterprises, and total factor productivity improvement is achieved by improving the level of green practical technology innovation rather than green invention technology innovation. From the analysis of the mechanism effect model, it can be seen that the implementation of China's carbon emissions trading makes Chinese agricultural enterprises give more attention to the improvement of their own green innovation level, resulting in an increase in the output of green innovation represented by green patents, especially the improvement of the level of green practical technology innovation. These patent achievements have also been used extensively in practice, which has led to the improvement of the internal production process of Chinese agricultural enterprises, and it also means that a professional energy-saving and emission-reduction technology service industry is being cultivated and formed, creating a channel for carbon emissions trading, which significantly promotes the improvement of agricultural total factor productivity in the pilot areas.

6. Further Research

6.1. Grouping by Enterprise Size

A large number of studies have shown that the size of an enterprise affects the cost of emission reduction, which in turn has an impact on the environmental protection decision of the enterprise. To investigate whether the difference in the effect of carbon emission trading truly exists under different enterprise scale characteristics, we set up a virtual variable of enterprise scale and divided the sample enterprises into large-scale enterprises and small-scale enterprises. Basic regression was performed on the two groups of samples. The regression results of Columns (1) and (2) in Table 7 show that the carbon emission trading pilot has significantly increased the total factor productivity of large-scale agricultural enterprises by about 0.137% on average, while it has no significant effect on small-scale agricultural enterprises. The possible reason for this situation is that large enterprises not only have the advantage of economies of scale but can also obtain government funding subsidies and low-cost financing by virtue of a good social reputation to make up for the cost of regulatory compliance brought by the carbon emission trading mechanism. At the same time, the strong financial strength of large enterprises can help them resist greater risks and embark on a path of independent transformation with the help of central environmental regulations.

Table 7. The first set of tests for heterogeneity.

Variable	TFP					
	(1) Large Scale	(2) Small Scale	(3) State Owned	(4) Nonstate Owned	(5) High Debt	(6) Low Debt
Treat * Time	0.137 ***	0.159	0.097 **	0.224 ***	0.227 ***	0.032
	(3.75)	(0.44)	(2.25)	(4.46)	(4.13)	(0.73)
Size	0.322 ***	0.389	0.245 ***	0.361 ***	0.269 ***	0.480 ***
	(14.58)	(0.57)	(7.63)	(12.89)	(8.69)	(13.65)
Roa	1.049 ***	1.763	0.842 ***	0.975 ***	0.453 **	1.505 ***
	(7.48)	(0.50)	(3.94)	(5.36)	(2.03)	(8.00)
Lev	0.627 ***	0.968	0.205 *	0.801 ***	0.362 **	1.305 ***
	(7.49)	(0.68)	(1.75)	(7.27)	(2.42)	(7.49)
Agencost	−0.749 ***	−14.822	−3.700 ***	−0.577 ***	−1.039 ***	−0.231 ***
	(−11.19)	(−0.95)	(−14.33)	(−8.44)	(−9.72)	(−2.65)
Cflow	0.450 ***	0.346	0.313 **	0.520 ***	0.316 **	0.389 ***
	(4.16)	(0.28)	(2.33)	(3.37)	(2.11)	(2.61)
Capital	−1.641 ***	−1.206	−1.592 ***	−1.518 ***	−1.923 ***	−1.404 ***
	(−13.47)	(−0.72)	(−10.01)	(−9.34)	(−8.90)	(−9.68)
Top1	−0.009 ***	0.015	−0.011 ***	−0.006 ***	−0.010 ***	−0.010 ***
	(−5.76)	(0.99)	(−4.03)	(−3.12)	(−4.19)	(−4.03)
Constant	7.020 ***	6.142	8.139 ***	6.467 ***	7.806 ***	5.484 ***
	(39.18)	(1.14)	(29.33)	(29.73)	(29.16)	(19.64)
Time effect	control	control	control	control	control	control
Individual effect	control	control	control	control	control	control
Observations	602	605	547	663	590	599
R-squared	0.948	0.998	0.956	0.953	0.946	0.965
F	2.485	2.485	100.4	100.4	86.71	86.71

Note: *, **, *** indicate significance at the 10%, 5%, and 1% levels, respectively.

6.2. Grouping by Enterprise Ownership

The different natures of property rights of state-owned holding enterprises and private holding enterprises lead to different paths and characteristics in political functions, development goals, market competition and other aspects, and different factors that are considered when making decisions. Therefore, state-owned enterprises and nonstate-owned enterprises may respond differently to the implementation of carbon emission trading policies. We construct the virtual variable of enterprise ownership nature, divided the sample enterprises into state-owned enterprises and nonstate-owned enterprises, and regressed the two samples separately using the differences-in-differences method. The regression results of Columns (3) and (4) in Table 7 show that the carbon emission trading pilot has significant positive effects on total factor productivity in both state-owned and nonstate-owned agricultural enterprises. However, the estimated interaction term coefficient of state-owned agricultural enterprises was 0.097 and significant at the 5% level, and the estimated coefficient of nonstate-owned agricultural enterprises was 0.224 and significant at the 1% level. The impact of the carbon emission trading policy on the total factor productivity of nonstate-owned enterprises is greater than that of state-owned enterprises. This may be because state-owned enterprises assume political functions, and the degree of innovation does not completely depend on their operating capacity. In contrast, private enterprises can adapt to the development of the market in environmental rights and interests in trading policies and independently choose the behaviors conducive to their profit maximization in fierce market competition. Therefore, the carbon trading market has a stronger incentive effect on the green technology innovation of private enterprises.

6.3. Grouping by Financial Structure

According to the principle of financial leverage, debt can reduce the total cost of capital and improve the value of enterprises. In addition, when the debt ratio increases, the equity concentration of management becomes larger, and a larger proportion of profits can be obtained in the project. A higher debt ratio also makes firms more willing to invest in riskier projects, such as innovation activities. Enterprises with lower debt levels have a stronger chance of launching research. Therefore, according to the median value of the enterprise asset-liability ratio, this paper divides the sample into high-debt enterprises and low-debt enterprises to test whether the effect of the carbon emission trading policy on the total factor productivity of agricultural enterprises is heterogeneous due to the difference in debt level. It can be seen from the regression results of Columns (5) and (6) in Table 7 that the carbon emission trading pilot significantly increased the total factor productivity of high-debt agricultural enterprises by about 0.137% on average, while it had no significant effect on low-debt agricultural enterprises, most likely because debt, as a signal to the outside world, is often used by management, and a high debt ratio shows management's confidence in future expectations and, for debtors, a willingness to invest in such companies, thus allowing firms to have sufficient capital for green innovation activities and thus contributing to the total factor productivity of highly indebted agribusinesses.

6.4. Grouping by Enterprise Region

The development level of the eastern region and the central and western regions may differ to some extent. The pilot policy of carbon emission trading may have different roles in promoting the total factor productivity of enterprises in different regions. This paper divides the samples into three subsamples: eastern, central and western, according to the different regions where the enterprises are located. As seen from the review results of Columns (1)–(3) in Table 8, the promotion effect of carbon emission trading pilot policies on the total factor productivity of enterprises in the eastern, central and western regions shows a downward trend. The total factor productivity of agricultural enterprises in the eastern, central and western regions increased by about 0.171%, 0.169%, and 0.082%, respectively. Among them, the promotion effect on the total factor productivity of enterprises in the eastern region is the most obvious. The promoting effects on the central and western regions were relatively weak, respectively. The possible reason is that carbon emission trading, as a market-motivated regulatory tool, relies on a unified, open, and orderly competitive market system to play its full role. The eastern region has an active market economy and a developed economic level, so the incentive effect of the carbon emission trading mechanism is more efficient. However, the economic development level of the central and western regions is lagging behind, and their primary goal is to achieve economic development. Therefore, the compliance cost of carbon emission trading will increase the costs and decrease the profits of enterprises in the central and western regions, resulting in a lack of motivation to improve the total factor productivity of enterprises.

Table 8. The first set of tests for heterogeneity.

Variables	TFP				
	(1) East	(2) Central	(3) West	(4) Government Subsidy	(5) Anarchy Subsidy
Treat * Time	0.171 ***	0.169	0.082	1.973 ***	0.150 ***
	(5.02)	(0.88)	(0.62)	(4.12)	(7.15)
Size	0.395 ***	0.333 ***	0.256 ***	0.296 ***	0.363 ***
	(12.44)	(6.73)	(6.50)	(11.88)	(5.07)
Roa	1.228 ***	0.573	0.543 *	1.246 ***	0.706 ***
	(6.85)	(1.64)	(1.77)	(7.70)	(3.00)
Lev	0.559 ***	1.101 ***	0.516 ***	0.680 ***	0.693 ***
	(5.45)	(5.61)	(2.91)	(7.33)	(3.82)
Agencost	−1.008 ***	−0.384 ***	−2.677 ***	−0.538 ***	−1.898 ***
	(−11.02)	(−3.58)	(−7.72)	(−7.22)	(−11.66)
Cflow	−0.036	0.303	0.913 ***	0.461 ***	0.714 ***
	(−0.25)	(1.22)	(4.65)	(3.95)	(3.39)
Capital	−1.491 ***	−1.727 ***	−1.580 ***	−1.501 ***	−1.417 ***
	(−10.35)	(−4.96)	(−6.72)	(−10.72)	(−6.24)
Top1	−0.007 ***	−0.012 ***	−0.010 ***	−0.009 ***	−0.010 ***
	(−3.63)	(−3.45)	(−3.05)	(−4.48)	(−2.69)
Constant	6.380 ***	6.928 ***	7.760 ***	7.096 ***	6.279 ***
	(25.85)	(18.60)	(21.04)	(34.81)	(10.36)
Time effect	control	control	control	control	control
Individual effect	control	control	control	control	control
Observations	642	266	302	907	266
R-squared	0.955	0.919	0.963	0.953	0.987
F	41.71	41.71	41.71	36.89	36.89

Note: *, *** indicate significance at the 10%, and 1% levels, respectively.

6.5. Grouping by Government Subsidies

Enterprises with government subsidies usually have more "exogenous resources", which gives them more opportunities to innovate and invest more, thus gaining a competitive advantage and improving their total factor productivity. To investigate whether the difference in government subsidies in carbon trading is real, we set up a virtual variable for government subsidies by referring to the practices of others and extracted the data of energy saving, emission reduction, green, environmental protection, clean energy, environment, waste gas, carbon emission, and carbon trading fields from the CSMAR by taking the logarithm, and if the value was null, then it was 0. The basic regressions were conducted for the two groups of samples obtained. The results are shown in Columns (4) and (5) of Table 8. The total factor productivity of agricultural enterprises with and without government subsidies is significantly increased under the influence of the carbon trading rights policy. The pilot carbon emissions trading policy significantly increased the total factor productivity of agricultural enterprises without government subsidies by about 0.150% on average, while the total factor productivity of agricultural enterprises with government subsidies increased by about 1.973% on average. The estimated coefficient of nongovernment subsidies is 0.150 and that of nongovernment subsidies is 1.973, which is greater than that of nongovernment subsidy enterprises. The possible reason is that government subsidies can provide enterprises with external resources to deal with environmental uncertainties, enabling enterprises to turn opportunities brought by environmental changes into an innovation impetus, forming a synergistic effect with innovation input and promoting the improvement of enterprise internationalization performance.

7. Conclusions and Policy Suggestions

7.1. Conclusions

The carbon emission trading mechanism is an important policy tool in using market mechanisms to promote corporate carbon emission reduction, an important institutional innovation to promote low-carbon and green development, and an important institutional arrangement to promote the "carbon peak in 2030 and carbon neutral in 2060". Therefore, this paper empirically examines the impact of carbon emission trading rights on the total factor productivity of agricultural enterprises using a double-difference model and a mediating effect model using data from listed agricultural companies in Shanghai and Shenzhen A-shares and GEM from 2010 to 2020 and investigates the mechanism of its impact in depth. The main conclusions are as follows.

(1) Carbon emission trading rights significantly increase the total factor productivity of agricultural enterprises.
(2) Green innovation plays a mechanistic role in the influence of carbon emission trading rights on the total factor productivity of agricultural enterprises.
(3) Heterogeneity analysis shows that the improvement effect of carbon emission trading rights on the total factor productivity of agricultural enterprises mainly exists in large-scale, nonstate-owned enterprises; enterprises with high debt levels; enterprises in the eastern region; and enterprises with government subsidies.

Limitations. First, due to the serious lack of relevant data before 2010, in order to ensure the accuracy of the results of the article, the data used in this empirical test starts from 2010. Second, China's current carbon emission trading is still in the pilot stage, and the transaction price is subject to excessive government control. At present, there is no continuous and large amount of transaction data, and it is impossible to conduct effective research on the entire market. Third, the total factor productivity of agricultural enterprises is a complex project. This paper only conducts empirical tests from the perspective of the green innovation effect, and other potential impact mechanisms and paths still need to be identified. Subsequent research can include all possible influencing factors, continue to improve the intermediate action mechanism of carbon emission trading policy on the total factor productivity of agricultural enterprises, and clarify their respective weights in the driving of total factor productivity of agricultural enterprises.

7.2. Policy Suggestions

Based on the above conclusions, we can give the following recommendations.

(1) We will improve and optimize China's rules and regulations on carbon emission trading, ensure that the transactions in the trading market are carried out legally and in an orderly manner, play a role in promoting green innovation in agricultural enterprises and promoting total factor productivity, and help agricultural enterprises transform and upgrade. At the same time, individuals trading in the carbon emission trading market should consciously abide by the market order, create a good trading market environment, and further promote the total factor productivity of agricultural enterprises.
(2) Green innovation is an effective way to realize the leap-forward of total factor productivity of agricultural enterprises and the long-term goal of continuously deepening the carbon trading mechanism. The government should strengthen green innovation compensation, enhance the capacity of independent research and development of enterprises and cooperative innovation, optimize the structure of green industry, and improve the support of environmental protection standards and management norms, inducing enterprises to complete the transformation of "innovation compensation". At the same time, we should further improve the incentive system of government rewards and punishments and green innovation, give full play to the incentive effect of government reward and punishment, fully encourage enterprises to engage

in green technology innovation, and guide enterprises to achieve improvements in profitability in the stage of "following the cost".

(3) According to the current situation and characteristics of agricultural enterprises with different scales, ownership properties, regions, and debt levels in China, differentiated regulation strategies should be implemented to avoid the adoption of "one-size-fits-all" regulation orders. At the same time, different types of enterprises should be treated equally to create a favorable competitive environment and to promote environmental regulatory instruments to maximize policy effects.

(4) Enterprises are encouraged to properly respond to carbon emission trading policies through R&D and innovation to achieve "decoupling" between high production capacity and high carbon emissions as soon as possible. At the same time, we should speed up the establishment of a national carbon emissions trading system to avoid transregional carbon emissions transfer, facilitate China's transition to a zero-carbon economy, and make positive contributions to leading global climate governance.

Author Contributions: Conceptualization, J.H. and Y.J.; data curation, D.Z.; formal analysis, J.H., D.Z. and Y.J.; funding acquisition, J.H. and Y.J.; methodology, D.Z., J.H. and Y.J.; software, D.Z.; supervision, J.H. and Y.J.; writing—original draft, D.Z. and J.H.; writing—review and editing, D.Z., Y.J., and J.H. All authors have read and agreed to the published version of the manuscript.

Funding: This work was supported by grants from Henan Science and Technology Think Tank Project (No. HNKJZK-2022-21B); Strategic Research Project of the Education and Science Commission of the Ministry of Education (No. 2021-29); and The General Project of Educational Science of Henan Province (No. 2021 YB0050).

Institutional Review Board Statement: Not applicable.

Informed Consent Statement: Not applicable.

Data Availability Statement: The data presented in this study are openly available in National Bureau of Statistics, reference numbers 978-7-5037-9120-8, 978-7-5037-8770-6, 978-7-5037-8432-3, 978-7-5037-8082-0, 978-7-5037-7706-6, 978-7-5037-7350-1, 978-7-5037-7019-7, and 978-7-5037-6754-8.

Conflicts of Interest: The authors declare no conflict of interest. The funders had no role in the design of the study; in the collection, analyses, or interpretation of data; in the writing of the manuscript, or in the decision to publish the results.

References

1. Xia, Q.Y.; Li, L.; Dong, J.; Zhang, B. Reduction Effect and Mechanism Analysis of Carbon Trading Policy on Carbon Emissions from Land Use. *Sustainability* **2021**, *13*, 9558. [CrossRef]
2. Lachaud, M.A.; Bravo-Ureta, B.E.; Ludena, C.E. Economic effects of climate change on agricultural production and productivity in Latin America and the Caribbean (LAC). *J. Agric. Econ.* **2021**, *53*, 321–332. [CrossRef]
3. Domazlicky, B.R.; Weber, W.L. Does environmental protection lead to slow reproductivity growth in the chemical Industry? *J. Environ. Resour. Econ.* **2004**, *283*, 301–324. [CrossRef]
4. He, G.J.; Wang, S.D.; Zhang, B. Watering Down Environmental Regulation in China*. *Q. J. Econom.* **2020**, *135*, 2135–2185. [CrossRef]
5. Cai, W.G.; Ye, P.Y. How does environmental regulation influence enterprises' total factor productivity? A quasi-natural experiment based on China's New Environmental Protection Law. *J. Clean. Prod.* **2020**, *276*, 124105. [CrossRef]
6. Tang, H.L.; Liu, J.M.; Wu, J.G. The impact of command-and-control environmental regulation on enterprise total factor productivity: A quasi-natural experiment based on China's "Two Control Zone" policy. *J. Clean. Prod.* **2020**, *254*, 120011. [CrossRef]
7. Ai, H.S.; Hu, S.L.; Li, K.; Shao, S.A. Environmental regulation, total factor productivity, and enterprise duration: Evidence from China. *J. Bus. Strategy Environ.* **2020**, *29*, 2284–2296. [CrossRef]
8. De, S.R.; Esposito, P.; Lasinio, C.J. Environmental regulation and productivity growth: Main policy challenges. *J. Int. Econ.* **2021**, *165*, 264–277.
9. Li, M.J.; Du, W.J. Opening the black box of capacity governance: Environmental regulation and capacity utilization of microcosmic firms in China. *J. Econ. Model.* **2022**, *108*, 105766. [CrossRef]
10. Fan, M.Y.; Ping, L.Q. Impact of environmental regulation on green total factor productivity: A new perspective of green technological innovation. *J. Environ. Sci. Pollut. Res. Int.* **2022**, 1–16. [CrossRef]
11. Silvia, A.T.; Kozluk, V.Z. Environmental policies and productivity growth: Evidence across industries and firms. *J. Environ. Econ. Manag.* **2016**, *6*, 2.

12. Zhao, X.M.; Liu, C.J.; Yang, M. The effects of environmental regulation on China's total factor productivity: An empirical study of carbon-intensive industries. *J. Clean. Prod.* **2018**, *1*, 325–334. [CrossRef]
13. Vargas, A.S.; Sanchez, R.M.; Ibarra, A.A. An Empirical Analysis of the Nonlinear Relationship Between Environmental Regulation and Manufacturing Productivity. *J. Appl. Econ.* **2019**, *16*, 357–371. [CrossRef]
14. Liu, S.M.; Hou, P.; Gao, Y.K.; Tan, Y. Innovation and green total factor productivity in China: A linear and nonlinear investigation. *J. Environ. Sci. Pollut. Res. Int.* **2020**, *29*, 12810–12831. [CrossRef] [PubMed]
15. Peng, J.Y.; Xie, R.; Ma, C.B.; Fu, Y. Market-based environmental regulation and total factor productivity: Evidence from Chinese enterprises. *J. Econ. Model.* **2020**, *3*, 6. [CrossRef]
16. Zhao, L.; Chen, L.Y. Research on the Impact of Government Environmental Information Disclosure on Green Total Factor Productivity: Empirical Experience from Chinese Province. *Int. J. Environ. Res. Public Health* **2022**, *19*, 729. [CrossRef]
17. Arjan, T.; Machiel, M.; Bert, S. An Efficiency Perspective on Carbon Emissions and Financial Performance. *J. Ecol. Econ.* **2020**, *176*, 106632.
18. Zheng, Y.; Zhou, M.; Wen, F.H. Asymmetric effects of oil shocks on carbon allowance price: Evidence from China. *J. Energy Econ.* **2021**, *97*, 105183. [CrossRef]
19. Sun, R.T.; Wang, K.Q.; Wang, X.J.; Zhang, J. China's Carbon Emission Trading Scheme and Firm Performance. *J. Emerg. Mark. Financ. Trade* **2022**, *58*, 837–851. [CrossRef]
20. Li, C.; Li, X.Y.; Song, D.Y.; Tian, M. Does a carbon emissions trading scheme spur urban green innovation? Evidence from a quasi-natural experiment in China. *J. Energy Environ.* **2022**, *33*, 640–662. [CrossRef]
21. Li, R.; Tang, B.J. Initial carbon quota allocation methods of power sectors: A China case study. *J. Nat. Hazards* **2016**, *84*, 1075–1089. [CrossRef]
22. Wang, F.Q.; Li, H.M.; Cao, Y.C.; Zhang, C.Y.; Yunlong, R. Knowledge Sharing Strategy and Emission Reduction Benefits of Low Carbon Technology Collaborative Innovation in the Green Supply Chain. *J. Front. Environ. Sci.* **2022**, *751*, 783835. [CrossRef]
23. Imma, B.; Hacer, S.; Ana, S. Gaps in Regulation and Policies on the Application of Green Technologies at Household Level in the United Kingdom. *Sustainability* **2022**, *14*, 4030.
24. Zhao, Z.; Liu, Z.; Peng, T.Q.; Li, L.L.; Zhao, Y.J.; Li, Y. Evaluation of Low-Carbon Scientific and Technological Innovation-Economy-Environment of High Energy-Consuming Industries. *J. Sens.* **2022**, *2022*, 2908447. [CrossRef]
25. Lentz, R.; Mortensen, D.T. An Empirical Model of Growth through Product Innovation. *J. Econom.* **2008**, *76*, 1317–1373.
26. Wu, Q.; Kanittha, T.; Pongsa, P. Examining the Impact and Influencing Channels of Carbon Emission Trading Pilot Markets in China. *Sustainability* **2021**, *13*, 5664. [CrossRef]
27. Dylan, G.R.; Dietrich, E. Does the Porter Hypothesis Explain Expected Future Financial Performance? The Effect of Clean Water Regulation on Chemical Manufacturing Firms. *J. Environ. Resour. Econ.* **2010**, *45*, 353–377.
28. Li, D.D.; Li, D.D. Comparison and Analysis of Measurement Methods of Total Factor Productivity. *Int. J. Front. Eng. Technol.* **2020**, *2*, 18–30.
29. Czyzewski, B.; Majchrzak, A. Economic size of farms and adjustments of the total factor productivity to the business cycle in Polish agriculture. *J. Agric. Econ.* **2017**, *64*, 93–102.
30. Liu, J.M.; Jiang, Y.L.; Gan, S.D.; He, L.; Zhang, Q.F. Can digital finance promote corporate green innovation? *J. Environ. Sci. Pollut. Res. Int.* **2022**, *29*, 35828–35840. [CrossRef]
31. Petia, T. Factor Immobility and Regional Impacts of Trade Liberalization: Evidence on Poverty from India. *Am. Econ. J. Appl. Econ.* **2010**, *2*, 1–41.
32. Wu, J.; Yang, J.J.; Zhou, Z.X. How does environmental regulation affect environmental performance? A case study of China's regional energy efficiency. *J. Expert Syst.* **2020**, *37*, e12326. [CrossRef]

International Journal of
Environmental Research and Public Health

MDPI

Article

How Policy Mix Choices Affect the COVID-19 Pandemic Response Outcomes in Chinese Cities: An Empirical Analysis

Chunyu Shi [1], Tao Xu [2], Zhihang Ying [2] and Huan Li [2,*]

[1] Department of Public Administration, School of Public Management, Zhejiang Gongshang University, Hangzhou 310018, China; shichunyu@zjgsu.edu.cn
[2] Department of Land Resources Management, School of Public Management, Zhejiang Gongshang University, Hangzhou 310018, China; 1920040103@pop.zjgsu.edu.cn (T.X.); 2020100135@pop.zjgsu.edu.cn (Z.Y.)
* Correspondence: lihuan2039@163.com

Abstract: Since January 2020, the COVID-19 pandemic has caused millions of deaths and has posed a major public health threat worldwide. Such a massive and complex crisis requires quick and comprehensive policy responses. We developed an empirical dataset of policy mixes that included 4915 policies across 36 Chinese cities and investigated the relationships between the policy design choices and the COVID-19 pandemic response outcomes of a city. Using topic modeling and ordinary least squares regression analysis, we found considerable variation among cities in the compositions and design features of their policy mixes. Our analysis revealed that restriction measures did not significantly influence limiting the spread of the pandemic, but they were negatively correlated with the economic growth rate. By contrast, health protection measures greatly contributed to controlling viral spread. Intensive socioeconomic support reduced the occurrence of secondary disasters. The most effective policy strategy to deal with the COVID-19 pandemic appears to be a comprehensive policy design with a mix of restrictions, health protection measures, and socioeconomic support policies accompanied by a timely lockdown. Our empirical findings can help to improve pandemic policy design and contribute to generating broader lessons for how local governments should deal with similar crises in the future.

Keywords: policy mix; policy design; COVID-19; pandemic management; policy outcomes; compound crisis

Citation: Shi, C.; Xu, T.; Ying, Z.; Li, H. How Policy Mix Choices Affect the COVID-19 Pandemic Response Outcomes in Chinese Cities: An Empirical Analysis. *IJERPH* **2022**, *19*, 8094. https://doi.org/10.3390/ijerph19138094

Academic Editors: Jie Chen, Qian Zhou and Ting Zhang

Received: 27 April 2022
Accepted: 29 June 2022
Published: 1 July 2022

1. Introduction

The coronavirus disease 2019 (COVID-19) pandemic has caused millions of deaths since January 2020 and is a major public health threat worldwide. Such a massive and complex crisis has exposed differences in the capacities of governments around the world to integrate and coordinate different policy tools to manage the pandemic and to deal with its consequences [1,2]. The pandemic offers a natural experiment wherein the crisis that governments faced was broadly the same, but the policy solutions that they enacted were different [2], creating a unique opportunity for understanding associations between policy responses and their consequences; thus, lessons can be learned to improve similar public health risk response capacity [3].

Previous studies have mostly focused on the comparison of state-level pandemic policy responses among countries [2]. They have characterized the "standard" portfolio of national pandemic responses and have discussed the similarities and differences between the various policy tools deployed [2,4]. Scholars have examined these COVID-19 policy responses from institutional and political perspectives [5]. Some studies have included a large-N sample, cataloging the policy tools adopted by governments around the world, and have analyzed the sequence, intensity, and balance of different policy mixes [6–8]. However, these studies did not assess how the policy choices impacted the pandemic management outcomes. Other studies have been more comprehensive. They have assessed governments' responses in detailed case studies [9–11], investigating not only how national responses differed but also how these choices were shaped by specific political systems and administrative traditions such as the nature of national leadership; the organization of central and local governments; and the relationships between decision-makers, elites, epistemic communities, and others [12–14].

These studies have provided a general understanding of the variety of policy choices among countries and have made important contributions to enriching our knowledge of the various COVID-19 pandemic responses. However, these studies have mostly focused on national policies, and to date, we lack an appreciation of how local governments managed to coordinate their policy tools to deal with the crisis; the consequences of their different policy choices also remain unclear [2,15,16]. The COVID-19 pandemic has been most acutely felt at the local level, especially in cities, where the response policies have been impactful and have significantly affected the COVID-19 crisis management outcomes [17]. For instance, within a country with standardized national response policy guidelines, why did some locations experience recurrent outbreaks while others did not? How did local authorities differ in the attention they gave to other issues that occurred during the pandemic? To clarify what happened in local areas and understand why there were differences in outcomes, we need to closely study local-level policies [18] to supplement and enrich existing findings based on investigations of national-level responses to COVID-19.

This study selected 36 Chinese cities to empirically assess and gain insights into local-level responses to the COVID-19 pandemic. Through the conceptual lens of a policy mix [19–22], we analyzed 4915 policies that were adopted by these cities between 23 January 2020 (after the lockdown of Wuhan) and 1 April 2022. Following Nauwelaers et al. [19], we defined "policy mix" as a combination of policy tools that interact to produce a specific policy response to resolve complex problems. We investigated how different municipal governments coordinated and integrated their policy tools in mixes to deal with the pandemic, explored links between policy design choices and the cities' COVID-19 pandemic response outcomes, and discussed how policy mix design can affect the crisis management outcomes in a city.

2. Materials and Methods

2.1. Data Collection and Sample

Data on COVID-19 response policies were compiled by collecting information from each municipal government's official website, which provides information on the municipality's pandemic response measures. The number of outbreaks and that of high-risk areas were retrieved from each city's Center for Disease Control (CDC) website. As there are no specific official criteria for COVID-19 outbreaks in China, when the virus spreads across administrative jurisdictions, specifically city districts, and the municipal government adopts a full-scale lockdown, we take that as the occurrence of an outbreak. High-risk areas are defined as counties or urban districts having more than 50 cumulative cases or clustered infections in the past 14 days (see the Guidelines on COVID-19 Prevention and Control issued by the Joint Prevention and Control Mechanism of the State Council, 17 February 2020).

The total number of secondary accidents caused by the pandemic control measures (including food shortages, accidental deaths due to refusal of access to medical treatment, the killings of dogs and cats, violent confrontations between officials and citizens, and other immediate damage) in each city were collected from a website where people can see daily trends in micro-blog topics in China (www.weibotop.cn/2.0/#, accessed on 2 April 2022). This is a palliative due to the lack of official statistics on this issue. Thus, these data are approximate and reflect the overall severity rather than the true total numbers of secondary accidents.

Information on the cities' 2-year average economic growth rates, gross domestic product (GDP), total population, and universities were collected from the National Bureau of Statistics of China website (https://data.stats.gov.cn, accessed on 21 March 2022). The cities' digital city rankings were obtained from a China Center for Information Industry Development (CCID) report published in June 2021 [23].

2.2. City Selection

The 36 cities (Figure 1) included in this study were selected mainly for the following reasons:

1. All 36 cities are municipal-level cities (divided into districts). According to the current Law on the Prevention and Treatment of Infectious Diseases, the municipal government is the agency responsible for responding to infectious diseases within its jurisdiction. It is the key decision-making body for pandemic management. The central or provincial governments only intervene when the municipal government is incapable of controlling the crisis. In that case, the higher levels of government primarily act as coordinators and supervisors but do not replace the municipal government in directly managing the crisis.
2. These 36 cities represent different geographical locations, population sizes, economic and technological development levels, and administrative and cultural traditions; they are located in eastern, central, and western China. Among them, there are 4 municipalities directly under the central government; another 14 are provincial capitals, and the other 18 are important transportation hubs, with active international economic and trade exchange. These hubs are close to mega-cities or are border cities. Although the cities differ considerably, they all face high pressure to prevent and control the COVID-19 pandemic.
3. The cities have relatively independent discretion to deal with the pandemic. Thus, our sample cities are comparable yet representative for examining the relationships between the different policy strategies that were chosen and the pandemic management outcomes of those choices.

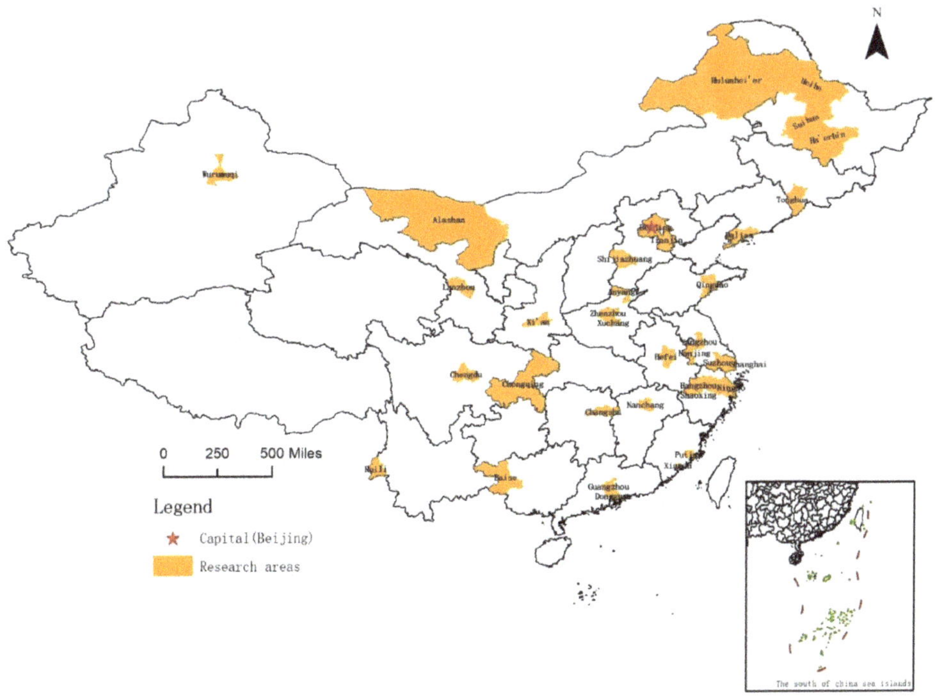

Figure 1. The locations of the 36 cities investigated in this study.

2.3. Analysis Methods

This study adopted a comparative methodology to shed light on the link between policy design and the cities' pandemic response outcomes. First, we used structural topic modeling to identify the topics around which the COVID-19 policy responses were clustered. Topic modeling is a machine learning technique for discovering latent common topics in text documents [24,25]. The topics resulting from this analysis were interpreted as types of policy tools adopted by municipal governments to deal with the COVID-19 pandemic. We applied the topic modeling in the following steps: (1) we collected documents related to municipal pandemic prevention and control policies and compiled them into a policy dataset; (2) we processed the word segmentation, then removed stop words in the Chinese language as well as frequently occurring words in this dataset (for example, "announce", "COVID-19", "policy"); and (3) we employed collocations to create a model for phrase extraction and for optimizing the word segmentation results. (4) After preprocessing the text, we selected the number of topics ($k = 28$) based on the assessment of models with 4–30 topics. Running the topic model, we obtained the prevalence of each policy tool, and the sum of the prevalence of the overall types of policy is always 1. The topic prevalence refers to the proportion of each topic in the corpus after clustering, and the calculation results can reflect the dependence of municipal governments on specific policy tools. The topic prevalence is calculated with Formula (1):

$$P_k = \frac{\sum_i^N \theta_{ki}}{N} \tag{1}$$

In Formula (1), P_k represents the prevalence of topic k, N is the total number of policy texts, and θ_{ki} refers to the probability of the topic k in the overall policy texts.

Second, we examined the balance of policy mixes across cities. In this way, we identified different configurations that represented the building blocks of policy tools designed to deal with the pandemic. We examined the balance of policy mixes by assessing the distributions of the policy tools included in each mix [22,26].

Third, we employed an ordinary least squares (OLS) regression model (Formula (2)) to investigate the relationship between a policy mix and a city's pandemic response outcomes. The dependent variables were measures of the immediate outcomes of a city's policy strategy: the number of major outbreaks in a city, the number of high-risk areas in a city, the number of secondary accidents in a city, and the city's 2-year average economic growth rate. Given the fact that except the case of Wuhan, the mortality from the COVID-19 is insignificant in Chinese cities (for example, from 17 May 2020 to 1 April 2022, only 4 death cases were reported in total by 3 different cities; see www.nhc.gov.cn, accessed on 21 March 2022), which does not constitute a major concern in public opinion. In contrast with international practice, in the four dimensions we considered in this study, outbreaks, high-risk areas, secondary accidents, and economic consequences, we did not include mortality in the dependent variables. The independent variables were the policy tools used to deal with the pandemic, which were measured by the prevalence of each tool in the policy mix of that city. The city's GDP, permanent population, number of universities, and digital city ranking were the control variables:

$$dependent_i = \alpha + \sum \beta_i independent_i + \sum \gamma_i control_i + \varepsilon_i \tag{2}$$

3. Results

3.1. Identifying Policy Tools

Applying topic modeling, we obtained 28 topics that outlined the basic parameters of the municipal-level COVID-19 pandemic responses. In decreasing order of prevalence, these 28 policy tools are shown in Table 1.

Table 1. Key policy tools adopted by the cities.

Policy Tool	Illustrative Action	Prevalence
1. Information management	Providing public information; requiring residents to report to their communities if they had been to risk areas	0.104059
2. Monitoring population health	Measuring temperatures; checking health QR codes and travel codes	0.085552
3. Mask requirements	Mask requirements in public places and collective locales such as workplaces, buses, subways, and taxis	0.069997
4. Sanitizer policies	Disinfections in public places and collective locales; frequent hand-washing campaigns	0.069543
5. Public testing	Mandated nucleic acid testing for urban residents every one to three days	0.067159
6. Quarantines	Mandated isolation for close and indirect contacts; isolation or home quarantine for travelers	0.066421
7. Gathering restrictions	Restrict gatherings to a maximum of five people; ban all social gatherings	0.064547
8. Travel restrictions	Inner city traffic restrictions; cancel interregional travels	0.064093
9. Contact tracing	Epidemiological survey professionals question individuals and analyze travel information using big data methods to determine virus spread paths and identify close and indirect contacts	0.061482
10. Social distancing	Keep one meter distance in public or collective places	0.052455
11. Vaccination campaigns	Set up free vaccination sites in individual communities; require local cadres, social workers, and medical professionals to visit households to mobilize people for COVID-19 vaccine uptake	0.040704
12. Work and production resumption supports other than economic support	Facilitate permit approval for logistics vehicles; simplify administrative examination and approval procedures; provide employment recruitment services for enterprises	0.029407
13. Humanitarian assistance other than access to medical facilities	Open psychological comfort hotlines; local cadres and social workers visit vulnerable groups such as elders, disabled, and migrants	0.026284
14. Supply chain management	Enacting material supply plans; ensuring smooth transportation of medical materials and life supplies	0.021913
15. Emergency investment in health care	Booster medical supplies; purchase protective equipment for health staff; support manufacturing of testing equipment	0.021459
16. Improving the local risk response system	Require local governments or enterprises to improve emergency plans; enhance emergency drills and local risk screening	0.018904
17. Restrictions on commercial activities	Limiting customer or visitor flow in shopping malls, supermarkets, cinemas, parks, and tourist spots	0.01669
18. Social mobilization	Appeal to the voluntary participation of individuals and businesses to help fight the pandemic	0.015782

Table 1. *Cont.*

Policy Tool	Illustrative Action	Prevalence
19. Funding or fiscal stimulus	Release funds to alleviate the economic impact of COVID-19; tax reduction and exemption	0.015441
20. Cancelling public events	Postpone sporting competitions; cancel expositions and festivities	0.01442
21. Promoting e-government services	Provide online government services such as social insurance and online administrative examination and approval	0.013057
22. Workplace and retail shops closures	Close retail outlets until further notice; permit only delivery and take-out at restaurants	0.012433
23. Living or income support	Distribute daily necessities to elders, disabled persons, and migrants; distribute consumption coupons	0.011467
24. Lockdowns	Full-scale lockdowns; district (partial) lockdowns	0.009878
25. Supporting public access to normal medical treatment;	Open green channels for dialysis patients, cancer patients, and pregnant women for medical treatment; inform doctors to prescribe adequate medication for particular patients during the period of lockdown	0.009424
26. Debt/contract relief for households and enterprises	Postpone households' and enterprises' debt and rent payments for three months; rent exemption in the period of lockdown	0.007777
27. School closures	Close schools and universities in the period of lockdown	0.005166
28. Restrictions on government services	Close petition reception; close marriage registration services	0.004485

The above 28 topics were divided into 3 categories based on the policy goals they were intended to accomplish:

1. Restrictions: These are policy tools that impose obligations, limitations, and prohibitions on individuals and collective actors [27]. These coercive measures aim to control the spread of the virus by reducing contacts and interactions. However, they can have negative effects [2] such as seriously impacting economic activity, supply chains, and public access to normal medical treatment. The restriction-based policy tools are as follows: lockdowns, quarantines, school closures, workplace and retail shop closures, canceling public events, gathering restrictions, travel restrictions, commercial activity restrictions, social distancing, mask requirements, and restrictions on government services.
2. Health protection measures: These are policies aiming to protect people from the direct effects of COVID-19. These proactive measures can alter and reduce the magnitude of a pandemic [27]. Compared with restrictions, which are obligations imposed on individuals and enterprises, health protection measures are responsive policy investments by the government. This category includes the following tools: information management, public testing, contact tracing, emergency investment in health care, sanitizer policies, vaccination services, monitoring population health, social mobilization, and improving the local risk response systems.
3. Socioeconomic support measures: These are policies that aim to protect the affected populations from the negative socioeconomic impacts of the pandemic and the secondary effects caused by restrictions [2]. This category consists of living/income support, debt or contract relief for households and enterprises, funding or fiscal stimulus, other work and production resumption support besides economic support, supply chain management, support for public access to normal medical treatment,

other humanitarian assistance besides access to medical facilities, and the provision of e-government services.

No city relied exclusively on only one or two policy tools to deal with the pandemic; most deployed all of the 28 tools over the last 2 years with different distributions of these measures. Eleven cities (including Shanghai, Guangzhou, Hefei, and Baise) have tried to guarantee a minimum level of government services by not closing some service locations, such as petition reception and administrative approval services. Two cities (Chongqing and Xi'an) did not provide any public access to normal medical treatment facilities. Xi'an encountered a severe secondary medical disaster during its major outbreak in January 2022. Several uninfected people died owing to a lack of timely access to medical treatment.

3.2. Policy Mixes' Tool Type Balance

The balance of a policy mix is measured by the distribution of policy tools within the mix. At the global level, the balance of the policy mixes is illustrated by the above sequential list. From this list, we identified three general trends.

First, the municipal governments opted for a preventive approach [28] to deal with the COVID-19 pandemic. This was indicated by the five most intensively used policy tools: information management, monitoring population health, mask requirements, sanitizer policies, and public testing. Second, social mobilization was not a prevalent policy tool; it ranked 18th among the 28 policies. This finding agrees with the low level of public participation in fighting the COVID-19 pandemic in China. Chinese crisis management has long been characterized by a government-led style, which heavily depends on state responses and investments [11]. The important role of social capital and resources has been minimized in the current Chinese crisis response policy design [29,30]. Third, lockdowns (ranking 24th) were not an important policy tool for cities, nor were economic supports (ranking 12th, 19th, and 26th) or supporting normal medical access for uninfected people (ranking 25th).

Although there were similarities, the distribution of these policy tools varied widely among the cities. The balance of policy mixes for the 36 cities is shown in Figure 2. The value of each color bar represents the proportion of that policy tool in the policy mix of the city. The proportion is measured by the prevalence of each policy tool in the policy mix of that city (for the results data, please see Table S1).

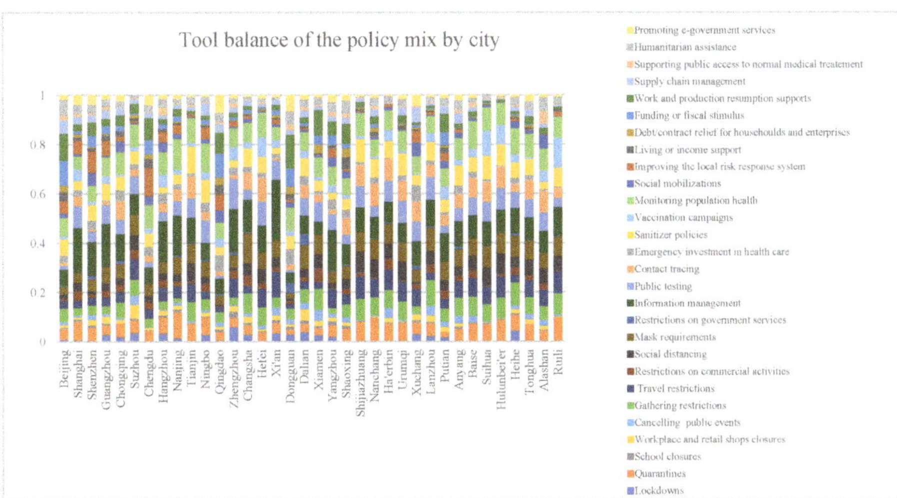

Figure 2. Tool balance of the policy mixes by city.

To further explore how the cities incorporated different policy tools to deal with the pandemic, we analyzed distinguishing combinations of the three policy tool categories discussed above. The proportion of policy tools (the sum of the proportion of each tool belonging to the same category) in each group (i.e., restrictions, health protection measures, and socioeconomic supports) was calculated for each city (Figure 3). Based the result obtained, the integration of the three policy tool clusters could be categorized into five patterns representing the different policy choice strategies.

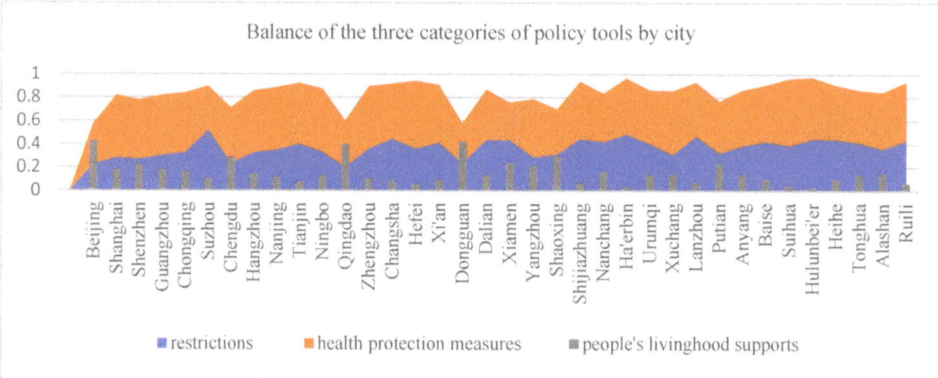

Figure 3. Balance of the three categories of policy tools by city.

Integrated health protection and socioeconomic support. In this strategy, municipal governments attached more importance to people's health and livelihoods. The policy responses centered on measures to protect people from the socioeconomic impacts of the pandemic. There was less emphasis on restrictions. Beijing, Chengdu, Dongguan, and Qingdao showed this pattern.

Integrated restriction and health protection measures. This strategy combined intensive restrictions with high-level health protection policy investments to protect the population from contracting COVID-19. Socioeconomic supports were less important in this policy mix. The following 15 cities showed this pattern: Changsha, Xi'an, Dalian, Shijiazhuang, Nanchang, Har'erbin, Urumqi, Lanzhou, Anyang, Baise, Hulunbei'er, Heihe, Tonghua, Alasha, and Ruili.

Restriction-oriented response. This policy strategy centered on restrictions and coercive measures to limit individual and business activities. Public health protection was less important, and socioeconomic supports were little utilized. Suzhou and Xiamen showed this pattern.

Health protection-oriented response. This policy mix emphasized investments in health protection measures that would protect people from contracting COVID-19. This strategy placed less emphasis on restrictions. It only slightly utilized socioeconomic supports, such as alleviating economic difficulties and the demands of daily life (such as procuring food supplies and access to normal medical treatment) during the outbreak. Shanghai, Shenzhen, Guangzhou, Chongqing, Hangzhou, Nanjing, Tianjin, Ningbo, Zhengzhou, Hefei, Yangzhou, Xuchang, and Suihua showed this pattern.

Comprehensive policy mix. This strategy used a balanced distribution of restrictions, health protection measures, and socioeconomic support policies. Shaoxing and Putian showed this pattern.

Maggetti and Trein (2022) found that politico-administrative arrangements did not markedly influence governments' policy choices when dealing with the COVID-19 pandemic. Similarly, we did not observe any significant correlations between a city's characteristics (i.e., economic, cultural, demographic, and geographic) and its policy design choices. For example, similar cities, such as Suzhou and Hangzhou, adopted very different policy strategies, while different cities, such as Beijing and Dongguan, adopted similar policy strategies. The policy decisions in many cases might simply be related to the local leaders' personal preferences.

3.3. Effects of Policy Mix on a City's Pandemic Response Outcomes

The R^2, F, and p values obtained from the OLS model (Formula (1)) indicated that the model passed the stability test and is highly representative. The results can be summarized as follows (Table 2):

1. Among the policy tools, lockdowns, school closures, canceling public events, travel restrictions, social distancing, contact tracing, vaccination campaigns, improving the local risk-response systems, and supply chain management had significant negative impacts on cities' 2-year average economic growth rates. By contrast, mask requirements, public testing, emergency investment in health care, debt/contract relief for households and enterprises, and support for public access to normal medical treatment did not have negative effects on the 2-year average economic growth rate.
2. Restriction-based tools did not significantly influence the number of major outbreaks or of high-risk areas.
3. Emergency investment in health care, vaccination campaigns, improving the local risk-response systems, supply chain management, and public access to normal medical treatment were negatively correlated with the numbers of major outbreaks, high-risk areas, and secondary accidents. Additionally, except for supply chain management, the others were positively correlated with the 2-year average economic growth rate.
4. By comparing these three policy tool categories, we found that restrictions and socioeconomic support measures did not significantly influence the control of the pandemic. In contrast, health protection measures strongly contributed to controlling the spread of the virus. Socioeconomic support measures particularly contributed to reducing the occurrence of secondary accidents.

Table 2. The effects of policy mix on the pandemic response outcomes.

		N-Outbreak	N-High Risk_Areas	N-SEC. Accidents	ECO_RATE
Restrictions	Lockdowns	0.152	1.975	1.010	−0.006 **
		(0.195)	(1.551)	(0.807)	(0.002)
	Quarantines	−0.036	0.038	−0.095	−0.000
		(0.045)	(0.360)	(0.188)	(0.000)
	School closures	−0.391	−4.433	0.560	−0.032 **
		(1.071)	(8.530)	(4.439)	(0.009)
	Workplace and retail shops closures	−0.231	−0.606	−0.806	0.001
		(0.158)	(1.258)	(0.655)	(0.001)
	Cancelling public events	0.042	0.912	1.171	−0.006 **
		(0.211)	(1.682)	(0.875)	(0.002)
	Gathering restrictions	−0.039	−0.676	−0.151	−0.001
		(0.094)	(0.748)	(0.389)	(0.001)
	Travel restrictions	0.100	0.412	0.039	−0.004 **
		(0.131)	(1.047)	(0.545)	(0.001)
	Restriction on commercial activities	0.011	−0.125	−0.533	0.003
		(0.168)	(1.339)	(0.697)	(0.001)

Table 2. *Cont.*

		N-Outbreak	N-High Risk_Areas	N-SEC. Accidents	ECO_RATE
	Social distancing	−0.042	−0.551	0.753	−0.009 **
		(0.324)	(2.578)	(1.342)	(0.003)
	Mask requirements	0.110	−0.086	−0.611	0.009 **
		(0.263)	(2.096)	(1.091)	(0.002)
	Restrictions on government services	0.323	−0.171	0.547	0.003
		(0.188)	(1.494)	(0.778)	(0.002)
Health protection Measures	Information management	−0.024	0.026	0.057	0.000
		(0.028)	(0.226)	(0.118)	(0.000)
	Public testing	0.011	−0.204	−0.214	0.003 **
		(0.104)	(0.826)	(0.430)	(0.001)
	Contact tracing	−0.117	0.133	0.546	−0.007 **
		(0.238)	(1.895)	(0.986)	(0.002)
	Emergency investment in health care	−0.184	−0.434 ***	−0.373 **	0.005 **
		(0.129)	(1.031)	(0.537)	(0.001)
	Sanitizer policies	−0.000	0.815	−0.252	0.002
		(0.151)	(1.200)	(0.625)	(0.001)
	Vaccination campaigns	−0.016	−0.230 **	−0.062 ***	−0.012 **
		(0.032)	(0.256)	(0.133)	(0.000)
	Monitoring population health	0.068	−0.046	−0.053	0.000
		(0.052)	(0.411)	(0.214)	(0.000)
	Social mobilizations	0.119	0.826	0.211	0.002
		(0.188)	(1.497)	(0.779)	(0.002)
	Improving the local risk response system	−0.080	−0.558 **	−0.293 **	−0.003 *
		(0.164)	(1.307)	(0.680)	(0.001)
Socioeconomic supports	Living or income support	0.022	−0.911	0.378	−0.003
		(0.161)	(1.282)	(0.667)	(0.001)
	Debt/contract relief for households and enterprises	0.171	0.853	−0.715	0.014 **
		(0.449)	(3.577)	(1.862)	(0.004)
	Funding or fiscal stimulus	−0.022	−0.547	−0.209	−0.001
		(0.099)	(0.785)	(0.409)	(0.001)
	Work and production resumption supports other than economic support	−0.005	0.848	0.201	0.000
		(0.101)	(0.808)	(0.420)	(0.001)
	Supply chain management	−0.003	−0.236	−0.032 **	−0.009 **
		(0.282)	(2.243)	(1.167)	(0.002)
	Supporting public access to normal medical treatment	−0.046	−0.052 ***	−1.108 **	0.010 **
		(0.297)	(2.369)	(1.233)	(0.002)

Table 2. *Cont.*

		N-Outbreak	N-High Risk_Areas	N-SEC. Accidents	ECO_RATE
	Humanitarian assistance other than access to medical facilities	0.000	−0.169	−0.396	0.000
		(0.063)	(0.503)	(0.262)	(0.001)
	Promoting e-government services	0.142	1.002	−0.222	0.000
		(0.115)	(0.918)	(0.478)	(0.001)
Control Variables	GDP	0.000	0.000	0.000	0.000
		(0.000)	(0.001)	(0.000)	(0.000)
	Permanent population	−0.001	−0.005	−0.005	0.000
		(0.001)	(0.009)	(0.005)	(0.000)
	University	0.015	0.154	0.098	0.000
		(0.035)	(0.279)	(0.145)	(0.000)
	Digital_city	0.017	0.069	−0.094	0.001 ***
		(0.027)	(0.214)	(0.111)	(0.000)
	_cons	−1.385	−10.244	5.165	−0.014
		(2.613)	(20.818)	(10.835)	(0.021)
	p	0.346	0.878	0.716	0.102
	r2	0.951	0.836	0.890	0.982
	F	1.830	0.479	0.757	5.071

Note: *, **, and *** represent the 10%, 5%, and 1% significance levels, respectively. N-outbreak: The total number of major outbreaks; N-high risk areas: The total number of high-risk areas; N-Sec.accidents: the total number of secondary accidents; Eco-rate: 2-year average economic growth rate.

4. Discussion

This study investigated how policy mixes affected cities' pandemic management outcomes under the context that pandemic prevention and control measures have become normalized in China. The situations of the 36 studied cities differ from that of Wuhan, which was the first city to face a COVID-19 outbreak. The included cities were more prepared and were able to rely on information and practical experiences from previously affected cities. There were relatively fewer uncertainties and cognitive blind spots about the COVID-19 virus characteristics. Therefore, the effects and effectiveness of different policy mixes were comparable among the studied cities.

4.1. Relation between Policy Mix and Pandemic Response Outcomes

The logistic regression analysis results showed that restriction policies had no significant influence on controlling the pandemic. However, health protection measures were associated with controlling the spread of the virus. The results revealed a negative correlation between restriction measures and the economic growth rate. Restrictions and socioeconomic support policies had opposite effects on the number of secondary disasters. The more frequently and stringently restriction policy tools were used, the more secondary accidents and disasters occurred. Conversely, more frequent and intense use of socioeconomic supports led to fewer secondary disasters.

Based on these findings, we established a correlative relationship between a city's policy mix pattern and its pandemic response outcomes (Table 3). Strategies 1 and 5 are the preferred policy choices for managing the pandemic. They are effective strategies for preventing or controlling the virus spread while avoiding the occurrence of serious negative socioeconomic consequences. Strategy 4 is suboptimal because although it is effective in controlling the spread of the virus, its consequences for secondary disaster prevention and economic protection are uncertain. Strategy 2 can control viral spread, but it might generate high levels of secondary disasters and have negative economic consequences. Strategy 3 is the worst choice because the restriction-oriented strategy cannot effectively control viral spread, but it negatively impacts secondary disasters and economic development.

Table 3. The relationships between policy mixes and pandemic response outcomes.

Policy Strategy \ Policy Outcomes	Virus Spread Controlling	Secondary Disasters	Economic Consequences
1. Integrated health protection and people's livelihood support	Positive	Negative	Negative
2. Integrated restrictions and health protection measures	Positive	Positive	Positive
3. Restriction-oriented policy response	No correlation	Positive	Positive
4. Health protection-oriented strategy	Positive	No correlation	No correlation
5. Comprehensive policy mix	Positive	Negative	Negative

4.2. The Importance of a Timely Lockdown

COVID-19 is highly contagious and can be spread through asymptomatic transmission; therefore, it is very difficult to prevent outbreaks. Many Chinese cities have been hit by the COVID-19 pandemic over the past 2 years. However, these cities have differed in the scale of outbreaks. Some cities have had a large number of cases across widely affected areas and have taken a long time to control the outbreak. Other cities have succeeded in controlling outbreaks in a short time with fewer cases and smaller affected areas. The implementation of timely lockdowns might be the key explanatory factor for these differences. A comparison between Shenzhen and Shanghai helps illustrate this hypothesis. The two cities are both international metropolia. The economic ranking of Shenzhen was the third (with 2.77 trillion yuan), and Shanghai is classified as the first (with 3.87 trillion yuan), among 337 Chinese municipal cities in 2020; Shenzhen is the fifth most populous city (with18 million permanent population in 2020) in China, and Shanghai is the second most populous city (with 25 million permanent population in 2020). Neither Shenzhen nor Shanghai had been hit by the COVID-19 outbreak until the arrival of the omicron virus in January 2022. Omicron is less dangerous but much more contagious than the previous variants such as alfa and delta.

Contrary to popular belief, not all Chinese cities implemented severe restrictions such as lockdowns to control viral spread. This is evidenced by lockdown policies ranking 24th among the 28 most often used policy tools (Figure 1), indicating that many municipal governments were reluctant to impose these measures. Some cities, including Shenzhen and Shanghai, refrained from adopting stringent restrictions to avoid their negative economic consequences. During the most recent outbreaks in the two cities in March 2022, in the early phase, both cities hesitated to impose lockdown measures for economic reasons. When the number of cases significantly increased for three consecutive days, Shenzhen imposed a lockdown policy, and the outbreak was under control one week later. In early March, the outbreak situation in Shanghai was similar to that in Shenzhen, but the authorities in Shanghai delayed the implementation of lockdown measures; they announced a lockdown policy 3 weeks after Shenzhen. As a result, Shanghai missed the optimal timing for initiating a lockdown. At present, the outbreak in Shanghai remains out of control (Table 4).

An appropriate and timely lockdown might be more effective than other restriction policies for controlling the spread of an outbreak, especially for severe viruses with a relatively high R0 (basic reproduction number) [2,31]. It might also be the least costly strategy, because when an outbreak is out of control, more cases and secondary disasters take place, resulting in more deaths and increased socioeconomic damage.

Table 4. Case comparison between Shenzhen and Shanghai.

Cases \ Date	12 March	13 March	14 March	15 March	16 March	20 March	21 March	28 March	1 April	26 April
Shenzhen	66	86	60	92	91	44	28	9	2	0
Shanghai	65	169	139	202	158	758	896	4477	24,943	16,980
Lockdown			Shenzhen, start			Shenzhen, end			Shanghai, start	

Note: date was retrieved from the two cities' CDC website (www.shenzhencdc.cn; www.scdc.sh.cn, accessed on 21 March 2022).

4.3. A Comprehensive Policy Mix for Compound Crises

The COVID-19 pandemic is a compound disaster in nature. It threatens not only public health but also multiple life-sustaining systems, functions, and infrastructure [32], such as economic activity, the supply of everyday necessities, the function of medical facilities, and logistics and transport systems. A pandemic is not a single negative event; rather, it is a concatenation of related negative events, generating multiple effects that become apparent on various time scales [32,33]. Pandemics are often accompanied by a variety of secondary disasters such as economic crisis, increased poverty, shortages of necessities, and excess mortality.

Studies have partly revealed the immediate negative effects that have arisen during the COVID-19 pandemic from medical, psychological, and social perspectives [34–37]. For instance, according to a recent study, during January–March 2020, in Wuhan, mortality from chronic noncommunicable diseases increased by 21%; there was an 83% increase in deaths from diabetes and a 66% increase in suicides [36]. The current study also found high incidence rates of secondary disasters during the pandemic period. In addition, larger outbreaks resulted in a greater number of secondary accidents. During the outbreaks in Tonghua, Xi'an, and Shanghai, a shortage of everyday necessities and excess deaths caused by restriction policies or the lack of medical access constituted two types of prominent immediate secondary disasters caused by ineffective supply chain management and a rigid "one size fits all" approach to pandemic control.

The complexity of the pandemic requires decision-makers to take a comprehensive approach rather than a single-event management approach to deal with the COVID-19 crisis [32,38]. Pandemic prevention and control are certainly the core aims, but decision-makers should also seriously consider the prospect of secondary disasters and enact compensatory measures to prevent the potential negative consequences of pandemic control measures, particularly restrictions [2,39]. It is necessary to implement a comprehensive and coherent policy mix with an appropriate distribution of the different types of policy tools available [40,41].

4.4. Study Limitations

This study has some limitations that should be addressed in future research. First, we examined only some of the serious immediate outcomes brought about by the different policy design choices. These outcomes were the most resounding concerns in Chinese public opinion. As such, we did not examine other issues such as the direct and indirect mortality caused by the COVID-19, which is an important concern at the international level. More comprehensive studies are necessary to provide a more in-depth assessment of the policy response outcomes and identify the optimal policy mix, as well as latent policy blind spots and mistakes. Such an in-depth study would better inform decision-makers and improve their policy responses when dealing with severe pandemics such as the COVID-19 crisis.

Second, given the complexity of our study (we investigated the effectiveness of the different combinations of 28 policy tools adopted by 36 cities), and for technical feasibility, we did not examine how the sequence and stringency of different policy tools affects the pandemic response outcomes. This limitation might be complemented by small-N cases with a limited number of policy tools or by detailed case studies.

Third, the completeness of the collected data regarding municipal policies was largely influenced by the amount of information that was made publicly available by the local governments. We were unable to discern precisely how many and what types of policies have been implemented in the form of internal governmental documents without informing the public. Moreover, since there was no central registry from which all data were collected using the same methodology, potential bias might have been introduced into the research. Although the results of our analysis are in agreement with our empirical observations, we recommend that future studies use integrated research methods [42,43] to overcome the limitations of the quantitative approach when investigating complex issues such as pandemic management.

5. Conclusions

This study investigated the relationship between the policy design of a city and its pandemic response outcomes. It contributes to the literature on comparative policy responses to a pandemic by offering a novel, local-level perspective.

Our analysis revealed that restriction measures did not significantly influence the spread of the virus, but they were negatively correlated with a city's economic growth rate. In contrast, health protection measures strongly contributed to controlling viral spread. Intensive socioeconomic support measures, such as improving supply chain management and public access to normal medical treatment, reduced the occurrence of secondary disasters. The most effective policy strategy to deal with the COVID-19 pandemic appears to be a comprehensive policy design with a mix of restrictions, health protection measures, and socioeconomic support policies accompanied by a timely lockdown.

Our empirical findings can help to improve policy design by highlighting diverging patterns of policy strategies and their consequences, thereby generating useful lessons for how local governments should deal with similar crises in the future. We suggest that decision-makers take a comprehensive approach rather than a single-event management approach to deal with compound crises such as the COVID-19 pandemic. They should seriously consider the prospect of secondary disasters and enact compensatory measures to prevent the potential negative consequences caused by crisis control measures. Given the specific cultural and political characteristics of the investigated cities, these findings might not be applicable to cities beyond mainland China. We suggest further in-depth studies to investigate the relationships between policy strategies and their consequences by considering the specific local or national sociocultural and political contexts.

Supplementary Materials: The following supporting information can be downloaded at: https://www.mdpi.com/article/10.3390/ijerph19138094/s1, Table S1: The distribution of policy tools by city.

Author Contributions: Conceptualization, C.S.; data curation, C.S. and T.X.; statistical analysis, C.S., H.L., T.X. and Z.Y.; Methodology, C.S., H.L., T.X. and Z.Y.; writing-original draft, C.S. and H.L.; writing-review, H.L. All authors have read and agreed to the published version of the manuscript.

Funding: This research was funded by the National Social Science Foundation of China (Grant No. 19BZZ082) and Zhejiang Science Foundation for Distinguished Young Scholars (Grant No. LR21G030001).

Institutional Review Board Statement: This study was conducted according to the guidelines of the Declaration of Helsinki and followed the Ethics Committee of Zhejiang Gongshang University standards.

Informed Consent Statement: Not applicable.

Data Availability Statement: The data presented in this study are available on request from the corresponding author.

Acknowledgments: We also thank Katherine Thieltges for editing the English text of a draft of this manuscript. We also thank Lu Lili and Mao Yimin for their constructive comments on earlier versions of this paper.

Conflicts of Interest: The authors declare no conflict of interest.

References

1. Maggetti, M.; Trein, P. Policy integration, problem-solving, and the coronavirus disease crisis: Lessons for policy design. *Policy Soc.* **2022**, *41*, 53–67. [CrossRef]
2. Capano, G.; Howlett, M.; Jarvis, D.S.L.; Ramesh, M.; Goyal, N. Mobilizing Policy (In) Capacity to Fight COVID-19: Understanding Variations in State Responses. *Policy Soc.* **2020**, *39*, 285–308. [CrossRef] [PubMed]
3. Triggle, C.R.; Bansal, D.; Abu Farag, E.A.; Ding, H.; Sultan, A.A. COVID-19: Learning from Lessons To Guide Treatment and Prevention Interventions. *Msphere* **2020**, *5*, e00317-20. [CrossRef] [PubMed]
4. Cairney, P. The UK government's COVID-19 policy: Assessing evidence-informed policy analysis in real time. *Br. Politics* **2021**, *16*, 90–116. [CrossRef]
5. Maor, M.; Howlett, M. Explaining variations in state COVID-19 responses: Psychological, institutional, and strategic factors in governance and public policy-making. *Policy Des. Pract.* **2020**, *3*, 228–241. [CrossRef]
6. Cheng, C.; Barcelo, J.; Hartnett, A.S.; Kubinec, R.; Messerschmidt, L. COVID-19 Government Response Event Dataset (CoronaNet v.1.0). *Nat. Hum. Behav.* **2020**, *4*, 756–768. [CrossRef]
7. Toshkov, D.; Carroll, B.; Yesilkagit, K. Government capacity, societal trust or party preferences: What accounts for the variety of national policy responses to the COVID-19 pandemic in Europe? *J. Eur. Public Policy* **2021**, *29*, 1009–1028. [CrossRef]
8. Gonzalez-Bustamante, B. Evolution and early government responses to COVID-19 in South America. *World Dev.* **2021**, *137*, 105180. [CrossRef]
9. Yan, B.; Zhang, X.M.; Wu, L.; Zhu, H.; Chen, B. Why Do Countries Respond Differently to COVID-19? A Comparative Study of Sweden, China, France, and Japan. *Am. Rev. Public Adm.* **2020**, *50*, 762–769. [CrossRef]
10. Woo, J.J. Policy capacity and Singapore's response to the COVID-19 pandemic. *Policy Soc.* **2020**, *39*, 345–362. [CrossRef]
11. Mei, C.Q. Policy style, consistency and the effectiveness of the policy mix in China's fight against COVID-19. *Policy Soc.* **2020**, *39*, 309–325. [CrossRef] [PubMed]
12. Migone, A.R. The influence of national policy characteristics on COVID-19 containment policies: A comparative analysis. *Policy Des. Pract.* **2020**, *3*, 259–276. [CrossRef]
13. Knill, C.; Steinebach, Y. What has happened and what has not happened due to the coronavirus disease pandemic: A systemic perspective on policy change. *Policy Soc.* **2022**, *41*, 25–39. [CrossRef]
14. Capano, G. Policy design and state capacity in the COVID-19 emergency in Italy: If you are not prepared for the (un)expected, you can be only what you already are. *Policy Soc.* **2020**, *39*, 326–344. [CrossRef] [PubMed]
15. Capano, G.; Howlett, M.; Jarvis, D.S.L.; Ramesh, M. Long-term policy impacts of the coronavirus: Normalization, adaptation, and acceleration in the post-COVID state. *Policy Soc.* **2022**, *41*, 1–12. [CrossRef]
16. Hale, T.; Angrist, N.; Goldszmidt, R.; Kira, B.; Petherick, A.; Phillips, T.; Webster, S.; Cameron-Blake, E.; Hallas, L.; Majumdar, S.; et al. A global panel database of pandemic policies (Oxford COVID-19 Government Response Tracker). *Nat. Hum. Behav.* **2021**, *5*, 529–538. [CrossRef]
17. OECD. *The Territorial Impact of COVID-19: Managing the Crisis across Levels of Government*; OECD Publishing: Paris, France, 2020. [CrossRef]
18. Bouckaert, G.; Galli, D.; Kuhlmann, S.; Reiter, R.; Van Hecke, S. European Coronationalism? A Hot Spot Governing a Pandemic Crisis. *Public Adm. Rev.* **2020**, *80*, 765–773. [CrossRef]
19. Nauewelaers, C.; Boekholt, P.; Mostert, B.; Cunningham, P.; Guy, K.; Hofer, R.; Rammer, C. *Policy Mixes for R&D in Europe*; European Commission—Directorate—General for Research: Maastricht, The Netherlands, 2009.
20. Rogge, K.S.; Reichardt, K. Policy mixes for sustainability transitions: An extended concept and framework for analysis. *Res. Policy* **2016**, *45*, 132–147. [CrossRef]
21. Rogge, K.S.; Kern, F.; Howlett, M. Conceptual and empirical advances in analysing policy mixes for energy transitions. *Energy Res. Soc. Sci.* **2017**, *33*, 1–10. [CrossRef]
22. Schmidt, T.S.; Sewerin, S. Measuring the temporal dynamics of policy mixes—An empirical analysis of renewable energy policy mixes' balance and design features in nine countries. *Res. Policy* **2019**, *48*, 103557. [CrossRef]
23. China Center for Information Industry Development (CCID). White Paper on China's Top 100 Digital Cities (2020). Available online: www.mtx.cn/#/report?id=684403 (accessed on 27 February 2022).
24. Roberts, M.E.; Stewart, B.M.; Tingley, D. stm: An R Package for Structural Topic Models. *J. Stat. Softw.* **2019**, *91*, 1–40. [CrossRef]
25. R Core Team. R: A Language and Environment for Statistical Computing. R Foundation for Statistical Computing. 2020. Available online: https://www.R-project.org/ (accessed on 13 March 2022).
26. Goyal, N.; Howlett, M. "Measuring the Mix" of Policy Responses to COVID-19: Comparative Policy Analysis Using Topic Modelling. *J. Comp. Policy Anal.* **2021**, *23*, 250–261. [CrossRef]
27. Howlett, M. *Designing Public Policies: Principles and Instruments*; Routledge: London, UK; New York, NY, USA, 2010; pp. 1–236.

28. Cairney, P.; Denny, E.S. Prevention Policy as the Ultimate 'Wicked' Problem. In *Why Isn't Government Policy More Preventive?* Cairney, P., Denny, E.S., Eds.; Oxford University Press: Oxford, UK, 2020.
29. Cai, C.K.; Jiang, W.Q.; Tang, N. Campaign-style crisis regime: How China responded to the shock of COVID-19. *Policy Stud.* **2022**, *43*, 599–619. [CrossRef]
30. Zhao, Z.H.; Zhou, Y.; Li, W.H.; Fan, X.H.; Huang, Q.S.; Tang, Z.H.; Li, H.; Wang, J.X.; Li, J.L.; Wu, J. Discussion on China's anti-epidemic response based on the Protocol on Prevention and Control of Coronavirus Disease 2019 from Chinese Authority. *Int. J. Health Plan. Manag.* **2022**, *37*, 1205–1220. [CrossRef] [PubMed]
31. OECD. First Lessons from Government Evaluations of COVID-19 Responses: A Synthesis. 2022. Available online: www.oecd.org/coronavirus/policy-reponses/ (accessed on 12 April 2022).
32. Ansell, C.; Boin, A.; Keller, A. Managing Transboundary Crises: Identifying the Building Blocks of an Effective Response System. *J. Contingencies Crisis Manag.* **2010**, *18*, 195–207. [CrossRef]
33. Alkan, M.L. Viral Epidemics: Past and Future. In *Managing Crises: Threats, Dilemmas, Opportunities, Springfield: Charles C Thomas;* Rosenthal, U., Boin, R.A., Comfort, L.K., Eds.; Charles C Thomas: Springfield, IL, USA, 2001; pp. 267–280.
34. Yuan, Z.; Dai, Z.; Chen, Y. Modelling the effects of Wuhan's lockdown during COVID-19, China. *Bull. World Health Organization. Suppl.* **2020**, *98*, 484–494. [CrossRef]
35. Phillipson, C.; Yarker, S.; Lang, L.; Doran, P.; Goff, M.; Buffel, T. COVID-19, Inequality and Older People: Developing Community-Centred Interventions. *Int. J. Environ. Res. Public Health* **2021**, *18*, 8064. [CrossRef]
36. Liu, J.; Zhang, L.; Yan, Y.; Zhou, Y.; Yin, P.; Qi, J.; Wang, L.; Pan, J.; You, J.; Yang, J. Excess mortality in Wuhan city and other parts of China during the three months of the covid-19 outbreak: Findings from nationwide mortality registries. *BMJ* **2022**, *372*, n415. [CrossRef]
37. McAlearney, A.S.; Gaughan, A.A.; MacEwan, S.R.; Gregory, M.E.; Rush, L.J.; Volney, J.; Panchal, A.R. Pandemic Experience of First Responders: Fear, Frustration, and Stress. *Int. J. Environ. Res. Public Health* **2022**, *19*, 4693. [CrossRef]
38. OECD. The Changing Face of Strategic Crisis Management. In *OECD Reviews of Risk Management Policies;* OECD Publishing: Paris, France, 2015. [CrossRef]
39. OECD. Tackling the mental health impact of the COVID-19 crisis: An integrated, whole-of-society response. In *OECD Policy Responses to Coronavirus (COVID-19);* OECD Publishing: Paris, France, 2021. [CrossRef]
40. Howlett, M.; Rayner, J. Design Principles for Policy Mixes: Cohesion and Coherence in 'New Governance Arrangements'. *Policy Soc.* **2007**, *26*, 1–18. [CrossRef]
41. Howlett, M.; How, Y.P.; Rio, P.D. The parameters of policy portfolios: Verticality and horizontality in design spaces and their consequences for policy mix formulation. *Environ. Plan.* **2015**, *33*, 1233–1245. [CrossRef]
42. Tonon, G. Integrated Methods in Research. In *Handbook of Research Methods in Health Social Sciences;* Liamputtong, P., Ed.; Springer Singapore: Singapore, 2019; pp. 681–694.
43. Dooren, W.V.; Noordegraaf, M. Staging Science: Authoritativeness and Fragility of Models and Measurement in the COVID-19 Crisis. *SocArXiv* **2020**, *80*, 610–615. [CrossRef] [PubMed]

International Journal of
Environmental Research and Public Health

MDPI

Article

A Complex Hybrid Model for Evaluating Projects to Improve the Sustainability and Health of Regions and Cities

Miroslav Kelemen [1], Beata Gavurova [2,*] and Volodymyr Polishchuk [3]

1 Faculty of Aeronautics, Technical University of Kosice, 041 21 Košice, Slovakia; miroslav.kelemen@tuke.sk
2 Faculty of Mining, Ecology, Process Control and Geotechnologies, Technical University of Košice, Letná 9, 042 00 Košice, Slovakia
3 Faculty of Information Technologies, Uzhhorod National University, 88000 Uzhhorod, Ukraine; volodymyr.polishchuk@uzhnu.edu.ua
* Correspondence: beata.gavurova@tuke.sk

Abstract: The main goal of the study is to develop a complex hybrid model for evaluating projects to improve the sustainability and health of regions and cities within the European Green Deal and Industry 5.0 concepts. The complex model is a comprehensive evaluation system that considers various influencing factors, the investor's intentions regarding the need and financing of projects, as well as expert opinion on the possibility of achieving sustainability and health of regions and cities by implementing this project with the investor. The model is based on modern theory of intellectual knowledge analysis, fuzzy set theory, and systems approach. Furthermore, we have an initial quantitative assessment and the linguistic significance of the level of the project financing decision with a reliability assessment. The knowledge from the repository of 896 project plans in the field of transport submitted for implementation and financing in the period 2021–2027 was used for the creation of the model. The results of the study were tested on the examples of evaluation of five real projects and demonstrated the applied value of the methodology for evaluating the level of decision-making feasibility of project financing in uncertainty and the importance of making correct management decisions based on expert opinions.

Keywords: urban sustainability; healthy cities; projects; risks; expert evaluation; fuzzy sets; European Green Deal; Industry 5.0; decision-making; transport; medical infrastructure

Citation: Kelemen, M.; Gavurova, B.; Polishchuk, V. A Complex Hybrid Model for Evaluating Projects to Improve the Sustainability and Health of Regions and Cities. *IJERPH* **2022**, *19*, 8217. https://doi.org/10.3390/ijerph19138217

Academic Editors: Jie Chen, Qian Zhou and Ting Zhang

Received: 11 June 2022
Accepted: 3 July 2022
Published: 5 July 2022

1. Introduction

Society recognizes the importance of addressing the resilience and health of regions and cities in implementing global strategic development plans at the regional and local levels, for example, through the efforts of each EU Member State to reduce regional disparities between the levels of development of European regions and to improve living standards in the least-favored regions [1].

The paper, using a multilateral interdisciplinary approach, is an effort to create a mathematical expert hybrid model based on fuzzy logic to support the decision-making processes of evaluation commissions at the state and local government levels, as well as decision-makers for implementing sustainable development policy and healthy regions and cities, improving the governance of cities and regions, in the context of the forthcoming implementation of the European Green Deal and the European Industry 5.0 concept, within the Member States. Addressing the issue also contributes to supporting efforts to become a candidate country and subsequently a full member of the European Union in meeting the EU's long-term strategic goals and commitments.

The research topic is related to the objective and transparent evaluation of projects based on criteria set by experts in the field to which the call for proposals relates.

The research problem is the quantitative and qualitative evaluation of the proposed solution content and risks in the field of resilience and health of regions and cities within the current societal challenges of climate change elimination expressed in the European Green Deal and the European Industry 5.0 concept.

The research question is focused on researching and creating an innovative algorithm for expert evaluation of projects to strengthen the resilience and health of regions and cities within the European Green Deal and the Industry 5.0 concept submitted in the competition, based on a neuro-fuzzy framework to support decision-making processes. On this basis, the paper proposes Hypotheses 1 and 2.

Hypothesis 1 (H1). *Project developers in strengthening the resilience and health of regions and cities who meet the grant provider's intentions in accordance with the European Green Deal and Industry 5.0 concept will get a better result based on a fuzzy expert assessment of the project's innovation ecosystem potential than project developers who do not meet the grant provider's intentions in the field of strengthening the resilience and health of regions and cities in line with the European Green Deal and the Industry 5.0 concept or only partially meet them.*

Hypothesis 2 (H2). *If the developed algorithm of the comprehensive hybrid model evaluation of resilience and health projects of regions and cities is applicable for the evaluation of projects within the European Union, then the algorithm will be applicable to the evaluation of resilience and health projects of regions and cities outside the European Union.*

The main goal of the study is to develop a complex hybrid model for evaluating projects to improve the sustainability and health of regions and cities, within the concepts of the European Green Deal and Industry 5.0. The model focuses on supporting the decision-making processes of evaluation commissions at the level of public administration and self-government and entities empowered to implement regional policy and local self-government with support for specialized, targeted projects and programs. Secondly, the results of scientific research are also used in the education and support of young scientists and professionals with social responsibility, which is usually expressed in the creation of social responsibility of companies, institutions, or public associations in an open civil society. The common goals are expressed in the intention of the model to maximize the potential of the innovation ecosystem of the project, bringing together different stakeholders in the idea and decision-making process to improve and enhance the sustainability and health of regions and cities according to European Green Deal and Industry 5.0 time, with the accepted level of project implementation risks and the level of required public funds (support from global sources, EU, state support), as well as co-financing of projects from private or corporate sources.

The key result of the paper is a comprehensive approach to evaluating projects to improve the sustainability and health of regions and cities, within the concepts of the European Green Deal and Industry 5.0, for practical use by evaluation commissions and decision-makers at state and local levels private sector. The output is the basis for further research work on the development of a web analytics tool on this topic. The acquired knowledge and algorithm can be transferred to the evaluation of projects outside the European Union, and the problem-solving methodology will allow repeating the procedure to other scientists and experts/evaluators of projects aimed at strengthening the sustainability and health of regions and cities.

1.1. Literature Review

The Europe Green Agreement and the Industry 5.0 concept are in line with the global implementation of the 2030 Agenda for Sustainable Development, under the auspices of the United Nations, which reflects the policies and responsibilities of all stakeholders [2].

The EU's long-term budget, together with the temporary NextGenerationEU instrument (NGEU, €806.9 billion), dedicated to supporting recovery, is the largest stimulus package ever funded in Europe [3].

One third of the €1.8 trillion investment from the NextGenerationEU recovery plan will go to the European Green Agreement and will also be funded by the EU's seven-year budget to ensure zero net greenhouse gas emissions by 2050, resource-independent economic growth, and no individual or region will be forgotten [4]. Industry 5.0. complements the existing "Industry 4.0" approach by specifically putting research and innovation at the service of the transition to a sustainable, human-centric, and resilient European industry [5].

The implementation of the strategic plans will be supported by various grant schemes for which research and project teams will compete at regional and local level. For example, the budget for financing EU development goals for Slovakia is provisionally at the level of more than 18.6 billion. In addition, Slovakia may have another 7.5 billion at its disposal. EUR for the implementation of the EU Recovery Plan, so the total budget envelope with co-financing of 2.9 billion. The Euro may be at the level of 29.0 billion Euro [6].

Many OECD (Organization for Economic Co-operation and Development) and EU Member States have adopted integrated investment strategies and integrated investment packages as their implementation tool and have put in place mechanisms to coordinate cross-sectoral public investment. More than two thirds of them have developed an integrated national investment strategy like the draft Agenda SK30 (Slovakia's Development Strategy until 2030) and the National Investment Plan of the Slovak Republic. However, cross-sectoral coordination for investment planning is a major challenge at sub-national level. The lack of cross-sectoral coordination is one of the six main challenges identified by EU Member State authorities, with almost 80% saying it was a major challenge [7]. Based on the analysis presented in the EC's Eighth Cohesion Report, the main changes in territorial disparities over the last decade and how policies have affected these disparities are set out [8].

Knowledge for solving problems and ideas for projects entered in the competition can also be drawn from the scientific works of the authors, whose results show that climate policy goals can be achieved not only directly but also indirectly by facilitating the implementation of other Sustainable Development Goals (SDGs), these include SDG9 (innovation and infrastructure), SDG5 (gender equality), SDG11 (sustainable cities and communities), and SDG17 (environmental taxation) [9]. Researchers Schwarz et al. [10] recommend building alliances among community, policy, businesses, and science professionals and leveraging connections among organizations, individuals, and agencies that are focused on this agenda, and in adaptive urban planning and design as in Ahern et al. [11]. The findings of scholars, as in the study of Sarwar et al., have significant practical implications for policymakers to introduce economic and non-economic reforms simultaneously to overcome environmental degradation effectively [12]. According to Zang et al., health shocks caused by air pollution are seriously affecting people's economic lives [13].

The work of Saniuk et al. provides an insight into the process of globalization and marginalization of Europe in world production, which prompted the German economy to implement the concept of Industry 4.0 called the Fourth Industrial Revolution [14]. The author Gajdzik examines the need for digitalization of processes in companies moving towards Industry 4.0 [15]. According to Štefko et al., Industry 4.0 and related automation and digitization significantly impact competition between companies. They must deal with the lack of financial resources to apply digital solutions in their businesses [16]. In relation to the Industry 5.0 concept, there is strong scientific interest. For example, the greatest value of selected scientific work of Madddikunta et al. [17] is that it discusses the perspectives of smart healthcare, cloud manufacturing, supply chain management, manufacturing, and various other applications as application development to be developed and run in Industry 5.0. Xu et al. [18] emphasize the importance and values of the transition from Industry 4.0 to Industry 5.0. The aim of another scientific study of Sindhwani at al. [19] is to analyze the factors of Industry 5.0 to achieve sustainability by integrating human values with technology. Moreover, the following work of Yin et al. [20] examines and proves the need to create digital green knowledge in the Industry 5.0 concept.

The empirical results of the studies can contribute to supporting environmental and economic policies in EU countries in achieving their sustainable development and the objectives of the European Green Agreement, as well as the sustainability of small and medium-sized enterprises [21–24]. Ferre-Comala et al. [25] represent the first step in introducing fuzzy logic into models of economic growth, respectively. In the work of Valla-Lloser et al. [26] we find data analyzed using multimethod models estimated as models of structural equations with mean and covariance structure. Vochozka et al. examine IoT-based systems of things, sustainable Industry 4.0 wireless networks, and digitized mass production in cyber-physical intelligent production [27]. As innovation enables Small and Medium-Sized Enterprises (SMEs) to be more competitive with their competitors, more innovative activities can force SMEs to overcome these challenges [28]. According to Tobisova et al. investment is a challenging and threatening indicator for businesses not only in times of depression, such as the current coronavirus pandemic, but also under normal market conditions. They present the methodology of financial risk assessment and investment development as an effective tool for corporate sustainability [29]. Optimization of financial costs to maintain the reliability of systems, assuming the estimated level of optimization of unexpected costs for the operator, is a crucial parameter [30]. Rehak et al. draw attention to the critical infrastructure system, which identifies the subsystems necessary for the functioning of the state (such as energy, transport, and emergency services). These issues are important for the resilience and health of the state and the regions [31]. In the work of Haškova et al. (2021), we find inspiring ideas for using the advantages of fuzzy logic in project evaluation, when we often encounter uncertainty in connection with randomness or ambiguity [32]. These tools have also been used innovatively in the field of safe and sustainable air transport [33] or in the expert evaluation of selected components of the smart city concept [34].

However, to date, no comprehensive approach to evaluating projects to improve the resilience and health of regions and cities based on a fuzzy set theory using hybrid methods has been implemented. In response to all these facts, it was decided to conduct a topical study to develop a complex hybrid model for evaluating projects to improve the sustainability and health of regions and cities, within the concepts of the European Green Deal and Industry 5.0. The hybrid integrated model determines the level of funding opportunities for the project, considering the target needs of investors and expert opinions on the possibility of achieving goals to improve the sustainability and health of regions and cities through the implementation of this project. The hybrid integrated model focuses on the unbiased evaluation of grant applicants and increases the security of their funding.

The comprehensive model is a complex system of functioning that considers various factors of influence, such as the importance of the project idea to improve the sustainability and health of regions and cities; risk-oriented factors of influence that potentially lead to the success of the project; factors of human influence and the team of project implementers, their experience, and knowledge in the field of sustainability and health of regions and cities. It also considers the investor's goals regarding the need and possibility of financing projects, as well as expert opinion on the possibility of achieving the goal of improving the sustainability and health of regions and cities by implementing this project with the support of investors. In addition, to adequately support the decision-making and processing of information obtained from experts, the model is based on the modern theory of intellectual analysis of knowledge, fuzzy set theory, and a systems approach.

1.2. Formal Formulation of the Evaluation Problem

Today, many innovative projects address the challenges of increasing the sustainability and health of regions and cities. The implementation of such projects allows to reduce the negative impact of human activities effectively and quickly on the environment, improve monitoring and improve the health of citizens. It is no secret that start-up (innovative) projects or grant projects provide faster and better solutions than government projects that involve complex bureaucratic actions and procedures. In addition, there are many problems in an emergency, the solution of which is important and necessary in a critically short period of time. Proof of this is the work of the municipality/region/state in the context of the COVID-19 pandemic. For example, the amount of garbage in quarantine has increased by an average of six times, as well as the big problem of disposing of personal protective equipment and others.

The resilience of regions and cities is characterized by biodiversity, versatility, multi-level networks, modularity, and adaptive design [11], as well as not only the concept of prevention and mitigation of regional and urban disasters (crisis situations) [35]. In this context, the following definitions are given for our study:

Definition 1. *Projects to increase the sustainability and health of regions and cities are projects based on innovative technologies and aimed at reducing the negative impact of human activities on the environment and/or improving the health of citizens, within the concepts of the European Green Deal and Industry 5.0. These are projects that affect sociocultural, political, economic, environmental, security and health, decision-making processes, policies, and activities aimed at improving health, lifestyle, equality, and equity of affordable health, services, and tools in regions and cities.*

Definition 2. *Sustainability of regions (cities) is the ability of regions (cities) to withstand unknown risks and recover from a disaster.*

The resilience of regions and cities is also inherently perceived in connection with public health issues. Sometimes these projects are also presented as so-called SMART Region or SMART City projects, investment project packages, etc. Objective and transparent expert evaluation of projects, especially in the specific area of strengthening the resilience and health of regions and cities within the European Green Deal and the Industry 5.0 concept, requires experience and complexity in evaluation. There is a need to finance such projects for their implementation and introduction on the market. Financing innovative projects is a risky activity. To minimize risks, it is necessary to have adequate decision support systems for evaluating the projects themselves, the teams implementing the project, and the risks. Therefore, the model is called hybrid, because, on the one hand, it uses project data from the project application, which is structured, poorly structured, or unstructured, and on the other hand combines the experience and knowledge of experts. The obtained level, which is a complex indicator, increases the degree and guarantees the security of financing of such projects.

Since the task for the solution is the area of expert evaluation, the following subjects of management are presented: Experts—persons who analyze and evaluate the project application; Investors are entities that are willing to finance evaluated projects; Project analyst is a person who adjusts the whole evaluation process, considering the needs of investors.

Let the system theoretical-multiple model problem of project evaluation to improve the sustainability and health of regions and cities, within the concepts of the European Green Deal and Industry 5.0, be presented as follows:

$$\{P, K_P, K_R, K_T, M_P, M_R, M_T, G_P, G_R, G_T, L, M_A | Y(f)\}, \quad (1)$$

where:

- $P = (p_1; p_2; \ldots; p_n)$—a set of projects submitted to some experts for funding by investors;
- K_P—information models of criteria (groups of criteria) to assess the importance of the project idea to improve the sustainability and health of regions and cities;
- K_R—information models of criteria for assessing risk-oriented factors of influence that will potentially lead to the failure of the project;
- K_T—information models of criteria (groups of criteria) for assessing human factors and the team of project implementers, their experience, and knowledge in the field of sustainability and health of regions and cities;

- M_P—fuzzy project evaluation model to improve the sustainability and health of regions and cities;
- M_R—fuzzy model for assessing the risks of project implementation to improve the sustainability and health of regions and cities;
- M_T—fuzzy model for assessing the competencies of the project implementation team;
- G_P—the goal of the importance of the region where the project will be implemented;
- G_R—the goal of acceptable risks;
- G_T—the goal of the competence of the project implementation subjects;
- L—expert opinions on the possibility of achieving the goal of improving the sustainability and health of regions and cities, by implementing this project with the support of investors and considering their goals;
- M_A—the model of aggregation of output data for deriving the level of decision-making expediency of project financing.

As a result, the output estimate is obtained $f = \mu_Y(f(\varphi_e))$ and level Y, which contains the feasibility of project financing, within the concepts of the European Green Deal and Industry 5.0, considering the goal needs of investors G and expert opinions L, thereby increasing funding projects security.

The complex hybrid model of project evaluation is shown in the form of a block diagram (Figure 1).

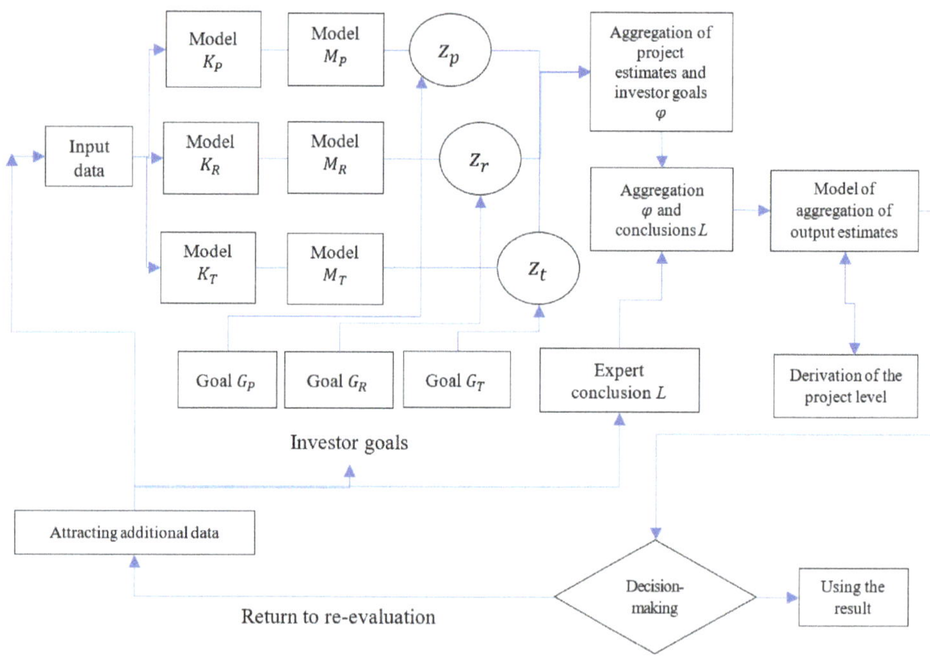

Figure 1. Block diagram of the complex hybrid model.

This study is arranged as follows: In Section 2, we describe the formal formulation of the problem, the hybrid complex model, and the information models for input processing. In Section 3, we will outline a simulation experiment, perform verification, and test the developed model on the example of five project evaluation. In Section 4, we discuss the results of the study and the advantages and disadvantages of the developed hybrid model. In Section 5, we conclude and present the main results that have been achieved for the first time. Ideas for future work and improvements are presented in conclusions of paper, namely the development of information technology and its support in the form of software for project evaluation with the specific focus.

2. Materials and Methods

The stages of designing a complex hybrid model will be presented in terms of the fuzzy mathematical models for obtaining project estimates for different information models, and the model of aggregation of initial estimates to determine the level of project funding.

M_P—fuzzy project evaluation model to increase the sustainability and health of regions and cities.

This model is based on the opinions of experts in a range of values of project quality for certain indicators. At the first stage of X evaluation projects, the expert analyzes the project application based on his own experience and expresses his views according to K_P—information model of criteria (groups of criteria) to assess the importance of the project idea to improve the sustainability and health of regions and cities. Information indicators $K_P = (K_{11}, K_{12}, \ldots, K_{ij}, \ldots, K_{ck_c})$ are divided into several groups $C = (C_1, C_2, \ldots, C_c)$. Without reducing the generality and visual presentation of the material, we will consider one project for this model. The calculations are similar for any number of projects.

In practice, experts most often express their opinions not in clear discrete values, but in intervals, for example: "project evaluation according to a certain criterion should be close to a certain number", or "project evaluation according to a certain criterion is likely, to be within certain limits", etc. Therefore, it is advisable to estimate x for each criterion in some range of numbers $x \in [a_0; b_0]$. The value of the interval is set by the project analyst of the organization that evaluates projects.

For the study, 7 experts with more than 15 years of experience in project management were invited to express their opinion on some criterion K_c according to one of the fuzzy statements $RL = \{A; B; C; D\}$, where: A = {project evaluation according to a certain criterion is in the range from a_1 to b_1}; B = {project evaluation according to a certain criterion is close to the number b_1}; C = {project evaluation according to a certain criterion is not greater than the number b_1}; D = {project evaluation according to a certain criterion is not less than the number b_1}. Set fuzzy statements are open. If necessary, the project analyst can supplement or change it.

Next, all fuzzy statements will be described using the model of presentation of fuzzy knowledge [36], using the functions of belonging criteria.

Fuzzy statement A = {project evaluation according to a certain criterion is in the range from a_1 to b_1} consider it as a fuzzy set and describe it using the trapezoidal membership function:

$$\mu_A(x) = \begin{cases} 0, & x \le a_0; \\ \frac{x-a_0}{a_1-a_0}, & a_0 \le x < a_1; \\ 1, & a_1 \le x < b_1; \\ \frac{b_0-x}{b_0-b_1}, & b_1 \le x < b_0; \\ 0, & x \ge b_0. \end{cases} \quad (2)$$

Statement B = {project evaluation according to a certain criterion is close to the number b_1}, correctly describe using the triangular membership function:

$$\mu_B(x) = \begin{cases} 0, & x \le a_0; \\ \frac{x-a_0}{b_1-a_0}, & a_0 < x \le b_1; \\ \frac{b_0-x}{b_0-b_1}, & b_1 < x < b_0; \\ 0, & x \ge b_0. \end{cases} \quad (3)$$

Next, consider the statement C = {project evaluation according to a certain criterion is not greater than the number b_1}, which is characterized in fuzzy sets by the Z-shaped type of membership function. Here we offer a Z-line:

$$\mu_C(x) = \begin{cases} 1, & 0 < x \le b_1; \\ \frac{b_0 - x}{b_0 - b_1}, & b_1 < x \le b_0; \\ 0, & x > b_0. \end{cases} \quad (4)$$

Statement D = {project evaluation according to a certain criterion is not less than the number b_1} represents an uncertainty of type S-like membership function, we propose an S-linear function:

$$\mu_D(x) = \begin{cases} 0, & x \le a_0; \\ \frac{x - a_0}{b_1 - a_0}, & a_0 < x \le b_1; \\ 1, & x > b_1. \end{cases} \quad (5)$$

Thus, the statements of experts on project indicators will not be discrete values, but intervals of values, according to the chosen statement RL = {A; B; C; D}.

At the next stage, we will pass from intervals of indistinct estimations of the project according to criteria of one group, to one-point estimation within group $C = (C_1, C_2, \ldots, C_c)$.

To do this, let the design analyst set the weights for each evaluation criterion w_{ij}, $i = \overline{1,c}; j = \overline{1,k_c}$, for example, from the interval $[1;10]$. If there is no need to set weights, then we can take them as equally important. For further calculations, we perform their rationing within the relevant group:

$$\alpha_{ij} = \frac{w_{ij}}{\sum_{j=1}^{k_c} w_{ij}}, \ i = \overline{1,c}; \ \alpha_{ij} \in [0;1], \quad (6)$$

where the condition is met $\sum_{j=1}^{k_c} \alpha_{ij} = 1$.

To fuzzification the data, we will find a weighted sum to determine the aggregate expert opinion within some group of criteria $C = (C_1, C_2, \ldots, C_c)$:

$$\overline{\varepsilon_i}(x) = \sum_{j=1}^{k_c} \mu_{RL\ ij}(x) \cdot \alpha_{ij}, \ i = \overline{1,c}. \quad (7)$$

Thus, they were obtained for each group $C_1, C_2, \ldots, C_c$ criteria a continuous set of values $\overline{\varepsilon_1}(x), \ \overline{\varepsilon_2}(x), \ldots, \overline{\varepsilon_c}(x); \ \overline{\varepsilon}(x) \in [0;1]$ on the interval of evaluation points $x \in [a_0; b_0]$. For the aggregate assessment of the expert opinion $x_i \in [a_0; b_0]$ of the corresponding group of criteria $i = \overline{1,c}$, the maximum value of the membership function of the weighted sum has been collected $\max_x \overline{\varepsilon_i}(x)$. Thus, we obtain an aggregated conclusion of the expert's opinions on the criteria for each group $(x_1, x_2, \ldots, x_c) \in [a_0; b_0]$. That is, for a group of criteria that have a common meaning, from the expert opinion, expressed in the range of values, the aggregate conclusion was reached, which is a numerical value from the range $[a_0; b_0]$.

In the third stage, the aggregated conclusions of the experts on the groups of criteria will be combined into a general assessment, which will represent the normalized value of the level of the project idea to improve the sustainability and health of regions and cities. To do this, let the project analyst set the weights for each group of criteria $C = (C_1, C_2, \ldots, C_c)$, w_i, $i = \overline{1,c}$, for example, from the interval $[1;10]$. If there is no need to set weights for groups of criteria, then we can take them as equally important. For further calculations we carry out their rationing:

$$\alpha_i = \frac{w_i}{\sum_{i=1}^{c} w_i}, \ i = \overline{1,c}; \alpha_i \in [0;1]. \quad (8)$$

For data defuzzification, we construct an aggregate estimate using the convolution model. For example, take a weighted average convolution:

$$m_p = \frac{1}{b_0} \sum_{i=1}^{c} x_i \cdot \alpha_i. \tag{9}$$

The obtained estimate $m_p \in [0;1]$ characterizes the importance of the level of the project idea to improve the sustainability and health of regions and cities. The higher the score, the better the project application and good opportunities for its implementation.

Estimates of other projects from the set are calculated similarly $P = (p_1; p_2; \ldots; p_n)$.

Thus, from the linguistically vague conclusions of the expert to the input descriptive (textual) data obtained from the project application to the quantitative assessment was transferred. Adequate use of the apparatus of fuzzy sets increases the degree of validity of future decisions.

M_R—fuzzy model for assessing the risks of project implementation to improve the sustainability and health of regions and cities.

The authors have already developed several fuzzy project risk assessment models for both investment and innovation projects, but they have not been verified for the evaluation of sustainability and health projects in regions and cities.

Let the set of projects $P = (p_1; p_2; \ldots; p_n)$, be submitted to some experts for funding by their investors. Projects will be evaluated according to the proposed information model of criteria for assessing risk-oriented factors influencing K_R, according to the criteria $\widetilde{K_R} = (K_{R1}, K_{R2}, \ldots, K_{Rk_R})$.

Each risk-oriented impact factor (risk criterion) will be assessed in a hybrid way, namely:

- Conclusions on the level of probability of occurrence of the risk situation described by the relevant criterion $\widetilde{K_R}$. We propose to unify such conclusions with the help of one of the terms of the following term set: T = {t_1(low level of risk); t_2(below average level of risk); t_3(average level of risk); t_4(above average level of risk); t_5(high level of risk)};
- Number confidence Δ of the expert's reasoning from the interval [0; 1], for each conclusion according to the corresponding criterion $\widetilde{K_R}$. Assuming the following content: 0—minimum confidence in their conclusions, and 1, respectively—maximum.

We present a fuzzy model for assessing the risks of project implementation in the form of an operator:

$$\epsilon(t;\Delta) \to m_r, \tag{10}$$

where ϵ—the operator that corresponds to the initial normalized value of the risks of the project m_r, with input variables $t;\Delta$.

Here are the stages to obtain the initial estimate m_r for some project p. In the case of multiple projects, the evaluation procedure will be repeated for all projects.

At the first stage we will carry out fuzzification of input hybrid data.

Let the term set of linguistic variables T be represented on some numerical interval, for delimitation of terms $[a_1; a_6]$, where $t_1 \in [1;20]$, $T_1 \in [a_1; a_2]$, $t_2 \in (20;40]$, $T_2 \in [a_2; a_3]$, $T_3 \in [a_3; a_4]$, $T_3 \in [a_3; a_4]$. The presented numerical interval is argued by the fact that the indicators characterize the level of probability of a risk event. Then it is natural to consider this level of risk as a percentage. If necessary, the interval partition values can be adjusted and changed by the project analyst.

To fuzzification the input hybrid data $(t_u; \Delta_u)$, $u = \overline{1, k_R}$ use the model of presentation of fuzzy knowledge in multidimensional space [4]. We use the cone-like membership function of belonging of two variables to combine conclusions on the level of probability of occurrence of a risk situation and the number confidence of the expert's opinions on providing his opinion:

$$\mu(K_{Ru}) = \begin{cases} 1 - \varepsilon_u, \; if \; \varepsilon_u < 1, \\ 0, \quad \varepsilon_u \geq 1. \end{cases}$$

$$O_u = \begin{cases} 100 - 20 \cdot \Delta_u, & \textit{if the conclusion } t_1; \\ 100 - 40 \cdot \Delta_u, & \textit{if the conclusion } t_2; \\ 100 - 60 \cdot \Delta_u, & \textit{if the conclusion } t_3; \\ 100 - 80 \cdot \Delta_u, & \textit{if the conclusion } t_4. \\ 100 - 100 \cdot \Delta_u, & \textit{if the conclusion } t_5. \end{cases} O_i = \begin{cases} a_2 \cdot q_i, & \text{if} \quad t_i \in T_1; \\ a_3 \cdot q_i, & \text{if} \quad t_i \in T_2; \\ a_4 \cdot q_i, & \text{if} \quad t_i \in T_3; \\ a_5 \cdot q_i, & \text{if} \quad t_i \in T_4; \\ a_6 \cdot q_i, & \text{if} \quad t_i \in T_5. \end{cases} \quad (11)$$

$$\varepsilon_u = \sqrt{\frac{(O_u - 100)^2}{100^2} + (\Delta_u - 1)^2}$$

O_u, Δ_u—the value of the u-th criterion $u = \overline{1, k_R}$.

The content of the membership function $\mu(K_{Ru})$ shows the level of the criterion, is the greater the value of $\mu(K_{Ru})$ the higher the level.

Without reducing the generality, the project analyst can also use other known methods to aggregate qualitative data. Presentation of input data in the form of linguistic assessment and the certainty of its assignment allows you to better reveal the views of experts.

In the second stage, the project analyst introduces weighting factors for each risk-oriented factor of influence (criterion) on the project implementation.

Denote the weights v_u, $u = \overline{1, k_R}$, from some interval [1; 10]. Otherwise, risk criteria may be equally important. Because it works in the space of assessments [0; 1], then, similarly, you need to normalize the weights:

$$\overline{v_u} = \frac{v_u}{\sum_{u=1}^{k_R} v_u}, u = \overline{1, k_R}. \quad (12)$$

In the third stage, we derive an aggregate risk assessment. To do this, build a membership function, as one of the proposed convolutions, depending on the wishes of the project analyst. Without reducing the generality, for example, take the middle convolution:

$$m_r = \sum_{u=1}^{k_R} \overline{v_u} \cdot \mu(K_{Ru}). \quad (13)$$

The obtained value has the following meaning: the larger the aggregate estimate $m_r \in [0; 1]$, the lower the risks of the project.

Thus, from the conclusions on the level of probability of the risk situation and the number of confidences of the expert's opinions on this issue, a quantitative assessment has been made, which increases the degree of validity of future decisions. Estimates of other projects from the set are calculated similarly $P = (p_1; p_2; \ldots; p_n)$.

The advantages of the model are argued by the fact that based on input; hybrid data reveals the vagueness of input estimates. Improves the efficiency of obtaining input assessments using the experience, knowledge, and expertise of experts. The model can derive a quantitative normalized output value of the risks of the project, which increases the degree of validity of further management decisions.

M_T—fuzzy model for assessing the competencies of the project implementation team.

Here it is proposed to use one of the models already developed by the authors, which at the output we obtain the normalized value $m_t \in [0; 1]$, o separately for the set of projects P, namely: Information model of evaluation and output rating of start-up projects development teams; Model of evaluation and selection of the expert group members; Model of evaluation and selection of expert group members for Smart Cities, Green Transportation and Mobility: from safe times to pandemic times [34].

Thus, normalized estimates of projects were obtained $m_p(x_e)$, $m_r(x_e)$, $m_t(x_e)$, $e = \overline{1, n}$, according to the proposed fuzzy evaluation models M_P, M_R, M_T.

The peculiarity of the complex hybrid model is that the investor has some goals in terms of the need and ability to finance projects to improve the sustainability and health of regions and cities. Such goals are correlated according to the models M_P, M_R, M_T. This is because in the future we will look for the closest distance between the estimates of models and objectives. Therefore, they must have the same meaning. Based on the experience of the authors in the subject area, the following goals are proposed:

G_P—the goal of the importance of the region where the project will be implemented.

Here we propose to use the categorization of regions, according to the Ministry of Transport and Construction of the Slovak Republic, as follows:

- Category 1—regions of international importance;
- Category 2—regions of national importance (national);
- Category 3—regions of supraregional importance;
- Category 4—regions of predominant importance at the regional level.

Without reducing the generality, the categories of project regions analysts can easily change according to needs and conditions.

G_R—the goal of acceptable risks is the level of risk that an investor can afford by investing in a project to increase the sustainability and health of regions and cities.

G_T—the goal of the competence of the project implementation subjects.

Since the problem of evaluating alternative projects consists of three goals, then the vectors $m_p(p) = \{m_p(p_1), m_p(p_2), \ldots, m_p(p_n)\}$, $m_r(p) = \{m_r(p_1), m_r(p_2), \ldots, m_r(p)\}$ and $m_t(p) = \{m_t(p_1), m_t(p_2), \ldots, m_t(p_n)\}$, we project on the three-dimensional coordinate system x, y, z respectively. For each project we get the coordinates of the goals G_P, G_R, G_T, which we present in the form: $(m_p(p_1), m_r(p_1), m_t(p_1)), (m_p(p_2), m_r(p_2), m_t(p_2)), \ldots,$ $(m_p(p_n), m_r(p_n), m_t(p_n))$.

Furthermore, a three-dimensional vector of investor goals was considered $T^* = (A_1, A_2, A_3)$, which considers the wishes of investors regarding the importance of alternative projects according to the goals G_P, G_R, G_T. The vector of investor goals was modeled as follows [37].

Let us analyze an object with 3 inputs and one output:

$$U = (A_1, A_2, A_3), \tag{14}$$

where U—the vector of the initial estimate (u_1, u_2, u_3), and its components may have values from the interval [0; 1], and A_1, A_2, A_3 are input linguistic variables.

To evaluate the linguistic variables A_1, A_2, A_3 qualitative terms from such term sets were used:

$$A_1 = (a_{11}, a_{12}, \ldots, a_{1t}), A_2 = (a_{21}, a_{22}, \ldots, a_{2t}),\ A_3 = (a_{31}, a_{32}, \ldots, a_{3t}). \tag{15}$$

Knowledge of the vector of investors' goals $T = (t_1, t_2, t_3)$ is obtained from the base of fuzzy knowledge, consisting of systems of logical expressions—"If—Then, Else", which link the values of input variables A_1, A_2, A_3 with one of the possible values U.

$$\text{IF } A_1 = a_{1t} \text{ and } A_2 = a_{2t} \text{ and } A_3 = a_{3t} \text{ THEN } U = (u_1, u_2, u_3) \text{ ELSE} \ldots \tag{16}$$

Thus, the project analyst sets the linguistic wish of the vector of investors' goals, which is translated into the vector of the initial quantitative and normalized assessment (u_1, u_2, u_3), which is denoted accordingly $(u_1, u_2, u_3) = (t_1, t_2, t_3)$.

The vague knowledge base for project evaluation to improve the sustainability and health of regions and cities is offered as follows:

IF we have goals:

G_P—the goal of the importance of the region where the project will be implemented:
a_{11} there are 4 categories of the region then $u_1 = 0.4$;
a_{12} there are 3 categories of the region then $u_1 = 0.6$;
a_{13} there are 2 categories of the region then $u_1 = 0.8$;
a_{14} there are 1 category of the region then $u_1 = 1$.

AND G_R—the goal of acceptable risks:

a_{21} high risk then $u_2 = 0.2$;

a_{22} average risk then $u_2 = 0.4$;
a_{23} low risk then $u_2 = 0.6$;
a_{24} very low risk then $u_2 = 0.8$;
a_{25} minimal risk then $u_2 = 1$.

AND G_T—the goal of the competence of the project implementation subjects:
a_{31} not interested in competence then $u_3 = 0.2$;
a_{32} may even be low competencies then $u_3 = 0.5$;
a_{33} are interested in average competencies then $u_3 = 0.7$;
a_{34} need the best competencies then $u_3 = 1$.

THEN logical statement can be formulated as follows:

If the investor needs the importance of the region where the project will be implemented A_1, the acceptable risk A_2 and the competence of the project implementation subjects A_3 then $U = (u_1, u_2, u_3)$.

A project analyst can change quantitative levels, or rules in goals. Therefore, the knowledge base is open, and the number of goals can be increased if necessary.

For all projects we find the values $Z_e = (z_{pe}, z_{re}, z_{te}), e = \overline{1,n}$, which characterize the relative estimates of the proximity of the evaluated projects to the vector of investor goals for each goal G_P, G_R, G_T, removing the question of different rating scales [37]:

$$z_{pe} = 1 - \frac{|u_1 - m_p(p_e)|}{max\left\{u_1 - \min_e m_p(p_e);\ \max_e m_p(p_e) - u_1\right\}}, \tag{17}$$

$$z_{re} = 1 - \frac{|u_2 - m_r(p_e)|}{max\left\{u_2 - \min_e m_r(p_e);\ \max_e m_r(p_e) - u_2\right\}}, \tag{18}$$

$$z_{te} = 1 - \frac{|u_3 - m_t(p_e)|}{max\left\{u_3 - \min_e m_t(p_e);\ \max_e m_t(p_e) - u_3\right\}}. \tag{19}$$

If one project is submitted for evaluation, then the investor does not need to comment on their own goals and this stage is skipped. To find the vector of values Z_e for projects must be at least two projects.

Furthermore, to aggregate the values of Z_e, it is proposed to use modeling of uncertainties of the form "average value" in three-dimensional space, using the cone-like membership function in the estimation space [0; 1]. Moreover, the value of the center of the base of the cone will be a unit vector $(x_1^0; x_2^0; x_3^0) = (1;1;1)$, and the experimentally obtained scaling by the coordinates of the vector Z_e will be $(3;3;3)$. Then, the three-dimensional cone-like membership function will be given by the formula:

$$\varphi_e = \begin{cases} 1 - \vartheta_e, & if\ \vartheta_e < 1, \\ 0, & otherwise. \end{cases}, \quad \text{where}: \ \vartheta_e = \frac{1}{3}\cdot\sqrt{(z_{pe}-1)^2 + (z_{re}-1)^2 + (z_{te}-1)^2}, e = \overline{1,n}. \tag{20}$$

Thus, the initial estimates φ_e will be obtained from the interval [0; 1] on n projects to increase the sustainability and health of regions and cities. The vector of investors' goals provides the construction of a ranking of alternatives given by the vectors of assessments and increases the security of choosing alternatives according to the target needs. The initial assessment is based on the assessment of the importance of the project idea, potential risks of the project, the competence of development teams, and considers the goals of investors on the importance of the region where the project will be implemented, risk acceptability, competence of the project implementation subjects.

Next, let the experts evaluating the projects express their conclusions on the possibility of achieving the goal of improving the sustainability and health of regions and cities by implementing this project with the support of investors and considering their goals. For this conclusion we introduce the linguistic variable $L = \{L_1;\ L_2; \ldots ; L_5\}$, where: L_1—high possibility of project implementation taking into account the goals of investors; L_2—the possibility of project implementation taking into account the goals of investors above average; L_3—average possibility of project implementation taking into account the goals of investors; L_4—low possibility of project implementation taking into account the goals of investors; L_5—very low possibility of project implementation taking into account the goals of investors.

Next, M_A—the model of aggregation of output data is proposed for deriving the level of decision-making expediency of project financing. A graphical interpretation of the M_A model is presented in Figure 2.

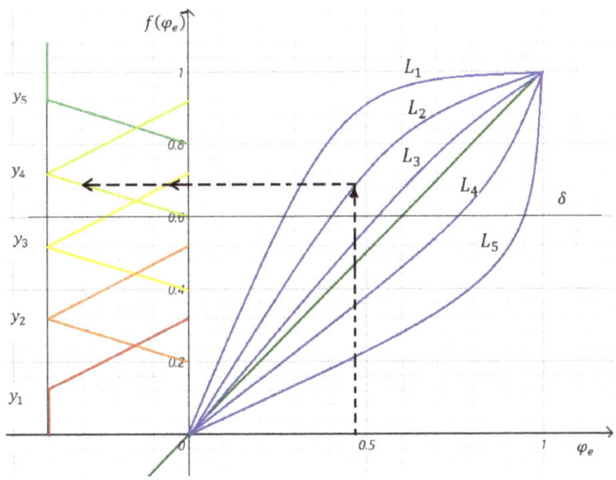

Figure 2. Graphic interpretation of the model M_A (y—levels of decision-making; L—expert opinion; φ_e—initial estimates; $f(\varphi_e)$—aggregate normalized estimate; δ—degree of decision making).

To interpret the dependence of the initial assessment φ_e and expert opinion L on the possibility of achieving the goal of improving the sustainability and health of regions and cities, by implementing this project with the support of investors, we offer the following membership function:

$$f(\varphi_e) = \begin{cases} 0, & \varphi_e < 0; \\ (\varphi_e)^k, & 0 \leq \varphi_e < 1;\ e = \overline{1,n}, \\ 1, & \varphi_e \geq 1. \end{cases} \tag{21}$$

where k is the threshold for the possibility of achieving the project goal with the support of investors' goals. The value of this threshold varies depending on the expert opinion L. This threshold can be obtained by learning from the test data of projects, having a history of projects, and investigating errors of the first and second kind. Mistakes of the first kind occur in cases where the project has good performance, receives funding, and the project does not implement. The second kind of error occurs when the project does not receive funding but implements it in another way. For example, we experimentally set: $k = \frac{2}{9}$ when we have an expert opinion L_1; $k = \frac{7}{9}$ when we have an expert opinion L_2; $k = \frac{4}{9}$—expert opinion L_3; $k = \frac{5}{9}$—expert opinion L_4; $k = \frac{3}{2}$—expert opinion L_5.

Thus, we obtained aggregated normalized estimates $f(\varphi_e)$, $e = \overline{1,n}$ from the interval [0; 1], on project evaluation models, investor goals and expert opinions that evaluate projects.

Levels Y of feasibility of project financing taking into account goals of investors and conclusions of experts, we will present as follows: y_1—very low level of feasibility of project financing; y_2—low level of feasibility of project financing; y_3—average level of feasibility of project financing; y_4—high level of feasibility of project financing; y_5—very high level of feasibility of project financing.

Levels of decision-making Y are correctly considered using triangular membership functions. This is because they will have intersections of the original values, and this will expand the ability to make decisions:

$$\mu_{y_1}(f(\varphi_e)) = \begin{cases} 1, & f(\varphi_e) \le \delta - \frac{\delta}{2}; \\ \frac{3\delta - 4 \cdot f(\varphi_e)}{\delta}, & \delta - \frac{\delta}{2} < f(\varphi_e) \le \delta - \frac{\delta}{4}. \end{cases} \quad (22)$$

$$\mu_{y_2}(f(\varphi_e)) = \begin{cases} \frac{4 \cdot f(\varphi_e) - 2\delta}{\delta}, & \delta - \frac{\delta}{2} < f(\varphi_e) \le \delta - \frac{\delta}{4}; \\ \frac{4\delta - 4 \cdot f(\varphi_e)}{\delta}, & \delta - \frac{\delta}{4} < f(\varphi_e) \le \delta. \end{cases} \quad (23)$$

$$\mu_{y_3}(f(\varphi_e)) = \begin{cases} \frac{4 \cdot f(\varphi_e) - 3\delta}{\delta}, & \delta - \frac{\delta}{4} < f(\varphi_e) \le \delta; \\ \frac{5\delta - 4 \cdot f(\varphi_e)}{\delta}, & \delta < f(\varphi_e) \le \delta + \frac{\delta}{4}. \end{cases} \quad (24)$$

$$\mu_{y_4}(f(\varphi_e)) = \begin{cases} \frac{4 \cdot f(\varphi_e) - 4\delta}{\delta}, & \delta < f(\varphi_e) \le \delta + \frac{\delta}{4}; \\ \frac{6\delta - 4 \cdot f(\varphi_e)}{\delta}, & \delta + \frac{\delta}{4} < f(\varphi_e) \le \delta + \frac{\delta}{2}. \end{cases} \quad (25)$$

$$\mu_{y_5}(f(\varphi_e)) = \begin{cases} \frac{4 \cdot f(\varphi_e) - 5\delta}{\delta}, & \delta + \frac{\delta}{4} < f(\varphi_e) \le \delta + \frac{\delta}{2}; \\ 1, & f(\varphi_e) \ge \delta + \frac{\delta}{2}. \end{cases} \quad (26)$$

Depending on the range in which the value of $f(\varphi_e)$, falls, one or another membership function μ_y is chosen with respect to the degree δ of decision-making. The degree δ belongs to the interval $[0;1]$ and is adjusted by the project analyst, and if necessary, it can be changed. This setting has the advantage that the model is easily adapted for a variety of grant projects and competitions, from student to multimillion H2020. Since the constructed membership functions (22)–(26) have intersections, for the evaluated projects p_e, $e = \overline{1,n}$ we obtain either one or two levels of decision-making Y and, accordingly, the same number of reliabilities for them.

As a result of the calculation, we obtain the linguistic significance of the level of decision-making of the feasibility of financing project Y and its assessment of reliability. That is, the reliability of the fact that the evaluation of the project belongs to one or another level. Based on the initial data, investors make decisions on the appropriateness of financing projects to improve the sustainability and health of regions and cities, considering the goals of investors G and the conclusions of experts L. If a situation arises where investors are not satisfied with any of the solutions, it is recommended to re-evaluation with additional data.

3. Results

The project evaluation criteria (proposed by experts) in the individual steps for quantitative evaluation as well as for project risk assessment must correspond to the problems to which the submitted projects are directed: the resilience and health of regions and cities within the European Green Deal and the European Industry 5.0 concept. Expert criteria will allow evaluating the content and the following benefits and impacts of the proposed projects (alone or in combination).

K_P—information models of criteria (groups of criteria) to assess the importance of the project idea to improve the sustainability and health of regions and cities.

A set of criteria is offered for assessing the importance of the project idea to improve the sustainability and health of regions, which is divided into five groups $C = (C_1, C_2, \ldots, C_5)$. The evaluation criteria in each group C are presented in the form of a question to justify the importance of the project idea, where the expert, based on the read project application, scores from the interval [1; 20] for each criterion according to the proposed fuzzy rules.

Group C_1—relevance, innovation, uniqueness of the project:

K_{11}—How does the project relate to the priorities for improving the resilience and health of the regions, namely:

- Sociocultural (activities or technologies that contribute to the preservation of cultural heritage, to the increase of citizens education in the regions or in cities, down extremism, racism and religious tolerance, support for marginalized groups, gender equality, equal treatment of men and women at work, in community and in the separation of labor, and other similar projects);
- Political (project activities to support the development of civil society and active citizen participation in public affairs, activities supporting citizen co decision in regional and urban development plans, activities supporting citizen participation in the implementation of policies at regional and local level, activities supporting and improving regional and urban management, support for the resilience of society and citizens against misinformation in the public and digital space, support for corporate social responsibility and active citizenship programs to meet the objectives of the European Green Deal and the European Industry 5.0 concept, strengthening the influence of the third sector, volunteering and cities, and other similar projects);
- Economic (project impact on job creation in the region and cities, improving the business environment and business development in regions and cities, impact on local taxes, project investments in regional and urban development—global resources, regional resources, local resources, private funding sources, development and investment projects, technologies and procedures reducing energy intensity, operation, and maintenance of buildings and infrastructure in regions and cities within the public and private sector, reducing the financial costs of regional and city administration, support for citizens' financial literacy programs, and other similar projects);
- Environmental (type, number, and extent of green technologies and applied procedures for green regions and cities, projects for the application of alternative energy sources, impact on water supply and water pollution in regions/cities on the climate, impact on soil decontamination, reduction of air pollution sources in regions and cities, projects with an impact on food safety and food self-sufficiency, projects to increase companies' awareness of their impact on the environment, projects to improve the quality of the indoor environment of public and private buildings, and other similar projects);
- Security (aspects of the project strengthening the resilience of the region and cities for security periods also in crisis situations, in preparing citizens for crisis situations, in preparing and improving the quality of human, material, and technical resources for crisis situations in regions and cities, benefits of business and non-business entities, civic associations and charities in regions and cities to prepare citizens and society for crisis situations, and other similar projects);
- Health (climate change also increases the risk of future pandemics and endangers the quality of life of citizens, therefore we evaluate the benefits and impacts of proposed projects to improve lifestyle health, equality, and equity of available health services and facilities in regions and cities, improve infrastructure of health facilities in regions and cities, or modernization projects to improve their services to citizens, non-investment projects to improve services to citizens under, and other similar projects).

K_{12}—completeness of definition, originality, and validity of the main ideas, proposals, sequence of development, which can be meaningful, original, and justified based on world experience; meaningful, original, and justified based on national experience; reasonable, but mostly consider the experience of performers; declarative, but not justified.

K_{13}—novelty of expected results, their difference from existing developments, completeness of disclosure and analysis of analogues and prototypes, namely in the application: well-defined expected results, revealed their differences from existing world analogues; novelty of results only at the national level; novelty of project results only at the local level.

K_{14}—the validity of the importance of the project for the applicant organization and partners, given the main/strategic activities. It considers the previous experience of the applicant and the partner for the project.

Group C_2—goals, objectives, short-term results of the project:

K_{21}—the application demonstrates the logical principle of the causal link between the definition of the purpose, objectives, objectives, and results of the project. In the application, all components are interdependent and subordinate; indicates how the partner is involved in the implementation of goals and objectives.

K_{22}—the results of the project achievement can be tracked within the project or immediately after its completion, the intermediate and final goals of the achievement are related to the defined objectives of the project.

K_{23}—the quality of the work plan of the project, which is identical to the application and estimate without factual differences. The work plan reflects in detail and in a strict logical sequence all the main stages of project implementation, indicates the activities of the partner organization, contains all the necessary components such as implementation stages, results, responsible persons, organizational and economic forms of stage executors.

Group C_3—is the target audience of the project:

K_{31}—target groups are clearly defined and correctly described through quantitative and qualitative indicators. Their needs have been identified in advance, or information on the existence of these needs that has been properly substantiated, possibly with reference to research. Target audiences of the project meet the goals, objectives, relevance of the project is confirmed by the needs and interests of target audiences.

K_{32}—the value of the project to the target audiences is clearly defined, it explains how the project meets the cultural needs and interests of the target audiences, identifies stakeholders, and describes how stakeholders will interact with the project or its results; the uniqueness and innovation of the project is confirmed by the needs and interests of the target audiences. It indicates how the applicant will work with stakeholders.

K_{33}—the communication plan of the project helps to draw attention to the results of the project on improving the resilience and health of regions, forming a sense of target audiences to the importance of sustainability and health, both at local and regional levels.

Group C_4—long-term project results:

K_{41}—What long-term results will be achieved through the project implementation? What will confirm the achievement of the project goal? The applicant aims to achieve the effect of long-term impact on its target audiences, environment, is the impact that can be fully realized in three to five years, this impact is adequately described through the indicators of project results.

K_{42}—the applicant provides measures for public presentation of project results in accordance with the project objectives and selected target audiences.

K_{43}—further activities are planned to prolong the long-term impact of the project: free access to project results, free access to project information.

K_{44}—the applicant organization plans to share its experience with other organizations, plans to establish partnerships with other organizations outside the project to further develop the idea.

Group C_5—quality of the project estimate:

K_{51}—the quality of cost estimates for compliance with the specified project objectives and investor requirements.

K_{52}—compliance of the budget with the stated objectives of the project. The project work plan, tasks and specific results are correlated with the estimate, as well as with the expected results.

K_{53}—cost-effectiveness is that the ratio between costs and expected results is satisfactory and rational, this one that confirms the efficient and transparent use of funds for project implementation.

K_{54}—the validity of costs is that all budget items are written in the form of formal records: price per unit, number of units, number of months, kilometers, number of participants, etc., as a result—the formation of prices for a single item of expenditure is transparent, reasonable. For example, travel expenses, attraction of material and technical base, administrative and other expenses are motivated by the goals and objectives of the project, contribute to their implementation, and do not contradict the requirements and restrictions of investors.

The above set of criteria is open, and the model does not depend on the number of groups. Investors can always add their own indicators when considering specific projects to improve the resilience and health of regions.

K_R—information models of criteria for assessing risk-oriented factors of influence that will potentially lead to the failure of the project.

The issue of assessing risk-oriented factors influencing project implementation is very complex. Depending on the project, the region, and the stages of project implementation, different risk indicators need to be adjusted. There are many classification approaches to risk assessment for both classic and innovative and start-up projects. Here are some criteria by which the expert can assess the risks that may arise in the implementation of projects to improve the sustainability and health of regions and cities:

K_{R1}—risks of insufficient consideration of environmental factors of the project, prospects for its completion and development; K_{R2}—risks of insufficient consideration of factors of behavior of competitors;

K_{R3}—risks of unforeseen expenses and reduced income;

K_{R4}—risks of project failure due to unforeseen budget changes and changes in funding levels;

K_{R5}—risks associated with innovations declared in the project implementation plans to increase the sustainability and health of regions and cities;

K_{R6}—risks are related to insufficient awareness of staffing with the scope of the project;

K_{R7}—environmental risks associated with not achieving the goals within the Green Deal concept;

K_{R8}—marketing risks at different stages of project implementation;

K_{R9}—marketing risks at the stage of presentation of results (sales of work results) of the project;

K_{R10}—risks of similar competitive projects in the region of project implementation;

K_{R11}—risks associated with securing property rights to innovations, patents.

The above set of criteria is completely open and inexhaustible. For example, if a thematic project selection competition is held, then project analysts must adapt this set of criteria to the theme of this competition.

According to K_T—information models of criteria (groups of criteria) for assessing human factors and the team of project implementers, their experience, and knowledge in the field of sustainability and health of regions and cities, we propose to use information models already developed by the authors. For example, if the project is submitted by a team of developers, then you can use the information model of evaluation and rating of the team of developers of start-up projects [38]. If the project is represented by an organization, then one of the approaches can be used [37].

The result of the study, the algorithm of the model, was tested on the example of the evaluation of five submitted projects $P = (p_1; p_2; \ldots; p_5)$ to improve the sustainability and health of regions and cities, which will be implemented by the Regional Development Agency of the Transcarpathian Region (Ukraine). For the creation of the model algorithm, the knowledge and good practice of the authors were used as experts and evaluators of the 896 projects from the stock of projects of the Partnership Council of the Trnava self-governing region in Slovakia, submitted under the plan of economic development and social development for implementation and financing in 2021–2027.

The calculations will be performed based on the developed complex hybrid model of project evaluation to improve the sustainability and health of regions and cities. To do this, we will evaluate separately on fuzzy models M_P, M_R, M_T, and M_A—the model of aggregation of output data for deriving the level of decision-making expediency of project financing. The evaluation was conducted by the authors of the article, who are experts in various commissions and competitions for the evaluation of grants, scientific, technical, and start-up projects.

For example, consider in more detail the evaluation of the project p_1, which is a sociocultural project that was successfully implemented in 2021 in Ukraine—"Showcase of Zakarpattia" [39], on models M_P and M_R.

M_P—fuzzy project evaluation model to improve the sustainability and health of regions and cities.

At the first stage of the project p_1 we get input data for each evaluation criterion according to K_P—information models of criteria (groups of criteria) to assess the importance of the project idea to improve the sustainability and health of regions and cities. Suppose that the expert sets his statements on some interval of numbers $x \in [1; 20]$ using one of the fuzzy statements $RL = \{A; B; C; D\}$. For each criterion and group of criteria, the project analyst determined the weights. Input data and weights are given in Table 1.

Table 1. Input data on expert evaluation according to K_P.

Group Criteria	Name Criteria	Fuzzy Statements	Evaluation Limits x	Weight Groups	Weight Criteria
C_1	K_{11}	A	from 17 to 19	10	10
	K_{12}	C	not more than 15		9
	K_{13}	D	not less than 13		9
	K_{14}	B	close to 18		7
C_2	K_{21}	A	from 18 to 19	8	7
	K_{22}	A	from 10 to 19		8
	K_{23}	B	close to 13		8
C_3	K_{31}	D	not less than 18	9	9
	K_{32}	C	not more than 16		8
	K_{33}	A	from 13 to 19		6
C_4	K_{41}	A	from 10 to 13	10	9
	K_{42}	D	not less than 18		7
	K_{43}	B	close to 15		8
	K_{44}	C	not more than 17		8
C_5	K_{51}	A	from 12 to 14	9	10
	K_{52}	C	not more than 15		9
	K_{53}	D	not less than 15		8
	K_{54}	A	from 15 to 20		9

At the next stage, we will move from the intervals of fuzzy project evaluations according to the criteria of one group, to one-point evaluation within the group. To do this, first, based on the input data, using the membership functions of criteria (2)–(5) we construct graphs of expert opinions. Next, the weights were divided within the corresponding group, according to Formula (6). The result is presented in the form of a vector: α_1= (0.28; 0.26; 0.26; 0.2), α_2= (0.35; 0.35; 0.3), α_3= (0.39; 0.35; 0.26), α_4= (0.28; 0.22; 0.25; 0.25), α_5= (0.28; 0.25; 0.22; 0.25). To fuzzification the data, we find the weighted sum by Formula (7). The results of the calculation, separately for the groups of criteria, will be illustrated on the graphs of functions that are built using our designed software (Figure 3).

For the aggregate assessment of the expert opinion $x_i \in [1; 20]$ of the corresponding group of criteria i, we take the maximum value of the membership function of the weighted sum: $\max_x \overline{\varepsilon_1}(x) = 0.93$ then $x_1 = 15$; $\max_x \overline{\varepsilon_2}(x) = 0.91$ then $x_2 = 13$; $\max_x \overline{\varepsilon_3}(x) = 0.95$ then $x_3 = 16$; $\max_x \overline{\varepsilon_4}(x) = 0.9$ then $x_4 = 13$; $\max_x \overline{\varepsilon_5}(x) = 0.97$ then $x_5 = 14$.

Thus, an aggregate conclusion of the expert's opinions on the criteria for each group was obtained.

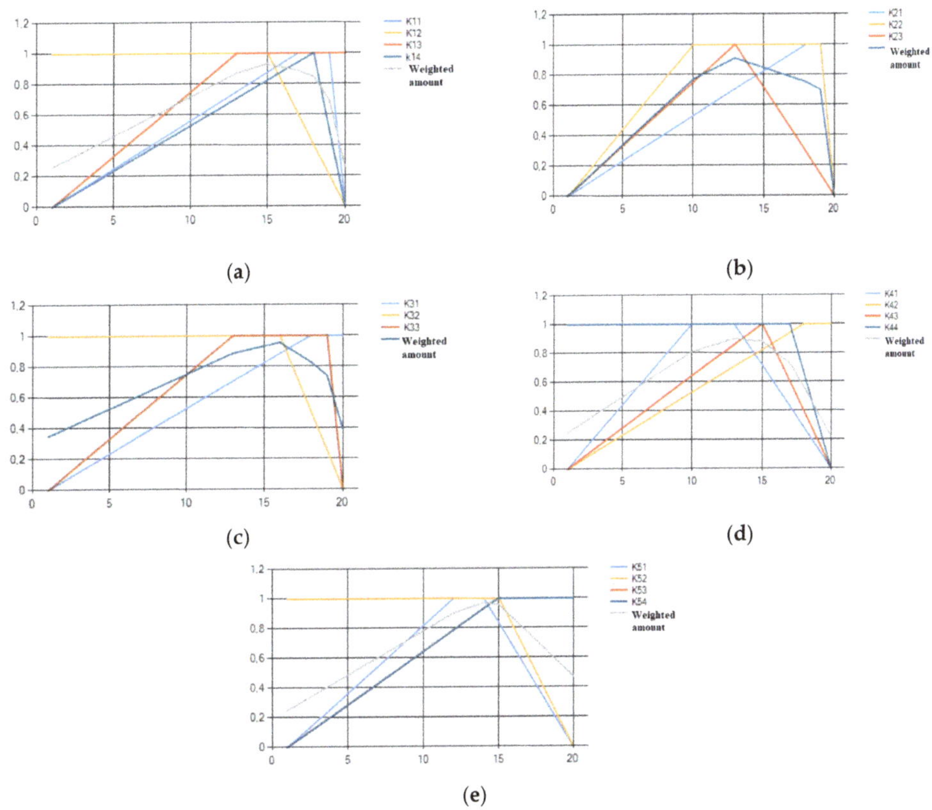

Figure 3. The result of the calculation of the project p_1 according to the model M_P: (**a**) the weighted amount for a group of criteria C_1; (**b**) the weighted amount for a group of criteria C_2; (**c**) the weighted amount for a group of criteria C_3; (**d**) the weighted amount for a group of criteria C_4; (**e**) the weighted amount for a group of criteria C_5.

In the third stage, the aggregated conclusions of the experts on the groups of criteria will be combined into a general assessment. To do this, calculate the normalized weights for each group of criteria, according to the Formula (8): $\alpha_1 = 0.22$; $\alpha_2 = 0.16$; $\alpha_3 = 0.2$; $\alpha_4 = 0.22$; $\alpha_5 = 0.2$. For defuzzification data, we construct an aggregate estimate using a weighted average convolution according to the Formula (9): $m_p = \frac{1}{20}(15{\cdot}0.22 + 13{\cdot}0.16 + 16{\cdot}0.2 + 13{\cdot}0.22 + 14{\cdot}0.2) = 0.71$.

M_R—fuzzy model for assessing the risks of project implementation to improve the sustainability and health of regions and cities.

At the first stage of the project p_1 we receive input from the expert on each evaluation criterion, according to the proposed K_R—information models of criteria for assessing risk-oriented factors of influence that will potentially lead to the failure of the project. Input data and weights according to the criteria determined by the project analyst are given in Table 2.

Table 2. Input data on expert evaluation according to K_R.

Name Criteria	Conclusions Experts	Confidence of the Expert's Reasoning	Weight Criteria
K_{R1}	t_1	0.8	10
K_{R2}	t_2	0.9	9
K_{R3}	t_1	0.7	9
K_{R4}	t_1	0.9	7
K_{R5}	t_3	0.7	10
K_{R6}	t_3	0.7	9
K_{R7}	t_1	0.8	10
K_{R8}	t_3	0.9	9
K_{R9}	t_2	0.9	8
K_{R10}	t_2	0.8	8
K_{R11}	t_1	0.8	9

In the first stage, we will carry out fuzzification of input hybrid data. To do this, the values of O_u, ε_u and $\mu(x_u)$ were calculated by the Formula (11). In the second stage, we calculate the normalized weights by Formula (12). The results of the calculation of the first and second stages are shown in Table 3.

Table 3. Calculation results for the model M_R.

Name Criteria	Value O_u	Value ε_u	Membership Function $\mu(K_{Ru})$	Normalized Weight Criteria $\overline{v_u}$
K_{R1}	84	0.256	0.744	0.102
K_{R2}	64	0.374	0.626	0.092
K_{R3}	86	0.331	0.669	0.092
K_{R4}	82	0.206	0.794	0.071
K_{R5}	58	0.516	0.484	0.102
K_{R6}	58	0.516	0.484	0.092
K_{R7}	84	0.256	0.744	0.102
K_{R8}	46	0.549	0.451	0.092
K_{R9}	64	0.374	0.626	0.082
K_{R10}	68	0.377	0.623	0.082
K_{R11}	84	0.256	0.744	0.092

In the third stage, we derive an aggregate risk assessment according to the Formula (13): $m_r = 0.63$.

M_T—fuzzy model for assessing the competencies of the project implementation team.

The team of project implementers p_1, their experience and knowledge in the field of sustainability and health of regions and cities are proposed to evaluate according to the Information model of evaluation and output rating of start-up projects development teams where all data on the calculation procedure are given in [37]. After the expert evaluation, we received that the teams implementing the p_1 project received the following number of points: $m_t = 0.74$.

Thus, normalized estimates of the project x_1 according to fuzzy estimation models were obtained $m_p(p_1) = 0.71,\ m_r(p_1) = 0.63,\ m_t(p_1) = 0.74$.

Similarly, the other projects are calculated, for which we obtain the following estimates: $m_p(p_2) = 0.62,\ m_r(p_2) = 0.87,\ m_t(p_2) = 0.42;\ m_p(p_3) = 0.77,\ m_r(p_3) = 0.82,$ $m_t(p_3) = 0.52; m_p(p_4) = 0.51, m_r(p_4) = 0.58, m_t(p_4) = 0.74; m_p(p_5) = 0.81, m_r(p_5) = 0.56,$ $m_t(p_5) = 0.36$.

Let the investor have his own goals regarding the need and possibility of financing projects to improve the sustainability and health of regions and cities.

If the investor needs the importance of the region where the project will be implemented $A_1 = \{2 \text{ category of the region}\}$, the acceptable risk $A_2 = \{\text{low risk}\}$ and the competence of the project implementation subjects $A_3 = \{\text{interested in average competencies}\}$ then $U = (0.8,\ 0.6,\ 0.7)$.

Next, for all projects the values of $Z_e = (z_{pe}, z_{re}, z_{te}),\ e = \overline{1,5}$ were found, which characterize the relative estimates of the proximity of the evaluated projects to the vector of investors' goals, for (17)–(19). For example, for a project p_1: $z_{p1} = 1 - \frac{|0.8-0.71|}{max\{0.8-0.51;0.81-0.8\}} = 0.69$, $z_{r1} = 1 - \frac{|0.6-0.63|}{max\{0.6-0.56;0.87-0.6\}} = 0.889$, $z_{t1} = 1 - \frac{|0.7-0.74|}{max\{0.7-0.36;0.74-0.7\}} = 0.882$.

Next, to aggregate the values of Z_e we use the three-dimensional cone-like membership function by the Formula (20).

After that, the experts evaluating the projects express their conclusions on the possibility of achieving the goal of improving the sustainability and health of regions and cities, by implementing this project with the support of investors and considering their goals.

Next, the dependencies of the initial assessment φ_e and of the expert opinion L on the possibility of achieving the goal of improving the sustainability and health of regions and cities, by implementing this project with the support of investor goals according to the Formula (21) were interpreted.

All the results of calculations and conclusions of experts L are presented in Table 4.

Table 4. Calculation results and expert opinions L.

	p_1	p_2	p_3	p_4	p_5
Evaluation z_p relative to the goal G_P	0.690	0.379	0.897	0	0.966
Evaluation z_r relative to the goal G_R	0.889	0	0.185	0.926	0.852
Evaluation z_t relative to the goal G_T	0.882	0.176	0.471	0.882	0
Output estimates φ_e	0.883	0.521	0.674	0.663	0.663
Expert opinions L	L_1	L_4	L_4	L_1	L_4
Aggregate normalized estimates $f(\varphi_e)$	0.969	0.443	0.611	0.903	0.598

Thus, aggregate normalized estimates $f(\varphi_e),\ e = \overline{1,5}$. for project evaluation models, investor goals, and expert opinions evaluating projects were obtained.

Next, consider M_A—the model of aggregation of output data for deriving the level of decision-making expediency of project financing. To obtain the output estimate $f = \mu_Y(f(\varphi_e))$ and the decision−making level Y, which contains the content of the feasibility of project financing, considering the goals of investors G and the conclusions of experts L, we use triangular membership functions (22)–(26). Let the project analyst determine the degree $\delta = 0.6$, then we get the following levels for the five evaluated projects:

- p_1: decision-making level y_5 with output estimate $\mu_{y_5}(0.969) = 1$;
- p_2: decision-making level y_1 with output estimate $\mu_{y_1}(0.443) = 0.05$ or decision-making level y_2 with output estimate $\mu_{y_2}(0.443) = 0.95$;
- p_3: decision-making level y_3 with output estimate $\mu_{y_3}(0.611) = 0.93$ or decision-making level y_4 with output estimate $\mu_{y_4}(0.611) = 0.07$;
- p_4: decision-making level y_5 with output estimate $\mu_{y_5}(0.903) = 1$;
- p_5: decision-making level y_2 with output estimate $\mu_{y_2}(0.598) = 0.01$ or decision-making level y_3 with output estimate $\mu_{y_3}(0.598) = 0.99$.

Based on the output data, investors decide on the feasibility of financing projects to improve the sustainability and health of regions and cities, within the concepts of the European Green Deal and Industry 5.0, considering the goals of investors G and expert opinions L.

As shown, two projects p_1 and p_4 received y_5—a very high level of feasibility of financing the project with a reliability of 1. Project p_1 has already been successfully funded and implemented, in line with the objectives of the European Green Deal. The knowledge gained because of the p_1 project became a model of succession and was also the basis for the presentation of subsequent innovative projects for other regions.

4. Discussion

The paper presents a comprehensive hybrid model for evaluating projects to improve the sustainability and health of regions and cities, within the concepts of the European Green Deal and Industry 5.0. To this end, the following have been developed: information models of input data for the evaluation of projects to improve the sustainability and health of regions and cities; fuzzy project evaluation model; fuzzy model for assessing the risks of project implementation; model of aggregation of output data for deriving the level of decision-making expediency of project financing.

The complex hybrid model can adequately determine the level of feasibility of project financing, considering the goals of investors and expert opinions on the possibility of achieving goals to improve the sustainability and health of regions and cities through the project. The study is based on the apparatus of fuzzy sets based on estimation intervals, showing the corridor of values of forecast parameters. This allows for increasing the degree of validity of decisions, as it considers all possible development scenarios, depicting a continuous spectrum. For the processing of expert information and fuzzy input data, intelligent analysis of knowledge is also used based on the membership functions to the evaluation criteria, one, and many variables, considering any type of input data. Intellectual analysis of knowledge allows revealing the subjectivity of experts and to obtain a quantitative assessment of an informal applied problem. The models developed in the work reveal the vagueness of the incoming expert opinions and increase the degree of validity of further decisions by investors on the choice of project for its financing. The value of the model is that it allows obtaining a comprehensive quantitative assessment of the project based on descriptive input (text) data obtained from the project application. For the expert, the evaluation procedure remains classic and well-known, he examines the project application, then on several issues expresses his views on the importance of the idea and quality of the project. After that, the data are processed by appropriate fuzzy and hybrid models, revealing the subjectivity of experts, and adjusting the parameters of the models and the target needs of investors to prevent the subjective influence of participants in the evaluation process on the result. At the end of the model, is the output quantitative assessment and linguistic significance of the level of decision-making expediency of project financing with the assessment of reliability.

The advantages of a complex hybrid model for evaluating projects to increase the sustainability and health of regions and cities, within the concept of the European Green Deal and Industry 5.0, stem from the advantages of the developed models. The hybrid model is based on various information models of input data, adapted to evaluate projects to improve the sustainability and health of regions and cities, and fuzzy models to assess various aspects of the presented projects, from the idea, and implementation risks to the contractors. The set of criteria is open, the model does not depend on their number, and project analysts can always adapt the set of criteria to highly specialized project topics. The model considers the investor's goals regarding the need and possibility of financing projects, namely: the purpose of the importance of the region where the project will be implemented, the purpose of acceptable risks, and the purpose of competence of project participants. The developed fuzzy knowledge base for evaluating projects to improve the resilience and health of regions and cities can be easily adapted to different goals of investors. The quality of the final decision is improved by involving an expert opinion on the possibility of achieving the goal of improving the sustainability and health of regions and cities, by implementing this project with the support of investors, and by considering their goals. The hybrid model determines the level of expediency of project financing, and there is a possibility, depending on the need, to change the degree of decisions. Models reveal the vagueness of input estimates, increase the degree of validity of future decisions, and focus on the impartial evaluation of projects, which in turn increases the security of their financing.

The key result of the presented paper is a comprehensive approach to the evaluation of projects to improve the sustainability and health of regions and cities, within the European

Green Deal and Industry 5.0 concepts, for practical use by evaluation commissions and decision-makers at national and local level, or private sector levels. The final algorithm of the hybrid model and its verification of applicability for the evaluation of projects in the selected area of interest of the grant provider confirmed the validity of hypothesis H1 and also confirmed the validity of hypothesis H2. In the context of the European Green Deal goal to reduce the net greenhouse gas emissions to zero by 2050, the novelty of Simionescu et al.'s paper [16] is related to the effective proposal of measures to improve quality of governance to achieve this goal in the Central and Eastern European countries (represented by Bulgaria, Czech Republic, Estonia, Hungary, Latvia, Lithuania, Poland, Romania, Slovak Republic, and Slovenia). The resulting hybrid model is a practical tool to support the implementation of state policy in the framework of objective, the transparent and anti-corruption policy at the regional level in the expert evaluation of projects to strengthen the resilience and health of regions and cities. The study by Fidlerová et al. [22] provides evidence of the perception of the business world from six countries (Finland, Slovakia, Italy, Austria, Spain, and Turkey) of their intention to identify business opportunities through sustainable development goals in different countries and sectors through strategy and practice. The created hybrid model enables the evaluation of such a potential of the innovative ecosystem of companies in business opportunities within the framework of strengthening the resilience and health of regions and cities. Multi-criteria analysis of Chovancova et al. [24] has thrown a spotlight on the Achilles heel of the EU country's disregard which might cause serious problems in the future for ensuring universal access to modern energy services, improving energy efficiency, and increasing the share of renewable energy. The created hybrid model based on fuzzy expert evaluation of projects allows obtaining high ratings in innovative proposals for strengthening regional resilience in the field of energy security and diversity of resources and solutions, with minimal negative impacts on public health and the environment. A survey by a team of authors Maddikunta et al. [17] on supporting technologies and potential applications in Industry 5.0 provides a discussion of smart healthcare, cloud manufacturing, supply chain management and manufacturing, some supporting technologies for Industry 5.0, such as edge computing, digital twins, collaborative robots, the Internet of all things, blockchain and 6G networks and beyond. The created hybrid model based on fuzzy expert evaluation of projects allows obtaining high ratings in innovative proposals for strengthening the health of regions and cities, developing health infrastructure and improving the quality of health services provided using artificial intelligence for prevention, individual health counseling and evidence-based medicine support. In a study by Xu et al. [18] Industry 4.0 is considered to be a technology-based industry, while Industry 5.0 is a value-based industry. The coexistence of two industrial revolutions raises questions and therefore requires discussion and clarification. The resulting hybrid model is a practical tool to support decision-making processes in the expert evaluation of projects to strengthen the resilience and health of regions and cities, appreciating solutions to human and technological aspects of transfer to the Industry 5.0 concept and the potential to manage them. The study by Sindhwani et al. [19] notes that the Industry 5.0 revolution is a challenge to put the ideas of sustainability into practice, to integrate human values with technology and is considered a step forward in achieving the goals of sustainable development. This study therefore proposes a framework for analyzing the factors that enable Industry 5.0 to achieve sustainability integration of human values with technology. The study inspires the creators of the hybrid model with the main focus criteria in Industry 5.0, which support resilience and societal value creation, and a new framework that combines the four steps needed to solve any Multi-Criteria Decision-Making problem: selection, weight, ranking, and verification. The created hybrid model based on fuzzy expert evaluation of projects allows obtaining high ratings in proposals to strengthen the resilience and health of regions and cities, which is an innovative way to address the integration of human values with advanced technologies.

The disadvantages (limitations) of this model include the use of different types of membership functions, namely: for fuzzy *RL* statements, to combine conclusions about the level of probability of risk situation and the number of confidences of the expert's opinions on providing their opinion, to aggregate Z_e, o interpret the dependence estimates φ_e and expert opinion L. The choice of the type of membership functions and the use of different types of convolutions can lead to ambiguity in the results.

The rationality of the obtained assessment of the level of expediency of project financing proves the advantages of the developed model. The reliability of the obtained results is ensured by the reasonable use of the apparatus of fuzzy sets, intellectual analysis of knowledge, and systematic approach, which is also confirmed by the results of the research.

5. Conclusions

To develop a complex hybrid model for evaluating projects to strengthen the resilience and health of regions and cities, the authors used their experience with a team of researchers and members, respectively: chairman of the working groups for transport and health infrastructure within the activities and plans for economic development and social development of the selected regions. Findings from the stack of project intentions, 896 projects in the field of transport, influenced the creation of an algorithm for solving the problem. Seven invited experts with more than 15 years of experience in project management helped determine the evaluation criteria. The algorithm of the expert model was verified using five real projects. The gained experience enables the transfer of knowledge and the methodology of solving the problem has the potential for repetition by other researchers, resp. project evaluators in practice. The new contributions and new understanding in the field based on the research of the topic are as follows:

- For the first time developed information models of input data for evaluation of projects to improve the sustainability and health of regions and cities. The set of criteria is open, and the model does not depend on their number. Project analysts can always adapt many criteria to highly specialized project topics;
- The model uses an adequate apparatus of fuzzy sets and allows obtaining a quantitative assessment of the project based on input descriptive (textual) data obtained from the project application, which increases the degree of validity of future decisions;
- The model reveals the vagueness of input estimates and can derive a quantitative normalized initial value of the risks of the project, which increases the degree of validity of further management decisions;
- The model determines the level of feasibility of project financing, considering the target needs of investors and expert opinions on the possibility of achieving goals to improve the sustainability and health of regions and cities through the implementation of this project. The hybrid complex model focuses on the impartial evaluation of projects and increases the security of their financing;
- The model is easily adapted for different size grant projects and competitions;
- The results demonstrate the applied value of the methodology for assessing the level of decision-making, the feasibility of project financing in conditions of uncertainty, and the importance of making sound management decisions based on expert opinions and unclear conditions.

The created hybrid model has the potential for implementation in the following key areas. The model can be used to support the decision-making processes of evaluation commissions at the level of public administration and self-government and entities authorized to implement regional policy and local self-government with the support of specialized, targeted projects, resp. programs. Second, the model can be used in the environment of small and medium enterprises, respectively, in the non-commercial sphere. Third, the results of scientific research can also be used to educate and support young scientists and professionals with social responsibility, which is usually reflected in the creation of social responsibility of companies, institutions or public associations in an open civil society.

The following research will focus on the development of information technologies for the evaluation of projects to improve the sustainability and health of regions and cities, within the concepts of the European Green Deal and Industry 5.0. The integration of human values with advanced technologies remains a major challenge. Information technologies will be based on the created hybrid model and software for project evaluation. Information technology, the hybrid model and software will together support decision-making on the security of grant funding. The developed model and its software support will be a useful tool for project analysts in preventing inefficient project financing and supporting the European Green Deal and Industry 5.0 concepts. Addressing this issue is also of great importance for countries applying for membership of the European Union, such as Ukraine. A state devastated by the war will have to rebuild society and the economy, while transparency of processes and independent expert evaluation of projects remain a constant challenge.

Author Contributions: Conceptualization, M.K. and V.P.; methodology, M.K. and V.P.; software, V.P.; validation, M.K., B.G. and V.P.; formal analysis, M.K. and V.P.; investigation, M.K., B.G. and V.P.; resources, M.K.; data curation, V.P.; writing—original draft preparation, M.K., V.P. and B.G.; writing—review and editing, M.K., B.G. and V.P.; visualization, V.P.; supervision, M.K.; project administration, B.G.; funding acquisition, B.G. All authors have read and agreed to the published version of the manuscript.

Funding: This research was funded by the Scientific Grant Agency of the Ministry of Education, Science, Research, and Sport of the Slovak Republic and the Slovak Academy Sciences as part of the research project VEGA 1/0590/22: "Exploration of natural, social and economic potential of areas with environmental burdens in the Slovak Republic for the development of specific forms of domestic tourism and quantification of environmental risks".

Institutional Review Board Statement: Not applicable.

Informed Consent Statement: Not applicable.

Data Availability Statement: The data presented in this study are available on request from the corresponding author.

Conflicts of Interest: The authors declare no conflict of interest.

References

1. The European Regional Development Fund. Available online: https://www.europarl.europa.eu/factsheets/en/sheet/95/europsky-fond-regionalneho-rozvoja-efrr- (accessed on 1 June 2022).
2. Department of Economic and Social Affairs, United Nations. Sustainable Development Goals. Available online: https://sdgs.un.org/goals (accessed on 1 June 2022).
3. NextGenerationEU. Available online: https://europa.eu/next-generation-eu/index_en (accessed on 1 June 2022).
4. Delivering the European Green Deal. Available online: https://ec.europa.eu/info/strategy/priorities-2019-2024/european-green-deal/delivering-european-green-deal_en (accessed on 1 June 2022).
5. Industry 5.0. Available online: https://ec.europa.eu/info/research-and-innovation/research-area/industrial-research-and-innovation/industry-50_en (accessed on 1 June 2022).
6. Unified Methodological Framework for the Preparation of Integrated Territorial Strategies and Investments in the Slovak Republic in the Programming Period 2021–2027 (Jednotný Metodický Rámec pre Prípravu Integrovaných Územných Stratégií a Investícií v SR v Programovom Období 2021–2027). Available online: https://www.mirri.gov.sk (accessed on 1 June 2022).
7. Example of an Integrated Project Package (Príklad Integrovaného Projektového Balíčka). Available online: http://mastripruty.sk/wp-content/uploads/2020/09/IntegProjektBalicky.pdf (accessed on 1 June 2022).
8. Cohesion in Europe towards 2050: 8th Cohesion Report. Available online: https://ec.europa.eu/regional_policy/en/information/publications/communications/2022/cohesion-in-europe-towards-2050-8th-cohesion-report (accessed on 1 June 2022).
9. Kluza, K.; Ziolo, M.; Postula, M. Climate Policy Development and Implementation from United Nations Sustainable Development Goals Perspective. *Res. Sq.* **2022**, 1–24. [CrossRef]
10. Schwarz, K.; Wohldmann, E.L.; Chen, Y.; Pouyat, R.V.; Gonzalez, A.; Mao, S.; Day, S.D. Community Knowledge and Concerns about Urban Soil Science, Practice, and Process: Perspectives from the Healthy Soils for Healthy Communities Initiative in Los Angeles, CA, United States. *Front. Ecol. Evol.* **2022**, *9*, 781587. [CrossRef]
11. Ahern, J.; Cilliers, S.; Niemelä, J. The concept of ecosystem services in adaptive urban planning and design: A framework for supporting innovation. *Landsc. Urban Plan.* **2014**, *125*, 254–259. [CrossRef]
12. Sarwar, S.; Shahzad, U.; Chang, D.; Tang, B. Economic and non-economic sector reforms in carbon mitigation: Empirical evidence from Chinese provinces. *Struct. Change Econ. Dyn.* **2019**, *49*, 146–154. [CrossRef]

13. Zhang, Y.; Shi, T.; Wang, A.-J.; Huang, Q. Air Pollution, Health shocks and Labor Mobility. *Int. J. Environ. Res. Public Health* **2022**, *19*, 1382. [CrossRef]
14. Saniuk, S.; Saniuk, A. Challenges of Industry 4.0 for Production Enterprises Functioning within Cyber Industry Networks. *Manag. Syst. Prod. Eng.* **2018**, *26*, 212–216. [CrossRef]
15. Gajdzik, B. Key Directions in Changes from Steelworks 3.0 to Steelworks 4.0 with Analysis of Selected Technologies of Digitalizing the Steel Industry in Poland. *Manag. Syst. Prod. Eng.* **2022**, *30*, 46–53. [CrossRef]
16. Štefko, R.; Vašaničová, P.; Jenčová, S.; Pachura, A. Management and Economic Sustainability of the Slovak Industrial Companies with Medium Energy Intensity. *Energies* **2021**, *14*, 267. [CrossRef]
17. Maddikunta, P.K.R.; Pham, Q.V.; Prabadevi, B.; Deepa, N.; Dev, K.; Gadekallu, T.R.; Ruby, R.; Liyanage, M. Industry 5.0: A survey on enabling technologies and potential applications. *J. Ind. Inf. Integr.* **2022**, *26*, 100257. [CrossRef]
18. Xu, X.; Lu, Y.; Vogel-Heuser, B.; Wang, L. Industry 4.0 and Industry 5.0—Inception, conception and perception. *J. Manuf. Syst.* **2021**, *61*, 530–535. [CrossRef]
19. Sindhwani, R.; Afridi, S.; Kumar, A.; Banaitis, A.; Luthra, S.; Singh, P.L. Can industry 5.0 revolutionize the wave of resilience and social value creation? A multi-criteria framework to analyze enablers. *Technol. Soc.* **2022**, *68*, 101887. [CrossRef]
20. Yin, S.; Yu, Y. An adoption-implementation framework of digital green knowledge to improve the performance of digital green innovation practices for industry 5.0. *J. Clean. Prod.* **2022**, *363*, 132608. [CrossRef]
21. Simionescu, M.; Strielkowski, W.; Gavurova, B. Could quality of governance influence pollution? Evidence from the revised Environmental Kuznets Curve in Central and Eastern European countries. *Energy Rep.* **2022**, *8*, 809–819. [CrossRef]
22. Fidlerová, H.; Starecek, A.; Vranaková, N.; Bulut, C.; Keaney, M. Sustainable Entrepreneurship for Business Opportunity Recognition: Analysis of an Awareness Questionnaire among Organisations. *Energies* **2022**, *15*, 849. [CrossRef]
23. Virglerova, Z.; Ivanova, E.; Dvorsky, J.; Belas, J.; Krulický, T. Selected factors of internationalisation and their impact on the SME perception of the market risk. *Oeconomia Copernic.* **2021**, *12*, 1011–1032. [CrossRef]
24. Chovancová, J.; Vavrek, R. On the Road to Affordable and Clean Energy: Assessing the Progress of European Countries toward Meeting SDG 7. *Pol. J. Environ. Stud.* **2022**, *31*, 1587–1600. [CrossRef]
25. Ferrer-Comalat, J.C.; Linares-Mustarós, S.; Rigall-Torrent, R. Incorporating Fuzzy Logic in Harrod's Economic Growth Model. *Mathematics* **2021**, *9*, 2194. [CrossRef]
26. Vall-Llosera, L.; Linares-Mustarós, S.; Bikfalvi, A.; Coenders, G. A Comparative Assessment of Graphic and 0–10 Rating Scales Used to Measure Entrepreneurial Competences. *Axioms* **2020**, *9*, 21. [CrossRef]
27. Wade, K.; Vochozka, M. Artificial Intelligence Data-driven Internet of Things Systems, Sustainable Industry 4.0 Wireless Networks, and Digitized Mass Production in Cyber-Physical Smart Manufacturing. *J. Self-Gov. Manag. Econ.* **2021**, *9*, 48–60. [CrossRef]
28. Ključnikov, A.; Civelek, M.; Fialova, V.; Folvarčná, A. Organizational, local, and global innovativeness of family-owned SMEs depending on firm-individual level characteristics: Evidence from the Czech Republic. *Equilib. Q. J. Econ. Econ. Policy* **2021**, *16*, 169–184. [CrossRef]
29. Tobisova, A.; Senova, A.; Izarikova, G.; Krutakova, I. Proposal of a Methodology for Assessing Financial Risks and Investment Development for Sustainability of Enterprises in Slovakia. *Sustainability* **2022**, *14*, 5068. [CrossRef]
30. Sedláčková, A.N.; Kurdel, P.; Mrekaj, B. Synthesis criterion of ergatic base complex with focus on its reliability. In Proceedings of the 2017 IEEE 14th International Scientific Conference on Informatics, Poprad, Slovakia, 14–16 November 2017; pp. 318–321. [CrossRef]
31. Rehak, D.; Patrman, D.; Foltin, P.; Dvořák, Z.; Skrickij, V. Negative Impacts from Disruption of Road Infrastructure Element Performance on Dependent Subsystems: Methodological Framework. *Transport* **2021**, *36*, 510–524. [CrossRef]
32. Hašková, S.; Šuleř, P.; Krulický, P. Advantages of fuzzy approach compared to probabilistic approach in project evaluation. *Entrep. Sustain. Issues* **2021**, *9*, 446–456. [CrossRef]
33. Kelemen, M.; Polishchuk, V.; Gavurová, B.; Andoga, R.; Szabo, S.; Yang, W.; Christodoulakis, J.; Gera, M.; Kozuba, J.; Kal'avský, P.; et al. Educational Model for Evaluation of Airport NIS Security for Safe and Sustainable Air Transport. *Sustainability* **2020**, *12*, 6352. [CrossRef]
34. Gavurova, B.; Kelemen, M.; Polishchuk, V. Expert model of risk assessment for the selected components of smart city concept: From safe time to pandemics as COVID-19. *Socio-Econ. Plan. Sci.* **2022**, *82*, 101253. [CrossRef] [PubMed]
35. Chen, Y.; Su, X.; Zhou, Q. Study on the Spatiotemporal Evolution and Influencing Factors of Urban Resilience in the Yellow River Basin. *Int. J. Environ. Res. Public Health* **2021**, *18*, 10231. [CrossRef] [PubMed]
36. Polishchuk, V.; Kelemen, M.; Włoch, I.; Polishchuk, A.; Sharkadi, M.; Mlavets, Y. Conceptual Model of Presentation of Fuzzy Knowledge. In Proceedings of the II International Scientific Symposium "Intelligent Solutions" (IntSol-2021), X International School-Seminar "Decision Making Theory" (IntSol-2021), Kyiv-Uzhhorod, Ukraine, 28–30 September 2021; Volume 3018, pp. 1–12. Available online: https://ceur-ws.org/Vol-3018/Paper_1.pdf (accessed on 1 June 2022).
37. Polishchuk, V. Technology to Improve the Safety of Choosing Alternatives by Groups of Goals. *J. Autom. Inf. Sci.* **2019**, *51*, 66–76. [CrossRef]
38. Kelemen, M.; Polishchuk, V. Model of Evaluation and Output Rating of Start-Up Projects Development Teams. In Proceedings of the Second International Workshop on Computer Modeling and Intelligent Systems (CMIS-2019), Zaporizhzhia, Ukraine, 15–19 April 2019. Available online: http://ceur-ws.org/Vol-2353/paper54.pdf (accessed on 1 June 2022).
39. Showcase of Zakarpattia. Available online: https://www.vitrina-zakarpattya.com.ua/en/home/ (accessed on 6 June 2022).

International Journal of
Environmental Research and Public Health

MDPI

Article

A Conceptual Framework for Blockchain Enhanced Information Modeling for Healing and Therapeutic Design

Zhen Liu [1], Zulan Yang [1,*], Mingjie Liang [1,*], Yi Liu [2], Mohamed Osmani [3] and Peter Demian [3]

[1] School of Design, South China University of Technology, Guangzhou 510006, China; liuzjames@scut.edu.cn
[2] School of Innovation, Guangzhou Academy of Fine Arts, No. 257 Changgang Road, Guangzhou 510261, China; liuyi@gzarts.edu.cn
[3] School of Architecture, Building and Civil Engineering, Loughborough University, Loughborough LE11 3TU, UK; m.osmani@lboro.ac.uk (M.O.); p.demian@lboro.ac.uk (P.D.)
* Correspondence: 201921052616@mail.scut.edu.cn (Z.Y.); mjliang@scut.edu.cn (M.L.)

Abstract: In the face of the health challenges caused by the COVID-19 pandemic, healing and therapeutic design (HTD) as interventions can help with improving people's health. It is considered to have great potential to promote health in the forms of art, architecture, landscape, space, and environment. However, there are insufficient design approaches to address the challenges during the HTD process. An increased number of studies have shown that emerging information modeling (IM) such as building information modeling (BIM), landscape information modeling (LIM), and city information modeling (CIM) coupled with blockchain (BC) functionalities have the potential to enhance designers' HTD by considering important design elements, namely design variables, design knowledge, and design decision. It can also address challenges during the design process, such as design changes, conflicts in design requirements, the lack of design evaluation tools and frameworks, and incomplete design information. Therefore, this paper aims to develop a conceptual BC enhanced IM for HTD (BC-HTD) framework that addresses the challenges in the HTD and promotes health and well-being. The structure of BC-HTD framework is twofold: (1) a conceptual high-level framework comprising three levels: user; system; and information, (2) a conceptual low-level framework of detailed content at the system level, which has been constructed using a mixed quantitative and qualitative method of literature analysis, and validated via a pre-interview questionnaire survey and follow-up interviews with industry experts and academics. This paper analyzes the process of BC enhanced HTD and the knowledge management of HTD to aid design decisions in managing design information. This paper is the first attempt to apply the advantages of BC enabled IM to enhance the HTD process. The results of this study can foster and propel new research pathways and knowledge on the value of design in the form of non-fungible token (NFT) based on the extended advantages of BC in the field of design, which can fully mobilize the healing and therapeutic behaviors of designers and the advantage potential of HTD to promote health, and realize the vision of Health Metaverse in the context of sustainable development.

Keywords: healing and therapeutic design; blockchain; building information modeling (BIM); landscape information modeling (LIM); city information modeling (CIM); art therapy; mental health; sustainable development; non-fungible token (NFT); Health Metaverse

Citation: Liu, Z.; Yang, Z.; Liang, M.; Liu, Y.; Osmani, M.; Demian, P. A Conceptual Framework for Blockchain Enhanced Information Modeling for Healing and Therapeutic Design. *IJERPH* **2022**, *19*, 8218. https://doi.org/10.3390/ijerph19138218

Academic Editors: Jie Chen, Qian Zhou and Ting Zhang

Received: 12 June 2022
Accepted: 3 July 2022
Published: 5 July 2022

1. Introduction

The coronavirus disease 2019 (COVID-19) has triggered a global mental health crisis [1]. Recent studies reported that several population groups, such as children [2], the elderly [3], caregivers [4], and medical staff [5], have suffered various mental health issues, including mood disorder, depression, anxiety, and stress. In the face of the impact of the COVID-19 epidemic, the World Health Organization has put forward a series of recommendations for epidemic prevention, such as home isolation, social distancing, and wearing masks [6]. However, prolonged isolation measures have had significant psychological consequences [7]. Amerio et al. point out that the built environment of housing can affect people's mental health when staying home for a long period [8]. Moreover, environmental factors such as landscape quality and planting in the home space also affect people's mental health [9]. Therefore, it is critical to devise measures to deal with the health threat brought by the COVID-19 to various groups.

Facing the health challenges posed by the COVID-19 pandemic, applications of healing and therapeutic design (HTD) in the field of art, architecture, landscape, space, and environment to overcome health barriers through the enhancement of aesthetics in design process have shown a positive effect on promoting health [10]. Moreover, the process of HTD based on information modeling (IM) can make better use of design information, strengthen design communication, and promote healing behavior [11]. In addition, faced with the problem of data privacy of patients under the COVID-19, blockchain (BC) has the advantage of protecting data privacy in the field of health care [12]. However, although HTD can help with improving people's health, there are design challenges in the whole process of HTD, such as changes and conflicts in design requirements [13], and incomplete consideration of design features [14,15]. Furthermore, BC and IM pay little attention to the application of HTD aiming at promoting health and addressing the challenges of HTD more generally. Therefore, this paper aims to explore the potential positive effects of integrating both HTD and the BC enhanced IM, and develop a conceptual BC enhanced IM for HTD (BC-HTD) framework that provides application value in the context of the COVID-19 pandemic.

2. Healing and Therapeutic Design (HTD) Potential for Addressing Health Problems of COVID-19

A variety of non-drug treatments, art, and design have shown a positive role in promoting mental health [16]. Art therapy is a non-verbal therapeutic approach [17] that promotes health by expressing and communicating [18] through psychotherapy [19] and artistic creative processes [20], such as drama [21], music [22], and painting [23]. Art therapy has been considered a valuable way of expression, and art shows great hope in the future of sustainable development [24]. Recent research on the COVID-19 pandemic reports that art therapy supports the psychosocial needs of children and young adults [25]; prevents depressive symptoms [26]; relieves anxiety in hospitalized patients [27]; and promotes people's physical, mental, and social health [28].

In the field of design, HTD refers to the use of design as an intervention to positively impact people's physical and psychological well-being, prevent diseases, and improve health [29], reduce stress and anxiety, and improve patient satisfaction [30]. Healing and therapeutic architecture can help with exploring emotional and spiritual issues [31] and promoting mental health [16]. Healing and therapeutic landscape has been associated with improving individuals' mental and physical health [32] and accelerating the recovery process of patients [33]. Healing and therapeutic space contributes to the well-being of patients [34] and relieves stress in an improved overall environment [35]. Additionally, it was argued that healing and therapeutic environment based on psychological stress theory and psychological development theory is a non-invasive method to reduce stress [36], which improves people's quality of life, sense of freedom, anxiety level, sleep pattern, and weight loss [37]. Hence, considering the impact of the COVID-19 pandemic, using art, architecture, landscape, space, and the environment as a HTD medium can promote well-being and healthy lifestyles for all ages [38], and build inclusive, safe, resilient, and sustainable buildings [39] in line with the United Nations Sustainable Development Goals (SDGs), namely SDG 3 (Good Health and Well-Being) and SDG 11 (Sustainable Cities and Communities).

3. HTD and Blockchain (BC) Enhanced Information Modeling (IM)

With the advent of the digital age, the application of intelligent IM, such as BC, building information modeling (BIM), landscape information modeling (LIM), and city information modeling (CIM), to promote sustainable development has shown potential to promote health in different fields. BC is a decentralized trading and data management technology, which allows digital information to be distributed without copying or modifying [40,41]. A tracking system established for the COVID-19 pandemic can be further augmented using artificial intelligence and BC technologies [42]. The application of BC for health data, health information technology, and health care related studies promote the development of precision medicine [43] and improve health care services through shared distributed health data views [44]. Moreover, the application of BIM has embodied a new paradigm of environmental sustainability in the design concept of 'healthy buildings' [45]. BIM in health monitoring of building structures [46] eventually facilitates the health and well-being of building occupants [47]. With the rapid development of BIM, many studies explored the adaptability of IM in the field of landscape, and proposed the concept of LIM related to the discipline of landscape architecture [48]. Landscape design improves many climate and health issues [49]. It uses LIM for visualization [50] to help create sustainable cities with using fewer resources to mitigate environmental impacts [51]. Furthermore, applying the principles of BIM at a city level to build a CIM can serve as an analyzing and planning tool for future sustainable cities [52]. When implementing sustainability concepts in cities, CIM is used to improve public services and life quality for their citizens [53].

The integration of BC and BIM in information management during the life cycle of buildings brings two main benefits: (1) the transition process from BIM to BC will be easier and more efficient; and (2) data security can also be ensured during the construction phase of real estate [54]. Moreover, BIM enhanced by BC improves the security of information system across the whole life cycle of a building [55–57]. BC also has the potential to solve problems and challenges in the integration of LIM and CIM. BC, BIM, LIM, and CIM are complementary, and their integration can overcome their own defects and produce more advantages. Thus, the IM of BIM, LIM, and CIM driven by BC enhance the sustainable development in architecture, landscape, and city, which could be used as auxiliary tools to promote the attention to health problems, and improve the sustainability of architecture, landscape, and city design throughout the whole life cycle of design via applications of digital health.

In the face of the impact of the COVID-19 epidemic, it is necessary to think about how to effectively respond to the reality of global public health emergencies through design. While COVID-19 has created health challenges, it has also brought unprecedented opportunities for innovation [58]. With the development of science and technology, digital technology has stimulated the potential of design innovation, changed traditional design approaches [59], and enhanced the healing and therapeutic effect of art [60]. The HTD medias, such as art, architecture, landscape, space, and environment, and the BC enhanced IM shows great potential in promoting health. In general, art therapy and HTD not only improve health, but also have potential association to achieve sustainable development. Liu et al. (2021) argue that the application of HTD in the fields of architecture, landscape, space, and environment facilitates the achievement of the SDGs, and lays the foundation for the integration of BC and IM in the design process to drive the promotion of HTD as a healthy and well-being enabler [10].

4. Method

This paper adopts a mixed quantitative and qualitative method of literature analysis to develop the conceptual BC-HTD framework, which was validated via a pre-interview questionnaire survey and follow-up interviews with industry experts and academics. Using the quantitative bibliometric method, i.e., the Network Visualization of keyword co-occurrence generated by VOSviewer version 1.6.15, which has been developed by Nees Jan van Eck and Ludo Waltman at Leiden University's Centre for Science and Technology Studies (CWTS) in the Netherlands, can reflect the relationship between different keywords, the frequency of occurrence, and different clusters [61,62]. Therefore, this paper conducts quantitative analysis based on the visual keyword co-occurrence network graph via VOSviewer software, which firstly analyzes keywords connections between BC, HTD, art therapy, and

COVID-19, and then discusses the keywords connections between BC, BIM, and design. In qualitative literature content analysis, this paper analyzes the Double Diamond model of the British Design Council [63] as the classic design process of HTD. As among the various human-centered design thinking models, the Double Diamond model [64] has been regarded as one of the most efficient and persuasive design thinking process models since it was proposed by the UK Design Council in 2005 [65], which facilitates with discovering problems and finding solutions through the 'vergence' and 'convergence' thinking in the four design stages, i.e., Discover, Define, Develop, and Deliver [66]. Based on the design process of the Double Diamond model, the conceptual BC-HTD framework has been developed to address challenges during the HTD process one by one in the four design stages, which has been further validated by industry experts and academics at the "2021 China Society of Industrial and Applied Mathematics Blockchain Technology and Application Summit Forum" (CSIAM-BTAF 2021) [67]. The validation was conducted with five participants through pre-interview questionnaire survey and follow-up interviews. The participants are asked to use a score of 1–4 (1 = strongly disagree, 2 = disagree, 3 = agree, 4 = strongly agree) to assess the structural clarity of the conceptual framework, the appropriateness of the content, and the clarity of the process, which are used as the evaluation criteria to verify the conceptual BC-HTD framework based on the average score of all the participants.

As shown in Figure 1, the method flow chart in this paper is divided into four parts: (1) using quantitative bibliometrics analysis via VOSviewer software to analyze the keyword co-occurrence relationship between BC, HTD, art therapy, and COVID-19; and BC, BIM, and design to determine the relationship between HTD and BC enhanced IM; (2) based on the results of quantitative bibliometric analysis, selecting relevant articles for qualitative analysis of specific content, and laying a theoretical foundation that underpins the conceptual BC-HTD framework in the field of digital health; (3) constructing the conceptual BC-HTD framework based on the quantitative and qualitative analysis; and (4) validating the conceptual BC-HTD framework.

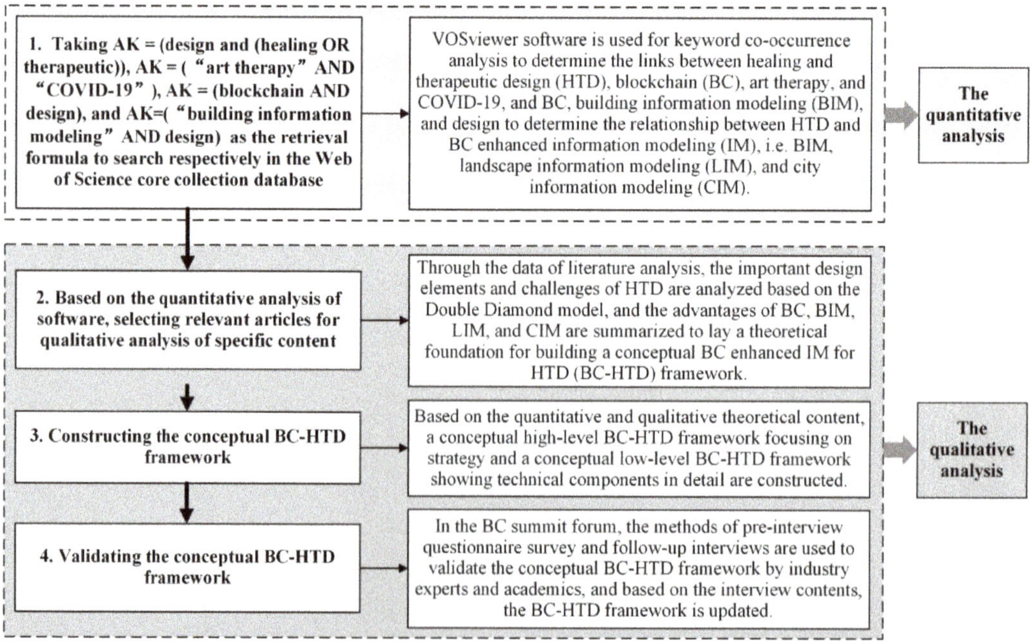

Figure 1. The flow chart of the research methodology.

5. Results

5.1. Quantitative Analysis Results

It can be seen from Figure 2 that the themes centered on HTD are mainly related to 'healing environment', 'therapeutic landscapes', 'healing garden', 'built environment', and 'architecture'; and the themes centered on BC are mainly related to 'architecture', 'information', 'management', 'framework', and 'smart contract'. In Figure 3, the themes on BC are associated with 'smart contract', 'big data', 'internet', 'architecture', and 'sustainable design'; and the themes centered on BIM are mainly related to 'building design', 'architecture', 'big data', 'internet', and 'environment'. Interestingly, both Figures 2 and 3 uncover that 'architecture' has been utilized as a bridge between HTD and BC; BC and BIM, respectively. This echoes the potential connection between HTD and BC enhanced IM, and also indicates the possibility of the integration of BC integrating and BIM, LIM, and CIM to solve the challenges in the HTD process.

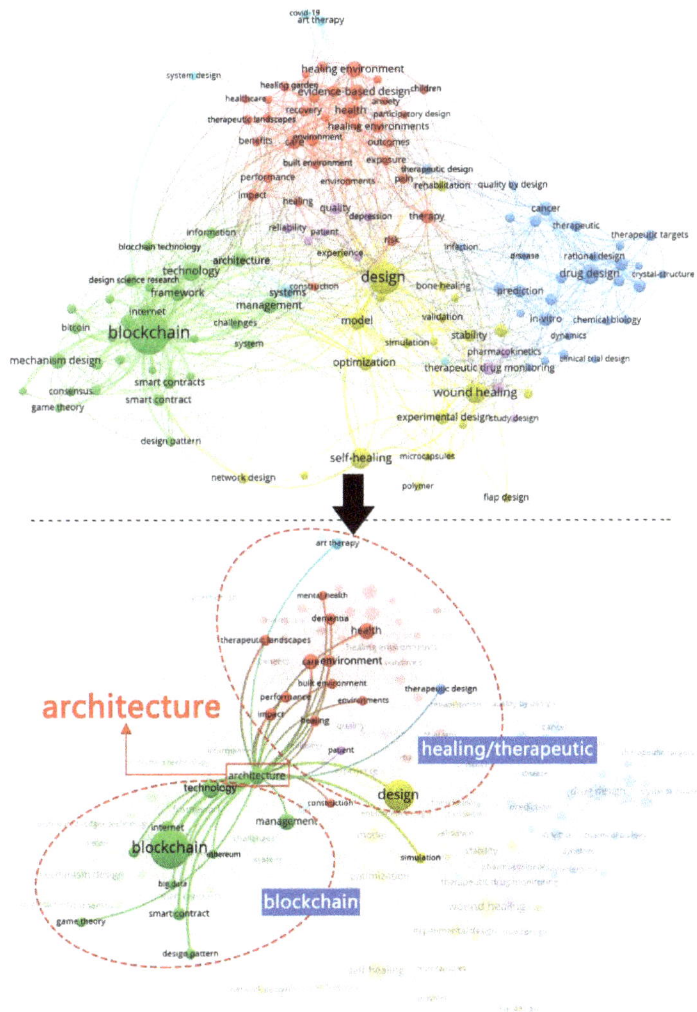

Figure 2. The relationship between healing and therapeutic design (HTD) and blockchain (BC) via VOSviewer software (generated by authors).

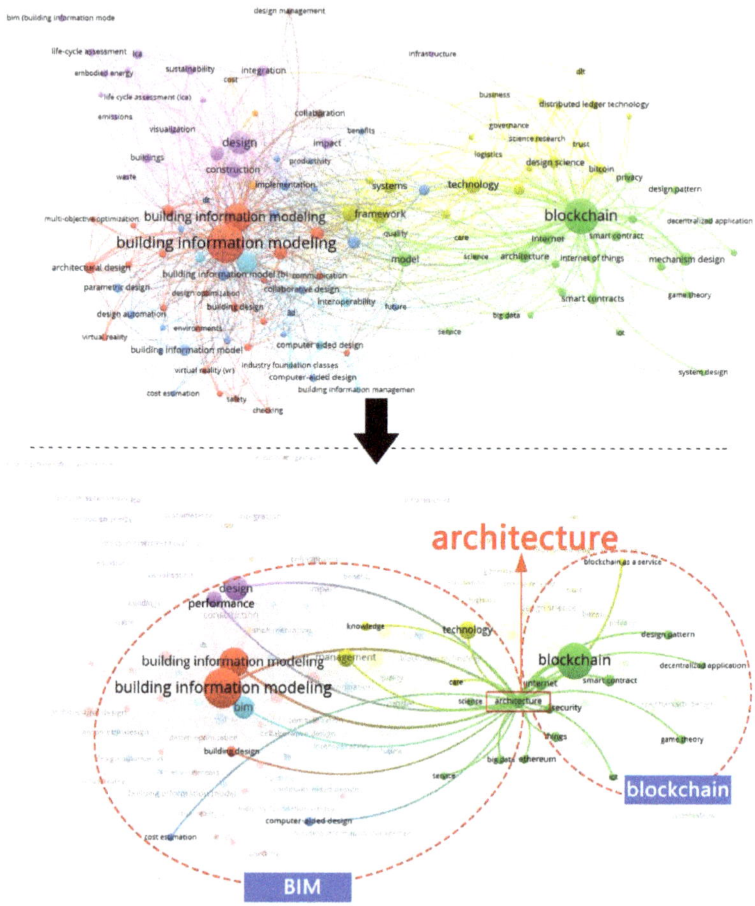

Figure 3. The relationship between BC, building information modeling, and design via VOSviewer software (generated by authors).

5.2. Qualitative Analysis Results

Based on the quantitative analysis results of visual keywords by the VOSviewer software, the following studies are selected for qualitative analysis of specific content. First, the important design elements of HTD and the challenges in the design process are analyzed from the design point of view. Then, the advantages of BC and IM are summarized from the design perspective.

5.2.1. The Important Design Elements and Challenges of HTD

The HTD studies are mainly associated with the healing and therapeutic architecture [31,68,69], spaces [70–72], environment [36,73,74], and healing and therapeutic landscape design based on gardens [33,75,76]. In addition, HTD studies are focused on dementia patients to improve their environments and their quality of life [77,78]. Based on the application field of HTD, the healing and therapeutic architectural design is largely associated with BIM; and the healing and therapeutic landscape design corresponds to LIM. Furthermore, the design fields of comprehensive healing and therapeutic architecture, landscape, space, and environment indicate a strong link with CIM. BC has also been linked to LIM and CIM, to enhance HTD.

The HTD emphasizes important design elements in the presentation of architecture, landscape, space, and environment in promoting health via two means:

(1) Understanding and differentiating between different design variables. The change of design variables and the action mechanism of health impact can facilitate the individual and collective reflection of design variables in the overall design suggestions [68];
(2) Design decision-making process based on different forms of knowledge of stakeholders. Transforming the implicit knowledge of stakeholders into explicit knowledge in the design-driven process of healing and therapeutic architecture enhances communication among stakeholders, and avoids arbitrary decision-making to facilitate the design of healing and therapeutic architecture [79]. Additionally, healing and therapeutic designers need to make correct design decisions based on evaluations from the stakeholders, such as architects, patients, and healthcare providers [80]. Furthermore, the stakeholders' judgments and decisions on the design of the healing and therapeutic built environment must be based on reliable evidence and knowledge [81].

Although HTD can promote human health through the medium of art, architecture, landscape, space, and environment, it also faces the following five challenges in the design process, such as hospital design:

(i) The changes and conflicts in design requirements. For example, due to the lack of consensus between hospital space design and nursing mode, it is easy to have conflicting design needs with nursing mode when designing the healing and therapeutic landscape of the hospital. It takes a long time to plan the design of the hospital from the perspective of architectural environment, which is difficult to flexibly respond to the changing needs over time [13].
(ii) Inconsistent design research framework and methodology. Although there are many studies on the healing and therapeutic environment with diverse methodologies, there is a lack of a unified research framework, which makes further research difficult [82].
(iii) Incomplete consideration of design features. The interrelationships between various design features are easily overlooked when there is HTD for the built and physical environments in which people with dementia live [14]. In addition, there are many issues related to aging that are not adequately addressed in the HTD for the environment in which people with dementia live, and environmental factors have not been considered comprehensively when intervening in the environment [15].
(iv) Lack of design evaluation tools and frameworks. Facing the dynamic needs of residents for the new generation of buildings, there is a lack of more comprehensive and informed tools to evaluate the effectiveness of the design and use of healing and therapeutic buildings, as well as a framework to clarify people-centered issues [83].
(v) Incomplete collection of design data. When there is HTD through art in the medical environment that are characterized by a diversity of intervention measures and results, the data collection is not comprehensive, data results are difficult to synthesize, and the evaluation of design results becomes difficult [16]. In addition, it is difficult to determine in the field of medical care whether the healing and therapeutic physical and social environment design results effectively improve the quality of life of patients, which reflects that the data on the impact of design on treatment results are inconclusive [34,84].

In order to further explore the challenges of HTD across all the design stages, this paper maps the five challenges during the HTD process one by one in the four design stages of Discover, Define, Develop, and Deliver in the Double Diamond model, as shown in Figure 4. In the Stages of Discover and Define, HTD is faced with the challenges of changes and conflicts in design requirements, and inconsistent design research frameworks and methodologies. In the Stage of Develop, HTD faces the challenge of incomplete consideration of design features. In the Stage of Deliver, HTD is challenged by the lack of tools and frameworks for design evaluation. Furthermore, HTD faces the challenge of incomplete collection of design data across all the design stages.

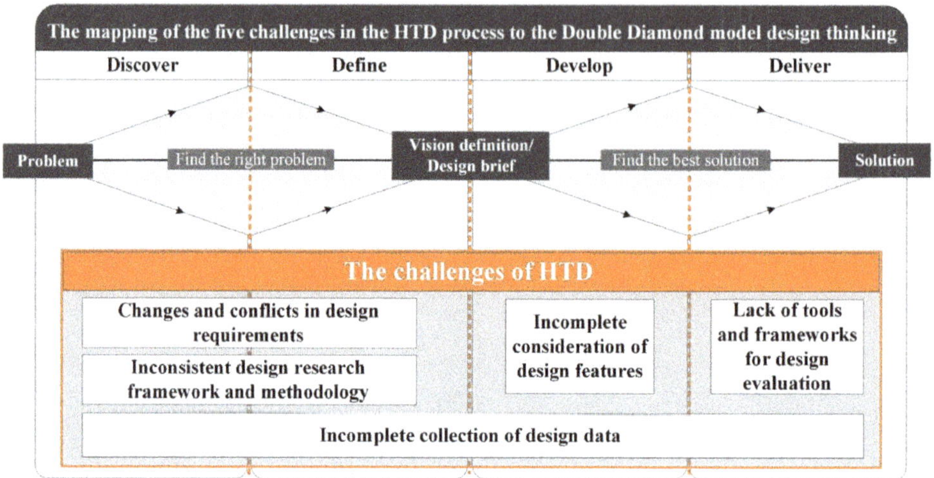

Figure 4. The mapping of the five challenges in the HTD process to the Double Diamond model design thinking (generated by authors).

5.2.2. The Advantages of BC

The BC technology, with its features of disintermediation, immutability, and trust, has become one of the most promising and potentially transformative technologies in many industries, which contributes to the SDGs of the United Nations and produces extensive changes in some established industries and practices [85]. BC has key properties of transparency, security, and traceability [55,86–88]. In addition, decentralization is the most prominent and essential feature of BC technology [89]. In a data-driven world, BC technology potentially brings benefits to individuals and organizations that lack information infrastructure or have no access to reliable integrated data [90]. Furthermore, using BC technology as a reliable and secure decentralized information system can potentially improve the sustainability of building assets by providing transparent and comprehensive information to all stakeholders at different life cycle stages of an asset [91]. To designers, BC technology advances the collaborative design process in a novel way of working [92].

In the fields of art and healthcare, BC technology embodies the advantages of promoting the art economy, protecting intellectual property (IP) rights, and enabling data sharing. First, since BC technology brings efficiency and transparency, and adds value to products and services in different fields, the art world has begun to utilize BC technology to promote the art economy [93]. Moreover, the development of BC technology and smart contracts provides artists with a form of digital copyright management and creates a new tradable digital asset; such a trend means that IP operates differently in digital culture [94]. In the field of health care, when the health care system needs to be patient-centered to connect different systems and improve the accuracy of electronic medical records, BC technology provides a stable framework for health care data with the functions of data sharing, health record management, and access control [95]. In terms of information sharing, BC technology solves the problem of information sharing in the supply chain composed of the stakeholders, and the information sharing supported by BC can add value to strengthen the collaborative work of different types of supply chains, such as health and medical treatment, construction, and smart city [96].

In the field of information technology, BC is a shared data or information database that is unfalsifiable, untraceable, open and transparent, and collectively maintained [97]. Therefore, the adoption of BC technology can make the development of communities and enterprises more transparent, efficient and scalable, which accelerates the model of sustainable development [98]. In addition, BC technology, as an immutable digital record tool, allows different people and organizations to collaborate and create shared value, which solves increasingly complex problems in global value chains in pursuit of sustainable development [99,100]. Facing the three-tier new value system of value production, value recording, and value realization [101], BC provides democratized information access opportunities for the stakeholders through a new form of value delivery architecture [102]. Furthermore, BC has the following contributions in creating public value and promoting sustainable development: (1) building an authorization environment; (2) helping the design process to produce innovative solutions; (3) improving operation capacity; and (4) legalizing the final results [103]. In general, there are a number of advantages of BC technology, such as decentralization, openness, transparency, collective maintenance, and efficient sharing of databases, which lay the groundwork for facilitating the HTD process.

5.2.3. The Advantages of Building Information Modeling (BIM), Landscape Information Modeling (LIM), and City Information Modeling (CIM)

In architectural design, BIM is a digital technology that uses a three-dimensional (3D) model to establish a set of project databases, which aid to achieve the SDGs of the project's entire life cycle through the retrieval and application of information [104]. Based on the sustainable and transparent BIM collaborative work environment, the information of components can be copied and verified in the environment, so that all the participants communicate in time across the whole life cycle of the construction project, and every participant conducts scientific analysis and makes corresponding decisions through the design information shared by different design professionals [105]. Designers use BIM for visual design that intuitively helps with understanding the space of key parts and arranging corresponding parts reasonably, so as to make better use of limited space and effectively improve design efficiency and quality [106]. Moreover, the use of innovative BIM technology facilitates with realizing end-to-end communication, data exchange and information sharing among collaborators, and improving the cooperation among stakeholders [107]. The application of BIM in architectural design has the potential to improve the quality of information for key design decisions, and the visual technology provided by BIM helps designers to predict changes in the construction industry [108]. Furthermore, the BIM automatically associates with updating the design information in the healing building to avoid manual insertion that takes a lot of time [109]. As such, the BIM can be used as a shared knowledge resource of equipment information to ensure the integrity and accuracy of information and data exchange in the design process [110].

In addition, the rapid development of BIM technology provides a mature foundation for the development of LIM that is related to the design of landscape architecture, which expands the application objects of BIM. The difference between LIM and BIM is that the LIM has the core elements of terrain, vegetation, water, and the environment [111]. Based on accessible data stored in LIM for design creation, realization and management phases, landscape designers can be enhanced in decision-making and presentation of design outcomes, where reliable exchange of information increases efficiency, reduces errors, and minimizes the risk of corrections [112]. In addition, the visual design process provided by LIM improves participation and cognitive response of the stakeholders [113]. Furthermore, the use of LIM technology brings obvious benefits to the design process: (1) standardizing the knowledge of landscape design; (2) supporting the design information of different participants; and (3) improving information exchange between landscape, architecture, and urban design [114].

Furthermore, with the rapid development of BIM technology in cities, CIM is also flourishing in city research. The CIM is a technology based on BIM, geographic information system, and internet of things, which can realize the co-growth of digital cities and physical cities, and is also a necessary way to realize smart cities [115]. Integrating geographic information system and BIM systems to create CIM optimizes the management and monitoring of urban maintenance works and makes more efficient use of the allocated economic resources [116]. Moreover, the CIM is a digital 3D model of a city, which includes different types of information data [117]. The application of CIM technology helps to improve information management processes and control, and understand data in different domains [118]. Using CIM to build a visual 3D dynamic maintenance management platform brings the benefits of less intervention, high efficiency, and high precision in the new concept of 'Community intelligent modeling' [119]. By connecting BIM and CIM, users can be provided with an interactive and rich 3D city model environment in which data can be accessed, analyzed, and shared anytime and anywhere [120]. Furthermore, the CIM is an emerging research field [121], which adds value to urban space construction and its management [122]. Hence, the latest progress of BIM research plays a key role in the application of CIM [123].

In general, since the CIM includes the information of natural landscape, architecture, and infrastructure [124], BIM technology is the basis of LIM technology, and the LIM is the bridge between BIM and CIM, which integrates the design between city and architecture. The advantages of BIM, LIM, and CIM mainly include: (1) strengthening the communication and coordination of design work; (2) visualizing 3D design model of architecture, landscape, and city; (3) verifying the design results with the simulation of 3D model; (4) sharing common 3D models and coordination information; and (5) standardizing the design knowledge of architecture, landscape, and the city.

6. The Development of Conceptual BC Enhanced IM for HTD (BC-HTD) Framework

6.1. The Process of HTD Enhanced by BC

As shown in Figure 5, the exchange of information within the context of sustainable development between stakeholders during HTD will be linked through IM driven by BC, which assists to understand and differentiate between different design variables. In terms of information flow, BC integrates data for health information management, as well as data and tools for visualizing 3D models provided by BIM, LIM, and CIM. Subsequently, the corresponding design data and tools driven by BC are obtained in the four design stages of Discover, Define, Develop, and Deliver within the Double Diamond design process. Additionally, the information in the design process is fed back to the design information management system via the BC technology—thus forming an interlocking and progressive relationship, and constantly enriching the data content of the design information management process. Finally, the management of HTD information for SDGs 3 and 11 to promote health and well-being and sustainable living can be realized.

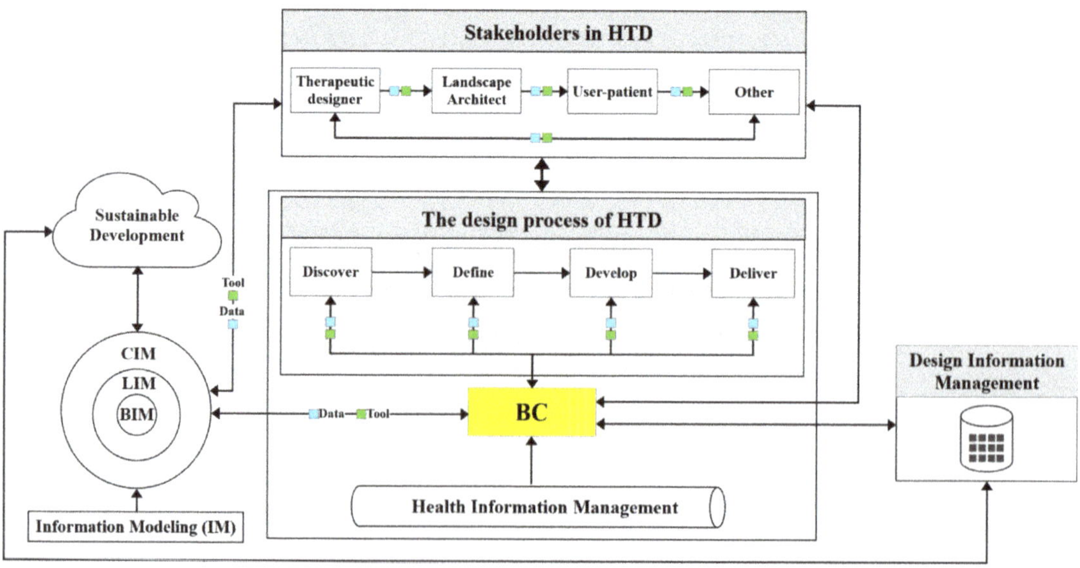

Figure 5. The process of HTD enhanced by BC (generated by authors).

6.2. The Knowledge Management for HTD Driven by BC

In the process of BC-driven HTD, the knowledge management of the HTD, such as design information and health information, can inform the knowledge utilization process between the environment, organizations, and individuals from the inflow and outflow of knowledge, as shown in Figure 6. In the whole process of knowledge flow, the IM enhanced by BC is used to record and store the value of the HTD knowledge in art, architecture, landscape, space, and environment, which forms a set of available knowledge systems to achieve relevant indicators of sustainable development, and improves the generation and utilization of knowledge life cycle across the whole knowledge management stages. In addition, the IM driven by BC is used to transform tacit knowledge achievements of stakeholders into explicit knowledge to solve the accumulation, security, inheritance, repetition, sharing, and management problems of the HTD knowledge. Hence, the knowledge management of HTD through innovation driven digital transformation enables design decision-makers to carry out the decision-making process based on various forms of knowledge of stakeholders, which aids in realizing sustainable development in terms of knowledge flow.

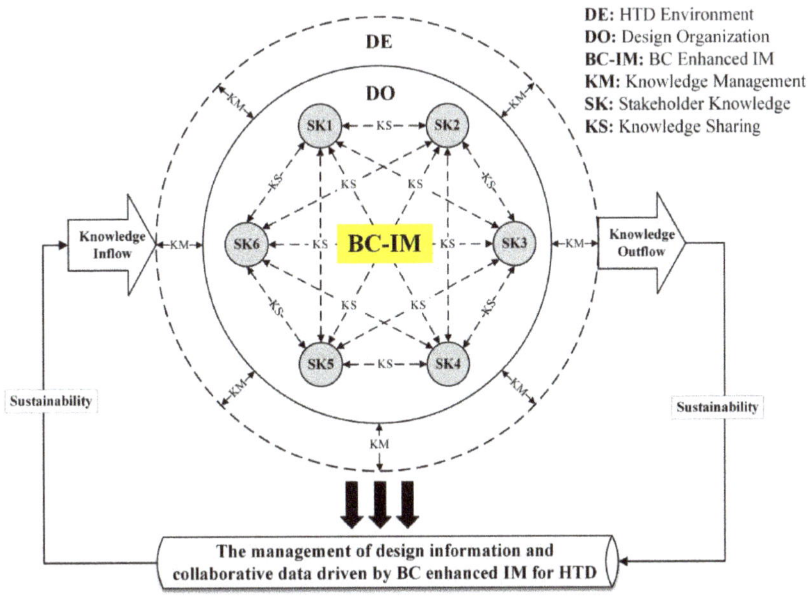

Figure 6. The knowledge management of HTD driven by BC (generated by authors).

6.3. The Potential Role of BC Enhanced IM in Addressing HTD Challenges

The potential roles of BC to enhance IM in line with the five identified challenges of HTD are:

(1) Responding flexibly to changes and conflicts in design requirements. Based on the advantages of BC in Section 5.2.2, the traceability database network of BC is used to summarize common information in healthcare, such as hospital design, and collaborative information for stakeholders in different time periods, which increases the consensus of design research and reflects the changing needs of users over time. For example, Wan et al. find that BC uses trusted ledgers to identify and understand information communicated between different stakeholders to achieve information consensus [96]. In addition, based on the advantages of BIM, LIM, and CIM in Section 5.2.3, the IM can gather the existing knowledge and information in art, ar-

chitecture, landscape, and other related fields, strengthen the communication and coordination among stakeholders, and promote the collaborative design process.

(2) Unified design research framework and methodology. The results in Sections 5.2.2 and 5.2.3 indicate that the traceable information database of BC enhanced IM facilitates with reviewing the past HTD cases, in which the most commonly used and most effective research methodology can be understood by sharing the common architectural, landscape, and city information.

(3) Fully considering the design characteristics. The BC enhanced IM directly transmits and uses design information collaboratively, and fully considers the interrelationship between various design features of the virtual built environment and physical environment. The IM presents the virtual 3D model to communicate design concepts and improve the quality of HTD. For instance, Lee et al. point out that digital manufacturing based on BIM provides instant design information and increases work efficiency, which avoids the problem of incomplete consideration of design characteristics caused by traditional paper documents [106].

(4) Improving design evaluation tools. The 3D models presented by the IM are used to simulate and verify the design results, and plan and analyze the elements of sustainable city development. Based on dynamic needs, the IM is facilitated to comprehensively and objectively evaluate the effectiveness of the design and the use of healing and therapeutic buildings, and clarify the human-centered problem framework. Furthermore, the consensus mechanism of the BC aids with design evaluation results. For example, Dantas et al. suggest that BIM and CIM can help city managers make assessments and decisions with simple and accurate data [53].

(5) Comprehensive collection of design data. BIM, LIM, and CIM enhanced by BC can bring seven main benefits to data collection: (a) BC provides transparent and comprehensive information to all the stakeholders at different stages of the HTD life cycle to improve design sustainability. For instance, Shojaei et al. show that BC stores and disseminates data information in different stages of asset construction, such as collection, verification, and extraction, which assists with achieving asset sustainability [91]. (b) BC establishes an open, transparent, collective maintenance, comprehensive and efficient design sharing information and database. (c) Design information for past, present, and future traceability is established through the traceability database network of BC. (d) The IM enables end-to-end communication, data exchange, and information sharing among stakeholders. (e) In the 3D models provided by the IM, accessing, analyzing, and sharing the data anytime and anywhere standardize the design knowledge and strengthen the information exchange.

Figure 7 illustrates the potential role of data and tools provided by BC enhanced IM in stakeholders and design process. From the user's point of view, BC enhanced IM facilitates the communication between the stakeholders during the HTD and gathers the dynamic needs of users through the traceability database network. From the perspective of design, the IM enhanced by BC establishes document data flow within the HTD process based on the domains of art, architecture, landscape, space, and environment, and uses design information and design tools throughout the four design stages of Discover, Define, Develop, and Deliver of the Double Diamond design thinking to solve the design challenges in the HTD process. As such, building design information management and collaborative data with BC enhanced IM for HTD strengthen the connection of HTD stakeholders and digitally drive the design process.

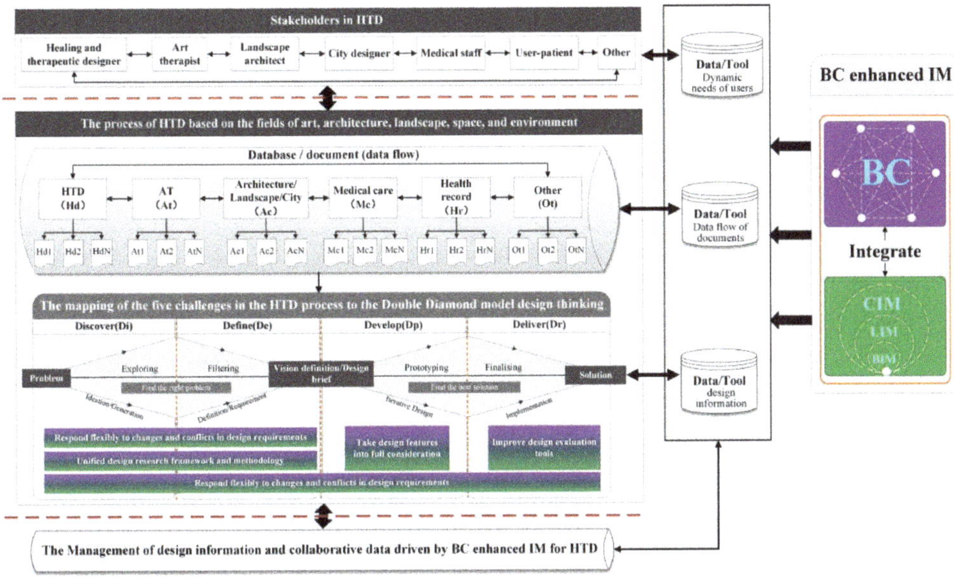

Figure 7. The potential roles of BC enhanced information modeling (IM) in addressing HTD challenges (generated by authors).

6.4. The Conceptual BC-HTD Framework for Sustainable Development

The development of the conceptual BC-HTD framework is based on the findings of the quantitative and qualitative analysis and the important design elements of HTD and associated challenges, as shown in Figure 8. The rationale of the conceptual BC-HTD framework is to use the BC enhanced IM, as tools to drive the design process during the HTD, and assist the flow of design knowledge and decision-making. The conceptual BC-HTD framework consists of a strategic high-level framework and a detailed low-level framework. The red coded numbers represent the important process actions of BC enhanced IM at different stages to identify the potential roles of the BC integrated IM (BC + BIM/LIM/CIM) in the whole life cycle of HTD, highlight the importance of design elements, and address HTD challenges.

6.4.1. High-Level BC-HTD Framework

Based on the relationship between the important design elements, HTD challenges, and the advantages of the BC enhanced IM, the conceptual high-level BC-HTD framework encompasses three levels comprising user, system, and information, as shown in Figure 9.

In the user level, BC + BIM/LIM/CIM consolidates the relationship between stakeholders of HTD; emphasizes information exchange, communication and coordination among stakeholders; and stores data of users' dynamic needs. At the system level, the advantages of BC, such as openness, transparency, collective maintenance, comprehensive and efficient sharing of database, and traceability, address HTD challenges across the four stages of Discover, Define, Develop, and Deliver of the Double Diamond design process model. Additionally, the advantages of communication, collaboration, coordination, and visual 3D model of the IM assist the whole HTD process based on the fields of art, architecture, landscape, space, and environment. In the information level, BC + BIM/LIM/CIM enable the interaction between the user and the system to be transmitted to the design information level and interacting within the level. Moreover, the process totally contributes the HTD information to facilitate with achieving sustainable development via research framework, design requirements, design characteristics, evaluation framework, and design data. As such, design driving and design decision-making process are carried out based on the

HTD information. In addition, the distributed network of BC + BIM/LIM/CIM expands the application of sustainable HTD information in different fields, such as art therapy, healthcare, architectural design, and landscape design, in which the BC + BIM/LIM/CIM is used as sustainable technology to promote sustainable development aimed at promoting health and well-being.

6.4.2. Low-Level BC-HTD Framework

A conceptual low-level BC-HTD framework is shown in Figure 10. At the system level of the HTD, the advantages of the BC enhanced IM (B-1) highlighted in the design processes of HTD. In particular, the B-2 at system level reflects the databases/documents of HTD, art therapy, architectural/landscape/city design, health records, and medical care integrated before the design process of the Double Diamond model of HTD. These data at B-3 related to HTD summarize the research consensus in various fields, unify the research framework and methodology, and comprehensively collect the data over time. In addition, the B-4 at a system level promotes the potential role of data and tools in realizing the sustainability throughout the four design stages of Discover, Define, Develop, and Define with an intelligent application scenario based on the BC + BIM/LIM/CIM. Through the flow and use of data, the B-5 at the system level is to judge whether the outcomes of HTD promote health by unifying data on design outcomes, a human-centered framework, and comprehensive and objective assessment tools. If the outcome of the HTD promotes health, the design information and collaborative data used will be managed in the BC enhanced IM at B-6. If the results of the HTD do not promote health, the relevant data of the HTD will be reintegrated and returned to the Double Diamond design process of the HTD.

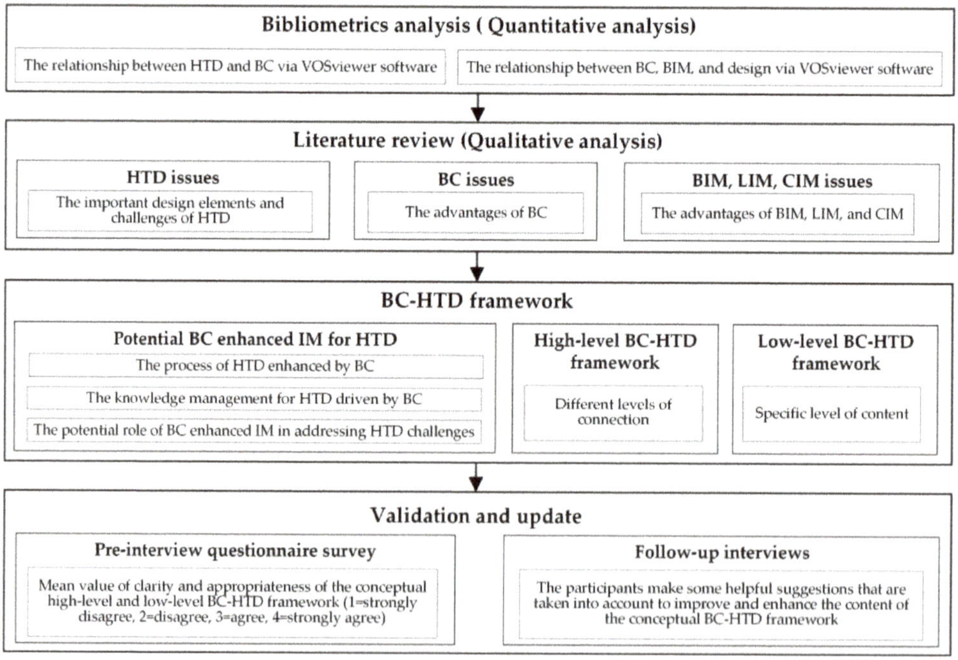

Figure 8. The conceptual BC-HTD framework design and development flow chart (generated by authors).

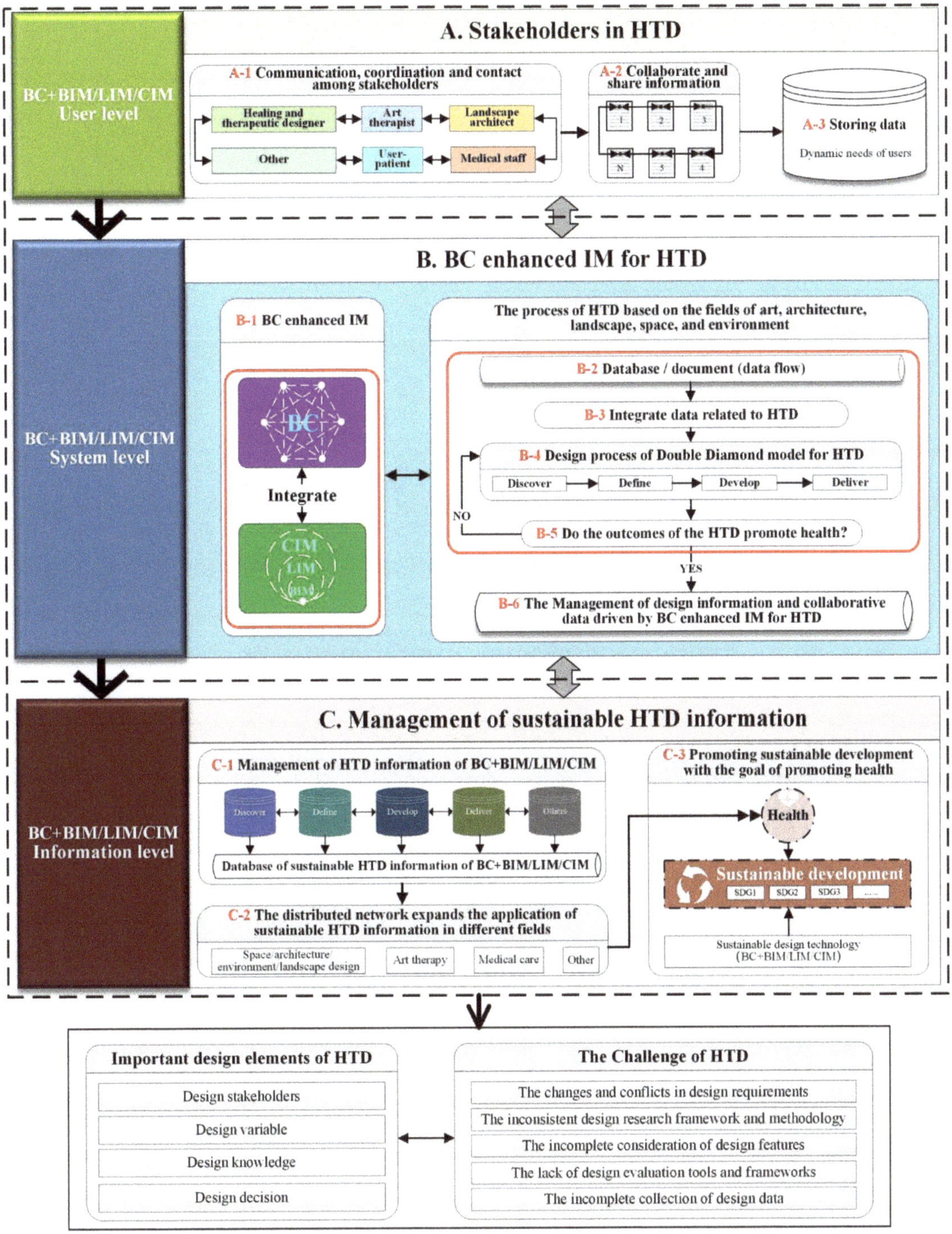

Figure 9. High-level BC-HTD framework (generated by authors).

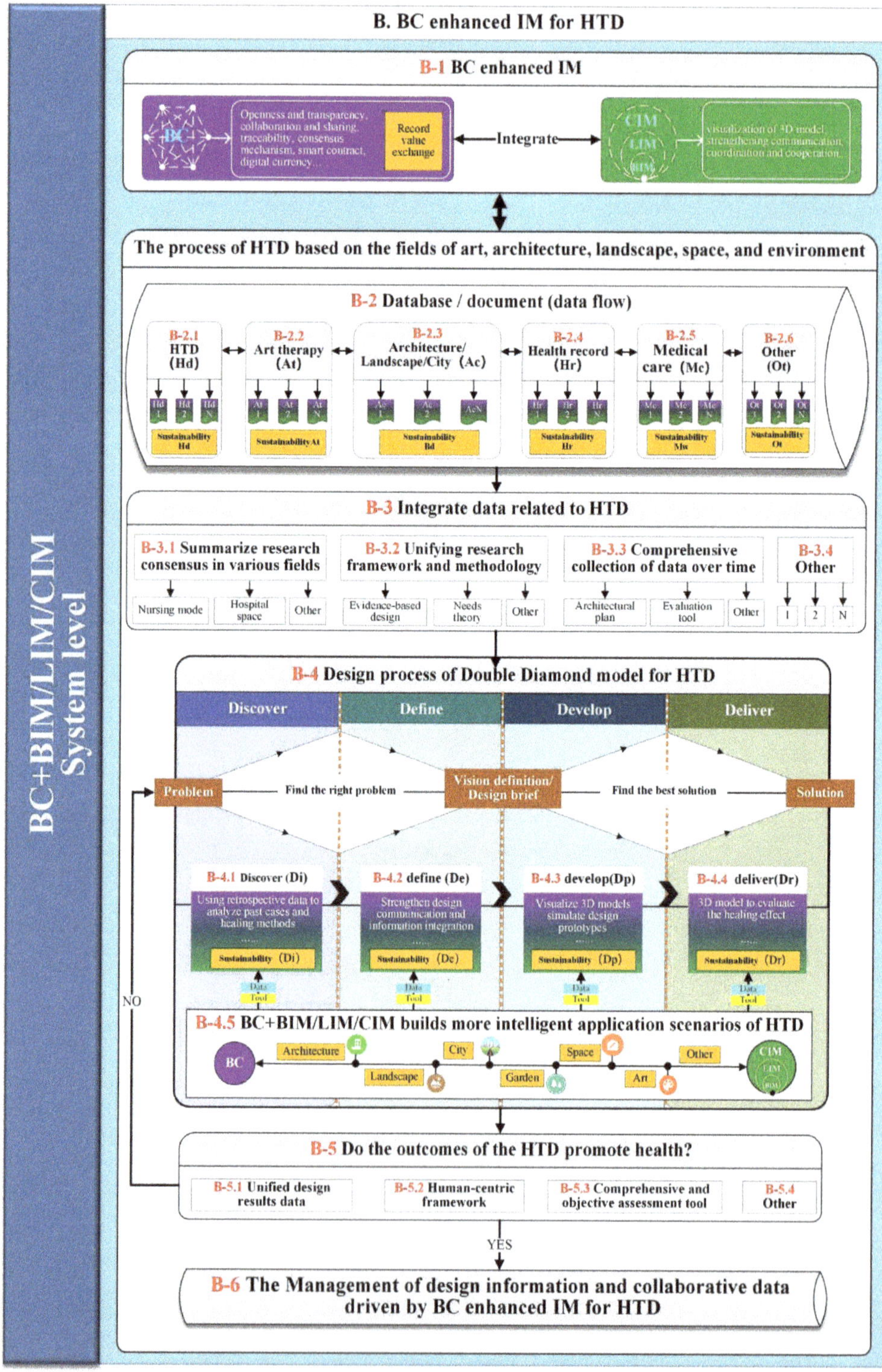

Figure 10. Low-level BC-HTD framework (generated by authors).

7. Validation and Update of the Conceptual BC-HTD Framework

The conceptual BC-HTD framework for digital health, as illustrated in Figures 8 and 9, was accepted and invited to present [125], and validated by industry experts and academics at the CSIAM-BTAF 2021 [67]. All the participants involved in the validation agreed that the conceptual BC-HTD framework is clear, as shown in Table 1. In addition, the participants put forward their views to BC driven HTD based on the conceptual high-level and low-level BC-HTD frameworks, and pointed out that BC has a great potential in fully considering the important design elements of HTD and solving the challenges in the process of the HTD. Furthermore, the participants made some helpful suggestions that are taken into account to improve and enhance the content of the conceptual BC-HTD framework, which are:

(1) In the part of stakeholders, the BC can be used for multi-party trust connection, such as interconnection, mutual trust, and alliance chain.
(2) The approach of establishing incentives based on the BC encourages the stakeholders to fully contribute their own data.
(3) For the challenge of HTD, since the BC technology may not be able to work between multiple stakeholders for pure design behavior, the BC technology must have business collaboration, commercial behavior, and transaction behavior to cooperate.
(4) The pure function of the BC can be applied to the protection of IP rights. For example, the design draft and phased achievements of the designers can be recorded via the BC, which can be confirmed uniquely with digital assets on the BC technology to ensure non-infringement and measure the designer's value by transaction behavior.
(5) The advantages of the BC, i.e., traceability, consensus mechanism, and smart contract, can help address the challenges of incomplete data collection during the HTD process.
(6) Building a real-time design knowledge base with BC enhanced IM is helpful to design decision-making.

Table 1. Mean value of clarity and appropriateness of the conceptual high-level and low-level BC-HTD framework (responses of industry experts and academics).

Evaluation Criteria	High-Level	Low-Level
Clarity of the structure	3.70	3.50
Appropriateness of content	3.15	3.00
Clarity of flow	3.40	3.20

Furthermore, in line with the suggestions of the participants, the conceptual BC-HTD framework was updated on the user layer in the high-level BC-HTD framework, as shown in Figure 11, where the A1 was added in "The alliance chain of stakeholders establishes business collaboration/transaction behavior", and A5 has been refined as "Digital assetization of data information pure IP rights and measure the value of design". In addition, A2 was updated as "Stakeholders enhance communication and coordination in interconnection and mutual trust", and the A3 is rewording as "Reward mechanism driven collaboration and information sharing". Furthermore, the participants' suggestions have been added to the user layer of the BC-HTD framework to establish business collaboration and transaction behaviors with stakeholder alliance chains, which ensure interconnection and mutual trust, encourage the stakeholders to contribute HTD data based on a reward mechanism, and quantify the design value of IP for digital assetization.

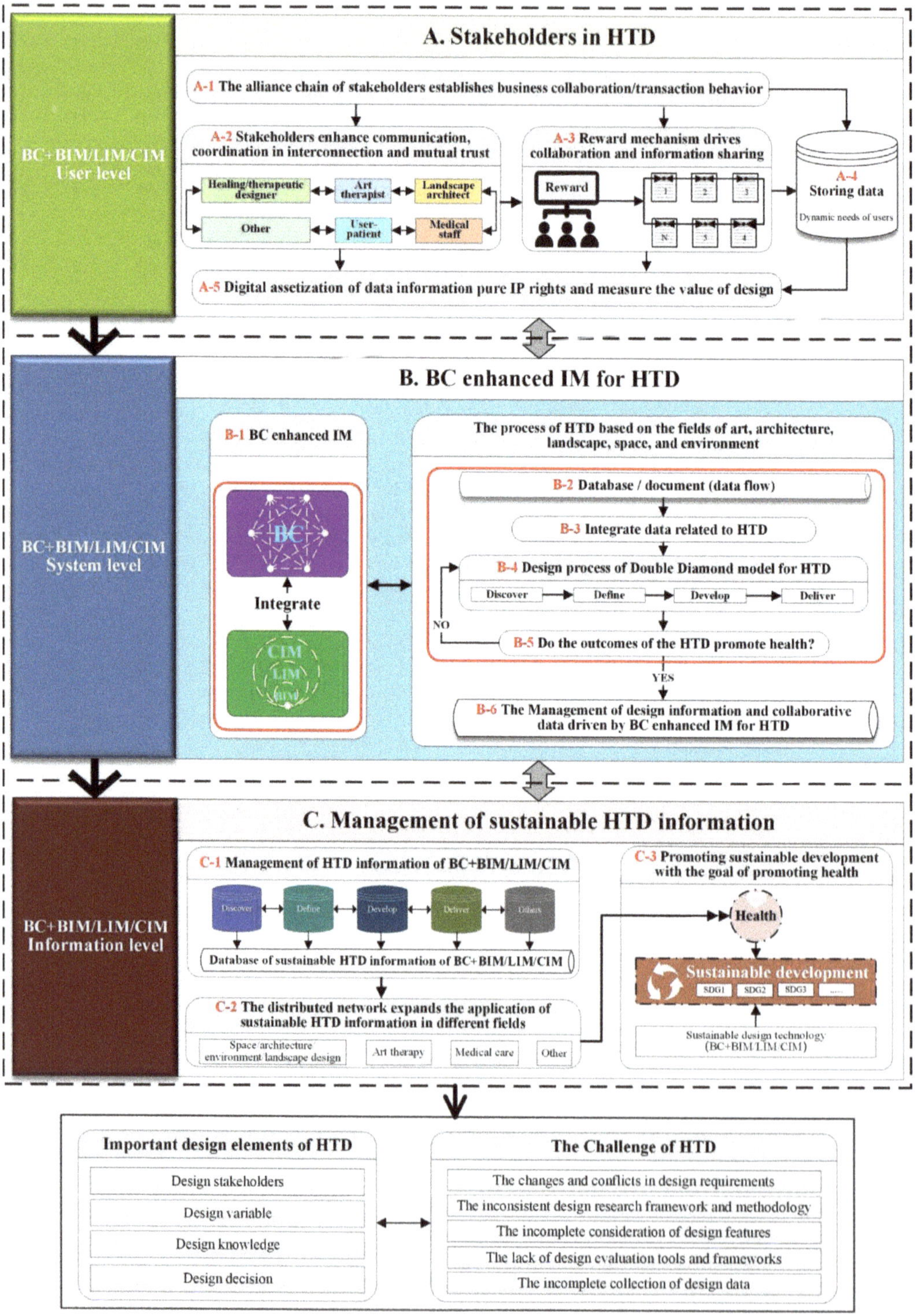

Figure 11. Updated high-level BC-HTD framework (generated by authors).

8. Discussion

8.1. Quantifying the Value of Design with BC Enhanced IM in HTD

The results in Section 5.2.2 indicate that the BC can assist to digitize IP and record value contributions in the process of information sharing. As such, BC has potential advantages in measuring the value of design. In the field of design, the value of designers cannot always simply be gauged from design works. This is because value is generated not only from suppliers (designers), but also from the experience services used by different participants and users throughout the whole design process [126]. Moreover, the concept of value in project management has changed from 'value management' to 'understanding how the stakeholders evaluate the value of different things [127]. Therefore, when the value of designers cannot be measured by design works, the BC represents a huge advantage. Based on the decentralization, transparency, and security characteristics of BC, the BC is a good value management method, where the BC encapsulates qualitatively different data and improves management efficiency, effectiveness, and performance of participants [128]. For enterprises, the real value of the enterprise can be assessed using the automatic decision-making value system of the BC [129]. Furthermore, the BC serves as a record that effectively determines the value of participants' contributions and functions as a true sharing economy [130]. As healing and therapeutic gardens play a key role in reducing the emotional impact of hospitalization in the field of health care, future research should quantify and monetize the therapeutic benefits of HTD [131].

The BC tracks the contribution of network participants to measure the value brought with adequately fine granularity [132] and protect the corresponding IP rights based on the BC consensus mechanism contributed by participants [133]. Additionally, the IP value of each designer is recorded, managed, quantified, transmitted, and protected in the consensus mechanism of BC technology, which can stimulate the original motivation of designers, disseminate knowledge and drive the design behavior, as shown in Figure 12. In the HTD stages of Discover, Define, Develop, and Deliver, the decentralized fine-grained provenance tracking and consensus mechanism of BC are used to distinguish the attribution objects of data, realize the traceability of data, and convert the design documents into digital assets, which can record, manage, transmit, and quantify the IP value of designers. Thence, the future research could use BC to distinguish the ownership of data in different design stages and digitalize design information.

8.2. BC-Based Non-Fungible Token to Quantify the Value of Art Therapy

Moreover, the results of the quantitative analysis presented in Section 5.1 suggest that there is a certain connection between art therapy and BC, with architecture as a bridge. When using the artistic medium for HTD, the outcome of artworks, such as paintings and music, can represent their value to HTD. In the field of art, BC can facilitate solving the problem of transparency of artworks, and the use of new forms of non-fungible token (NFT) in the BC, which secures the rights of art works, allows precise control of copyright and ownership, and highlights new technologies addressing IP issues in digital art [134]. With analyzing the keyword co-occurrence relationship between art therapy and NFT in the context of COVID-19 in the Web of Science core collection database via VOSviewer, it can be seen that the COVID-19 is a bridge between art therapy and NFT, as shown in Figure 13, which indicates a potential association in measuring the value of art therapy in the way of NFT. When quantifying the value of an artwork, NFT can bring greater certainty to issues of ownership and authenticity of artwork [135]. In the application of digital assets, NFT has gained obvious public attention by recording the ownership of digital assets such as images, music, videos, and virtual works through smart contracts of the BC [136]. Based on the unique properties of BC's distributed and immutable records, NFT creates a record of the source of digital artworks in the BC and operate the copyright management of artworks [137]. Additionally, each uniquely identifiable entity can be mapped to the NFT's transfer by tying each entity to the BC [138]. Therefore, future research could use the approach of NFT in the BC to quantify the value of art-mediated healing and therapeutics, and drive the healing and therapeutic behavior of art therapists in the form of digital assets to promote people's health and well-being.

Furthermore, BC presents a great potential in the tokenization of digital assets [139]. BC technology creates a trusted environment based on the essence of transparency, and makes information publicly used in the whole network in a trusted environment, which can maintain the integrity and invariance of data, promote stakeholders in different chains to jointly create value, ensure the availability of information, and provide a coordination mechanism [140]. Therefore, quantifying the value of design with BC enhanced IM drives HTD behavior and promotes achievement of SDGs. Interestingly, since new digital technologies contribute to the concept of the Metaverse in which resources connect the virtual digital world to the physical world [141], the properties of BC in the sharing economy creates sustainable business models in the Metaverse [142]. The future development trend of Health Metaverse is prospected in the way of quantifying the design value of BC enhanced IM including BIM, LIM, and CIM, and NFT management of digital art assets, which has certain social significance to achieve sustainable development from the field of digital health.

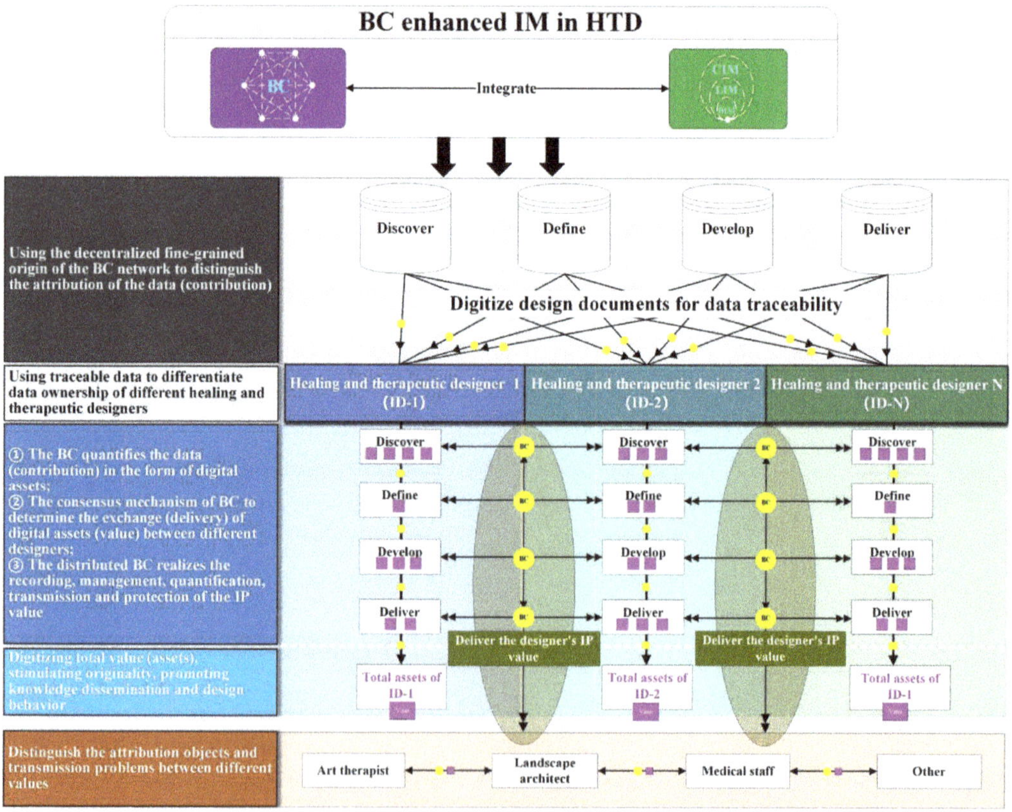

Figure 12. Quantifying the value of design with BC enhanced IM in HTD (generated by authors).

Figure 13. The relationship between art therapy and non-fungible tokens in the context of COVID-19 (generated by authors).

9. Conclusions

At present, the HTD, which promotes health to achieve sustainable development, faces design-related challenges in the fields of art, architecture, landscape, space, and the environment. The development of emerging IM, such as BIM, LIM, and CIM, is enhanced by BC to promote sustainable development, bringing immediate advantages in solving the challenges of HTD in the field of digital health. Therefore, this paper is the first attempt to apply the advantages of BC to IM with a view to enhancing the HTD process in line with the Double Diamond model of the British Design Council, considering important elements and challenges in the design process. From a research perspective, in the aftermath of the COVID-19 epidemic, this study investigates the application of integration of BC with BIM, LIM, and CIM in HTD, which is aimed at promoting health and well-being heading to the sustainable development. In terms of research content, this paper proposes a BC-driven HTD process and a management process of design knowledge. Moreover, the conceptual BC-HTD framework driven by BC + BIM/LIM/CIM has a high-level framework of three levels, i.e., user, system, and information, and a low-level framework of detailed content at the system level, which has been constructed using a mixed quantitative and qualitative method of literature analysis, and validated and updated via pre-interview questionnaire and follow-up interviews with industry experts and academics. This paper analyzes the process of BC enhanced HTD and the knowledge management of HTD to aid design decisions in managing design information. The potential of BC to quantify the HTD value is constantly being tapped. The results of this study can help future research to quantify the value of design in the form of NFT based on the extended advantages of BC in the field of design, which can fully mobilize the advantage potential of HTD to promote health, and realize the vision of Health Metaverse in future digital health. In addition, the form of NFT based on the BC facilitates mobilizing the healing and therapeutic behaviors of designers in the use of the advantage potential of HTD to promote health in achieving the SDG 3 (Good Health and Well-Being) and SDG 11 (Sustainable Cities and Communities). However, the quantitative analysis based on VOSviewer software in this paper focuses on the WOS core collection database. The conceptual BC-HTD framework is validated by industry experts and academics. As such, the follow-up research could conduct quantitative analysis of multiple databases, such as Scopus and ScienceDirect, and explore a practice approach for BC enhanced IM for HTD to promote health in the context of COVID-19 based on the conceptual BC-HTD framework.

Author Contributions: Conceptualization, Z.L., Z.Y., M.L. and Y.L.; methodology, Z.L., Z.Y., M.L., Y.L., M.O. and P.D.; software, Z.Y.; formal analysis, Z.L. and Z.Y.; investigation, Z.L., Z.Y. and M.L.; resources, Z.L., M.L. and Y.L.; data curation, Z.L. and Z.Y.; writing—original draft preparation, Z.L., Z.Y. and M.L.; writing—review and editing, Z.L., Z.Y., M.L., Y.L., M.O. and P.D.; validation, Z.L., Z.Y., M.L., M.O. and P.D.; visualization, Z.Y.; supervision, Z.L.; project administration, Z.L. and M.L.; funding acquisition, Z.L. All authors have read and agreed to the published version of the manuscript.

Funding: This research was funded by the Guangdong Provincial Department of Science and Technology 2021–2022 Overseas Famous Teacher Project: "Carbon Neutral Goal Oriented Sustainable Development Design Course (SUDEC)".

Institutional Review Board Statement: Not applicable.

Informed Consent Statement: Not applicable.

Data Availability Statement: Publicly available datasets were analyzed in this study. These data can be found here: https://login.webofknowledge.com/ (accessed on 30 April 2022).

Acknowledgments: The authors would like to thank all the people who are involved in this research including anonymous reviewers for their putting forward constructive suggestions to this paper. Z.L. would like to thank two-year Isabella who is the future blockchain enhanced healing and therapeutic design to him, and his student Yang for her hard work to make this project so meaningful with the end of the trilogy. Z.Y. would like to thank her supervisor for his continuous output of research topics that keep pace with the times, which let her harvest accumulated academic achievements while broadening her horizons, herself for her perseverance in the academic path, which makes her gain double happiness in the process of graduation, and the School of Design, South China University of Technology, for providing rich data resources and learning environment.

Conflicts of Interest: The authors declare that there is no conflict of interest.

References

1. Vowels, L.M.; Carnelley, K.B.; Stanton, S.C. Attachment anxiety predicts worse mental health outcomes during COVID-19: Evidence from two studies. *Pers. Individ. Differ.* **2022**, *185*, 111256. [CrossRef] [PubMed]
2. Jiao, W.Y.; Wang, L.N.; Liu, J.; Fang, S.F.; Jiao, F.Y.; Pettoello-Mantovani, M.; Somekh, E. Behavioral and Emotional Disorders in Children during the COVID-19 Epidemic. *J. Pediatr.* **2020**, *221*, 264–266. [CrossRef] [PubMed]
3. Yang, Y.; Zhao, Y.; Zhang, F.; Zhang, L.; Lingjian, Z. COVID-19 in Elderly Adults: Clinical Features, Molecular Mechanisms, and Proposed Strategies. *Aging Dis.* **2020**, *11*, 1481–1495. [CrossRef]
4. Wang, C. Mental health and social support of caregivers of children and adolescents with ASD and other developmental disorders during COVID-19 pandemic. *J. Affect. Disord.* **2021**, *6*, 100242. [CrossRef]
5. Qiu, Y.; Wu, Q.; Chen, R.; Guan, C. Research on psychological stress and mental health of medical staff in COVID-19 prevention and control. *Int. J. Disaster Risk Reduct.* **2021**, *65*, 102524. [CrossRef]
6. Coronavirus Disease (COVID-19) Pandemic. Available online: https://www.who.int/emergencies/diseases/novel-coronavirus-2019 (accessed on 23 October 2021).
7. Mumtaz, F.; Khan, M.I.; Zubair, M.; Dehpour, A.R. Neurobiology and consequences of social isolation stress in animal model—A comprehensive review. *Biomed. Pharmacother.* **2018**, *105*, 1205–1222. [CrossRef] [PubMed]
8. Amerio, A.; Brambilla, A.; Morganti, A.; Aguglia, A.; Bianchi, D.; Santi, F.; Costantini, L.; Odone, A.; Costanza, A.; Signorelli, C.; et al. COVID-19 Lockdown: Housing Built Environment's Effects on Mental Health. *Int. J. Environ. Res. Public Health* **2020**, *17*, 5973. [CrossRef]
9. Akbari, P.; Yazdanfar, S.-A.; Hosseini, S.-B.; Norouzian-Maleki, S. Housing and mental health during outbreak of COVID-19. *J. Build. Eng.* **2021**, *43*, 102919. [CrossRef]
10. Liu, Z.; Yang, Z.; Osmani, M. The Relationship between Sustainable Built Environment, Art Therapy and Therapeutic Design in Promoting Health and Well-Being. *Int. J. Environ. Res. Public Health* **2021**, *18*, 10906. [CrossRef]
11. Pinkerton, P.J.; Johnson, J.L. Design practices contribute to stabilization unit safety: Providing safety and dignity in facility design can be beneficial to the healing process. *Behav. Healthc. Exec.* **2017**, *37*, 53–56.
12. Tan, L.; Yu, K.; Shi, N.; Yang, C.; Wei, W.; Lu, H. Towards Secure and Privacy-Preserving Data Sharing for COVID-19 Medical Records: A Blockchain-Empowered Approach. *IEEE Trans. Netw. Sci. Eng.* **2021**, *9*, 271–281. [CrossRef]
13. Curtis, S.; Gesler, W.; Fabian, K.; Francis, S.; Priebe, S. Therapeutic Landscapes in Hospital Design: A Qualitative Assessment by Staff and Service Users of the Design of a New Mental Health Inpatient Unit. *Environ. Plan. C Gov. Policy* **2007**, *25*, 591–610. [CrossRef]
14. Day, K.; Carreon, D.; Stump, C. The therapeutic design of environments for people with dementia: A review of the empirical research. *Gerontologist* **2000**, *40*, 397–416. [CrossRef] [PubMed]
15. van Hoof, J.; Kort, H.H.; Van Waarde, H.; Blom, M. Environmental Interventions and the Design of Homes for Older Adults with Dementia: An Overview. *Am. J. Alzheimer's Dis. Other Dement.* **2010**, *25*, 202–232. [CrossRef] [PubMed]
16. Daykin, N.; Byrne, E.; Soteriou, T.; O'Connor, S. The impact of art, design and environment in mental healthcare: A systematic review of the literature. *J. R. Soc. Promot. Health* **2008**, *128*, 85–94. [CrossRef] [PubMed]
17. Kometiani, M.K.; Farmer, K.W. Exploring resilience through case studies of art therapy with sex trafficking survivors and their advocates. *Arts Psychother.* **2020**, *67*, 101582. [CrossRef]
18. David, I.A.B.; Or, M.B.; Regev, D.; Snir, S. Changes over time in therapeutic and art therapy working alliances in simulated art therapy sessions. *Arts Psychother.* **2021**, *75*, 101804. [CrossRef]
19. Virago, M.-C. Art psychotherapy and public health. *Public Health* **2021**, *196*, 150–157. [CrossRef]
20. Gruber, H.; Weiß, J. Therapeutic action in art therapy: Results of an empirical study. *Eur. J. Integr. Med.* **2010**, *4*, 179. [CrossRef]

21. Orkibi, H. The user-friendliness of drama: Implications for drama therapy and psychodrama admission and training. *Arts Psychother.* **2018**, *59*, 101–108. [CrossRef]
22. Wang, C.Y.; Xiao, R.S. Music and art therapy combined with cognitive behavioral therapy to treat adolescent anorexia patients. *Am. J. Transl. Res.* **2021**, *13*, 6534–6542. [PubMed]
23. Mehl, A.; Brauer, D.; Didwiszus, A.; Gelin-Kroz, B.; Pranga, D.; Zerm, R.; Gutenbrunner, C.; Reif, M.; Kröz, M. The Anthroposophic Art Therapy Assessment Paint (AART-ASSESS-P): A peer-report instrument to assess patients' pictorial expression during Anthroposophic Painting Therapy. *Explore-J. Sci. Health* **2021**, *17*, 541–548. [CrossRef] [PubMed]
24. Wright, T.; Liang, Y. Examining the Scholarly Literature: A Bibliometric Study of Journal Articles Related to Sustainability and the Arts. *Sustainability* **2019**, *11*, 3780. [CrossRef]
25. Nagra, A.; Stubbs, E.; Shameti, S.; Haq, S.; Gilbert, R. 1754 Virtual art therapy: Meeting the psychosocial needs of children and young people with a long term health condition during the COVID-19 pandemic. *Arch. Dis. Child.* **2021**, *106*, A479.
26. Renzi, A.; Verrusio, W.; Evangelista, A.; Messina, M.; Gaj, F.; Cacciafesta, M. Using drawings to express and represent one's emotional experience during the coronavirus disease 2019 pandemic: A case report of a woman living in a nursing home. *Psychogeriatrics* **2020**, *21*, 118–120. [CrossRef]
27. Khademi, F.; Rassouli, M.; Rafiei, F.; Moayedi, S.; Torres, M.; Marzban, N.; Haji, E.; Golitaleb, M. The effect of mandala colouring on anxiety in hospitalized COVID-19 patients: A randomized controlled clinical trial. *Int. J. Ment. Health Nurs.* **2021**, *30*, 1437–1444. [CrossRef]
28. Gupta, N. Singing Away the Social Distancing Blues: Art Therapy in a Time of Coronavirus. *J. Humanist. Psychol.* **2020**, *60*, 593–603. [CrossRef]
29. Shin, Y.; Hyoung, S.E.; Hong, J. A basic study on extraction of healing design elements for silver generation. *J. Digit. Interact. Des.* **2013**, *12*, 9–20.
30. Schweitzer, M.; Gilpin, L.; Frampton, S. Healing spaces: Elements of environmental design that make an impact on health. *J. Altern. Complement Med.* **2004**, *10*, S-71–S-83. [CrossRef]
31. Chalfont, G.E. Connection to Nature at the Building Edge: Towards a Therapeutic Architecture for Dementia Care Environments. Ph.D. Thesis, University of Sheffield, Sheffield, UK, May 2006.
32. Bergeman, J.A. Evaluating the Healing Effects of Design Elements in Therapeutic Landscapes: A Case Study of Rosecrance Healing Garden. Master's Thesis, University of Colorado, Denver, CO, USA, 11 May 2012.
33. Belčáková, I.; Galbavá, P.; Majorošová, M. Healing and therapeutic landscape design—Examples and experience of medical facilities. *Archnet-IJAR Int. J. Arch. Res.* **2018**, *12*, 128–151. [CrossRef]
34. Papoulias, C.; Csipke, E.; Rose, D.S.; McKellar, S.; Wykes, T.H. The psychiatric ward as a therapeutic space: Systematic review. *Br. J. Psychiatry* **2014**, *205*, 171–176. [CrossRef] [PubMed]
35. Keum, J. A Study on the Healing Space Planning of High School Based on Biophilic Design. *Youth Facil. Environ.* **2021**, *19*, 65–76.
36. Oh, J.Y.; Park, H.K. A Study on the Healing Effect of the Design Elements of the Healing Environment from the Environmental Stress Point of View. *Korean Soc. Sci. Art* **2019**, *37*, 215–226. [CrossRef]
37. Cioffi, J.M.; Fleming, A.; Wilkes, L.; Sinfield, M.; Le Miere, J. The effect of environmental change on residents with dementia: The perceptions of relatives and staff. *Dementia* **2007**, *6*, 215–231. [CrossRef]
38. Health—United Nations Sustainable Development. Available online: https://www.un.org/sustainabledevelopment/health/ (accessed on 23 October 2021).
39. Cities—United Nations Sustainable Development Action 2015. Available online: https://www.un.org/sustainabledevelopment/cities/ (accessed on 23 October 2021).
40. Wang, J.; Wu, P.; Wang, X.; Shou, W. The outlook of blockchain technology for construction engineering management. *Front. Eng. Manag.* **2017**, *4*, 67–75. [CrossRef]
41. Yang, R.; Wakefield, R.; Lyu, S.; Jayasuriya, S.; Han, F.; Yi, X.; Yang, X.; Amarasinghe, G.; Chen, S. Public and private blockchain in construction business process and information integration. *Autom. Constr.* **2020**, *118*, 103276. [CrossRef]
42. Kim, H.; Song, J. Simulation Algorithms for The Transmissibility to Evaluate Novel Coronavirus Pandemic. *J. Med. Biomed. Appl. Sci.* **2020**, *8*, 392–408.
43. Linn, L.A.; Koo, M.B. Blockchain for health data and its potential use in health it and health care related research. In *ONC/NIST Use of Blockchain for Healthcare and Research Workshop*; ONC/NIST: Gaithersburg, MD, USA, 2016.
44. Xie, Y.; Zhang, J.; Wang, H.; Liu, P.; Liu, S.; Huo, T.; Duan, Y.-Y.; Dong, Z.; Lu, L.; Ye, Z. Applications of Blockchain in the Medical Field: Narrative Review. *J. Med. Internet Res.* **2021**, *23*, e28613. [CrossRef]
45. D'Amico, A.; Bergonzoni, G.; Pini, A.; Currà, E. BIM for Healthy Buildings: An Integrated Approach of Architectural Design based on IAQ Prediction. *Sustainability* **2020**, *12*, 10417. [CrossRef]
46. Panah, R.S.; Kioumarsi, M. Application of Building Information Modelling (BIM) in the Health Monitoring and Maintenance Process: A Systematic Review. *Sensors* **2021**, *21*, 837. [CrossRef]
47. Jutraž, A.; Kukec, A.; Otorepec, P.; Lampič, L.; Pohleven, J.; Sandak, J.; Malovrh, K.; Sajn, M.V. Monitoring Environmental and Health Impact Data in BIM Models to Assure Healthy Living Environments. In Proceedings of the 37th Conference on Educa-tion-and-Research-in-Computer-Aided-Architectural-Design-in-Europe (eCAADe)/23rd Conference of the Iberoamerican-Society-Digital-Graphics (SIGraDi), Porto, Portugal, 11–13 September 2019.

48. Yang, C.; Han, F.; Wu, H.; Chen, Z. Heritage landscape information model (HLIM): Towards a con-textualised framework for digital landscape conservation in China. In *International Archives of the Photogrammetry, Remote Sensing and Spatial Information Sciences*; GonzalezAguilera, D., Remondino, F., Toschi, I., Rodri-guezGonzalvez, P., Stathopoulou, E., Eds.; Intl Soc Photogrammetry & Remote Sensing-Isprs: Hannover, Germany, 2019; Volume 42, pp. 1221–1227.
49. Langenheim, N.; White, M.; Tapper, N.; Livesley, S.J.; Ramirez-Lovering, D. Right tree, right place, right time: A visual-functional design approach to select and place trees for optimal shade benefit to commuting pedestrians. *Sust. Cities Soc.* **2020**, *52*, 101816. [CrossRef]
50. Zhao, L.; Zhou, Z. Research on Landscape Information Model Construction Based on Visualization Technology. In Proceedings of the 2020 3rd International Conference on Computer Information Science and Artificial Intelligence (CISAI) 2020, Hulunbuir, China, 25–27 September 2020.
51. White, M.G.; Haeusler, M.H.; Zavoleas, Y. Simulation of Plant-Agent Interactions in a Landscape Information Model. *J. Digit. Landsc. Archit.* **2020**, 188–197. [CrossRef]
52. Schaufler, C.; Schwimmer, E. City Information Modeling–an expedient tool for developing sustainable, responsive and resilient cities? *IOP Conf. Ser. Earth Environ. Sci.* **2020**, *588*, 032005. [CrossRef]
53. Dantas, H.S.; Sousa, J.M.M.S.; Melo, H.C. The Importance of City Information Modeling (CIM) for Cities' Sustainability. *IOP Conf. Ser. Earth Environ. Sci.* **2019**, *255*, 012074. [CrossRef]
54. Ganter, M.; Lützkendorf, T. Information management throughout the life cycle of buildings—Basics and new approaches such as blockchain. *IOP Conf. Ser. Earth Environ. Sci.* **2019**, *323*, 012110. [CrossRef]
55. Suliyanti, W.N.; Sari, R.F. Blockchain-based building information modeling. In Proceedings of the 2019 2nd International Conference on Applied Engineering (ICAE), Batam, Indonesia, 2–3 October 2019.
56. Erri Pradeep, A.S.; Yiu, T.W.; Amor, R. Leveraging blockchain technology in a BIM workflow: A literature review. In Proceedings of the International Conference on Smart Infrastructure and Construction 2019, ICSIC 2019: Driving Data-Informed Decision Making, Cambridge, UK, 8–10 July 2019.
57. Suliyanti, W.N.; Sari, R.F. Blockchain-based implementation of building information modeling information using hyperledger composer. *Sustainability* **2020**, *13*, 321. [CrossRef]
58. Harkness, A.; Gattamorta, K.A.; Estrada, Y.; Jimenez, D.; Kanamori, M.; Prado, G.; Behar-Zusman, V. Latinx health disparities research during COVID-19: Challenges and innovations. *Ann. Behav. Med.* **2020**, *54*, 544–547. [CrossRef] [PubMed]
59. Feng, Y. Innovative digital technology design and game healing-Serious Game's innovative design for children with special needs. In Proceedings of the 3rd International Conference on Energy Resources and Sustainable Development (ICERSD 2020), Harbin, China, 25–27 December 2020.
60. Liu, Z.; Yang, Z.; Xiao, C.; Zhang, K.; Osmani, M. An Investigation into Art Therapy Aided Health and Well-Being Research: A 75-Year Bibliometric Analysis. *Int. J. Environ. Res. Public Health* **2021**, *19*, 232. [CrossRef]
61. Chen, S.; Lu, Q.; Bai, J.; Deng, C.; Wang, Y.; Zhao, Y. Global publications on stigma between 1998–2018: A bibliometric analysis. *J. Affect. Disord.* **2020**, *274*, 363–371. [CrossRef]
62. Kim, M.; Kwon, S. Analysis of Research Trends in the Rock Blasting Field Using Co-Occurrence Keyword Analysis. *Explos. Blasting* **2022**, *40*, 1–16.
63. What is the Framework for Innovation? Design Council's Evolved Double Diamond | Design Council. Available online: https://www.designcouncil.org.uk/news-opinion/what-framework-innovation-design-councils-evolved-double-diamond (accessed on 10 January 2022).
64. Design Council | About Design | Managing Design | The Design Process. Available online: https://webarchive.nationalarchives.gov.uk/ukgwa/20080728102250mp_/http://www.designcouncil.org.uk/en/About-Design/managingdesign/The-Study-of-the-Design-Process/ (accessed on 10 January 2022).
65. Zhang, X.; Zhang, H.; Zhang, L.; Zhu, Y.; Hu, F. Double-Diamond Model-Based Orientation Guidance in Wearable Human–Machine Navigation Systems for Blind and Visually Impaired People. *Sensors* **2019**, *19*, 4670. [CrossRef]
66. Liu, J.; Nah, K. Design Collaboration Mode of Man–Computer Symbiosis in the Age of Intelligence. In *Advances in Intelligent Systems and Computing*; Ahram, T., Karwowski, W., Vergnano, A., Leali, F., Taiar, R., Eds.; Springer: Cham, Switzerland, 2020; Volume 1131, pp. 640–645.
67. Website of China Society of Industrial and Applied Mathematics (csiam. Org. CN). Available online: https://www.csiam.org.cn/home/article/detail/id/1532.html (accessed on 26 May 2022).
68. Gaminiesfahani, H.; Lozanovska, M.; Tucker, R. A Scoping Review of the Impact on Children of the Built Environment Design Characteristics of Healing Spaces. *HERD Health Environ. Res. Des. J.* **2020**, *13*, 98–114. [CrossRef] [PubMed]
69. Dovjak, M.; Shukuya, M.; Krainer, A. User-Centred Healing-Oriented Conditions in the Design of Hospital Environments. *Int. J. Environ. Res. Public Health* **2018**, *15*, 2140. [CrossRef] [PubMed]
70. Kim, M.; Lee, J. A Study on Healing Spatial Design Based on Multi-Sensory Stimulation Environment. *J. Korea Intitute Spat. Des.* **2021**, *16*, 69–80.
71. Liddicoat, S.; Badcock, P.; Killackey, E. Principles for designing the built environment of mental health services. *Lancet Psychiatry* **2020**, *7*, 915–920. [CrossRef]
72. Seo, J.; Cho, M. Analyzing Therapeutic Design Characteristics in the Indoor Atrium of the Outpatient Areas in Children's Hospitals Overseas. *J. Archit. Inst. Korea Plan. Des.* **2019**, *35*, 65–75.

73. Chun, M.Y.; Hwang, J.; Yun, J.Y.; Sim, G.Y.; Choi, G.-S.; Kim, G.H.; Jeong, J.H. The Effect of Seoul Dementia Healing Design Project on Cognition and Social Engagement. *Dement. Neurocogn. Disord.* **2020**, *19*, 140–151. [CrossRef]
74. Tan, J.; Jhin, S.Y. Healing Environment Design Research Trend—Focusing on analysis of domestic prior research. *J. Basic Des. Art* **2021**, *22*, 113–127. [CrossRef]
75. Mariana, Y.; Wijaya, Y. Healing garden implementation in rehabilitation centre at Jakarta as a concept of eco-architecture design. In Proceedings of the 3rd International Conference on Eco Engineering Development, Solo, Indonesia, 13–14 November 2019.
76. Iswoyo, H.; Yanti, C.W.B.; Jackson, S. Therapeutic landscape: Its virtue and suggestion for its application. *Enfermería Clínica* **2020**, *30*, 279–284. [CrossRef]
77. Chaudhury, H.; Cooke, H.A.; Cowie, H.; Razaghi, L. The influence of the physical environment on residents with dementia in long-term care settings: A review of the empirical literature. *Gerontologist* **2018**, *58*, e325–e337. [CrossRef]
78. The Physical Environment for People with Dementia. Available online: https://www.ncbi.nlm.nih.gov/books/NBK464816/pdf/Bookshelf_NBK464816.pdf (accessed on 10 January 2022).
79. Lundin, S. A Consciously Applied, Design-Driven Dialogue Can Improve Healing Architecture. *HERD Health Environ. Res. Des. J.* **2021**, *14*, 61–70. [CrossRef] [PubMed]
80. Lundin, S. Can healing architecture increase safety in the design of psychiatric wards? *Herd-Health Env. Res. Des. J.* **2021**, *14*, 106–117. [CrossRef] [PubMed]
81. Park, J.G.P. A study on healing environments and evidence-based design-Focused on healthcare environments in the United States. *J. Korea Inst. Healthc. Archit.* **2011**, *17*, 41–50.
82. Huisman, E.; Morales, E.; van Hoof, J.; Kort, H. Healing environment: A review of the impact of physical environmental factors on users. *Build. Environ.* **2012**, *58*, 70–80. [CrossRef]
83. Barnes, S.; Design, I.C.E.S. The design of caring environments and the quality of life of older people. *Ageing Soc.* **2002**, *22*, 75–789. [CrossRef]
84. Frazee, K.D. The Impact of Therapeutic Design on Social Engagement among Residents with Dementia during Programmed Activities in Dementia Care Units. Master's Thesis, Simon Fraser University, Burnaby, BC, Canada, 6 December 2010.
85. Hughes, L.; Dwivedi, Y.K.; Misra, S.K.; Rana, N.P.; Raghavan, V.; Akella, V. Blockchain research, practice and policy: Applications, benefits, limitations, emerging research themes and research agenda. *Int. J. Inf. Manag.* **2019**, *49*, 114–129. [CrossRef]
86. Foth, M. The promise of blockchain technology for interaction design. In Proceedings of the OzCHI '17: 29th Australian Conference on Human-Computer Interaction, Brisbane, QLD, Australia, 28 November–1 December 2017.
87. Lapointe, C.; Fishbane, L. The Blockchain Ethical Design Framework. *Innov. Technol. Gov. Glob.* **2019**, *12*, 50–71. [CrossRef]
88. Moosavi, J.; Naeni, L.M.; Fathollahi-Fard, A.M.; Fiore, U. Blockchain in supply chain management: A review, bibliometric, and network analysis. *Environ. Sci. Pollut. Res.* **2021**, 1–15. [CrossRef]
89. Guo, W.; Xiong, N.; Chao, H.-C.; Hussain, S.; Chen, G. Design and Analysis of Self-Adapted Task Scheduling Strategies in Wireless Sensor Networks. *Sensors* **2011**, *11*, 6533–6554. [CrossRef]
90. Vladimirova, A.V. Blockchain Revolution in Global Environmental Governance: Too Good to Be True? In *Internet Science*; Svetlana, S., Bodrunova, S.S., Koltsova, O., Følstad, A., Halpin, H., Kolozaridi, P., Kolozaridi, L., Smoliarova, A., Niedermayer, H., Eds.; Springer: Cham, Switzerland, 2019; Volume 11551, pp. 212–223.
91. Shojaei, A.; Wang, J.; Fenner, A. Exploring the feasibility of blockchain technology as an infrastructure for improving built asset sustainability. *Built Environ. Proj. Asset Manag.* **2019**, *10*, 184–199. [CrossRef]
92. Davidova, M.; McMeel, D. Codesigning with Blockchain for Synergetic Landscapes—The CoCreation of Blockchain Circular Economy through Systemic Design. In *CAADRIA 2020 ReAnthropocene—Des. Age Humans*; Holzer, D., Nakapan, W., Globa, A., Koh, I., Eds.; Association for Computer Aided Architectural Design in Asia: Bangkok, Thailand, 2020; Volume 2, pp. 333–342.
93. Suvajdzic, M.; Stojanovic, D.; Appelbaum, J. Blockchain art and blockchain facilitated art economy: Two ways in which art and blockchain collide. In Proceedings of the 2019 4th Technology Innovation Management and Engineering Science International Conference (TIMES-iCON), Bangkok, Thailand, 11–13 December 2019.
94. O'Dwyer, R. Limited edition: Producing artificial scarcity for digital art on the blockchain and its implications for the cultural industries. *Converg. Int. J. Res. New Media Technol.* **2018**, *26*, 874–894. [CrossRef]
95. Hölbl, M.; Kompara, M.; Kamišalić, A.; Nemec Zlatolas, L. A Systematic Review of the Use of Blockchain in Healthcare. *Symmetry* **2018**, *10*, 470. [CrossRef]
96. Wan, P.K.; Huang, L.; Holtskog, H. Blockchain-Enabled Information Sharing Within a Supply Chain: A Systematic Literature Review. *IEEE Access* **2020**, *8*, 49645–49656. [CrossRef]
97. Wang, P.; Qiao, S. Emerging Applications of Blockchain Technology on a Virtual Platform for English Teaching and Learning. *Wirel. Commun. Mob. Comput.* **2020**, *2020*, 6623466. [CrossRef]
98. Mora, H.; Morales-Morales, M.R.; Pujol-López, F.A.; Mollá-Sirvent, R. Social cryptocurrencies as model for enhancing sustainable development. *Kybernetes* **2021**, *50*, 2883–2916. [CrossRef]
99. Nikolakis, W.; John, L.; Krishnan, H. How Blockchain Can Shape Sustainable Global Value Chains: An Evidence, Verifiability, and Enforceability (EVE) Framework. *Sustainability* **2018**, *10*, 3926. [CrossRef]
100. Tseng, C.-T.; Shang, S. Exploring the Sustainability of the Intermediary Role in Blockchain. *Sustainability* **2021**, *13*, 1936. [CrossRef]
101. Pazaitis, A.; De Filippi, P.; Kostakis, V. Blockchain and value systems in the sharing economy: The illustrative case of Backfeed. *Technol. Forecast. Soc. Chang.* **2017**, *125*, 105–115. [CrossRef]

102. Chong, A.Y.L.; Lim, E.T.K.; Hua, X.; Zheng, S.; Tan, C.-W. Business on Chain: A Comparative Case Study of Five Blockchain-Inspired Business Models. *J. Assoc. Inf. Syst.* **2019**, *20*, 1308–1337. [CrossRef]
103. Tavares, E.C.; Meirelles, F.D.S.; Tavares, E.C.; Cunha, M.A.; Schunk, L.M. Blockchain in the Amazon: Creating public value and promoting sustainability. *Inf. Technol. Dev.* **2021**, *27*, 579–598. [CrossRef]
104. Liu, Z.; Osmani, M.; Demian, P.; Baldwin, A. A BIM-aided construction waste minimisation framework. *Autom. Constr.* **2015**, *59*, 1–23. [CrossRef]
105. Sun, H.; Fan, M.; Sharma, A. Design and implementation of construction prediction and management platform based on building information modelling and three-dimensional simulation technology in Industry 4.0. *IET Collab. Intell. Manuf.* **2021**, *3*, 224–232. [CrossRef]
106. Lee, J.-S.; Kwon, N.; Ham, N.-H.; Kim, J.-J.; Ahn, Y.-H. BIM-Based Digital Fabrication Process for a Free-Form Building Project in South Korea. *Adv. Civ. Eng.* **2019**, *2019*, 4163625. [CrossRef]
107. Lokshina, I.V.; Greguš, M.; Thomas, W.L. Application of integrated building information modeling, IoT and blockchain technologies in system design of a smart building. In *Procedia Computer Science*; Shakshuki, E., Yasar, A., Malik, H., Eds.; Elsevier Science BV: Amsterdam, The Netherlands, 2019; Volume 160, pp. 497–502.
108. Saoud, L.A.; Omran, J.; Hassan, B.; Vilutienė, T.; Kiaulakis, A. A method to predict change propagation within building information model. *J. Civ. Eng. Manag.* **2017**, *23*, 836–846. [CrossRef]
109. Schreuder, E.; Lebesque, L.; Bottenheft, C. Healing environments: What design factors really matter according to patients? An exploratory analysis. *Herd-Health Environ. Res. Des. J.* **2016**, *10*, 87–105. [CrossRef] [PubMed]
110. Li, Y.-W.; Cao, K. Establishment and application of intelligent city building information model based on BP neural network model. *Comput. Commun.* **2020**, *153*, 382–389. [CrossRef]
111. Ervin, S.; Hasbrouck, H. *Landscape Modeling—Digital Techniques for Landscape Visualisation*; McGraw-Hill: New York, NY, USA, 2001; pp. 221–223.
112. Zahrádková, V.; Achten, H. Required components for Landscape Information Modelling (LIM): A literature review. In *Peer Reviewed Proceedings of Digital Landscape Architecture 2015 at Anhalt University of Applied Sciences*; Buhmann, E., Ervin, S.M., Pietsch, M., Eds.; Vde Verlag GMBH: Berlin/Offenbach, Germany, 2015; pp. 284–288.
113. Gill, L. A 3D Landscape Information Model. Ph.D. Thesis, University of Sheffield, Sheffield, UK, 13 December 2013.
114. Zajíčková, V.; Achten, H. Landscape Information Modeling. In *eCAADe 2013 Computation and Performance*; Stouffs, R., Sariyildiz, S., Eds.; eCAADe (Education and research in Computer Aided Architectural Design in Europe) and Faculty of Architecture, Delft University of Technology: Delft, The Netherlands, 2013; Volume 2, pp. 515–523.
115. Wang, Z.; Jiang, H.; Zhang, W.; Liu, L. The Problem Analysis and Solution Suggestion in the Process of City Information Model Construction. In Proceedings of the 2020 4th International Conference on Smart Grid and Smart Cities (ICSGSC), Osaka, Japan, 18–21 August 2020.
116. Acampa, G.; Battisti, F.; Di Pietro, G.; Parisi, C.M. City information model for the optimization of urban maintenance cost. *AIP Conf. Proc.* **2021**, *2343*, 090002. [CrossRef]
117. Bott, H.; Grassl, G.; Anders, S. *Nachhaltige Stadtplanung: Lebendige Quartiere—Smart Cities—Resilienz*; DETAIL: München, Germany, 2018. [CrossRef]
118. Melo, H.C.; Tomé, S.; Silva, M.H.; Gonzales, M.M.; Gomes, D. Implementation of City Information Modeling (CIM) concepts in the process of management of the sewage system in Piumhi, Brazil. In Proceedings of the IOP Conference Series: Earth and Environmental Science, Brussels, Belgium, 5–7 February 2019.
119. Qian, Y.; Leng, J. CIM-based modeling and simulating technology roadmap for maintaining and managing Chinese rural traditional residential dwellings. *J. Build. Eng.* **2021**, *44*, 103248. [CrossRef]
120. Faltejsek, M.; Kocurova, P. Geographical information systems and monitoring of climatic conditions in cities. *IOP Conf. Ser. Earth Environ. Sci.* **2020**, *444*, 012016. [CrossRef]
121. da Silva Almeida, F.A.; Andrade, M.L.V.X. Considerações sobre o conceito de City Information Modeling. *InSitu São Paulo* **2018**, *4*, 21–38.
122. Xu, X.; Ding, L.; Luo, H.; Ma, L. From building information modeling to city information modeling. *J. Inf. Technol. Constr.* **2014**, *19*, 292–307.
123. Pereira, A.P.; Buzzo, M.; Zimermann, I.; Neto, F.H.; Malgarezi, H. A Descriptive 3D City Information Model Built from Infrastructure BIM: Capacity Building as a Strategy for Implementation. *Int. J. E-Plan. Res.* **2021**, *10*, 138–151. [CrossRef]
124. Kruglikov, S.V.; Zakharova, G.B. Multi-Agent Analysis of Scenarios for ldquoArctic Smart Cityrdquo. In Proceedings of the Computer-Aided Technologies in Applied Mathematics, Tomsk, Russia, 7–9 September 2020.
125. Wonderful Sharing of "Student Forum". Available online: https://mp.weixin.qq.com/s/A0N1AqBKykt-UZM_hmLpgg (accessed on 26 May 2022).
126. Aarikka-Stenroos, L.; Jaakkola, E. Value co-creation in knowledge intensive business services: A dyadic perspective on the joint problem solving process. *Ind. Mark. Manag.* **2012**, *41*, 15–26. [CrossRef]
127. Oliomogbe, G.O.; Smith, N.J. Value in megaprojects. *Organ. Technol. Manag. Constr. Int. J.* **2012**, *4*, 617–624. [CrossRef]
128. Chen, K. Value management in Blockchain technology related projects. In Proceedings of the 13th International Conference on Business Excellence (ICBE)—Sustainable Business Models and Innovation in the Knowledge Economy, Bucharest, Romania, 21–22 March 2019.

129. Liu, X.; Cai, S. An automatic decision-making value system with pharmaceutical manufacturing industry based on block-chain. In Proceedings of the 2018 11th International Symposium on Computational Intelligence and Design (ISCID), Hangzhou, China, 8–9 December 2018.
130. Chen, K.; Stegerean, R.; Nistor, R.L. Value Creation and Value Added in Blockchain Technology. In *International Management Conference*; Popa, I., Dobrin, C., Ciocoiu, C.N., Eds.; EDITURA ASE: Bucharest, Romania, 2018; pp. 862–878.
131. Reeve, A.; Nieberler-Walker, K.; Desha, C. Healing gardens in children's hospitals: Reflections on benefits, preferences and design from visitors' books. *Urban For. Urban Green.* **2017**, *26*, 48–56. [CrossRef]
132. Chakraborty, S.; Vishwanathan, B.; Jayachandran, P. Value attribution through provenance tracking in blockchain networks. In Proceedings of the 2019 IEEE International Conference on Web Services (ICWS), Milan, Italy, 8–13 July 2019.
133. Song, H.; Zhu, N.; Xue, R.; He, J.; Zhang, K.; Wang, J. Proof-of-Contribution consensus mechanism for blockchain and its application in intellectual property protection. *Inf. Process. Manag.* **2021**, *58*, 102507. [CrossRef]
134. Kharitonova, Y.S.; Rahmatulina, R.S. Technological Convergence and the Future of Copyright. In *Lecture Notes in Networks and Systems*; Popkova, E.G., Ed.; Springer: Cham, Switzerland, 2020; Volume 368, pp. 267–274.
135. Mackenzie, S.; Bērziņa, D. NFTs: Digital things and their criminal lives. *Crime Media Cult. Int. J.* **2021**, 1–16. [CrossRef]
136. Dowling, M. Is non-fungible token pricing driven by cryptocurrencies? *Financ. Res. Lett.* **2022**, *44*, 102097. [CrossRef]
137. van Haaften-Schick, L.; Whitaker, A. From the Artist's Contract to the blockchain ledger: New forms of artists' funding using equity and resale royalties. *J. Cult. Econ.* **2022**, *46*, 287–315. [CrossRef]
138. Lee, J.; Kwon, T. Distributed Watchdogs Based on Blockchain for Securing Industrial Internet of Things. *Sensors* **2021**, *21*, 4393. [CrossRef]
139. Hong, S.; Noh, Y.; Hwang, J.; Park, C. Fabasset: Unique digital asset management system for hyperledger fabric. In Proceedings of the 2020 IEEE 40th International Conference on Distributed Computing Systems (ICDCS), Singapore, Singapore, 29 November–1 December 2020.
140. Goyal, S.; Sanjith, K.; Sisodia, A.; Suhaas, N.M.; Akram, S. Transactions Process in Advanced Applications on Ethereum Blockchain Network. In Proceedings of the 2020 International Conference on Recent Trends on Electronics, Information, Communication & Technology (RTEICT), Bangalore, India, 12–13 November 2020.
141. Zhang, L. MRA: Metaverse Reference Architecture. In *Lecture Notes in Computer Science*; Tekinerdogan, B., Wang, Y., Zhang, L.J., Eds.; Springer: Berlin, Germany, 2021; Volume 12993, pp. 102–120.
142. Tan, T.M.; Salo, J. Ethical Marketing in the Blockchain-Based Sharing Economy: Theoretical Integration and Guiding Insights. *J. Bus. Ethic.* **2021**, 1–28. [CrossRef]

International Journal of
Environmental Research and Public Health

MDPI

Article

Air Pollution and Workplace Choice: Evidence from China

Tao Lin [1], Wenhao Qian [2,*], Hongwei Wang [2] and Yu Feng [2]

[1] School of Economics, Shanghai University of Finance and Economics, 777 Guoding Rd., Shanghai 200433, China; lintao@163.sufe.edu.cn
[2] School of Public Economics and Administration, Shanghai University of Finance and Economics, 777 Guoding Rd., Shanghai 200433, China; wangjue@mail.shufe.edu.cn (H.W.); fengyu101296@outlook.com (Y.F.)
* Correspondence: qianwenhao@163.sufe.edu.cn

Abstract: Understanding the impacts of air pollution on public health and individual behavior is crucial for optimal environmental policy design. Using 2015 census microdata in China, this paper examined the causal effect of air pollution on working place choice. The research design relies on a regression discontinuity design based on China's Huai River Policy. The discontinuity in air pollution caused by the Huai River Policy provides a natural experiment to estimate the impact of air pollution. The results show that air pollution significantly increases the possibility of individuals working near home. The positive effect of air pollution on working near home is more significant for women, the elderly, urban individuals and those individuals working in secondary and tertiary industries. This study improves our understanding of the health effects and avoidance behavior associated with environmental hazards, discusses the negative impact of air pollution on labor mobility and mismatch by making individuals work nearby, and emphasizes that strengthening air pollution control should be a long-term policy.

Keywords: air pollution; workplace; avoidance behavior; public health; regression discontinuity design; China

Citation: Lin, T.; Qian, W.; Wang, H.; Feng, Y. Air Pollution and Workplace Choice: Evidence from China. *IJERPH* **2022**, *19*, 8732. https://doi.org/10.3390/ijerph19148732

Academic Editors: Jie Chen, Qian Zhou and Ting Zhang

Received: 7 June 2022
Accepted: 15 July 2022
Published: 18 July 2022

1. Introduction

Air pollution is considered as a major issue for the community in China. In recent years, the problem of air pollution caused by China's rapid, extensive, and low-quality economic development has attracted great attention from the government and society. According to the 2019 China Ecological Environment Status Bulletin, a total of 218 days of severe and serious pollution have occurred in 337 prefecture-level and above cities across the country, of which the number of days of haze with $PM_{2.5}$ as the primary pollutant accounted for 78.8%. In 2019, the World Health Organization (WHO) has announced ten major threats to human health, among which air pollution ranks first. Epidemiological studies show that inhaling polluted air will lead to pathological changes in the lung and respiratory system, chronic damage to organs such as the heart and brain, resulting in cancer, stroke, heart and brain diseases [1].

Theoretically, there has been a growing body of economic literature on the impact of air pollution on human capital, including physical health [2–4], mental health [5,6], cognitive performance [7,8], and productivity [9–11]. Chen et al. [2] and Ebenstein et al. [12] provided the first quasi-experimental evidence of the impacts of sustained exposure to air pollution focused on China. They examined the impact of sustained pollution exposure on life expectancy, based on China's central winter heating system, and found that the winter heating policy raised PM_{10} levels by 46 percent in the region north of the Huai River between 2004 and 2012, causing a reduction in life expectancy of 3.4 years. Chang et al. [11] studied workers in the service sector, where jobs may be more cognitively demanding than those in the manufacturing sector. Using daily performance data for workers in two call centers in China, the authors estimated that a 10-unit increase in the Air Pollution Index (API) decreases the number of daily calls handled by a worker by 0.35 percent. These studies have reached the consensus that there exist negative effects of air pollution on human capital and productivity.

Facing high levels of pollution, individuals can take preventive measures to reduce exposure and mitigate the impact, such as defensive spending (e.g., face masks and air purifiers) [13,14] and migration [15,16]. Using sales indices for face masks and air purifiers from China's largest ecommerce platform, Taobao, Sun et al. [13] showed that people buy more face masks and air purifiers when ambient pollution levels exceed key alert thresholds. However, risk-compensating and avoidance behaviors in mitigation and adaptation are not adequately considered due to data limitations and identification problems. Increasing defense spending is not the only, nor is it a major preventive measure [17]. Due to the household registration system and high housing prices, it is difficult to migrate to cleaner cities in China [17]. Therefore, it is of theoretical and practical significance to explore how to avoid the impact of air pollution when air pollution is difficult to be controlled in the short term.

On the other hand, workplace choice is not only an important individual behavior, but also an important economic concept in labor economics. Choosing where to live and work will affect the welfare of individuals [18,19]. Whether the labor force can freely choose the place of work not only affects labor mobility, but also has an important impact on economic development [20]. Existing studies have studied the determinants of workplace choice from various aspects, such as income, education, and preference [21–23]. Using data of 833 knowledge-workers in high-technology and financial services, Frenkel et al. [23] investigated the residential location and workplace choice of knowledge-workers at the intra-metropolitan level by applying discrete choice models. They found that the most important factors are municipal socioeconomic level, housing affordability, and commuting time, while substantial secondary factors are cultural and educational land-use and culture-oriented lifestyle. However, there is little literature on the relationship between environment and workplace choice. Especially, when the environmental quality is deteriorating, workplace selection may become a way to avoid pollution risks. To reduce exposure, does air pollution affect people's workplace choice? We provide an answer to this question in the context of China.

This paper examined the causal effect of air pollution on working place choice. The data link the 2015 census microdata at the individual level with air pollution at the county level. We estimated the effect of air pollution on working near home using a regression discontinuity design (RD) based on China's Huai River Policy [2,12,14]. The policy dictates that areas to the north of the Huai River receive free or highly subsidized coal for indoor heating. This has led to the construction of a coal-powered centralized heating infrastructure only in cities north of the Huai River, with no equivalent system in cities to the south. The central heating system generates considerable air pollutants during coal combustion. The Huai River Policy provides a compelling natural experiment to estimate the causal effects of air pollution on working near home.

We obtained several findings. First, there is strong evidence that the air quality is deteriorating north of the Huai River. On average, the Huai River Policy increases PM_{10} concentrations in the north by 13.2 percent. Second, we found that the Huai River Policy has a large and statistically significant positive impact on working near home. The Huai River Policy increases the probability of working near home in the north by 5.6 percent on average. Third, we found that an additional 10 $\mu g/m^3$ of PM_{10} significantly increases the probability of working near home by 13.6 percent. Fourth, the positive effect of air pollution on working near home is more significant for women, the elderly, urban respondents, and those individuals who work in secondary industries. These findings are consistent with the existing literature that higher air pollution is associated with poorer health, higher mortality, and better self-protection [5,6,14].

We make two contributions to the literature. First, we contribute to a new but growing body of literature that identifies the coping strategies for environmental shocks. Relevant work in this body of literature has detected the role of risk-compensating behaviors, such as pollution information, household location choices, avoidance actions, and defensive spending (e.g., face masks and air purifiers), in helping households and individuals to cope with environmental shocks and reduce pollution exposure [13,14,24]. To our knowledge, our paper is the first to provide evidence on how changes in pollution levels affect work site selection. Individuals facing high levels of pollution may choose to work near home to reduce exposure and mitigate the impact. Although some empirical evidence confirms that households choose locations to seek a better environmental quality (i.e., sorting, migration) [15,25–31], migration is a long-term choice of a family and limited by many socio-economic factors (e.g., housing prices and health care). We argue that working near home may be a more common choice to avoid pollution than migration, especially due to China's generally high house prices and hukou restrictions. Our study extends the literature on pollution avoidance behavior.

Second, we contribute to the literature on labor mobility. This directly connects to the existing studies on the factors that drive labor mobility and cause labor spatial mismatch. Many scholars have studied this problem from many aspects (e.g., human capital and migration cost) [32–35]. We try to answer this question from a new perspective. We argue that outdoor air pollution reduces the cross-city mobility of labor and the possibility of cross-regional work. Our empirical results also verify this. In areas with more serious pollution, the labor force tends to work in local cities rather than across regions, which means that in areas with more serious air pollution, there is lower labor mobility. This may be an important reason for labor spatial mismatch [36,37] and market segmentation [38,39], as well as further widening of the income gap and unbalanced development among regions [20,40].

The rest of this paper is organized as follows. Section 2 provides background on the Huai River Policy and its recent reform. Section 3 introduces the data sources and variable design. Section 4 introduces the empirical strategy. Section 5 discusses the causal impact of air pollution on working near home. Section 6 presents the heterogeneity analysis. Section 7 discusses our results. Section 8 concludes this paper.

2. Institutional Background: Huai River Policy

As northern China is very cold in winter, respondents use various forms of heating. The traditional heating method in China is to burn loose coal in a stove. China's central heating system began in the 1950s. Referring to the heating mode of the Soviet Union, China initially established a central heating system mainly using coal as fuel.

Due to resource and budget constraints, central heating gives priority to the cold northern region, which is limited to cities in north, northeast and northwest China. Specifically, the Qinling Mountains and Huai River are the dividing line (the average temperature of this line in January is about 0 °C). Cities north of the Huai River have central heating, while cities south of the Huai River do not have heating. This is also known as the Huai River Policy.

Before 1978, subject to the level of economic development, the development speed of urban central heating was quite slow. Since the reform and opening up in 1978, China has gradually transitioned from a planned economy to a market economy. Many private sectors began to be born on a large scale, and the central heating system also entered a period of great development. By 2003, most northern cities in China had built central heating systems.

With the rapid growth of the urban central heating area, the financial burden of northern cities is increasing. The commercialization reform of heating implemented by the government in 2003 also changed the original free heating system [41]. The government abolished the welfare policy of free heating and began to charge for heating. In terms of charge management, the government still provides heating subsidies for employees of state-owned enterprises and institutions, but employees of non-state-owned enterprises do not enjoy the benefits. The commercialization of heating increases the heat cost of respondents. However, with the growth of urban construction and personal income, China's urban central heating area still maintains a stable and rapid growth. Due to the reform of the heating policy, coal consumption in northern China continues to grow [12,14]. Since 2003, although the central heating system has increased the household heating cost, it has not significantly reduced the household heating demand. Central heating in the northern regions in winter is still dominated by coal-fired heating.

However, with the rapid growth of the urban heating area, the heating mode with coal as the main fuel means that the air pollutants (soot, sulfur dioxide, etc.) produced by coal combustion also increase synchronously. Based on the quasi-natural experiment of the central heating policy in northern China, some scholars have found, through an RD design, that central heating leads to more serious air pollution in northern China [2,12,14,42]. This seems to be a contradiction and trade-off between heating and air quality. Figure 1 shows the locations of the Huai River (red line) and the air quality. It is clear that counties in northern China are much more polluted than those in southern China.

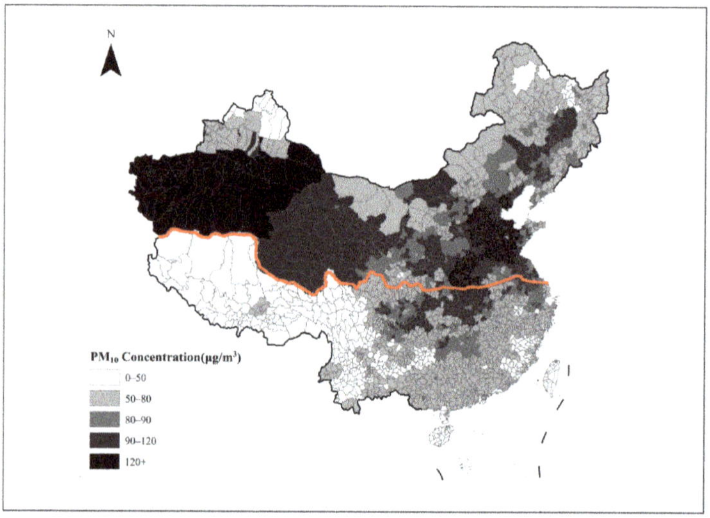

Figure 1. Huai River Policy line and PM_{10} concentrations. Note: The red line is China's Huai River/Qinling Mountain Range winter heating policy line. The polygons represent counties, the third level of the administrative hierarchy in China. The coloring of the polygons corresponds to average PM_{10} concentrations from 2014 to 2015.

In order to protect the environment and reduce the impact of pollution on respondents' health, the government has implemented many projects and policies to reduce the emission of pollutants. One of the biggest is the replacement of coal with natural gas or electricity as primary fuels for heating [43]. In 2013, Beijing first proposed and implemented the coal-to-gas policy, replacing coal with natural gas or electricity for central heating in urban areas, and providing subsidies to encourage families to replace coal-fired heating in rural areas. Later, other regions such as Tianjin and Hebei also launched the coal-to-gas policy in 2015 and 2016. It should be noted that despite the policy of changing coal to gas, the northern region still mainly depends on coal combustion to realize central heating in winter [43].

3. Data

3.1. Population Sample Survey Data

We mainly used the sampling survey data of 1% of China's population in 2015. These are nationwide data. China's National Bureau of Statistics conducted a national 1% population sampling survey at 0:00 on 1 November 2015. The survey takes the whole country as the whole and prefecture-level cities (regions, leagues, and prefectures) as the subpopulation. The stratification, two-stage, probability proportion and cluster sampling methods were adopted. The final sample size was 21.31 million, accounting for 1.55% of the total population of the country. The census takes the individual as the unit, and counts a number of indicators (e.g., gender and education). Additionally, it also counts a number of indicators of the family characteristics (e.g., hukou and family registration). The individual work information and characteristic data used in this paper are from this population sample survey.

3.2. Air Pollution

We collected the historical data of 1482 air monitoring stations in China from the air quality online monitoring and analysis platform (The real-time data are published on the following website: http://www.aqistudy.cn/ (accessed on 1 May 2021)). The platform is the largest real-time air quality monitoring network ever built in China, implementing the full coverage of municipalities, provincial capitals, cities with independent planning, all prefecture-level cities, key environmental protection cities, and environmental protection model cities. The data include the PM_{10} concentration per hour from 1 November 2014 to 30 October 2015. We calculated the pollution data of each county according to the monitoring information of each monitoring station. First, we averaged the hourly data of each monitoring station to obtain the daily monitoring results of each monitoring station. Then, taking the county as the center, we calculated the weighted average of air quality variable at each air monitoring station within 100 km to obtain the pollution index of each county every day. Among them, the reciprocal of the distance from each monitoring station to the county center was taken as the weight. Finally, we calculated the mean value of air quality indicators in each county during the sample period and finally obtained the PM_{10} concentration of 2501 counties in China.

3.3. Heating City

The list of heating cities is mainly from the statistical yearbook of China's urban construction. In order to be consistent with the statistical range of household mortality, we mainly used the list of heating cities in 2014. Among 295 prefecture-level and above cities in China, 130 northern cities had central heating, and the other 165 southern cities had no central heating system. Although the list of heating cities will change every year, the change is very small, only increasing or decreasing by one or two cities. Overall, the list of urban heating in China remains basically unchanged.

3.4. Control Variable

We controlled some individual characteristics, including gender, age, marriage, ethnicity, and type of hukou. We also controlled the meteorological conditions. The meteorological data come from the China meteorological data network (see http://data.cma.cn (accessed on 10 May 2021)). The original data are the observation data of 840 meteorological stations in China, including rainfall, average wind speed, air pressure, and minimum and maximum temperatures. We mainly used temperature, precipitation, relative humidity, and wind speed for control since they are the main meteorological factors affecting air pollutants. In order to calculate the above four variables of each county, we first interpolated the meteorological station data according to the inverse distance weighting (IDW) method to obtain a $1\text{km}\times1\text{km}$ grid layer across the country. Then, we extracted the above four variables of each county center based on this layer. Finally, we obtained the average temperature, precipitation, relative humidity, and wind speed of each county. The descriptive statistics of the variables are shown in Appendix A Table A1.

4. Empirical Strategy

Formally, a linear regression equation for the impact of air pollution on working near home was estimated as shown below:

$$Work_{ci} = \beta_0 + \beta_1 Pollution_c + \varphi X_{ci} + \varepsilon_{ci} \quad (1)$$

where subscripts c and i represent counties and respondents, respectively; the dependent variable *Work* is an indicator variable that equals one if respondent i works and lives on the same street, and zero otherwise; *Pollution* is the PM_{10} concentration of county c; X is the vector of observable features that may affect working place selection; ε is the disturbance term; and the coefficient β_1 measures the effect of PM_{10} exposure on working place selection after controlling for the available covariates.

The key challenge in estimating the causal impact of air pollution on working place choice is that variations in air pollution could be endogenous. Consistent estimation of β_1 requires that the unobserved determinants of working place selection do not covary with *Pollution* after adjustment for the observed covariates, but the validity of this assumption has been questioned by previous research. For example, air pollution levels are often associated with complex meteorological processes that can directly affect human health, and it is difficult to control for all these factors [12,17]. Other unobserved socio-economic factors (e.g., income) could also confound the impact of air pollution on working near home. Furthermore, pollution concentrations are prone to measurement error, which will attenuate the coefficient associated with PM_{10}. Therefore, the OLS estimate of β_1 is likely to be biased.

We addressed the potential endogeneity issue by constructing a regression discontinuity (RD) design based on the Huai River Policy (akin to existing studies such as Chen et al. [2], Ito and Zhang [14], and Ebenstein et al. [12]). As shown in Section 2, this policy provides free or heavily subsidized coal for heating north of the river but no subsidies to the south. This has led to the construction of a coal-powered centralized heating infrastructure only in cities north of the Huai River, with no equivalent system in cities to the south. Therefore, northern cities face more serious air pollution [12]. Near the Huai River boundary, the counties in the south become the opposite of the counties in the north. By comparing the difference in local air pollution caused by the Huai River Policy, we can estimate the local average treatment effect (LATE) of air pollution on individual workplace selection [2]. RD design is a quasi-experimental research design which could address the previous literature's limitations and provide a clear identification. Following Chen et al. [2] and Ebenstein et al. [12], we examined whether the Huai River Policy causes discontinuous changes in PM_{10} concentrations and the probability of working near home north of the river using the following specifications:

$$Pollution_c = \alpha_0 + \alpha_1 D_c + \alpha_2 f(Dist_c) + \kappa X_{ci} + \nu_{ci} \quad (2)$$

$$Work_{ci} = \delta_0 + \delta_1 D_c + \delta_2 f(Dist_c) + \gamma X_{ci} + \mu_{ci} \quad (3)$$

where *Dist* is the running variable, representing the shortest distance (in km) from each county to the Huai River, taking positive values for counties to the north of the Huai River and negative values for counties to the south; D is an indicator variable equal to one for counties with a positive value of *Dist*; $f(Dist)$ is a local regression function in *Dist* that allows the relationship between outcomes and the running variable (*Dist*) to vary on either side of the cutoff; in all our specifications, we also controlled for a vector of covariates (X), including demographic variables and meteorological conditions such as gender, ethnicity, age, marriage, hukou type, temperature, precipitation, relative humidity, and wind speed; μ and ν are the error terms.

The parameters of interest are α_1 and δ_1, which provide an estimate of whether there exist discontinuities in PM_{10} and the probability of working near home north of the river, after flexible adjustment for the covariates. If the key assumptions of the RD are satisfied, the estimated α_1 and δ_1 reveal the causal effect of the Huai River Policy on *Pollution* and *Work*.

The parameters α_1 and δ_1 can be identified by both non-parametric and parametric methods. In this paper, we emphasize the results using the non-parametric approach, as the parametric RD approach is found to have several undesirable statistical properties [43,44]. In practice, the key of the RD design is to select the optimal bandwidth to localize the regression fit near the cutoff. The choice of bandwidth involves balancing the conflicting goals of focusing comparisons close to the cutoff (for the "bias" concern) and having a large enough sample for reliable estimation (for the "precision" concern). We used the mean squared error (MSE) optimal and data-driven bandwidth selection methods (following Calonico et al. [45]; Calonico et al. [46]) and different kernel functions (i.e., triangular, epanech., and uniform) to calculate the optimal bandwidth. For all RD estimations, we estimated local linear regressions using observations within an optimal bandwidth. All standard errors were clustered at the county level.

There are two key assumptions for RD designs. One is that the treatment status is determined by a random assignment or forcing variable and cannot be manipulated [47]. In our design, the forcing variable is the shortest distance (in km) from each county to the Huai River, which cannot be manipulated, but we still give some evidence. Appendix A Figure A6 shows the histogram of county distance with a kernel density estimate, and Appendix A Figure A7 shows the McCrary test [48] (the McCrary test is an important test used to check whether there is any jump in the density of the forcing variable). We found that the density of *Dist* moves smoothly around the threshold. The second assumption is that any unobserved determinants of PM_{10} or whether respondents work near home may change smoothly as they cross the Huai River. In the Result section, we show that a variety of work- and pollution-related local characteristics (i.e., covariates) (we include two main sets of covariates that might be related to the outcome variables; the first set is a vector of weather variables, and the second set is a vector of the demographic characteristics) are smooth functions across the threshold. Additionally, we used non-parametric RD estimation involving additional covariates to increase the efficiency of the estimator (if the relevant assumption is not fully satisfied, adjustment for control variables could remove potential sources of bias and allow for causal inference. In addition, including balanced covariates in RD estimation could also increase the precision of the RD estimator) [49].

Next, we used a fuzzy RD approach [46,49,50] to estimate the impact of air pollution on working near home. This approach is used to assess the impact of an imperfect binary treatment where the probability of treatment rises at some threshold, but being above or below the threshold does not fully determine treatment status (i.e., imperfect compliance). In our context, exposure to PM_{10} increases significantly to the north of the Huai River, but pollution exists both north and south of the river, making our context naturally analogous to a fuzzy RD [51].

The fuzzy RD estimates can be estimated by taking the ratio of the estimated discontinuity in the probability of working near home to the estimated discontinuity in PM_{10}, by local linear regression at the Huai River (see Calonico et al. [51]). Actually, this result is an instrumental variable method, in which PM_{10} is instrumented by the Huai River Policy. The fuzzy RD estimates of the impact of PM_{10} on working near home are analogous to the 2SLS estimates [46,49,50]. Specifically, if the Huai River Policy only influences respondents working near home through its impact on PM_{10}, an important appeal of the results is that they produce estimates of the impact of units of PM_{10}, so the results are applicable in other settings (e.g., other developing countries with comparable impacts of units of PM_{10} concentrations).

5. Results

5.1. Summary Statistics and Graphical Analysis

Table 1 presents the summary statistics for the main variables and provides evidence on the validity of the RD design. Columns (1) and (2) report the mean values and SDs to the north and south of the Huai River. Column (3) documents the mean difference between the north and the south along with the standard error, and column (4) reports the discontinuous changes and standard errors along the Huai River using local linear regression.

Table 1. Summary statistics, means, and standard deviations/errors.

Variable	South	North	Difference in Means	Adjusted Difference
	(1)	(2)	(3)	(4)
		Panel A: Air pollution exposure at survey counties		
PM10	82.748	118.072	35.324 ***	11.225 ***
	(14.116)	(25.527)	(0.044)	(3.459)
		Panel B: Working place selection of respondents		
Working near home	0.646	0.758	0.112 ***	0.053 **
	(0.478)	(0.428)	(0.001)	(0.027)
		Panel C: Individual characteristics of respondents		
Gender	0.489	0.488	−0.002	−0.016
	(0.500)	(0.500)	(0.001)	(0.024)
Nation	0.057	0.021	−0.036 ***	−0.015
	(0.232)	(0.144)	(0.000)	(0.010)
Age	38.870	36.790	−2.080 ***	−2.281
	(20.570)	(20.799)	(0.045)	(1.599)
Marriage	0.742	0.750	0.008 ***	−0.007
	(0.438)	(0.433)	(0.001)	(0.010)
Hukou	0.435	0.308	−0.127 ***	−0.246
	(0.496)	(0.462)	(0.001)	(0.146)
		Panel D: Meteorological conditions at survey counties		
Temperature	16.510	13.569	−2.940 ***	0.094
	(1.201)	(1.653)	(0.003)	(0.154)
Precipitation	9.498	8.879	−0.619 ***	−0.205
	(0.290)	(0.182)	(0.001)	(0.131)
Relative humidity	77.127	65.521	−11.607 ***	0.776
	(2.916)	(5.033)	(0.009)	(0.657)
Wind speed	1.862	2.225	0.362 ***	−0.291
	(0.489)	(0.462)	(0.001)	(0.273)

Note: SDs for means and standard errors for mean differences are in parentheses. Adjusted differences in column (4) are the estimated discontinuity along the Huai River using local linear regression discontinuity with a triangular kernel and the MSE bandwidth selection method. ** Significant at 5%; *** significant at 1%.

We begin the analyses with an assessment of the Huai River Policy's impact on PM_{10}. Panel A shows large differences in PM_{10} concentrations between the south and the north of the Huai River. According to the local linear RD estimates, the north-south difference in PM_{10} along the Huai River is 11.2 $\mu g/m^3$. In Figure 2, we plot the binned averages of county-level PM_{10} concentrations against the distance from the county centroid to the Huai River. We also plot the polynomial fit of PM_{10} against the running variable. It is clear that PM_{10} has a discontinuous jump to the north of the river.

Similarly, we observed a large decline in the probability of working near home along the Huai River. Column (3) in Panel B of Table 1 shows that the share of respondents working near home in the north is much higher than in the south by 0.112. Column (4) shows that the local linear adjusted differences are 5.3 percent. In Figure 3, we plot the binned averages of working near home against the distance from the county centroid to the Huai River and its polynomial fit. An upward jump in the share of working near home is observed to the north of the river.

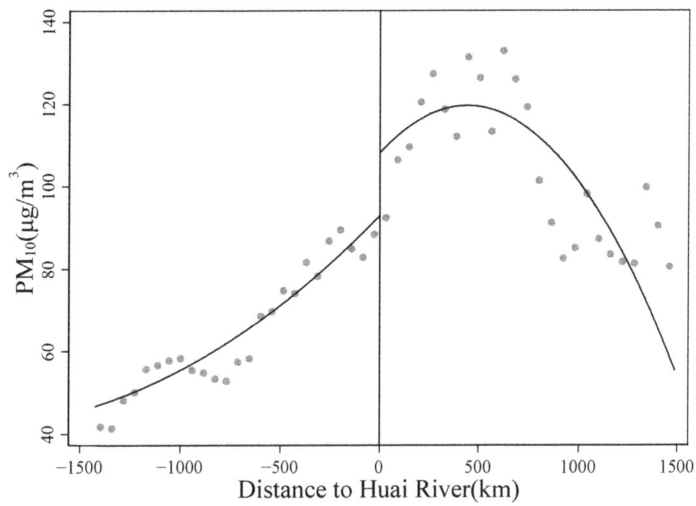

Figure 2. RD plot for PM_{10}. Note: The figure plots the binned averages of county-level PM_{10} concentrations against the running variable. The solid line represents a quartic polynomial fit of PM_{10} on each side of the threshold.

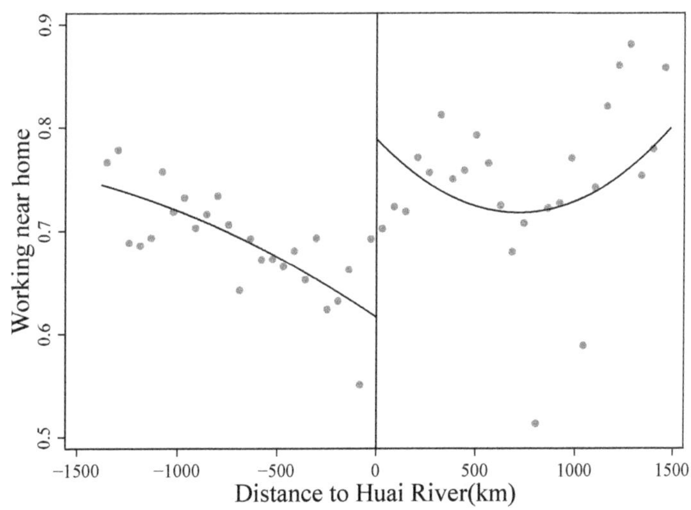

Figure 3. RD plot for work. Note: The figure shows the binned averages of working near home against the running variable. The solid line represents a quartic polynomial fit of working near home on each side of the threshold.

Additionally, though the RD design's identification assumption that unobservables change smoothly at the boundary is impossible to be tested directly, it would be reassuring if observable determinants change smoothly at the boundary. We tested a rich set of demographic characteristics and weather variables and present them in Panels C and D of Table 1. We found that, though there are differences between the south and north of the Huai River, the differences from the local linear regressions are much smaller and statistically insignificant at the boundary.

5.2. Impact of the Huai River Policy

Table 2 presents the RD estimates of PM_{10} and working near home along the Huai River using local linear regression. We used the mean squared error optimal bandwidth method (MSE) proposed by Calonico et al. [49] and Calonico et al. [46]. Each RD estimate also has the optimal bandwidth for both sides of the threshold and all standard errors are clustered at the county level. Columns (1)–(3) report the RD results using the three different kernel functions without inclusion of any other control variables. In Columns (4)–(6), we present the results for the same three regressions but with demographic and weather controls.

Table 2. RD estimates of the impacts of the Huai River Policy.

Variables	RD Estimates					
	(1)	(2)	(3)	(4)	(5)	(6)
	Panel A: Impact of the Huai River Policy on PM10					
PM10	11.225 ***	12.137 ***	12.213 ***	11.784 ***	12.603 ***	12.258 ***
	(3.459)	(3.447)	(4.750)	(3.367)	(3.360)	(4.706)
Bandwidth	538.312	500.452	455.471	546.285	507.273	452.124
	Panel B: Impact of the Huai River Policy on working near home					
Working near home	0.053 **	0.058 **	0.064 **	0.056 **	0.059 **	0.059 **
	(0.027)	(0.028)	(0.030)	(0.026)	(0.028)	(0.029)
Bandwidth	274.914	241.226	208.783	279.352	250.149	218.813
Observations	802,178	802,178	802,178	802,178	802,178	802,178
Controls	N	N	N	Y	Y	Y
Kernel	Triangular	Epanech.	Uniform	Triangular	Epanech.	Uniform

Note: Each cell in the table represents a separate RD estimate along the Huai River using local linear regressions with different kernel functions. Robust standard errors in parentheses are clustered at the county level. Controls include weather information and sociodemographic variables defined in Table 1. ** Significant at 5%; *** significant at 1%.

Different kernel functions and the inclusion of control variables did not significantly change the estimate. We emphasize the estimates from the most comprehensive specification in Column (4). Panel A of Table 2 shows that the impact of the Huai River Policy on PM_{10}. We found that the Huai River Policy increases PM_{10} concentrations in the north by 11.8 $\mu g/m^3$ on average, which is equivalent to an increase of 13.2 percent in the mean in the regression sample (given the average PM_{10} is 89.2 $\mu g/m^3$).

Panel B of Table 2 reports the RD estimates for working near home. We found that the Huai River Policy has a large and statistically significant positive impact on working near home. Specifically, the Huai River Policy increases the probability of working near home in the north by 5.6 percent on average, which is equivalent to an increase of 8 percent (given the sample mean is 0.702). These regression results echo the graphical results that the Huai River Policy causes a significant deterioration in the air quality and an increase in the probability of working near home in northern China.

5.3. Impact of PM_{10} on Work

Table 3 presents the estimated effects of an additional 10-$\mu g/m^3$ increase in PM_{10} exposure on respondents working near home. Panel A reports the fuzzy RD estimates using three different kernel functions. To make sure that our analyses are not sensitive to different specifications, we estimated the fuzzy RD results without and with weather and demographic characteristics. We found that the RD results are reasonably robust for different kernel functions and control variables. We present the results in Column (4), where the triangular kernel function is used and both demographic and weather conditions are controlled. Panel A shows that an additional 10 $\mu g/m^3$ in PM_{10} significantly increases the probability of working near home by 13.6 percent. This observation is consistent with the results in the previous section and indicates that the Huai River Policy affects the probability of respondents working near home via its impact on PM_{10}.

Table 3. Fuzzy RD and OLS estimates of the impacts of PM_{10} on work.

Variables	Panel A: Fuzzy RD Estimates						Panel B: OLS Estimates	
	(1)	(2)	(3)	(4)	(5)	(6)	(1)	(2)
PM10 (per 10 points)	0.132 ***	0.157 ***	0.152 **	0.136 ***	0.155 ***	0.151 **	0.005 ***	0.005 ***
	(0.043)	(0.046)	(0.068)	(0.043)	(0.042)	(0.064)	(0.001)	(0.001)
Bandwidth	401.273	396.563	374.286	412.204	415.305	345.638		
Observations	802,178	802,178	802,178	802,178	802,178	802,178	802,178	802,178
Controls	N	N	N	Y	Y	Y	N	Y
Kernel	Triangular	Epanech.	Uniform	Triangular	Epanech.	Uniform		

Note: Each cell in the table represents a separate estimate or regression. Columns (1)–(6) report the fuzzy RD results estimating the impact of 10 $\mu g/m^3$ of PM_{10} on work, treating distance from the Huai River as the forcing variable and PM_{10} as the treating variable, with the Huai River representing a "fuzzy" discontinuity in the level of air pollution exposure. Column (1) and (2) in Panel B report the OLS estimates of the association between PM_{10} and work. Robust standard errors in parentheses are clustered at the county level. Controls include weather information and sociodemographic variables defined in Table 1. ** Significant at 5%; *** significant at 1%.

Panel B reports the OLS results for comparison. The estimate in Column (2) of Panel B implies that a 10-point increase in PM_{10} is associated with a 0.5% increase in the probability of working near home. In addition, it is worth emphasizing that, relative to the OLS estimates, the fuzzy RD estimates are more stable and larger in magnitudes, suggesting that OLS estimates are biased downward possibly due primarily to omitted variables and/or measurement errors. These findings are remarkably stable and are not affected by the inclusion of different controls and alternative ways to estimate the RD coefficient and standard errors.

5.4. Robustness Checks

We conducted several robustness checks to help assess the validity of our results. First, we used the air quality index (AQI) as an independent variable and re-estimate. We used the PM_{10} concentration in the main tables because PM_{10} is the main pollutant produced by coal-fired heating. Coal combustion produces a variety of pollutants. We used the overall measure of ambient air quality, the AQI, to measure pollution. Six air pollutants (i.e., $PM_{2.5}$, PM_{10}, SO_2, NO_2, CO, and O_3) were used to compute the AQI (the Ministry of Environmental Protection: http://www.mee.gov.cn/ (accessed on 10 May 2021)). In reality, the Ministry of Environmental Protection (MEP) often uses it to inform the public of pollution levels [43]. The larger the AQI score, the higher the air pollution level. Appendix A Table A2 reports the results using the AQI. In general, we found that the results are similar in sign and magnitude to those in Tables 2 and 3.

Second, we constructed two alternative measures for respondents working near home: whether respondents drive to work (Yes = 1) and the time required for going to work (in minutes). If one works near home, this means that they are less likely to drive to work, and that the time required to go to work should be shorter. Appendix A Figures A1 and A2 present the RD plots. Table A3 reports the estimated results. We found air pollution significantly decreases the probability of respondent driving to work and the time required for going to work. These results support our findings in the main analysis.

Third, we conducted a placebo test to assess the significance of these findings, exploring whether discontinuities are observed in other regions of China. We estimated the discontinuities in PM_{10} and working near home at 100 km intervals north and south of the Huai River across China as well as at the actual Huai River (which is reported as the 0 km displacement). Figure A3 presents estimates and shows that the only statistically significant discontinuous changes in PM_{10} and working near home occur at the actual Huai River. In all other instances, the estimated effect of zero is within the 95% confidence interval.

Fourth, we then examined the sensitivity of our RD estimates to small changes in bandwidths. We set the bandwidths to range from 100 km to 1000 km. For each bandwidth, we estimated the discontinuities in PM_{10} and working near home by local linear regression and second-order polynomial regression, respectively. As shown in Figures A4 and A5 in the Appendix A, the estimate results remain reasonably robust to alternative bandwidths.

Finally, given that air pollution may be responsible for migration in China [15], we explored the potential impact of migration on the results in two ways. One way was to test whether air pollution causes respondents to migrate. We defined migration equal to one if the respondent migrated in the past two years, and zero otherwise, and then investigated the impact of the Huai River Policy and PM_{10} on migration using an RD design. The RD estimates are shown in Table A4. The results in Panel A show that there is no difference in mobility between the north and the south. The results in Panel B show that air pollution has no effect on population migration. This result is consistent with the results of Ebenstein et al. [12]. They assessed migration patterns in China and found that migration did not appreciably alter people's lifetime exposure to air pollution. There is little evidence that there are many environmental migrations in China. The second way was to exclude those samples with a residence duration of less than 5 years at the same prefecture city level and re-estimate the models (following Ding et al. [52]). Appendix A Table A5 reports the results of the RD estimates. In general, we found that the results are similar in sign and magnitude to those in Tables 2 and 3.

6. Heterogeneity Analysis

To better understand the effect of air pollution on working place choice, we examined different subgroups based on respondents' demographic characteristics. It is helpful for researchers to further study the research topic and for policy makers to design appropriate policies.

6.1. Gender Difference

We examine the gender difference in Table 4. We compared males and females and found that exposure to PM_{10} had a greater positive effect on females working near home than males in general. Panel A summarize the RD estimates of the Huai River Policy on working near home for both men and women. We estimated that the increase in the probability of working near home at the Huai River boundary is around 5.1% and 6.2% (statistically significant) for males and females, respectively. Panel B summarizes the fuzzy RD estimates of PM_{10} on the probability of respondents working near home for both men and women. A 10-unit increase in PM_{10} will significantly increase the probability of working near home for males and females by 9.8% and 11.1%, respectively. These results indicate that females suffer from air pollution more than males. This is consistent with existing studies which show that women have a higher risk for cognitive and health declines associated with increased exposure to air pollution (e.g., Kim et al. [53]; Zhang et al. [7]; Ding et al. [52]).

Table 4. The impacts of PM_{10} on work by gender.

Variables	Panel A: Impacts of Huai River Policy on Work				Panel B: Impacts of PM10 on Work			
	Males		Females		Males		Females	
	(1)	(2)	(3)	(4)	(1)	(2)	(3)	(4)
Working near home	0.051 **	0.045 *	0.062 **	0.087 ***	0.098 *	0.079 *	0.111 **	0.090 *
	(0.026)	(0.024)	(0.029)	(0.033)	(0.051)	(0.043)	(0.054)	(0.052)
Bandwidth	311.742	264.165	278.618	297.873	307.526	229.815	291.463	233.927
Observations	463,585	463,585	338,593	338,593	463,585	463,585	338,593	338,593
Controls	Y	Y	Y	Y	Y	Y	Y	Y
Kernel	Triangular	Uniform	Triangular	Uniform	Triangular	Uniform	Triangular	Uniform

Note: Each cell in the table represents a separate estimate or regression. Panel A reports the RD results estimating the impact of the Huai River Policy on work. Panel B reports the fuzzy RD results estimating the impact of 10 $\mu g/m^3$ of PM_{10} on work, treating distance from the Huai River as the forcing variable and PM_{10} as the treating variable, with the Huai River representing a "fuzzy" discontinuity in the level of air pollution exposure. Robust standard errors in parentheses are clustered at the county level. Controls include weather information and sociodemographic variables defined in Table 1. * Significant at 10%; ** significant at 5%; *** significant at 1%.

6.2. Age Group Difference

Second, in Table 5, we investigate the impact of air pollution on working place choice for different age groups. We divided the sample into two age groups: young people (aged < 50 years) and old people (aged ≥ 50 years). Panel A summarizes the RD estimates of the Huai River Policy on working near home for both elderly and young people. We found that the Huai River Policy has a positive and statistically significant impact on working near home for the elderly. The increase in the probability of the elderly working near home at the threshold is around 6.8%. In contrast, the magnitude of the estimates is much smaller and statistically insignificant for the young group. Based on the fuzzy RD results in Panel B, a 10-unit increase in PM_{10} will increase the probability of the elderly working near home by 14.8%. Since the elderly suffer from air pollution resulting from the Huai River Policy [43], they are more sensitive to air pollution and are more likely to choose to work near home to mitigate the negative impact of air pollution on health.

Table 5. The impacts of PM_{10} on work by age.

Variables	Panel A: Impacts of Huai River Policy				Panel B: Impacts of PM10 on Work			
	Age < 50		Age ≥ 50		Age < 50		Age ≥ 50	
	(1)	(2)	(3)	(4)	(1)	(2)	(3)	(4)
Working near home	0.048	0.049	0.068 ***	0.093 ***	0.100	0.115	0.148 **	0.144 **
	(0.030)	(0.033)	(0.020)	(0.020)	(0.133)	(0.327)	(0.074)	(0.065)
Bandwidth	291.291	206.563	241.578	319.535	279.627	167.415	284.219	314.158
Observations	600,252	600,252	201,926	201,926	600,252	600,252	201,926	201,926
Controls	Y	Y	Y	Y	Y	Y	Y	Y
Kernel	Triangular	Uniform	Triangular	Uniform	Triangular	Uniform	Triangular	Uniform

Note: Each cell in the table represents a separate estimate or regression. Panel A reports the RD results estimating the impact of the Huai River Policy on work. Panel B reports the fuzzy RD results estimating the impact of 10 $\mu g/m^3$ of PM_{10} on work, treating distance from the Huai River as the forcing variable and PM_{10} as the treating variable, with the Huai River representing a "fuzzy" discontinuity at the level of air pollution exposure. Robust standard errors in parentheses are clustered to the county level. Controls include weather information and sociodemographic variables defined in Table 1. ** Significant at 5%; *** significant at 1%.

6.3. Rural–Urban Difference

We also examined how air pollution affects workplace choice behavior between rural and urban individuals. Samples were divided into two groups by the type of hukou (i.e., household registration): urban group and rural group. Table 6 reports the RD estimates for each group. In Panel A, we find that the Huai River Policy significantly increases the probability of working near home by 18.7% for urban respondents, but insignificantly for rural respondents. The fuzzy RD results in Panel B show that a 10-unit increase in PM_{10} will increase the probability of urban respondent working near home by 25.1%. There are three reasons. First, air pollution in urban areas is more serious than in rural areas [43], because there are more pollution emissions (e.g., industrial emissions) and higher implementation intensities for the Huai River Policy in urban areas. Second, air pollution information is readily available in urban areas, but the same information is difficult to obtain in rural areas. Air pollution information is a key determinant of pollution avoidance and associated health impacts [24,43]. Third, due to the nature of the work and transportation cost, the work of rural individuals is relatively fixed (e.g., work on the field). In urban areas, the traffic is relatively perfect and individuals have more job choices. Thus, the effect of air pollution on working near home for the urban group is more significant than that for the rural group.

Table 6. The impacts of PM_{10} on work by rural–urban.

Variables	Panel A: Impacts of Huai River Policy				Panel B: Impacts of PM10 on Work			
	Rural		Urban		Rural		Urban	
	(1)	(2)	(3)	(4)	(1)	(2)	(3)	(4)
Working near home	0.025	0.027	0.187 ***	0.197 ***	0.045	0.034	0.251 **	0.185 *
	(0.025)	(0.025)	(0.043)	(0.046)	(0.055)	(0.048)	(0.128)	(0.098)
Bandwidth	293.338	238.894	310.852	251.616	276.526	204.354	285.683	352.119
Observations	554,756	554,756	247,422	247,422	554,756	554,756	247,422	247,422
Controls	Y	Y	Y	Y	Y	Y	Y	Y
Kernel	Triangular	Uniform	Triangular	Uniform	Triangular	Uniform	Triangular	Uniform

Note: Each cell in the table represents a separate estimate or regression. Panel A reports the RD results estimating the impact of the Huai River Policy on work. Panel B reports the fuzzy RD results estimating the impact of 10 $\mu g/m^3$ of PM_{10} on work, treating distance from the Huai River as the forcing variable and PM_{10} as the treating variable, with the Huai River representing a "fuzzy" discontinuity in the level of air pollution exposure. Robust standard errors in parentheses are clustered at the county level. Controls include weather information and sociodemographic variables defined in Table 1. * Significant at 10%; ** significant at 5%; *** significant at 1%.

6.4. Occupation Difference

Last, we examined the occupation difference. Samples were divided into three groups by the type of occupation of respondents: primary industry, secondary industry, and tertiary industry. Table 7 reports the RD estimates for each group. Panel A summarizes the RD estimates of the Huai River Policy for the three groups. We found that the Huai River Policy has a negative and statistically significant impact on working near home for those respondents who work in secondary and tertiary industries. Specifically, the increase in the probability of working near home at the threshold is around 16.1% and 14.7% for those respondents who work in secondary and tertiary industries, respectively. Correspondingly, a 10-unit increase in PM_{10} will increase the probability of working near home by 23.5% and 16.9%, respectively. However, this effect does not exist for those respondents who work in primary industries. This is due to the nature of the primary industries. Primary industries depend on natural conditions (e.g., land and trees), which are immovable. Thus, for those respondents who work in the primary industries, work and workplace cannot be changed at will.

Table 7. The impacts of PM_{10} on work by occupation.

Variables	Panel A: Impacts of Huai River Policy			Panel B: Impacts of PM10 on Work		
	Ind1	Ind2	Ind3	Ind1	Ind2	Ind3
	(1)	(2)	(3)	(1)	(2)	(3)
Working near home	0.003	0.161 ***	0.147 ***	0.001	0.235 ***	0.169 ***
	(0.004)	(0.040)	(0.030)	(0.004)	(0.067)	(0.055)
Bandwidth	399.085	342.017	379.282	315.258	349.973	373.902
Observations	263,564	235,168	303,446	263,564	235,168	303,446
Controls	Y	Y	Y	Y	Y	Y
Kernel	Triangular	Triangular	Triangular	Triangular	Triangular	Triangular

Note: Each cell in the table represents a separate estimate or regression. Panel A reports the RD results estimating the impact of the Huai River Policy on work. Panel B reports the fuzzy RD results estimating the impact of 10 $\mu g/m^3$ of PM_{10} on work, treating distance from the Huai River as the forcing variable and PM_{10} as the treating variable, with the Huai River representing a "fuzzy" discontinuity in the level of air pollution exposure. Robust standard errors in parentheses are clustered at the county level. Controls include weather information and sociodemographic variables defined in Table 1. *** Significant at 1%.

7. Discussion

Our RD analysis showed that an additional 10 $\mu g/m^3$ in PM_{10} significantly increases the probability of working near home by 13.6 percent. This implies that, facing high levels of pollution, individuals would choose to work nearby to reduce pollution exposure given that migration is restricted. As far as its mechanism and theoretical framework is concerned, the main explanation for our findings may be that air pollution has a significant negative impact on physical and mental health, and this impact is well known [8,12,17]. This mechanism is supported by many related literature reports. Using the same identification strategy as this article, Chen et al. [2] and Ebenstein et al. [12] found that the winter heating policy raised PM_{10} levels by 46 percent in the region north of the Huai River between 2004 and 2012, causing a reduction in life expectancy of 3.4 years. Individuals can take preventive measures to reduce exposure and mitigate the negative impact of air pollution. Based on sales data on air purifiers, Ito and Zhang [14] estimated that a household is willing to pay \$13.40 annually to remove 10 mg/m^3 of PM_{10} and \$32.70 annually to eliminate the increased pollution caused by China's winter heating policy. Willingness to pay for air quality is one of the risk aversion behaviors. Our findings are consistent with the above literature. To mitigate this negative impact of outdoor air pollution, individuals choose to work near home. If one works near home, which means that they are less likely to drive to work and need a shorter amount of time to get to work, they can be less exposed to air pollution. This is a natural and instinctive response to air pollution. Our findings confirm and expand the conclusions of the existing literature. After 2013, China's real-time pollution monitoring and disclosure program (henceforth, the information program) was launched and marked a turning point in pollution information access and awareness [24]. Therefore, individuals can more easily obtain air quality information and pay attention to health. Based on personal welfare and utility maximization, individuals are more likely to choose to work near home to reduce pollution exposure.

On the other hand, in terms of workplace choice behavior, our results show that in areas with more serious pollution, the labor force tends to work in local cities rather than across regions. A natural question is, what does that mean? A direct result and interpretation is that outdoor air pollution reduces the cross-regional flow of labor and reduces the possibility of labor working across regions. In areas with more serious pollution, the labor mobility is lower, which is an important reason for labor spatial mismatch and market segmentation, as well as further widening of the income gap and unbalanced development among regions [20,40]. In fact, air pollution is aggravating the segmentation of the labor market as a new natural factor [54]. This is a clue that has not been fully studied in the previous literature. The existing studies mainly believe that rivers and terrain are the natural determinants of labor market segmentation [55,56]. In other words, our results show that if air pollution is controlled and reduced, individuals can choose to work further away. This can promote labor mobility and balanced development. These are the theoretical and practical implications of the paper. Our theoretical implication is to build a bridge between environmental economics and labor economics from the perspective of labor mobility. The practical implication is that we have emphasized the necessity of pollution control and that environmental regulation policies should be implemented for a long time.

8. Conclusions

Air pollution is considered as a major issue for the community in China. Understanding how changes in pollution levels affect public health and avoidance behaviors is crucial for optimal environmental policy design. We used China's Huai River Policy as an RD design to evaluate the causal impact of air pollution on working place choice. The Huai River Policy led to the construction of a coal-powered centralized heating infrastructure only in cities north of the Huai River, with no equivalent system in cities to the south. The discontinuity in air pollution caused by the Huai River Policy provides a natural experiment to estimate the impact of air pollution. The data link the 2015 census microdata at the individual level with air pollution at the county level.

Our results show that the Huai River Policy has increased PM_{10} concentrations by 13.2 percent and caused a 5.6 percent increase in the probability of individuals working near home. This implies that an additional 10 $\mu g/m^3$ in PM_{10} would significantly increase the probability of working near home by 13.6 percent in China, which means that individuals would choose to work nearby to reduce pollution exposure and mitigate the negative impact of pollution on health. Heterogeneity analyses showed that the positive effect of air pollution on the choice to work nearby is more significant for women, the elderly, urban respondents and those respondents who work in secondary and tertiary industries. Following the rich literature, we provided several explanations for our results and discussed the negative impact of air pollution on labor mobility and mismatch by making individuals work nearby.

The results provide new evidence on how people protect themselves against pollution. Individuals facing high levels of pollution would choose to work nearby to reduce exposure and mitigate the impact. This paper deepens our understanding of coping strategies and avoidance behaviors to environmental shocks and highlights a negative impact on labor mobility and regional balanced development. This is crucial for the regional balanced development policy and environmental policy design in many developing countries. Our results go beyond the trade-off between the economy and environment, and show that worsening air pollution could reduce the potential for economic growth. One policy implication is that to improve the economic quality, air pollution must be further controlled. If air pollution decreases significantly, the resulting rise in labor mobility will promote productivity and achieve a win-win situation for the economy and the environment. One limitation of this paper is that, in recent years, China's air quality has been continuously improved and the household registration system has been relaxed, and thus people's risk aversion behavior may change (e.g., migration), which may make the estimation of this paper a higher bound. In future research, we will use updated data and clearer identification strategies to verify the above problems.

Author Contributions: Conceptualization, T.L. and H.W.; formal analysis, T.L. and W.Q.; funding acquisition, T.L. and W.Q.; methodology, W.Q.; software, H.W. and Y.F.; visualization, W.Q.; writing—original draft, T.L. and W.Q.; writing—review and editing, T.L., W.Q., H.W. and Y.F. All authors have read and agreed to the published version of the manuscript.

Funding: This paper was supported by two funds: 1. Graduate Innovation Fund of School of Economics, Shanghai University of Finance and Economics: Market integration and high-quality development of regional economy: theory and empirical study, no. kycx-2020-05. 2. Graduate Innovation Fund of Shanghai University of Finance and Economics: Does buying a marriage house for children lead to poverty: From the perspective of intergenerational transfer in rural families, no. CXJJ-2021-342.

Institutional Review Board Statement: Not applicable.

Informed Consent Statement: Not applicable.

Data Availability Statement: 3rd Party Data. Restrictions apply to the availability of these data. Data was obtained from National Bureau of Statistics in China and are available with the permission of School of Economics, Shanghai University of Finance and Economics.

Acknowledgments: The authors would like to express their gratitude to the National Bureau of Statistics team for collecting the data. The authors would like to thank the School of Economics, Shanghai University of Finance and Economics, for providing the datasets.

Conflicts of Interest: The authors declare no conflict of interest.

Appendix A

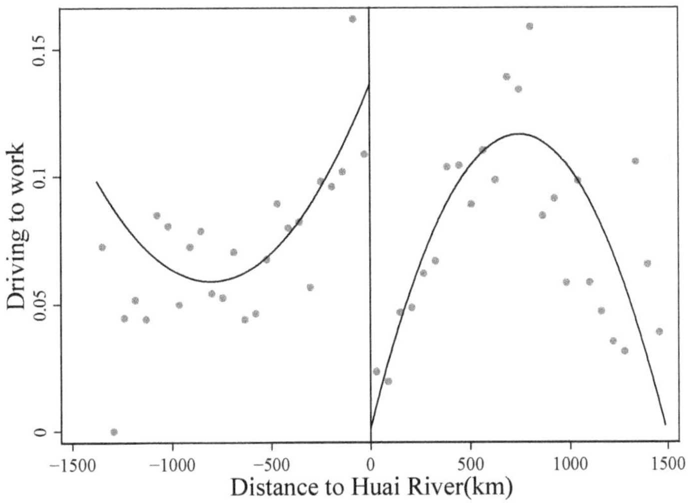

Figure A1. RD plot for driving to work. Notes: The figure shows the binned averages of driving to work against the running variable. The solid line represents a quartic polynomial fit of driving to work by car on each side of the threshold.

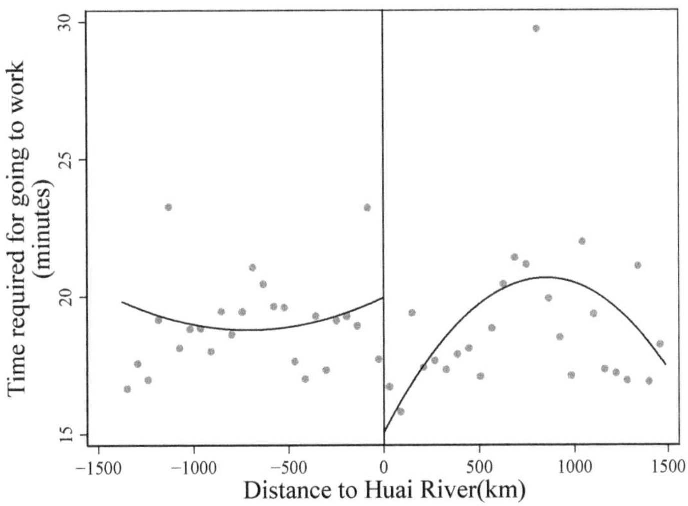

Figure A2. RD plot for the time required for going to work. Notes: The figure shows the binned averages of the time required for going to work against the running variable. The solid line represents a quartic polynomial fit of time on each side of the threshold.

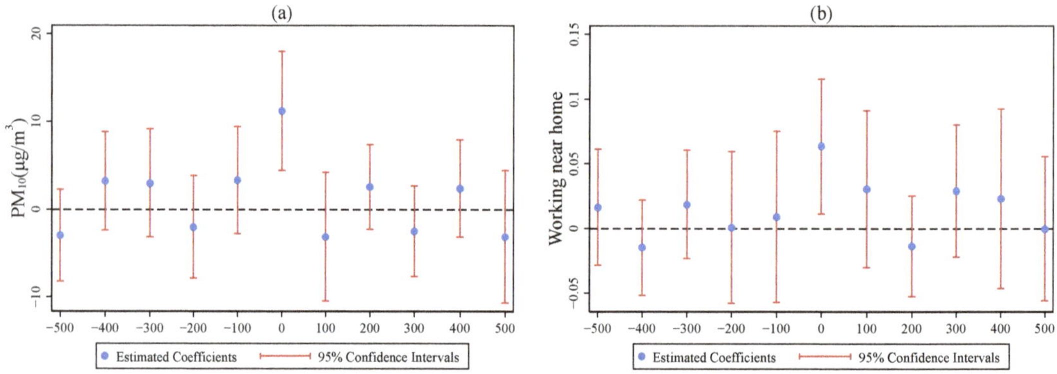

Figure A3. Placebo testing: estimated discontinuity in pollution at displaced Huai River boundaries. Notes: In (**a**), each point plots the point estimate of a separate estimation of α_1 in Equation (2) along with the 95 percent confidence interval at the displaced Huai River boundaries. In (**b**), each point plots the point estimate of a separate estimation of δ_1 in Equation (3) along with the 95 percent confidence interval at the displaced Huai River boundaries. Each RD estimates is based on the MSE bandwidth selection method and triangular kernel function.

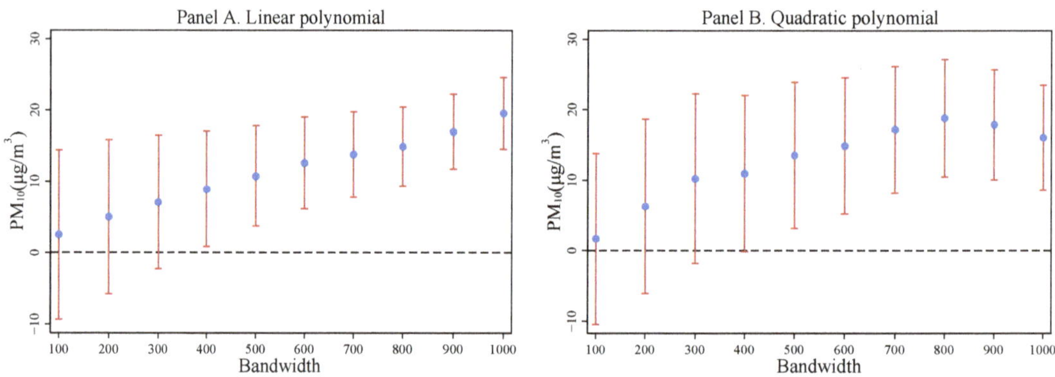

Figure A4. Robustness to alternative bandwidths for the impact of the Huai River Policy on PM_{10}. Notes: Each point plots the point estimate of a separate estimation of α_1 in Equation (2) along with the 95 percent confidence interval, ranging from 100 km to 1000 km bandwidths. (**Panel A**) plots estimates using linear polynomials in distance. (**Panel B**) plots estimates from equivalent regressions but using second-order polynomials in distance. Each RD estimate is based on the MSE bandwidth selection method and triangular kernel function.

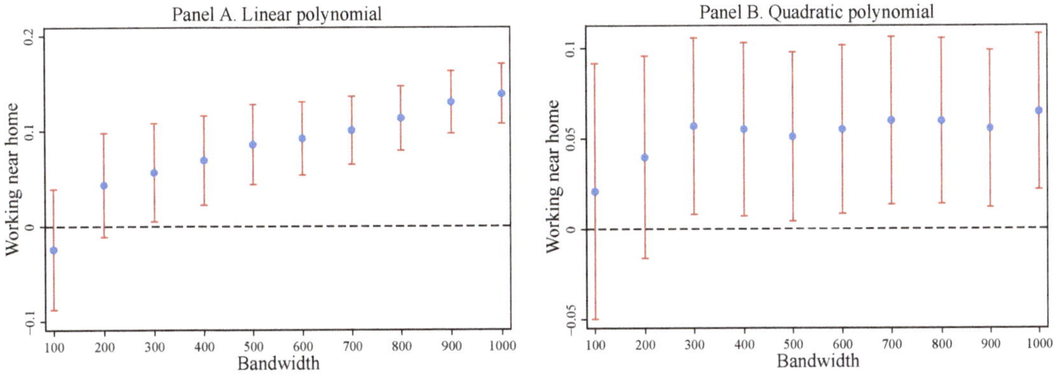

Figure A5. Robustness to alternative bandwidths for the impact of the Huai River Policy on work. Notes: Each point plots the point estimate of a separate estimation of δ_1 in Equation (3) along with the 95 percent confidence interval, ranging from 100 km to 1000 km bandwidths. (**Panel A**) plots estimates using linear polynomials in distance. (**Panel B**) plots estimates from equivalent regressions but using second-order polynomials in distance. Each RD estimate is based on the MSE bandwidth selection method and triangular kernel function.

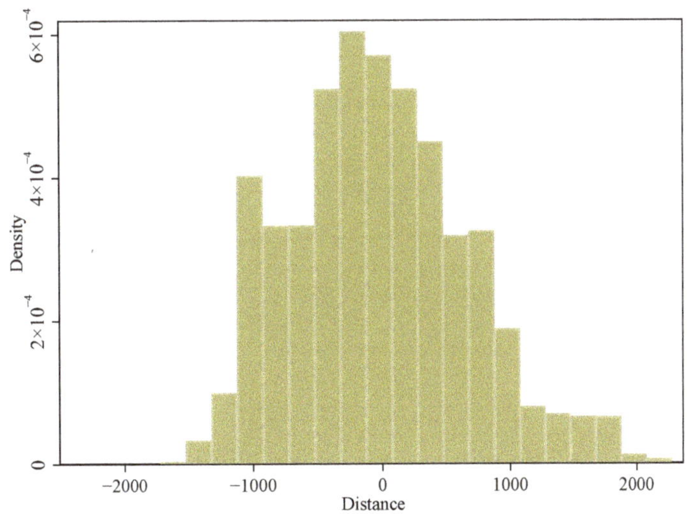

Figure A6. Distributions of distances of counties from the Huai River.

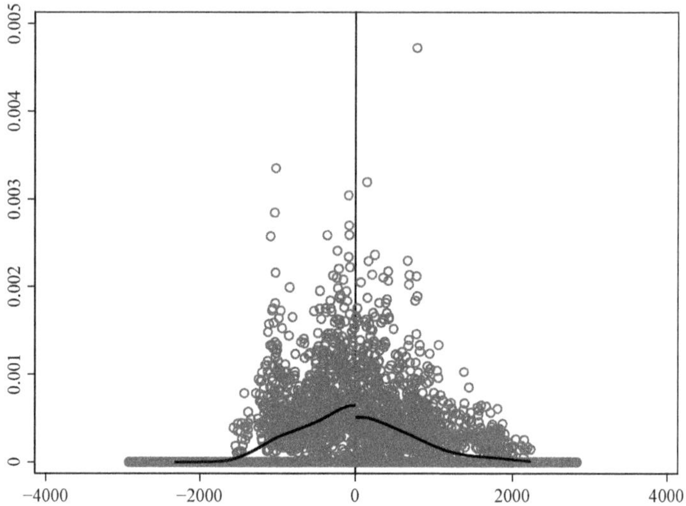

Figure A7. McCrary test of the discontinuity in distances of counties from the Huai River. Notes: The hollow circles represent the point estimates within bins. Solid lines are the density curve estimates.

Table A1. Descriptive statistics.

Variables	Obs	Mean	Std. Dev	Min	Max
Working place selection					
Working near home (Yes = 1)	802,178	0.702	0.458	0.000	1.000
Air pollution					
PM_{10} concentration (μg/m^3)	802,178	89.241	30.496	25.192	181.676
Individual characteristics					
Gender (Male = 1)	802,178	0.487	0.500	0.000	1.000
Nation (Han = 1)	802,178	0.086	0.281	0.000	1.000
Age	802,178	37.364	20.593	0.000	111.000
Marriage (Yes = 1)	802,178	0.735	0.441	0.000	1.000
Type of hukou (Urban = 1)	802,178	0.410	0.492	0.000	1.000
Meteorological conditions					
Temperature of county (°C)	802,178	3.627	3.883	24.473	3.627
Precipitation of county (mm)	802,178	0.508	0.000	10.118	0.508
Relative humidity	802,178	9.008	34.465	86.018	9.008
Wind speed (m/s)	802,178	0.515	0.931	5.845	0.515

Note: This table reports the summary statistics for the main variables used in the analysis.

Table A2. Robustness to using the alternative air pollution measure (AQI).

Variables	RD Estimates					
	(1)	(2)	(3)	(4)	(5)	(6)
Panel A: Impact of the Huai River Policy on AQI						
AQI	13.241 ***	12.781 ***	12.238 ***	13.331 ***	11.942 ***	12.852 ***
	(3.032)	(3.103)	(4.328)	(4.219)	(3.534)	(3.163)
Bandwidth	494.842	503.716	467.435	473.853	482.471	453.289
Panel B: Impact of the AQI on working near home						
Working near home	0.142 **	0.148 **	0.161 **	0.136 **	0.141 **	0.157 **
	(0.061)	(0.065)	(0.067)	(0.063)	(0.064)	(0.062)
Bandwidth	478.537	486.562	469.364	459.817	467.384	439.715
Observations	802,178	802,178	802,178	802,178	802,178	802,178
Controls	N	N	N	Y	Y	Y
Kernel	Triangular	Epanech.	Uniform	Triangular	Epanech.	Uniform

Note: Each cell in the table represents a separate RD estimate along the Huai River using local linear regressions with different kernel functions. Robust standard errors in parentheses are clustered at the county level. Controls include weather information and sociodemographic variables defined in Table 1. ** Significant at 5%; *** significant at 1%.

Table A3. RD estimates of the impacts on the alternative work measure.

Variables	Panel A: Impact of the Huai River Policy on Work		Panel B: Impacts of PM10 on Work	
	(1)	(2)	(1)	(2)
Driving to work	−0.128 ***	−0.124 ***	−0.244 **	−0.242 **
	(0.013)	(0.014)	(0.113)	(0.119)
Bandwidth	365.666	316.909	296.336	297.601
Time required	−3.709 ***	−3.781 ***	−7.186 ***	−7.499 **
	(1.263)	(1.251)	(2.195)	(2.927)
Bandwidth	354.039	356.565	233.738	229.445
Observations	802,178	802,178	802,178	802,178
Controls	N	Y	N	Y
Kernel	Triangular	Triangular	Triangular	Triangular

Note: Each cell in the table represents a separate estimate or regression. Panel A reports the RD results estimating the impact of the Huai River Policy on work. Panel B reports the fuzzy RD results estimating the impact of 10 $\mu g/m^3$ of PM_{10} on work, treating distance from the Huai River as the forcing variable and PM_{10} as the treating variable, with the Huai River representing a "fuzzy" discontinuity in the level of air pollution exposure. The triangular kernel function is used. Robust standard errors in parentheses are clustered at the county level. Controls include weather information and sociodemographic variables defined in Table 1. ** Significant at 5%; *** significant at 1%.

Table A4. RD estimates of the impacts on migration.

Variables	Panel A: Impact of the Huai River Policy on Migration		Panel B: Impacts of PM10 on Migration	
	(1)	(2)	(1)	(2)
Migration	0.053	0.070	0.146	0.195
	(0.122)	(0.123)	(0.216)	(0.271)
Bandwidth	219.60	243.68	218.91	228.66
Observations	802,178	802,178	802,178	802,178
Controls	N	Y	N	Y
Kernel	Triangular	Triangular	Triangular	Triangular

Note: Each cell in the table represents a separate estimate or regression. Panel A reports the RD results estimating the impact of the Huai River Policy on migration. Panel B reports the fuzzy RD results estimating the impact of 10 $\mu g/m^3$ of PM_{10} on migration, treating distance from the Huai River as the forcing variable and PM_{10} as the treating variable, with the Huai River representing a "fuzzy" discontinuity in the level of air pollution exposure. The triangular kernel function is used. Robust standard errors in parentheses are clustered at the county level. Controls include weather information and sociodemographic variables defined in Table 1.

Table A5. RD estimates for samples with a residence duration at the same prefecture-level city of more than 5 years.

Variables	Panel A: Impact of the Huai River Policy on Work		Panel B: Impacts of PM10 on Work	
	(1)	(2)	(1)	(2)
Working near home	0.051 **	0.054 **	0.128 ***	0.124 ***
	(0.022)	(0.027)	(0.041)	(0.042)
Bandwidth	277.742	279.925	431.48	427.57
Observations	698,504	698,504	698,504	698,504
Controls	N	Y	N	Y
Kernel	Triangular	Triangular	Triangular	Triangular

Note: Each cell in the table represents a separate estimate or regression. Panel A reports the RD results estimating the impact of the Huai River Policy on work. Panel B reports the fuzzy RD results estimating the impact of 10 $\mu g/m^3$ of PM_{10} on work, treating distance from the Huai River as the forcing variable and PM_{10} as the treating variable, with the Huai River representing a "fuzzy" discontinuity in the level of air pollution exposure. The triangular kernel function is used. Robust standard errors in parentheses are clustered at the county level. Controls include weather information and sociodemographic variables defined in Table 1. ** significant at 5%; *** significant at 1%.

References

1. Sørensen, M.; Daneshvar, B.; Hansen, M.; Dragsted, L.O.; Hertel, O.; Knudsen, L.; Loft, S. Personal PM2.5 exposure and markers of oxidative stress in blood. *Environ. Health Perspect.* **2003**, *111*, 161–166. [CrossRef]
2. Chen, Y.; Ebenstein, A.; Greenstone, M.; Li, H. Evidence on the impact of sustained exposure to air pollution on life expectancy from China's Huai River policy. *Proc. Natl. Acad. Sci. USA* **2013**, *110*, 12936–12941. [CrossRef]
3. Ebenstein, A.; Fan, M.; Greenstone, M.; He, G.; Yin, P.; Zhou, M. Growth, pollution, and life expectancy: China from 1991–2012. *Amer. Econ. Rev.* **2015**, *105*, 226–231. [CrossRef]
4. Lai, W. Pesticide use and health outcomes: Evidence from agricultural water pollution in China. *J. Environ. Econ. Manag.* **2017**, *86*, 93–120. [CrossRef]
5. Zhang, X.; Zhang, X.; Chen, X. Happiness in the air: How does a dirty sky affect mental health and subjective well-being? *J. Environ. Econ. Manag.* **2017**, *85*, 81–94. [CrossRef]
6. Chen, S.; Oliva, P.; Zhang, P. *Air pollution and Mental Health: Evidence from China*; National Bureau of Economic Research: Cambridge, MA, USA, 2018.
7. Zhang, X.; Chen, X.; Zhang, X. The impact of exposure to air pollution on cognitive performance. *Proc. Natl. Acad. Sci. USA* **2018**, *115*, 9193–9197. [CrossRef]
8. Lai, W.; Li, S.; Li, Y.; Tian, X. Air Pollution and Cognitive Functions: Evidence from Straw Burning in China. *Am. J. Agric. Econ.* **2022**, *104*, 190–208. [CrossRef]
9. Graff Zivin, J.; Neidell, M. The impact of pollution on worker productivity. *Am. Econ. Rev.* **2012**, *102*, 3652–3673. [CrossRef]
10. Chang, T.; Graff Zivin, J.; Gross, T.; Neidell, M. Particulate pollution and the productivity of pear packers. *Am. Econ. J. Econ. Policy* **2016**, *8*, 141–169. [CrossRef]
11. Chang, T.Y.; Graff Zivin, J.; Gross, T.; Neidell, M. The effect of pollution on worker productivity: Evidence from call center workers in China. *Am. Econ. J. Appl. Econ.* **2019**, *11*, 151–172. [CrossRef]
12. Ebenstein, A.; Fan, M.; Greenstone, M.; He, G.; Zhou, M. New evidence on the impact of sustained exposure to air pollution on life expectancy from China's Huai River Policy. *Proc. Natl. Acad. Sci. USA* **2017**, *114*, 10384–10389. [CrossRef] [PubMed]
13. Sun, C.; Kahn, M.E.; Zheng, S. Self-protection investment exacerbates air pollution exposure inequality in urban China. *Ecolog. Econ.* **2017**, *131*, 468–474. [CrossRef]
14. Ito, K.; Zhang, S. Willingness to pay for clean air: Evidence from air purifier markets in China. *J. Polit. Econ.* **2020**, *128*, 1627–1672. [CrossRef]
15. Chen, S.; Oliva, P.; Zhang, P. *The Effect of Air Pollution on Migration: Evidence from China*; National Bureau of Economic Research: Cambridge, MA, USA, 2017.
16. Freeman, R.; Liang, W.; Song, R.; Timmins, C. Willingness to pay for clean air in China. *J. Environ. Econ. Manag.* **2019**, *94*, 188–216. [CrossRef]
17. Greenstone, M.; He, G.; Li, S.; Zou, E.Y. China's war on pollution: Evidence from the first 5 years. *Rev. Environ. Econ. Policy* **2021**, *15*, 281–299. [CrossRef]
18. Monheit, A.C.; Vistnes, J.P. Health Insurance Availability at the Workplace: How Important are Worker Preferences? *J. Hum. Resour.* **1999**, *34*, 770–785. [CrossRef]
19. Wiswall, M.; Zafar, B. Preference for the Workplace, Investment in Human Capital, and Gender. *Q. J. Econ.* **2017**, *133*, 457–507. [CrossRef]
20. Roca, J.D.L.; Puga, D. Learning by working in big cities. *Rev. Econ. Stud.* **2017**, *84*, 106–142. [CrossRef]
21. Batabyal, A.A.; Nijkamp, P. Workplace choice, commuting costs, and wage taxation in urban and adjacent rural regions. *Ann. Reg. Sci.* **2020**, *65*, 775–786. [CrossRef]
22. El Koussa, M.; Atun, R.; Bowser, D.; Kruk, M.E. Factors influencing physicians' choice of workplace: Systematic review of drivers of attrition and policy interventions to address them. *J. Glob. Health* **2016**, *6*, 020403. [CrossRef]
23. Frenkel, A.; Bendit, E.; Kaplan, S. Residential location choice of knowledge-workers: The role of amenities, workplace and lifestyle. *Cities* **2013**, *35*, 33–41. [CrossRef]
24. Barwick, P.J.; Li, S.; Lin, L.; Zou, E. *From Fog to Smog: The Value of Pollution Information*; National Bureau of Economic Research: Cambridge, MA, USA, 2019.
25. Kahn, M.E. Smog reduction's impact on California county growth. *J. Reg. Sci.* **2000**, *40*, 565–582. [CrossRef]
26. Chay, K.Y.; Greenstone, M. Does air quality matter? Evidence from the housing market. *J. Polit. Econ.* **2005**, *113*, 376–424. [CrossRef]
27. Banzhaf, H.S.; Walsh, R.P. Do people vote with their feet? An empirical test of Tiebout. *Am. Econ. Rev.* **2008**, *98*, 843–863. [CrossRef]
28. Greenstone, M.; Gallagher, J. Does hazardous waste matter? Evidence from the housing market and the superfund program. *Q. J. Econ.* **2008**, *123*, 951–1003. [CrossRef]
29. Bayer, P.; Keohane, N.; Timmins, C. Migration and hedonic valuation: The case of air quality. *J. Environ. Econ. Manag.* **2009**, *58*, 1–14. [CrossRef]
30. Xue, S.; Zhang, B.; Zhao, X. Brain drain: The impact of air pollution on firm performance. *J. Environ. Econ. Manag.* **2021**, *110*, 102546. [CrossRef]

31. Khanna, G.; Liang, W.; Mobarak, A.M.; Song, R. *The Productivity Consequences of Pollution-Induced Migration in China*; National Bureau of Economic Research: Cambridge, MA, USA, 2021.
32. Harris, J.R.; Todaro, M.P. Migration, unemployment and development: A two-sector analysis. *Am. Econ. Rev.* **1970**, *60*, 126–142.
33. Fu, Y.; Gabriel, S.A. Labor migration, human capital agglomeration and regional development in China. *Reg. Sci. Urban Econ.* **2012**, *42*, 473–484. [CrossRef]
34. Poncet, S. Provincial migration dynamics in China: Borders, costs and economic motivations. *Reg. Sci. Urban Econ.* **2006**, *36*, 385–398. [CrossRef]
35. Tombe, T.; Zhu, X. Trade, migration, and productivity: A quantitative analysis of china. *Am. Econ. Rev.* **2019**, *109*, 1843–1872. [CrossRef]
36. Kain, J.F. Housing segregation, negro employment, and metropolitan decentralization. *Q. J. Econ.* **1968**, *82*, 175–197. [CrossRef]
37. Lehmann, E.; Ledezma, P.L.M.; Van der Linden, B. Workforce location and equilibrium unemployment in a duocentric economy with matching frictions. *J. Urban Econ.* **2016**, *91*, 26–44. [CrossRef]
38. Piore, M.J. Labor market segmentation: To what paradigm does it belong? *Am. Econ. Rev.* **1983**, *73*, 249–253.
39. Barnichon, R.; Figura, A. Labor market heterogeneity and the aggregate matching function. *Am. Econ. J. Macroecon.* **2015**, *7*, 222–249. [CrossRef]
40. Ma, L.; Tang, Y. A tale of two tails: Wage inequality and city size. 2016; *Unpublished manuscript*.
41. World Bank. *China—Heat Reform and Building Energy Eciency Project*; Technology Report; World Bank: Washington, DC, USA, 2005.
42. Almond, D.; Chen, Y.; Greenstone, M.; Li, H. Winter heating or clean air? Unintended impacts of China's Huai river policy. *Am. Econ. Rev.* **2009**, *99*, 184–190. [CrossRef]
43. Fan, M.; He, G.; Zhou, M. The winter choke: Coal-fired heating, air pollution, and mortality in China. *J. Health Econ.* **2020**, *71*, 102316. [CrossRef]
44. Gelman, A.; Imbens, G. Why high-order polynomials should not be used in regression discontinuity designs. *J. Bus. Econ. Stat.* **2019**, *37*, 447–456. [CrossRef]
45. Calonico, S.; Cattaneo, M.D.; Farrell, M.H.; Titiunik, R. rdrobust: Software for regression-discontinuity designs. *Stata J.* **2017**, *17*, 372–404. [CrossRef]
46. Calonico, S.; Cattaneo, M.D.; Farrell, M.H. Optimal bandwidth choice for robust bias-corrected inference in regression discontinuity designs. *Econom. J.* **2020**, *23*, 192–210. [CrossRef]
47. Lee, D.S.; Lemieux, T. Regression discontinuity designs in economics. *J. Econ. Lit.* **2010**, *48*, 281–355. [CrossRef]
48. McCrary, J. Manipulation of the running variable in the regression discontinuity design: A density test. *J. Econom.* **2008**, *142*, 698–714. [CrossRef]
49. Calonico, S.; Cattaneo, M.D.; Farrell, M.H.; Titiunik, R. Regression discontinuity designs using covariates. *Rev. Econ. Statist.* **2019**, *101*, 442–451. [CrossRef]
50. Calonico, S.; Cattaneo, M.D.; Farrell, M.H. On the effect of bias estimation on coverage accuracy in nonparametric inference. *J. Am. Stat. Assoc.* **2018**, *113*, 767–779. [CrossRef]
51. Calonico, S.; Cattaneo, M.D.; Farrell, M.H. Coverage error optimal confidence intervals for local polynomial regression. *arXiv* **2018**, arXiv:1808.01398.
52. Ding, L.; Fan, M.; Nie, P. Pollution and the Decline in Human Cognition: Evidence from China. Available online: https://ssrn.com/abstract=3792594 (accessed on 24 August 2021).
53. Kim, H.; Noh, J.; Noh, Y.; Oh, S.S.; Koh, S.-B.; Kim, C. Gender difference in the effects of outdoor air pollution on cognitive function among elderly in Korea. *Front. Public Health* **2019**, *7*, 375. [CrossRef]
54. Bian, Y.; Song, K.; Bai, J. Market segmentation, resource misallocation and environmental pollution. *J. Clean. Prod.* **2019**, *228*, 376–387. [CrossRef]
55. Zhao, D.; Yu, A.; Guo, J. Judicial institutions, local protection and market segmentation: Evidence from the establishment of interprovincial circuit tribunals in China. *China Econ. Rev.* **2022**, 101829. [CrossRef]
56. Xu, F.; Li, Q.; Yang, M. The impacts of high-speed rail on the transformation of resource-based cities in China: A market segmentation perspective. *Resour. Policy* **2022**, *78*, 102807. [CrossRef]

International Journal of
Environmental Research and Public Health

MDPI

Article

Air Pollution and Migration Intention: Evidence from the Unified National Graduate Entrance Examination

Chao Xu [1] and Xiulei Wang [2,*]

[1] School of Public Finance & Taxation, Shandong University of Finance and Economics, Jinan 250002, China; xuchaode@126.com
[2] School of Economics & Trade, Hunan University, Changsha 410006, China
* Correspondence: wxl20180705@163.com

Abstract: Using a unique dataset of applicants for the Unified National Graduate Entrance Examination (UNGEE) of 76 double first-class universities in China, this paper evaluates the causal impact of air pollution on the migration intentions of highly educated talents by exploiting an instrumental variable approach based on annually average wind speed. We find that a 1 μg/m^3 increase in the annually average $PM_{2.5}$ concentration in destination cities decreases the number of applicants for the UNGEE of elite universities by about 250, but better university quality and more abundant educational resources can weaken the effect partially. A heterogeneity analysis indicates that the university-city choices of applicants are shifting from north to south. Our findings suggest that air pollution may lead to the loss of high human capital.

Keywords: air pollution; migration intention; high human capital; instrumental variable

Citation: Xu, C.; Wang, X. Air Pollution and Migration Intention: Evidence from the Unified National Graduate Entrance Examination. *IJERPH* **2022**, *19*, 8813. https://doi.org/10.3390/ijerph19148813

Academic Editors: Jie Chen, Qian Zhou and Ting Zhang

Received: 30 June 2022
Accepted: 18 July 2022
Published: 20 July 2022

1. Introduction

Air pollution has become increasingly deteriorated and attracted widespread attention worldwide, and is a major health hazard. According to the World Bank Report, air pollution is responsible for millions of deaths and creates economic loss which amounts to trillions of dollars in Asia and Sub-Saharan Africa (see http://www.yicai.com/news/5097668.html (accessed on 9 September 2016)). Mounting research has investigated the causal health effects of air pollution in both developed countries [1,2] and developing countries [3,4]. These studies find that acute exposure to air pollution can cause damage to physical and mental health, such as increasing mortality [5], increasing overweight and obesity rates [6], reducing life expectancy [7], and reducing hedonic happiness [8]. A growing body of literature also finds that people may adopt avoidance strategies, and even re-locate and migrate to reduce air pollution exposure in highly polluted areas [9–11]. Due to higher incomes and greater knowledge of the harmful effects of air pollution, elites are more sensitive to air pollution and have a higher willingness to pay for avoiding pollution [12,13]. However, little is known about the influence of air pollution on migration intentions of highly educated talents in developing countries.

Data on the applicants for the UNGEE of double first-class universities in China provide an opportunity to study the effects of air pollution on the migration intentions of highly educated talents. First, the UNGEE, or kaoyan, is a selective examination organized by the education authorities and admissions agencies for the selection of graduate students. The UNGEE is becoming more and more difficult as the number of applicants increases year by year. (In the past five years, the number of applicants for the UNGEE has increased rapidly. In 2017, for the first time, the number of applicants exceeded 2 million. In 2021, the number of applicants reached 3.77 million with an increase of 360,000 from 3.41 million in 2020, which has reached a record high. The number of applicants was 4.57 million in 2022. See http://www.moe.gov.cn/jyb_xwfb/s5147/202012/t20201228_507808.html (accessed on 26 December 2020)). The requirements and difficulties of the UNGEE of double first-class universities, China's elite universities, are much greater than those of ordinary universities. Most applicants of double first-class universities are about to obtain or have already obtained bachelor's degrees, which allows us to focus on highly educated talents. Second, the dataset on applicants only includes the number of applicants for full-time master's degree students. If applicants are admitted as full-time postgraduate students, they must study for master's degrees in university for the next two to three years. Therefore, the university-city choices represent their intentions to move over the next few years. In addition, compared with college-city choices after the National College Entrance Examination (gaokao), applicants are more likely to work and live in cities in which they apply for their master's degrees in the future. Using a unique manually collected dataset on the applicants for UNGEE of 76 double first-class universities in China, this paper estimates the causal effects of air pollution on the migration intentions of highly educated talents. We exploit an instrument variable (IV) for air pollution to correct the estimated bias of the ordinary least square estimation (OLS) from omitted variables and measurement errors. The IV estimation results show that a 1 $\mu g/m^3$ increase in $PM_{2.5}$ concentration in destination cities significantly decreases the number of applicants by 250. This effect is equivalent to 2.2%, given the average 11,547 applicants. The magnitude of the result is consistent with the research on the job location decisions [14]. The reduction in the number of applicants in social science due to air pollution is larger than that in natural science. The results are consistent across different specifications and alternative samples. Moreover, heterogeneous effects show that air pollution decreases more applicants for the UNGEE of first-class discipline universities, which reveals that better university quality can remedy the negative effects partially. Furthermore, we also find that the university-city choices of applicants are shifting from north to south.

This paper makes three contributions to the existing literature. First, to the best of our knowledge, it is among the first to investigate the causal impacts of destination cities' air pollution on migration intentions in highly polluted developing countries, using unique university-level applicant data. A large literature in environmental economics explores the negative effects of original and destination cities' air pollution on job location decisions [12,14], and net-outmigration rates in China [11]. However, little is known about the relationship between air pollution and migration intentions. This paper is closest to that of Qin and Zhu (2018) and Jia and Chen (2021). They find that increases in original cities' air quality index (AQI) increase the settlement intentions of floating migrants and emigration interests in China. We study the same linkage between air pollution and migration intentions, but we focus on the effects of different pollutants ($PM_{2.5}$ versus AQI) on migration intentions of different groups (highly educated talents versus potential international migrants and floating migrants). Using an online search index on "emigration" to construct a daily measurement of city-level people's emigration interests, Qin and Zhu (2018) examine the effects of air pollution on emigration interests with the Poisson regression model. Jia and Chen (2021) study the effects of air pollution on migrants' settlement intentions with an instrumental variable approach using the ventilation coefficient. Based on survey questions from the 2017 National Migrant Population Dynamic Monitoring Survey, a dummy variable is constructed to measure the settlement intentions of floating migrants by Jia and Chen (2021). However, we exploit an instrumental variable based on wind speed and use the number of applicants for UNGEE of double first-class universities to measure short-term migration intentions of highly educated talents.

Second, this paper also adds to the literature on the determinants of migration decisions. A large body of studies have focused on economic and environmental factors such as income [15], wage [16], labor market demand [17] and housing prices [18]. There is some evidence of the causal relationship between air pollution and migration choices and the intentions of floating migrants [11] and the general population [19]. Few research studies have focused solely on highly educated groups. This study confirms previous findings that air pollution is associated with brain drain, not only from the perspective of job location choices of graduate students, but also from the perspective of location choices of studying for master's degrees. Relative to previous literature on the job location choices of Tsinghua graduates and general college graduates [12,14], we focus on the applicants for UNGEE of 76 double first-class universities. Our sample includes more elite universities than Zheng et al. (2019) and is more concentrated on high quality universities than Lai et al. (2021).

Third, although many studies find that air pollution has negative effects on economic and social welfare from the perspective of productivity [20], human capital [21], crime [22], and physical and mental health [23,24], evidence of the causal relationship between air pollution exposure and talent loss is insufficient because of data availability. Highly educated talents are the core competitiveness of development in the future. The economic and social costs of the loss of talents are becoming increasingly apparent. Policy makers should focus on environmental amenities to attract talents, who are more sensitive to air pollution and climate change.

The rest of this paper is structured as follows. The Section 2 presents data and empirical strategy. Section 3 introduces the baseline results and provides robustness checks. Section 4 discusses the heterogeneous effects of air pollution on the quantity of applicants across the quality, type, and region of universities. Section 5 compares the results with the existing literature. Section 6 concludes.

2. Methodology

2.1. Data and Variables Analysis

It is plausible for us to define the applicants who apply for 76 double first-class universities of UNGEE as the elites. According to the requirements of the China Graduate Admission Information Network, the applicants for UNGEE must be the people who are about to obtain or have already obtained bachelor's degrees, or have graduated from vocational college for over 2 years (see https://yz.chsi.com.cn/kyzx/jybzc/202109/20210903/2105941509.html (accessed on 3 September 2021)). However, for the applicants who graduated from vocational college, the aimed universities that they choose require them to have academic achievements in the journals of the Chinese Science Citation Database or Chinese Social Sciences Citation Index in the past 3 years, additionally. Therefore, most of the applicants who apply for UNGEE successfully are those who are about to or have obtained bachelor's degrees. According to the data that was released by the National Bureau of Statistics of China, until 2019, the number of undergraduates in China accounted for only about 3.8% of the total population (see http://www.stats.gov.cn/ (accessed on 2 December 2020)). No matter the education degree or the population proportion, applicants who apply for UNGEE can be treated as elites in China. Under this premise, based on 137 double first-class universities that are listed in China's fourth round of subject evaluation (see http://www.cdgdc.edu.cn/xwyyjsjyxx/xkpgjg/ (accessed on 28 December 2017)), and further considering whether the schools' official websites have published the application data of past years for UNGEE, 76 universities are finally determined as the research sample (The specific list of 76 universities is shown in Table A1 in the Appendix A. Some universities have different campuses in different cities; in this paper, the campuses of the same universities in different cities are regarded as different universities). We manually crawl the data that include the quantity of applicants for 2010–2021, the number of students to be enrolled in the admission brochure for 2010–2021, and the enrollment ratio for 2009–2020. The amount of universities that we choose holds for 55.5% of all double first-class universities, and the geographical distributions of them cover 34 prefecture-level cities of 25 provinces in China. Figure 1 plots the specific regional distribution and number of double first-class university for every city. From the layout, the universities are locating in Shihezi of Xinjiang in the west, Ningbo of Zhejiang in the east, Harbin of Heilongjiang in the north, and Haikou of Hainan in the south, which have a generally representative in area. Owing to the fact that the data of some universities are missing in some years, the data that we use are an unbalanced panel data and the total amount is 585. Due to the need to examine the differences between applicants of different disciplines, and according to the "Catalogue of Disciplines and Majors for Granting Doctoral" and "Master's Degrees and Cultivating Postgraduates" that are issued by the Ministry of Education of the People's Republic of China (MOE of PRC) (see http://www.moe.gov.cn/srcsite/A08/moe_1034/s3882/201209/t20120918_143152.html (accessed on 14 September 2012)), we further divide the applicants into social science and natural science and then re-count the quantity of the different discipline applicants (social science includes: philosophy, economics, law, education, literature, history, military science, and management; natural science includes: science, engineering, agriculture, and medicine).

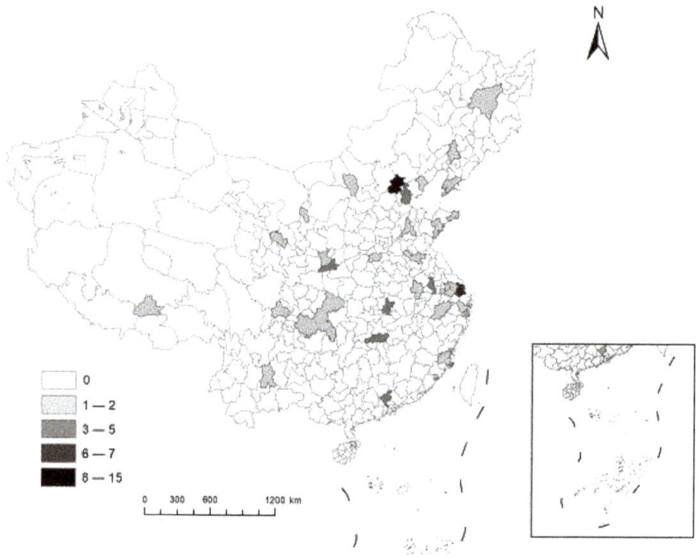

Figure 1. Regional distribution and quantity of sample universities in China. Note: This figure presents the regional distribution and quantity of all sample universities in China, and the different degrees of gray represent the different amounts of universities in each city.

To determine the variables, we select the number of applicants for UNGEE in each university as the dependent variable (Apply) and choose the average urban $PM_{2.5}$ concentration as the independent variable ($PM_{2.5}$). As for the control variables, we mainly consider the following three aspects. The first is the factors of the university: when applicants choose a university in applying for UNGEE, they refer to the expectedly admitted student number that is published in the admission brochures of the aimed university firstly. The more the quantity of students to be recruited, the higher the probability of admission, and the more intense the intentions of students to apply are. Therefore, we add the number of students to be enrolled into the model as the control variable in school (Enrollment). The second is the characteristics of the city: the applicants also take urban features of the city where the intended university is located into consideration. A better urban economic development, richer recreational life, and lower living cost will be more attractive to applicants. Hence, we add per capita GDP (Rj_gdp), third industry proportion (Industry 3_rate), and consumer price index (CPI) into the equation. In addition, applicants will also consider comfort, convenience of urban life, and educational resource. So, the density of the population (Popu), the number of buses and trams (Transpor), and per capita educational expenditure (Edu_cost) are also added into the model. Last is the climate conditions of the city: different growth backgrounds make applicants have different climatic adaptability. If the applicants are admitted by the intended university, they will study and live in the city where the intended university is located as "quasi-residents" for 2 or 3 years, so the applicants will also consider the climatic features of the city when apply for UNGEE. We put annually average rainfall (Avgrain) and annually average temperature (Avgtemp) into the model. The application for UNGEE of the corresponding year was completed in October of the previous year, so the explanatory variables, except the expectedly admitted student number, are introduced into the model with a lag of one term.

The data of the universities are from official websites of 76 double first-class universities. The other data such as per capita GDP, consumer price index (CPI), third industry ratio, and so on are from the 2009–2020 "China Urban Statistical Yearbook", and the urban $PM_{2.5}$ concentration data are from the 2009–2020 $PM_{2.5}$ density map released by Columbia University; the annually average temperature and annually average rainfall are from the China Meteorological Data Sharing Service System.

2.2. Descriptive Statistics

We use the "summary" command of Stata to perform the statistical analysis with the main variables that are used in this paper. The statistics include observation, mean, minimum, maximum, and standard deviation. Table 1 shows the summary statistics for the main variables used in the analysis. On average, the quantity of applicants for UNGEE in each university is about 11,547, and there is a big difference between various universities. Among them, there are relatively more applicants who major in social science, accounting for about 57.6%, and relatively fewer applicants for natural science, holding for around only 42.4%. The mean of urban $PM_{2.5}$ concentration is approximate 49.79 μg/m^3, and there are little differences between different cities.

Table 1. Descriptive statistics of main variables.

Variables		Obs	Mean	SD	Min	Max
Apply		585	11,547	7446	237	41,522
Rw_apply	Social science	585	6654	5654	6	28,297
Zr_apply	Natural science	585	4895	4097	0	21,627
$PM_{2.5}$		585	49.79	16.73	4.50	99.71
Enrollment		585	2809	1584	145	8737
Rj_gdp		585	133.73	64.84	16.91	462.95
Industry 3_rate		585	59.72	13.06	25.69	83.87
CPI		585	137.34	13.38	109.65	171.37
Popu		585	957.61	646.68	15.61	4119
Edu_cost		585	1573	2012	14.13	9623
Transpor		585	15.29	7.68	1.27	167.70
Avgtemp		585	14.49	4.05	3.10	25.53
Avgrain		585	26.57	13.96	4.03	71.97
Avgwindsp		585	2.23	0.41	1.08	4.13

Note: The consumer price index (CPI) is calculated with 100 based on 2008.

Before reporting the benchmark results, we preliminarily examine the relevance between $PM_{2.5}$ concentration and the number of applicants. From the fitting diagram (Figure 2), there is a strong negative correlation between $PM_{2.5}$ concentration and the quantity of applicants. In addition, the regression coefficient is −236.6853, and p-value is 0.00, which is significant at 1% level. It illustrates that the more severe the city air pollution, the fewer the number of applicants. Next, we will use a panel fixed-effect model to empirically test the specific impacts of air pollution on the applicants' university-city choices.

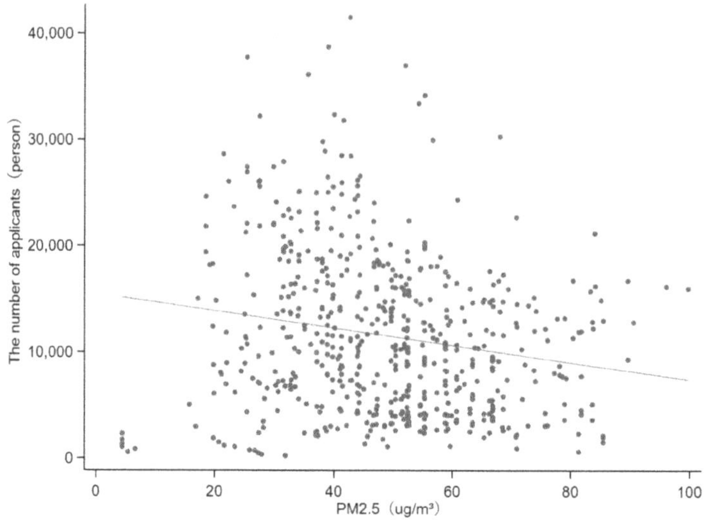

Figure 2. $PM_{2.5}$ concentration and the number of applicants. Note: This figure displays the relationship between $PM_{2.5}$ concentration and the number of applicants for all sample universities.

2.3. Empirical Strategy

Theoretically, we use Equation (1) to estimate the impacts of air pollution on the university-city choices of applicants.

$$Apply_{icpt} = \alpha_0 + \alpha_1 \mathrm{PM}_{2.5icpt} + \alpha_2 X_{icpt} + \lambda_i + \pi_t + \varepsilon_{icpt} \quad (1)$$

In Equation (1), $Apply_{icpt}$ denotes the number of applicants for UNGEE in each university; $\mathrm{PM}_{2.5icpt}$ is the annually average $PM_{2.5}$ concentration of the city where the intended university is located; X_{icpt} is a series of control variables; and λ_i represents the fixed effect of a school individual, which can control for time-invariant confounders specific to school; π_t is a time fixed effect, which can account for shocks common on all universities and cities in a particular year; and ε_{icpt} denotes the random error. In each variable, the subscript i denotes university, c means city, p is province, and t represents year. The α_1 depicts the average impacts of air pollution on the number of applicants in each university. If its estimated value is significantly negative, it means that air pollution has a negative impact on the quantity of applicants. Its amount indicates that the average $PM_{2.5}$ concentration changes by 1 $\mu g/m^3$, how many will change in the number of applicants in each university.

Based on this, this paper may meet endogenous challenges caused by omitted variables, measurement error, and reverse causation. The dependent variable of this paper measures applicants' choosing intentions rather than actual migration behaviors, so there is no need to consider the endogenous problems caused by simultaneity. In terms of omitted variables, although Equation (1) controls the fixed effect of university and avoids the omitted variables at schools, the factors affecting applicants' university-city selection at the city and province are more complex, and it is unfeasible to fully involve in the model, so there will exist unconsidered factors in the error term. Additionally, the data that we manually collected may exist with a measurement error. To overcome the challenges, we use the instrumental variable of air pollution to perform a two-stage least squares (2SLS) estimation based on Equations (2) and (3).

The first stage:

$$\mathrm{PM}_{2.5icpt} = \beta_0 + \beta_1 Avgwindsp_{icpt} + \beta_2 X_{icpt} + \lambda_i + \pi_t + \mu_{icpt} \quad (2)$$

The second stage:

$$Apply_{icpt} = \gamma_0 + \gamma_1 \widehat{PM}_{2.5icpt} + \gamma_2 X_{icpt} + \lambda_i + \pi_t + \nu_{icpt} \quad (3)$$

To determine the instrumental variable, we mainly consider whether the selection of instrumental variable meets the restriction of relevance and exclusion restriction at the same time. The relevance restriction means that the instrumental variable has a clear effect on the endogenous variable ($PM_{2.5}$), and the exclusion restriction means that the only reason for the relationship between the instrument variable and dependent variable is the endogenous variable. The existing literature usually chooses meteorological indicators as the instrumental variable for air pollution. For example, based on the fact that the higher the altitude, the higher the atmospheric temperature will be, Arceo et al. (2016) and Chen et al. (2022) use thermal inversion as the instrumental variable of air pollution. Normally, the hot air rises and the cold air falls, which facilitate the diffusion of pollutants, but in turn, there is a thermal inversion, and the pollutants are not easy to diffuse. So, the more serious the thermal inversion, the more severe the air pollution. When studying the impacts of environmental regulation on the layout of polluting industries, based on the fact that the intensity of regulation is related to the degree of pollution, Broner et al. (2012) use the ventilation coefficient as the instrumental variable for environmental regulation [25]. Generally, the higher the wind speed, the lighter the pollution will be, and the better the condition of lateral diffusion. So, the smaller the ventilation index, the stronger the environmental regulation. Similar to this, we choose the annually average wind speed (Avgwindsp) as the instrumental variable of air pollution. In general, if the wind speed is higher, the lateral diffusion conditions of pollutants will be better, and the $PM_{2.5}$ concentration will be lower. Therefore, the $PM_{2.5}$ concentration and wind speed will have a negative relationship. Figure 3 depicts the fitting scatter diagram of the instrumental variable (annually average wind speed) and endogenous variable ($PM_{2.5}$ concentration). The regression coefficient is -10.5289, and the p-value is 0.00, which is significant at 1% level. It discloses that two variables are changing conversely, which satisfies the relevance restriction, and the wind speed is usually determined by the city's meteorological conditions, which is not directly related to other factors that affect applicants' university-city selection, so it also meets the exclusion restriction.

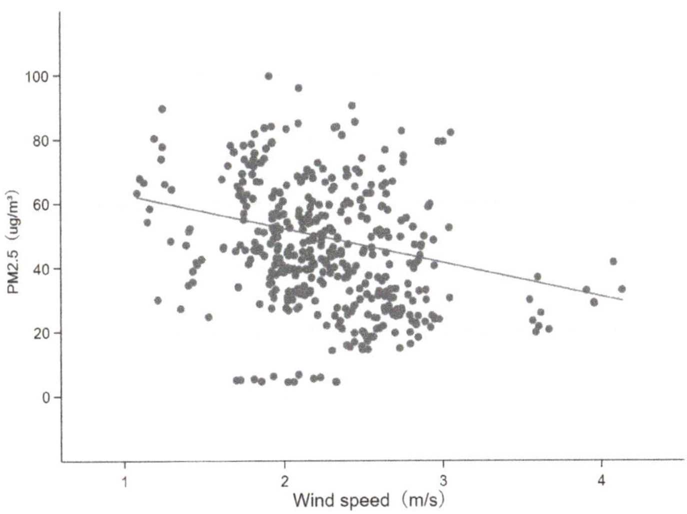

Figure 3. Wind speed and $PM_{2.5}$ concentration. Note: This figure displays the relationship between annually average wind speed and the $PM_{2.5}$ concentration of all sample cities.

3. Empirical Results

3.1. The Baseline Results

As a reference, the ordinary least squares (OLS) estimation is first performed based on Equation (1), and the variables of university, urban, and climate are added to the equation step by step. The columns (1)–(3) of Table 2 show the regression results.

Table 2. Impact of air pollution on applicants' number (OLS estimates).

Variables		OLS	
Apply	**(1)**	**(2)**	**(3)**
$PM_{2.5}$	−58.5446 **	−58.6956 **	−56.5464 **
	(23.10)	(23.82)	(23.71)
Enrollment	2.0565 ***	2.1590 ***	2.1918 ***
	(0.26)	(0.26)	(0.26)
Rj_gdp		−12.4473	−10.0484
		(8.94)	(9.95)
Industry_3rate		−49.3432	−42.9970
		(57.23)	(56.97)
CPI		296.9077 **	293.5499 **
		(126.15)	(126.12)
Popu		−0.8787 **	−0.9502 **
		(0.45)	(0.45)
Transpor		8.6109	−5.2994
		(21.06)	(21.90)
Edu_cost		0.1588	0.1245
		(0.13)	(0.13)
Avgtemp			−906.4734 **
			(396.44)
Avgrain			−53.6604 **
			(24.49)
School FE	Yes	Yes	Yes
Year FE	Yes	Yes	Yes
N	585	585	585
R^2	0.5340	0.5396	0.5453

Note: Standard errors clustered at city level are reported in the brackets. *** $p < 0.01$, ** $p < 0.05$.

Column (1) is the estimated result of adding only the variable of university. The estimated coefficient of $PM_{2.5}$ is significantly negative, and the estimated coefficient of the number of students to be enrolled is significantly positive. Columns (2) and (3) are the regression results of adding the variables of city and climate in turn. From the column (3) that adds all the control variables, the estimated coefficient of $PM_{2.5}$ is still significantly negative, revealing that the $PM_{2.5}$ concentration has a negative impact on the university-city selection of applicants. The higher the $PM_{2.5}$ concentration in the city where the aimed at university is located, the smaller the number of applicants to the university will be. The estimated coefficient of the number of students to be enrolled is still significantly positive at the 1% level, demonstrating that the number of applicants will increase with the increase of students' number to be enrolled. From the perspective of the control variables, the estimated coefficient of the consumer price index (CPI) is significantly positive, which is inconsistent with our expectation, and the estimated coefficient of population density is significantly negative, indicating that the applicants may dislike a city of high population density. Lastly, the estimated coefficients of the annually average temperature and annually average rainfall are significantly negative, showing that the applicants may escape from the city of high temperature and rainy climate.

Next, we use the annually average wind speed as an instrumental variable of air pollution to estimate Equations (2) and (3). To be consistent with the OLS estimation, the variables of university, city, and climate are added to the equations in turn, and the estimation results are shown in columns (1)–(3) of Table 3.

Table 3. Impact of air pollution on applicants' number (2SLS estimates).

Second Stage			
Variables		**2SLS**	
Apply	**(1)**	**(2)**	**(3)**
$PM_{2.5}$	−250.4749 **	−324.9521 ***	−250.4680 **
	(104.96)	(103.45)	(97.61)
Enrollment	2.2718 ***	2.5286 ***	2.4464 ***
	(0.30)	(0.33)	(0.31)
Rj_gdp		1.7623	−0.2087
		(11.35)	(10.68)
Industry_3rate		−115.8101 *	−90.9361
		(68.81)	(65.07)
CPI		153.2544	194.7881
		(151.26)	(142.80)
Popu		−1.4972 ***	−1.3889 ***
		(0.55)	(0.52)
Edu_cost		0.0296	0.0336
		(0.16)	(0.15)
Transpor		13.6354	1.2228
		(23.67)	(23.57)
Avgtemp			−733.7366 *
			(431.00)
Avgrain			−54.7615 **
			(26.12)
School FE	Yes	Yes	Yes
Year FE	Yes	Yes	Yes
N	585	585	585
R^2	0.5491	0.5152	0.5680
First Stage			
Avgwindsp	−7.4706 ***	−8.7096 ***	−9.2802 ***
	(1.39)	(1.47)	(1.57)
F	41.18	35.22	30.77
N	585	585	585

Note: Standard errors clustered at city level are reported in the brackets. *** $p < 0.01$, ** $p < 0.05$, * $p < 0.1$.

From column (1), the first stage shows that the estimated coefficient of average wind speed (Avgwindsp) is significantly negative at the 1% level, indicating that the faster the wind speed, the lower the $PM_{2.5}$ concentration will be. And the F value (41.18) is larger than 10, there is no risk of a weak instrumental variable. In the second stage, the estimated coefficient of $PM_{2.5}$ is significantly negative at the 5% level but compared with the result estimated by the ordinary least squares (OLS) (column 1 of Table 2), the absolute value becomes larger, revealing that the OLS estimated result could be underestimated. Columns (2) and (3) are the estimated results of adding urban and climatic variables in turn. From column (3), the coefficient of $PM_{2.5}$ is still significantly negative, indicating that the increase in $PM_{2.5}$ concentration by an average 1 $\mu g/m^3$ will generate a reduction of applicants' quantity by about 250, which accounts for 2.2% of the average quantity of all applicants. The estimated coefficient of the number of students to be enrolled is still significantly positive; specifically, the number of students to be enrolled increases by 1, and the amount of applicants increases by around 2. Additionally, the estimated coefficients of population density, annually average temperature, and annually average rainfall are significantly negative too. One exception is the consumer price index (CPI), although the result is still positive, but it is no longer significant, demonstrating that the consumer price index (CPI) may have few causal effects on applicants' university-city choices. Meanwhile, the first stage shows that the estimated coefficient of average wind speed is still significantly negative, and the F value (30.77) is still higher than 10, further certifying that our determination of the instrumental variable is plausible.

Due to different majors, the attention to the air information of applicants for different disciplines may be differential, and the ratio of gender between different disciplines are also distinguishing. Existing studies have shown that compared with males, females are more concerned about air quality [26,27]. Taking the difference into consideration, we further investigate the effect of air pollution on different subjects' applicants. The estimation result is shown in columns (1) and (2) of Table 4.

Table 4. Different discipline applicants.

	Second Stage	
	2SLS	
Variables	**(1)**	**(2)**
Apply	**Social Science**	**Natural Science**
$PM_{2.5}$	−200.0694 ***	−50.1722
	(73.80)	(44.07)
University	Yes	Yes
Urban	Yes	Yes
Climate	Yes	Yes
School FE	Yes	Yes
Year FE	Yes	Yes
N	585	585
R^2	0.4359	0.5507
	First Stage	
Avgwindsp	−9.2802 ***	−9.2802 ***
	(1.57)	(1.57)
F	30.77	30.77
N	585	585

Note: Standard errors clustered at city level are reported in the brackets. University control includes number of students to be recruited; urban controls include GDP per capita, the proportion of the tertiary industry, consumer price index, population density, education expenditure per capita, number of buses and trams (per 10,000 people); climate controls include annually average temperature, annually average rainfall. *** $p < 0.01$.

Column (1) is the estimated result of social science. The estimated coefficient of $PM_{2.5}$ is −200.0694, which means that the average $PM_{2.5}$ concentration increases for 1 $\mu g/m^3$, and the number of applicants for social science decreases by about 200. Column (2) is the estimated result of natural science: for every 1 $\mu g/m^3$ increase in $PM_{2.5}$ concentration, the number of applicants for natural science will decrease by about 50, but it is statistically insignificant, demonstrating that air pollution may have few significant effects on the choices of natural science applicants. It is consistent with our anticipation that the applicants of social science may pay more attention to air quality and have a higher standard for life, due to the professional knowledge that they are exposed to every day. In addition, social science has a larger scale of female students who are more sensitive to air pollution than male students, so the sensitivity to it is higher.

3.2. Robustness Checks

In order to further verify the robustness of benchmark regression results, we mainly consider replacing the independent variable, control variable, and excluding other affecting factors to test the results.

3.2.1. Alternative Air Pollution Indicators

China's outdoor pollutants of air pollution mainly include $PM_{2.5}$ and SO_2 [28–30]. SO_2 is easily soluble in human body fluids, and the long-run existence can lead to upper respiratory tract infections, chronic bronchitis, emphysema, and other diseases, so it may also affect the university-city choices of applicants. We substitute $PM_{2.5}$ with SO_2, re-estimate Equations (2) and (3), and the regression result is shown in column (2) of Table 5.

Table 5. Robustness check results.

		Second Stage			
			2SLS		
Variables	(1)	(2)	(3)	(4)	(5)
Apply	Baseline	Replace Independent Variable	Replace University Control Variable	Exclude Agglomeration of Double First-Class Universities	Add Non-Double First-Class Universities
$PM_{2.5}$	−250.4680 ** (97.61)		−215.1581 ** (97.44)	−526.1274 ** (190.00)	−135.2575 * (73.75)
SO_2		−57.2924 * (30.24)			
University	Yes	Yes	Yes	Yes	Yes
Urban	Yes	Yes	Yes	Yes	Yes
Climate	Yes	Yes	Yes	Yes	Yes
School FE	Yes	Yes	Yes	Yes	Yes
Year FE	Yes	Yes	Yes	Yes	Yes
N	585	585	585	288	1117
R^2	0.5680	0.2077	0.5780	0.4578	0.5679
		First Stage			
Avgwindsp		−40.5707 ** (15.90)	−9.1943 *** (1.57)	−11.4495 *** (3.00)	−6.9300 *** (1.23)
F		16.30	30.82	28.64	30.64
N		585	585	288	1117

Note: Standard errors clustered at city level are reported in the brackets. University control of column (3) includes ratio of enrollment, university control of other columns includes number of students to be recruited; urban controls include GDP per capita, the proportion of the tertiary industry, consumer price index, population density, education expenditure per capita, number of buses and trams (per 10,000 people); climate controls include annually average temperature, annually average rainfall. *** $p < 0.01$, ** $p < 0.05$, * $p < 0.1$.

The result shows that the estimated coefficient of SO_2 is negative at the 10% level; a rise in SO_2 concentration by one unit on average causes a reduction of applicants' numbers by about 57. It further demonstrates that air pollution does have a negative impact on the university-city choices of applicants, which verifies the robustness of the benchmark regression results.

3.2.2. Alternative University Control Variable

In the baseline regression, we choose the number of students to be enrolled that published in their intended university's admission brochure as the university control variable. However, when applying for UNGEE, applicants also focus on the admission ratio of recent years, as the admission proportion can reflect the competition and difficulty of target university. In view of this, we displace the number of students to be recruited with one year lag of admission ratio to re-regress Equations (2) and (3); the result is reported in column (3) of Table 5. It shows that the estimated coefficient of $PM_{2.5}$ is −215.1581 at a 5% significant level, which is analogous to the estimated coefficient of benchmark regression (−250.4680), indicating that the baseline regression result is stable.

3.2.3. Excluding the Agglomeration of Double First-Class Universities

Some double first-class universities exist as an agglomeration in partial Chinese cities; the agglomeration in a single city may underestimate the impact of air pollution on applicants' university-city choices. During the data collection process, we notice that Beijing, Shanghai, Wuhan, Nanjing, and other traditional first-tier and second-tier cities have more than 5 double first-class universities. In order to eliminate the impact, we exclude cities with more than 5 double first-class universities in the sample and re-regress the equations. Column (4) of Table 5 reports the regression result. After moving partial cities, although the absolute value of the estimated coefficient in $PM_{2.5}$ becomes larger, it is still significantly negative, showing that the benchmark regression result is steady. Specifically, for every 1 $\mu g/m^3$ increase in $PM_{2.5}$ concentration on average, the number of applicants applying for UNGEE decreases by about 526, which is greater than the benchmark result (250). The reason is that these excluding cities such as Beijing, Shanghai, Wuhan, Nanjing, and so on are the traditional preferred city for study. Furthermore, the gathering of double first-class universities represents more abundant educational resources, which can bring more opportunities and growth to applicants, and may increase the attractiveness to applicants. Thereby, these advantages can weaken the negative impact of air pollution on applicants' choosing intentions. Therefore, after removing these sample cities, the regression coefficient becomes larger.

3.2.4. Considering the Non-Double First-Class Universities

The sample that we use in the baseline regression is the data of 76 double first-class universities. During the data collection process, we note that the official websites of some non-double first-class universities have also published application data over these years. Therefore, we add the data that we manually crawl from the website of 82 non-double first-class universities into the sample to re-regress the equations, and the result is shown in column (5) of Table 5. It shows that the coefficient of $PM_{2.5}$ is significantly negative, so the benchmark conclusion still holds. For every 1 $\mu g/m^3$ increase in $PM_{2.5}$ concentration on average, the number of applicants decreases by about 136. Compared with the benchmark result (250), the absolute value decreases, illustrating that the sample of non-double first-class universities lowers the sensitivity. Generally speaking, applicants who apply for non-double first-class universities usually are the group that did not perform very well in gaokao and usually have a relatively poor starting point during their undergraduate degree, so the range of universities they can choose from is limited. Therefore, compared with air quality, they may pay more attention to other factors such as who is more likely to be admitted when make their university-city choices.

4. The Heterogeneous Effects

In addition to the average effects, we further investigate how the effects differ in terms of university. Firstly, according to the results of China's fourth round of subject evaluation, we divide the universities into different qualities, and investigate the heterogeneity between world-class universities and first-class discipline universities. Secondly, according to the division of university by the MOE of PRC, the heterogeneity between comprehensive and non-comprehensive universities is examined. Finally, we take the location of universities into consideration, and we estimate the heterogeneity between northern and southern universities.

4.1. Different Quality Universities

The attractiveness of a different quality university for applicants has certain differences. Compared with first-class discipline universities, world-class universities are more likely to be pursued by applicants. Therefore, the air pollution sensitivity between applicants who apply for different quality universities may be distinguishing. China's fourth round of subject evaluation divided double first-class universities into world-class universities and first-class discipline universities. Generally speaking, world-class universities usually have a better quality than first-class discipline universities. According to the result, we separate 76 universities into world-class universities and first-class discipline universities and examine the heterogeneity between them. We define the dummy variable for the world-class university and its interaction with the air pollution measure in Equations (2) and (3) to estimate the heterogeneous effect. The regression result is shown in column (1) of Table 6.

The result reveals that air pollution has a significantly negative impact on applicants for double first-class universities. However, compared with first-class discipline universities, the world-class universities lower the sensitivity of air pollution for applicants. It demonstrates that air pollution indeed affects the choices of applicants, but the quality of the university can weaken the effect. The world-class universities are those at the top in China, which are also the targets that all students pursue, so applicants will only take air pollution a little into account when faced with a better-quality university choice. The result is similar with our conclusion in the robustness checks of excluding the agglomeration of double first-class universities, which further illustrates the potential importance of university quality and educational resources in the university-city selection of applicants.

Table 6. The heterogeneous effects on migration intentions.

Second Stage			
	2SLS		
Variables / Apply	(1)	(2)	(3)
$PM_{2.5}$	−431.7390 **	−404.8751 *	−33.6891
	(196.27)	(218.04)	(132.13)
$PM_{2.5}$ × World-class university	420.1479 **		
	(189.89)		
$PM_{2.5}$ × Comprehensive university		348.2737	
		(336.12)	
$PM_{2.5}$ × Northern university			−186.2481 *
			(98.38)
University	Yes	Yes	Yes
Urban	Yes	Yes	Yes
Climate	Yes	Yes	Yes
School FE	Yes	Yes	Yes
Year FE	Yes	Yes	Yes
N	585	585	585
R^2	0.3631	0.3281	0.5856
First Stage			
Avgwindsp	−6.2735 ***	−11.1137 ***	−5.4436 ***
	(1.84)	(1.91)	(1.40)
F	29.52	30.42	29.68
N	585	585	585

Note: Standard errors clustered at city level are reported in the brackets. University control includes number of students to be recruited; urban controls include GDP per capita, the proportion of the tertiary industry, consumer price index, population density, education expenditure per capita, number of buses and trams (per 10,000 people); climate controls include annually average temperature, annually average rainfall. *** $p < 0.01$, ** $p < 0.05$, * $p < 0.1$.

4.2. Different Types of Universities

The university of a different type contains different majors, and comprehensive universities usually contain more sorts of majors than non-comprehensive universities. So, the number of applicants who apply for comprehensive universities may be larger than non-comprehensive universities, and there may be differences in air pollution sensitivity among them. Based on this, according to the sort of university from the MOE of PRC (Search each university in https://www.baidu.com/, accessed on 26 December 2020), we divide 76 double first-class universities into comprehensive and non-comprehensive, and then define the dummy variable for the comprehensive university and its interaction with the air pollution measure in Equations (2) and (3) to estimate the heterogeneous effect. The estimated result is presented in column (2) of Table 6. The result discloses that air pollution has a significantly negative impact on the choices of applicants, but there is no significant difference in applicants for the two types of universities. It demonstrates that there is no significant difference in the sensitivity of applicants to air pollution among different types of universities.

4.3. Different Regions of Universities

The Qinling-Huaihe geographical line divides China into the two parts of the south and north. Due to the cold climate in winter, the Chinese government provides a free heating system for all households and indoor places in the north, and the supply of heating requires a large amount of fossil fuels such as coal, which emits a lot of pollutants, but it does not exist in the south. The policy difference causes an initial difference in air pollution between the two regions [3,7]. In view of this, we divide 76 double first-class universities into southern and northern according to the Qinling-Huaihe boundary, and then define the dummy variable for northern university and its interaction with air pollution measure in Equations (2) and (3) to estimate the heterogeneous effect. Column (3) of Table 6 represents the regression result.

The result shows that air pollution has little impact on applicants for southern universities, but the universities of the north significantly aggravate the negative effect on applicants, which is consistent with our anticipation. The applicants who live or study in China have a full recognition that air pollution in the north (the average $PM_{2.5}$ concentration is 51.41 $\mu g/m^3$) is more serious than in the south (the average $PM_{2.5}$ concentration is 47.99 $\mu g/m^3$). Worse air quality may affect their physical and mental health during the study period for a master's degree, and the inherent awareness may drive them to evade a northern university when other reference factors such as university quality are identical.

To verify the above conclusion of different regions, we analyze the application data and $PM_{2.5}$ concentration data and then draw the trend graphs (Figure 4). The left side of Figure 4 shows the trend of northern air pollution deterioration ratio (deterioration ratio = (average northern $PM_{2.5}$ concentration − average national $PM_{2.5}$ concentration)/average national $PM_{2.5}$ concentration), and the right side of Figure 4 is the trend of the proportion that the applicants of northern and southern universities account for the whole country from 2010 to 2021. From the left side, we can find that the ratio has gradually increased during the period, manifesting that compared with the whole country, northern air pollution is aggravating. From the right, the proportion of the number of applicants to northern universities is gradually decreasing, while the ratio of southern universities is gradually increasing, summarizing that with the deterioration of northern air quality, the university-city choosing intentions of applicants are shifting from north to south. The factual analysis confirms our above conclusion reasonably.

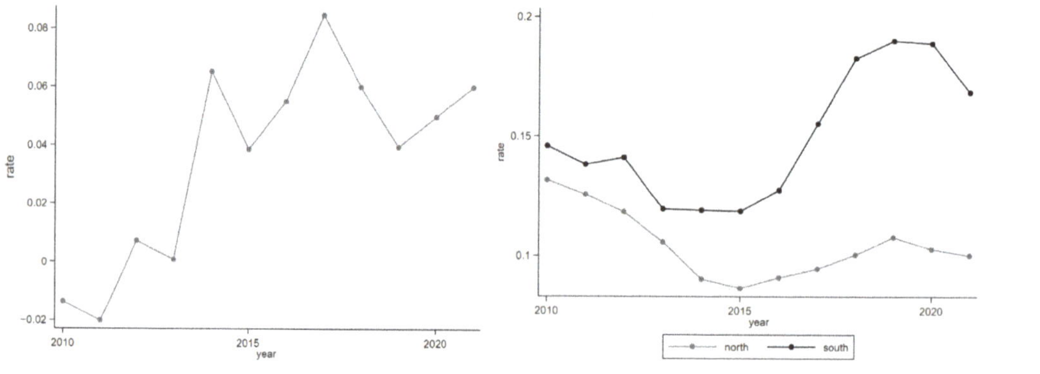

Figure 4. Northern $PM_{2.5}$ concentration ratio and northern-southern ratio of applicants' number. Note: The (**left**) figure displays the ratio that northern $PM_{2.5}$ concentrations are higher than all of the country, and the (**right**) figure displays the ratio that northern and southern applicants' number account for the whole country.

5. Comparison with Existing Literature

Ultimately, we summarize the estimates of the effects of air pollution on migration or migration intention in the existing literature in Table 7. Firstly, some literature focuses topics on talents [13,14,31]. Based on the same perspective of college or university graduates and the same pollutant of air pollution as us, Lai et al. (2021) find that with a 1 $\mu g/m^3$ increase in $PM_{2.5}$ concentration in the original city, the probability of college graduates to leave the city increases by 1%, which is lower than our result (2.17%). From the view of corporations, Wang and Wu (2021) disclose that with a 1 $\mu g/m^3$ increase in $PM_{2.5}$ concentration in the original city, the stock of technologically innovative professionals decreases by 0.15%. Using

AQI as a pollutant of air pollution, Xue et al. (2021) conclude that with a 100-point increase in AQI in a destination city, the search volume index of choosing a destination city as the intended work place for corporate human capital decreases 2.74%, and the magnitude is similar with our result (2.17%).

Table 7. Summary of the estimated air pollution impacts on migration or migration intention in existing literature.

Paper	Country	Type of Migration	Pollutants	Factor of Dependent Variable	Increase in Pollutant Concentration	Change in Migration or Migration Intention
This study	China	Applicants of UNGEE	$PM_{2.5}$	The quantity of applicants (move into destinational city)	1 μg/m³ (destinational city)	−2.17%
Qin and Zhu (2018)	China	Emigration interests in prefecture cities	AQI	Baidu search index on "emigration" (move into destinational city)	100-point (destinational city)	−2.30–4.80%
Li et al. (2020)	China	Children's migration	$PM_{2.5}$	Probability of children's migration with parents (move into destinational city)	1 μg/m³ (destinational city)	−5.18%
Liu and Yu (2020)	China	Urban migration	AQI	Migrants' interest in settling down in current city (stay in original city)	100-point (original city)	−15.1%
Lai et al. (2021)	China	College graduates	$PM_{2.5}$	Probability to leave current city (move out of original city)	1 μg/m³ (original city)	+1.00%
Wang and Wu (2021)	China and India	Technological innovative professionals (TIP)	$PM_{2.5}$	Stock of TIP (move out of original city)	1 μg/m³ (original city)	+0.15%
Jia and Chen (2021)	China	Floating migrants	AQI	Migrants' settlement intentions (move into destinational city)	100-point (destinational city)	−33.2%
Xue et al. (2021)	China	Corporate human capital (executives)	AQI	Search volume index of intended work places (move into destinational city)	100-point (destinational city)	−2.74%
Chen et al. (2022)	China	Migration in China's counties	$PM_{2.5}$	Net-outmigration ratio (move out of original city)	1μg/m³ (original city)	+0.53%

In this paper, we use the application of UNGEE to measure migration intention, and some existing literature also measures migration intention from other perspectives. Treating the Baidu search index on "emigration" as the migration intention, Qin and Zhu (2018) reveal that the increase of 100-point in the AQI of the destination city decreases 2.3–4.8% emigration interests to the destination city, which is lower than the urban or floating migration interest in settlement [32,33]. Apart from migration intention, some literature also pay attention to actual migration. Liu and Yu (2020) and Chen et al. (2022) disclose that the net outflow of population increases 15.1% and 0.53% with the increase of 100-point in AQI and 1 $\mu g/m^3$ in the $PM_{2.5}$ concentration of the original city. Lastly, using children migration data, Li et al. (2020) detect that the probability of children migration with parents decreases 5.18% with a 1 $\mu g/m^3$ increase in the $PM_{2.5}$ concentration in the destination city [34]. Based on the same pollutant of air pollution, the result is larger than ours, which reveals that the children who are identified as the vulnerable group are more sensitive to air pollution than teenagers.

6. Conclusions

Based on the merging of application data for UNGEE of 76 double first-class universities and urban $PM_{2.5}$ concentration data in China, this paper uses wind speed as the instrumental variable of air pollution and exploits the two-stage least squares (2SLS) method to empirically investigate the effect of air pollution on applicants' university-city choices. We find that air pollution has a negative impact on the university-city choices of applicants: the average increase in urban $PM_{2.5}$ concentration by 1 $\mu g/m^3$ reduces the number of applicants for each university of a destination city by about 250. Among them, the number of applicants for social science decreases significantly by 200, and the number of applicants for natural science decreases by 50. Compared with previous research, our conclusions are subtly different. Additionally, the impacts of air pollution on applicants are highly heterogeneous. Air pollution has more significantly negative effects on applicants of first-class discipline universities than world-class universities. The reason is that the quality of university can weaken the negative effects of air pollution on applicants. However, the impacts have no significant difference in comprehensive and non-comprehensive universities. Lastly, due to the reason that air pollution in the north is more deteriorated than in the south, the universities located in the north aggravate the negative effects of air pollution on applicants, which results in the fact that university-city selecting intentions of applicants have a tendency that shift from north to south.

This paper provides evidence for studies on the effects of air pollution on high human capital migration intention from developing countries. Furthermore, by comparing with previous studies, we disclose a differential completion from the perspective of university. The conclusions of this paper show that applicants who apply for UNGEE are highly sensitive to air pollution, and the applicants of social science are more sensitive than natural science. There are also differences between different qualities and regions of the universities. All of the above conclusions can be further extended to the working location decisions of graduates, or flowing orientation of talents, and provide practical recommendations for the introduction of talents in a number of cities. In the mature development stage, governments should prioritize economic development, but also try to trade off the environment condition, and take measures to build an "environmentally friendly, resource-saving, and livable" city to attract a "knowledge-based and innovative" labor force to join in. In addition, taking heterogeneous effects into consideration, policy makers should implement differentiated policies for different groups and regions.

This study also has some limitations: the first is that we do not have more microscopic individual data, such as personal information for each applicant, which can track the migration origin and destination of each applicant. We can only use the quantity of applicants for every university to measure migration intentions. The second is that we do not have the physical and mental health data of the Chinese university students at our sample universities, so we cannot analyze the mechanism of impact from physical and mental health channels. And so we can't know that how air pollution affects applicants' university-city choices.

Author Contributions: Conceptualization, X.W.; methodology, C.X.; software, C.X.; validation, C.X.; formal analysis, C.X.; investigation, X.W.; resources, X.W.; data curation, X.W.; writing—original draft preparation, X.W.; writing—review and editing, C.X.; visualization, X.W.; supervision, C.X.; project administration, C.X. All authors have read and agreed to the published version of the manuscript.

Funding: This research received no external funding.

Institutional Review Board Statement: Not applicable.

Informed Consent Statement: Not applicable.

Data Availability Statement: No new data were created or analyzed in this study. Data sharing is not applicable to this article.

Conflicts of Interest: The authors declare no conflict of interest.

Appendix A

Table A1. List of 76 double first-class universities.

Beijing (15)	Beijing University, Renmin University of China, Beijing University of Aeronautics and Astronautics, China Agricultural University, Beijing Normal University, Minzu University of China, Central University of Finance and Economics, University of International Business and Economics, China University of Political Science and Law, Beijing University of Posts and Telecommunications, Beijing Forestry University, Capital Normal University, Beijing Foreign Studies University, China University of Mining & Technology (Beijing), University of Chinese Academy of Sciences
Tianjin (4)	Nankai University, Hebei University of Technology, Tianjin Medical University, Tiangong University
Shanghai (7)	Tongji University, Shanghai Jiao Tong University, East China Normal University, Donghua University, Shanghai International Studies University, Shanghai University of Finance and Economics, Shanghai University
Chongqing (1)	Southwest University
Guangzhou (4)	Sun Yat-sen University, South China University of Technology, Jinan University, South China Normal University
Nanjing (5)	Nanjing University, Southeast University, Nanjing University of Posts and Telecommunications, Nanjing Forestry University, Nanjing Agricultural University
Wuxi (1)	Jiangnan University
Suzhou (1)	Soochow University
Xuzhou (1)	China University of Mining and Technology (Xuzhou)
Hangzhou (1)	Zhejiang University
Ningbo (1)	Ningbo University
Wuhan (5)	Wuhan University, China University of Geosciences (Wuhan), Huazhong Agricultural University, Zhongnan University of Economics and Law, Central China Normal University
Changsha (3)	Central South University, Hunan University, National University of Defense Technology
Hefei (1)	Anhui University
Fuzhou (1)	Fuzhou University
Xiamen (1)	Xiamen University
Zhengzhou (1)	Zhengzhou University
Kunming (1)	Yunnan University
Shihezi (1)	Shihezi University
Tibet (1)	Tibet University
Xian (4)	Xidian University, Shaanxi Normal University, Northwest University, Chang'an University
Xianyang (1)	Northwest A&F University
Chengdu (2)	Sichuan University, Southwestern University of Finance and Economics
Dalian (1)	Dalian University of Technology
Shenyang (2)	Northeastern University (Shenyang), Liaoning University
Harbin (1)	Harbin Engineering University
Haikou (1)	Hainan University
Yinchuan (1)	Ningxia University
Lanzhou (1)	Lanzhou University
Qinhuangdao (1)	Northeastern University (Qinhuangdao)
Jinan (1)	Shandong University (Jinan)
Weihai (1)	Shandong University (Weihai)
Qingdao (2)	Ocean University of China, China University of Petroleum (East China)
Inner mongolia (1)	Inner Mongolia University

References

1. Schlenker, W.; Walker, W.R. Airports, air pollution, and contemporaneous health. *Rev. Econ. Stud.* **2015**, *83*, 768–809. [CrossRef]
2. Arceo, E.; Hanna, R.; Oliva, P. Does the Effect of Pollution on Infant Mortality Differ between Developing and Developed Countries? Evidence from Mexico City. *Econ. J.* **2016**, *126*, 257–280. [CrossRef]
3. Ebenstein, A.; Fan, M.; Greenstone, M.; He, G.; Zhou, M. New Evidence on the Impact of Sustained Exposure to Air Pollution on Life Expectancy from China's Huai River Policy. *Proc. Natl. Acad. Sci. USA* **2017**, *114*, 10384–10389. [CrossRef] [PubMed]
4. He, G.; Liu, T.; Zhou, M. Straw burning, PM2. 5, and death: Evidence from China. *J. Dev. Econ.* **2020**, *145*, 102468. [CrossRef]
5. Fan, M.; He, G.; Zhou, M. The winter choke: Coal-fired heating, air pollution, and mortality in China. *J. Health Econ.* **2020**, *71*, 102316. [CrossRef]
6. Deschenes, O.; Wang, H.; Wang, S.; Zhang, P. The effect of air pollution on body weight and obesity: Evidence from China. *J. Dev. Econ.* **2020**, *145*, 102461. [CrossRef]
7. Chen, Y.; Ebenstein, A.; Greenstone, M.; Li, H. Evidence on the Impact of Sustained Exposure to Air Pollution on Life Expectancy from China's Huai River Policy. *Proc. Natl. Acad. Sci. USA* **2013**, *110*, 12936–12941. [CrossRef]
8. Zhang, X.; Zhang, X.; Chen, X. Happiness in the air: How does a dirty sky affect mental health and subjective well-being? *J. Environ. Econ. Manag.* **2017**, *85*, 81–94. [CrossRef]
9. Zhang, Z.; Hao, Y.; Mu, Z.N. Does environmental pollution affect labor supply? An empirical analysis based on 112 cities in China. *J. Clean. Prod.* **2018**, *190*, 378–387. [CrossRef]
10. Ito, K.; Zhang, S. Willingness to pay for clean air: Evidence from air purifier markets in China. *J. Political Econ.* **2020**, *128*, 1627–1672. [CrossRef]
11. Chen, S.; Oliva, P.; Zhang, P. The Effect of Air Pollution on Migration: Evidence from China. *J. Dev. Econ.* **2022**, *156*, 102833. [CrossRef]
12. Zheng, S.; Zhang, X.; Sun, W.; Lin, C. Air Pollution and Elite College Graduates' Job Location Choice: Evidence from China. *Ann. Reg. Sci.* **2019**, *63*, 295–316. [CrossRef]
13. Xue, S.; Zhang, B.; Zhao, X. Brain Drain: The Impact of Air Pollution on firm Performance. *J. Environ. Econ. Manag.* **2021**, *110*, 102546. [CrossRef]
14. Lai, W.; Song, H.; Wang, C.; Wang, H. Air pollution and brain drain: Evidence from college graduates in China. *China Econ. Rev.* **2021**, *68*, 101624. [CrossRef]
15. Clark, W.A.; Ledwith, V. How much does income matter in neighborhood choice? *Popul. Res. Policy Rev.* **2007**, *26*, 145–161. [CrossRef]
16. So, K.S.; Orazem, P.F.; Otto, D.M. The effects of housing prices, wages, and commuting time on joint residential and job location choices. *Am. J. Agric. Econ.* **2001**, *83*, 1036–1048. [CrossRef]
17. Wozniak, A. Are college graduates more responsive to distant labor market opportunities? *J. Hum. Resour.* **2010**, *45*, 944–970.
18. Plantinga, A.J.; Détang-Dessendre, C.; Hunt, G.L.; Piguet, V. Housing prices and inter-urban migration. *Reg. Sci. Urban Econ.* **2013**, *43*, 296–306. [CrossRef]
19. Qin, Y.; Zhu, H. Run away? Air Pollution and Emigration Interests in China. *J. Popul. Econ.* **2018**, *31*, 235–266. [CrossRef]
20. Fu, S.; Viard, V.B.; Zhang, P. Air Pollution and Manufacturing Firm Productivity: Nationwide Estimates for China. *Econ. J.* **2021**, *131*, 3241–3273. [CrossRef]
21. Zivin, J.G.; Liu, T.; Song, Y.; Tang, Q.; Zhang, P. The unintended impacts of agricultural fires: Human capital in China. *J. Dev. Econ.* **2020**, *147*, 102560. [CrossRef]
22. Burkhardt, J.; Bayham, J.; Wilson, A.; Carter, E.; Berman, J.D.; O'Dell, K.; Pierce, J.R. The effect of pollution on crime: Evidence from data on particulate matter and ozone. *J. Environ. Econ. Manag.* **2019**, *98*, 102267. [CrossRef]
23. Chen, C.; Li, C.; Li, Y.; Liu, J.; Meng, C.; Han, J.; Xu, D. Short-term effects of ambient air pollution exposure on lung function: A longitudinal study among healthy primary school children in China. *Sci. Total Environ.* **2018**, *645*, 1014–1020. [CrossRef] [PubMed]
24. Shepherd, A.; Mullins, J.T. Arthritis diagnosis and early-life exposure to air pollution. *Environ. Pollut.* **2019**, *253*, 1030–1037. [CrossRef] [PubMed]
25. Broner, F.; Bustos, P.; Carvalho, V.M. Sources of Comparative Advantage in Polluting Industries. NBER Working Paper Series. 2012. No.18337. Available online: https://www.nber.org/papers/w18337 (accessed on 1 August 2012).
26. Arias-Ortiz, N.E.; Icaza-Noguera, G.; Ruiz-Rudolph, P. Thyroid Cancer Incidence in Women and Proximity to Industrial Air Pollution Sources: A Spatial Analysis in a Middle Size City in Colombia. *Atmos. Pollut. Res.* **2018**, *9*, 464–475. [CrossRef]
27. Dutta, S.; Banerjee, S. Exposure to Indoor Air Pollution & AMP.; Women Health. *Environ. Urban. Asia* **2014**, *5*, 25–89.
28. Maji, K.J.; Sarkar, C. Spatio-Temporal Variations and Trends of Major Air Pollutants in China during 2015–2018. *Environ. Sci. Pollut. Res. Int.* **2020**, *27*, 33792–33808. [CrossRef]
29. Guo, H.; Gu, X.; Ma, G.; Shi, S.; Wang, W.; Zuo, X.; Zhang, X. Spatial and Temporal Variations of Air Quality and Six Air Pollutants in China during 2015–2017. *Sci. Rep.* **2019**, *9*, 15201. [CrossRef]
30. Ren, L.; Yang, W.; Bai, Z. Characteristics of Major Air Pollutants in China. *Ambient. Air Pollut. Health Impact China* **2017**, *2017*, 7–26.
31. Wang, F.; Wu, M. Does Air Pollution Affect the Accumulation of Technological Innovative Human Capital? Empirical Evidence from China and India. *J. Clean. Prod.* **2021**, *285*, 124818. [CrossRef]
32. Liu, Z.; Yu, L. Stay or leave? The Role of Air Pollution in Urban Migration Choices. *Ecol. Econ.* **2020**, *177*, 106780. [CrossRef]

33. Jia, K.; Chen, S. Escaping from Pollution: Air Pollution and the Settlement Intentions of Floating Migrants in Chinese Cities. *Migr. Stud.* **2021**, *9*, 1480–1498. [CrossRef]
34. Li, X.; Chen, H.; Li, Y. The Effect of Air Pollution on Children's Migration with Parents: Evidence from China. *Environ. Sci. Pollut. Res.* **2020**, *27*, 12499–12513. [CrossRef] [PubMed]

International Journal of
Environmental Research and Public Health

MDPI

Article

What Affects the Economic Resilience of China's Yellow River Basin Amid Economic Crisis—From the Perspective of Spatial Heterogeneity

Liangang Li [1], Pingyu Zhang [2,3] and Chengxin Wang [1,*]

1 College of Geography and Environment, Shandong Normal University, Jinan 250358, China; llg911208@163.com
2 Northeast Institute of Geography and Agroecology, Chinese Academy of Sciences, Changchun 130002, China; zhangpy@iga.ac.cn
3 College of Resources and Environment, University of Chinese Academy of Sciences, Beijing 100049, China
* Correspondence: 110105@sdnu.edu.cn

Abstract: This paper contributes to the study of regional economic resilience by analyzing the dynamic characteristics and influence mechanisms of resilience from the perspective of spatial heterogeneity. This paper focuses on the resistance and recoverability dimensions of resilience and analyzed the dynamic changes in economic resilience in China's Yellow River Basin in response to the 2008 economic crisis. The multi-scale geographical weighted regression model was utilized to examine the effect of key factors on regional economic resilience. Our findings show the following: (1) The resistance of the Yellow River Basin to the financial crisis was high; however, the recoverability decreased significantly over time. (2) The spatial heterogeneity of driving factors was significant, and they had different effect scales on economic resilience. Related variety, government agency, environment, and opening to the global economy had a significant effect on economic resilience only in a specific small range. Specialization, unrelated variety, and location had opposite effects in different regions of the Yellow River Basin. (3) Specialization limited the area's resistance to shock but enhanced the recoverability. Related variety improved regional economic resilience. Unrelated variety was not conducive to regional resistance to shock and had opposite effects on the recoverability in different regions. (4) Government agency and financial market promoted regional economic resilience. Environment pollution and resource-based economic structure limited regional economic resilience. Opening to the global economy and urban hierarchy limited regional resistance to shock, but strong economic development had the opposite effect of improved regional resistance. The location in the east of the Yellow River Basin enhanced the recoverability; however, the location in the west limited the recoverability.

Keywords: regional economic resilience; spatial heterogeneity; spatiotemporal evolution; influence mechanism; Yellow River Basin; China

Citation: Li, L.; Zhang, P.; Wang, C. What Affects the Economic Resilience of China's Yellow River Basin Amid Economic Crisis—From the Perspective of Spatial Heterogeneity. *IJERPH* **2022**, *19*, 9024. https://doi.org/10.3390/ijerph19159024

Academic Editors: Jie Chen, Qian Zhou and Ting Zhang

Received: 19 May 2022
Accepted: 18 July 2022
Published: 25 July 2022

1. Introduction

As complex dynamic systems, regional economic systems are frequently affected by uncertain shocks such as international financial crisis and COVID-19 [1–3]. How to deal with uncertain shocks, resist the impact of the shocks, and quickly restore development has become the key to maintaining the healthy and sustainable development of cities in the current highly uncertain shock environment [4–6]. However, regional (urban) economic systems show significant spatial differences in coping with shocks. Specifically, some regions have been seriously affected by shocks, resulting in stagnation of or a decline in economic development. Interestingly, some cities can resist the negative impact of shocks and achieve rapid economic recovery in a short time through adjustment [7–9]. The different performances of urban response to shocks have led to extensive discussions in economic geography and regional science on how to cope with shocks and to what extent regional economic systems can recover or even transform [10–13]. Regional economic resilience is considered to be the key to explaining such differences [14,15]. Especially under the COVID-19 epidemic shock, regional economic resilience has become a buzzword in the current academic and policy circles both in developed and emerging economies [3,16–18]. Regional economic resilience addresses the regional ability to resist and recover from external shocks and, broadly speaking, to adapt to uncertain contexts for maintaining the evolving abilities for economic development and growth [4,6,10]. Regional economic resilience provides a new perspective for analyzing the evolution mechanism of regional systems under uncertain shock environments [3].

The Yellow River Basin is an important ecological region and major economic zone in China. It spans eight provinces and has significant differences in different scale units within the region. The Yellow River Basin includes the eastern coastal areas and the central and western regions of China. Regional economic development has long depended on resource-based industries and opening to the outside world [1,19], and investment has a great pulling effect on regional development. This has played an important role in the economic development of the Yellow River Basin, but it has also caused serious environmental pollution. However, in the context of the financial crisis, this over-reliance on specific investment and poor environments may limit the regional economic resilience to the shock [20]. This is mainly because, under the influence of the financial crisis, foreign trade declined, foreign capital began to withdraw capital to reduce losses, and the desire for domestic capital investment declined. After the shock, China entered a high-quality development stage, and the environmental situation has since become an important force to support economic development. The reduction in investment and the weak environment limit the ability of the Yellow River Basin to cope with the shock, and the economic development is slow.

The weak ecological environment and extensive development model of the Yellow River Basin lead to its extreme vulnerability to external shocks such as the financial crisis [21], resulting in the interruption of the regional development path and falling into the recession track. The Yellow River Basin is a typical vulnerable area to the financial crisis. Under the background of China's national strategy of ecological protection and high-quality development of the Yellow River Basin in 2019, how to deal with uncertain shocks and maintain stable economic development in the Yellow River Basin has become the key to high-quality development. There is an urgent need to study the characteristics of economic resilience in the Yellow River Basin and explore the differences in the influence mechanism of regional economic resilience from the perspective of basin heterogeneity. This paper attempts to explore ways to improve the ability of the Yellow River Basin to deal with external shocks so as to maintain the sustainable economic development of the Yellow River Basin in the event of uncertain shocks in the future.

Therefore, in this paper, we attempt to contribute to the study of regional economic resilience in terms of dynamic measurement of regional economic resilience and the spatial heterogeneity of the influence mechanism. Based on the dynamic perspective, we took the prefecture-level cities in the Yellow River Basin of China as the research object. We conducted a dynamic analysis on the level of economic resilience of the Yellow River Basin in the face of the 2008 international financial crisis. We tried to explore the spatiotemporal evolution law of regional economic resilience. On this basis, we comprehensively considered structural factors, agency-based factors, resource-based economic structure, environment, and urban hierarchy factors and provide empirical analysis on the spatial differences in influencing factors of regional economic resilience under different spatial scales. This paper attempted to explore the influence mechanism of regional economic resilience so as to provide a theoretical reference for the sustainable and stable development of the Yellow River Basin under uncertain shocks.

The remainder of this paper is organized as follows. Section 2 reviews the relevant literature. Section 3 introduces the study area, methodology, and influence factors of regional economic resilience. After showing the spatiotemporal evolution characteristics of regional economic resilience in Section 4, Section 5 discusses the determinants of regional economic resilience in the Yellow River Basin. Section 6 concludes the paper.

2. Review of Literature

At present, the world is facing various uncertainties. Such uncertain events may cause serious consequences and eventually lead to the emergence of shocks or risks such as a financial crisis [22,23]. The shocks or risks will have an important impact on the investment decisions of different actors. The shocks may lead to expected investment failure and limit regional sustainable development [20]. Regional economic resilience is considered to be the key factor to explain a region's response to uncertain shocks or risks. How to reduce the possibility of occurrence of uncertain risks, mitigate the negative impact of risks, reduce the vulnerability of the economic system, and improve the regional economic resilience to cope with future shocks is the key to maintaining regional sustainable and stable development under the current highly uncertain environment [20,23,24].

Resilience was first used to represent the rebound of physical systems after experiencing shocks. Holling introduced the concept of resilience into ecology, indicating the ability of ecosystems to recover to a single equilibrium state after a shock [25]. Subsequently, the connotation of resilience was extended to multiple equilibrium states, indicating the ability of a region to return to the original stable state or enter a new stable state after a shock [26,27]. From the perspective of evolution, the concept of evolutionary resilience was put forward [6,10,28]. Evolutionary resilience emphasizes that the system is always in the never-ending process of nonlinear dynamic change, and resilience reflects the long-term adaptation process of the system in the uncertain shock environment [11,29]. Regional economic resilience refers to the ability of a regional economic system to resist shocks in the face of external shocks, to mitigate the impact of shocks, and to recover the pre-shock development trajectory of the region or shift to a new and better development trajectory through adaptation [3,26].

The concept of regional economic resilience involves the discrimination of adaptation and adaptability. Adaptation starts from the path dependence and emphasizes the structure and mode formed by the regional economic system in its long-term historical development process. This historical shaping has strong adaptation. In a short time, when a region is subject to external shocks, the path dependence of the regional system can maintain the original development path of the region or the path renewal based on the original foundation and emphasize the resistance, recovery, and renewal of the region from the shock [11,17]. Additionally, adaptability is more about path breakthrough, emphasizing that when the regional economic system is subject to external shocks, under the agency of the state and other governments, it can break the original development path, establish a new development path, achieve path breakthrough, and maintain the new development of the region in the long term, thus emphasizing the re-orientation [10,30]. Therefore, the explanation of regional economic resilience in our paper is more from the perspective of adaptation in a short period of time, emphasizing the resistance and recovery of the region to the shock.

Resilience measurement is mainly based on two methods: constructing a single index or an indicator system. A resilience index is mainly aimed at "sudden shocks" (especially the 2008 international financial crisis). It is measured through core variables such as GDP and employment [31–33]. However, most of the existing studies chose provincial units for research, and this ignores the urban differences within province [34,35]. Most of the studies were analyzed from the static perspective [29,36]. Resilience is measured by the variables at the beginning and end of the shock, which only reflects the final resilience in this period. However, the economic resilience at different times in this period is not measured, and the change process of economic resilience in this period cannot be reflected. There are few studies from the dynamic perspective, which cannot fully reflect the influence process of external shocks on regional economy [37]. The index system method is mainly aimed at the measurement of regional economic resilience under "slow-burn" shocks [38,39], involving crisis contexts such as resource depletion and population contraction. However, there is no consensus on indicators, resulting in large differences in index systems [40].

The influencing factors of regional economic resilience are the focus of empirical research. Influenced by the evolutionary economic geography, the influencing factors of regional economic resilience mainly focus on structural factors such as industrial structure and industrial development models [10,12,37]. They also focus on the impact of regional basic industry composition, diversification, and specialization on regional economic resilience. It is generally believed that regions with more significant manufacturing industries are seriously affected by financial crisis [29]. Specialized structures will accelerate shock diffusion. Diversified structures can play the role of "shock absorber" and reduce the influence [3,6,8,37]. Diversified structures also involve the discussion of related diversification and unrelated diversification [17]. In addition, the role of agency-based factors such as entrepreneurship and government support has been paid an increasing amount of attention. It is found that agency-based factors can affect economic resilience through adjusting the structural factors [3,4,12,41], but the role of government agency is often ignored in the existing research [3,17].

There are few studies on economic resilience at the watershed scale [1]. Watershed units cover a wide range, and the existing studies did not pay attention to the spatial heterogeneity of watershed-scale objects. Goodchild believes that scale is the most important topic in geographic information science [42]. The influence mechanism of a certain socio-economic phenomenon is often determined by multiple spatial processes of different scales. However, the existing studies ignored the spatial heterogeneity of influencing factors and often assumed that all influencing factors play a role in the whole study area [34,37]. It should be noted that some influencing factors may only have a significant impact in a small area but not in other areas. Some influencing factors have positive effects in a certain area but negative effects in another specific area. This is also the focus of our paper.

Based on the framework of regional economic resilience proposed by Martin [8,13,26] combined with the characteristics of our study area and considering spatial heterogeneity, we put forward the theoretical analysis framework of this paper. Regional economic resilience is the ability of a region to adapt to external uncertain shocks such as a financial crisis. It is mainly reflected in two dimensions: resistance and recoverability. Resistance reflects the vulnerability of a region to a financial crisis and the depth of impact. High resistance indicates that the region is less affected by the shock. Recoverability reflects the regional recovery after the financial crisis. High recoverability indicates that the region can actively adapt to the environmental changes after the shock and achieve recovery development through path adjustment and transformation.

3. Study Area and Possible Influencing Factors

3.1. Study Area and Period Division

The Yellow River Basin in China mainly covers eight provinces and regions (Figure 1), including 91 prefecture-level cities [43]. In 2018, the population of the Yellow River Basin accounted for 23.8% of China, while the GDP accounted for only 20.35% of China, and the economic development was slow. Moreover, there are many resource-based cities in the Yellow River Basin, accounting for 46%.

Considering data availability and administrative consistency, we used the GDP growth rate to divide the economic development stages of the Yellow River Basin before and after the 2008 financial crisis, providing a basis for the measurement of regional economic resilience [12,29]. The GDP growth rate of China and the eight provinces is shown in Figure 2.

It can be found that, before the 2008 financial crisis (2004–2007), the GDP rate showed a continuous upward trend and reached its peak in 2007, which was the recovery period of the region facing the last shock. However, after the 2008 international financial crisis, the GDP rate declined rapidly, reaching the first trough in 2009, and the international financial crisis basically ended after 2010. Therefore, the period 2008–2009 was the contraction period of the Yellow River Basin facing the financial crisis. The "4 trillion" support policy proposed by China in response to the financial crisis played an important role in the economic recovery development, making the GDP rate rise briefly in 2010. However, China then ended the high-speed growth trend, paid attention to the high-quality development of the economy, and stepped into a medium–high-speed growth trend. After 2010, the GDP rate showed a downward trend. This downward trend was mainly due to the influence of environmental change caused by the 2008 financial crisis and transformation of China's economic development mode, which still belongs to the recovery period after the financial crisis. Therefore, we believe that 2010–2018 is the recovery period of the Yellow River Basin after the financial crisis.

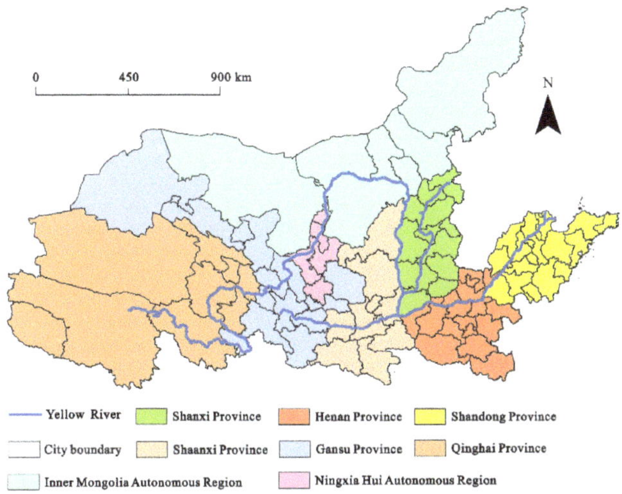

Figure 1. The location of the Yellow River Basin in China.

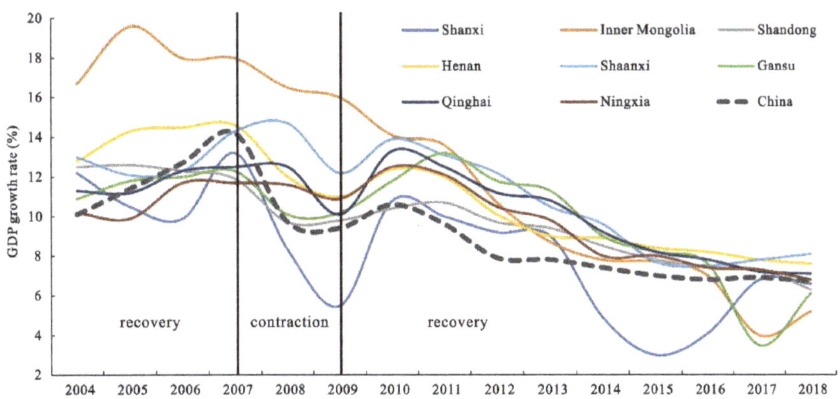

Figure 2. The GDP growth rate in 2004–2018.

3.2. Research Methods

3.2.1. Measurement of Regional Economic Resilience

In this paper, the regional economic resilience is measured by constructing the resistance and recoverability index [8,12], which is calculated by comparing the change of urban GDP with the expected change.

The calculation of the expected change of urban economic output in the contraction (2007–2009) or recovery (2009–2018) period is as follows:

$$\left(\Delta R_i^{t+k}\right)^{expected} = \sum_{j}^{n} R_{ij}{}^{t} \times G_n{}^{t+k} \quad (1)$$

where $\left(\Delta R_i^{t+k}\right)^{expected}$ represents the expected change of economic output of city i in the contraction or recovery period ($t + k$), $R_{ij}{}^{t}$ represents the economic output of industry j of city i at starting time t, and $G_n{}^{t+k}$ represents the change rate of national economic output in $t + k$ time.

The calculation of resistance and recoverability is as follows:

$$Resistance = \frac{\left(\Delta R_i^{contraction}\right) - \left(\Delta R_i^{contraction}\right)^{expected}}{\left|\left(\Delta R_i^{contraction}\right)^{expected}\right|} \quad (2)$$

where $\left(\Delta R_i^{contraction}\right)$ represents the actual change of economic output of city i during the contraction period, and $\left(\Delta R_i^{contraction}\right)^{expected}$ represents the expected change of economic output of city i during the contraction period.

$$Recoverability = \frac{\left(\Delta R_i^{restore}\right) - \left(\Delta R_i^{restore}\right)^{expected}}{\left|\left(\Delta R_i^{restore}\right)^{expected}\right|} \quad (3)$$

where $\left(\Delta R_i^{restore}\right)$ represents the actual change of economic output of city i during the recovery period, and $\left(\Delta R_i^{restore}\right)^{expected}$ represents the expected change of economic output of city i during the recovery period.

Resistance (recoverability) greater than 0 means that the resistance (recoverability) of the city in the face of shock is higher than the national average.

3.2.2. Multi-Scale Geographical Weighted Regression (MGWR)

MGWR considers the problem of spatial heterogeneity and improves the geographic weighted regression by allowing different bandwidths of each variable [44]. At the same time, it provides the influence scale of different variables, which can analyze the effect of each variable on the dependent variable at different scales and obtain more reliable estimation results. The MGWR model can reflect whether an independent variable has a significant impact on the dependent variable in the whole study area, whether an independent variable has a significant impact on the dependent variable in a specific range within the study area, and whether an independent variable has opposite or different impacts on the dependent variable in different ranges within the study area. The calculation of the MGWR model is as follows:

$$y_i = \sum_{j=1}^{k} \beta_{bwj}(u_i, v_i)x_{ij} + \varepsilon_i \quad (4)$$

where β_{bwj} represents the regression coefficient of the j-th variable, b_{wj} represents the bandwidth used by the regression coefficient of the j-th variable, (u_i, v_i) represents the spatial coordinates of region i, x_{ij} represents the observed value of the j-th variable of region i, and ε_i is the random perturbation term.

3.3. Possible Influencing Factors of the Yellow River Basin's Economic Resilience

Regional economic resilience is affected by many factors. The industrial structure is considered to be a key factor affecting regional economic resilience and has been widely discussed [27,45]. However, the role of government agency is often ignored [3,6]. The proportion of state-owned enterprises is significant, and the regional economic development is seriously affected by the government's macro-control. Therefore, the economic resilience of the Yellow River Basin to cope with uncertain shocks may be more deeply affected by government agency. However, the influence mechanism of regional economic resilience is not clear. It is urgent to further explore the role of different structural and agency-based factors in regional economic resilience [12]. According to the literature, we summarize the main factors affecting regional economic resilience as follows.

3.3.1. Industrial Structure

The industrial structure is a key factor affecting regional economic resilience, and a change in the industrial structure will affect the resistance and recoverability of a regional economy to shocks [26,46]. The specialized structure is more likely to be exposed to shocks, which is prone to the shock diffusion of "pulling one hair and moving the whole body" [17]. The vulnerability of regional economic systems is high, meaning that rapid fluctuations in the regional economy can be easily caused. However, in the recovery stage, the specialized industrial structure may be more conducive to regional recovery, mainly because the specialized structure can help to improve the implementation effect of specific policies and guide the rapid transformation of specific industries to achieve recovery and development.

A diversified structure plays the role of "shock absorber" [3,17,47]. When the shock has a specific industrial orientation, other types of industries are less affected and can complement and maintain economic development [12,29]. However, the effect of diversified structures on regional economic resilience is not clear, which mainly involves the discussion of related variety and unrelated variety. Related variety focuses on the technology substitution or complementarity between different industries, and different industries have similar knowledge or capability bases [6,8]. Related variety takes into account industrial cooperation while dispersing the shock, which is considered to be the core of developing long-term economic resilience [11,26]. Unrelated variety can block the spread of specific shocks due to the lack of industrial linkages. In the short term, it may be conducive to the dispersion of shocks, but in the long term, it is not conducive to industrial innovation and economic resilience [29].

3.3.2. Opening to the Global Economy

The degree of openness to the global economy includes the degree of cooperation outside the region and can also represent the degree of embedding in the global economy or participating in the global division of labor. A high degree of openness to the global economy means that the region can attract external funds and technologies, export products and services to the outside world, and improve the efficiency of the regional economic system. After the shock, it can adapt to the new environment in time and improve the regional ability to deal with the shock [34,48,49]. However, opening to the global economy plays a double-edged sword role in regional economic resilience. When the shock seriously affects the regional import and export departments, the regions with a high degree of openness to the global economy may be more seriously impacted, which limits the regional ability to deal with the shock [4,31].

3.3.3. Government Agency

As a key factor affecting regional economic resilience, government agency can even determine regional economic resilience [3,17,50]. Government agency, such as regulation and control, can guide the optimization and adjustment of the regional industrial structure to change the development mode and attract high-quality talents and then affect the level of regional economic resilience to cope with the shock [4,40,51]. After the shock, the government support or investment play can limit the negative influence of the shock to the greatest extent. The government can provide support for the recovery and development of enterprises or industries [26]. Government agency can provide policy support for the regional economic system to update the development path or create a new path and improve the regional economic resilience to the shock [3,52].

3.3.4. Financial Market

The financial market of the regional economic system is an important variable to deal with the financial crisis. It determines the development of the regional economy under uncertain shocks through the process of investment or resource utilization [20]. Regions with a good financial market may have a better ability to cope with shocks. This is mainly because a good financial market helps to attract capital. After the shock, it can provide enough capital support for enterprises to cope with the shock, help the industry through the difficult period, and then enhance the regional resilience. At the same time, a good financial market can provide stable capital investment for industrial adjustment, improve or transform resource utilization efficiency, promote regional innovation output and the pace of industrial transformation, and then enhance regional resilience [26,34,48].

3.3.5. Resource-Based Economy

Resource-based cities in the Yellow River Basin account for 46%. Studies have shown that compared with other cities, resource-based cities have high vulnerability and poor adaptability to shocks [3,11,12]. The development of cities in the Yellow River Basin mostly depends on resource-based industries, which are greatly affected by market prices. Under the 2008 international financial crisis, the price of raw materials seriously declined. The development path of the Yellow River Basin relying on resource-based industries may limit the ability of the region to resist shocks. With China entering a high-quality development stage and the intensification of resource depletion, the development of the resource-based economy in the Yellow River Basin has been severely restricted. Strong path dependence has hindered the industrial breakthrough and transformation, which may limit the regional recovery and transformation. In a word, the resource-based economy in the Yellow River Basin may limit the resilience [3,12,37].

3.3.6. The Environmental Condition of the Yellow River Basin

The ecological environment of the Yellow River Basin is relatively fragile, facing serious resource and environmental problems. As China enters the stage of high-quality development, the environment has become the key to restricting the sustainable development of regional economy [1,19,53]. The development mode of the Yellow River Basin over-relying on resource-based industries has aggravated environmental pollution and restricted the entry of high-end talents and high-tech industries. There are many industries with high energy consumption and high pollution, which are more vulnerable to fluctuations in the international market, which may lead to the low ability of the region to cope with the financial crisis. With the transformation of the regional development mode, the regions with improved environmental conditions after the shock have realized industrial adjustment and transformation, attracting talents, new technologies, and new industries. The regions can adapt to the new environment and achieve rapid recovery and development.

3.3.7. Urban Hierarchy

The Yellow River Basin covers a large area, and the urban hierarchy varies greatly. The hierarchy difference between cities may be a factor affecting the resilience. In the context of economic globalization, cities with a high degree participate more in the regional division of labor and have close external relations. The negative impact of the international financial crisis may have a more serious influence on the economy of high-grade cities through the process of economic globalization. However, after the shock, high-grade cities may attract talents and capital through their attraction, actively participate in the regional division of labor in the post-financial crisis era, and quickly restore regional economic development.

In addition, regional economic resilience is also related to the level of economic development. It is generally believed that areas with good economic development can provide funds, infrastructure, and technical support for the region to cope with shocks [4]. Areas with a high urbanization level can attract the agglomeration of resource elements, and their modern industrial structure and development mode may help the region adapt to the transformation in time after the shock [54].

Based on the existing literature, we selected industrial specialization, industrial diversification, degree of openness, government agency, environment, resource-based economy, and urban hierarchy as key elements and took economic development level and modernization level as control variables to explore the influence mechanism of economic resilience in the Yellow River Basin. The connotation and calculation method of each variable are shown in Table 1.

Table 1. Description of influencing factors.

Variable	Definition	Unit
Regional economic resilience	Resistance and recoverability index	
Specialization	Specialization index (SPC)	
Related variety	Related variety index (RV)	
Unrelated variety	Unrelated variety index (U-RV)	
Openness	Total import and export/GDP (OPE)	%
Government agency	Fixed asset investment/GDP (GOV)	%
Financial market	Deposits of banking system national/GDP (FIN)	%
Resource-based economy	Proportion of employed persons in mining industry (REB)	%
Environment	Carbon emissions (ENV)	Million tons
Urban hierarchy	0 for urban population less than 0.5 million, 1 for urban population between 0.5 and 1 million, and 2 for urban population greater than 1 million (CDG)	
Urban development	Per capita GDP (GDP)	CNY
Urbanization	Ratio of urban population to total population (URB)	%

Specialization (SPC) and diversification (RV, U-RV) are calculated by the number of employed persons in urban units by industry in various regions. The calculation of specialization index is:

$$SPC_i = \sum_{j=1}^{k} \left| V_{i,j} - V_j \right| \tag{5}$$

where $V_{i,j}$ represents the proportion of the employment of industry j in region i in the total employment of the region. V_j represents the proportion of the employment of industry j in the total employment of the Yellow River Basin.

Economic diversification is represented by related variety (RV) and unrelated variety (U-RV) respectively. The calculation of related variety is as follows:

$$RV_{i,t} = \sum_{j=1}^{k} P_{i,j} \times E_{i,j}; E_{i,j} = \sum_{s=1}^{n} \left({P_{i,s}} \middle/ {P_{i,j}} \right) \times ln\left({P_{i,j}} \middle/ {P_{i,s}} \right) \tag{6}$$

where $P_{i,s}$ is the proportion of employment in the s-th industry of city i at time t, and n is the number of all industries. In the paper, n is 19, $P_{i,j}$ is the proportion of employment in the j-th major department of city i at time t, and k is the number of major departments, which is divided into six major departments on the basis of 19 industries in the paper.

The calculation of unrelated variety is:

$$U - RV_{i,t} = \sum_{j=1}^{k} P_{i,j} \times ln(1 / P_{i,j}) \quad (7)$$

Considering the serious lack of data in some cities, only 87 cities were selected for analysis in the influencing factor analysis part.

3.4. Data Sources

Our data were derived from the China City Statistical Yearbook for 2004–2018 and the relevant province's statistical yearbook.

4. Spatiotemporal Evolution Characteristics of Regional Economic Resilience

4.1. Temporal Evolution Characteristics

Based on Equations (2) and (3), we dynamically measured the resistance and recoverability levels of the Yellow River Basin in the face of the 2008 international financial crisis. At the same time, in order to compare the economic resilience of the Yellow River Basin to this shock, we also measured the recoverability of the region to the previous shock before 2008. In order to further reflect the temporal evolution of the overall economic resilience of the Yellow River Basin, we calculated the average value of the resistance and recoverability levels of the Yellow River Basin and eight provinces from 2005 to 2018. The results are shown in Figure 3.

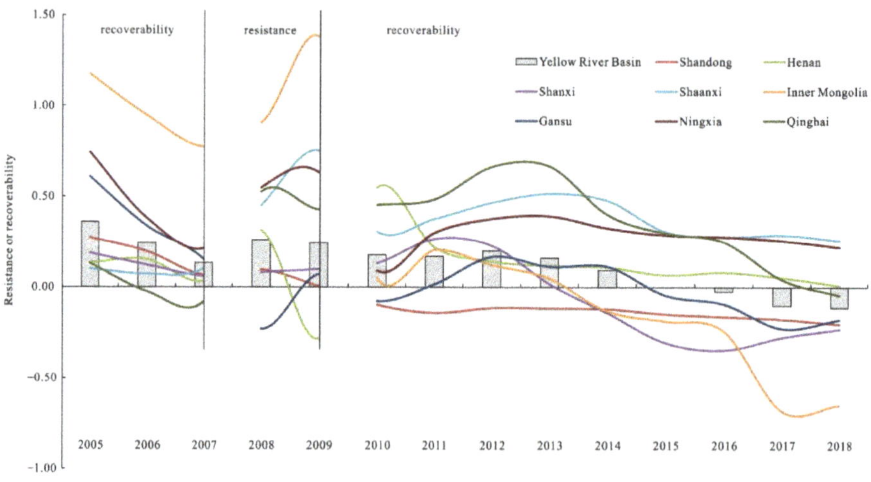

Figure 3. Average economic resilience of the Yellow River Basin.

The results show that before the 2008 financial crisis, that is, during the period of 2005–2007, the average recoverability of the Yellow River Basin and most provinces was greater than 0, indicating that the economy of the Yellow River Basin had recovered. In the stage of resistance to the 2008 financial crisis (2008–2009), the average resistance of the Yellow River Basin and most provinces was greater than 0, indicating that the Yellow River Basin was less affected by the shock than the national average level, and the regional economy had high resistance to the shock except for Henan. This is mainly because of the "4 trillion" support policy put forward by the state in response to the international financial crisis, which buffered the impact of the shock on the Yellow River Basin during this period.

During the recovery phase (2010–2018), the recoverability of the Yellow River Basin and all provinces showed a downward trend, and in recent years, the average recoverability of the Yellow River Basin has been less than 0. From 2010 to 2018, the recoverability level of the Yellow River Basin decreased by 163%. This shows that in the recovery stage, under the background of "three periods superimposed" and China's entry into the high-quality development stage compared with the national average level, the recoverability of the Yellow River Basin was weak, the ability of the regional economy to adapt to the new environment was weak, and the regional transformation and development were slow. Except for Shaanxi, Ningxia, and Henan, the average recoverability of the other provinces was less than 0 in 2018. For a long period of time, the Yellow River Basin could not adapt to the new environment during the recovery period, making it difficult to update or break through the path of regional economic development, and the speed of regional economic development was lower than the national average.

There were significant differences in economic resilience among different provinces. This spatial difference in economic resilience may lead to spatial differences in the mechanism of influencing factors.

4.2. Spatial Evolution Characteristics

The level of resistance or recoverability of the Yellow River Basin in 2005, 2007, 2008, 2009, 2010, and 2018 was selected for visual expression to reflect the spatial evolution characteristics of economic resilience in the Yellow River Basin. The specific results are shown in Figure 4.

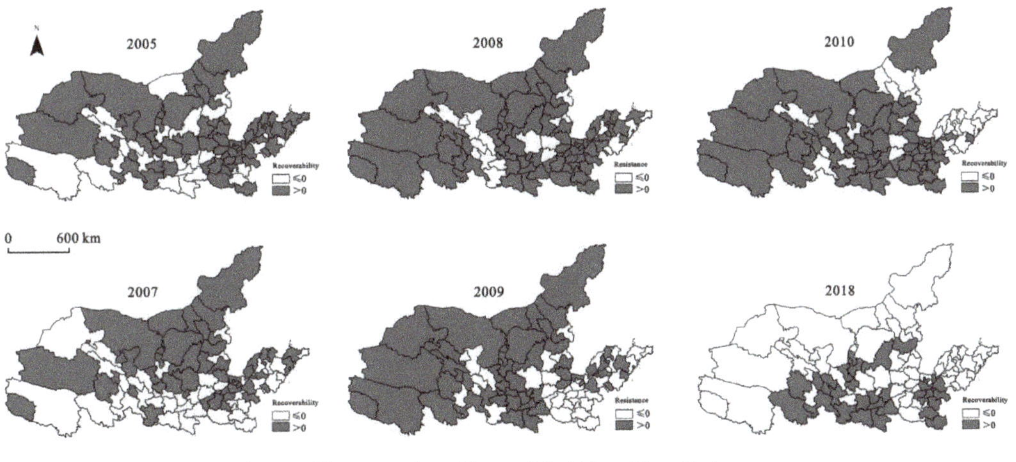

Figure 4. The economic resilience of the Yellow River Basin.

Figure 4 shows that the recoverability of the Yellow River Basin was high from 2005 to 2007 but showed a downward trend. The proportion of cities with recoverability less than 0 rose from 31% in 2004 to 47% in 2007. From 2008 to 2009, the resistance of the Yellow River Basin to the financial crisis was higher than the national average, with average resistances of 0.26 and 0.24, respectively, but the resistance level in the eastern part of the Yellow River Basin decreased significantly. Cities with high resistances showed significant characteristics of spatial agglomeration. From 2008 to 2009, the proportion of cities with resistance less than 0 rose from 22% to 44%. From 2010 to 2018, the recoverability of the Yellow River Basin showed a significant downward trend. The recovery and development of the Yellow River Basin were slow after the shock. The average recoverability decreased from 0.18 to −0.11, decreasing by 162.9%. From 2010 to 2018, the proportion of cities with recoverability less than 0 rose from 33% to 65%. Cities with high recoverability were mainly concentrated in the south of the Yellow River, while other regions had low recoverability over time. The regional development path after the shock could not adapt to the new environment. At the same time, it was found that the resistance or resilience of the Yellow River Basin showed characteristics of spatial differences.

5. Determinants of Economic Resilience in the Yellow River Basin

5.1. Model Comparison and Scale Analysis

Before the regression of the model, we carried out variance inflation factor (VIF) test on the selected influencing factors. The results show that the VIF values of all variables were less than 4, indicating that there was no multicollinearity among the influencing factors, so regression analysis could be carried out. Table 2 shows the regression results of the OLS model and MGWR model in the 2008–2009 resistance period and 2010–2018 recovery period, respectively. The results show that the goodness-of-fit R^2 and log-likelihood (log-L) values of the MGWR model were higher than those of OLS model, and the Akaike information criterion (AIC) value was lower than that of OLS, indicating that the regression result of the model was more accurate after considering spatial heterogeneity. At the same time, it was found that the heterogeneity scale plays an extremely important role in the influence mechanism of regional economic resilience. Some variables only had an impact on economic resilience within a specific range. Once the specific range was exceeded, the impact of the variable disappeared. In other words, the action process of different factors on regional economic resilience runs on different spatial scales.

Table 2. Statistical description of regression coefficient.

	OLS		MGWR	
	Coefficient (2008–2009)	**Coefficient (2010–2018)**	**Bandwidth (2008–2009)**	**Bandwidth (2010–2018)**
Constant	0.000	0.000	85	44
SPC	0.069	−0.075	44	81
RV	0.124	0.252 *	53	79
U-RV	−0.084	−0.113	85	44
OPE	−0.336 **	0.036	57	85
GOV	0.443 ***	0.109	55	83
FIN	0.181	0.312 ***	85	85
REB	−0.122	−0.268 **	85	85
ENV	0.064	−0.086	72	81
CDG	−0.273 **	0.047	85	85
GDP	0.273 *	−0.147	48	85
URB	0.225	−0.244 *	85	85
R^2	0.418	0.408	0.727	0.696
Log-L	−99.901	−100.624	−66.952	−71.678
AIC	223.802	225.247	191.099	193.483

*** $p < 0.01$; ** $p < 0.05$; * $p < 0.1$.

The MGWR results show that in the resistance stage (2008–2009), the bandwidth of specialization, related variety, opening to the outside world, government agency, and GDP were small. They had high spatial heterogeneity. Beyond this scale, the regression coefficient changed dramatically. In the recovery stage (2010–2018), the bandwidth of constant and unrelated variety were small. The constant represents the impact of different locations on regional economic resilience when other independent variables are determined. Its bandwidth was 44, indicating that the recoverability of the Yellow River Basin was the most sensitive to location and had a great impact in a local range. The impact of influencing factors on economic resilience can be shown by the coefficient spatial distribution map below.

5.2. Spatial Pattern Analysis of Influencing Factors

5.2.1. Resistance in 2008–2009

The regression coefficient of each significant variable is shown in Figure 5. Industrial structure variables had significant effects on resistance, and the characteristics of spatial heterogeneity were obvious. The SPC variable significantly limited regional economic resistance (Figure 5a). The specialized structure had a significant impact on the economic resistance mainly in the central and southern regions of the Yellow River Basin. The value range of this variable was −0.263~−0.235. The negative impact of the financial crisis quickly spread to all industries due to excessive linkages between industries, causing regional economic recession.

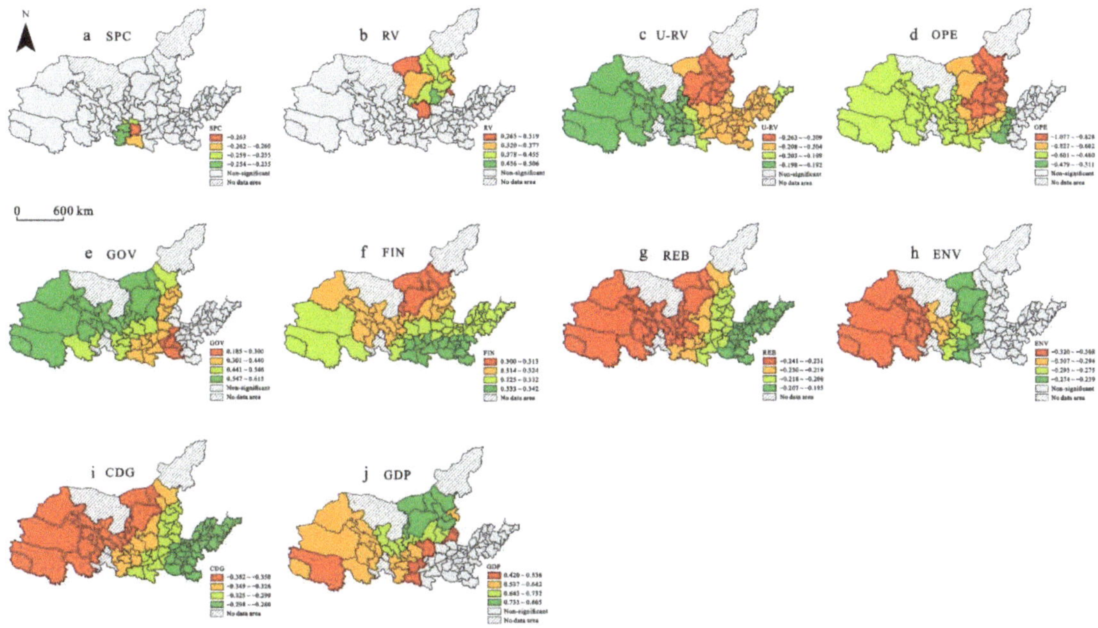

Figure 5. Spatial coefficient distribution of significant variables in 2008–2009.

The RV variable significantly promoted economic resistance (Figure 5b). RV played a significant role mainly in the central and northern regions of the Yellow River Basin. The improvement in related variety improved the ability of the region to cope with the shock. The value range of the RV was 0.269~0.506. This is mainly because related variety strengthened the connection between different departments. Firstly, related variety dispersed the impact of the shock, avoiding the influence quickly spreading to other industries so as to maintain economic development. Secondly, related diversified industries absorbed the personnel and resource elements of the affected industries, which is conducive to accelerating industrial adjustment and resource reuse.

The U-RV variable had a significant negative effect on regional economic resistance (Figure 5c). The unrelated variety structure in the northeast of the Yellow River Basin had a higher restrictive effect on regional economic resistance. The value range of the U-RV was −0.217~−0.192. The economic development of the Yellow River Basin has long relied on resource-based industries, which were seriously affected by the shock. The proportion of industries unrelated to resources was low. Even though these industries were less affected by the shock, they had less impact on economic development. At the same time, the unrelated variety structure is not conducive to the flow of talents and resources. After the shock, the efficiency of resource utilization was reduced, which is not conducive to economic development.

The OPE variable significantly limited regional economic resistance (Figure 5d). The role of OPE in the east was not significant. The negative effect of OPE was greater in the central area. The value range of the OPE regression coefficient was −1.077~−0.311. This is mainly because the foreign trade of the central and western regions of the Yellow River Basin mainly depends on natural resources. The financial crisis led to a decline in the price and demand of the international resource market, which had an important impact on the resource export industry. This limited the resistance of the central and western regions to the financial crisis.

The GOV variable significantly promoted regional economic resistance (Figure 5e) and showed a spatial heterogeneity characteristic. The regression coefficient increased gradually from the center and south of the Yellow River Basin to the west. The value range of this variable was 0.185~0.615. The results show that in the face of the international financial crisis, government agency helped cities actively resist the shock. There are many resource-based cities in the center and west of the Yellow River Basin, and the state-owned economy accounts for a large proportion. Government agency plays a profound role in the choice of investment and development mode. Government agency can provide funds and policy support for industrial adjustment and help expand the domestic market to digest resource products, thus maintaining economic development and enhancing economic resistance.

The FIN variable had a significant positive effect on regional economic resistance on a global scale (Figure 5f). The regression coefficient increased gradually from the north of the Yellow River Basin to the south. The value range of the FIN regression coefficient was 0.300~0.342. This is mainly because a good financial market can provide enough financial support for industrial adjustment or overcoming difficulties and avoid capital withdrawal after the shock. The government can also attract funds into the market through a series of financial support measures to improve resource utilization efficiency and maintain economic development.

The REB variable significantly limited economic resistance on a global scale (Figure 5g). The regression coefficient decreased gradually from the east of the Yellow River Basin to the west. The value range of the REB regression coefficient was −0.241~−0.195. The financial crisis led to a decline in the price and demand of the international resource market, which had a profound impact on the resource-based industries. There are many resource-based cities in the center and west of the Yellow River Basin, and their economic development depends on resource-based industries, which hindered the ability of the regional economy to resist the shock.

The ENV variable significantly limited regional economic resistance (Figure 5h) and showed a spatial heterogeneity characteristic. The regression coefficient decreased gradually from the center of the Yellow River Basin to the west. The value range of the ENV regression coefficient was −0.320~−0.239. The environmental conditions in these regions play a more significant role in limiting regional resistance to shocks. This is mainly because these regions have long relied on traditional resource industries, which has exacerbated environmental pollution in the process of development. After the financial crisis, the development of traditional resource industries was restricted, and environmental pollution restricted the entry of talents and high-tech industries, resulting in an insufficient foundation for industrial adjustment in these regions, thus limiting the ability to resist the shock.

The CDG variable had a significant negative effect on regional economic resistance on a global scale (Figure 5i). The value range of the CDG regression coefficient was −0.382~−0.208. The urban hierarchy in the west of the Yellow River Basin was more sensitive to economic resistance. This is mainly because high-level cities have more participation in the global division of labor, and the Yellow River Basin is mostly at the supply and processing ends in the global division of labor. After the financial crisis, the international market was depressed, and the high-level cities that participated in the global division of labor were more seriously affected, which hindered the economic resistance.

The GDP had a significant positive effect on regional economic resistance (Figure 5j) and showed a spatial heterogeneity characteristic. The value range of the GDP regression coefficient was 0.420~0.865. Economic development was more sensitive to economic resistance in the north of the Yellow River Basin. A series of supporting measures taken by the region to resist the shock needed the support of local economic development, especially in the center and west of the Yellow River Basin, where economic development is slow.

5.2.2. Recoverability in 2010–2018

The regression coefficient of each significant variable is shown in Figure 6. The location reflected by the constant term had a significant effect on the regional economic recoverability on a certain scale (Figure 6a). The location in the west of the Yellow River Basin had a significant negative effect on the recoverability, while the location in the east of the Yellow River Basin had a significant positive effect on the recoverability. The value range of the constant coefficient was −0.379~0.580. This is mainly because the west of the Yellow River Basin has a large proportion of resource industries, the regional environment is poor, and the economic development is relatively slow. This location hindered the adaptation and transformation of the region in the recovery period. However, the east of the Yellow River Basin is a coastal area with good economic development. This location promoted the transformation process of the region in the new environment, and the regional recoverability.

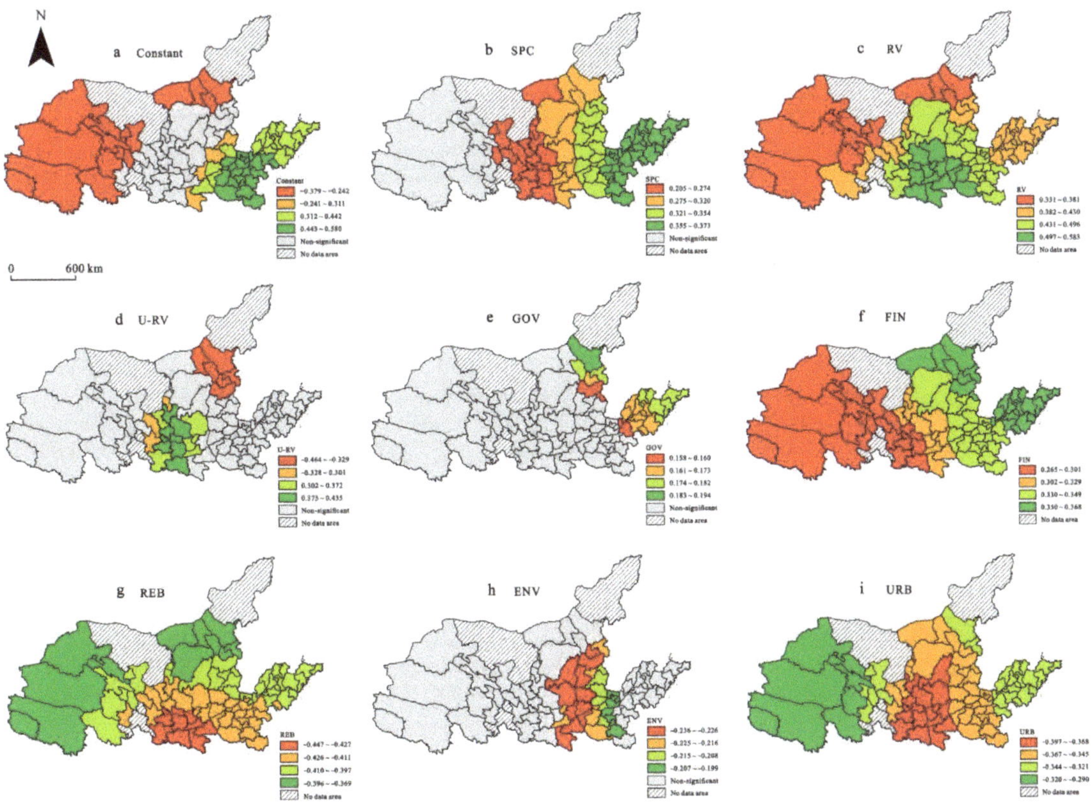

Figure 6. Spatial coefficient distribution of significant variables in 2010–2018.

Industrial structure variables had significant effects on recoverability, and the characteristics of spatial heterogeneity were also obvious. The SPC variable significantly promoted regional economic recoverability in the center and east of the Yellow River Basin (Figure 6b); this is contrary to the regression result of resistance. The regression coefficient increased gradually from the center of the Yellow River Basin to the east. The value range of this variable was 0.205~0.373. In the recovery stage, the specialized industrial structure was conducive to the implementation of specific industrial policies, accelerating industrial transformation and improving resource utilization efficiency.

The RV variable significantly promoted economic recoverability on a global scale (Figure 6c). The regression coefficient increased gradually from the northwest of the Yellow River Basin to the southeast. The value range of RV was 0.331~0.583. This is mainly because related variety can promote the generation of innovation activities. When external shocks occur, it can actively adapt to the external environment through inter-industry exchanges, update existing departments, or cultivate new industrial departments.

The U-RV variable had a significant effect on regional economic recoverability on a certain scale (Figure 6d). The unrelated variety structure in the northeast of the Yellow River Basin had a negative effect on recoverability, but it had a positive effect in the center and south of the Yellow River Basin. The value range of U-RV was −0.464~0.435. As China enters the stage of high-quality development, unrelated variety can break the path dependence of regions, achieve path breakthrough, and create new development paths to recover economic development. However, the unrelated variety structure may ignore the role of existing industries, and the cost of cultivating completely unrelated new industries is high, which may have the opposite effect on some regions.

The GOV variable significantly promoted regional economic recoverability in the northeast of the Yellow River Basin (Figure 6e). The value range of this variable was 0.158~0.194. Government agency provided financial and policy support for the breakthrough development of the industry and played an important role in guiding industrial adjustment and accelerating the transformation of the development mode. Especially in the eastern coastal areas, the policy inclination was greater, the economic development was better, and the government's supporting role was more significant.

The FIN variable had a significant positive effect on regional economic recoverability on a global scale (Figure 6f). The regression coefficient increased gradually from the west of the Yellow River Basin to the east. The value range of the FIN regression coefficient was 0.265~0.368. The good financial market provided enough funds for industrial adjustment and supported the industry in adapting to the new environment.

The REB variable significantly limited economic recoverability on a global scale (Figure 6g). The regression coefficient decreased gradually from the center and south of the Yellow River Basin to the surrounding areas. The value range of the REB regression coefficient was −0.447~−0.369. At this stage, great changes took place in China's development mode, focusing on the quality of economic development. The past development model based on resource consumption could no longer adapt to the new environment. The large proportion of traditional resource-based industries limited the recovery and development of the regional economy.

The ENV variable significantly limited regional economic recoverability in center of the Yellow River Basin (Figure 6h). The value range of the ENV regression coefficient was −0.236~−0.199. Most of these areas were concentrated in Shaanxi, Shanxi, and Henan. There are many resource-based cities. The past development model seriously damaged the environment. In the recovery stage, this poor environmental condition restricted the investment in industrial technology upgrading, hindered the introduction of high-tech industries, and led to the slow development of the regional transformation.

The URB variable had a significant negative effect on regional economic recoverability on a global scale (Figure 6i). The value range of the URB regression coefficient was −0.397~−0.290. The regression coefficient decreased gradually from the center of the Yellow River Basin to the surrounding areas. This may be related to the measurement of urbanization. We measured urbanization based on the proportion of the non-agricultural population, which cannot fully reflect the quality of urbanization.

6. Conclusions

Regional economic resilience is considered to be an important factor to explain and understand the differences in regional performance in coping with and adapting to external shocks [8,26]. Especially under the environment of the COVID-19 epidemic shock, regional economic resilience has attracted an increasing amount of attention from academia and politics [3,17]. In the existing studies, spatial heterogeneity was considered less, and the influence of structural factors on regional economic resilience was mostly analyzed at the macro overall scale. There was less analysis of the elements of agency-based factors. At the same time, the effect of various factors on regional economic resilience has a scale effect; that is, the effect of some influencing factors may only be significant on the local spatial scale, and beyond this scale, it has little effect. Therefore, we took the Yellow River Basin as the research object. We analyzed the spatiotemporal evolution process of economic resilience in the face of the international financial crisis in 2008. On this basis, considering the characteristics of spatial heterogeneity, we analyzed the influence factors of economic resilience in the Yellow River Basin by integrating structural factors, agency-based factors, resource-based economy, and environment and urban hierarchy factors.

Based on our results, we draw the following conclusions:

(1) The resistance of the Yellow River Basin to the financial crisis was high, and it was less affected by the shock in the early stage, but it showed a small decline. The recoverability of the Yellow River Basin after the shock was weak, showing a significant downward trend with the evolution of time. In the long run, the Yellow River Basin could not adapt to the new environment. The economic resilience of the Yellow River Basin showed significant spatial agglomeration and difference characteristics.

(2) In the resistance period and recovery period, the influence mechanism of economic resilience in the Yellow River Basin was significantly different. However, spatial heterogeneity played a significant role in different periods. Related variety, government agency, environment, and opening to the global economy had a significant effect on economic resilience only in a specific small range, beyond which the impact was small. Specialization, unrelated variety, and location had opposite effects in different regions of the Yellow River Basin.

(3) Structural factors still played a significant role in regional economic resilience, but the influence mechanism was changed in different periods. Specialization limited the area's resistance to shock but enhanced the recoverability after the shock. Related variety significantly improved the regional ability to cope with the shock by giving full play to the "shock absorber". Unrelated variety was not conducive to regional resistance to the shock and had opposite effects on the recoverability in different regions.

(4) Government agency and financial market significantly promoted the regional economic resistance and recoverability. Environment pollution and resource-based economic structure significantly limited the regional economic resistance and recoverability. Opening to the global economy and urban hierarchy limited the regional resistance to the shock, but strong economic development had the opposite effect of improved regional resistance. The location in the east of the Yellow River Basin enhanced the recoverability; however, the location in the west limited the recoverability.

7. Discussion

From the perspective of evolutionary economic geography, considering the dynamic evolution and spatial heterogeneity of basin-scale economic resilience, we discussed the economic resilience mechanism in the face of 2008 international financial crisis by using the MGWR model. For this special scale unit of the Yellow River Basin, we needed to consider the characteristics of spatial heterogeneity and explore the effect of different factors on regional economic resilience at different spatial scales in order to provide a policy reference for the Yellow River Basin to deal with uncertain shocks in the future.

The structural factor is an important factor of regional economic resilience, which has been verified again. In the process of high-quality development of the Yellow River Basin, we need to pay attention to the connection and cooperation between different industries not only to ensure decentralized shocks but also to ensure innovation spillover. Governments should play their role in macro-control and provide policy support for the high-quality development of the Yellow River Basin. Government agency should promote the pace of industrial transformation, accelerate the renewal or creation of regional development paths and promote the transformation process of resource-based cities. The government should enhance the regional specialization of high-tech industries and improve the efficiency of resource utilization. The Yellow River Basin should reasonably control the level of cities, enhance the status of cities in the global division of labor, pay attention to foreign and domestic market, and enhance regional resistance. In view of the unfavorable location conditions such as Qinghai and Gansu, local governments should formulate development strategies considering regional characteristics in future planning. It is worth noting that in the future, we need to implement different development policies on different scales according to the actual urban situation.

Our research also has deficiencies. Due to data limitations, our paper only discussed the economic resilience of the Yellow River Basin in the face of the international financial crisis from the dimensions of resistance and recoverability. At the same time, this paper only selected some key elements to analyze the influence mechanism. In fact, the resilience of the regional economy is affected by many factors. We ignored factors such as innovation and entrepreneurship.

Author Contributions: Conceptualization, L.L. and C.W.; methodology, L.L.; software, L.L.; formal analysis, L.L. and P.Z.; writing—review and editing, L.L. and P.Z.; supervision, C.W.; funding acquisition, L.L. All authors have read and agreed to the published version of the manuscript.

Funding: This work was funded by the National Natural Science Foundation of China (42101161, 42071162); National Social Science Foundation of China (20BJY070); Project funded by China Postdoctoral Science Foundation (2020M672113); Shandong Postdoctoral Innovation Project (202003021); Project funded by Shandong Humanities and Social Sciences (2021-YYGL-29).

Institutional Review Board Statement: Not applicable.

Informed Consent Statement: Not applicable.

Data Availability Statement: Not applicable.

Conflicts of Interest: The authors declare no conflict of interest.

References

1. Chen, Y.; Su, X.; Zhou, Q. Study on the Spatiotemporal Evolution and Influencing Factors of Urban Resilience in the Yellow River Basin. *Int. J. Environ. Res. Public Health* **2021**, *18*, 10231. [CrossRef] [PubMed]
2. Giannakis, E.; Bruggeman, A. Economic crisis and regional resilience: Evidence from Greece. *Pap. Reg. Sci.* **2017**, *96*, 451–476. [CrossRef]
3. Li, L.; Liu, S.; Li, C.; Zhang, P.; Lo, K. What Matters for Regional Economic Resilience Amid Multi Shock Situations: Structural or Agency? Evidence from Resource-Based Cities in China. *Sustainability* **2022**, *14*, 5701. [CrossRef]
4. Martin, R.; Gardiner, B. The resilience of cities to economic shocks: A tale of four recessions (and the challenge of Brexit). *Pap. Reg. Sci.* **2019**, *98*, 1801–1832. [CrossRef]
5. McCartney, G.; Pinto, J.; Liu, M. City resilience and recovery from COVID-19: The case of Macao. *Cities* **2021**, *112*, 103130. [CrossRef]
6. Boschma, R. Towards an Evolutionary Perspective on Regional Resilience. *Reg. Stud.* **2015**, *49*, 733–751. [CrossRef]
7. Balland, P.; Rigby, D.; Boschma, R. The technological resilience of US Cities. *Camb. J. Reg. Econ. Soc.* **2015**, *8*, 167–184. [CrossRef]
8. Martin, R.; Sunley, P.; Gardiner, B.; Tyle, P. How Regions React to Recessions: Resilience and the Role of Economic Structure. *Reg. Stud.* **2016**, *50*, 561–585. [CrossRef]
9. Shi, T.; Qiao, Y.; Zhou, Q.; Zhang, J. The regional differences and random convergence of urban resilience in China. *Technol. Econ. Dev. Econ.* **2022**, *28*, 979–1002. [CrossRef]
10. Martin, R. Regional economic resilience, hysteresis and recessionary shocks. *J. Econ. Geogr.* **2012**, *12*, 1–32. [CrossRef]

11. Hu, X.; Hassink, R. Exploring adaptation and adaptability in uneven economic resilience: A tale of two Chinese mining regions. *Camb. J. Reg. Econ. Soc.* **2017**, *10*, 527–541. [CrossRef]
12. Tan, J.; Hu, X.; Hassink, R.; Ni, J. Industrial structure or agency: What affects regional economic resilience? Evidence from resource-based cities in China. *Cities* **2020**, *106*, 102906. [CrossRef]
13. Martin, R.; Sunley, P. Regional economic resilience: Evolution and evaluation. In *Handbook on Regional Economic Resilience*; Bristow, G., Healy, A., Eds.; Edward Elgar: Cheltenham, UK, 2020; pp. 10–35.
14. Hassink, R. Regional resilience: A promising concept to explain differences in regional economic adaptability? *Camb. J. Reg. Econ. Soc.* **2010**, *3*, 45–58. [CrossRef]
15. Reggiani, A.; De Graaff, T.; Nijkamp, P. Resilience: An Evolutionary Approach to Spatial Economic Systems. *Netw. Spat. Econ.* **2002**, *2*, 211–229. [CrossRef]
16. Martin, R.; Gardiner, B. The resilience of Britain's core cities to the great recession (with implications for the COVID recessionary shock). In *Economic Resilience in Regions and Organisations*; Wink, R., Ed.; Springer: Berlin/Heidelberg, Germany, 2021; pp. 57–89.
17. Hu, X.; Li, L.; Dong, K. What matters for regional economic resilience amid COVID-19? Evidence from cities in Northeast China. *Cities* **2021**, *120*, 103440. [CrossRef] [PubMed]
18. Shi, T.; Qiao, Y.; Zhou, Q. Spatiotemporal evolution and spatial relevance of urban resilience: Evidence from cities of China. *Growth Chang.* **2021**, *52*, 2364–2390. [CrossRef]
19. Liu, K.; Qiao, Y.; Shi, T.; Zhou, Q. Study on coupling coordination and spatiotemporal heterogeneity between economic development and ecological environment of cities along the Yellow River Basin. *Environ. Sci. Pollut. Res.* **2021**, *28*, 6898–6912. [CrossRef]
20. Drozdowski, G. Economic calculus qua an instrument to support sustainable development under increasing risk. *J. Risk Financ. Manag.* **2021**, *14*, 15. [CrossRef]
21. Chen, Y.P.; Fu, B.J.; Zhao, Y.; Wang, K.B.; Zhao, M.M.; Ma, J.F.; Wu, J.H.; Xu, C.; Liu, W.G.; Wang, H. Sustainable development in the Yellow River Basin: Issues and strategies. *J. Clean. Prod.* **2020**, *263*, 121223. [CrossRef]
22. Aven, T.; Renn, O. On risk defined as an event where the outcome is uncertain. *J. Risk Res.* **2009**, *12*, 1–11. [CrossRef]
23. Klinke, A. Public understanding of risk and risk governance. *J. Risk Res.* **2021**, *24*, 2–13. [CrossRef]
24. Zhou, Q.; Zhu, M.; Qiao, Y.; Zhang, X.; Chen, J. Achieving resilience through smart cities? Evidence from China. *Habitat Int.* **2021**, *111*, 102348. [CrossRef]
25. Holling, C. Resilience and Stability of Ecological Systems. *Annu. Rev. Ecol. Syst.* **1973**, *4*, 1–23. [CrossRef]
26. Martin, R.; Sunley, P. On the notion of regional economic resilience: Conceptualization and explanation. *J. Econ. Geogr.* **2015**, *15*, 1–42. [CrossRef]
27. Simmie, J.; Martin, R. The economic resilience of regions: Towards an evolutionary approach. *Camb. J. Reg. Econ. Soc.* **2010**, *3*, 27–43. [CrossRef]
28. Hu, X.; Yang, C. Institutional change and divergent economic resilience: Path development of two resource-depleted cities in China. *Urban Stud.* **2019**, *56*, 3466–3485. [CrossRef]
29. Li, L.; Zhang, P.; Li, X. Regional Economic Resilience of the Old Industrial Bases in China—A Case Study of Liaoning Province. *Sustainability* **2019**, *11*, 723. [CrossRef]
30. Kurikka, H.; Grillitsch, M. Resilience in the periphery: What an agency perspective can bring to the table. In *Economic Resilience in Regions and Organisations*; Wink, R., Ed.; Springer: Berlin/Heidelberg, Germany, 2021; pp. 147–171.
31. Di Pietro, F.; Lecca, P.; Salotti, S. Regional economic resilience in the European Union: A numerical general equilibrium analysis. *Spat. Econ. Anal.* **2021**, *16*, 287–312. [CrossRef]
32. Ringwood, L.; Watson, P.; Lewin, P. A quantitative method for measuring regional economic resilience to the great recession. *Growth Chang.* **2019**, *50*, 381–4022. [CrossRef]
33. Sensier, M.; Devine, F. Understanding regional economic performance and resilience in the UK: Trends since the global financial crisis. *Natl. Inst. Econ. Rev.* **2020**, *253*, 18–28. [CrossRef]
34. Eraydin, A. Attributes and characteristics of regional resilience: Defining and measuring the resilience of Turkish regions. *Reg. Stud.* **2016**, *50*, 600–614. [CrossRef]
35. Fingleton, B.; Garretsen, H.; Martin, R. Recessionary shocks and regional employment: Evidence on the resilience of UK regions. *J. Reg. Sci.* **2012**, *52*, 109–133. [CrossRef]
36. Giannakis, E.; Bruggeman, A. Regional disparities in economic resilience in the European Union across the urban-rural divide. *Reg. Stud.* **2020**, *54*, 1200–1213. [CrossRef]
37. Tan, J.; Lo, K.; Qiu, F.; Zhang, X.; Zhao, H. Regional economic resilience of resource-based cities and influential factors during economic crises in China. *Growth Chang.* **2020**, *51*, 362–381. [CrossRef]
38. Bruneckiene, J.; Palekienė, O.; Simanavičienė, Ž.; Rapsikevičius, J. Measuring regional resilience to economic shocks by index. *Eng. Econ.* **2018**, *29*, 405–418. [CrossRef]
39. Zhang, Y.; Zhang, J.; Wang, K.; Wu, X. An Empirical Perception of Economic Resilience Responded to the COVID-19 Epidemic Outbreak in Beijing–Tianjin–Hebei Urban Agglomeration, China: Characterization and Interaction. *Int. J. Environ. Res. Public Health* **2021**, *18*, 10532. [CrossRef]
40. Li, L.; Zhang, P.; Lo, K.; Liu, W.; Li, J. The evolution of regional economic resilience in the old industrial bases in China: A case study of Liaoning Province, China. *Chin. Geogr. Sci.* **2020**, *30*, 340–351. [CrossRef]
41. Bristow, G.; Healy, A. Regional resilience: An agency perspective. *Reg. Stud.* **2014**, *48*, 923–935. [CrossRef]

42. Goodchild, M. Models of scale and scales of modelling. In *Modelling Scale in Geographical Information Science*; Tate, N.J., Atkinson, P.M., Eds.; John Wiley and Sons: Hoboken, NJ, USA, 2001; pp. 3–10.
43. Song, C.; Yin, G.; Lu, Z.; Chen, Y. Industrial ecological efficiency of cities in the Yellow River Basin in the background of China's economic transformation: Spatial-temporal characteristics and influencing factors. *Environ. Sci. Pollut. Res.* **2022**, *29*, 4334–4349. [CrossRef]
44. Yu, H.; Fotheringham, A.; Li, Z.; Oshan, T.; Wei, K.; Wolf, L. Inference in multiscale geographically weighted regression. *Geogr. Anal.* **2019**, *52*, 87–106. [CrossRef]
45. Angulo, A.; Mur, F.; Trivez, F. Measuring resilience to economic shocks: An application to Spain. *Ann. Reg. Sci.* **2018**, *60*, 349–373. [CrossRef]
46. Elmqvist, T.; Andersson, E.; Frantzeskaki, N.; McPhearson, T.; Olsson, P.; Gaffney, O.; Takeuchi, K.; Folke, C. Sustainability and resilience for transformation in the urban century. *Nat. Sustain.* **2019**, *2*, 267–273. [CrossRef]
47. Mazzola, F.; Pizzuto, P.; Ruggieri, G. The role of tourism in island economic growth and resilience: A panel analysis for the European Mediterranean countries (2000–2015). *J. Econ. Stud.* **2019**, *46*, 1418–1436. [CrossRef]
48. Di Caro, P. Testing and explaining economic resilience with an application to Italian regions. *Pap. Reg. Sci.* **2017**, *96*, 93–113. [CrossRef]
49. Wang, Z.; Wei, W. Regional economic resilience in China: Measurement and determinants. *Reg. Stud.* **2021**, *55*, 1228–1239. [CrossRef]
50. Ezcurra, R.; Rios, V. Quality of government and regional resilience in the European Union. Evidence from the Great Recession. *Pap. Reg. Sci.* **2019**, *98*, 1267–1290. [CrossRef]
51. Kitsos, T. Economic resilience in Great Britain: An empirical analysis at the local authority district level. In *Handbook on Regional Economic Resilience*; Bristow, G., Healy, A., Eds.; Edward Elgar: Cheltenham, UK, 2020; pp. 190–207.
52. Giannakis, E.; Bruggeman, A. Determinants of regional resilience to economic crisis: A European perspective. *Eur. Plan. Stud.* **2017**, *25*, 1394–1415. [CrossRef]
53. Zhou, Q.; Zhong, S.; Shi, T.; Zhang, X. Environmental regulation and haze pollution: Neighbor-companion or neighbor-beggar? *Energy Policy* **2021**, *151*, 112183. [CrossRef]
54. Ženka, J.; Slach, O.; Pavlik, A. Economic resilience of metropolitan, old industrial, and rural regions in two subsequent recessionary shocks. *Eur. Plan. Stud.* **2019**, *27*, 2288–2311. [CrossRef]

International Journal of
Environmental Research and Public Health

MDPI

Article

Local Disproportions of Quality of Life and Their Influence on the Process of Green Economy Development in Polish Voivodships in 2010–2020

Grzegorz Drozdowski and Paweł Dziekański *

Department of Economics and Finance, Jan Kochanowski University in Kielce, Uniwersytecka 15 Str., 25-406 Kielce, Poland; gdrozdowski@ujk.edu.pl
* Correspondence: pawel.dziekanski@ujk.edu.pl

Abstract: Voivodships are centres of economic, social, and cultural life—they gather economic and social activities. This research aimed to evaluate the spatial differentiation of the quality of life in voivodships in Poland with the use of a synthetic measure. To achieve the research objective, the research methods used were literature analysis, statistical analysis, and synthetic measure. The Technique for Order Preference by Similarity to an Ideal Solution method was used to build synthetic measures. The choice of variables in 2010–2020 was largely conditioned by the availability of data collected in the regional system at the level of voivodships at the Local Data Bank of the Central Statistical Office. As a result of the analysis of voivodships in Poland, based on the quality of life measure, four groups were distinguished (according to the value of quartiles). In the group of the best voivodeships there were: Pomerania, Masovia, Lower Silesia, and West Pomeranian in 2010, and Masovia, Pomerania, Greater Poland, Lower Silesia, and Lesser Poland in 2020, and in the IV, the weakest group: Lodz Province, Podlasie Province, Lubusz Province, and Holy Cross in 2010, and Lodz Province, Podlasie Province, Holy Cross, and Lublin Province in 2020. The synthetic quality of life ranged from 0.37 to 0.56 in 2010 and from 0.39 to 0.64 in 2020. Regional authorities, taking care to improve economic potential, cause increasing the attractiveness of the area and attracting new entrepreneurs, create new jobs, and improve the quality of life of the inhabitants. Quality of life is shaped by economic activity and working conditions, health, education, free time and social relations, economic and physical security, and the quality of the natural environment. The results of the research conducted allow local governments to make comparisons. The conclusions drawn may allow them to identify potential directions for developing policy optimization.

Keywords: quality of life; healthy region; healthy environment; spatial; synthetic measure; voivodship

Citation: Drozdowski, G.; Dziekański, P. Local Disproportions of Quality of Life and Their Influence on the Process of Green Economy Development in Polish Voivodships in 2010–2020. *IJERPH* **2022**, *19*, 9185. https://doi.org/10.3390/ijerph19159185

Academic Editors: Jie Chen, Qian Zhou and Ting Zhang

Received: 23 June 2022
Accepted: 22 July 2022
Published: 27 July 2022

1. Introduction

The existing connection among the economy, the existing networks of dependence and cooperation, and the increasing unification of markets has become one of the causes of the contemporary crisis [1]. It is not only a financial and economic crisis but also a social, ecological, and political crisis. The growing interconnection of regional economies creates the threat of transferring negative phenomena to related economies in the tightening cooperative network and the global system of flows (resources, factors of production, capital, goods and services, etc.) [2,3]. Development problems should be considered, inter alia, in the area of restrictions and barriers to doing business, or taking advantage of opportunities for further development.

The modern economic system is facing the challenge of responding to increasing needs while facing changes in the quality of life and climate, and the depletion of raw materials and the deterioration of our global environment [4]. A green economy allows for the harmonious management of local resources. It is an economy that contributes to improving human wellbeing and increasing social justice, while significantly reducing environmental risks and resource scarcity. It stands for a low carbon, resource sparing, and socially solid economy. A green economy means a restructuring of economic activity and infrastructure to ensure greater returns on natural, human, and economic capital. The green economy is indicated as a new model of management in which the range of ecological solutions is increased. As emphasized, this is the way to achieve sustainable development; it is not an alternative concept.

One of the tasks of local government administration units is to care for the process of sustainable development and to improve the quality of life (as the sum of a healthy region (city, commune) and a healthy environment (natural and human functioning and enterprises)), and to improve competences and social cohesion, effectively manage local resources (such as the environment, people, infrastructure, and financial resources), provide residents and economic entities with a feeling of stability, reducing the uncertainty of company operations. In the economic sphere, the priority should be building a modern industry, supporting entrepreneurship, and investing in innovations and new technologies. The indicated areas can be achieved while maintaining sustainable development consistent with environmental protection and sustainable management of resources [5].

The undeniable determinant of socioeconomic development and the quality of life is the natural environment, the resources of which constitute the foundation of economic activity and the integrity of societies. The natural environment is both the basis for the broadly understood development and is also a barrier due to the exhaustion of resources. The limitation of environmental resources in combination with the unlimited needs of people makes it necessary to manage its resources rationally. Because of this, it is possible to use the natural environment, and thus satisfy human needs, which results in obtaining an appropriate quality of life [6].

J. Piasny defines the standard of living as the entirety of the real living conditions of people, the degree of satisfaction of their material and cultural needs by a stream of goods and services, financed both from private and social funds [7]. J. Drewnowski and W. Scott define the standard of living of the population as the level of satisfaction of needs per unit of time, following as a result of goods, services, and living conditions enjoyed by the population during that unit of time [8].

Considering the issue of the quality of life, the authors decided to formulate the following research questions: What is the spatial differentiation of the quality of life in terms of regions in Poland? Does the level of quality of life depend on the level of variables characterizing the development process (endogenous socioeconomic variables)? The following questions were assessed in turn: Which endogenic potential variables shape the level of quality of life? To what extent does the financial situation shape the quality of life?

2. Literature Review

The European Union and numerous international organizations have included the green economy in the developed strategies. The European Union wants to create its competitive advantage in the economy, production, technological development, research and innovation by using the concept of sustainable development. The United Nations Conference on Sustainable Development RIO + 20 in June 2012 was also focused on the concept of green economy, where it was emphasized that it is necessary to redefine the economy and adopt a new model of socioeconomic development (green economy), in which special attention is given to environmental issues. Contrary to the current model (brown economy), largely based on the use of fossil fuels and other nonrenewable resources, the new model should learn from the experiences of the environmental economy and ensure the right relationship between the economy and ecosystems [9]. It is worth emphasizing that the concept of green growth is in line with the assumptions of the Europe 2020 strategy, which is based on three main pillars: smart, sustainable, and inclusive growth. Europe needs to strengthen the synergies between smart and green growth to cope with climate change, environmental and energy challenges, and increasing resource scarcity [10].

The green economy is a way of obtaining and using resources. The related structural changes in the economy are caused by the emergence of new industries of waste recycling, emission-free energy production, absorption of greenhouse gas emissions, and green urban planning. These changes should be accompanied by a parallel increase in the quality of life of the inhabitants [11]. However, a real transition to a green economy is only possible with sustainable development. The green economy includes green products and services, investments, green sectors of the economy, public procurement, and jobs. In the concept of a green economy, on the one hand, there is a certain restriction to economic processes, and on the other hand, the adjective green suggests a constant presence of ecological criteria. A new aspect of defining a green economy is the inclusion of social references and environmental aspects in every decision and production process. The concept of a green economy becomes multidimensional, pointing to the economic, social, and environmental dimensions. The green economy is more than the sum of the commitments already made: it has the potential to introduce us to a new development paradigm and a new business model where growth, development, and the environment are seen as reinforcing each other [12]. Increasing resource efficiency, promoting sustainable consumption and production, combating climate change, protecting biodiversity, combating desertification, reducing pollution, and managing natural resources and ecosystems responsibly is imperative and at the same time driving the transformation towards a green economy [13]. The indicated processes should also have a positive impact on the quality of life of the inhabitants.

The benefits of a circular green economy include better resource and ecological efficiency, a lower carbon footprint, less dependence on fossil resources, and the valorization of byproducts and waste materials from multiple sources (e.g., agroindustrial). This concept focuses on the idea of recycling, reusing, remanufacturing and maintaining a sustainable production process. A sustainable and environmentally friendly way of disposing the waste is crucial for the protection of the environment and human health. In this respect, the waste biorefinery is an example of its potential. Environmental, social, and economic problems are closely intertwined, complex and complex [14,15]. The multifaceted nature of the problems becomes a serious challenge for governments, politicians, and decision-makers [16,17]. The concept of a green economy has been criticized for significant overlap with or an attempt to replace sustainable development. Deterioration of the natural environment affects the quality of life of the population. The quality of life assessment can be positive or negative (low, medium, high quality of life; better, worse, more or less developed). The essence of nonvaluing (descriptive) interpretation consists in determining the separateness (differences) or similarities of the quality of life [18,19].

Quality of life is a complex, multifaceted category. High quality of life as the overriding goal of the concept of sustainable development should be the result of the development policy at all levels of management (national, regional, and local) [20]. Quality of life refers to the degree of satisfaction of material and nonmaterial needs of individuals and social groups, and it is defined both by objective indicators, e.g., life expectancy, the extent of poverty, the level of enrollment, and subjective indicators, e.g., the degree of satisfaction with living conditions and its various aspects, level of happiness, stress, meaning in life. The concept of quality of life is defined as multidisciplinary due to its complexity and internal connections [21]. Quality of life can be viewed in terms of human health, the state of the economy, employment, infrastructure development, crime, and the environment, both at an individual and a social level [22,23].

J. Berbeki (2005) in his works pointed to a subjective assessment of the quality of life of the inhabitants of the Małopolskie voivodship. A. Zborowski raised the issue of the level and quality of life in the space of an urban region (based on the example of Krakow). A. Sobali-Gwosdz (2004) draws attention to the size of cities, their rank and their functions in the assessment of the quality of life. M. Gotowska and A. Jakubczak (2012) emphasize the influence of local authorities on the lives of residents [24–27]. Most often, the quality of life is interpreted as the degree of satisfaction concerning material and spiritual human needs. It is shaped by many factors, the most important of which are: housing situation, employment security, health and life protection, the possibility of learning and improving qualifications, access to culture, access to commercial establishments, the condition of technical infrastructure, and the degree of satisfaction of individual needs. J. Rutkowski includes general satisfaction with life, expectations, prospects, aspirations (subjective factors), and the social and economic conditions we live in (objective factors) as factors influencing the shaping of the quality of life [28,29].

High quality of life is of particular importance in local territorial systems. How we perceive and evaluate our lives is strongly influenced by local (regional) aspects. It is the responsibility of local (regional) authorities to use the forces inherent in economic and spatial systems, i.e., social capital, together with environmental and economic potential [30,31]. Increasing the quality of life is the main goal of sustainable development. The quality of life is assessed using the housing dimension (quality of housing and housing environment) and is one of the main issues influencing the quality of life [32]. The level and quality of life of the population are influenced by numerous microeconomic factors (including human, material, and financial resources, which create a closed environment for households and the population) and macroeconomic factors (development policy, fiscal policy, unemployment, and inflation) [33,34]. Institutional factors (administration, social infrastructure and social assistance, public safety) influencing the quality of life are a relatively new area of measurement [35]. When discussing the quality of life, the most frequently analysed factors include health protection, life safety, the condition of the natural environment, the standard of living of the inhabitants, the condition of public transport and communication, the housing situation, education and training opportunities, and access to culture. An important area of the quality of life is social infrastructure and social assistance, which is the base of the social policy of the state.

Circular economy (green economy or bioeconomy—including economic activities in materials and the field of energy) shows the need for the new global society and economy to be based on renewable processes, favouring biodiversity, bringing benefits (tangible and intangible) to all people (their quality of life) now and in the future [36]. The key element is the management of limited natural resources [37]. The green economy is interpreted as '4R'—i.e., reduction, reuse, recycling, and recovery. These relate to reducing resource consumption and preserving natural capital, energy resource recovery (e.g., burning waste for heating), and consumption based on continuous growth and increasing resource capacity by decoupling economic growth from environmental pressures [38,39].

3. Materials and Methods

This research aimed to evaluate the spatial differentiation of the quality of life in voivodships in Poland with the use of a synthetic measure. This enables the ranking and grouping of voivodeships from the point of view of the main criterion, together with examining whether and to what extent the variables of its structure determine it, and indicating the importance of local research and the information obtained as part of the research carried out at various stages of decision-making in a territorial unit. The synthetic measure (built using the Technique for Order Preference by Similarity to an Ideal Solution method) facilitates the comparison of objects in multidimensional spaces but also allows them to be organized in terms of the phenomenon under study. The factor analysis and the coefficient of variation were used to delimit the variables, and the correlation analysis was used to determine the relationships between the variables. The scatter diagrams and maps of spatial differentiation of the studied phenomenon are presented. The method of descriptive analysis was also used, together with a literature study on the quality of life and its determinants.

Empirical (measurable) data were collected in the spatial terms of Polish voivodships. The choice of variables was conditioned by the availability of secondary data collected in the Local Data Bank of the Central Statistical Office (BDL GUS) for the years 2010–2020. The research was carried out dynamically, determining the values of min $\{x_{ij}\}$ and max $\{x_{ij}\}$ for the entire research period. A voivodship should be understood as a local government unit, i.e., a regional self-government community (all inhabitants), the highest level of the basic territorial division of the country, established to perform public administration. The analysis was made on the NUTS 2 level, in Poland—voivodships.

When examining spatial differentiation in terms of the main criterion (quality of life), a certain number of diagnostic variables should be distinguished that characterize the level of the analysed phenomenon, which can be written using a multidimensional data matrix [40]. As a complex phenomenon, the quality of life was characterized based on variables illustrating, among others, social, economic, infrastructural, environmental, financial, and green economy aspects. The spatial (intraregional) polarization of the quality of life variables in the modern economy occurs primarily between cities (regions of growth in the region) and peripheral areas [41].

The selection of diagnostic variables and their verification in terms of content and/or statistics allowed for the definition of the observation matrix, which consists of objects and features. It was written as X_{ij}:

$$X_{ij} = \begin{bmatrix} x_{11} & x_{12} & \dots & x_{1m} \\ x_{21} & x_{22} & \dots & x_{2m} \\ \dots & \dots & \dots & \dots \\ x_{n1} & x_{n2} & \dots & x_{nm} \end{bmatrix}, \quad (1)$$

where: X_{ij}—denotes the values of the j-th variable for the i-th object, matrix of data objects, i—object number (i = 1, 2, ... , n), j—variable number (j = 1, 2, ... , m).

The determinants characterizing the quality of life are interactive. They are a tangle of interrelated variables that create a multidimensional space. The following variables presented in Table 1 were distinguished in the study (selected after statistical and content evaluation).

Table 1. List of variables describing the quality of life.

	Variables	Unit	S/D *
X3	Dwellings equipped with sanitary facilities—water supply	%	s
X4	Dwellings equipped with sanitary facilities—bathroom	%	s
X6	Dwellings equipped with installations—gas mains	%	s
X7	Uses the system—water supply system	%	s
X8	Uses the system—sewage system	%	s
X9	Persons using the system—gas network	%	s
X10	Total migration balance per 1000 population	Osoba	d
X11	Total average monthly disposable income per 1 person	PLN	s
X16	Deaths per 1000 population	-	d
X17	Natural increase per 1000 population	-	s
X18	Total employed per 1000 population	Osoba	s
X22	Population per bed in general hospitals	Osoba	s
X25	Total industrial and municipal wastewater requiring treatment discharged to water or land during the year	Dam^3/km^2	d
X26	Industrial and municipal wastewater requiring treatment discharged to water or land during the year—treated	Dam^3/km^2	d
X27	Total waste collected during the year	T	d
X27	Share of the area of active landfills in the total area	%	d
X29	% Population using sewage treatment plants	%	s
X31	Share of green areas in the total area	%	s
X33	Gross enrolment rate—primary schools	-	s
X34	Average gross monthly salaries	PLN	s
X36	Own income per capita	PLN PC	s
X37	Property expenditures per capita	PLN PC	s
X38	Income from personal income tax (PIT)	PLN PC	s

Table 1. *Cont.*

	Variables	Unit	S/D *
X39	Income from corporate income tax (CIT)	PLN PC	s
X40	Expenditure on transport and communications PLN	PLN PC	s

For the construction of the synthetic measure, a set of 42 potential diagnostic variables collected by public statistics and related to the analysed phenomenon was originally adopted; the table shows the number of those selected for the construction of the synthetic measure as a result of the analysis. The variables were removed based on the correlation coefficient, coefficient of variation, and factor analysis; * S stimulant/D destimulant/. Source of data: a study based on the BDL CSO data.

Difficulties related to the implementation of the research (selection of variables in the structure of the synthetic measure) are related, among others, to changes in legal regulations regarding the income system, the scope of tasks performed by territorial units, budget reporting, changes in the administrative division, changes in the socioeconomic situation, random events, or the lack of data collected as part of public statistics at the level of municipalities (or points, or provinces; some data were incomplete, data did not cover all voivodeships).

After determining and collecting data on the initial set of features, verification activities were undertaken according to the statistical criterion. This allowed for the elimination of quasi-constant variables. For this purpose, the coefficient of variation was used, given by the formula:

$$V_i = \frac{S_i}{\overline{x}} \tag{2}$$

where: V_i—coefficient of variation for the i-th variable, S_i—standard deviation for the i-th variable, and $\overline{x}$ is the arithmetic mean of the i-th variable. Diagnostic features should show sufficient spatial variability, i.e., they should be the carrier of information differentiating the examined objects. From the set of variables, the features satisfying the inequality were eliminated $|V_i| \leq V^*$, where V^* denotes the critical value of the coefficient of variation. The value $V^* = 0.10$ was adopted as the critical value [42].

Variables strongly correlated with each other as carriers of similar information were also eliminated. It is assumed that in the case of identifying too high a value of the correlation index, a representative should be selected. The choice can be made based on the merits. The value $r^* = 0.75$ is also taken as the threshold level of the correlation coefficient [43]. According to K. Kukuła and K. Kukuła and L. Luty, the correlation between the features does not rule out the correctness of their selection for the study, because the linear ordering of objects is based on the value of a synthetic variable. It is obtained by summing unified diagnostic variables considered important from the substantive point of view [44,45].

The selection of variables was also made based on factor analysis performed in the Statistica program (Statistica 13, TIBCO Software Inc., StatSoft Polska, Kraków, Polska). The indicated method allows for the transformation of the original set of objects into a set of their groups, using orthogonal transformations of the original data matrix (e.g., factor analysis, principal components method) [46]. It allows for a reduced number of analysed variables and transforms the old system of variables into a new system consisting of the main factors. Factor analysis is a method of studying the structure of internal relationships in multivariate observations [47–49].

The eigenvalues of the reduced correlation matrix, defining the variances of subsequent factors and their percentage share in the overall variability of the entire set, are presented in Table 2. After finding the presence of strong and statistically significant correlations between the analysed features, the number of factors was determined. Five factors were selected, four of them individually explain more than 10% of the total variance; the fifth explains 6.786%. Together, they explain 89.56% of the total variance.

Table 2. Groups of factors and their eigenvalues describe the quality of life.

Factor	Own Value	% of Total (Variance)	Cumulative (Own Value)	Cumulative (%)
1	9.577473	39.90614	9.57747	39.90614
2	4.196891	17.48705	13.77436	57.39318
3	3.181361	13.25567	16.95573	70.64885
4	2.912074	12.13364	19.86780	82.78250
5	1.628870	6.78696	21.49667	89.56946

Data source: own study based on the CSO BDL data, in the Statistica program.

Based on the scree criterion, the five most important factors that make up the 'slope' were identified as the most important. The factor loadings, similar to the coefficients included in the eigenvector, reflect the influence of individual variables on a given principal component. These are the values showing what part of the variance of a given component is constituted by the original variables.

Based on the information included in Tables 2 and 3, it can be seen that the first main factor, exhausting 39.90614% of the total variability resource, and its eigenvalue is 9.577473. It is identified by the variables X10, X11, X18, X33, X34, X36, X38, X39, characterized by positive factor loadings.

Table 3. Values of factor loadings after rotation with the 'Varimax' method.

Variables	Factor (1)	Factor (2)	Factor (3)	Factor (4)	Factor (5)
X3	0.146035	**0.926340**	0.184745	0.208493	0.108775
X4	0.225769	**0.837793**	0.260945	0.372442	−0.045131
X6	0.153575	0.283894	**0.793697**	0.313021	0.217332
X7	0.017929	**0.766253**	−0.490532	−0.305696	0.136024
X8	0.101065	**0.905829**	0.191370	0.227639	−0.092560
X9	0.139483	0.216800	**0.831425**	0.305760	0.164121
X10	**0.789840**	0.265765	0.137077	0.410081	0.159171
X11	**0.795852**	0.274948	0.013686	−0.329413	−0.265372
X16	−0.048288	−0.172561	−0.198620	**−0.869399**	0.253781
X17	0.363022	0.067732	0.189999	**0.832429**	−0.146957
X18	**0.840321**	0.297020	0.251333	0.027656	0.248020
X22	−0.003097	0.396936	−0.102618	**0.775106**	0.109800
X25	0.273933	0.231362	**0.720062**	−0.410569	0.056443
X26	0.292836	0.234781	**0.724555**	−0.358166	0.089340
X27	0.348106	**0.838415**	0.037944	−0.219797	0.172228
X29	0.092625	**0.882838**	0.203478	0.143047	−0.074970
X31	−0.040598	−0.029420	**0.943407**	0.138305	0.007733
X33	**0.814294**	−0.036575	0.163372	0.017195	0.212391
X34	**0.920246**	0.080156	0.147446	−0.033572	0.160096
X36	**0.929814**	0.030116	−0.003919	0.215951	0.045051
X37	−0.296295	−0.068217	−0.070475	0.125170	**−0.904070**
X38	**0.950249**	0.230411	0.085565	0.008273	0.165767
X39	**0.937224**	0.053138	0.001038	0.151287	0.192889
X40	−0.248796	−0.008971	−0.182734	0.096070	**−0.924675**
War.wyj.	6.821100	5.182818	3.939372	3.326612	2.226768
Udział	0.284212	0.215951	0.164141	0.138609	0.092782

Extract: Principal components; Marked loads are >0.700000. Source: own study based on the CSO BDL data, in the Statistica program.

The second factor consists of the variables X3, X4, X7, X8, X27, X29. It explains 17.48705% of the total variation resources, and the eigenvalue of this factor is 4.196891; therefore, its importance in presenting the diversity of the entire set from the mathematical point of view is the most important.

The third factor (formed by X6, X9, X25, X26, X31) accounts for 13.25567% of the common varieties of all variables, and its eigenvalue is 3.181361. The fourth factor is identified by the variables X16 (with a negative factor load), X17, X22. It exhausts 12.13364% of the common varieties of all variables, and its eigenvalue is 2.912074. The last fifth factor is characterized by negative factor loadings (variables X37, X40) exhausts 6.78696 resources of common variation, and its eigenvalue is 1.628870.

The analysis of the level of the coefficient of variation and correlation leads to the conclusion that the selected input variables are slightly correlated with other variables. The value of the coefficient of variation ranged from 0.02 (X33), −2.78 (X10) to 1.99 (X17) in 2010, and from X33 (0.02), −4.26 (X10) to 0.95 (X25) in 2020; in 2010, for the variables X17 (1.99), X25 (0.92), X26 (0.89), the lowest X3 (0.03), X33 (0.02), X10 (−2.78), and in 2020, respectively, X25 (0.95), X26 (0.84), X31 (0.74) and X33 (0.02), X17 (−0.5), X10 (−4.26). It should also be noted that the variables are positive (15 in 2010, 16 in 2020) and negative (9 and 8 variables, respectively). asymmetry W in the case of stimulants (19 variables in both extremes for the years presented) is not a favourable situation, as it means that a greater number of communes have values of these variables lower than their average.

In the next stage of the research, the direction of variable preferences regarding the general criterion under consideration was determined, dividing them into stimulants and destimulants [50,51]. Most of the variables are obvious and their determination is intuitive. In doubtful cases, it is worth using Grabiński's procedure, which uses the fact that stimulants should be positively correlated with stimulants (the same is true for destimulants) and negatively correlated with destimulants [52]. The correctness of determining the nature of the variables can be verified by specifying the direction of correlation of individual variables with the decision variable. For a stimulant, this direction should be positive, and for a destimulant, the direction should be negative [53].

Diagnostic variables usually have different titers and different ranges of variation, which makes it impossible to compare and add them directly [54–56]. To make the variables comparable, the unitarization procedure was used, the purpose of which is to replace the different ranges of the variability of individual variables with a constant range [57,58].

The normalization of diagnostic variables, by the zeroed unitarization procedure, was performed depending on their types, according to the following formulas [42]:

$$Z_{ij} = \frac{x_{ij} - \min_i x_{ij}}{\max_i x_{ij} - \min_i x_{ij}}, \text{ when } x_i \in S, \tag{3}$$

$$Z_{ij} = \frac{\max_i x_{ij} - x_{ij}}{\max_i x_{ij} - \min_i x_{ij}}, \text{ gdy } x_i \in D \tag{4}$$

where: S—stimulant, D—destimulant; i = 1, 2 . . . n; j = 1, 2 . . . m,

$\max x_{ij}$—maximum value of the j-th variable,

$\min x_{ij}$—minimum value of the j-th variable,

x_{ij}—is the value of the j-th variable for this object,

Z_{ij}—the normalized value of the jth variable for this object (belongs to the interval [0; 1]) [59–63].

All variables are standardized concerning the range of variability and their location in the observation space. As a result of unitarization, we obtain a matrix of feature values:

$$Z_{ij} = \begin{bmatrix} z_{11} & z_{12} & \cdots & z_{1m} \\ z_{21} & z_{22} & \cdots & z_{2m} \\ \cdots & \cdots & \cdots & \cdots \\ z_{n1} & z_{n2} & \cdots & z_{nm} \end{bmatrix}, \tag{5}$$

where Z_{ij} is the unitary value of j-th variables for the i-th object.

A synthetic measure based on the Technique for Order Preference by Similarity to an Ideal Solution (TOPSIS) method was used to assess the spatial differentiation of the quality of life in voivodships in Poland. This measure allowed for a multidimensional and comprehensive examination at the level of the phenomenon in individual examined objects, conducting comparative analyses of objects (in spatial and time terms), and their linear ordering [64,65]. The first synthetic measure of development was proposed by Z. Hellwig to evaluate the economic development of selected countries. The synthetic measure made it possible to order the examined objects according to the level of phenomena (which cannot be measured with one measure). It provides the basis for the evaluation and comparison of multifeature objects according to the established criteria, and a comparative image between the analysed objects allows for indicating weaker and better areas of the unit's operation. Moreover, it enables the grouping of the analysed territorial units. It can be a helpful tool for assessing the accuracy of past decisions and the effectiveness of past regional management instruments [66].

The TOPSIS linear ordering method is a reference method in which two reference points of objects in multidimensional space are determined—a pattern and an antipattern [67,68]. Their coordinates are as follows:

(a) for the pattern:

$$z_j^+ = \begin{cases} \max\{z_{ij}\} \text{ for stimulant variables} \\ \min\{z_{ij}\} \text{ for destimulant variables} \end{cases} \tag{6}$$

(b) for the antipattern:

$$z_j^- = \begin{cases} \min\{z_{ij}\} \text{ for stimulant variables} \\ \max\{z_{ij}\} \text{ for destimulant variables} \end{cases} \tag{7}$$

The Euclidean distances of individual objects from the pattern and antipattern were successively calculated, according to the formulas:

(a) distances of objects from the pattern:

$$d_i^+ = \sqrt{\frac{1}{n}\sum_{j=1}^{m}\left(z_{ij} - z_j^+\right)^2} \tag{8}$$

(b) distances of objects from the antipattern:

$$d_i^- = \sqrt{\frac{1}{n}\sum_{j=1}^{m}\left(z_{ij} - z_j^-\right)^2} \tag{9}$$

where: n—is the number of variables forming the pattern or antipattern, z_{ij}—is the unitized value of the j feature for the tested unit (or the normalized value of the jth variable of the ith object), and z_j^+/z_j^-—is the pattern or antipattern object [69,70].

The synthetic measure for individual objects according to the TOPSIS method was determined based on the formula:

$$q_i = \frac{d_i^-}{d_i^- + d_i^+}, \text{ gdzie } 0 \le q_i \le 1,\ i = 1, 2, \ldots, n; \tag{10}$$

with the proviso that: $q_i \in [0; 1]$; d_i^-—is the distance of the object from the antipattern (from 0) and d_i^+ is the distance of the object from the pattern (from 1). A higher value of the measure indicates a better situation for an individual in the analysed area. The TOPSIS method enables the assessment to be made with the use of an unlimited number of criteria, the readability of the obtained results is high, and it allows for a linear ordering of objects (e.g., building a ranking of units in spatial terms). A significant advantage of the TOPSIS method is its computational simplicity, the indication of a positive and negative model, and a large number of alternative criteria that can be used in the evaluation process [71–76].

In the last stage of research, the division into typological groups was used to interpret the obtained measures. The first, second, and third quartiles were adopted as threshold values. The size of the synthetic measure in the first group means a better unit, and weaker units for the groups that follow [77].

The next step was to test the strength of the relationship between the variables. For this purpose, Pearson's linear correlation coefficients were used, expressed by the formula:

$$r_{xy} = \frac{\sum_{i=1}^{n}\left(x_i - \overleftarrow{x}\right)\left(y_i - \overleftarrow{y}\right)}{\sqrt{\sum_{i=1}^{n}\left(x_i - \overleftarrow{x}\right)^2 \sum_{i=1}^{n}\left(y_i - \overleftarrow{y}\right)^2}} \quad (11)$$

where, r_{xy}—Pearson's linear correlation coefficient, x and y are measurable statistical features x = (1,2, ... n), y = (1,2, ... n), and $\overleftarrow{x}, \overleftarrow{y}$ are the arithmetic average of the x and y features. The Pearson linear correlation coefficient takes the value from the interval, where, when $r_{xy} = 0$, there is no linear relationship, and when $r_{xy} = 1$ or $r_{xy} = -1$, there is an exact linear relationship between the features (positive or negative).

Additionally, a dendrogram is presented, a scatter plot with a fit line, and linear regression analysis and autocorrelation analysis were performed [78].

In the assessment of the synthetic measure, the cluster analysis using Ward's minimal variance method with the Euclidean distance was also used. Its results are presented in the form of a dendrogram. This method is a hierarchical and agglomeration approach. Owing to it, it was possible to designate groups of voivodeships similar in terms of the quality of life. Hierarchical rankings of homogeneous clusters were developed for comparative purposes for the years 2010–2020. The necessary calculations were performed using the Statistica program.

To assess the impact of endogenous potentials of Polish voivodeships on the spatial differentiation of the synthetic quality of life measure, a regression model describing the dependence of the variables was estimated. Regression analysis (implemented in the Gretl program) examines the relationship between the variables of interest to us. It allows describing the relationships between the explanatory variables (Y) and the explained variables (X), between which there are more or less clear linear relationships. Linear regression analysis aims to calculate regression coefficients such that the model predicts the value of the dependent variable as well as possible so that the error of estimation is as small as possible. We describe a linear regression model by the following formula:

$$y_i = b\, x_i + a,\ i = 1, 2, \ldots, n, \quad (12)$$

In the case of the multiple regression model, when we have a larger number of variables, we use the following formula:

$$y = b_1 x_1 + b_2 x_2 + \ldots + b_i x_i + a,\ i = 1, 2, \ldots, n, \quad (13)$$

where:

b—is the regression coefficient calculated for the individual variables of the model;
x—explanatory variable;
y—is the dependent variable;
a—is an intercept.

In the process of building a regression model, high autocorrelation of variables should be excluded, and the fit of the model should be checked using the analysis of variance. Next, we move on to reading the beta standardized coefficients and their significance level. Then, we determine the percentage of the variance explained by reading the (preferably corrected) R2 statistic. The coefficient of determination determines the degree to which the estimated regression function explains the variability of the variable y. It takes values from 0 to 1. The closer to 1, the better the regression function fits the empirical data [79–84].

Spatial autocorrelation means that the values of geographically close objects are more similar to each other than distant ones. This phenomenon causes the formation of spatial clusters with similar values [85–87]. Positive spatial autocorrelation occurs when we observe the spatial accumulation of high or low values of the observed variables. Negative autocorrelation means neighbouring high values with low values in the space, and low values with high values. Lack of spatial autocorrelation means spatial randomness, i.e., high and low values of the observed variables are distributed independently [85]. By analysing the result of autocorrelation, it is possible to determine clusters of objects similar to each other. Knowing and understanding the structures of space enables better anticipation of changes and facilitates taking actions in development policy [88,89].

Global Moran, I statistics can be used to investigate spatial relationships [90,91]. The statistics check whether adjacent parcels form clusters with similar synthetic measure values. It was determined based on the formula [92]:

$$I = \frac{\sum_{i=1}^{n} \sum_{j=1}^{n} w_{ij} (x_i - \bar{x})(x_j - \bar{x})}{S_o \, \sigma^2}. \quad (14)$$

Local Moran statistics are negative when a given area is surrounded by regions with significantly different values of the studied variable. Positive values of the statistics should be interpreted as follows: the region is surrounded by similar regions. Owing to this, it is possible to determine clusters with low or high values of the studied variable [93,94]. The local version of the Moran statistics is the most popular analysis and is known as LISA (Local Indicators of Spatial Association). The local form of the I Moran coefficient for observations, which determines the similarity of the spatial unit to its neighbours and the statistical significance of this relationship, is determined by the formula:

$$I_i = \frac{(x_i - \bar{x}) \sum_{j=1}^{n} w_{ij} (x_j - \bar{x})}{\sigma^2}, \quad (15)$$

where:

n—number of spatial objects (number of points or polygons);
x_i, x_j—values of the variable for the compared objects;
$\bar{x}$—average value of the variable for all objects;
w_{ij}—elements of the spatial weight matrix (weights matrix standardized with rows to one),
$s_o = \sum_{i=1}^{n} \sum_{j=1}^{n} w_{ij}$,
$\sigma^2 = \frac{\sum_{j=1}^{n} (x_i - \bar{x})^2}{n}$,—variance [95].

The Moran I statistic takes a value from the interval (−1, 1), where the value '0' means no spatial autocorrelation, negative values are negative autocorrelation (<−1, 0; units with different values appear next to each other in space, differentiation of the examined objects), positive values signal a positive spatial correlation (0, >1; units with similar values occur next to each other, forming clusters) [96,97].

To illustrate the spatial dependence of the quality of life distribution in voivodships in Poland, the I Moran statistics were calculated using the Queen matrix standardized by rows to one. The calculations were made in the PQStat program.

4. Results

Figure 1 presents the results of the classification of voivodeships in Poland obtained based on the synthetic measure of the quality of life. Four influences were identified, numbered, respectively, 4, 6, 2, 4 (in groups I, II, III, IV) of the voivodship in 2010 and 5, 3, 4, 4 in 2020. The best voivodships were in the group I: Pomerania, Masovia, Lower Silesia, and West Pomeranian in 2010 (Masovia, Pomerania, Greater Poland, Lower Silesia, and Lesser Poland in 2020), and in IV—the weakest: Lodz Province, Podlasie Province, Lublin Province, and Holy Cross in 2010 (Lodz Province, Podlasie Province, Holy Cross, and Lublin Province in 2020), in the light of the variables and linear ordering methods included in the study. The synthetic measure of the quality of life ranged from 0.37 (Lublin

Province and Holy Cross) to 0.56 (Pomerania) in 2010 and from 0.39 (Lublin Province) to 0.64 (Masovia) in 2020. From 2020 to 2010, all voivodships recorded an increase in the value of the quality of life measure (Lesser Poland, Greater Poland, and Masovia to the highest degree). The classification of voivodships was carried out based on quartiles, which were threshold values for subsequent groups. Figure 1 shows the classification of Polish voivodeships according to the synthetic measure of the quality of life. Black indicates the group of voivodeships characterized by a better condition in the main criterion under study, the lighter the grey showing increasingly weaker units.

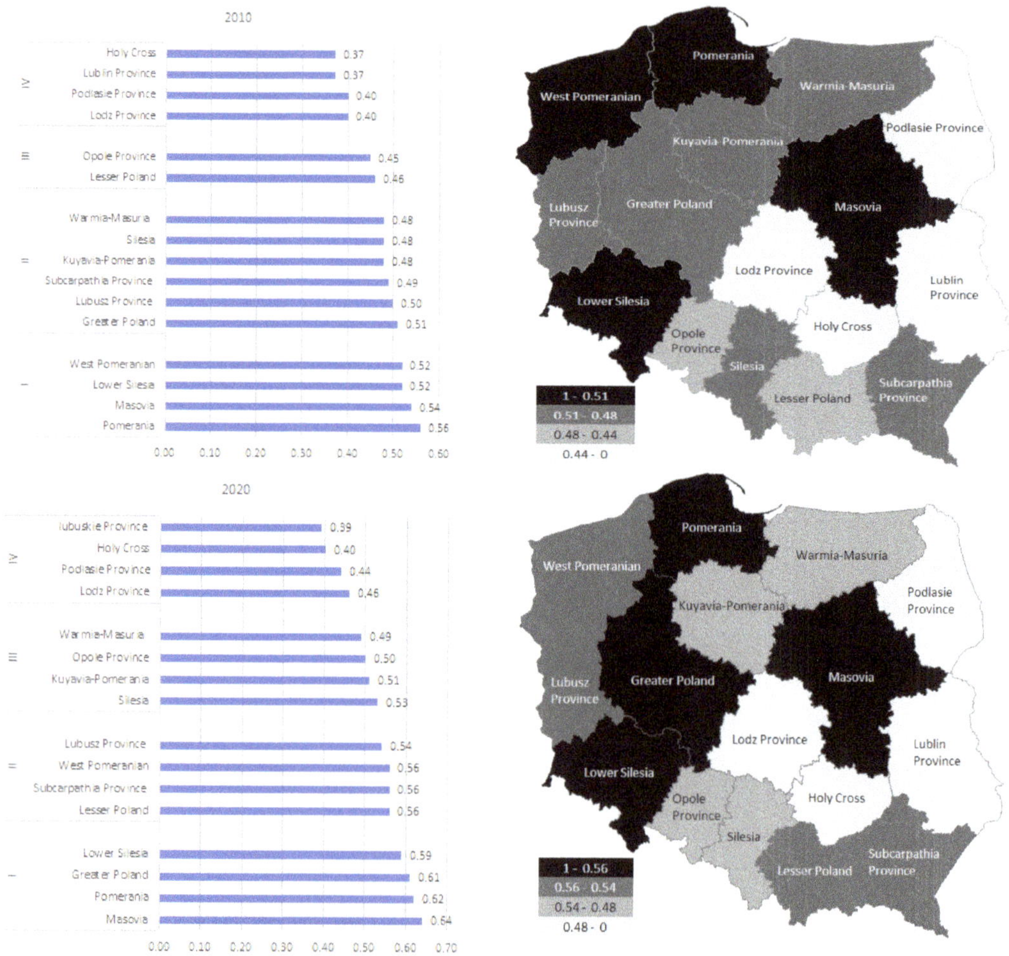

Figure 1. *Cont.*

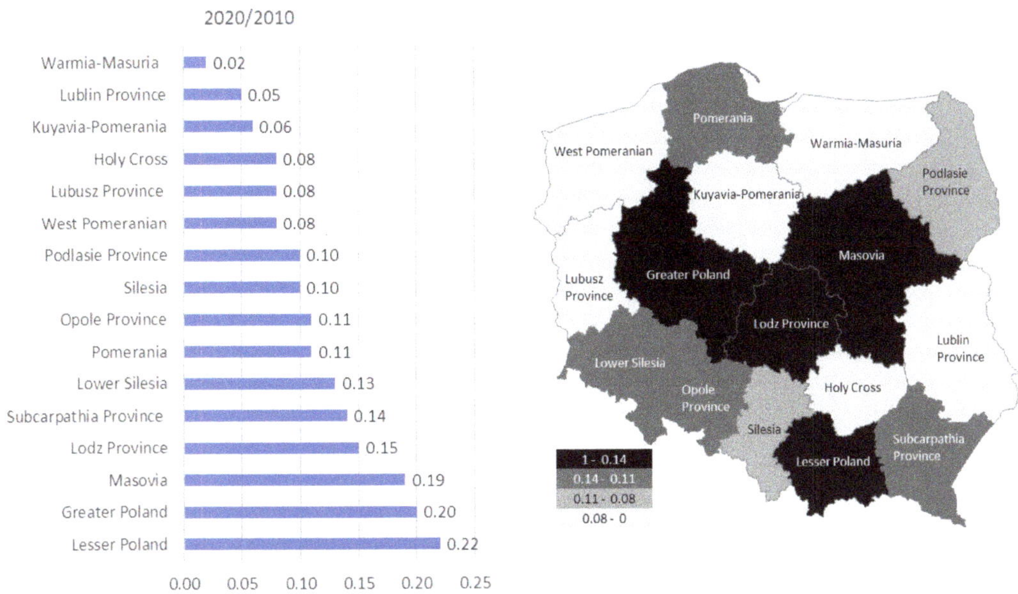

Figure 1. Groups and spatial differentiation of the synthetic measure of the quality of life in voivodships in Poland in 2010 and 2020. Source: own study based on the BDL CSO data.

Figure 2 shows the number of observations and the model of the distribution of the synthetic measure of the quality of life in 2010 and 2020. The synthetic measure ranged from 0.37 to 0.56 in 2010 and from 0.39 to 0.64 in 2020. Both in 2010 and 2020 we observe lefthand skewness (As < 0). Left skew indicates that a greater number of units have values for these variables greater than their mean. The most numerous range in 2010 is 0.46–0.48 and 0.50–0.52; in both cases it was made up of three voivodeships (19%). In 2020, the most numerous range is 0.54–0.56 (three units, 19%), which means that there is a dominant feature in this range.

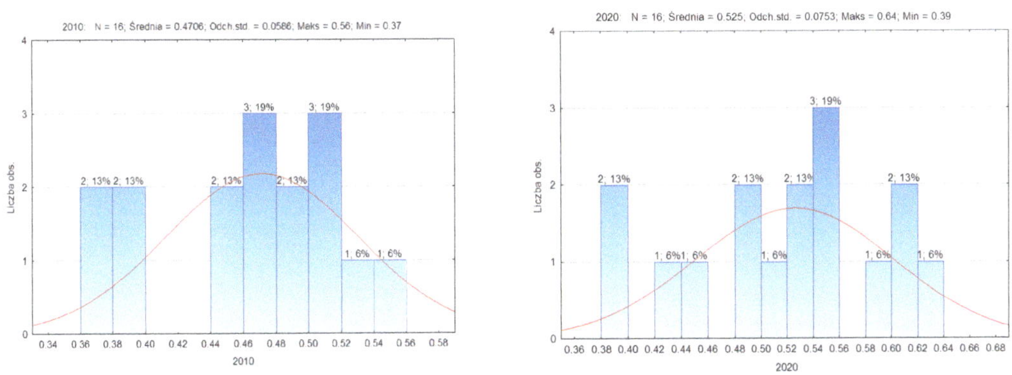

Figure 2. Distribution diagram showing the synthetic measure of the quality of life in voivodships in Poland in 2010 and 2020. Source: own study based on the BDL CSO data.

Statistical characteristics of the synthetic quality of life measure (Table 4) in voivodships in Poland in 2010 compared to 2020 show differentiation of the studied phenomenon. The standard deviation was 0.06 and 0.07. It indicates a slight differentiation of units in the examined aspect. The coefficient of variation (0.13–0.14) shows slight disproportions. The range (0.20–0.25) indicates the size of the dispersion between the smallest and the largest value of the variable in the studied area.

Table 4. Measures differentiating the synthetic measure of the quality of life in voivodships in Poland in 2010 and 2020.

	2010	2020
min	0.37	0.39
max	0.56	0.64
range	0.20	0.25
average	0.47	0.53
median	0.48	0.54
standard deviation	0.06	0.07
quartile deviation	0.04	0.04
coefficient of variation	0.13	0.14
positional coefficient of variation	0.08	0.08
quartile range	0.08	0.08
skewness (asymmetry)	−0.53	−0.41
kurtosis (measure of concentration)	−0.58	−0.59

Source: own study based on the BDL CSO data.

Pearson's correlation coefficient between the value of the synthetic measure in 2010 to 2020 according to the quality of life measure was 0.942. Outliers (Lublin Province and Holy Cross) were characterized by a peripheral location, agricultural function, and a weak labour market (Figure 3a). The bag chart (Figure 3b) shows statistically similar groups of the voivodship, pointing to Pomerania, Lesser Poland, and Warmia-Masuria as outliers. These are voivodships characterized by an industrial function and a good labour market.

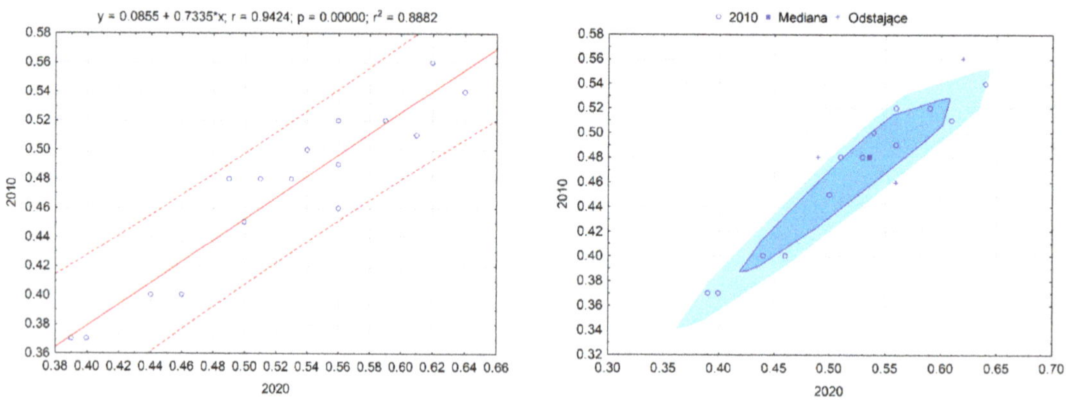

(a) (b)

Figure 3. Scatter plot with the fit line (**a**) and bag chart (**b**) of the synthetic measure of the quality of life of voivodships in Poland. Source: own study based on the BDL CSO data.

Development is a multidimensional process that combines social, economic, cultural, political, and technical processes together with the interdependencies between them. The relations between its components are not constant and are subject to change. It is spatially diversified, which results from the location rent, i.e., the specificity of the resources, including specific natural and non-natural conditions. The location rent refers to the spatial location and endogenous territorial potential, therefore its recognition is extremely important for building social and economic cohesion [98–100].

The endogenous potential of an individual (including the quality of life) is built, among others, by the professional activity of inhabitants, the local labour market, entrepreneurship, infrastructure, and the condition of the natural environment. Appropriate potential contributes to an increase in the standard of living, a better social situation, and greater public safety. The level of development is not uniform. Its spatial diversity results in different conditions for running a business, or a different level and living conditions of the inhabitants [101]. Each voivodeship has its endogenous potential, which, in connection with the exogenous potential and the ability to respond to changes in the environment, may constitute an opportunity for development. Endogenous factors (specific, unique, and corresponding to a given local system [102]) are the main driving force of regional development [103,104].

The quality of life measure in the case of Polish voivodeships in the analysed years was correlated with variables in the economic, infrastructural, demographic, and natural environment. In particular, the measure of the quality of life to its structure variables was correlated with: flats equipped with water supply systems (0.7372), bathroom (0.81), network gas (0.6607), using the sewage system (0.7474) and gas network (0.6183), migration (0.7238), average monthly disposable income (0.5137), number of employees (0.7515), population per bed in general hospitals (0.5054), total waste collected during the year (0.7176), population using sewage treatment plants (0.6865), and average monthly salary (0.5363).

Quality of life is a complex process relating to many different aspects of human functioning. It is determined by many different elements, including the condition of the natural environment; access to education and culture; health and social care; safety in terms of health, loss of property, and economic terms; the quality of infrastructure; and the natural environment.

In the analysis of the green economy, elements shaping the quality of life can be found. The development of the region should be related to concern for the environment, preserving the ability of ecosystems to provide specific services and ensuring good-quality elements of the environment, which should have a positive impact on the quality of life of the inhabitants. In the area of variables describing the green economy, the quality of life measure was correlated with electricity consumption (0.2525), the share of agricultural area (−0.3907), loess (0.2767), legally protected areas (−0.2186) in the total area, waste collected selectively (0.2125) or the total annual (0.3644), mixed waste (0.6604), household waste per capita (0.6847), and the area of wild landfills (−0.2042).

An important goal of sustainable development is to improve the quality of life. Conceptually, high quality of life is the overriding goal of sustainable development [105]. The quality of life measure is also correlated with the elements shaping sustainable development, i.e., entities entered in the register (0.7921), natural persons running a business (0.727), sold production of industry (0.727), and using sewage systems (0.7474).

Another area influencing the quality of life is the financial situation. Financial resources are an essential element for the effective achievement of the unit goals in terms of current or development tasks. There is a feedback loop between the socioeconomic and financial variables [106,107]. The financial situation is the state of its finances that allows it to cover: current bills, expenses without incurring debts in a given budget period, all costs of running a business in the long term, and services at a level ensuring the safety and quality of life of residents [108]. X. Wang, L. Dennis, and Y. Sen believe that the socioeconomic environment is only one of the factors that should be taken into account when analysing the financial situation [109]. M.P. Rodríguez Bolivar and coauthors identified the main factors shaping the financial situation as the state and changes in the size of the population, the conditions of the local labour market, the needs of the local community, the size of the supply and directions of distribution of local public goods and services, and the wealth of the society, among others [110]. In the area of financial situation, the quality of life was correlated with the share of own income in total income (0.6586), the level of transfers from the state budget per capita (−0.4258), burdening own income with debt-servicing expenses (−0.3133), share in taxes constituting state budget income 0.6444, own income per capita (PC) (0.7068), income from tax of natural persons MS (0.6514), legal persons MS (0.6857), and general subsidy (−0.5289).

As a result of the use of hierarchical methods, we obtain a dendrogram that illustrates the hierarchical structure of voivodships in terms of the quality of life measure. Based on the adopted features, clustering was performed using Ward's method, taking into account the Euclidean distance between units. The result of clustering voivodeships for the analysed years, at the level of 0.5, are three groups of voivodeships most similar to each other, i.e.,

- Group I: Lower Silesia, Greater Poland, Masovia, and Pomerania (the group includes units with the highest level of synthesis and the best sizes of diagnostic plots);
- Group II: Kuyavian-Pomeranian, Warmian-Masurian, Opole Province, Lubusz, Subcarpathian, Silesian, Lesser Poland, and West Pomeranian;
- Group III: Lublin Province, Holy Cross, Lodz Province, and Podlasie Province (Figure 4).

The results of clustering may be a stimulus for further, in-depth research aimed at determining which variables had a decisive impact on the assignment of regions to individual clusters.

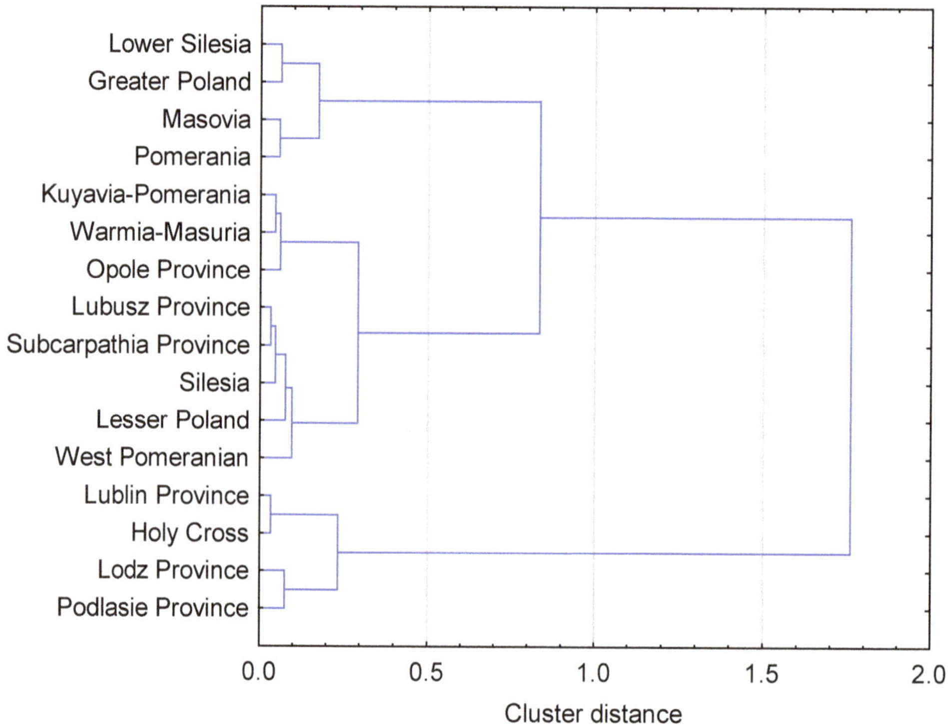

Figure 4. Clusters of Polish voivodships with a similar level of the synthetic measure of the quality of life. Source: own study based on the BDL CSO data.

The impact of spatial factors on changes in the quality of life results from their location in the economic system of the region and its existing network connections. Autocorrelation makes it possible to learn about the spatial structure of the dependence of units and the interaction between the values of the studied variable in different locations. The statistics of I Moran make it possible to determine the similarities and differences between communes in general terms. By analysing the result of spatial autocorrelation, it is possible to determine clusters of objects similar to each other, but also to find objects or groups of objects that differ from their neighbourhoods.

Table 5 presents the evolution of the values of global Moran I statistics, which inform about the existence of spatial autocorrelation. A positive autocorrelation was recorded in 2010, and a slight negative spatial relationship in 2020. Based on the global values of Moran's I obtained, it can be noticed that in the discussed period there is a decrease in autocorrelation. The decreasing value of the analysed statistics informs about the progressing process of weakening spatial dependence. This means that any observed quality of life level can appear anywhere with equal probability.

Table 5. Values of the global Moran's I statistics for the synthetic measure of the quality of life in voivodeships in Poland (in 2010 and 2020).

Variables	2010	2020
Moran's I	0.132925	−0.04291
Expected I	−0.06667	−0.06667
	Under the assumption of normality	
Variance I	0.022125	0.022125
Z statistic	1.341839	0.159703
p-value	0.179648	0.873115
	Assuming randomness	
Variance I	0.023059	0.023033
Z statistic	1.314393	0.156522
p-value	0.188714	0.875621

Source: own study based on the BDL CSO data.

Another aspect of spatial autocorrelation analysis is the study of the shaping of variable values to neighbouring locations. Such an analysis is made possible by local statistics. The values of local statistics allow stating the existence of the so-called outliers (voivodships 'in plus' or 'in minus' from their neighbours), or clustering of objects with similar measure values. Figure 5 shows the results obtained. Significant and positive values of local Moran's I statistics were obtained in the following voivodships: West Pomeranian (0.7581), Pomerania (0.6997), Lublin Province (0.6046), Holy Cross (0.4091), Lubusz Province (0.3940), Lower Silesia (0.2307), Greater Poland (0.2222), Podlasie Province (0.1500), Kuyavia-Pomerania (0.0748), Lesser Poland (0.0742), and Warmia-Masuria (0.0666) in 2010 (West Pomeranian 0.4015, Lublin Province 0.3574, Pomerania 0.2934, Lower Silesia 0.2868, Podlasie Province 0.2750, Greater Poland 0.2250, Lubusz Province 0.16328, and Holy Cross 0.16328 in 2020). These voivodships are surrounded by units with similar levels of potential within the studied area. Negative values of the I Moran measure were observed in the following voivodeships: Lodz Province −0.0214, Opole Province −0.0413, Silesia −0.1383, Subcarpathia Province −0.3986, and Masovia −1.0904 in 2010 (Silesia −0.0397, Lodz Province −0.0765, Opole Province −0.0993, Kuyavia-Pomerania −0.1032, Warmia-Masuria −0.1699, Lesser Poland −0.1750, Subcarpathia Province −0.4632, and Masovia −1.5559 in 2020).

To assess the impact of variables describing the quality of life area (taking into account the variables describing the green economy, waste policy, sustainable development, and financial aspect), a regression model was estimated (Table 6). The model shows the importance of the share of legally protected areas, residential areas in the total area, using the sewage system, the demographic dependency ratio for the elderly, the share of own income in total income, and personal income tax MS in the process of shaping and quality of life in voivodships in Poland. These are the variables that shape the endogenous economic base of the region. Their impact on the quality of life is varied. Their appropriate level increases the standard of living, improves the social situation, and enhances the natural environment. It can be concluded that the model fits well. (R-square determining coefficient 0.883110, corrected R-square 0.878960. The F statistic ((6, 169) 212.8002) is statistically significant (*p*-value), which means that the construction of the linear model is correct.

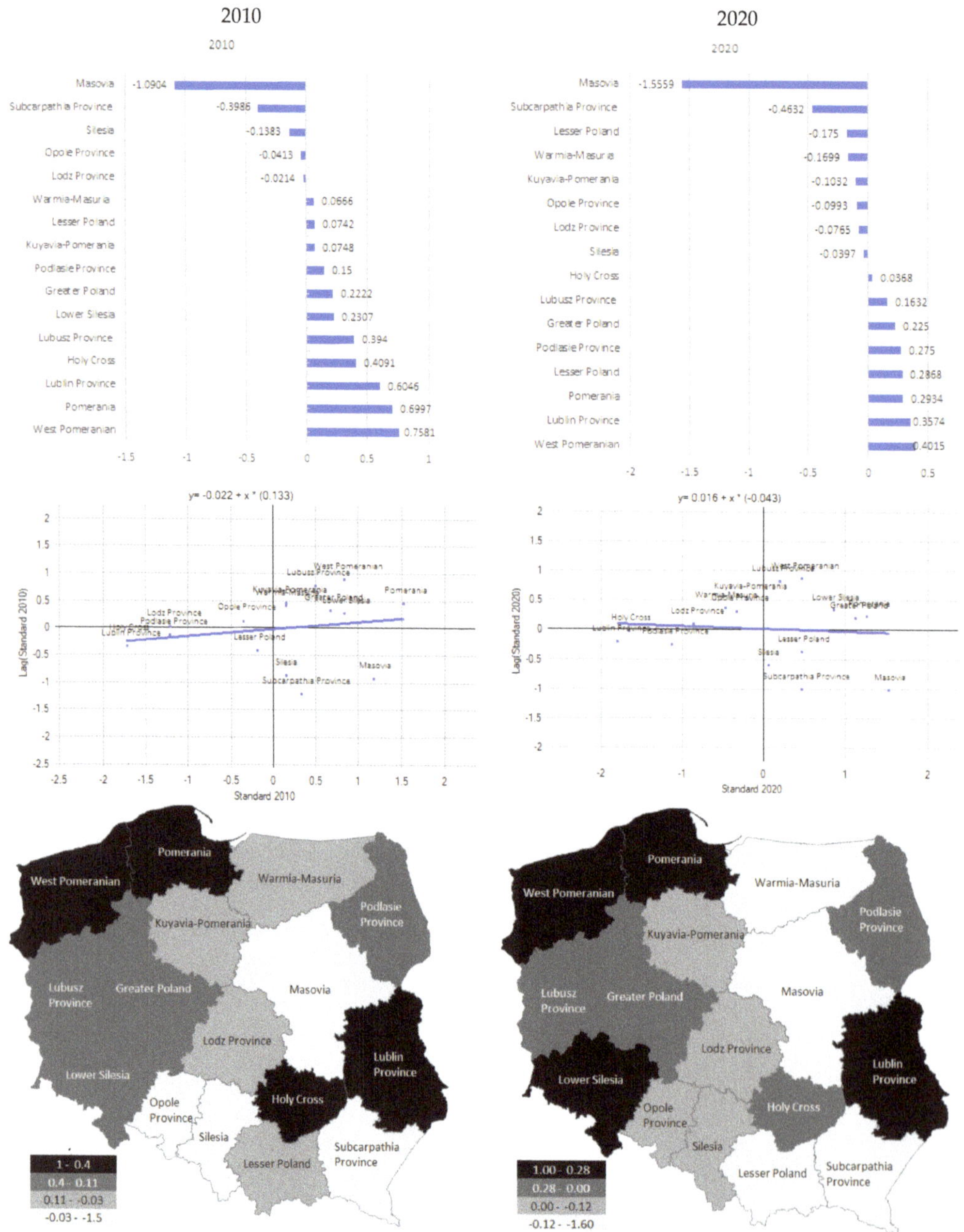

Figure 5. Spatial differentiation of the local value of the Moran I statistics for the synthetic measure of the quality of life in voivodships in Poland (in 2010 and 2020). Source: own study based on the BDL CSO data.

Table 6. Results of the regression analysis of the synthetic measure of the quality of life in voivodships in Poland.

	Coefficient	Standard Error	t-Student's	p-Value
Const.	0.289516	0.0270921	10.69	<0.0001
Share of legally protected areas in total area	0.000470627	0.000155975	3.017	0.0029
% Usage of sewage network	0.00390254	0.000260736	14.97	<0.0001
Old age dependency ratio	−0.00992326	0.000858840	−11.55	<0.0001
Residential areas in the total area	−0.0100945	0.00258376	−3.907	0.0001
Share of own income in total income	0.0762585	0.0221662	3.440	0.0007
Income tax from individuals	0.00445128	0.000461540	9.644	<0.0001
Arithmetic mean of the dependent variable	0.496080	Standard deviation of dependent variable		0.066676
Sum of squares residuals	0.090940	Residual standard error		0.023197
Coefficient of determination R-square	0.883110	Adjusted R-square		0.878960
F (6, 169)	212.8002	p-values for F-test		4.88×10^{-76}
Logarithm of credibility	416.2543	Inrom. Crit. Akaike'a		−818.5086
Crit. Bayes. Schwarza	−796.3152	Crit. Hannana–Quinna		−809.5071

Observations 1–176 used; dependent variable (Y): synthetic measure quality of life. Source: own study based on the BDL CSO data.

5. Discussion

Development is interpreted in terms of economic growth, but terms of demographic, social, cultural and environmental development are also important. It is to take into account one of the basic goals, which is to increase the level and quality of life, which occurs owing to positive changes in the living environment as a place to meet the needs of individuals. Systematic research on the quality of life of local and territorial communities should provide the information necessary for the authorities to evaluate and establish the regional policy. The increase or decrease in quality of life should be treated as a way of assessing the effects of local development management [111,112].

The responsibility for the conditions in which we live lies with ourselves and with the regional (local) authorities in the areas in which we live. The authorities collect funds for various reasons, and most of all for improving the quality of life. The pace of changes in the quality of life area may be decisive for some people from the point of view of migration and professional plans. The definitions of the standard of living functioning today are extremely broad and complex, which results from the combination of both measurable and nonmeasurable, objective and subjective, and quantitative and qualitative features of life, which indicates its multidimensionality (the multidimensionality of the phenomenon under study can be indicated by the number of variables in Table 1) [113].

The issues of sustainable development (or green economy) have a huge impact on all aspects of human life in economic, social, environmental, and political terms. The processes of structural transformations in economies are accompanied by an increase in the unevenness of their development [114]. Both the green economy and sustainable development are aimed at improving the quality of life by ensuring that human needs are met, and by protecting the environment, natural and social resources, and protecting the integrity of society [115].

The results obtained confirmed the spatial differentiation of the quality of life of residents and the influence of elements of the green economy on its formation. The assessment further indicates the strong influence of social and economic conditions on quality of life.

The green economy is a means to achieve sustainable development in terms of effective and purposeful use of endogenous factors of development (and activity). It helps to achieve integration between the dimensions of sustainable development (environmental, social, economic, and spatial or institutional (political)). This strengthens the context of the protection of the natural environment (conditioning socioeconomic development) and the quality of life. The green economy (which reduces carbon emissions and increases resource efficiency) must recognize state sovereignty over natural resources and must be based on resource efficiency and sustainable consumption and production patterns. The environment is the main source of resources that make life easier and foster development [116].

The sustainability (or green economy) orientation around the 'three E's' (environmental protection, economic growth, and social justice) is also correlated with quality of life considerations. Quality of life refers to people's perception of their position in life about their culture, values, and expectations. Achieving quality of life progress through sustainable development, particularly at the city level, requires careful planning that is both site- and culture-specific, and that includes contributions from communities and citizens. Improving the quality of life and meeting the needs of the present through sustainable development—introducing a green economy—should help ensure a greater probability of meeting the needs of future generations [117].

The adoption of a green economy can be useful for economic and social reasons as it has helped to reduce environmental pollution and, together with the inappropriate use of scarce resources, shapes the quality of life of the inhabitants. It benefits the region's economy both socially and environmentally, ensuring better resource use, reducing the misuse of scarce resources, eliminating environmental pollution, and improving the region's ecological growth [118].

The appropriate quality and structure of endogenous potential (endogenous territorial capital) ensures sustainable dynamics of regional processes and affects the level of development differentiation of individual provinces. Geographical, social, and economic conditions make the various provinces of the country characterized by a different economic situation, and thus a different level of development and quality of life.

The analysis of intraregional diversification (West Pomeranian Voivodeship) in terms of quality of life shows the need to create a system of incentives for the involvement of the private sector and the social economy in the development of social welfare, education, and social assistance—better integration and coordination of public services to increase the effectiveness of social services provided [119]. The results of quality of life research should be available to employees of city offices, city councillors, and housing estates councils, and constitute a starting point for spatial and transport planning, urban greenery and public spaces management, and revitalization activities. The diagnosis should also be available to nongovernmental organizations and socially active residents so that it can become the basis for public discussion and public participation in making decisions on budget expenditures during public consultations and submitting projects to civic budgets. In this way, systematic quality of life surveys can be an important element of knowledge-based and participatory decision-making in cities [120].

Quality of life is an interdisciplinary concept (numerous tasks and features that shape it), which makes it difficult to evaluate and define it, and indicates the need for multidimensional evaluation. The voivodship ratings obtained depend on what feature and specific quality of life symptom we take into account. However, it should be remembered that the results of the analysis depend on the diagnostic features adopted for the study (their structure and quantity) and may change when a different set is used. The selection of features is one of the tasks of particular importance because it largely determines the final results of the study, the accuracy of assessments and analyses, the accuracy of predictions, and the accuracy of decisions made on their basis. It is very difficult to collect reliable and comparable statistical data, especially in the analysis of the quality of life, which is a very complex phenomenon (also indicated by the presented studies by the authors, which indicates numerous variables characterizing the studied phenomenon) [121].

The minimum necessary condition for ecologically sustainable development is to maintain the total natural capital stock at the current level or above. The aim of ecologically sustainable development (green economy) is the wise use of natural resources in the short term so that these resources are available in the long term. Ecological sustainability cannot occur when people can deplete natural resources, leaving only polluted water and barren soil for future generations. Instead, ecological sustainability is the belief that all people must use resources wisely and efficiently, so that the resources are never exhausted or excessively polluted, which undoubtedly affects the quality of life at the current time [122,123].

Assessing the various economic, social and natural variables thus helps to explain the challenges of sustainable development (or the green economy) and highlights opportunities by linking different action plans. The indicated factors have an impact, in addition to inequality, and the development of the population, shaping the paths of economic development [124,125].

The proposed set of variables (methodology) of the quality of life analysis should make it possible to determine the quality of life measure for any country. Its use allows for quick diagnostics and identification of further trends in changes in the quality of life of residents, and comparative analysis of the quality of life in selected regions, both statically and dynamically. It should be remembered that the active cooperation of state and regional (and local) authorities with the inhabitants is needed to improve the infrastructure and create attractive living conditions [126].

6. Conclusions

The quality of life of the inhabitants is built, among others, by the professional activity of inhabitants, local labour market, entrepreneurship, infrastructure, and the condition of the natural environment. The appropriate potential increases the standard of living, increases production, improves the social situation, and provides greater public safety. The quality of life level is not uniform. Each voivodeship has its endogenous potential (all elements important for the economy of a given area, often of a specific and unique nature, corresponding only to a given local system), which, in conjunction with the exogenous potential and the ability to respond to changes in the environment, may constitute an opportunity for the development of a given area and quality of life.

As a result of the analysis of voivodships in Poland, based on the quality of life measure, four groups were distinguished (according to the value of quartiles). The best voivodeships were included in group I: Pomerania, Masovia, Lower Silesia, and West Pomeranian in 2010 (Masovia, Pomerania, Greater Poland, Lower Silesia, and Lesser Poland in 2020), and in group IV—the weakest: Lodz Province, Podlasie Province, Lubusz Province, and Holy Cross in 2010. (Lodz Province, Podlasie Province, Holy Cross, and Lublin Province in 2020), in the light of the variables and methods of linear ordering included in the study. The synthetic measure of the quality of life ranged from 0.37 (Lublin Province and Holy Cross) to 0.56 (Pomerania) in 2010, and from 0.39 (Lublin Province) to 0.64 (Masovia) in 2020. Quality of life as a category is complex and multifaceted; it is an interdisciplinary concept.

It is shaped by economic activity and working conditions, health, education, free time and social relations, economic and physical security, and quality of the natural environment. The epidemic state declared in Poland in 2020 as a result of the COVID-19 pandemic has affected many areas of our social and professional life. Numerous restrictions in aspects of society's functioning have translated into a deepening of social inequalities, including perceptions of quality of life. COVID-19 also exacerbated inequalities in terms of opportunities, earned income, health care, and social security.

Systematic research on the quality of life should provide the information necessary for the authorities to evaluate and correct the manner in which social policy is conducted. The increase or decrease in synthetic measures should be treated as a way of assessing the effects of the current management of the region. The results obtained may constitute an important source of information for local government authorities on disproportions between units. The procedure described may be applied in other regions (countries). For comparison between regions, it should cover the same variables in the research areas indicated.

The results indicate the directions of new research, which include, among others, comparing the results of order based on a larger number of variables and conducting a dynamic analysis in a specific extended period to learn about the trends of changes. The results also indicate the need to analyse outliers and determine their impact on the situation of the studied area.

The added value of the article is the results of the research focused on the assessment of the quality of life of the inhabitants of voivodships in Poland in the years 2010–2020.

Author Contributions: Conceptualization, G.D., P.D.; methodology, G.D., P.D.; software, G.D., P.D.; validation, G.D., P.D. formal analysis, G.D., P.D.; investigation, G.D., P.D.; resources, G.D., P.D.; data curation, G.D., P.D.; writing—original draft preparation, G.D., P.D.; writing—review and editing, G.D., P.D.; visualization, G.D., P.D.; supervision, G.D., P.D.; project administration, G.D., P.D.; funding acquisition, G.D., P.D. All authors have read and agreed to the published version of the manuscript.

Funding: This research was funded by [Jan Kochanowski University of Kielce] grant number [SUPB.RN.22.006]. The extent of using skills to improve the efficiency of companies in an environment of high capital volatility.

Institutional Review Board Statement: Not applicable.

Informed Consent Statement: Not applicable.

Data Availability Statement: Data sharing not applicable.

Conflicts of Interest: The authors declare no conflict of interest.

References

1. Krugman, P. *The Return of Depression Economics and the Crisis of 2008*; W.W. Norton & Company: New York, NY, USA; London, UK, 2009.
2. Gorzelak, G. *Geografia Polskiego Kryzysu. Kryzys Peryferii czy Peryferia Kryzysu?* RSA—Sekcja Polska: Warszawa, Poland, 2009.
3. Gorzelak, G. Kryzys finansowy w krajach Europy Środkowej i Wschodniej. In *Europejskie Wyzwania dla Polski i jej Regionów*; Tucholska, A., Ed.; Ministerstwo Rozwoju Regionalnego: Warszawa, Poland, 2010.
4. Heshmati, A. *An Empirical Survey of the Ramifications of a Green Economy*; IZA Discussion Papers, No. 8078; Institute for the Study of Labor (IZA): Bonn, Germany, 2014.
5. Binda, J.; Łapińska, H. The 2030 Agenda for Sustainable Development and improvements in quality of life in Poland. *ASEJ Sci. J. Bielsk. Sch. Financ. Law* **2019**, *22*, 13–16. [CrossRef]
6. Kryk, B. Środowiskowe uwarunkowania jakości życia w województwie zachodniopomorskim na tle Polski. *Ekon. Sr.* **2015**, *3*, 170–181.
7. Piasny, J. Poziom i jakość życia ludności oraz źródła i mierniki ich określania. *Ruch Praw. Ekon. Socjol.* **1993**, *2*, 73–92.
8. Drewnowski, J.; Scott, W. *The Level of Living Index*; Report No. 4; UNRISD: Geneva, Switzerland, 1966.
9. Towards a Green Economy: Pathways to Sustainable Development and Poverty Eradication—A Synthesis for Policy Makers 2011 (2012), United Nations Environmental Programm. Available online: www.unep.org/greeneconomy (accessed on 1 March 2022).
10. Kasztelan, A. Zielony wzrost jako nowy kierunek rozwoju gospodarki w warunkach zagrożeń ekologicznych. *Stud. Ekon.* **2015**, *2*, 185–208.
11. Loiseau, E.; Saikku, L.; Antikainen, R.; Droste, N.; Hansjürgens, B.; Pitkänen, K.; Leskinen, P.; Kuikman, P.; Thomsen, M. Green economy and related concepts: An overview. *J. Clean. Prod.* **2016**, *139*, 361–371. [CrossRef]
12. Ryszawska, B. Zielona gospodarka w dokumentach strategicznych Unii Europejskiej. *Ekon. Sr.* **2013**, *3*, 26–37.
13. UN Conference RIO+20, Contribution by the European Union and Its Member States, United Nations Conference on Sustainable Development 2012. Available online: www.unep.org (accessed on 1 March 2022).
14. Venkata Mohan, S.; Nikhil, G.N.; Chiranjeevi, P.; Nagendranatha Reddy, C.; Rohit, M.V.; Kumar, A.N.; Sarkar, O. Modele biorafinerii odpadów w kierunku zrównoważonej biogospodarki o obiegu zamkniętym: Krytyczny przegląd i perspektywy na przyszłość. *Bioresour. Technol.* **2016**, *215*, 2–12. [CrossRef]
15. Venkata Mohan, S.; Modestra, J.A.; Amulya, K.; Butti, S.K.; Velvizhi, G. Biogospodarka o obiegu zamkniętym z bioproduktami z sekwestracji CO_2. *Trendy Biotechnol.* **2016**, *34*.
16. OECD. *Applications of Complexity Science for Public Policy*; OECD: Paris, France, 2009.
17. Sterman, J.D. Sustaining Sustainability: Creating a Systems Science in a Fragmented Academy and Polarized World. Springer Science+Business Media. Available online: http://jsterman.scripts.mit.edu/docs/Sterman%20Sustaining%20Sustainability%2010-2.pdf (accessed on 1 March 2022).
18. Ostasiewicz, W. *Ocena i Analiza Jakości Życia*; Wydaw, A.E., Ed.; Wydawnictwo Akademii Ekonomicznej we Wrocławiu: Wrocław, Poland, 2004.
19. Borys, T.; Rogala, P. *Jakość Życia na Poziomie Lokalnym—Ujęcie Wskaźnikowe*; Program Narodów Zjednoczonych ds. Rozwoju (UNDP) w Polsce: Warszawa, Poland, 2008.
20. Kusterka-Jefmańska, M. Jakość życia a procesy zarządzania rozwojem lokalnym. *Pr. Nauk. Uniw. Ekon. Wrocławiu* **2015**, *391*, 202–210. [CrossRef]
21. Romney, D.M. A Structural Analysis of Health Related Quality of Life Dimensuins. *Hum. Relat.* **2002**, *45*, 165–176. [CrossRef]

22. Enăchescu, V.; Hristache, D.A.; Paicu, C. The interpretative valences of the relationship between sustainable development and the quality of life. *Rev. Appl. Socio-Econ. Res.* **2012**, *4*, 93–96.
23. Van de Kerk, G.; Manuel, A.R. A comprehensive index for a sustainable society: The SSI—The Sustainable Society Index. *Ecol. Econ.* **2008**, *66*, 228–242. [CrossRef]
24. Berbeka, J. Jakość życia ludności w województwie małopolskim: Ocena subiektywna. *Zesz. Nauk. Akad. Ekon. Krakowie* **2005**, *697*, 17–28.
25. Zborowski, A. *Przemiany Struktury Społeczno-Przestrzennej Regionu Miejskiego w Okresie Realnego Socjalizmu i Transformacji Ustrojowej (na Przykładzie Krakowa)*; Instytut Geografii i Gospodarki Przestrzennej UJ: Kraków, Poland, 2005.
26. Sobala-Gwosdz, A. Poziom życia w miastach województwa podkarpackiego a ich położenie, funkcje i pozycja w hierarchii. In *Zróżnicowanie Warunków Życia Ludności w Mieście, Konwersatorium Wiedzy o Mieście*; Jażdżewska, I., Ed.; Wydawnictwo Uniwersytetu Łódzkiego: Łódź, Poland, 2004; pp. 107–120.
27. Gotowska, M.; Jakubczak, J. Zastosowanie wybranych metod do oceny zróżnicowania poziomu życia ludności w Polsce. In *Modele Ustroju Społecnzo-Gospodarczego; Kontrowersje i Dylematy*; Mączynska, E., Ed.; PTE: Warszawa, Poland, 2015.
28. Rutkowski, J. Jak badać jakość życia. *Wiadomości Statystyczne* **1988**, *5*, 42.
29. Kud, K.; Woźniak, M. Percepcja środowiskowych czynników jakości życia na obszarach wiejskich w województwie podkarpackim. *Humanit. Soc. Sci.* **2013**, *18*, 63–74. [CrossRef]
30. Kusterka-Jefmańska, M. Wysoka jakość życia jako cel nadrzędny lokalnych strategii zrównoważonego rozwoju, Zarządzanie publiczne. *Zesz. Nauk. Inst. Spraw. Publicznych Uniw. Jagiellońskiego* **2010**, *12*, 115–123.
31. Kusterka-Jefmańska, M. Pomiar jakości życia na poziomie lokalnym—Wybrane doświadczenia europejskie i doświadczenia polskich samorządów. *Pr. Nauk. Uniw. Ekon. Wrocławiu* **2012**, *264*, 230–239.
32. Štreimikienė, D. Quality of Life and Housing. *Int. J. Inf. Educ. Technol.* **2015**, *5*, 140–145.
33. Papuć, E. Jakość życia—Definicje i sposoby jej ujmowania. *Curr. Probl. Psychiatry* **2011**, *12*, 141–145.
34. Rogala, P. Pomiar subiektywnej jakości życia na poziomie lokalnym—Studium przypadku. *Ekon. Wroc. Econ. Rev.* **2017**, *23*, 35–43. [CrossRef]
35. Borys, T. *Jakość Życia Jako Integrujący Rodzaj Jakości, w: Jakość Życia w Perspektywie Nauk Humanistycznych, Ekonomicznych i Ekologii*; Akademia Ekonomiczna we Wrocławiu: Jelenia Góra, Poland, 2003.
36. D'Amato, D.; Korhonen, J. Integrating the green economy, circular economy and bioeconomy in a strategic sustainability framework. *Ecol. Econ.* **2021**, *188*, 107143. [CrossRef]
37. Kuzior, A.; Arefieva, O.; Poberezhna, Z.; Ihumentsev, O. The Mechanism of Forming the Strategic Potential of an Enterprise in a Circular Economy. *Sustainability* **2022**, *14*, 3258. [CrossRef]
38. Ghisellini, P.; Cialani, C.; Ulgiati, S. A review on circular economy: The expected transition to a balanced interplay of environmental and economic systems. *J. Clean. Prod.* **2016**, *114*, 11–32. [CrossRef]
39. Murray, A.; Skene, K.; Haynes, K. The circular economy: An interdisciplinary exploration of the concept and application in a global context. *J. Bus. Ethics* **2017**, *140*, 369–380. [CrossRef]
40. Strahl, D. Możliwości wykorzystania miar agregatowych do oceny konkurencyjności regionów. *Pr. Nauk. Wrocławiu* **2000**, *860*, 106–120.
41. Szulc, E. *Ekonometryczna Analiza Wielowymiarowych Procesów Gospodarczych*; Wydawnictwo UMK: Toruń, Poland, 2007.
42. Kukuła, K. *Metoda Unitaryzacji Zerowanej*; s. 86. Powtórka; PWN: Warszawa, Poland, 2000.
43. Malina, A. *Wielowymiarowa Analiza Przestrzennego Zróżnicowania Struktury Gospodarki Polski Według Województw*; Wyd. Akademii Ekonomicznej w Krakowie: Kraków, Poalnd, 2004; pp. 96–97.
44. Kukuła, K.; Luty, L. O wyborze metody porządkowania liniowego do oceny gospodarki odpadami w Polsce w ujęciu przestrzennym. *Zesz. Nauk. Szkoły Głównej Gospod. Wiej. Warszawie* **2018**, *18*, 183–192. [CrossRef]
45. Malina, A.; Zeliaś, A. *O Budowie Taksonomicznej Miary Jakości Życia, Taksonomia 4*; Wydawnictwo Akademii Ekonomicznej we Wrocławiu: Wrocław, Polska, 1997.
46. Sobczak, E. Klasyfikacja podregionów Polski ze względu na stopień ochrony środowiska. *Pr. Nauk. Akad. Ekon. Wrocławiu* **2004**, *1009*, 107–119.
47. Czyż, T. Zastosowanie metody czynnikowej w badaniach przestrzenno-ekonomicznych. *Przegląd Geogr.* **1970**, *42*, 467–486.
48. Adamowicz, M.; Janulewicz, P. Wykorzystanie analizy czynnikowej do oceny rozwoju społeczno-gospodarczego w skali lokalnej. *Pr. Nauk. Uniw. Ekon. Wrocławiu* **2013**, *305*, 15–23.
49. Malina, A. Analiza czynnikowa jako metoda klasyfikacji regionów Polski. *Przegląd Stat.* **2006**, *53*, 33–48.
50. Wysocki, F. *Metody Taksonomiczne w Rozpoznawaniu Typów Ekonomicznych Rolnictwa i Obszarów Wiejskich*; Wyd. Uniwersytetu Przyrodniczego w Poznaniu: Poznań, Poalnd, 2010.
51. Łuczak, A.; Wysocki, F. *Wykorzystanie Metod Taksonometrycznych i Analitycznego Procesu Hierarchicznego do Programowania Rozwoju Obszarów Wiejskich*; Wydawnictwo Akademii Rolniczej im. Augusta Cieszkowskiego w Poznaniu: Poznań, Poland, 2005.
52. Grabiński, T. Metody określania charakteru zmiennych w wielowymiarowej analizie porównawczej. *Zesz. Nauk. Akad. Ekon. Krakowie* **1985**, *213*, 35–63.
53. Pluta, W. *Wielowymiarowa Analiza Porównawcza w Badaniach Ekonometrycznych*; PWN: Warszawa, Poland, 1986.
54. Walesiak, M. Problemy selekcji i ważenia zmiennych w zagadnieniu klasyfikacji. *Pr. Nauk. Wroc. Taksonomia* **2005**, *12*, 106–118.
55. Rogowski, W.; Krysiak, N. Zastosowanie metody wzorca do tworzenia klas ryzyka kredytowego. *Bank Kredyt* **1997**, *7–8*, 92–103.

56. Hellwig, Z.; Siedlecka, U.; Siedlecki, U. *Taksonometryczne Modele Zmian Struktury Gospodarczej Polski*; Instytut Rozwoju i Studiów Strategicznych: Warszawa, Poland, 1995; p. 16.
57. Özkan, B.; Özceylan, E.; Kabak, M.; Dikmen, A.U. Evaluation of criteria and COVID-19 patients for intensive care unit admission in the era of pandemic: A multi-criteria decision making approach. *Comput. Methods Programs Biomed.* **2021**, *209*, 106348. [CrossRef]
58. Hellwig, Z. Taksonometria ekonomiczna, jej osiągnięcia, zadania i cele. In *Taksonomia–Teoria i jej Zastosowania*; Pociecha, J., Ed.; Wydawnictwo Akademii Ekonomicznej w Krakowie: Kraków, Poland, 1990.
59. Wysocki, F.; Lira, J. *Statystyka Opisowa*; Wyd. AR: Poznań, Poland, 2005.
60. Młodak, A. *Analiza Taksonomiczna w Statystyce Regionalnej*; Centrum Doradztwa i Informacji Difin: Warszawa, Poland, 2006.
61. Prus, P.; Dziekański, P.; Bogusz, M.; Szczepanek, M. Spatial Differentiation of Agricultural Potential and the Level of Development of Voivodeships in Poland in 2008–2018. *Agriculture* **2021**, *11*, 229. [CrossRef]
62. Dziekanski, P.; Pawlik, A.; Wronska, M.; Karpinska, U. Demographic Potential as the Basis for Spatial Differentiation of the Financial Situation Communes of Eastern Poland in 2009-2018. *Eur. Res. Stud. J.* **2020**, *23*, 872–892. [CrossRef]
63. Dziekański, P.; Prus, P. Financial Diversity and the Development Process: Case study of Rural Communes of Eastern Poland in 2009–2018. *Sustainability* **2020**, *12*, 6446. [CrossRef]
64. Lenormand, M.; Deffuant, G. Generating a Synthetic Population of Individuals in Households: Sample-Free vs Sample-Based Methods. *J. Artif. Soc. Soc. Simul.* **2013**, *6*, 1–12. [CrossRef]
65. Malina, A. Analiza przestrzennego zróżnicowania poziomu rozwoju społeczno-gospodarczego województw Polski w latach 2005–2017. *Nierówności Społeczne Wzrost Gospod.* **2020**, *61*, 138–155. [CrossRef]
66. Hellwig, Z. Zastosowanie metody taksonomicznej do typologicznego podziału krajów ze względu na poziom ich rozwoju oraz zasoby i strukturę wykwalifikowanych kadr. *Przegląd Stat.* **1968**, *4*, 307–326.
67. Wójcik-Leń, J.; Leń, P.; Mika, M.; Kryszk, H.; Kotlarz, P. Studies regarding correct selection of statistical methods for the needs of increasing the efficiency of identification of land for consolidation—A case study in Poland. *Land Use Policy* **2000**, *87*, 104064. [CrossRef]
68. Bąk, A. Zastosowanie metod wielowymiarowej analizy porównawczej do oceny stanu środowiska w województwie dolnośląskim. *Wiad. Stat.* **2018**, *63*, 7–20.
69. Behzadian, M.; Khanmohammadi Otaghsara, S.; Yazdani, M.; Ignatius, J. A state-of the-art survey of TOPSIS applications. *Expert Syst. Appl.* **2012**, *39*, 13051–13069. [CrossRef]
70. Zalewski, W. Zastosowanie metody TOPSIS do oceny kondycji finansowej spółek dystrybucyjnych energii elektrycznej. *Ekon. Zarządzanie* **2012**, *4*, 137–145.
71. Hwang, C.L.; Yoon, K. *Multiple Attribute Decision Making. Methods and Applications*; Springer: Berlin, Germany, 1981.
72. Pietrzak, M.B. The problem of the inclusion of spatial dependence within the TOPSIS Method. *Montenegrin J. Econ.* **2016**, *12*, 69–86. [CrossRef] [PubMed]
73. Jahanshahloo, G.R.; Lotfi, F.H.; Izadikhah, M. An Algorithmic Method to Extend {TOPSIS} for Decision-Making Problems with Interval Data. *Appl. Math. Comput.* **2006**, *2*, 1375–1384.
74. Velasquez, M.; Hester, P.T. An Analysis of Multi-Criteria Decision Making Methods. *Int. J. Oper. Res.* **2013**, *2*, 56–66.
75. Gavurova, B.; Megyesiova, S. Sustainable Health and Wellbeing in the European Union. *Front. Public Health* **2022**, *10*, 851061. [CrossRef]
76. Bieniasz, A.; Gołaś, Z.; Łuczak, A. Zróżnicowanie kondycji finansowej gospodarstw rolnych wyspecjalizowanych w chowie owiec i kóz w krajach Unii Europejskiej. *Rocz. Ekon. Rol. Rozw. Obsz. Wiej.* **2013**, *100*, 168–181.
77. Kozera, A.; Wysocki, F. Problem ustalania współrzędnych obiektów modelowych w metodach porządkowania liniowego obiektów. *Res. Papka Wrocław Univ. Econ.* **2016**, *27*, 131–142.
78. Nowak, E. *Metody Taksonomiczne w Klasyfikacji Obiektów Społeczno—Gospodarczych*; PWE: Warszawa, Poland, 1990.
79. Prosto o Dopasowaniu Prostych, Czyli Analiza Regresji Liniowej w Praktyce. Available online: https://media.statsoft.pl/_old_dnn/downloads/analiza_regresji_liniowej_w_praktyce.pdf (accessed on 1 March 2022).
80. Górecki, T. *Podstawy Statystyki z Przykładami w R*; Wydawnictwo BTC: Legionowo, Poland, 2011.
81. Krzyśko, M. *Wielowymiarowa Analiza Statystyczna*; Wydawnictwo Naukowe UAM: Poznań, Poland, 2000.
82. Welfe, A. *Ekonometria*; Wyd. Naukowe PWN: Warszawa, Poland, 2009.
83. Gruszczyski, M. (Ed.) *Mikroekonometria. Modele i Metody Analizy Danych Indywidualnych*; Wolters Kluwer: Warszawa, Poland, 2010.
84. Conover, W.J.; Iman, R.L. Rank transformations as a bridge between parametric and nonparametric statistics. *Am. Stat.* **1981**, *35*, 124–129. [CrossRef]
85. Kopczewska, K. *Ekonometria i Statystyka Przestrzenna z Wykorzystaniem Programu R Cran (Econometry and Spatial Statistics Using Software R Cran)*; CEDEWU.PL: Warszawa, Poland, 2011.
86. Bivand, R. Autokorelacja przestrzenna a metody analizy statystycznej w geografii. In *Analiza Regresji w Geografii*; Chojnicki, Z., Ed.; PWN: Poznań, Poland, 1980; pp. 23–38.
87. Getis, A. A History of the Concept of Spatial Autocorrelation: A Geographer's Perspective. *Geogr. Anal.* **2008**, *40*, 297–309. [CrossRef]
88. Suchecki, B. *Ekonometria Przestrzenna. Metody i Modele Analizy Danych Przestrzennych*; Wydawnictwo, C.H., Ed.; Beck: Warszawa, Poland, 2010.

89. Sikora, J. Określenie siły i charakteru autokorelacji przestrzennej na podstawie globalnej statystyki I Morana infrastruktury rolniczej Polski południowej i południowo-wschodniej. *Infrastrukt. Ekol. Teren. Wiej.* **2009**, 217–227.
90. Longley, P.; Goodchild, M.F.; Maguire, D.J.; Rhind, D.W. *GIS. Teoria i Praktyka (gis. Theory and Practice)*; Wydawnictwo Naukowe PWN: Warszawa, Poland, 2006.
91. Cliff, A.D.; Ord, J.K. *Spatial Autocorrelation*; Pion: London, UK, 1973.
92. Upton, G.; Fingleton, B. *Spatial Data Analysis by Example*; Wiley: New York, NY, USA, 1985.
93. Statystyka Globalna Morana. Available online: http://manuals.pqstat.pl/przestrzenpl:autocorpl:gmoranpl (accessed on 1 March 2022).
94. Anselin, L. Local Indicators of Spatial Association—LISA. *Geogr. Anal.* **1995**, *27*, 93–115. [CrossRef]
95. Moran, P.A.P. Notes on Continuous Stochastic Phenomena. *Biometrika* **1950**, *37*, 17–23. [CrossRef]
96. Janc, K. Zjawisko autokorelacji przestrzennej na przykładzie statystyki I Morana oraz lokalnych wskaźników zależności przestrzennej (LISA)—Wybrane zagadnienia metodyczne. In *Idee i Praktyczny Uniwersalizm Geografii*; IGiPZ PAN; Komornicki, T., Podgórski, Z., Eds.; Dokumentacja Geograficzna: Warszawa, Poland, 2006; Volume 33, pp. 76–83.
97. Zeliaś, A. *Ekonometria Przestrzenna*; PWE: Warszawa, Poland, 1991.
98. Heffner, K. Typologia gmin wiejskich w Polsce pod kątem widzenia układów osadniczych. In *Lokalne Bariery Rozwoju Obszarów Wiejskich*; Rosner, A., Ed.; Fundacja Programów Pomocy dla Rolnictwa (FAPA): Warszawa, Poland, 2000.
99. Ossowska, L.; Poczta, W. *Endogenne Uwarunkowania Rozwoju Społecznogospodarczego Obszarów Wiejskich Pomorza Środkowego*; Wydawnictwo UP w Poznaniu: Poznań, Poland, 2009.
100. Rosner, A.; Stanny, M. Zróżnicowanie poziomu rozwoju obszarów wiejskich w Polsce według komponentu społecznego. In *Zróżnicowanie Poziomu Rozwoju Społeczno-Gospodarczego Obszarów Wiejskich a Zróżnicowanie Dynamiki Przemian*; Rosner, A., Ed.; Instytut Rozwoju Wsi i Rolnictwa PAN: Warszawa, Poland, 2007.
101. Capello, R. *Regional Economics. Routledge Advanced Texts in Economics and Finance*; Routledge Taylor & Francis Group: London, UK; New York, NY, USA, 2014.
102. Korenik, S. *Rozwój Regionu Ekonomicznego na Przykładzie Dolnego Śląska*; Wydawnictwo AE we Wrocławiu: Wrocław, Poland, 1999; p. 38.
103. Zupan, B.; Pustovrh, A.; Cankar, S.S. Does Decentralized Governance Lead to Less Scientific Output? A Fuzzy Set Analysis of Fiscal Decentralization and Determinants of National Innovation Capacity. *Lex Localis* **2017**, *15*, 647–668. [CrossRef]
104. Churski, P.; Kołsut, B. Potencjał rozwojowy gminy Powidz w okresie postępującej endogenizacji procesów rozwoju. *Rozw. Reg. Polityka Reg.* **2017**, *40*, 35–52.
105. Ostasiewicz, W. *Towards Quality of Life Imroviement*; The Publishing House of the Wrocław University of Economics: Wrocław, Poland, 2006.
106. Hendrick, R. Assessing and measuring the fiscal heath of local governments. *Urban Aff. Rev.* **2004**, *40*, 78–114. [CrossRef]
107. Stanny, M.; Strzelczyk, W. *Kondycja Finansowa Samorządów Lokalnych a Rozwój Społeczno-Gospodarczy Obszarów Wiejskich. Ujęcie Przestrzenne*; Wydawnictwo Naukowe SCHOLAR: Warszawa, Poland, 2018.
108. Groves, S.M.; Valente, M.G. *Evaluating Financial Condition: A Handbook for Local Government*; International City/County Management Association: Washington, DC, USA, 1994.
109. Wang, X.; Dennis, L.; Sen, Y. Measuring Financial Condition: A Study of U.S. States. *Public Budg. Financ.* **2007**, *27*, 1–21. [CrossRef]
110. Rodríguez-Bolívar, M.P.; Navarro-Galera, A.; Alcaide-Muñoz, L.; López-Subirés, M.D. Risk Factors and Drivers of Financial Sustainability in Local Government: An Empirical Study. *Local Gov. Stud.* **2016**, *42*, 29–51. [CrossRef]
111. Murawska, A. Zmiany w poziomie i jakości życia ludności na obszarach wiejskich w Polsce. *J. Agribus. Rural Dev.* **2012**, *3*, 169–180.
112. Heffner, K.; Rosner, A. Spatial variations in economic development of rural areas in Poland. In *Rural Development in the Enlarged European Union*; Zawalińska, K., Ed.; Instytut Rozwoju Wsi i Rolnictwa PAN: Warszawa, Poland, 2005.
113. Kalinowski, S. *Poziom Życia Ludności Wiejskiej o Niepewnych Dochodach*; PWN: Warszawa, Poland, 2015.
114. Gryshova, I.; Kyzym, M.; Khaustova, V.; Korneev, V.; Kramarev, H.V. Assessment of the Industrial Structure and its Influence on Sustainable Economic Development and Quality of Life of the Population of Different World Countries. *Sustainability* **2020**, *12*, 2072. [CrossRef]
115. Tapia-Fonllem, C.; Corral-Verdugo, V.; Fraijo-Sing, B. Sustainable Behavior and Quality of Life. In *Handbook of Environmental Psychology and Quality of Life Research*; International Handbooks of Quality-of-Life; Fleury-Bahi, G., Pol, E., Navarro, O., Eds.; Springer: Berlin/Heidelberg, Germany, 2017.
116. The Green Economy the "Cornerstone" of Sustainable Development. Available online: https://ali-hadadah.medium.com/the-green-economy-the-cornerstone-of-sustainable-development-4f89d1e49c1e (accessed on 1 March 2022).
117. Cusack, C. Sustainable Development and Quality of Life. In *Multidimensional Approach to Quality of Life Issues*; Sinha, B., Ed.; Springer: Singapore, 2019. [CrossRef]
118. Elimam, H. How Green Economy Contributes in Decreasing the Environment Pollution and Misuse of the Limited Resources. *Environ. Pollut.* **2017**, *6*, 10. [CrossRef]
119. Kryk, B. Zróżnicowanie jakości życia w zakresie infrastruktury socjalnej i opieki społecznej na przykładzie powiatów województwa zachodniopomorskiego. *Stud. Pr. Wydziału Nauk. Ekon. Zarządzania* **2014**, *37*, 79–89.
120. Czepkiewicz, M.; Jankowski, P. Analizy przestrzenne w badaniach nad jakością życia w miastach. *Ruch Praw. Ekon. Socjol.* **2015**, *77*, 101–117. [CrossRef]

121. Bąk, I.; Szczecińska, B. Jakość życia w ujęciu obiektywnym w województwach Polski. Analiza porównawcza. *Folia Pomeranae Univ. Technol. Stetinensis. Oeconomica* **2015**, *80*, 15–26.
122. Gazzola, P.; Querci, E. The Connection Between the Quality of Life and Sustainable Ecological Development. *Eur. Sci. J.* **2017**, *13*, 361–375.
123. Dobrowolski, Z.; Drozdowski, G. Does the Net Present Value as a Financial Metric Fit Investment in Green Energy Security? *Energie* **2022**, *15*, 353. [CrossRef]
124. Cibulka, S.; Giljum, S. Towards a Comprehensive Framework of the Relationships between Resource Footprints, Quality of Life, and Economic Development. *Sustainability* **2020**, *12*, 4734. [CrossRef]
125. Drozdowski, G. Economic Calculus Qua an Instrument to Support Sustainable Development under Increasing Risk. *J. Risk Financ. Manag.* **2021**, *14*, 15. [CrossRef]
126. Trunina, I.; Khovrak, I.; Pryakhina, K.; Usanova, O. Life quality as an indicator of sustainable development: International statistical research. *J. Geol. Geogr. Geoecol.* **2021**, *30*, 772–780. [CrossRef]

International Journal of
*Environmental Research
and Public Health*

MDPI

Article

Does the National Fitness Policy Promote National Health?—An Empirical Study from China

Jun-Yi Zheng [1], Li-Xia Luan [1] and Mei Sun [2,*]

[1] School of Physical Education, Huazhong University of Science & Technology, Wuhan 430074, China; jillz@hust.edu.cn (J.-Y.Z.); luanlixia@hust.edu.cn (L.-X.L.)
[2] College of Public Administration, Huazhong University of Science & Technology, Wuhan 430074, China
* Correspondence: d201781019@hust.edu.cn; Tel.:+86-173-2629-7368

Abstract: The influence of national health level in the stability and sustainable development of national society is increasingly prominent. The purpose of this study is to examine whether, when, and how national fitness policies exert influence on national health. Panel data from 2008 to 2017 of 30 Chinese provinces (cities) (except the Tibet autonomous region) were used to systematically reveal the direct impact of national fitness policies on national health and its characteristics in different regions, as well as the interaction mechanisms of human capital and finance health expenditures in public sports. This study found that first, national fitness policies had a positive effect on adult health. Second, sports human capital weakens the health effect of national fitness policies, while public finance health expenditures strengthen this effect. Lastly, the health effect of national fitness policies varies significantly across regions due to uneven regional economic development, and the differences in the effects on different age groups (adults and children) are equally pronounced. This study suggests that national fitness public service system and diverse national fitness plans improving national health level are important for a new dynamic balance and high quality coordinated development in both Chinese economic growth and social welfare.

Keywords: national fitness policy; national health; human capital; public finance health expenditures; regional differences

Citation: Zheng, J.-Y.; Luan, L.-X.; Sun, M. Does the National Fitness Policy Promote National Health?—An Empirical Study from China. *IJERPH* **2022**, *19*, 9191. https://doi.org/10.3390/ijerph19159191

Academic Editors: Jie Chen, Qian Zhou and Ting Zhang

Received: 24 May 2022
Accepted: 25 July 2022
Published: 27 July 2022

1. Introduction

Health is the most significant human capital and is an important means to promote sustainable socioeconomic development [1]. However, in the context of the COVID-19 pandemic and traditional social problems such as aging population and chronic diseases in the information age, public health faces escalating challenges. As a result, governments have incorporated improving national health into Sustainable Development Goals and has gradually gained prominence in global and national health policies. It effectively increases the life expectancy of the population and promote public health well-being and equity [2]. The most common non-medical intervention adopted by governments involves encouraging people to actively participate in physical fitness activities for the purpose of disease prevention and health promotion [3,4].

The Chinese government has always provided great importance to national health and considered it a people-oriented issue. Promoting national fitness activities is an important part of the "National Strategy for a Healthy China". In the fight against the COVID-19 pandemic, the Chinese government has emphasized that "the safety and health of the people should come first" [5], which highlights the importance of national health. At present, China has built a relatively complete medical and health care system, but given the population base, economic base, regional development, and other social problems, the overall public health supply is insufficient, and the health service providers are relatively fewer; hence, the national health needs cannot be guaranteed in an all-round and full life cycle.

Furthermore, the rapid urbanization brought by China's socioeconomic transformation has further intensified the conflicts between public health and social equality.

As a prerequisite for health practice, formulation, promulgation, and implementation of a national fitness policy are positive responses to the public service system of national fitness and macroeconomic regulation of health governance. In addition, it is an important initiative to meet national health needs and promote sustainable national economic development. Research in the area of public services for national health can enable policy-makers to optimize investments, promote policy foresight and rationality, and thereby achieve greater socioeconomic benefits [6]. Although existing studies have noted the positive association of national health promotion with fitness policies, they have not yet clarified their utility value and the pathways and mechanisms of their impact on people's well-being. Most studies have focused on environmental science, health economics, epidemiology, and demography [7,8]. Scholars have paid more attention to the group-differentiated characteristics of environmental pollution [9,10], health investments and returns in the human capital perspective, the mechanisms of different diseases [11,12], and health inequalities arising from social structures and institutions [13]. In fact, for public health services, the above-mentioned studies focus too much on micro-individual and group studies that intermingle environmental, organizational, and group distractions, ignoring the fact that mass sport behavior as a social behavior is more related to the influence of public health inputs and outputs at the national level. In general, positive national health outcomes are more likely to be attributed to health policy factors that create favorable conditions for the optimization of internal mechanisms and the improvement of the external environment. However, there is a lack of literature on this topic, which is not conducive to pioneering academic inquiry and future government practice.

Based on the literature review and analysis, this study concludes that there are still some issues that need further consideration in the study of the influencing factors on national health. First, most previous literature have used a linear framework to determine the direct relationship between environmental pollution, economic development, and public health [14–16]. A few studies have involved quantitative analysis of the causal relationship between public sports policies and health, and even fewer studies have explored the non-linear moderating effects. Second, most of the studies based on Chinese samples focus on the overall analysis of Chinese provinces and autonomous regions or a few key cities, ignoring the rapid but unbalanced economic development among regions; hence, an in-depth exploration of health policy effects among different regions in the overall national sample is necessary. It is important to consider the effects of the national fitness public service system, its policy effectiveness in promoting national health development, and its possible influential mechanisms, especially to increase the research on the differences in the health effects between regions.

This study differs from previous intuitive analyses in that instead of looking into environmental, health, medical, and economic perspectives of national health, it takes a cross-disciplinary approach, such as public administration and physical education. To our knowledge, this is the first study to use cross-provincial (municipal) level panel data in China from 2008–2017, which were validated by constructing an empirical model to deeply reveal the intrinsic mechanisms and paths of national fitness policies affecting national health levels; the resulting problem of equilibrium in the supply of public services for national fitness were discussed. The main contributions of this study are: first, based on the panel data of 30 provinces and autonomous regions (except Tibet) in China in the last decade, the effect of national fitness policy on national health is examined from a macro perspective, which provides a valuable and evidence-based reference for the development of the national strategy of "Healthy China". Second, the empirical analysis using individual fixed-effects models can help overcome the shortcomings of the traditional linear regression method to examine the effects of explanatory variables on the conditional expectations of the explanatory variables, and can reveal the effects of national fitness policies on national health in a comprehensive and stable manner. Third, the relationship between the national fitness policy and national health is discussed by region, making the research findings more consistent with the reality of regional unbalanced development in China. In addition, our study involves the relationship between policy intensity, mortality, human capital, and financial investment, reflecting from the side that national health is not only influenced by the environment but also by other related factors. This helps to better understand the related occurrence mechanism and provide empirical support, and also provides positive inspirational effects and important references for existing theoretical research and practical exploration.

The succeeding sections reviews the evolution of national fitness policies in China and the progress of domestic and international research; introduces the data, variables, and model construction of the study; analyzes and discusses the data results; and highlights the main findings of the study and recommendations for future research. We focus on the determinants of the national fitness policy intensity change that may promote or hinder the national health level and their ways of action.

2. Practical Development and Theoretical Basis of China's National Fitness Policy

2.1. The Evolution of China's National Fitness Policy in Practice

China's national fitness policy is an important institutional guarantee for improving national health and health literacy. The success of the 2008 Beijing Olympic Games shifted the public sports hotspot from competitive sports to national fitness, unveiling the prelude to a new era of comprehensive promotion of national fitness programs. Subsequently, national fitness and "Healthy China" became national strategies, and the government successively issued national fitness policies, such as the Regulations on National Fitness (State Decree No. 560), Guidance on Accelerating National Fitness into Families, and National Fitness Plan (2011–2015), National Fitness Plan (2016–2020), to construct a comprehensive range of basic public sports services. In particular, at the local government level, provinces in China have issued various forms of provincial Regulations on National Fitness (Promotion) in response to national policies, and conducted extensive national fitness sports activities. This study focuses on the national fitness policies in Chinese provinces during the booming period of national fitness since 2008, and analyzes the evolution of the intensity and content of national fitness policies from 2008 to 2017.

This paper mainly focuses on following types of national fitness policies from 2008 to 2017 in Chinese provinces: national fitness regulations which refers to those basic legal documents that set the direction of reform and development, service system and operation mechanism for national fitness, often with a certain strategic and holistic nature, such as sports law, national fitness regulations, regulations on public cultural and sports facilities, etc.; national fitness regulatory documents, which refers to guiding documents involving the design of the national fitness policy process and the implementation of responsibilities, they are the refinement of the national fitness regulations, such as the national fitness implementation plan, the implementation opinions on promoting the high-quality development of national fitness, the guidelines on the operation and maintenance management of national fitness venues and facilities, etc.; relevant national fitness work documents referring to the supporting specific national fitness work guidance, such as the road running sports events and activities safety management guide, notice on further strengthening the supervision and management of outdoor sports events and activities, the mass sports competition and the National Fitness Games competition regulations, etc.; and a small number of administrative license approvals and local government regulations involving national fitness, such as the Provincial Sports Bureau's notice on the main points of the province's mass sports work, etc.

First, we discuss the evolution and development of national fitness policies in Chinese provinces. China's national fitness policy system is a typical centrally led paradigm, with local governments in each province developing national fitness policies and refining rules in response to the central policies, and providing public sports services as well as scientific fitness guidance directly to the public [17]. In the manuscript, initial intensity of national fitness policies in China in 2008 and national fitness policy intensity and policy intensity accumulation of provinces in China in 2017 are national fitness policies in China for a specific year interval. These numbers are authentic since they are based on Chinese practice. In terms of Figure 1, more than half of the other provinces have not yet issued supporting national fitness regulations, so the minimum value is specified as 0. Thus, starting from 0, with 1 as the unit of measurement, each increase of one unit indicates that the true increment of the number of national fitness policies is 1. The largest number of initial policies is in Zhejiang province, with a policy intensity of 7. To facilitate comparison of the effects, the scale interval is therefore set to 0–8, i.e., the true number of initial intensity of national fitness policies in China in 2008 is 0–8. The intensity of national fitness policies in each province in 2008 shows that the introduction of national fitness policies in China is in the initial stage. Only a total of 14 provinces, including Zhejiang, Jiangsu, Anhui, Fujian, and Inner Mongolia, achieved zero breakthrough in national fitness policies. This result indicates that the construction and development of relevant policies in Chinese provinces are obviously insufficient. The 14 provinces that have issued national fitness policies and regulations include both economically developed and coastal provinces in the east such as Shanghai, Zhejiang, and Fujian province, which have a high level of health literacy among residents, as well as underdeveloped regions in the central and western parts of China that have quite ethnic characteristics and sufficient natural resources such as Chongqing, Inner Mongolia, and Yunnan province. In addition, the starting intensity of the national fitness policy in 2008 in economically developed regions such as Beijing, Tianjin and Guangdong and underdeveloped regions such as Liaoning, Qinghai and Gansu were all zero, which did not show full consistency with regional economic development or resource distribution, so their specific mechanisms of action and effects need to be further explored.

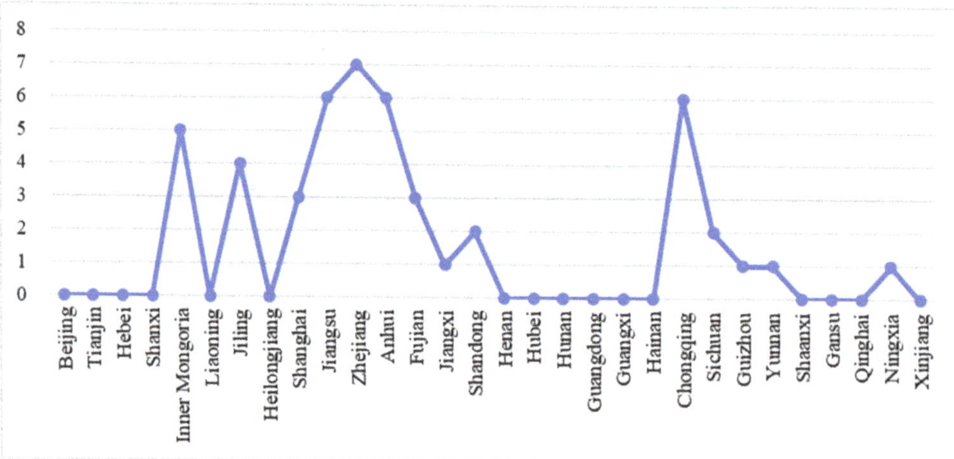

Figure 1. Initial intensity of national fitness policies in China in 2008.

This study plots the national fitness policies in each province in 2017 and the cumulative intensity of national fitness policies from 2008 to 2017 to present the changes in the intensity of national fitness policies in each province of China visually. As shown in Figure 2, there is a significant increase in the intensity of national fitness policies by provinces in China in 2017 compared to 2008. Same as the above, Figure 2 shows that national fitness policy intensity in China in 2017 involves a real policy quantity interval of 0–200, starting from 0, with 200 as the unit of measurement, and each increase of one unit indicates that the real increment of the number of national fitness policies is 200. Among them, there are still some provinces where the specification of the number of national fitness policies tends to be 0, such as Tianjin; Fujian province has the highest number of

200 policies. The real policy quantity interval of policy intensity accumulation of provinces in China from 2008 to 2017 starts from 0, with the lowest in Tianjin, where the number of policy accumulation is 0; the highest in Fujian, where the number of policies is 1084. After several debugging of the scale, it is found that contrast effect is the most obvious in the scale of 200. In addition, with a scale of 200, the number of provinces in the interval above 200 and below 200 is basically the same. Therefore, the true interval for the number of policy intensity accumulation of provinces in China from 2008 to 2017 is 0–1200. Overall, all provincial governments in China have basically achieved the coverage of national fitness policies. The analysis shows that the cumulative value of national fitness policy intensity exceeds 200 in more than half of the provinces, among which Fujian Province and Jiangsu Province even reach more than 800, and the construction of national fitness policies and related regulations has significantly accelerated. In addition, the unbalanced characteristics of national fitness policies among different regions are highlighted. For instance, the cumulative intensity of national fitness policies in Hainan Province in 2017 was 67, while the cumulative intensity of national fitness policies in Fujian Province in 2017 reached 1084. The reason for this is that although both the Hainan and Fujian Provinces are coastal cities, there are significant differences in their population density, economic development level, natural conditions, and resource carrying capacity. The specific mechanism and effect of the influence of different factors on the intensity difference of national fitness policies between regions need to be further explored.

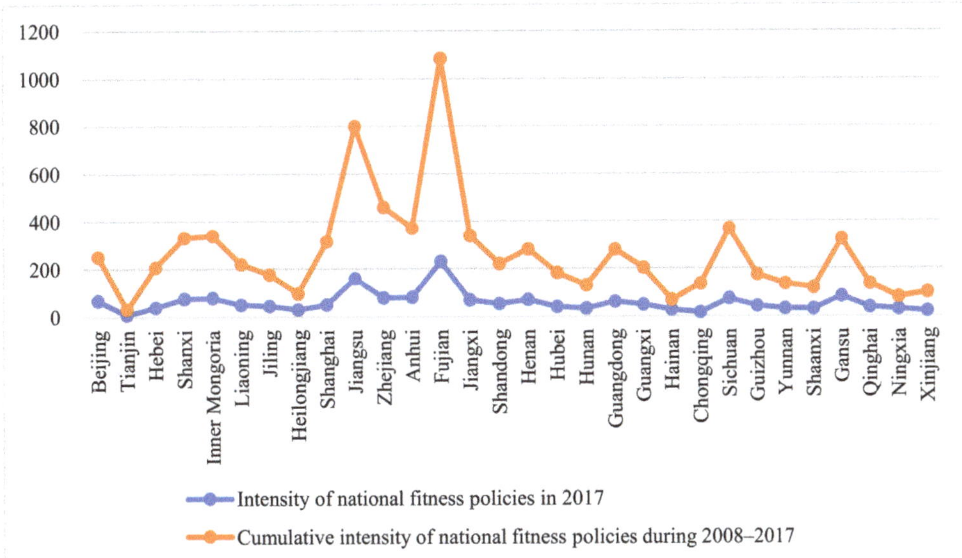

Figure 2. National fitness policy intensity and policy intensity accumulation of provinces in China in 2017.

Second, in terms of policy content, the focus of national fitness policy has shifted from the layout of infrastructure such as venue facilities, organization construction, fitness activities, scientific guidance, and physical fitness monitoring to the development and optimization of the public service system of national fitness. In August 2009, the Regulations on National Fitness was the first special regulation on national fitness in China which clarified the right of citizens to participate in national fitness and its legal status. National fitness became an essential livelihood project for national social development. Subsequently, central and local government policies on various elements of national fitness, such as social sports instructors, sports facility construction, fitness activities, fitness environment, social capital, and supervision services, have been continuously introduced to drive the construction of national fitness public service systems in all aspects [18]. For example, in 2011, the General Administration of Sports issued the Social Sports Instructor Development Plan (2011–2015), which clearly regulates the construction of social sports instructors. In 2015, Jiangsu Province issued the Implementation Opinions on Accelerating the Development of Sports Industry and Promoting Sports Consumption, which mobilizes social capital to strengthen the Jiangsu practice of national fitness, and takes the lead in the country to build a public sports service system demonstration area with clear functions, a sound network, and benefits for all.

Relying on the characteristic advantages of regional resources, several characteristic national fitness projects have emerged in some provinces and localities, such as the Guangdong Greenway Sports Project, Fujian Rainbow Trail Project, the Colorful Yunnan National Fitness Project, and the National Fitness Corridor along the Wei River in Shaanxi. The National Fitness Plan (2016–2020) proposes to deepen sports reform and create a new fashion of national fitness, and the coverage of national fitness policies has gradually achieved precise positioning, developing from universal policies to focus on compensation governance for disadvantaged groups. Considering the differences in health status and resource allocation of people at different levels, the sports rights and participation needs of key groups represented by women, people with disabilities, the elderly, farmers, and ethnic minorities are more urgent [19]. The national fitness policy has changed from a non-equal and biased supply under stratified segmentation to an integrated and coordinated development; the central and local governments have gradually established an institutional balance mechanism for resource allocation in the supply of public services for national fitness by increasing policy efforts, strengthening health promotion, and optimizing resource matching.

This study concludes that the differences in the number of national fitness policies in different regions of China during 2008–2017 mainly stem from the level of regional economic development (based on GDP per capita) and health literacy of its residents. Take the 2017 GDP per capita ranking of Chinese provinces and cities as an example, the top 10 regions in descending order are Beijing, Shanghai, Tianjin, Jiangsu, Zhejiang, Fujian, Guangdong, Shandong, Inner Mongolia, and Chongqing; the bottom 10 in descending order are Sichuan, Qinghai, Jiangxi, Anhui, Shanxi, Heilongjiang, Guangxi, Guizhou, Yunnan, and Gansu. Overall, the number of national fitness policies in economically developed coastal areas (such as Zhejiang, Fujian, etc.) is significantly higher than that in less developed areas (such as Hunan, Hainan, Ningxia, Heilongjiang, etc.). On this basis, with the conditions of economic development, some developed regions (such as Jiangsu, Guangdong, etc.) have made full use of the advantages of regional resources to strengthen the policy inclination of national fitness projects, and are committed to building a sound public service system of national fitness. At the same time, we notice that there are also some special provinces (such as Sichuan, Anhui, Jiangxi, Gansu, etc.) that still maintain relatively high accumulation of national fitness policies despite the lack of economic development level. They are aided by the advantages of locations, ethnic characteristics, natural resources and environmental carrying capacity, and also their attempts to attract talents and investments by improving residents' health environment and optimizing public service. We believe that the future of fitness policy will be a good one. Therefore, we believe that future research needs deep analysis on the specific elements of the differences in the number of national fitness policies in different regions through field research, expert interviews, and panel data to further supplement and improve existing research.

In summary, China's national fitness policies have achieved leapfrog development during the period 2008–2017. National fitness and national health have gradually achieved deep integration, and public sports services have entered an active construction phase. Furthermore, the national fitness policy intensity in Chinese provinces increased significantly during this period, and policy-led national fitness group activities are widely conducted; research has shown that during this period, public participation is high and individual health literacy is improved [20]. However, the analysis and evaluation of the effects of national fitness policies have been mainly based on objective allocation quantities such as sports facilities, venues, and funding scales [17], and these relatively one-sided evaluation approaches have neglected the substantive examination of national health-related impact indicators, especially the regional quantitative analysis under specific socioeconomic and lifestyle conditions.

2.2. Literature Review

Due to the high material living standards and better public awareness of sports and related education systems in developed countries such as Europe and the United States, as well as some medium-sized developed countries, sports are considered an important activity that governments must provide for their citizens, and the public is generally aware of the important role of national fitness in improving their health and quality of life. As early as the 1960s, national fitness became a major means to improving chronic diseases among occupational groups, relieve social medical pressure and maintain social stability in these countries. In 1985, the International Olympic Committee established the Mass Sports Commission to call for a World Congress of Mass Sports. In the following year, the first World Congress of Mass Sports was held in Cologne, Germany, to exchange experiences on the themes of practical and theoretical development of mass sports, stakeholder relations, health and social benefits, and future development, which further set off a worldwide boom in mass sports activities.

Since the 1990s, major western developed countries have promulgated national fitness and mass sports policies, and mass sports have basically achieved comprehensive popularity; the value of sports has been generally recognized and respected by the public in the integration of health values. The U.S. Healthy People Report is considered the beginning of the global Healthy People program, which is officially renamed as the National Fitness Program in 2010. The plan has a clear aim of "changing people's behavior through sports", and includes both universal national health promotion policies and specific prevention and control programs for some diseases (such as arthritis, heart disease, obesity, etc.), involving business and industry, education, health care, public fitness and recreation, urban transportation planning, volunteer organizations, and other fields. This emphasizes the transformation of basic health education, the professionalism of health institutions, and the operability of strategy implementation [21]. The British National Health Service system is characterized by high welfare and wide coverage. The government has introduced the National Health Insurance Act, the National Health Service Act, and the Health and Social Care Act to improve the health of the nation, establishing a unified framework and management system for the National Health Service. It has strengthened front-end preventive health care and community services through decentralization, entrusted purchase, quality control, and service integration, and guided the public to actively strengthen self-health management. The quality of Cuba's Fitness System is among the highest in the world for its community and family centered approach and emphasis on a preventive approach to health. The Cuban model aims to bring health care back to the community through a continuous effort to maintaining quality of service via the collection of health statistics from primary health care providers serving families and communities, and the regular review of health care quality by public health officials. This model of community-based, neighborhood-based, collective social structure for universal health care also provides valuable lessons and references for other countries. Other countries such as Norway, Sweden, Australia, and Japan have established relatively well-developed national fitness programs and mass sports regulations, combining sports activities with their related environment, public health, education, and media campaigns to create feasible conditions to make sports an important part of the public's daily life.

Based on the above management practices, research on trend prediction, group difference analysis, policy effect assessment and influencing factors, and policy process of national health have emerged from the academic community. For example, Porter et al. [22]

systematically assessed the relationship between exercise behaviors (physical activity, sedentary time, screen time) and cardiovascular health in adolescents based on the National Fitness Program guidelines using data from the 2012 NHANES Adolescent Health Survey. Based on public fitness and exercise registry data from the Fitness Registry and the Importance of Exercise National Database (FRIEND Registry), Nevill et al. [23] used multiple regression and anisotropic growth models to derive an updated predictive model of public cardiorespiratory fitness improvement in the U.S. Rolfe [24] developed a simple assessment tool to examine the state of urban public sport investment in regional Queensland, Australia, focusing on the potential economic and social benefits of public sport investment in infrastructure and project delivery. Polyakova and Ramchandani [25] examined regular users' perceptions of the quality of public sports centers in England and analyzed the possible challenges and obstacles of multifunctional public sports facilities in creating sustainable sports participation. Fernández-Martínez et al. [26] examined the satisfaction and loyalty of users of public sports and health services aged 12–16 years in Spain at different stages and the possible impact of different dimensions of service quality on them. Carrad et al. [27] used a multi-case study to explore the process of organizational change and its possible perceived facilitators and potential barriers in the implementation of a health promotion program in New South Wales, Australia, specifying that customized health promotion strategies in different contexts require the involvement of leaders and the organization of practical actions.

In summary, extant research focuses on two aspects: the overall assessment and analysis of the implementation process of national health promotion programs through case studies in different cultural contexts and social relationships, and the examination of the effectiveness of national fitness policy implementation on public health based on micro-individual health indicators. However, the direct health effects of national health policies at the regional level have not been sufficiently discussed. Based on this, this study examines the effects of national fitness programs on national health in China and its possible regional differences using panel data at a macro level. We try to reveal the direct correlation between national fitness policies and national health and explore the potential mechanisms that may influence national fitness policies to promote or inhibit national health.

3. Materials and Methods

3.1. Variable Selection

In order to explore the effect and mechanism of the influence of national fitness policy on national health through regression analysis, we conduct data selection and construct an econometric model. The data are obtained from the China Statistical Yearbook, China Health and Health Statistical Yearbook, China Environmental Yearbook, China Environmental Statistical Yearbook, some statistical yearbooks of Chinese provinces and cities, and the Legal Star database. The sample selection interval is 10 years from 2008 to 2017. Due to the lack of corresponding data in Tibet, the data from this region is excluded.

As far as the explanatory variables are concerned, this study uses adult mortality and child mortality to reflect the national health level. The mortality data in this study are obtained from a study by Zhou et al., (2019) [28], which is published in the prestigious medical journal The Lancet with high reliability, and applies methods in GBD (the Global Burden of Diseases, Injuries, and Risk Factors Study) to systematically analyze mortality, morbidity, and risk factors under the health model of provincial administrative units in China. The core national health surveillance indicators involved in the existing studies are diverse and complex, and no consensus has been reached. Scholars have used average life expectancy (ALE), neonatal mortality rate (NMR), infant mortality rate (IMR), maternal mortality ratio (MMR), and malaria incidence (MI) as important indicators to evaluate the health level of a given region based on regional differences and research purposes [29,30]. Based on the national population and the coverage of the population served, this study follows the study of Sun and Li (2017) [31] and takes population mortality rate to assess the national health level, aiming to explore the overall level of national health and possible regional differences in the local context of China. It has been established that child health and child mortality are important factors of health for all policies, according to Timmons et al., (2012) [4], Guo and Huang (2019) [5], and Zhou and Gao (2021) [18]. In the case of China, existing studies on health outcomes for all have mostly focused on adult health, neglecting to explore child health and child mortality. Currently, various forms of children's physical development centers have emerged in China during the promotion of the national fitness project, which increases the focus on children's health. The realistic development needs are consistent with the selection and setting of variables in this paper. Therefore, in order to analyze the health effects of national fitness policies on different groups, this study follows Zhou et al., (2017)'s [28] definition and further divides mortality rates into adult mortality (aged from 15 to 60) and child mortality (aged under 5). In general, the lower the adult mortality rate and child mortality rate, the higher the level of national health.

In terms of explanatory variables, this study uses the cumulative number of national fitness policies promulgated by each province in China over the years as an indicator of the national fitness policy intensity. The data are obtained from the Legal Star Database, which is the most authoritative, informative, and updated regulatory database in China, covering all kinds of existing laws, administrative regulations, departmental regulations, judicial interpretations, local regulations, rules, normative documents, etc., approved and promulgated by the central government and local governments in China, as well as the provincial governments' official websites. We conduct a comprehensive search of national fitness policies and regulations from 2008 to 2017 by province according to keywords, which are national fitness, (national) fitness program, (mass) sports, public sports, universal health, mass (sports) participation. Considering the cumulative effect of policies [32], it is generally believed that the greater the number of policies introduced within a certain period, the stronger the willingness and governance ability of local governments to treat specific issues [33]; thus, the cumulative effect of policies may have an important impact on the research results [34]. Accordingly, this study takes the cumulative number of policies in a specific period as a measure of the national fitness policy intensity.

Meanwhile, this study also includes two explanatory variables in the model, namely, practitioners and financial expenditures, to explore the key mechanisms of the relationship between national fitness policy intensity and national health. In practice, there are two ways to evaluate the supply efficiency of public goods, one is to measure it by calculating the input-output ratio, and the other is to establish relatively quantifiable indicators, i.e., efficiency criteria [35]. Since the former output is difficult to quantify accurately, most of the existing literature evaluates and analyzes financial expenditures through evaluation indicators. This study draws on Liu's [36] research on government sports investment indicators, and selects personnel and expenditures, i.e., the number of sports practitioners per 10,000 population and finance health expenditures per capita as indicators, which can better reflect the efficiency of public goods supply inputs and equilibrium outputs. Since information on China's finance is not easily accessible, it is difficult to collect independent data on sports finance expenditures. Thus, this study uses culture, sports, and media finance expenditures recorded in statistical yearbooks instead. Since China's reform and opening up, culture and media have become highly market-oriented and are much less dependent on the state funds than sports, so the vast majority of culture, sports, and media expenditures are still invested in sports, and it is reasonable to choose this expenditure to represent the state's financial expenditures in sports.

Finally, as far as the control variables are concerned, nine factors such as social environment, health care, economy, and population, which are closely related to national health, were selected in this study. Specifically, they include: health care expenditures per capita (total health care expenditures/total population), health education institutes/stations (number of public health care institutions, such as infirmaries, nursing stations, etc.), $PM_{2.5}$ (degree of air pollution), park green space per capita (area of urban green space/total population), urban sewage treatment rate (proportion of treated sewage to total sewage discharge), household waste harmless treatment rate (the proportion of harmlessly treated domestic waste to total waste intake), GDP per capita (gross domestic product per capita), urbanization rate (proportion of urban population), and population density (total population/land area).

Data on health care expenditures per capita and health education institutes/stations are obtained from the China Health Statistical Yearbook, data on $PM_{2.5}$, sewage treatment rate, garbage treatment rate, and park green space per capita are obtained from the China Environment Yearbook and the China Environment Statistical Yearbook, and data on per capita GDP, population density, and urbanization rate are obtained from the China Statistical Yearbook. Numerous studies have confirmed the negative impact of environmental problems on national health, and the spillover of air pollution is stronger compared with other environmental factors, and this study uses annual $PM_{2.5}$ emissions to measure the degree of air pollution [31]. Other environmental issues such as water pollution, waste disposal, and greening have also become important challenges that currently threaten people's lives and health and may have a confounding effect on national health [37,38]. Studies have also found that personal economic income as well as health care expenditures could significantly affect changes in national health status [39,40]. Further, in a study on the efficiency of public sports services in 31 provincial governments in China, Li et al. [41] have found that two GDP per capita indicators (sports stadium area per capita and sports expenditure per capita) have a positive effect on the efficiency of public sports services, while population density and educational literacy are significantly related to the services' efficiency. Hence, GDP per capita, population density, and educational literacy also become important factors that may influence national health. Moreover, in the context of intense urbanization and modernization, the health status of urban residents usually faces greater risks and challenges compared to rural residents.

3.2. Descriptive Statistics

The sample data in this study involves 30 provinces, cities, and autonomous regions in China except Tibet, which spans a 10-year period from 2008 to 2017, with a total of 300 samples. Table 1 reports the results of descriptive statistics and expected signs for each variable. The differences between the maximum and minimum values of culture, sports, and media practitioners per 10,000 population and financial expenditures on culture, sports, and media per capita are significant and may be important factors influencing the relationship between policy intensity and national health (adult mortality and child mortality).

3.3. Model Specifications

An econometric model is constructed in this study to analyze the effect of policy intensity on national health. Among them, y_{it} represents the explained variable, i.e., adult mortality or child mortality; $Policy_{it}$ is the main explanatory variable in this study, representing the policy intensity in each province in a specific year; X'_{it} represents the above-mentioned control variables; α_1 and β analysis represent the regression coefficients of the explanatory and control variables, and δ_i and ϵ_{it} represent the error terms.

$$y_{it} = \alpha_0 + \alpha_1 Policy_{it} + X'_{it}\beta + \gamma_t + \delta_i + \epsilon_{it} \quad (1)$$

In order to explore the specific mechanism of the effect of the policy intensity of national fitness on national health, this study constructs an econometric model with cross-sectional terms on the basis of the above econometric model. Among them, $Policy_{it}Employee_{it}$ is the interaction term between policy intensity and practitioners, and $Policy_{it}Expendit_{it}$ is the interaction term between policy intensity and financial expenditures. Through this model, we explore the interaction between the policy intensity on national fitness and the related practitioners and financial expenditures.

$$y_{it} = \alpha_0 + \alpha_1 Policy_{it} + \alpha_2 Policy_{it}Employee_{it} + \alpha_3 Policy_{it}Expendit_{it} + X'_{it}\beta + \gamma_t + \delta_i + \epsilon_{it} \quad (2)$$

Table 1. Descriptive statistics.

Variables	Unit	Obs	Mean	SD	Min	Max
Dependent variables						
Policy intensity	Accumulating policy number	300	3.423224	1.811232	0.000000	6.989335
Independent variables						
Adult mortality	%	300	0.000092	0.000023	0.000038	0.000162
Child mortality	%	300	0.016183	0.007370	0.005000	0.043000
Moderating variables						
Culture, sports, and media practitioners per 10,000 population	person	300	2.367759	0.508242	1.524408	4.471974
Financial expenditures on culture, sports, and media per capita	yuan	300	5.048278	0.622657	3.682046	6.869663
Control variables						
Health care expenditures per capita	yuan	300	6.629206	0.497882	5.071565	7.901217
Health education institutes/stations	institute	300	1.385850	0.892431	0.000000	3.526361
$PM_{2.5}$	ug/m^3	300	3.551505	0.477682	2.186051	4.423648
Park green space per capita	m^2	300	2.449364	0.233631	1.813195	2.984166
Urban sewage treatment rate	%	300	−0.189196	0.166759	−0.919045	−0.022246
Household waste harmless treatment rate	%	300	−0.191159	0.248369	−1.331049	0.000000
GDP per capita	yuan	300	10.541603	0.522224	9.195734	11.832077
Urbanization rate	%	300	−0.629852	0.229329	−1.234088	−0.109815
Population density	person per km^2	300	7.843010	0.440769	6.475433	8.694000

Note: Logarithms are taken for the independent and control variables.

Finally, considering that this study used multi-year panel data, based on the results of the Hausman test, we used an individual fixed-effects model in the regression analysis to effectively eliminate time-invariant factors.

4. Results and Analysis

4.1. Direct Effect of National Fitness Policy Intensity on National Health

Table 2 shows the influence of national fitness policy intensity on adult and child mortality. Among the control variables, health education institutes/stations (r = −0.000002, $p < 0.01$), and green space per capita (r = −0.000009, $p < 0.01$) are significantly negatively correlated with adult mortality, while other control variables are not. There is a significant negative correlation between the national fitness policy intensity and adult mortality (r = −0.000001, $p < 0.01$); the greater the national fitness policy intensity, the lower the adult mortality rate.

Among the control variables, health expenditure per capita (r = −0.002, $p < 0.01$), green space per capita (r = −0.003, $p < 0.001$), sewage treatment rate (r = −0.004, $p < 0.001$), urbanization rate (r = −0.018, $p < 0.001$) are significantly negatively correlated with child mortality. The larger the green space per capita, the higher the sewage treatment rate, the higher the urbanization rate, then the lower the child mortality rate. In addition, there is a significant positive correlation between population density and child mortality (r = 0.002, $p < 0.001$); the higher the population density, the higher the child mortality rate. There is also a significant positive correlation between national fitness policy intensity and child mortality rate (r = 0.0003, $p < 0.01$); the higher the national fitness policy intensity, the higher the child mortality rate.

Table 2. Regression results of equation.

	Adult Mortality			Child Mortality		
	Correlation Coefficient	SE	$p > t$	Correlation Coefficient	SE	$p > t$
Policy intensity	−0.000001	0.000000	0.009	0.000296	0.000105	0.005
Culture, sports, and media practitioners per 10,000 population	−0.000003	0.000003	0.176	0.001446	0.000651	**0.027**
Financial expenditures on culture, sports, and media per capita	−0.000003	0.000002	0.079	−0.000131	0.000428	0.760
Health care expenditures per capita	−0.000003	0.000002	0.112	−0.001719	0.000514	0.001
Health education institutes/stations	−0.000002	0.000001	0.098	−0.000363	0.000273	0.184
$PM_{2.5}$	0.000000	0.000002	0.859	−0.000252	0.000466	0.590
Park green space per capita	−0.000009	0.000003	0.002	−0.003014	0.000703	0.000
Urban sewage treatment rate	−0.000004	0.000003	0.209	−0.003749	0.000727	0.000
Household waste harmless treatment rate	0.000001	0.000002	0.628	0.000148	0.000548	0.788
GDP per capita	0.000000	0.000003	0.948	−0.001182	0.000834	0.158
Urbanization rate	0.000011	0.000008	0.182	−0.017875	0.002115	0.000
Population density	−0.000003	0.000002	0.086	0.001627	0.000400	0.000

4.2. Interactive Effects of Practitioners and Financial Expenditures

As shown in Table 3, there is a significant positive correlation ($p < 0.01$) between the interaction term between national fitness policy intensity and culture, sports, and media workers per 10,000 population and adult mortality. The main effect between policy intensity and adult mortality is significantly negatively correlated ($p < 0.01$), so there is a significant negative moderating effect of culture, sports, and media practitioners per 10,000 population between national fitness policy intensity and adult mortality. The more culture, sports, and media practitioners per 10,000 population, the weaker the relationship between national fitness policy intensity and adult mortality. Furthermore, there is a significant negative correlation ($p < 0.05$) between financial expenditures on culture, sports, and media per capita and adult mortality, i.e., the higher the financial expenditures, the lower the adult mortality. The interaction term between national fitness policy intensity and finance expenditures on culture, sports, and media per capita has a significant negative correlation ($p < 0.01$) with adult mortality. The main effect between policy intensity and adult mortality is significantly negatively correlated ($p < 0.01$), so there is a significant positive moderating effect of finance expenditures on culture, sports, and media per capita between national fitness policy intensity and adult mortality. The higher the finance expenditures on culture, sports, and media per capita, the stronger the relationship between national fitness policy intensity and adult mortality.

As shown in Table 3, there is a significant positive correlation between culture, sports, and media practitioners per 10,000 population and child mortality ($r = 0.001$, $p < 0.05$), but the interaction term between culture, sports, and media practitioners per 10,000 population and policy intensity has no significant correlation with child mortality ($p > 0.1$); the moderating effect of practitioners is not significant. There is a negative correlation between financial expenditures on culture, sports, and media per capita and child mortality, but its correlation is not significant ($p > 0.1$). Moreover, the interaction term between national fitness policy intensity and financial expenditures on culture, sports, and media per capita is also not significantly correlated with child mortality ($p > 0.1$), and the amount of financial expenditures has no significant effect on the relationship between national fitness policy intensity and child mortality.

Table 3. Regression results of equation.

	Adult Mortality			Child Mortality		
	Correlation Coefficient	**SE**	$p > t$	**Correlation Coefficient**	**SE**	$p > t$
Policy intensity	−0.000001	0.000000	0.004	0.000291	0.000118	0.014
Culture, sports, and media practitioners per 10,000 population	−0.000001	0.000003	0.791	0.001539	0.000688	0.026
Financial expenditures on culture, sports, and media per capita	−0.000004	0.000002	0.019	−0.000211	0.000433	0.627
Policy intensity * practitioners (interaction item)	0.000001	0.000000	0.005	0.000003	0.000105	0.977
Policy intensity * financial expenditures (interaction item)	−0.000001	0.000000	0.002	−0.000148	0.000097	0.127
Health care expenditures per capita	−0.000001	0.000002	0.806	−0.001238	0.000569	0.030
Health education institutes/stations	−0.000001	0.000001	0.194	−0.000342	0.000273	0.211
$PM_{2.5}$	−0.000001	0.000002	0.616	−0.000512	0.000481	0.289
Park green space per capita	−0.000008	0.000003	0.003	−0.002650	0.000720	0.000
Urban sewage treatment rate	−0.000004	0.000003	0.158	−0.003801	0.000723	0.000
Household waste harmless treatment rate	0.000000	0.000002	0.994	−0.000193	0.000567	0.734
GDP per capita	0.000000	0.000003	0.889	−0.001278	0.000831	0.125
Urbanization rate	0.000010	0.000009	0.277	−0.020361	0.002468	0.000
Population density	−0.000002	0.000002	0.221	0.001713	0.000403	0.000

Note: Interaction items are policy intensity and practitioners, and policy intensity and financial expenditures. The table has been marked with "*", the same below.

4.3. Comparison of Regional Differences

In this study, we divide the 30 provinces, cities, and autonomous regions of China based on the GDP per capita ranking in 2017, and mark the top 15 as developed regions and the bottom 15 as underdeveloped regions. We first conducted a comparison of the effects of the relationship between national fitness policies intensity and adult mortality, and the results of the analysis are shown in Table 4. In developed regions, there is a significant negative correlation ($p < 0.001$) between national fitness policy intensity and adult mortality, i.e., the higher the policy intensity, the lower the adult mortality in developed regions. On the other hand, in underdeveloped regions, there is no significant correlation ($p > 0.1$) between national fitness policy intensity and adult mortality.

Table 4. Regression results of equation.

	Adult Mortality in Developed Regions			Adult Mortality in Underdeveloped Regions		
	Correlation Coefficient	**SE**	$p > t$	**Correlation Coefficient**	**SE**	$p > t$
Policy intensity	−0.000001	0.000000	0.000	0.000000	0.000001	0.818
Culture, sports, and media practitioners per 10,000 population	−0.000007	0.000003	0.038	−0.000006	0.000003	0.094
Financial expenditures on culture, sports, and media per capita	0.000001	0.000001	0.374	−0.000008	0.000003	0.006
Health care expenditures per capita	0.000000	0.000002	0.929	−0.000003	0.000004	0.396
Health education institutes/stations	0.000001	0.000001	0.170	−0.000007	0.000002	0.001
$PM_{2.5}$	0.000001	0.000002	0.486	0.000000	0.000003	0.934
Park green space per capita	−0.000008	0.000002	0.001	−0.000005	0.000005	0.290
Urban sewage treatment rate	0.000003	0.000004	0.443	−0.000007	0.000004	0.060
Household waste harmless treatment rate	0.000000	0.000002	0.916	−0.000001	0.000003	0.725
GDP per capita	−0.000002	0.000003	0.509	0.000000	0.000005	0.975
Urbanization rate	−0.000006	0.000007	0.405	0.000022	0.000017	0.201
Population density	−0.000009	0.000001	0.000	0.000005	0.000003	0.085

As shown in Table 5, there is a significant negative relationship between culture, sports, and media practitioners per 10,000 population and adult mortality in developed regions ($p < 0.05$), i.e., the more practitioners, the lower the adult mortality in developed regions. The interaction term between national fitness policy intensity and culture, sports, and media practitioners per 10,000 population and adult mortality rate in developed regions is significantly positively correlated ($p < 0.001$). The main effect between policy intensity and adult mortality is significantly negatively correlated ($p < 0.01$), so there is a significant negative moderating effect of culture, sports, and media practitioners per 10,000 population between national fitness policy intensity and adult mortality in developed regions. On the other hand, in underdeveloped regions there is a significant negative correlation between culture, sports, and media practitioners per 10,000 population and adult mortality ($p < 0.05$), i.e., the more practitioners, the lower the adult mortality in underdeveloped regions. However, as there is no correlation between policy intensity and adult mortality, and the interaction term of policy intensity and practitioners and adult mortality in underdeveloped areas is also not established ($p > 0.1$), thus culture, sports, and media practitioners per 10,000 population cannot significantly influence the relationship between them.

Table 5. Regression results of equation.

	Adult Mortality in Developed Regions			Adult Mortality in Underdeveloped Regions		
	Correlation Coefficient	SE	$p > t$	Correlation Coefficient	SE	$p > t$
Policy intensity	−0.000002	0.000000	0.000	0.000000	0.000001	0.914
Culture, sports, and media practitioners per 10,000 population	−0.000003	0.000003	0.026	−0.000005	0.000004	0.019
Financial expenditures on culture, sports, and media per capita	0.000000	0.000001	0.088	−0.000008	0.000003	0.007
Policy intensity * practitioners	0.000001	0.000000	0.000	0.000000	0.000001	0.807
Policy intensity * financial expenditures	−0.000001	0.000000	0.000	0.000000	0.000001	0.804
Health care expenditures per capita	0.000003	0.000002	0.073	−0.000003	0.000004	0.464
Health education institutes/stations	0.000001	0.000001	0.111	−0.000007	0.000002	0.003
$PM_{2.5}$	0.000000	0.000002	0.929	0.000000	0.000003	0.982
Park green space per capita	−0.000008	0.000002	0.001	−0.000005	0.000005	0.301
Urban sewage treatment rate	0.000002	0.000004	0.626	−0.000007	0.000004	0.062
Household waste harmless treatment rate	0.000000	0.000002	0.941	−0.000001	0.000003	0.694
GDP per capita	−0.000004	0.000003	0.212	0.000000	0.000005	0.996
Urbanization rate	−0.000001	0.000008	0.892	0.000022	0.000018	0.226
Population density	−0.000008	0.000001	0.000	0.000005	0.000003	0.085

Table 5 also shows that there is a significant negative relationship between the interaction term of national fitness policy intensity and finance expenditures on culture, sports, and media per capita and adult mortality in developed regions ($p < 0.001$). The main effect between policy intensity and adult mortality is significantly negatively correlated ($p < 0.01$), so there is a significant positive moderating effect of finance expenditures between national fitness policy intensity and adult mortality in developed regions. On the other hand, in underdeveloped regions, there is a significant negative correlation between finance expenditures and adult mortality ($p < 0.01$), i.e., the higher the finance expenditures, the lower the adult mortality in underdeveloped regions. However, since there is no correlation between policy intensity and adult mortality and there is no significant correlation between the interaction term of finance expenditures and policy intensity and adult mortality in underdeveloped areas ($p > 0.1$), finance expenditures do not significantly affect the relationship between policy intensity and adult mortality in underdeveloped regions.

4.4. Heterogeneity Analysis of National Fitness Policy Intensity Affecting National Health

4.4.1. Group Heterogeneity Analysis

The results show that national fitness policy intensity has a differential impact on adult mortality and child mortality. It may be due to the increasing financial expenditure on public sports, as well as the increasing amount of health education institutes/stations and park green space per capita. Chinese government departments at all levels provide great importance to improving the national health level and widely publicize and educate the public, which makes the public pay increased attention to their own health conditions. As a result, their willingness, number, and frequency of participating in sports and fitness activities continue to increase, thus promoting adult health. This can be interpreted as the gradual emergence of the "herd effect" of national fitness, resulting in a decline in adult mortality. However, this health effect has not positively affected children's health. This study argues that this finding is a good clarification that the impact of established national fitness policies on children's health promotion is negligible. It implies that there may be other non-linear pathways of action for this relational process. This may be due to the content of the national fitness policy, which is geared more towards adults and is increasingly focused on middle and old age health issues and less on adolescent and child populations. In addition, increasing population density has resulted in fewer places for a large number of children to participate in physical activity per capita, which somewhat inhibiting child physical development and thus increasing child mortality. On the other hand, although Chinese society is aware of the important role of physical activity participation in children's physical and mental development, the implementation of health promotion policies generally lacks a good social awareness and supportive environment. Especially a passive physical education atmosphere from schools, communities, and families cannot meet children's increasing health development needs. Therefore, it is necessary to analyze the transmutation characteristics and existing dilemmas of children's sports health promotion policies from different perspectives and uses different methods in subsequent studies to explore more efficient paths for children's health. In addition, the practitioner variable does not play a facilitating role in the national fitness policies. This is due to the phenomenon of redundancy caused by the excessive number of sports practitioners, which may reduce administrative efficiency and thus weaken the positive promoting effect of the national fitness policies. However, the financial expenditures on public sports per capita reinforce the positive effect of national fitness policies in promoting adult health. Abundant material resources can provide a solid foundation for the venue facilities, technical guidance, and physical therapy and rehabilitation needed to enhance citizens' physical health.

4.4.2. Regional Heterogeneity Analysis

Heterogeneity in the impact of national fitness policies on national health is also reflected across regions. We first compare the differences in health outcomes across regions in terms of national fitness policy intensity. In terms of direct effects, developed regions had higher levels of adult health, while health outcomes in underdeveloped regions are not significant. This may be because the overall level of economic and social development in underdeveloped regions is relatively low, resulting in an inadequate supply of public services for national fitness. The specific manifestations are: first, the serious lack of sports facilities and fitness venues exposes the problems of insufficient total supply, uneven distribution of supply resources and unreasonable utilization of resources. Second, the lack of professional sports personnel makes it difficult to meet the public's demand for learning special sports skills, which in turn inhibits their enthusiasm for sports participation. Third, due to the limited regional openness and low overall health education level in underdeveloped regions, public awareness of participation in physical fitness activities needs to be enhanced.

Further, the inclusion of practitioners and financial expenditures exacerbates the regional variability in the health effects of national fitness policies. This study argues that although the public service system of national fitness in developed regions is more complete, there may still be a problem of redundant practitioners. The lack of reasonable human resource allocation increases manpower costs, which may result in wasted public sport resources, reduce the positive experience of public participation in physical fitness activities, and lead to limited benefits for policy recipients, which in turn affects adult health. In those regions where economic and social development is relatively lagging behind, public services for national fitness are ranked low in the weighting of government policy-making matters, so sports practitioners play a limited role in the process of national fitness policies influencing national health. It applies to the role of sports financial expenditure in the stage process of national fitness policy affecting national health. The state has introduced targeted special financial support to broaden the coverage of public services for national fitness, which to a certain extent has alleviated the contradiction of balanced supply and demand of diversified and multi-level public demand for physical fitness. However, for regions and cities with lower levels of economic development, government policy-makers and administrative departments are not sufficiently aware of the importance of public services for national fitness to promote national health and sustainable regional economic development, and there is a gap in the allocation of sports resources and other specific measures compared to developed regions. In addition, the rapid but extremely unbalanced regional economic development in China, as well as the lack of clear boundaries in social responsibilities between government, market and individual, have further caused the supply of national fitness resources in different regions to exhibit inequitable characteristics. Some of the less developed regions, especially the central and western regions and rural areas, still have some urgent problems in the provision of public services for national fitness.

4.5. Robust Analysis

In order to ensure the rationality of the model and ensure that the regression is not an accidental observation result of a sample estimation, the robustness test of this study is implemented by replacing dependent variables and independent variables respectively after completing the above tests and analyses. The results are shown in Table 6. First, annual policy intensity is used instead of cumulative policy intensity. The regression results show that the higher the policy intensity per year, the lower the adult mortality. The higher the policy intensity per year, the lower the child mortality. Although not significant, its direction is consistent with the original results for child mortality. The results of the regression analysis obtained after substitution show approximately the same results as above. Second, the health index is used to replace adult mortality and child mortality. Considering the size and demographic differences of the provinces, the health index also has strong explanatory power compared to adult and child mortality. The results of the regression analysis obtained after substitution are still consistent with the above.

Table 6. Regression results of robustness analysis.

	Adult Mortality			Child Mortality			Health Index		
	Correlation Coefficient	SE	$p > t$	Correlation Coefficient	SE	$p > t$	Correlation Coefficient	SE	$p > t$
Policy intensity	−0.000001	0.000000	0.007	0.000151	0.000114	0.187	0.002423	0.000290	0.000
Culture, sports, and media practitioner per 10,000 population	−0.000003	0.000003	0.176	0.001481	0.000659	0.025	−0.003226	0.001799	0.074
Financial expenditures on culture, sports, and media per capita	−0.000003	0.000002	0.058	0.000080	0.000425	0.852	−0.000399	0.001181	0.736
Health care expenditure per capita	−0.000004	0.000002	0.067	−0.001502	0.000513	0.004	0.017375	0.001420	0.000
Health education institutes/stations	−0.000002	0.000001	0.083	−0.000356	0.000276	0.200	−0.000944	0.000753	0.211
$PM_{2.5}$	0.000000	0.000002	0.803	−0.000167	0.000474	0.725	−0.005963	0.001288	0.000
Park green space per capita	−0.000009	0.000003	0.001	−0.002933	0.000710	0.000	0.003719	0.001941	0.056
Urban sewage treatment rate	−0.000003	0.000003	0.253	−0.003800	0.000737	0.000	−0.001509	0.002007	0.453
Household waste harmless treatment rate	0.000001	0.000002	0.623	0.000294	0.000554	0.596	−0.001017	0.001515	0.503
GDP per capita	−0.000001	0.000003	0.849	−0.000743	0.000827	0.370	0.013836	0.002304	0.000
Urbanization rate	0.000012	0.000008	0.137	−0.018021	0.002156	0.000	−0.022906	0.005843	0.000
Population density	−0.000003	0.000002	0.086	0.001619	0.000405	0.000	0.003401	0.001106	0.002

5. Conclusions

This study empirically examines the effect of national fitness policy intensity on population mortality in developed and underdeveloped regions by analyzing panel data on 30 Chinese provinces from 2008–2017 using an individual fixed effects model. Given that government investment in public sports in terms of personnel and funding may have important effects on national health, we take culture, sports, and media practitioner per 10,000 population and financial expenditures on culture, sports, and media per capita as moderating variables to assess the nonlinear relationship between national fitness policy intensity and national health. Based on data fitting and model derivation, the following main findings were obtained: First, the intensity of national fitness policy had a significant negative effect on adult mortality and child mortality, with a stable long-term equilibrium relationship in developed regions and a non-significant effect in underdeveloped regions. Second, culture, sports, and media practitioner per 10,000 population negatively moderates the relationship between national fitness policy intensity and adult mortality, but does not have a significant effect on the relationship between national fitness policy intensity and child mortality. When culture, sports, and media practitioner per 10,000 population increases significantly, the negative effect of national fitness policy intensity on adult mortality will be significantly weakened. Third, financial expenditures on culture, sports, and media per capita can significantly positively affect the relationship between national fitness policy intensity and adult mortality, but not with child mortality. The negative effect of national fitness policy intensity on adult mortality is significantly enhanced when financial expenditures on culture, sports, and media per capita increases. Finally, the relationships between policy intensity, culture, sports, and media practitioner per 10,000 population, financial expenditures on culture, sports, and media per capita, and adult mortality in developed regions are consistent with the national analysis, whereas sports, and media practitioner per 10,000 population, and financial expenditures on culture, sports, and media per capita, in underdeveloped regions do not exert significant effects. We speculate to some extent that there may be other factors that reinforce the effect of policy intensity on adult mortality. It further suggests that health research on public sports policies is still in its infancy in China, and thus there is a huge research space.

6. Discussion

This study comprehensively examines the efficiency of national fitness policies and their impact on national health in 30 Chinese provinces, and provides guidance for optimizing the current human resource allocation and financial investment patterns of China's national fitness public service system, as well as improving national physical fitness and health. These findings have important policy implications. First, the study shows that national fitness policy intensity can significantly reduce population mortality. Provincial governments need to provide great importance to the development of national fitness sports, especially in the economically underdeveloped areas, to increase the policy support and efficiency of national fitness public services according to the content needs of the national fitness programs in the territory. Second, provincial governments should focus on developing sports practitioners to meet the requirements of public sports in the new era, strictly implement and establish a long-term responsibility mechanism, and improve the management efficiency of sports practitioners. It is necessary to avoid the redundancy and confusion of practitioners, which may bring constraints to the implementation of national fitness policies or practical operations. Third, a stable growth mechanism of financial expenditures for national fitness public services can be established. It can provide sufficient financial guarantee for national fitness, and promote scientific, refined and rationalized financial expenditure management of China's national fitness public service system. Finally, the network effect, organizational effect, and scale effect of sports expenditures on national fitness should be examined, based on the impact of financial expenditures on national fitness public services. In-depth interviews should be conducted to explore the possible influence mechanisms of national fitness policy intensity in underdeveloped regions, ensuring that the development of national fitness in underdeveloped regions can also have sufficient public service resources for national fitness.

This study has some limitations that need to be improved and optimized in future studies. First, this study examines the impact of national fitness policy intensity on population mortality, and focuses on the efficiency of national fitness public services. However, only the quantitative dimension of policies is analyzed, and other dimensions such as quality, price, and acceptance of national fitness programs are not addressed. In future studies, we need to deepen the exploration of relevant impact mechanisms. Second, in terms of research sample and data analysis, other methods such as field questionnaires, face-to-face interviews, focus group discussions and small-scale policy experiments, can be introduced in future studies to further verify and expand the feasibility of existing findings. Research data of 30 provinces can also be refined for inter-provincial comparison studies to explore the stability and dispersion of provincial governments' national fitness policy efficiency. Finally, future research can explore the multi-subject utility of national fitness, further determine their transmission path and mechanism that affect public sports investment and national health, and refine indicators for public service investment in national fitness.

Author Contributions: J.-Y.Z.: conceptualization, writing—original draft preparation, software, and validation. L.-X.L.: investigation, resources, data curation, project administration, and funding acquisition. M.S.: writing—review and editing, formal analysis, methodology, visualization, and supervision. All authors have read and agreed to the published version of the manuscript.

Funding: This research was funded by the National Social Science Foundation of China, grant number 20BTY011.

Institutional Review Board Statement: This study used publicly available survey data, and did not involve ethical review and approval.

Informed Consent Statement: Not applicable. This study uses survey data that is publicly available, and does not involve any humans.

Data Availability Statement: Data used in this study are available from corresponding author, upon reasonable request.

Acknowledgments: The authors express sincere gratitude to Ya Sun and Yi-ming Xiao of Huazhong University of Science and Technology, China, for their technical support applied in this study.

Conflicts of Interest: The authors declare no conflict of interest.

References

1. Sen, A.; Ahmed, S.; Peter, F. *Why Health Equity*; Oxford University Press: Oxford, UK, 2004.
2. Reddock, J. Seeking Consensus on Universal Health Coverage Indicators in the Sustainable Development Goals. *J. Health Serv. Res. Policy* **2017**, *22*, 178–182. [CrossRef] [PubMed]
3. Timmons, B.W.; LeBlanc, A.G.; Carson, V.; Connor Gorber, S.C.; Dillman, C.; Janssen, I.; Kho, M.E.; Spence, J.C.; Stearns, J.A.; Tremblay, M.S. Systematic Review of Physical Activity and Health in the Early Years (Aged 0–5 Years). *Appl. Physiol. Nutr. Metab.* **2012**, *37*, 773–792. [CrossRef] [PubMed]
4. Janssen, I.; LeBlanc, A.G. Systematic Review of the Health Benefits of Physical Activity and Fitness in School-aged Children and Youth. *Int. J. Behav. Nutr. Phys. Act.* **2010**, *7*, 40. [CrossRef] [PubMed]
5. Guo, J.; Huang, Z.B. On Major Problems and Countermeasures of Health Governance in China. *Acad. J. Zhongzhou* **2019**, *6*, 68–72.
6. Mushkin, S.J. Health as an Investment. *J. Polit. Econ.* **1962**, *70*, 129–157. [CrossRef]
7. McMonagle, R.; Castellanos, I.; Sutaria Patel, S.S. Advancing Energy Justice as a Climate and Public Health Solution. *World Med. Health Policy* **2021**, *13*, 146–153. [CrossRef]
8. Wang, Y. The Mechanism of "Internet + State Governance" on Public Health Emergencies: Taking the Prevention of COVID-19 as an Example. *Inf. Stud. Theor. Appl.* **2021**, *44*, 64–70.
9. Miao, Y.Q.; Chen, W.J. Air Pollution and Health Needs: An Application of the Grossan Model. *World Econ.* **2010**, *33*, 140–160.
10. Li, Z.; Folmer, H.; Xue, J. To What Extent Does Air Pollution Affect Happiness? The Case of the Jinchuan Mining Area in China. *Ecol. Econ.* **2014**, *99*, 88–99. [CrossRef]
11. McShane, C.J.; Quirk, F.B.; Swinbourne, A. Development and Validation of a Work Stressor Scale for Australian Farming Families. *Aust. J. Rural Health* **2016**, *24*, 238–245. [CrossRef] [PubMed]

12. Albutt, A.; Berzins, K.; Louch, G.; Baker, J. Health Professionals' Perspectives of Safety Issues in Mental Health Services: A Qualitative Study. *Int. J. Ment. Health Nurs.* **2021**, *30*, 798–810. [CrossRef] [PubMed]
13. Cockerham, W.C. *The New Black-Well Companion to Medical Sociology*; Willey-Blackwell: Hoboken, NJ, USA, 2010.
14. Grossman, G.M.; Krueger, A.B. Economic Growth and the Environment. *Q. J. Econ.* **1995**, *110*, 353–377. [CrossRef]
15. Ebenstein, A.; Fan, M.; Greenstone, M.; He, G.; Yin, P.; Zhou, M. Growth, Pollution, and Life Expectancy: China From 1991–2012. *Am. Econ. Rev.* **2015**, *105*, 226–231. [CrossRef]
16. Chen, S.Y.; Chen, D.K. Air Pollution, Government Regulations and High-Quality Economic Development. *Econ. Res.* **2018**, *53*, 20–34.
17. Li, M.; Xu, W.X. Momentum for Governance: Driving Force for Effectively Implementing Sport-Related Public Policy in the Chinese Context: Based on a Review of Policy on the Sports Industry Over the Past 3 Decades. *J. Beijing Sport Univ.* **2021**, *44*, 38–50.
18. Zhou, J.Y.; Cao, H. Research on the Seven Main Logics in the Evolution of the Policy System of National Fitness Program. *J. Guangzhou Sport Univ.* **2021**, *41*, 25–35.
19. Yu, Y.H. Theoretical System and Policy Thinking of the National Fitness and Healthy China. *J. Beijing Sport Univ.* **2019**, *42*, 25–35.
20. Gao, K.T.; Chen, J.Q.; Li, L.H. The Evolution and Trends of China's Sports Public Service Policies Since the Founding of China 70 Years Ago. *J. Phys. Educ.* **2020**, *27*, 17–22.
21. NCPPA. Resources Plans. Available online: http://www.ncppa.org/resources/plans (accessed on 12 May 2010).
22. Porter, A.K.; Matthews, K.J.; Salvo, D.; Kohl, H.W. Associations of Physical Activity, Sedentary Time, and Screen Time with Cardiovascular Fitness in United States Adolescents: Results from the Nhanes National Youth Fitness Survey (NNYFS). *J. Phys. Act. Health* **2017**, *14*, 506–512. [CrossRef] [PubMed]
23. Nevill, A.M.; Myers, J.; Kaminsky, L.A.; Arena, R. Improving Reference Equations for Cardiorespiratory Fitness Using Multiplicative Allometric Rather Than Additive Linear Models: Data from the Fitness Registry and the Importance of Exercise National Database Registry. *Prog. Cardiovasc. Dis.* **2019**, *62*, 515–521. [CrossRef] [PubMed]
24. Rolfe, J. Simple Economic Frameworks to Evaluate Public Investments in Sporting Events in Regional Australia. *Econ. Anal. Policy* **2019**, *63*, 35–43. [CrossRef]
25. Polyakova, O.; Ramchandani, G. Perceived Service Quality Among Regular Users of Gyms in Public Sports Centres in the UK. *Manag. Sport Leis.* **2020**, 1–20. [CrossRef]
26. Fernández-Martínez, A.; Dueñas-Dorado, L.A.; Teva-Villén, M.R.; Nuviala, A. Consolidation, Stages of Change, and Loyalty Among Users of Public Sports and Health Services Aged 12–16. *Int. J. Environ. Res. Public Health* **2021**, *18*, 10113. [CrossRef] [PubMed]
27. Carrad, A.; Parrish, A.M.; Yeatman, H. Building Public Health Capacity Through Organizational Change in the Sport System: A Multiple-Case Study Within Australian Gymnastics. *Int. J. Environ. Res. Public Health* **2021**, *18*, 6726. [CrossRef] [PubMed]
28. Zhou, M.; Wang, H.; Zeng, X.; Yin, P.; Zhu, J.; Chen, W.; Li, X.; Wang, L.; Wang, L.; Liu, Y.; et al. Mortality, Morbidity, and Risk Factors in China and Its Provinces, 1990–2017: A Systematic Analysis for the Global Burden of Disease Study 2017. *Lancet* **2019**, *394*, 1145–1158. [CrossRef]
29. Cheng, M.M.; Yang, M.Z. Impact of Urbanization on the Health of Chinese Residents: An Empirical Study Based on Provincial Panel Data. *China Popul. Resour. Environ.* **2015**, *25*, 89–96.
30. Kaiser, R.; Johnson, N.; Jalloh, M.F.; Dafae, F.; Redd, J.T.; Hersey, S.; Jambai, A. The WHO Global Reference List of 100 Core Health Indicators: The Example of Sierra Leone. *Pan Afr. Med. J.* **2017**, *27*, 246. [CrossRef]
31. Sun, M.; Li, X.W. Air Pollution and Public Health: An Empirical Study Based on Provincial Panel Data. *Popul. J.* **2017**, *39*, 5–13.
32. Yi, H.T.; Liu, Y. Green Economy in China: Regional Variations and Policy Drivers. *Glob. Environ. Chang.* **2015**, *31*, 11–19. [CrossRef]
33. Schmidt, T.S.; Sewerin, S. Measuring the Temporal Dynamics of Policy Mixes—An Empirical Analysis of Renewable Energy Policy Mixes' Balance and Design Features in Nine Countries. *Res. Policy* **2019**, *48*, 103557. [CrossRef]
34. Zeng, Q.Q.; Tong, W.S. How Do Energy Policies Affect the Development of Industrial Green Economy? *China Popul. Resour. Environ.* **2018**, *28*, 20–28.
35. Afonso, A.; Fernandes, S. Assessing and Explaining the Relative Efficiency of Local Government. *J. Socio Econ.* **2008**, *37*, 1946–1979. [CrossRef]
36. Liu, C.H. Research on the Efficiency of Chinese Government Sports Based on DEA-Malmquist. *J. TUS* **2017**, *32*, 291–297.
37. Lu, H.Y.; Qi, Y. Environment Quality, Public Services and National Health: An Analysis Bases on Cross-County Data. *J. Fin. Econ.* **2013**, *39*, 106–118.
38. Allanson, P.; Petrie, D. Longitudinal Methods to Investigate the Role of Health Determinants in the Dynamics of Income-Related Health Inequality. *J. Health Econ.* **2013**, *32*, 922–937. [CrossRef] [PubMed]
39. Qu, W.H.; Yan, Z.J. The Influence of Environment Pollution, Economic Growth and Healthcare Services to Public Health Based on China's Provincial Panel Data. *Chin. J. Manag. Sci.* **2015**, *23*, 166–176.
40. Li, Y.L.; Liu, C.; Qiu, P.; Wang, Z. Efficiency Evaluation and Influencing Factors of Public Sports Service in 31 Provincial Governments in China. *J. TUS* **2018**, *33*, 305–310.
41. Peng, D.S. The Influence of Urbanization on Mass Sports Participation. *Urban Probl.* **2019**, *6*, 94–103.

International Journal of
Environmental Research and Public Health

MDPI

Article

A Novel Block Chain Method for Urban Digitization Governance in Birth Registration Field: A Case Study

Jihui Shi [1], Solomon Kwadwo Nyedu Danquah [2] and Wanhao Dong [3,*]

[1] Department of Management Science, Huzhou University, Huzhou 313000, China; sjh@zjhu.edu.cn
[2] School of Information Engineering, Huzhou University, Huzhou 313000, China; solodanq@gmail.com
[3] School of Public Finance & Administration, Shanghai Lixin University of Accounting and Finance, Shanghai 201209, China
* Correspondence: dongwanhao@lixin.edu.cn

Abstract: Even though digitization is widely recognized as one of the most imperative trends in achieving effective urban governance, digital infrastructure remains far from the global trend in many African countries. This paper proposes a novel, resilient data manipulation architecture model called the Birth Notification Verification Model (BNVM) using blockchain and smart contracts. The proposed solution was evaluated in a real-world use case scenario in Ghana. The model, which is based on the Ten Civil Registration and Vital Statistics (CRVS) Framework, focuses on the initial inputs for birth registration at the birth notification level. The approach presented in this study paves the way for the creation of decentralized, secure, transparent, and automated systems for civil registration. The application of a smart contract architecture that blends a centralized design with an on-chain and off-chain architecture is further supported by this, providing more evidence of its viability. It offers a safe verification framework for the Ghana Birth and Death Registry based on smart contract technology and can guarantee a birth notification as proof of birth certificate registration in accordance with international standards. The findings provide insight into the use of blockchain technology in public registry institutions. Furthermore, exploring its adoption and implementation in Sub-Saharan Africa contributes to the growing field of blockchain technology research and demonstrates how the concept will address long-standing issues with corruption and security in developing countries.

Keywords: civil registration; block chain; digitization governance; smart contract

Citation: Shi, J.; Danquah, S.K.N.; Dong, W. A Novel Block Chain Method for Urban Digitization Governance in Birth Registration Field: A Case Study. *IJERPH* **2022**, *19*, 9309. https://doi.org/10.3390/ijerph19159309

Academic Editors: Jie Chen, Qian Zhou and Ting Zhang

Received: 14 June 2022
Accepted: 24 July 2022
Published: 29 July 2022

1. Introduction

Digitization governance is one of the most significant current discussions in the urban governance field. Especially, with the spreading of Blockchain Technology (BCT), researchers have shown an increased interest in the application of the technology in solving birth registration challenges as a digital infrastructure in developing countries. According to [1], Blockchain technology enables the shared registry concept from distributed systems to be implemented in a variety of application domains, ranging from cryptocurrency to potentially any industrial system requiring decentralized, robust, trusted, and automated decision-making in a multi-stakeholder environment. The characteristics of the technology could lead to improvements in efficiency, transparency and therefore trust [2]. However, along with this growth in blockchain technological innovations, there is increasing concern over data security and the effectiveness of social systems like civil registrations. Many countries in low and middle-income countries are struggling to achieve adequate coverage and quality civil registrations [3]. Around one-third of all births are not registered. This disparity is most apparent and is known as the scandal of invisibility. In many nations, computerization of birth registration systems at all levels has substantially improved the management and maintenance of an effective system, which has helped to alleviate many of the urban governance difficulties involved.

However, there is little advice for urban governance at present as to how to manage existing or emerging technology pressures or guidance on cross-system coordination and interoperability for efficient and effective Civil Registration and Vital Statistics (CRVS) [4]. In their studies, [5] demonstrates that in countries with a continuous commitment to digital governance, substantial improvement in CRVS systems can be made very fast, particularly when modern Information and Communication Technologies (ICT) are used. Nations of this caliber have enormous potential for advancement, but lack proper access to modern technology, mostly due to a lack of infrastructure. Fundamentally, these nations want transparency, security, and accountability in their operations, all of which are cornerstones of BCT [6].

This study provides an exciting opportunity to make an important contribution to the growing area of urban digitization governance research by exploring the BCT adoption and implementation from the perspective of Sub-Sahara African challenges. The study further evaluates the extent and application of smart contract implementation in a real use case scenario. A blockchain-based system would lead to credible social identity, prevent identity fraud and ease the registration processes. From a broader perspective, robust civil registration and vital statistics systems will propel pursuits towards the achievement of sustainable governance by providing security, facilitating inclusion and access to social services.

It does not seem too difficult to register births with Ghana's Birth and Death Registry (BDR) even after many years when only an affidavit and a weighing card are required for registration to be completed. This poses a risk and opens the way for fraud [7]. Cases of unapproved amendments of data at the BDR in Ghana and unapproved fees charged by some officials to provide birth certificates to foreign nationals in Ghana have been reported. It can be assumed that an improvement in the security and integrity of the institution's information system to ensure process verification would curb the current governance challenges.

The main objective of the research is to develop a design model that implements the concepts of BCT to improve processes in birth registration at the Ghana Birth and Death Registry. Specifically, this study aims at achieving the following:

a. To investigate the current birth registration processes at the Ghana BDR.
b. To identify key pain points as well as relevant blockchain features that can be implemented.
c. To propose a new block-chain based solution to tackle identified pain points.
d. To test the application of a smart contract solution in the blockchain architecture.

2. Literature Review

2.1. Background

2.1.1. Civil Registry in Urban Governance

As a basic infrastructure of Urban Governance, civil registration involves the legal notification and recording of individual vital events, including births and deaths, by the government [8]. The office of the civil registrar maintains the records and registers that contain information about vital events, and issues legal certificates on-demand to entitled claimants. This legal data can be used to support further urban planning and digital governance [9]. Birth certificates establish the identity of a person. They also facilitate access to education, employment, economic resources, social protection systems and services, and legal rights and entitlements [10]. In many countries, computerization at all levels of a registration system has greatly facilitated the managing and maintaining of an effective registration system. This is largely due to the increasing use of relatively inexpensive information and communications technology (ICT) that helps to solve many of the issues involved. The use of ICT can also speed up the compilation and availability of vital statistics [11]. A civil registration system encompasses a range of practices involving many institutions. Activities include notifying and registering events and issuing certificates. The 'Ten CRVS Milestones' framework is designed to help CRVS stakeholder's policymakers, managers and development partners better understand how the systems function as a whole, from end to end, by describing the key processes that must be accomplished in any CRVS system to support better governance [3]. Each milestone represents the output or product of several activities that are logically grouped. It also encapsulates a set of requirements that every CRVS system should fulfil [12]. The systematic application of the CRVS Milestone framework exposes neglected aspects in many CRVS systems such as the importance of the anti-epidemic of COVID-19, where the health sector could play a crucial role [13]

2.1.2. Blockchain Technology

The characteristics of blockchain made it an important technology to solve many urban governance problems. Blockchain is a technology that makes the shared registry concept from distributed systems a reality for several application domains, from the cryptocurrency one to potentially any industrial system requiring decentralized, robust, trusted and automated decision-making in a multi-stakeholder situation [1]. Ensuring the trustworthiness of records is a requirement in a range of different contexts where systems of record provide the critical underlying infrastructure necessary to achieve development objectives. This includes organizations responsible for civil registries of births, deaths and marriages, land registries and repositories of financial transactions. Untrustworthy civil registration entries may mean that citizens are unable to prove their identities as a necessary precondition to accessing social protection benefits, or that opportunities for identity fraud emerge that undermine a country's immigration policies and national security [14]. The characteristics of blockchain technology could lead to improvements in efficiency, transparency and therefore trust [2]. It is characterized by the following features:

a. *Peer-to-Peer Network infrastructure*—In a P2P network, there is no centralized server, and each user is a node with server functionality. This layer embodies decentralization and network robustness [15]
b. *Cryptography*—Blockchain employs cryptography for authentication, permission enforcement, integrity verification, and other areas. It makes use of a variety of cryptographic techniques including cryptographic one-way hash functions, Merkle trees and public key (private-public key pairs) [16].
c. *Consensus Mechanism*—In a blockchain network, a consensus is used to prevent dishonest actors from writing potentially invalid information to the database [17].
d. *Timestamp*—The process of 'trusted timestamping' is an established approach for claiming that particular digital information existed at a particular 'point in time' in the past. It is assumed that the time-stamped information is not changeable by anyone in the future. The digital information can be time-stamped by using secure cryptographic methods [18].
e. *Ledger*—The ledger represents a list of bundled (data) transactions in cryptographically linked 'blocks'. Once the transaction data is verified a 'block' will be created. The 'blocks' in the chain are groups of transactions posted sequentially to the ledger by using a cryptographic signature—that is, added to the 'chain' [2].
f. *Validity Rule*—Common set of rules of the network (i.e., what transactions are considered valid, how the ledger gets updated, etc.) [12].

2.1.3. Smart Contracts and Time Stamp-Related Research

Zheng et al. classified significant smart contract applications into six groups based on their generalizations [19]. When the transaction request and verification related criteria and conditions are met, smart contracts allow for the transfer of value. Contracts in the actual world are identical to these contracts. The only difference between them is that they are fully digital, which means that they are comprised of a short programming code that is kept inside a distributed ledger system. For example, The use of BCT in trade finance to prove trade-related documents may minimize loan risk, and smart contracts can govern the execution of inter-organizational processes and openly automate delayed or instalment payments, among other things [20]. Smart contracts offer a wide range of potential applications, spanning from the Internet of Things to the sharing economy, among others.

Deth et al., introduced a free-to-use time-stamping service for online news articles. His proposed system uses secure technologies for saving the results of the time-stamped content for example embedding hashes into the Bitcoin blockchain (which is a cryptographically validated blockchain) [18]. Thus, information is present in a distributed blockchain network, making it impossible to get manipulated. Wouda also in his study, proposes an infrastructure for a blockchain-based application to improve the current way real estate is transacted [2]. In the first place, his proposed model could be deployed as a record-keeping tool (blockchain audit trail). Physical and contractual information, related to a property, is recorded and validated by means of blockchain features during the life cycle of a property (operation phase). Validation of related information is summarized in a framework, which is encrypted (hashed) and stored in the blockchain. Again, Lv et al. also designed and developed a catering safety tracing system to solve catering safety traceability problems [21]. Through blockchain technology, the proposed system can ensure the reliability of traceability information. Using a web application and a hybrid APP, users can manage and query trace information. The SSM (Spring + Spring MVC+ Mybatis) framework which was used in web application development simplifies the development and reduces the deployment difficulty. Furthermore, Elisa et al. proposed an e-government framework that can enforce security and privacy in the public sector by employing blockchain technology [22]. The theoretical and qualitative analysis of security and privacy of the framework showed that cryptography, immutability and the decentralized management and control offered by the blockchain technology can provide the required security and privacy in e-government systems. Their proposed system also has the potential of solving the interoperability issues between government departments which is one of the limitations of existing e-government systems. A growing body of literature has elucidated the enormous benefits that distributed ledger technologies like blockchain bring to the table of technological innovations, such as the high transparency on food traceability, high-level autonomy in school credit bank system etc. It is widely an acceptable phenomenon that it solves several verification challenges and thus can be applied to various domains, including CRVS systems [23]. Furthermore, a more appropriate blockchain design is said to be the hybrid architecture in smart contract implementation [24]. However, it is inadequate in terms of implementation and application in a variety of situations, for instance the CRVS system in Africa. Because of this shortcoming, the conclusion's generalizability is limited, necessitating its application over a wide range of fields. Little attention has been given to the application of blockchain technology in tackling issues related to civil registration and vital statistics. Even so, much of the research has been restricted to Europe and Asia without sufficient attention to its application in the context of Sub-Saharan countries like Ghana. This indicates a need to investigate and implement a blockchain-based solution to address the present verification challenges that exist in Ghana.

3. Methodology

3.1. Research Approach

For the first research question, an explorative approach is used to identify the current business process of the institution. This involved the use of documents and previous research detailing the process of the current CRVS System. De Savigny recommends a set of documents required for such enquiry [3]. Based on that, an entire process mapping and modelling exercise are subsequently done to describe and analyze the current processes as indicated in Table 1. The 'Ten CRVS Milestones' framework proposed by [3,25] as CRVS international standards and best practices is used as a basis for thematic content analysis. Subsequently, pain points in the process maps are identified. The information gathered was utilized to develop the implementation strategy. Its goal was to close the gaps in the present infrastructure and eliminate the pain points associated with verification. A future blockchain design in areas that could be streamlined to improve the performance of the system is proposed. A prototype is then proposed. A live-data prototype is suitable for this research to visualize the BPMN solution. Live-data prototypes are built with HTML, CSS, and JavaScript most of the time. Additionally, they are built on a Local Test Network to illustrate the designed BPMN solution as well as prove its value and motivate actors to implement the solution. The solution orientation can be evaluated by end-users in an early stage and is expected to lead to the improvement of the final design and reduce the chance of critical changes later in the process. The Ethereum platform was selected to develop the decentralized smart contract application for the following factors: It is now considered to be one of the most advanced blockchains available. A solidity programming language is supported, which allows designers to create stateful smart contracts of any complexity using a Turing–complete language.

Table 1. Research Design.

Research Question	Data Source	Data Analysis	End-Product
What does a birth registration process in Ghana look like?	Documents: • Comprehensive assessments reports • Standard operating procedures	• Thematic Analysis • Business Process Mapping and Notation (BPMN)	BPMN Diagram
What pain points occur during birth registration in Ghana?	BPMN Diagram	The Ten (10) CRVS Framework	Proposed BPMN Diagram
What does the proposed blockchain-based solution look like?	Blockchain Literature	Analysis based on the problem statement	Prototype: • Solidity • Node.js • React App • MongoDB • Ganache

3.2. Modeling

3.2.1. Thematic Content Analysis

Grant and Booth argue that, a qualitative systematic review is a method for integrating or comparing the findings from qualitative studies [26]. The explorative approach is used to identify the current business process of the institution, the author independently carried out the thematic content analysis. This involved the review of documents and previous research detailing the process of the current CRVS System including [7,27–29]:

a. Reports from previous comprehensive assessments
b. Strategic documents containing vision and mission statements, as well as aims and goals of the CRVS system
c. Relevant laws and regulations
d. Standard operating procedures and workflow diagrams.

Megel and Heermann explained that secondary qualitative data collected can be analyzed using different theories (e.g., grounded theory, interpretative phenomenological analysis, text interpretation (e.g., thematic coding) etc [30]. All the approaches mentioned here use preconceived categories in the analysis. They are ideographic, means they focus on the individual case without reference to a comparison group. Therefore, from the above-mentioned documents, a thematic content analysis method was employed to analyze the secondary data in juxtaposition to the 'Ten CRVS Milestones' framework.

3.2.2. Business Process Model and Notation (BPMN)

Process mapping can be used to describe, compare and visualize an organization, processes, workflows and functionality of a CRVS system [10]. We used BPMN to describe and analyze the business architecture of the current system for pain point identification and solution proposition.

4. BNVM Model and BPMN Process

4.1. The BNVM Model

Inspired by the Ten CRVS Framework, the model focuses on the initial inputs for birth registration at the birth notification level. A robust architecture that allows birth events to be automatically authenticated prior to birth registration is critical to ensuring a more secured registration system (Figure 1).

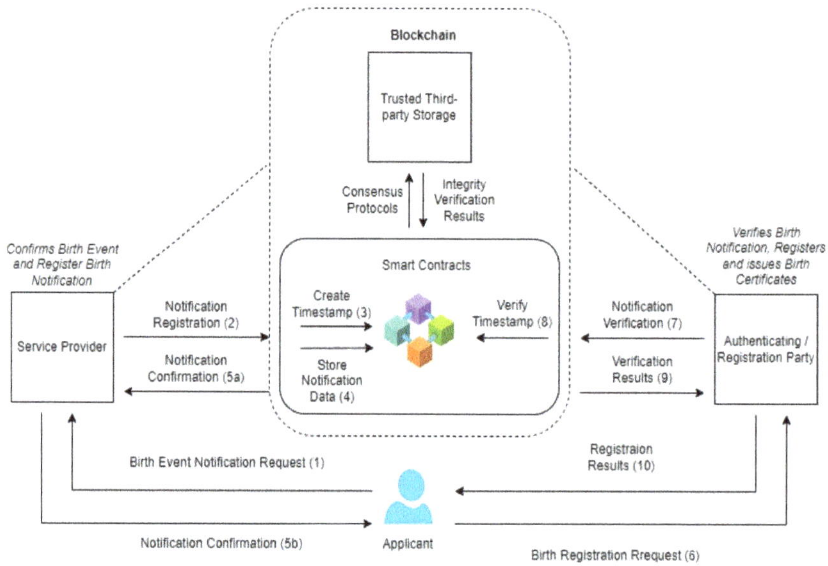

Figure 1. The Birth Notification Verification Model.

Within this model, a birth event is requested by an applicant to the Service Provider (SP) who could be a health professional at a hospital. The service provider registers the notification on the blockchain system that automatically triggers two smart contracts (1) Creation of a Timestamp and (storage of data). After a successful blockchain transaction, the service provider issues a notification confirmation receipt to the applicant for birth registration. Subsequently, a birth registration request is made at the Registration office that represents the authentication or registration party (ARP). They verify the notification receipt on the blockchain with an automatic trigger of the timestamp verification smart contract. After the necessary consensus and verification protocols execution on the blockchain, the verification results are produced for the final internal birth certificate registration processes. Feedback is then given to the applicant. Fundamentally, the blockchain component serves as the verification architecture for the Authenticating and Registration Parties prior to the actual birth registration. Without a successful authentication of the birth notification, the registration party cannot proceed with the issuance of a birth certificate. The model presupposes a dependent relationship between the blockchain, the registration party's systems and the service provider system.

The model functionality is given in Table 2 below:

Table 2. Explain of BNVM Functionality.

Functionality: Using Blockchain and Smart Contract Technology to guarantee data manipulation fraud in BNVM
Input: Birth Event Details **Output:** System Status **Step 1.** Birth Event is declared to a service provider **Step 2.** SP records details on the blockchain system **Step 3.** Event Creation Smart Contract (ECSC) is triggered. **Step 4.** Timestamp Creation Smart Contract (TCSC) is triggered. **Step 5.** ARP inputs timestamp ID upon birth registration request by applicant **Step 6.** Timestamp Verification Smart Contract (TVSC) is triggered. **Step 7.** Verification results is given. **Step 8.** A system update necessary for final registration steps and issuance of birth certificates

Table 2 depicts the algorithm for verifying data according to the proposed model. Firstly, the birth event is declared to a service provider. Secondly, the event details are inputted into the system. After that, ECSC is triggered to store notification data on the blockchain; TSC is further triggered to generate the trusted timestamp for the event. When the ARP inputs the timestamp ID, TVSC is triggered to verify the timestamp on the blockchain. There is an automatic system update after the successful timestamp verification.

4.2. Current Registration BPMN Process

The process is represented visually in the BPMN model. The procedure is divided into three steps: notification, validation/verification, and registration and storage (or archiving). Figure 2 depicts the phases in the process, as well as the activities and stakeholders that are linked with each step in the process.

A parent notifies a healthcare institution of a birth event and, under the current system, obtains a child welfare/weighing card for their kid. When a parent or informant takes their child to the registry to register for new birth, the registration process starts. A child's welfare or weighing card is required, and the Registration officer fills up Form A when the client provides the necessary information. Because this form is only accessible in English, the registration officer will translate any information submitted to the client into another language. The information on the form is then manually put into a local register, which is subsequently scanned, compiled, and sent to the central register in soft copy. As soon as the birth is recorded for free by the local registrar, the newborn is immediately awarded a birth certificate. The term "late registration" refers to the fact that birth is not documented until the kid reaches the age of 1. Late registrations are handled in the same way as early registrations, with a few exceptions. As with early registrations, the registration process begins at the district level and is overseen by the regional office; however, certificates are only issued in Accra, at the central registry/head office, and are then delivered to the location of registration for collection, unlike early registrations. The process is represented visually in the BPMN model. The procedure is divided into three steps: notification, validation/verification, and registration and storage (or archiving).

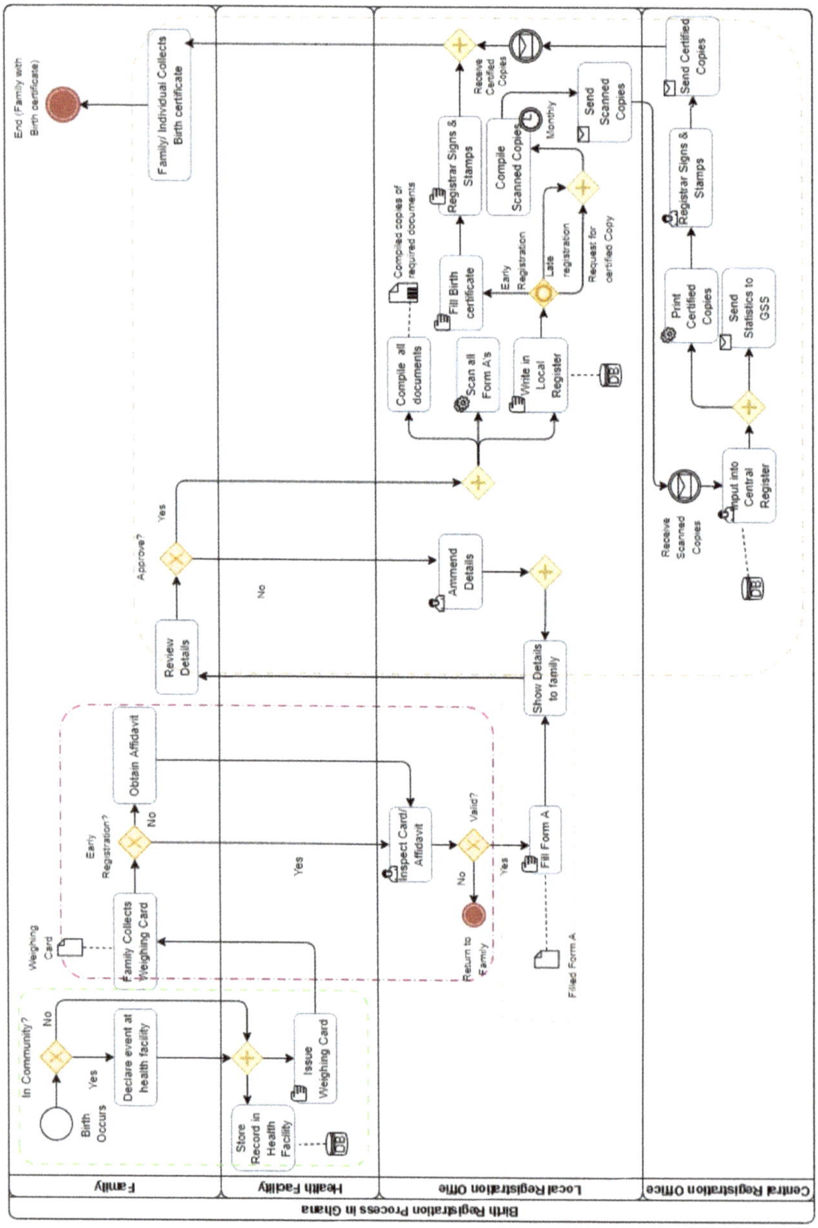

Figure 2. Current Birth Registration Process (BPMN Diagram).

4.2.1. Notifications

Table 3 shows the various activities carried out by actors during the notification stage. During the notification phase, the birth event must be declared at a health centre by the family. At the end of the notification process, a weighing card is issued.

Table 3. Notification Actors and Activities.

Involved Actors	Family, Health Facility
Task in BPMN	1. Declare Birth Event 2. Issue Weighing Card 3. Store Record

4.2.2. Verification/Validation

Table 4 shows the various activities carried out by actors during the verification stage. During the verification and validation phase, the family must collect a welfare or weighing card and an affidavit—if it is late registration. A local registration office would physically inspect these documents and allow you to fill out a Form A registration form.

Table 4. Verification/Validation Actors and Activities.

Involved Actors	Family, Local Registration Office
Task in BPMN	1. Obtain a welfare Card, Weighing Card and or an affidavit 2. Inspect Card

4.2.3. Registration and Storage

Table 5 shows the various activities carried out by actors in the registration phase. For the time being, families must submit a Form A registration form at a local registration office to proceed to the registration and storage stage. After all, parties have confirmed the information, the local office enters it into a local register, prints up a birth certificate, stamps it, and gives it to the family. Note that this is not a certified copy since it only includes the stamp of the local registrar, not the stamp of the national registrar general. Late registration or certified copy registration are handled by the local registrar who gathers and scans all form A documents once a month and sends them to the central registration office (CRO). A certified copy and a certificate for late registrations are only available from the CRO, which is the only body authorized to issue them. The central register is updated with the scanned information from the local offices, and certified copies are made, signed by the registrar general, and sent to the local offices, from where the family collects them. Following that, handwritten data are sent to the Ghana Statistical Service (GSS).

Table 5. Registration Actors and Activities.

Involved Actors	Family, Local Registration Office, Central Registration Office
Task in BPMN	1. Fill Form A 2. Show details to family 3. Review Details 4. Amend details if necessary 5. Compile all documents 6. Scan all Form A's 7. Write in the Local Register 8. Fill out Birth Certificate (Uncertified Copy) 9. Local Registrar Stamps 10. Compile scanned copies 11. Send scanned copies every month 12. Input details in a central register 13. Print certified copies 14. Registrar General Signs and Stamps 15. Send Certified Copies to Family 16. Family Collects Certified Copies at Local Office 17. Send Statistics to GSS

4.3. The Pain Points

The methodology presented above is used to establish and analyze the process's pain points by comparing them to the Ten CRVS Framework. Using this method, much more clarity and depth may be gained than a general explanation of the process's pain points. Additionally, by visualizing the present process, it's simple to understand how the suggested solution fits into it. The framework defines the numerous stages necessary for civil registration. This comparison demonstrates that the whole process is now encountering birth notice and data exchange challenges. The aforementioned pain points are crucial when it comes to confirming and verifying birth events before issuing birth certificates. In the absence of enhanced digitization of birth event notification and data exchange, there is a risk of oversight, as well as unlawful data collection and insertion. Additionally, information processing would be carried out manually, resulting in lengthy delays and inconsistencies throughout the process.

4.3.1. Birth Notifications

As seen in the preceding Figure 3, the system's persistent issues arise from the notification and verification methods. Among them are the following:

a. An undefined method and documentation for birth notification with separate notification information.
b. Inadequate integration of notification and registration procedures results in the lack of a centralized record of weighing cards.
c. As a result, there are no effective means to validate an individual's assertion that a weighing card provided as proof for late or delayed birth registration is authentic and correct.
d. Illegal modification of weighing card data is neither traceable nor verifiable.

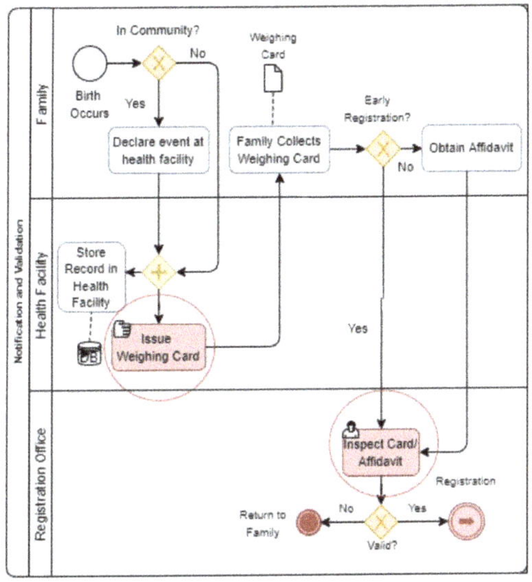

Figure 3. Sharing Pain Point (BPMN Diagram).

Birth notification, as defined by Cobos Muoz et al. is the collection and subsequent transmission of critical information about the fact of birth or death by a designated agent or official of the CRVS system via a CRVS-authorized notification form (paper or electronic), with the information transmitted being sufficient to support eventual registration and certification of the vital event [31].

4.3.2. Data Sharing

Another key problem faced by the system is seen in Figure 4. It was a lack of co-operation with the essential entities for data verification and sharing. Cobos Muoz et al. argues that Coordination across all ministries, agencies and administrative levels is critical to the success of any CRVS system, therefore, plays an extremely vital part in the CRVS Framework [31].

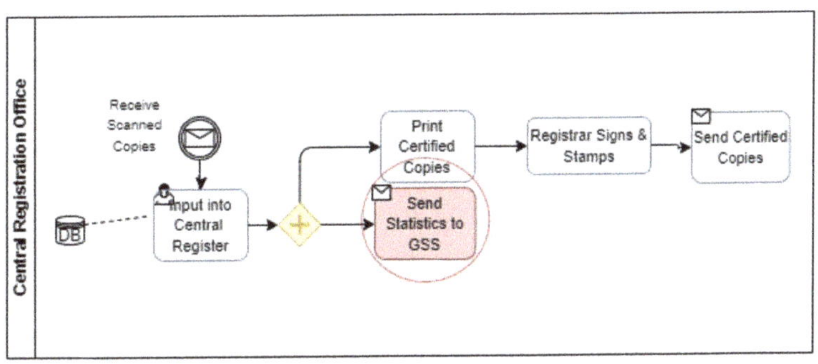

Figure 4. Notification and Verification Pain Points (BPMN Diagram).

5. Proposed Framework

5.1. Proposed Registration Process

According to the highlighted pain points throughout the registration process, the significant issue was the absence of a digital verification method for the registration system's main stakeholders, namely the health care workers responsible for birth notification and the

BDR Official. As a result, Figure 5 proposes the following workflow utilizing conventional BPMN rules.

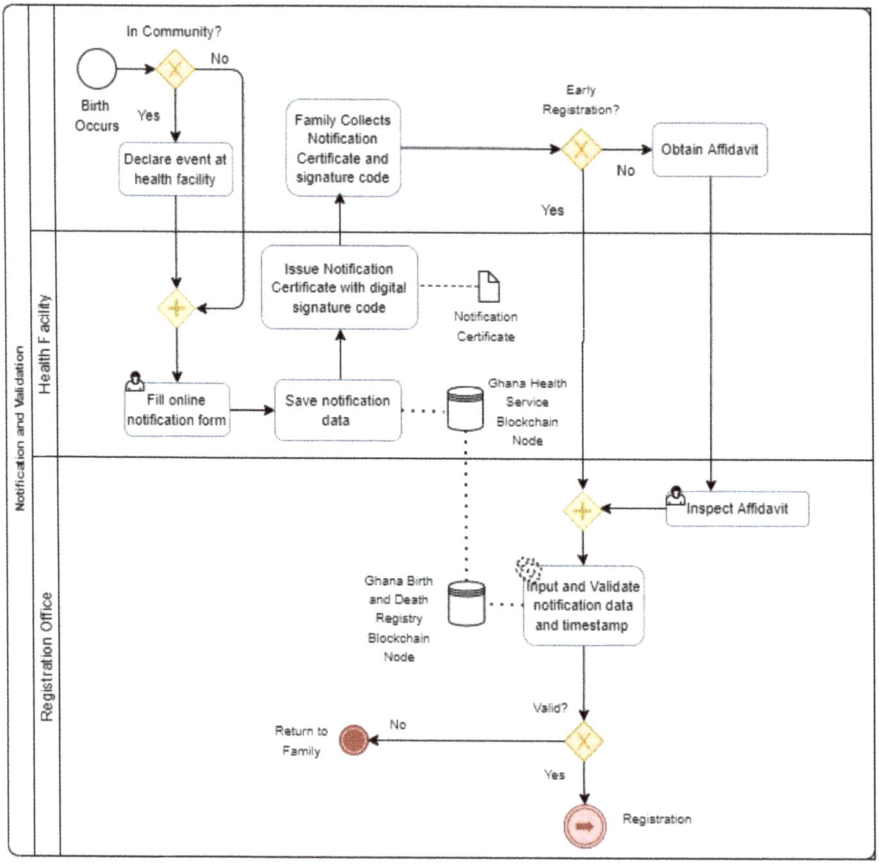

Figure 5. Proposed Notification and Registration Process (BPMN Diagram).

5.1.1. Within Each Actor

a. Family-The family will be responsible for notifying a health facility of the birth event and obtaining a notification certificate with a signature code instead of a weighing card as documentation of the event for birth registration purposes.

b. Health Facility-Certified Health Practitioners will be responsible for completing an online notification form and issuing notification certificates that include all pertinent information about the birth event. Unlike the previous procedure, digital records of the notice will be stored on a central server (GHS node) that acts as a node on a blockchain network.

c. Registration Office—In addition to a valid notification certificate (instead of a weighing card), birth registration will need an affidavit (when necessary). The notification data and signature code are entered, which results in automated verification of the data and timestamp, while background investigations are necessary to confirm the validity of an affidavit.

5.1.2. Between Actors

a. The approach evaluates two distinct scenarios: at-home delivery and birth in a health centre. Due to the lack of health facilities nationally, several births occur at home and so go unrecognized. In such cases, families must get notification certificates from a health provider within the appropriate birth registration time (usually one year).
b. Families are required to attend a local registration centre and provide notification certificates as proof of birth in addition to completing a registration form (Form A). Occasionally, campaigns for birth registration require volunteers from the BDR to travel directly to people's homes, particularly in remote regions, to register them.
c. Local Registration Center and Health Facility- Currently, local registration centres are located in a variety of places, including certain health facilities. In contrast to the existing approach, the BDR will use the blockchain network to share a database among hospitals. This will enable the verification of notification certificates before registration to be automated.

5.2. Architecture Overview

The suggested system is structured in such a way that it addresses the institution's notification and sharing challenges. As depicted in Figure 6, specific notification forms requesting information by international standards should be used instead of weighing cards as proof of registration notice. The Ghana Health Service, the Ghana Statistical Service, and the National Identification Authority are suggested as nodes on a blockchain network. A smart contract will be launched to store and validate timestamps. A secure timestamp of the date and time of birth event notification registration and subsequent change is critical for maintaining the validity of notification records and hence serves as the birth event verification element. A parent initiates birth notification by declaring a birth event at a hospital or health institution. A licensed health professional accesses the proposed web-based platform, logs in using their practitioner's license number or login credentials, and completes an online notification form. Once done, the system will generate a timestamp, save a copy of the data off-chain, generate a PDF of the record with a unique timestamp ID, and connect with the smart contract to add the record as a block.

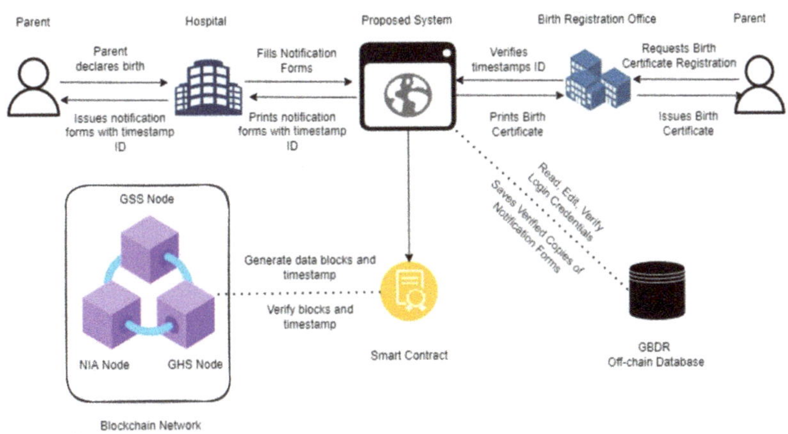

Figure 6. Architecture Overview.

A parent or informant must first seek registration at a local registration facility. A BDR official will be needed to access the site using their given ID/login credentials and complete a birth registration request form that requires just the event notification ID. The smart contract will be invoked in this situation to validate the record and timestamp. After approval, the record is updated to reflect the registration, and a birth certificate may be printed and stamped.

6. The Prototype and Evaluation

6.1. Design of the Architecture

Figure 7 illustrates the technologies utilized to build the solution using the Ethereum Blockchain. The contract is deployed using an Ethereum client linked to a Ganache-based private Ethereum network. The Solidity programming language is used to create the blockchain-based smart contract (SC). The Birth Notification System (BNS)—(a Java program)—makes use of the React App client, which serves as a web interface to the NodeJS server. The architecture was used to evaluate the implementation of a smart contract for verification. NodeJS Server communicates with the Ethereum client using the web3j library and Meta Mask.

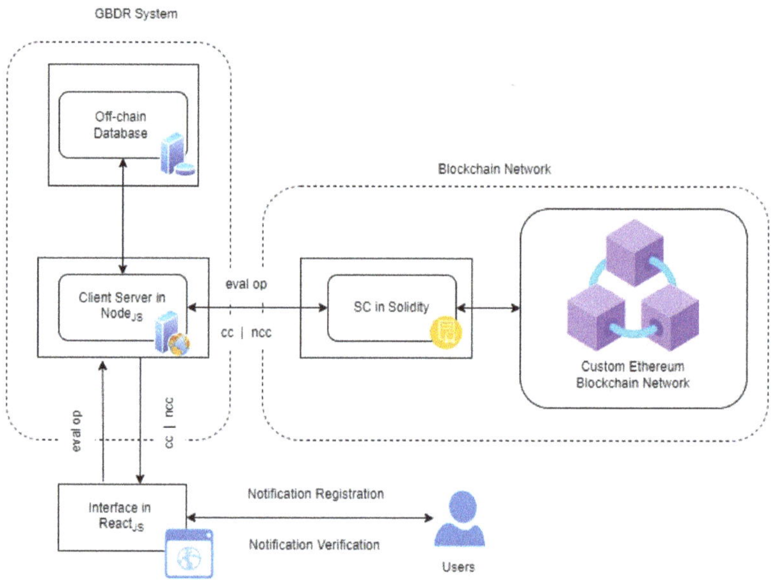

Figure 7. Application Development Components.

6.2. Smart Contract Deployment

6.2.1. Contract Events

To ensure that the contract executes smoothly, it divides the entire process into two states, corresponding to two events:

- When the HO fills a notification form, it is called to save the information on the blockchain network;
- This is executed when the LRO inputs the timestamp ID and clicks on verify. It is called to authenticate the timestamp ID on the blockchain network;

The contract code snippet above will be executed whenever a registration or verification event is triggered from the front end. This is made possible via the Meta Mask chrome plugin, which links the front end and back end Ethereum networks and provides access to information through the web3.js API.

6.2.2. Timestamp Verification

To further address the shortcomings of the process, we present an approach that automatically generates a publicly verifiable, tamper-proof timestamp for each registration record. This code snippet initiates the off-chain database system to allow the information to be saved. Following this initiation, then call for the execution of the smart contract as the variables within the contract. As long as the time values for the creation of the notification form match, a notification of a Successful Registration Pops Up.

6.3. *Evaluation and Analysis*

To further assess the proposed model, a privacy analysis is carried out on the proposed architecture overview, and a comparative analysis is carried out with the traditional registration process.

6.3.1. Privacy Analysis

Participants in the public Blockchain are free to enter and leave, so the on-chain data are visible to everyone. The privacy of the data cannot be protected. For the model proposed in this paper, consortium Blockchain can be used to authenticate all the participants, and the encryption function of the storage contract and the decryption function of the reading contract can be used to protect the data privacy stored in Blockchain. The multichain structure can protect the privacy of the data. At the same time, no one can view others' data without permission.

Based on the Novel BNVM, the proposed architecture used to ensure the privacy of patients or applicants and verification of notification records can strengthen the trust between the GBDR and GHS and reduce the running costs of registration and maintain the security of the whole system. It has the following advantages in terms of privacy and security.

a. Good fault tolerance. The decentralized system does not depend on a single service node and can effectively solve the single-point failure. Multiple service nodes depend on each other to reduce the possibility of errors. Decentralized, autonomous, and distributed nature will bring spontaneous innovation and new ways to coexist with efficiency.
b. Attack protection. The centralized system is easily attacked by a third party or becomes an attacker, while the decentralized system has no centralization. If malicious nodes attack all nodes on the whole system, they will pay a high cost, so the possibility of evil is very low.
c. It was preventing monopoly. Compared with the centralized system, it is difficult to use the information asymmetry to collude with each other in the decentralized system. A decentralized system allows all nodes to participate in the decision-making, ensuring the system's security and transparency. At the same time, it also can audit malicious behaviours.
d. They are improving the trust between participants. The decentralized system has no unified third party, so all participants do not have to bear the risk caused by trusting the third party. The system can automatically facilitate cooperation between the two parties.

6.3.2. Compared with the Current System

The proposed architecture combining blockchain and smart contract technology is different from the current system. Table 6 mainly compares this model with the current system from five aspects, including the data integrity of birth notification records, the data storage persistence of notification and registration records, The difficulty of verification, and compatibility. The proposed model provides a good foundation for the transformation of urban digital governance in future.

Table 6. Proposed architecture compared to the current system.

Index	Current System	Proposed Architecture
Data integrity	It is easy to destroy data integrity because of hardware failure, network failure, logic problems, unexpected catastrophic events, and human activity.	It dramatically reduces external interference and human-made damage. The Blockchain participants cannot arbitrarily destroy the integrity of the data because of the several reproductions existence.
Data storage persistence	The registration data is mainly stored in the server. If the server is damaged, the data is completely lost.	Registration data has multiple backups so data storage has better persistence.
The difficulty of Verification	It is challenging and complex to verify notification data because the information sources are not easily verifiable, so the verification process is not efficient.	It automatically verifies the existence of a birth event using timestamp smart contract, so it saves manpower and time.
Compatibility	Different third-party institutions have different civil registry data requirements. Because of the lack of a sharing system.	The connected blockchain notification system has the potential for further development of dashboard for different nodes to view data in real-time and meaningful ways.

7. Discussion

In light of the blockchain solution deployment lifecycle proposed by [32], this study discusses the solution in three areas: the benefits, deployment and feasibility.

7.1. The Benifits

As introduced in Section 5 and illustrated in Figures 5 and 6. The centralized nature of the proposed system has the potential of facilitating direct interactions between public institutions and citizens. Following the evidence by [32], the append-only way of updating the blocks ensures the irrevocability of a ledger and increases the integrity and verifiability of data. It reduces operational risk and transactional costs as well as increases compliance and trust in government institutions. Its security will ensure proper and efficient use of public funds, decrease the cost of human verification and expedite process coordination.

7.2. The Deployment

The deployment of smart contract is the key to gurantee the data security and privacy. Core requirements for deployment will involve considerations for technologies like cloud computing as demonstrated by [33,34]. The proposed architecture bridges the gap between the Ghana Health Service and the Ghana Births and Deaths Registry by demonstrating how a BNVM enhances the security and integrity of the information system. However, critical issues relating to data privacy and relevant policies to ensure the usage of the system by the necessary parties are paramount to the successful deployment of the solution. As a government system, data is expected to increase vastly over the years. As a result, an implementation should involve the use of side-chains and demand lightweight data to be stored on-chain for verification only. Laws and international standards for civil registration and vital statistics fully support the critical need for data sharing among the cited nodes [10,35,36]. Currently, the government is deploying a blockchain solution for the management of land registries [37]. Therefore, it can be assumed that the blockchain infrastructure experience would be present for the general deployment of the proposed solution.

7.3. The Feasibility

This research provides additional evidence of the applicability of a smart contract architecture that combines an Ethereum-based blockchain platform with a centralized database design [24]. It provides a secure and feasible verification framework for GBDR that is based on blockchain technology and can ensure a birth notification as proof of birth certificate registration per international standards as described by [35].

8. Conclusions

8.1. Theoretical Contribution

A large and growing body of literature has investigated the broad application of blockchain technology to solve different private and e-government challenges of reliability and traceability of data to ensure security [2,6,18,26]. However, little attention has been given to the tackling of issues related to civil registration and vital statistics. In their studies, Somaiman et al. presented and evaluated the performance of a novel hybrid architecture for the implementation of a smart contract [24]. However, much uncertainty still exists about the applicability of the architecture in solving e-government challenges especially in developing countries. This study introduced a resilient blockchain-based design solution, BNVM, for resolving birth registration verification difficulties to help in transforming the digital governance of Ghana. It provides additional evidence of the applicability of a smart contract architecture that combines an Ethereum-based blockchain platform with a centralized database design.

8.2. Practical Contribution

The findings and proposals from this study suggests several courses of action for practitioners. Government database architectures can now move closer to implementing a blockchain based system by offering a safe verification framework for the Ghana Birth and Death Registry based on smart contract technology. Additionally, by connecting civil registration with other government systems like identification and health, it will be possible to improve CRVS quickly and facilitate interoperability across all industries.

8.3. Study Limitations

The limitations of this research are inherent in its scope. The goal of this study is to optimise Ghana's civil registry's birth registration process. Although the proposed blockchain approach addresses the process's current pain points and difficulties, the study's depth is constrained. For instance, the data sources are restricted to published empirical research. An empirical inquiry could be conducted to affirm the validity of the processes discovered. Additionally, research on technical and legal subjects is not included in this study. These issues are left out of scope due to the author's insufficient knowledge of them. As is the case with all emerging technologies, the majority of research on blockchain technology is focused on designing frameworks.

8.4. Suggestions for Further Research

Future researchers could repeat this study by assessing the applicability of the framework in international settings. As the first study to concentrate on civil registry optimization using a blockchain framework, more study is required to test the concept using an application. Additionally, investigations into the legal and technical aspects of implementations could be conducted.

Author Contributions: Conceptualization, J.S., S.K.N.D. and W.D.; methodology, J.S., S.K.N.D.; validation, J.S. and W.D.; formal analysis, J.S., S.K.N.D. and W.D.; resources, J.S., S.K.N.D. and W.D.; writing—original draft preparation, J.S., S.K.N.D. and W.D.; writing—review and editing, J.S. and W.D.; visualization, J.S., S.K.N.D.; supervision, J.S. and W.D.; project administration, J.S. and W.D.; funding acquisition, J.S. and W.D. All authors have read and agreed to the published version of the manuscript.

Funding: The author(s) disclosed receipt of the following financial support for the research, authorship, and/or publication of this article: The first two authors (J.S. and D.S.K.N.) contributed equally to this study. This work was supported by the National Social Science Fund of China (grant number 19BTJ038) and Shanghai Pujiang Program (grant number 18PJC085).

Acknowledgments: This research was supported in part by the National Social Science Fund of China under Grant 19BTJ038 and Shanghai Pujiang Program 18PJC085.

Conflicts of Interest: The authors declared no potential conflict of interest with respect to the research, authorship, and/or publication of this article.

References

1. Belotti, M.; Božić, N.; Pujolle, G.; Secci, S. A Vademecum on Blockchain Technologies: When, Which, and How. *IEEE Commun. Surv. Tutorials* **2019**, *21*, 3796–3838. [CrossRef]
2. Wouda, H.P.H. *Blockchain in Office Building Transactions*; Eindhoven University of Technology: Eindhoven, The Netherlands, 29 March 2019.
3. De Savigny, D.C.M.D. *CRVS Best-Practice and Advocacy: Understanding CRVS Systems: The Importance of Process Mapping*; Bloomberg Philanthropies Data for Health Initiative, The University of Melbourne: Melbourne, Austrilia, 2018.
4. CRVS-ESEC. Current state of crvs. In Proceedings of the CRVS Innovations Conference, Ottawa, ON, Canada, 27–28 February 2018.
5. Mikkelsen, L.; Phillips, D.E.; Abouzahr, C.; Setel, P.W.; De Savigny, D.; Lozano, R.; Lopez, A.D. Counting Births and Deaths 3—A Global Assessment of Civil Registration and Vital Statistics Systems: Monitoring Data Quality and Progress. *Lancet* **2015**, *386*. [CrossRef]
6. Ahishakiye, E.; Wario, R.; Niyonzima, I. Developing Countries and Blockchain Technology: Uganda' s Perspective. *Int. J. Latest Res. Eng. Technol.* **2018**, *4*, 94–99.
7. Ghana Statistical Services; UNICEF; UNDP; UNFPA. *Civil Registration and Vital Statistics System in Ghana*; Ghana Statistical Services: Accra, Ghana, 2015.
8. Xiao, X.; Xie, C. Rational planning and urban governance based on smart cities and big data. *Environ. Technol. Innov.* **2021**, *21*, 101381. [CrossRef]
9. Buttazzoni, A.; Veenhof, M.; Minaker, L. Smart City and High-Tech Urban Interventions Targeting Human Health: An Equity-Focused Systematic Review. *Intern. J. Environ. Res. Public Health* **2020**, *17*, 2325. [CrossRef] [PubMed]
10. Richards, N.; Sorchik, R.; Brolan, C. *CRVS Best Practice and Advocacy: Why the Sustainable Development Goal Agenda Needs Strong Civil Registration and Vital Statistics Systems*; University of Melbourne: Carlton, VIC, Australia, 2018.
11. WHO. *Strengthening Civil Registration and Vital Statistics for Births, Deaths and Causes of Death*; WHO: Geneva, Switzerland, 2013.
12. Muñoz, D.C.; Abouzahr, C.; De Savigny, D. The 'Ten CRVS Milestones' Framework for Understanding Civil Registration and Vital Statistics Systems. *BMJ Glob. Health* **2018**, *3*, e000673. [CrossRef] [PubMed]
13. Liu, J.; Liu, S.; Xu, X.; Zou, Q. Can Digital Transformation Promote the Rapid Recovery of Cities from the COVID-19 Epidemic? An Empirical Analysis from Chinese Cities. *Intern. J. Environ. Res. Public Health* **2022**, *19*, 3567. [CrossRef] [PubMed]
14. Lemieux, V.L. Trusting Records: Is Blockchain Technology the Answer? *Rec. Manag. J.* **2016**, *26*, 110–139. [CrossRef]
15. Liu, Y.; He, D.; Obaidat, M.S.; Kumar, N.; Khan, M.K.; Raymond Choo, K.K. Blockchain-based identity management systems: A review. *J. Netw. Comput. Appl.* **2020**, *166*, 102731. [CrossRef]
16. Hileman, G.; Rauchs, M. Global Blockchain Benchmarking Study. 2017. Available online: https://www.jbs.cam.ac.uk/fileadmin/user_upload/research/centres/alternative-finance/downloads/2017-09-27-ccaf-globalbchain.pdf (accessed on 8 September 2021).
17. Sudhan, A.; Nene, M.J. Employability of blockchain technology in defence applications. In Proceedings of the Proceedings of the International Conference on Intelligent Sustainable Systems ICISS 2017, Palladam, India, 7–8 December 2017; pp. 630–637.
18. Detho, W. Developing a system for securely time-stamping and visualizing the changes made to online news content. *arXiv* **2018**, arXiv:1802.07285.
19. Zheng, Z.; Xie, S.; Dai, H.N.; Chen, W.; Chen, X.; Weng, J.; Imran, M. An Overview on Smart Contracts: Challenges, Advances and Platforms. *Futur. Gener. Comput. Syst.* **2020**, *105*, 475–491. [CrossRef]
20. Xu, X.; Weber, I.; Staples, M.; Xu, X.; Weber, I.; Staples, M. Design Process for Applications on Blockchain. In *Architecture for Blockchain Applications*; Springer: Cham, Switzerland, 2019; pp. 93–111.

21. Lv, T.; Gan, Z.; Wei, P.; Zhao, T. The Design and Implementation of Catering Safety Tracing System Based on Block Chain. In Proceedings of the 2nd International Conference on Safety Produce Informatization, IICSPI, Chongqing, China, 28–30 November 2019; pp. 371–374.
22. Elisa, N.; Yang, L.; Chao, F.; Cao, Y. *A Framework of Blockchain-Based Secure and Privacy-Preserving E-Government System*; Springer—Wireless Networks: Berlin/Heidelberg, Germany, 2018. [CrossRef]
23. Wild, J.; Arnold, M.; Stafford, P. Technology: Banks Seek the Key to Blockchain. Financial Times. Available online: https://www.ft.com/content/eb1f8256-7b4b-11e5-a1fe-567b37f80b64 (accessed on 2 March 2022).
24. Solaiman, E.; Wike, T.; Sfyrakis, I. Implementation and Evaluation of Smart Contracts Using a Hybrid On- and off-Blockchain Architecture. *Concurr. Comput.* **2021**, *33*, e5811. [CrossRef]
25. Suthar, A.B.; Khalifa, A.; Yin, S.; Wenz, K.; Fat, D.M.; Mills, S.L.; Nichols, E.; AbouZahr, C.; Mrkic, S. Evaluation of Approaches to Strengthen Civil Registration and Vital Statistics Systems: A Systematic Review and Synthesis of Policies in 25 Countries. *PLoS Med.* **2019**, *16*, e1002929. [CrossRef] [PubMed]
26. Grant, M.J.; Booth, A. A Typology of Reviews: An Analysis of 14 Review Types and Associated Methodologies. *Health Info. Libr. J.* **2009**, *26*, 91–108. [CrossRef] [PubMed]
27. Abouzahr, C.; De Savigny, D.; Mikkelsen, L.; Setel, P.W.; Lozano, R.; Nichols, E.; Notzon, F.; Lopez, A.D. Civil Registration and Vital Statistics: Progress in the Data Revolution for Counting and Accountability. *Lancet* **2015**, *6736*, 1–13, Series Counting Births and Deaths 1.
28. Peters, B.G.; Mawson, A. *Governance and Policy Coordination—The Case of Birth Registration in Ghana*; WP-2015-05; UN: Accra, Ghana, 2015.
29. UNICEF; GOG. Bottleneck Analysis—Birth Registration in Ghana. 2016, p. 54. Available online: https://www.unicef.org/ghana/media/1746/file/BottleneckAnalysis---BirthRegistrationinGhana.pdf (accessed on 17 July 2021).
30. Megel, M.E.; Heermann, J.A. Methods of Data Collection. *Plast. Surg. Nurs.* **1994**, *14*, 109–110. [CrossRef] [PubMed]
31. Cobos Muñoz, D.; Sant Fruchtman, C.; De Savigny, D. *Intervention: Improving Registration Practices*; Swiss Tropical and Public Health Institute, University of Basel: Basel, Switzerland, 2019; Volumes 1116–1201.
32. Tschorsch, F.; Scheuermann, B. Bitcoin and beyond: A Technical Survey on Decentralized Digital Currencies. *IEEE Commun. Surv. Tutorials* **2016**, *18*, 2084–2123. [CrossRef]
33. Ahram, T.; Sargolzaei, A.; Sargolzaei, S.; Daniels, J.; Amaba, B. Blockchain technology innovations. In Proceedings of the IEEE Technology and Engineering Management Society Conference, TEMSCON 2017, Santa Clara, CA, USA, 8–10 June 2017; pp. 137–141. [CrossRef]
34. Tapas, N.; Merlino, G.; Longo, F.; Puliafito, A. Blockchain-based publicly verifiable cloud storage. In Proceedings of the 2019 IEEE International Conference on Smart Computing, SMARTCOMP 2019, Washington, DC, USA, 12–15 June 2019; pp. 381–386. [CrossRef]
35. World Economic Forum. *Redesigning Trust: Blockchain Deployment Toolkit—Supply Chain Focus*; World Economic Forum: Colony, Switzerland, 2020; p. 244.
36. United Nations. *Handbook on Training in Civil Registration and Vital Statistics Systems*; United Nations: New York, NY, USA, 2002; p. 281.
37. Schmidt, K.; Sandner, P. *Solving Challenges in Developing Countries with Blockchain Technology*; FSBC Works Paper; FSBC: Rancho Cordova, CA, USA, 2017; pp. 1–22.

International Journal of
Environmental Research and Public Health

MDPI

Article

Career Development, Institutional Factors, Social Factors and Urban Young Returnees' Happiness in the Context of Healthy China

Feiwei Shen [1], Jing Zou [2,3,4,*], Xianhong Huang [5], Cong Wang [6] and Mingjie Zhao [4]

1 College of Public Administration, Hangzhou Normal University, Hangzhou 311121, China; zjsfw.hi@163.com
2 School of Public Affairs, Zhejiang University, Hangzhou 310058, China
3 Hangzhou International Urbanology Research Center and Zhejiang Urban Governance Studies Center, Hangzhou 311121, China
4 School of Finance, Zhejiang University of Finance and Economics, Hangzhou 310018, China; zhaomj00@163.com
5 Department of Health Policy and Management, School of Public Health, Hangzhou Normal University, Hangzhou 311121, China; hxh974291@163.com
6 School of Public Health, Hangzhou Normal University, Hangzhou 311121, China; wang11172021@163.com
* Correspondence: glss2008@163.com

Abstract: In the context of the Healthy China 2030 Plan, the importance of the happiness of urban young returnees should not be underestimated. Based on a large-scale social survey of social practices in China, this paper applies a hierarchical linear regression model (HLM) and a structural equation model (SEM) to investigate the determinants of urban young returnees' happiness. The results show that the happiness of urban young returnees in China is not only influenced by their socio-demographic characteristics, such as age and education, but mainly by their occupational development, institutional factors (especially the employment and entrepreneurship policy system) and social factors (physical environment and urban rural relationship), which are different from those of ordinary residents. Further study shows that occupational development indirectly affects the happiness of urban young returnees through relationship adaptation, collective adaptation and material adaptation, the indirect effects accounts for 42.18%, 21.64% and 36.18%, respectively. Institutional factors exert an indirect effect on the happiness of urban young returnees through relationship adaptation (46.80%) and material adaptation (53.20%). Social factors indirectly affect the happiness of urban young returnees through relationship adaptation (44.20%), collective adaptation (16.96%) and material adaptation (38.84%). Policies to improve the happiness of urban young returnees are suggested.

Keywords: urban young returnees; happiness; healthy China; HLM; SEM

Citation: Shen, F.; Zou, J.; Huang, X.; Wang, C.; Zhao, M. Career Development, Institutional Factors, Social Factors and Urban Young Returnees' Happiness in the Context of Healthy China. *IJERPH* **2022**, *19*, 9379. https://doi.org/10.3390/ijerph19159379

Academic Editor: Paul B. Tchounwou

Received: 29 June 2022
Accepted: 27 July 2022
Published: 31 July 2022

1. Introduction

Health is an indispensable condition for the comprehensive development of people and a basic condition for economic and social development. Today, countries around the world are gradually regarding improving people's quality of life and health as their top priority, and doing so has become a popular topic of research. Since 2014, China has gradually attached importance to "national health," which has become an important part of the national strategy. The outline of the Healthy China 2030 plan issued by the CPC Central Committee and the State Council proposes promoting the equalization of basic public health services; focusing on rural areas and grassroots units; gradually reducing the disparities in basic health services and health levels between urban and rural areas, regions and people; and promoting social equity. In improving the levels of basic public services in rural areas, we need to comprehensively promote the construction of healthy villages. Urban young returnees are the backbone of healthy rural construction, so their sense of happiness should not be ignored. Numerous studies focus on factors affecting people's happiness, such as socio-demographic characteristics [1], economic factors [2], social capital [3], social trust [4], migration and neighbourhood characteristics [5], but ignore the happiness of young returnees, especially the institutional and social factors in China. Due to the gap between urban and rural areas in terms of economy, culture and other aspects, urban young returnees have different degrees of psychological imbalance in rural life, which leads to short-term and long-term adaptation obstacles, thus affecting their happiness.

To fill the research gap, this paper contributes to the literature in three important ways. First, the particular advantage is that our unique data allow us to explore the determinants of urban young returnees' happiness in the context of a healthy China, where urban young returnees are a specific group that that does not receive enough attention. Second, HLM and SEM are applied to analyse the influencing factors of urban young returnees' happiness. Third, social adaptation theory is used to construct the theoretical framework, and material adaptation, collective adaptation, relationship adaptation and psychology adaptation are introduced as the underlying mechanisms.

1.1. Literature Review

1.1.1. The Concept of Urban Young Returnees and Happiness

With the increase of urban young returnees, increasing numbers of scholars are addressing them. Urban young returnees are usually defined as individuals who return to their hometown or other former place of residence. They are an important component of adult migration in the late 20s and 30s [6]. Happiness at the individual level has been studied and defined in several ways, for instance referring to individuals' overall evaluations of their lives [7] including their utility and subjective welfare [8]. There are a number of characteristics associated with happiness such as subjective well-being [9] and life satisfaction [10]. Happiness is a "positive emotional state", which expresses something more enduring than simply "feeling good", extending to a tendency toward positive feelings and moods [11]. In this framework, saying one is happy implies a general "psychic affirmation" of one's life. In terms of measuring happiness, some studies use a single question, such as, Overall, do you feel happy with your life? [12] Some studies use factor analysis to construct the feeling of happiness [13]. In this paper, in combination with the questions in the survey, the feeling of happiness was measured in four dimensions using factor analysis: (1) My life is close to my ideal in many ways. (2) My goal in life is enough to give me the motivation to struggle. (3) I feel happy when I devote myself to what I do. (4) I think my work can bring positive effect to the development of my hometown.

1.1.2. Previous Studies on Determinants of People's Happiness

Happiness, as a critical goal of human life, has been widely explored in the fields of psychology, sociology, economics and others [3,14]. At the same time, the determinants of happiness have also been discussed.

Previous research mainly focuses on socio-demographic factors affecting people's happiness such as gender, age, education and marital status. Some studies suggest that females are happier than males [15], while other studies show that there is no difference in happiness between men and women [16]. Some researchers concluded that age does not impact happiness [16], while others established a U-shaped relationship between age and happiness [17]. In general, married people are happier than single people [15,16]. Regarding education, there is no consensus. Some found that education is positively related to happiness [15,16], while others determined that the relationship is negative [18]. However, the personal factors mentioned above can only explain a small part of the differences [19].

The associations between economic and health factors and happiness has also been discussed. Most scholars believe that there is a positive but weak relationship between income and happiness [20]. However, some studies show that income is negatively associated with happiness [21,22]. If income matters mainly in a relative sense [23], migration to a wealthier country could hinder one's happiness, and unemployment can also have a negative impact on well-being [18]. However, health has a positive effect on happiness [24].

Social relationships are also an essential element that influences happiness [20,25,26]. Reflix (2003) [27] defines these as cooperative relationships among social actors promoting collective action. Their core components are civic participation and mutual trust among community members. People who surround themselves with friendly, helpful and trustworthy neighbours are happier than lonely people [28]. Social interaction with neighbours can promote people's happiness. In addition, socio-cultural features are associated with well-being [29], and the emotional experience of daily activities also has a significant impact on people's happiness [30]. Using an instrumental variable and two-stage residual inclusion, Lu et al. (2019) confirm the positive relationship between social trust and happiness in China [4].

The relationship between migration and happiness is also an important issue. The most commonly used method of measuring this relationship is to compare the happiness of migrants with that of local residents, and the common finding is that migrants are less happy than natives [31]. Bartram (2013) compares migrants with those who stayed in the country they left, and he finds that migrants from eastern to western Europe do not experience greater happiness [32]. However, for migrants from countries where the average happiness level is low, migrants seem to become happier after moving. Later, he finds that migrants are less happy than stayers when they move from wealthier to poorer countries in Europe [2]. On the contrary, migrants from Germany are happier than those who stay in Germany. Longitudinal analysis of the panel data indicates that migration to wealthier areas has a positive impact on happiness [33].

Until recently, some scholars have concentrated on the relationships between housing, neighbourhood and happiness, primarily examining the community's social attributes as the underlying mechanism. For example, residents feel happier in less deprived communities [20]. Community influences life satisfaction through community satisfaction, while community economic characteristics influence life satisfaction through housing and family satisfaction [34]. In addition, the community's social composition, such as race and ethnicity, can also affect residents' happiness. For instance, homogeneous groups are beneficial for the happiness of the people who live in them [1,35]. In China, most research focuses on the association between homeownership and happiness and finds that homeowners are happier than tenants [36–38]. In addition, Chen et al. (2021) find that Chinese urban residents' happiness is higher when the local government promises greater commitment to improving housing affordability [39]. Few studies focus on the role of the community, but using Guangzhou survey data, Liu et al. (2017) hypothesize that neighbourhood relationships directly improve migrants' happiness and that the correlation is more robust for locals than for migrants [40]. Migrants living in commercial housing, work unit housing, affordable housing and urban villages are happier than those living in old housing communities [5].

In summary, most research focuses on the determinants of people' happiness that arise from personal characteristics, economic factors, health status, social relations, migration, housing and community characteristics, but the factors that influence urban young returnees' happiness are ignored. As a very special group, urban young returnees come to the city and then return to the countryside and have experienced the dual influences of urban and rural life. Naturally, their psychological state is quite different from that of ordinary residents, and their adaptability to return to the countryside and their happiness also need to be reconsidered. Therefore, this paper will concentrate on this issue and explore the internal path of urban young returnees' happiness, so as to improve their well-being and present suggestions for the healthy China strategy.

1.2. Theoretical Framework

According to the seventh census published by the National Bureau of Statistics in 2021, there are more than 375 million migrants in China. More and more migrants are returning to their hometowns. In 2020, there will be 10.1 million entrepreneurs and innovators returning home. That is 1.6 million more than in 2019, the year with the largest and fastest growth in recent years. Returning youth have gone through two stages: rural to urban and urban to rural. The main reason for returning is the difficulty of finding a job [41], followed by family reasons such as caring for family members [42]. In addition, community and macro political factors affect returning behaviour [43].

As an amphibious group living in both the city and the countryside, urban young returnees vacillate between putting down roots in the city and returning to the countryside. Rural society has its own way of living working and communicating, as well as its own logic of living, surviving and operating. Today, great changes have taken place in rural areas, and the country attaches great importance to rural revitalization. There are both opportunities and challenges for urban young returnees returning to the countryside. When the urban young returnees return to the countryside, they may be confronted with the great divide between urban and rural life and the weakening of their past relationships with the countryside. Social adaptation is the process by which individuals' concepts and behaviours change with the social environment in order to adapt to it [44], and urban young returnees should constantly adjust their subjective adaptation to the rural society to improve their sense of happiness. Different scholars distinguish different types of social adaptation, including occupational adaptation [45], economic adaptation [46], social interaction [46], psychological adaptation [47] and cultural adaptation [48]. Here, based on the information in the questionnaire, social adaptation is divided into four types by factor analysis, including material adaptation, collective adaptation, relationship adaptation and psychological adaptation. Among them, material adaptation includes consumption patterns, employment structure and social security; collective adaptation includes living environment, social trust and social network; relationship adaptation contains genetic relationship, geographical relation and business relationship; and psychological adaptation refers to self-identity, self-efficacy and self-expectation. This should summarize the various adaptations of today's urban young returnees to the rural areas. The personal factors (career development), institutional factors (organizational culture and policy system) and social factors (physical environment and urban–rural relationship) perceived by urban young returnees will change and adjust through their various social adaptations and ultimately affect their happiness, and all the effects may be positive. The theoretical framework is proposed in Figure 1.

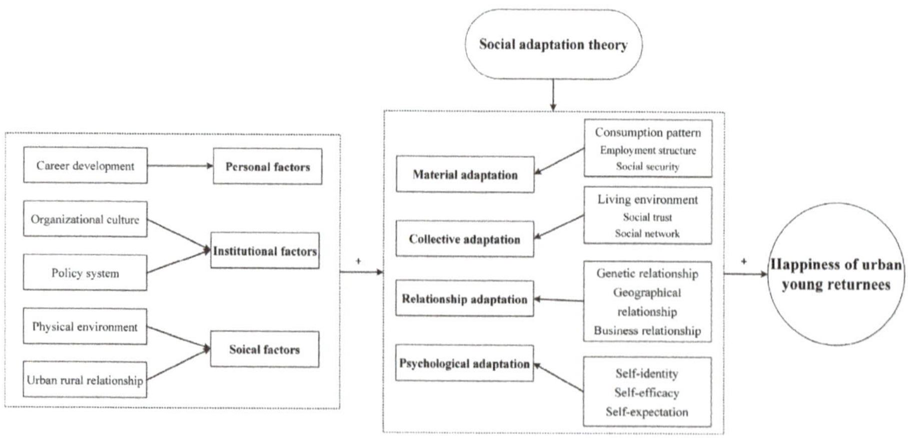

Figure 1. The theoretical framework of the study. Source: Authors.

2. Materials and Methods

2.1. Data

The data are from a large-scale professional social survey conducted by Hangzhou Normal University in January to February 2021. The respondents (urban young returnees) are residents registered in rural areas who have chosen to return to the countryside as their main place of production and living after a period of urban life, including migrant workers, entrepreneurs, Xin Xiangxian (people who have a love of hometown in contemporary villages, who once went away for an official reason but returned to the countryside to teach or took root in the countryside for a long time and served the countryside with their own knowledge and ability), young college students and retired servicemen. In conjunction with the theoretical framework and a literature review, preliminary questionnaire items were drawn up, and 60 urban young returnees were surveyed. Then, the reliability and validity of the data were tested, and the formal questionnaire was adjusted according to the results. Based on the large-scale special social practices organized by Hangzhou Normal University, nearly 800 volunteers were recruited to conduct research in four regions of east, middle, west and northeast China.Probability proportionate to size sampling (PPS) was used to select the samples. A total of 3140 questionnaires were sent out, and 2234 questionnaires were returned, representing a recovery rate of 71.1%. After eliminating the questionnaires with obvious rules and inconsistent answers, a total of 2202 valid questionnaires were obtained, an effective rate of 98.6%.

Table 1 displays the basic information of the respondents. Most urban young returnees are between 21 and 40 years old, about 55.2% of them are female and 56.3% of them have a bachelor's degree. The proportion of single urban young returnees accounts for 57.4%, and 56.4% of urban young returnees stay in the city for 3–5 years. Another 28.6% of them return for more than 5 years, while 21% of them return for 1 to 2 years. Most urban youth have no children or only one child. Comparing the change in salary between before and after returning to the hometown, the current income is higher than the previous income in the city. Looking at the change in occupation before and after returning to the hometown, the ratio of unemployed decreased significantly, from 33.9% to 15.7%. The proportion of urban young returnees engaged in science, education, culture, health and social security increased significantly, from 17.9% to 30.7%. The proportion of urban young returnees engaged in agriculture, forestry, husbandry and fishery also increased, from 4.3% to 8.6%.

Table 1. Descriptive information on the respondents.

Characteristics	Classification	Frequency	Rate	Characteristics	Classification	Frequency	Rate
Age	≤20	277	12.6	Living years in the city	3–5	1241	56.4
	21–30	1166	53.0		6–8	290	13.2
	31–40	469	21.3		9–11	132	6.0
	≥41	290	13.2		≥12	539	24.5
Education	Junior high school and below	173	7.9	Returning time	<1	634	28.8
	Senior school or technical secondary school	297	13.5		1–2	463	21.0
	Junior college	398	18.1		2–3	262	11.9
	Undergraduate	1240	56.3		3–4	213	9.7
	Master or above	94	4.3		≥5	630	28.6
Marital status	Unmarried	1263	57.4	Number of Children	0	1348	61.2
	Married	912	41.4		1	514	23.3
	Divorced	25	1.1		2	313	14.2
	Widowed	2	0.1		≥3	27	1.2
Monthly income in the city (yuan)	≤3000	860	39.1	Current monthly income	≤3000	501	22.8
	3001–6000	792	36.0		3001–6000	947	43.0
	6001–9000	358	16.3		6001–9000	495	22.5
	≥9001	192	8.7		≥9001	259	11.8

Table 1. *Cont.*

Characteristics	Classification	Frequency	Rate	Characteristics	Classification	Frequency	Rate
Occupation in the city	Agriculture, forestry, husbandry and fishery	95	4.3	Current occupation	Agriculture, forestry, husbandry and fishery	189	8.6
	Mining, manufacturing and construction	210	9.5		Mining, manufacturing and construction	192	8.7
	Production and supply of electricity, gas and water	56	2.5		Production and supply of electricity, gas and water	60	2.7
	Transportation, storage and postal services	97	4.4		Transportation, storage and postal services	87	4.0
	Information transmission, computer and software industry	143	6.5		Information transmission, computer and software industry	164	7.4
	Service industry	307	13.9		Service industry	321	14.6
	Financial industry	131	5.9		Financial industry	141	6.4
	Real estate industry	22	1.0		Real estate industry	28	1.3
	Science, education, culture, health and social security	394	17.9		Science, education, culture, health and social security	657	30.7
	Unemployment (including students)	747	33.9		Unemployment (including students)	345	15.7
Gender	Male	987	44.8	Total		2202	100
	Female	1215	55.2				

Source: A large-scale professional social survey conducted by Hangzhou Normal University; the following tables and figures are the same.

2.2. Variable

According to the theoretical framework, we identified the antecedents, mediators and outcome variables of this study. The antecedent variables include individual factors, institutional factors and social factors, the intermediary variables include individual adaptation, relationship adaptation, collective adaptation and material adaptation, and the outcome variable is the happiness of urban young returnees. Their specific meaning and the results of confirmatory factor analysis conducted using Amos software are shown in Table 2. According to the results, Cronbach's α are all above 0.9, indicating that the scale has good reliability. KMO and AVE were all above 0.7, indicating that the scale has good validity.

Table 2. The confirmatory factor analysis results.

Variable	Items [1]	KMO	Bartlett Spherical Test	Factor Load	α	AVE	CR	Total α
Career development	Q1	0.951	27,742.771	0.828	0.819	0.736	0.893	0.953
	Q2			0.858				
	Q3			0.886				
Organizational culture	Q4			0.917	0.914	0.853	0.946	
	Q5			0.933				
	Q6			0.920				
Policy system	Q7			0.920	0.918	0.859	0.948	
	Q8			0.934				
	Q9			0.927				
Physical environment	Q10			0.924	0.906	0.842	0.941	
	Q11			0.927				
	Q12			0.902				
Urban rural relationship	Q13			0.907	0.801	0.722	0.885	
	Q14			0.918				
	Q15			0.707				

Table 2. *Cont.*

Variable	Items [1]	KMO	Bartlett Spherical Test	Factor Load	α	AVE	CR	Total α
Psychological adaptation	Q16 Q17 Q18	0.979	40,132.592	0.883 0.930 0.920	0.898	0.830	0.936	0.972
Relationship adaptation	Q19 Q20 Q21 Q22 Q23			0.831 0.820 0.868 0.893 0.876	0.909	0.736	0.933	
Collective adaptation	Q24 Q25 Q26 Q27 Q28 Q29			0.839 0.854 0.843 0.837 0.871 0.833	0.920	0.716	0.938	
Material adaptation	Q30 Q31 Q32 Q33 Q34 Q35			0.841 0.788 0.879 0.889 0.842 0.865	0.923	0.725	0.940	
Happiness	Q36 Q37 Q38 Q39			0.867 0.904 0.911 0.892	0.915	0.799	0.941	

Note: all load values are significant at 0.001. α is the internal consistency reliability coefficient. CR is the combination reliability coefficient. AVE is the average amount of variance extracted. [1] Detailed information are presented in Table A1 in the Appendix A.

2.3. Methodology

First, to analyse the differences in happiness among urban young returnees in China, multivariate analysis of variance and *t* test are applied. In addition, correlation analysis is used to analyse the association between the independent variables and the happiness of urban young returnees.

For non-equilibrium nested data, the hierarchical linear model can decompose and estimate the variance and covariance components in the data and reveal their hierarchical differences. Therefore, this paper adopts the HLM model as the basic research method, and the specific settings of this model are as follows:

$$Happiness_i = \beta_0 + \beta_1 Socio\_demo_i + \varepsilon_i \quad (1)$$

$$Happiness_i = \beta_0 + \beta_1 Socio\_demo_i + \beta_2 Per_i + \beta_3 Inst_i + \beta_4 Soci_i + \varepsilon_i \quad (2)$$

$$Happiness_i = \beta_0 + \beta_i X_i + \varepsilon_i \quad (3)$$

Among them, $Happiness_i$ is the happiness of urban young returnees. $Socio\_demo_i$ is the social demography factors, including gender, age, education, returning time, current occupation and current monthly income. Per_i means personal factors such as career development. $Inst_i$ is institutional factors, containing organizational culture and policy system. $Soci_i$ represents the social factors, including physical environment and urban rural relationship. X_i represents all the control variables. ε_i is the random error term.

However, among the variables in this study, individual factors, institutional factors and social factors of urban returnees cannot be measured with a single index, and happiness refers to the subjective understanding and willingness of urban returnees and cannot be directly measured. These characteristics among variables make it difficult for traditional analysis methods to obtain more accurate results, while the structural equation model (SEM) can handle the related problems well. Therefore, this study uses Amos software to construct a structural equation model to analyse the relationship between the variables, which is widely used in the research fields of sociology, psychology, economics and behavioural sciences.

SEM is a multivariate statistical analysis method of analysing the relationships between variables based on the covariance matrix between variables, which integrates factor analysis and path analysis. It is mainly divided into a measurement model and a structure model. The measurement model mainly describes the relationships between latent variables and observed variables through factor analysis, while the structural model uses path relationship analysis to measure the relationship between variables. The measurement model is as follows:

$$X = \cap_x \zeta + \delta \tag{4}$$

$$Y = \cap_y \eta + \varepsilon \tag{5}$$

Below, ζ is the matrix of the exogenous latent variable, η is the matrix of the endogenous latent variable, Y is the endogenous observation variable, $\cap_x$ represents the load matrix of the exogenous observation variables with respect to the exogenous latent variables. $\cap_y$ represents the load matrix of the endogenous observation variables with respect to the endogenous latent variables. δ represents the measurement error of the exogenous observation variables, and ε is the measurement error of the endogenous observation variables. The structural model is as follows:

$$\eta = B\eta + \Gamma\zeta + \mu \tag{6}$$

B represents the coefficient matrix of the relationship between internal latent variables, Γ is the coefficient matrix of the influence of the exogenous latent variables on the endogenous latent variables and μ is the structural vector error.

Firstly, a conceptual model is constructed; then, the parameters of the model are estimated from the survey data to determine the correlation between the variables in the model; finally, the goodness of fit is tested to evaluate whether the model is supported by the actual data.

3. Results

3.1. The Difference of Happiness among the Urban Young Returnees in China

Table 3 shows that there are significant differences in the happiness of urban young returnees in terms of gender, age, education, time of returning home, current occupation and current monthly income but no significant difference in terms of length of stay in the city and occupation in the city. This suggests that the happiness of urban returnees is influenced more by how they live now in the countryside than by how they used to live in the city.

Table 3. The differences in happiness among urban young returnees in China.

Variable	Classification	Happiness	T(P)/F(P)
Gender	Male	15.24 ± 3.73	2.223 (0.026)
	Female	14.90 ± 3.34	
Age	≤20	14.40 ± 3.97	7.050 (<0.001)
	21–30	14.93 ± 3.54	
	31–40	15.45 ± 3.27	
	≥41	15.49 ± 3.27	
Education	Junior high school and below	14.23 ± 3.46	3.384 (0.009)
	Senior school or technical secondary school	14.95 ± 3.89	
	Junior college	14.97 ± 3.47	
	Undergraduate	15.18 ± 3.41	
	Master or above	15.55 ± 3.52	

Table 3. *Cont.*

Variable	Classification	Happiness	T(P)/F(P)
Marital status	Unmarried	14.93 ± 3.64	1.835 (0.139)
	Married	15.21 ± 3.36	
	Divorced	15.36 ± 3.09	
	Widowed	11.50 ± 2.12	
Number of Children	0	14.94 ± 3.61	1.422 (0.234)
	1	15.27 ± 3.34	
	2	15.20 ± 3.36	
	≥3	14.70 ± 4.26	
Length of stay in the city	3–5	15.11 ± 3.49	1.034 (0.376)
	6–8	15.00 ± 3.34	
	9–11	15.37 ± 3.49	
	≥12	14.86 ± 3.71	
Returning time	<1	14.63 ± 3.91	4.393 (0.002)
	1–2	15.21 ± 3.17	
	2–3	14.89 ± 3.60	
	3–4	15.62 ± 3.00	
	≥5	15.23 ± 3.45	
Occupation in the city	Agriculture, forestry, husbandry and fishery	14.83 ± 4.17	0.980 (0.455)
	Mining, manufacturing and construction	15.30 ± 3.75	
	Production and supply of electricity, gas and water	14.86 ± 3.78	
	Transportation, storage and postal services	14.92 ± 3.69	
	Information transmission, computer and software industry	15.48 ± 3.03	
	Service industry	14.96 ± 3.42	
	Financial industry	15.27 ± 3.63	
	Real estate industry	16,45 ± 2.46	
	Science, education, culture, health and social security	14.97 ± 3.40	
	Unemployment (including students)	14.95 ± 3.53	
Current occupation	Agriculture, forestry, husbandry and fishery	14.77 ± 4.28	2.934 (0.002)
	Mining, manufacturing and construction	15.64 ± 3.32	
	Production and supply of electricity, gas and water	14.58 ± 3.87	
	Transportation, storage and postal services	14.86 ± 3.64	
	Information transmission, computer and software industry	15.47 ± 3.14	
	Service industry	14.96 ± 3.41	
	Financial industry	14.66 ± 3.67	
	Real estate industry	15.79 ± 2.97	
	Science, education, culture, health and social security	15.31 ± 3.13	
	Unemployment (including students)	14.48 ± 3.94	
Monthly income in the city (yuan)	≤3000	14.84 ± 3.62	1.733 (0.158)
	3001–6000	15.17 ± 3.21	
	6001–9000	15.27 ± 3.42	
	≥9001	15.08 ± 4.39	
Current monthly income	≤3000	14.37 ± 3.86	9.80 (<0.001)
	3001–6000	15.10 ± 3.15	
	6001–9000	15.53 ± 3.36	
	≥9001	15.27 ± 4.18	

3.2. The Correlations between the Independent Variables and the Happiness of Urban Young Returnees in China

Table 4 indicates that all independent variables are positively associated with urban young returnees' happiness, and the correlation coefficients are more than 0.6. This shows that the variables we selected are suitable for the next regression.

Table 4. The correlations between the core variables and happiness.

Variables	Dimensions	SWB [1]
Personal factors	Career development	0.724 ***
Institutional factors	Organizational culture	0.601 ***
	Policy system	0.661 ***
Social factors	Physical environment	0.707 ***
	Urban rural relationship	0.716 ***
Psychological adaptation	Self-identity	0.668 ***
	Self-efficacy	0.689 ***
	Self-expectation	0.709 ***
Relationship adaptation	Genetic relationship	0.746 ***
	Geographical relation	0.786 ***
	Business relationship	0.707 ***
Collective adaptation	Living environment	0.765 ***
	Social trust	0.708 ***
	Social networks	0.776 ***
Material adaptation	Consumption pattern	0.754 ***
	Employment structure	0.760 ***
	Social security	0.752 ***

Note: *** represent significance at the 1% level. [1] SWB: Subjective well-being.

3.3. The Hierarchical Liner Regression Results of Urban Young Returnees' Happiness

Before applying the structural equation model, hierarchical linear regression is used for the benchmark regression, and the results are shown in Table 5. The variables of social demography, personal factors, institutional factors, social factors are gradually applied to the model. Based on the results of the above multivariate analysis and correlation analysis, we discarded variables such as the duration of residence in the city and occupation in the city because these variables had no significant correlations with the happiness of urban young returnees. The results indicate that the social demography variables, such as gender, monthly income, returning time, current occupation, have no significant effects on the happiness of urban young returnees. Only age and education have positive effects on the happiness of urban young returnees. The results are in contradiction with some previous studies [15,17,18], as urban young returnees are a special group different from common residents. With increasing age and higher education level, more wealth and resources are accumulated, which may improve the sense of happiness.

Table 5. Hierarchical linear regression results for urban young returnees' happiness.

Variable	Tier 1 [1]	Tier 2 [2]	Tier 3 [3]
	Beta	Beta	Beta
Gender (Female)			
Male	−0.050 *	−0.013	−0.017
Age (Aged below 20)			
Aged between 21 and 30	0.018	0.019	0.006
Aged between 31 and 40	0.093 *	0.071 **	0.047 *
Aged over 41	0.122 **	0.072 **	0.042 *
Education (Junior high school and below)			
Senior school or technical secondary school	0.112 **	0.039	0.023
Junior college	0.152 **	0.030	0.022
Undergraduate	0.250 **	0.064 *	0.046 *
Master or above	0.112 **	0.037 *	0.034 *
Returning time (Less than 1 year)			
Between 1 and 2 years	0.046	0.009	0.011
Between 2 and 3years	0.004	−0.012	−0.010
Between 3 and 4 years	0.062 **	0.011	−0.010
More than 5 years	0.014	−0.032	−0.026

Table 5. *Cont.*

Variable	Tier 1 [1]	Tier 2 [2]	Tier 3 [3]
	Beta	Beta	Beta
Current occupation (Agriculture, forestry, husbandry and fishery)			
Mining, manufacturing and construction	0.059 *	0.015	−0.001
Production and supply of electricity, gas and water	−0.020	0.002	−0.010
Transportation, storage and postal services	0.005	0.005	−0.016
Information transmission, computer and software industry	0.029	0.018	−0.008
Service industry	0.010	−0.010	−0.017
Financial industry	−0.022	−0.002	−0.019
Real estate industry	0.023	−0.004	−0.003
Science, education, culture, health and social security	0.031	0.024	−0.003
Unemployment	0.032	0.011	0.013
Current Monthly income (≤3000)			
3001–6000	0.083 *	0.001	0.007
6001–9000	0.096 *	0.004	0.007
≥9001	0.032	−0.008	−0.001
Personal factors			
Career development		0.306 **	0.161 **
Institutional factors			
Organizational culture		−0.035	−0.081 **
Policy system		0.121 **	0.017
Social factors			
Physical environment		0.210 **	0.020
Urban rural relationship		0.304 **	0.061 **
Psychological adaptation			
Self-identity			0.006
Self-efficacy			−0.025
Self-expectation			0.080 **
Relationship adaptation			
Genetic relationship			0.031
Geographical relation			0.186 **
Business relationship			0.034
Collective adaptation			
Living environment			0.089 **
Social trust			0.008
Social networks			0.098 **
Material adaptation			
Consumption pattern			0.092 **
Employment structure			0.116 **
Social security			0.107 **
R2	0.205	0.812	0.877
F	3.996	144.653	175.590
ΔR2	0.042	0.617	0.110
ΔF	3.996	785.258	86.064
VIFmax	4.903	5.022	5.093

Note: ** and * represent significance at the 5% and 10% levels, respectively. [1] Tier 1 refers to the social demography variables input into the model. [2] Tier 2 refers to the social demography, personal factor, institutional factor and social factor variables input into the model. [3] Tier 3 refers to all the control variables input into the model.

However, other factors such as career development, policy system, physical environment and urban–rural relationship all have significant positive effects on the happiness of urban young returnees, with the exception of organizational culture, which has a negative impact on urban young returnees' happiness. Urban young returnees have experienced different cultures in various cities. When they return to rural areas to participate in different organizational cultural activities, there may be short-term collisions and contradictions between the different cultures, which is not conducive to the improvement of their well-being.

3.4. The SEM Results of Urban Young Returnees' Happiness

In order to further analyse the relationships between the independent variables and happiness of urban young returnees, all Q variables are explicit and can be observed directly, and their definitions are shown in Table A1 in the Appendix A. Career development (X1), psychological adaptation (M1), relationship adaptation (M2), collective adaptation (M3) and material adaptation (M4) are used as the exogenous latent variables, and happiness (Y) was taken as the endogenous latent variable to construct a structural equation model. The maximum likelihood method was used to estimate the initial model.

The results of the test of the model fitting parameters show that the p-values of two paths, career development $\rightarrow$ happiness and psychological adaptation (M1) $\rightarrow$ happiness, are greater than 0.05. Consequently, they are deleted. The p-values of the other paths are less than 0.05 and thus statistically significant. The model is modified by the correction index by adding two residual paths [e1–e2] and [e1–e3]. The empirical results show good model fit: relative fit index (CFI) = 0.946, AGFI = 0.867, RMSEA = 0.065. CFI and AGFI exceed the suggested threshold, and RMSEA is lower than the threshold 0.08 (Byrne, 2015). The revised model of the influence mechanism of career development on the happiness of urban returnees is shown in Figure 2. The coefficient connecting the core variables (X1, M1–M4) and the explicit variable Q is the standardized load coefficient, and all coefficients are greater than 0.5, indicating that the model measurement relationship is good. Meanwhile, the coefficient between the latent variables is the standardized path coefficient, which shows the influence relationships between the latent variables. For example, the standardized path coefficient of X1 on M1 is 0.91. The explanation of Figures 3 and 4 is similar to that of Figure 2. Since the significance is not shown in Figure 2, we need to deepen the analysis via Table 6.

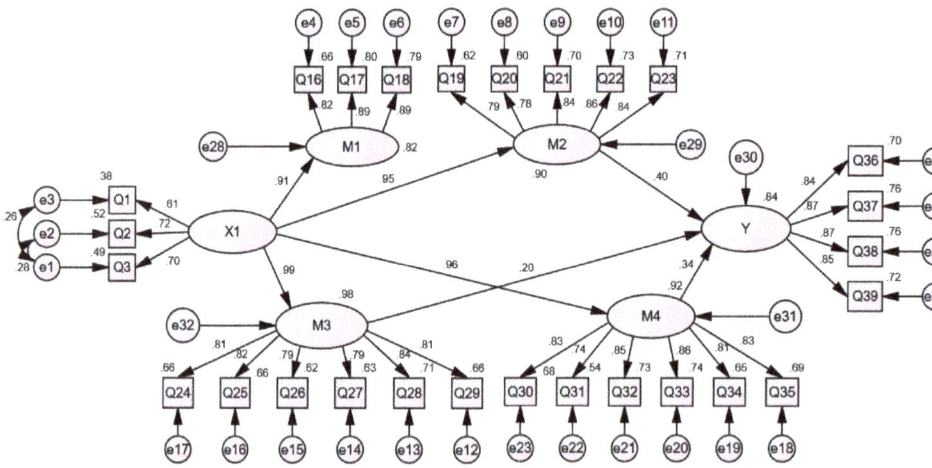

Figure 2. A revised model of the influence mechanism of career development on the happiness of urban young returnees.

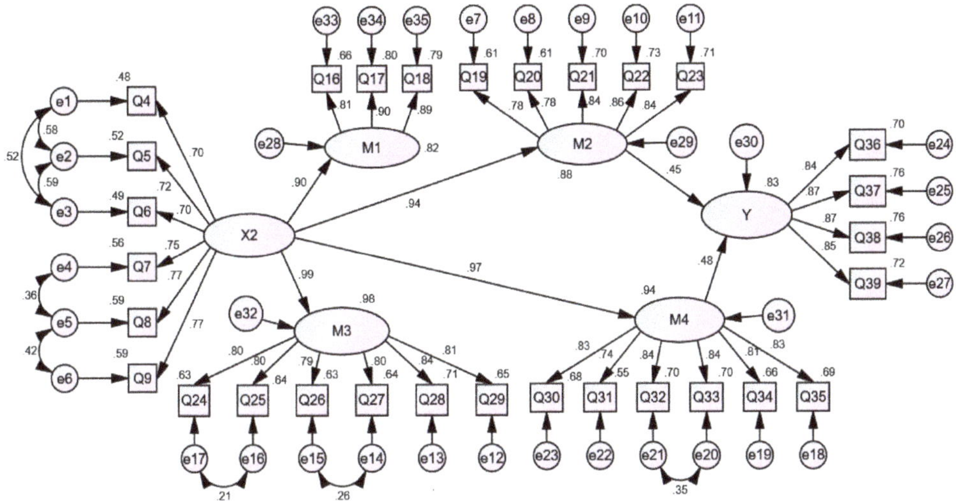

Figure 3. A revised model of the influence mechanism of institutional factors on the happiness of urban returnees.

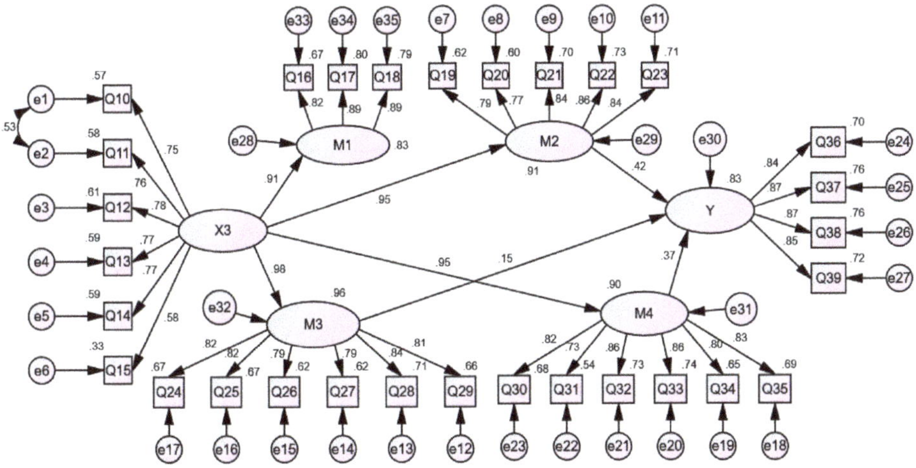

Figure 4. A revised model of the influence mechanism of social factors on the happiness of urban young returnees.

To further analyse the influencing mechanism of career development on happiness, the specific path is decomposed as shown in Table 6. From this, we find that career development can significantly affect the material adaptation, collective adaptation, psychological adaptation and relationship adaptation of urban young returnees. Moreover, the standardized indirect effect of Career development → Happiness is 0.901 ($p < 0.01$), and the standardized indirect effect of Career development → Relationship adaptation → Happiness is 0.380 ($p < 0.01$), the standardized indirect effect of Career development → Collective adaptation → Happiness is 0.195 ($p < 0.01$), the standardized indirect effect of Career development → Material adaptation → Happiness is 0.326 ($p < 0.01$). This means that career development does not directly affect the happiness of urban young returnees but indirectly affects their happiness through relationship adaptation, collective adaptation and material adaptation. The indirect effects account for 42.18% (0.380/0.901), 21.64% and 36.18%, respectively. Good career development can expand the network resources and social capital of urban young returnees, leading to the growth of wealth, thus increasing their happiness.

Table 6. The effects of career development on the happiness of urban young returnees.

Paths	Standardized Direct Effect	Standardized Indirect Effect	Standardized Total Effect	p
Career development → Psychological adaptation	0.907		0.907	***
Career development → Relationship adaptation	0.949		0.949	***
Career development → Collective adaptation	0.989		0.989	***
Career development → Material adaptation	0.960		0.960	***
Psychological adaptation → Happiness	/		/	/
Relationship adaptation → Happiness	0.400		0.400	***
Collective adaptation → Happiness	0.197		0.197	***
Material adaptation → Happiness	0.340		0.340	***
Career development → Happiness	/	0.901	0.901	***
Career development → Psychological adaptation → Happiness	/	/	/	/
Career development → Relationship adaptation → Happiness		0.380	0.380	***
Career development → Collective adaptation → Happiness		0.195	0.195	***
Career development → Material adaptation → Happiness		0.326	0.326	***

Note: *** represent significance at the 1% level.

Additionally, the model fitting parameter test results show that the p-values of the paths for institutional factors—(X2) → happiness, psychological adaptation (M1) → happiness and collective adaptation (M3) → happiness—are greater than 0.05. Consequently, they are deleted. The p-values of the other paths are less than 0.05 and thus statistically significant. The model is modified by the correction index by adding eight residual paths [e1–e2], [e1–e3], [e2–e3], [e4–e5], [e5–e6], [e16–e17], [e14–e15] and [e20–e21]. The empirical results show that the model fit is good: CFI = 0.937, AGFI = 0.859, RMSEA = 0.068. The revised model of the influence mechanism of institutional factors on the happiness of urban returnees is shown in Figure 3.

Table 7 indicates that institutional factors can also affect the material adaptation, collective adaptation, psychological adaptation and relationship adaptation of urban young returnees. In addition, the standardized indirect effect of Institutional factors → Happiness is 0.876 ($p < 0.01$), the standardized indirect effect of Institutional factors → Relationship adaptation → Happiness is 0.410 ($p < 0.01$), and the standardized indirect effect of Institutional factors → Material adaptation → Happiness is 0.466 ($p < 0.01$). This means that institutional factors do not directly affect the happiness of urban young returnees but rather indirectly affect the happiness of urban young returnees through relationship adaptation and material adaptation. The indirect effects accounts for 46.80% (0.410/0.876), 53.20%, respectively. Good systems and policies can create good business environments for urban young returnees; cultivate good business relations; and stimulate entrepreneurship, employment, consumption, etc., thus improving their happiness.

In addition, the model fitting parameter test results show that the p-values of social factors (X3) → happiness, psychological adaptation (M1) → happiness are greater than 0.05. Consequently, they are deleted. The p-values of the other paths are less than 0.05 and thus statistically significant. The model is modified by the correction index by adding one residual path, [e1–e2]. The empirical results show that the model fit is good: CFI = 0.924, AGFI = 0.824, RMSEA = 0.074. The revised model of the influence mechanism of social factors on the happiness of urban returnees is shown in Figure 4.

Table 7. The effects of institutional factors on the happiness of urban young returnees.

Paths	Standardized Direct Effect	Standardized Indirect Effect	Standardized Total Effect	p
Institutional factors → Psychological adaptation	0.904	/	0.904	***
Institutional factors → Relationship adaptation	0.938	/	0.938	***
Institutional factors → Collective adaptation	0.989	/	0.989	***
Institutional factors → Material adaptation	0.967	/	0.967	***
Psychological adaptation → Happiness	/	/	/	/
Relationship adaptation → Happiness	0.453		0.453	***
Collective adaptation → Happiness	/	/	/	***
Material adaptation → Happiness	0.482	/	0.482	***
Institutional factors → Happiness	/	0.876	0.876	***
Institutional factors → Psychological adaptation → Happiness	/	/	/	/
Institutional factors → Relationship adaptation → Happiness	/	0.410	0.410	***
Institutional factors → Collective adaptation → Happiness	/	/	/	***
Institutional factors → Material adaptation → Happiness	/	0.466	0.466	***

Note: *** represent significance at the 1% level.

Finally, Table 8 indicates that social factors can also affect the material adaptation, collective adaptation, psychological adaptation and relationship adaptation of urban young returnees. The standardized indirect effect of Social factors → Happiness is 0.896 ($p < 0.01$); the standardized indirect effect of Social factors → Relationship adaptation → Happiness is 0.396 ($p < 0.01$); the standardized indirect effect of Social factors → Collective adaptation → Happiness is 0.152 ($p < 0.01$); and the standardized indirect effect of Social factors → Material adaptation → Happiness is 0.348 ($p < 0.01$). This means that social factors do not directly affect the happiness of urban young returnees but indirectly affect the happiness of urban young returnees through relationship adaptation, collective adaptation and material adaptation. The indirect effects account for 44.20% (0.396/0.896), 16.96% and 38.84%, respectively. Social factors are conducive to urban young returnees' expanding their social resources and social relations and forming collective awareness and social trust, and this cumulative effect will promote their employment, entrepreneurship and consumption, thus increasing their sense of happiness.

Table 8. The effects of social factors on the happiness of urban young returnees.

Paths	Standardized Direct Effect	Standardized Indirect Effect	Standardized Total Effect	p
Social factors → Psychological adaptation	0.909		0.909	***
Social factors → Relationship adaptation	0.954		0.954	***
Social factors → Collective adaptation	0.978		0.978	***
Social factors → Material adaptation	0.949		0.949	***
Psychological adaptation → Happiness	/	/	/	/
Relationship adaptation → Happiness	0.415		0.415	***
Collective adaptation → Happiness	0.155		0.155	***
Material adaptation → Happiness	0.367		0.367	***
Social factors → Happiness	/	0.896	0.896	***
Social factors → Psychological adaptation → Happiness	/	/	/	/
Social factors → Relationship adaptation → Happiness	/	0.396	0.396	***
Social factors → Collective adaptation → Happiness	/	0.152	0.152	***
Social factors → Material adaptation → Happiness	/	0.348	0.348	***

Note: *** represent significance at the 1% level.

4. Discussion

The Healthy China 2030 Plan emphasizes that people's health should be prioritized in development, focusing on rural areas and grass-roots units. The happiness of urban young returnees is also an important form of mental health. The findings in this study differ significantly from those of previous studies. They mainly concentrated on the effects of gender, age, education and marital status on residents' happiness [16,49]. However, in our study, we focus on urban young returnees, a special group returning to their hometowns or other previous places of residence [6]. Their happiness is affected by career development, institutional factors (especially employment and the entrepreneurship policy system) and social factors (physical environment and the urban–rural relationship). They attach more importance to their career development, and they pay more attention to corporate systems related to their career development than to the household registration system [50]. This implies that today's urban young returnees have their own unique views and career concepts. Furthermore, urban young returnees focus on the urban–rural relationship. This also contradicts with previous studies [20,25,26] that concentrate on the social relationships. Our study focuses on the urban–rural relationship rather than the social relationships among community residents.

In addition, we introduce the theory of social adaptation to explain the underlying mechanism of urban young returnees' happiness [44], which includes material adaptation, collective adaptation, relationship adaptation and psychological adaptation [47]. The results of the study do not fully agree with the hypothesis. Another study concludes that career development indirectly affects the happiness of urban young returnees through relationship adaptation, collective adaptation and material adaptation. Institutional factors indirectly affect the happiness of urban young returnees through relationship adaptation and material adaptation. Social factors indirectly affect the happiness of urban young returnees through relationship adaptation, collective adaptation and material adaptation. The mediating effect of psychological adaptation is not significant in the above paths. On the one hand, this shows that psychological adaptation is a long-term process and does not constitute the mechanism of related factors on urban young returnees' happiness, such as personal factors, institutional factors and social factors. On the other hand, it may be related to the rationality of the preliminary questionnaire design. Despite some limitations, the above mechanisms should generally complement and innovate previous research.

Thus, the findings in this study have important policy implications for improving the well-being of urban young returnees in the context of the Healthy China 2030 Plan. From these data, we can see that the return of urban youth has brought vitality and new changes to their hometowns, which is helpful for rural revitalization and a healthy China. It would be beneficial for the government to promote urban young returnees' happiness in several aspects. First, a series of measures should be taken such as entrepreneurship and employment policies to encourage urban young returnees to start businesses and gain employment so that they can better adapt to their relationships and material environment and increase their happiness. In addition, the social security system in rural areas should be gradually improved including medical care, pensions, employment and so on. Second, rural infrastructure (roads, facilities, communications, waste disposal) and basic public services (health care and education environment) should be developed. Finally, there should be a breakthrough in the soft environment, for example, promoting integrated and harmonious development between urban and rural areas, strengthening interpersonal relationship and increasing support and encouragement for the urban young returnees from family and society. These can improve their material adaptation, collective adaptation and relational adaptation and thereby enhance their happiness, which in turn will benefit the construction of a healthy China.

This study enriches the literature by highlighting the importance of career development, entrepreneurship and employment policy, and social factors in influencing the happiness of urban young returnees and explaining the underlying mechanisms. However, there are some limitations. First, this paper uses the questionnaire survey method. The main drawback of this method is that we cannot assess the authenticity of the questionnaire completed by the respondents, which may affect the accuracy of the conclusions. In addition, due to the data constraints, only the effects of cross-sectional data are discussed, and the dynamic changes in the happiness of urban young returnees are not considered.

Moreover, there may be other paths that affect the happiness of urban young returnees. All of these need to be further explored in the future.

5. Conclusions

In the context of the Healthy China 2030 Plan, the happiness of urban young returnees cannot be ignored. Based on a large-scale social practice survey in China, this paper applies a hierarchical linear regression model (HLM) and a structural equation model (SEM) to discuss the influencing factors on the happiness of urban young returnees. The results show that the happiness of urban young returnees in China is less influenced by their socio-demographic characteristics, such as age and education, and more by career development, institutional factors and social factors, which are different from those of ordinary residents. Further study finds that career development indirectly affects the happiness of urban young returnees through relationship adaptation, collective adaptation and material adaptation. The indirect effects account for 42.18%, 21.64% and 36.18% respectively. Institutional factors indirectly affect the happiness of urban young returnees through relationship adaptation (46.80%) and material adaptation (53.20%). Social factors indirectly affect the happiness of urban young returnees through relationship adaptation (44.20%), collective adaptation (16.96%) and material adaptation (38.84%).

Author Contributions: Conceptualization and formal analysis, F.S.; writing-review and editing, J.Z.; methodology, X.H.; writing-original draft preparation, C.W. and M.Z. All authors have read and agreed to the published version of the manuscript.

Funding: This research was funded by the project of the post-doctoral research base of Hangzhou International Urbanology Research Center of Zhejiang University (22CYBHJD02), Leisure Empowers Common Prosperity of Zhejiang University (22CSX13), the Key Research Base of Humanities and Social Sciences in Colleges and Universities in Sichuan Province (SQZL2022A01) and the Postdoctoral Research Foundation of China (2021M692844).

Institutional Review Board Statement: Ethical review and approval were waived for this study due to the absence of sensitive data and to the processing of data with the assurance of the confidentiality and anonymization of the personal information of all the subjects involved in the study.

Informed Consent Statement: Informed consent was obtained from all subjects involved in the study.

Data Availability Statement: Restrictions apply to the availability of these data because the data were obtained from a third party. They can be made available by the first authors (F.-W.S. and J.Z.) with the permission of the third party.

Conflicts of Interest: The authors declare no conflict of interest.

Appendix A

Table A1. The detailed items.

Variable	Items
Career development	Q1 Always pay attention to and search for the information about the occupation I am interested in. Q2 The countryside provides me with a stage to give full play to my professional expertise. Q3 I am optimistic about the future of my current job.
Organizational culture	Q4 My village often holds cultural activities (village evening party, writing Spring Festival couplets, comparison of filial piety and morality, etc.). Q5 My village often carries out cultural publicity activities (lectures, broadcasting, door-to-door publicity, etc.). Q6 My village has various cultural organizations (Yangko team, square dance team, band, etc.).
Policy system	Q7 The village where I live lets young urban returnees know about relevant employment and entrepreneurship policies through various channels. Q8 The village where I live has supportive policies for entrepreneurship and employment. Q9 The village where I live has policies to attract young people from the cities to return to their hometowns to find jobs and start businesses.

Table A1. *Cont.*

Variable		Items
Physical environment		Q10 My village has complete infrastructure (roads, facilities, communications, waste disposal). Q11 The basic public service system (medical and health, education environment) in my village is sound. Q12 The economic development of my village is better.
Urban rural relationship		Q13 I prefer the way of life in the countryside. Q14 I prefer the pace of life in the countryside. Q15 I think there are development differences between urban and rural areas.
Psychological adaptation	Self-identity	Q16 I'm proud of being a rural person.
	Self-efficacy	Q17 In the countryside, I can give full play to my ability.
	Self-expectation	Q18 In the countryside, I can achieve my goals and ideals.
Relationship adaptation	Genetic relationship	Q19 My family and friends agreed with my choice of returning home. Q20 My family and friends have given me funds and contacts to start my business.
	Geographical relationship	Q21 I am willing to take part in the cultural construction or cultural activities of the village. Q22 I live in a harmonious village.
	Business relationship	Q23 I prefer the way I get along with people when I work in the countryside.
Collective adaptation	Living environment	Q24 I think the living environment is good now. Q25 I think the living standard is high now.
	Social trust	Q26 The public service expenditure in my village is high. Q27 My village has high financial transparency.
	Social networks	Q28 It's easy for me to get help from others or organizations. Q29 I have established close relationships with potential or existing friends.
Material adaptation	Consumption pattern	Q30 I think the proportion of basic living expenses in the total income is reasonable. Q31 I agree with the consumption mode that attaches importance to material life.
	Employment structure	Q32 I understand the social security system (medical, pension, employment, etc.) in my village. Q33 I am satisfied with the social security system (medical, pension, employment, etc.) in my village.
	Social security	Q34 I think the quality of the workers in the village is high. Q35 I think the non-agricultural industry in my village has absorbed more workers.
Happiness		Q36 My life is close to my ideal in many ways. Q37 My life goal is enough to give me the motivation to struggle. Q38 I feel happy when I devote myself to what I do. Q39 I think my work can bring positive influence to the development of my hometown.

References

1. Dekker, K.; de Vos, S.; Musterd, S.; van Kempen, R. Residential Satisfaction in Housing Estates in European Cities: A Multi-Level Research Approach. *Hous. Stud.* **2011**, *26*, 479–499. [CrossRef]
2. Bartram, D. Inverting the Logic of Economic Migration: Happiness among Migrants Moving from Wealthier to Poorer Countries in Europe. *J. Happiness Stud.* **2015**, *16*, 1211–1230. [CrossRef]
3. Arampatzi, E.; Burger, M.J.; Novik, N. Social Network Sites, Individual Social Capital and Happiness. *J. Happiness Stud.* **2018**, *19*, 99–122. [CrossRef]
4. Lu, H.; Tong, P.; Zhu, R. Longitudinal Evidence on Social Trust and Happiness in China: Causal Effects and Mechanisms. *J. Happiness Stud.* **2020**, *21*, 1841–1858. [CrossRef]
5. Zou, J.; Deng, X. The Complex Association between Migrants' Residential Community Choice and Subjective Well-Being: Evidence from Urban China. *Growth Chang.* **2021**, *52*, 1652–1679. [CrossRef]
6. Lichter, D.T.; Long, L. Migration and Residential Mobility in the United States. *Soc. Forces* **1990**, *68*, 991. [CrossRef]
7. Schultz, B.L.W. Sumner, Welfare, Happiness, and Ethics, Oxford, Clarendon Press, 1996, Pp. Xii + 239. *Utilitas* **2002**, *14*, 403–406. [CrossRef]
8. Cárdenas, M.; Mejía, C.; Di Maro, V. Education and Life Satisfaction: Perception or Reality? In *Paradox and Perception: Measuring Quality of Life in Latin America*; Graham, C., Ed.; Lora, E: Washington, DC, USA, 2009; ISBN 9780815703266.
9. Ryff, C.D. Psychological Well-Being Revisited: Advances in Science and Practice. *Psychother. Psychosom.* **2015**, *83*, 10–28. [CrossRef]

10. Bieda, A.; Hirschfeld, G.; Schönfeld, P.; Brailovskaia, J.; Lin, M.; Margraf, J. Happiness, Life Satisfaction and Positive Mental Health: Investigating Reciprocal Effects over Four Years in a Chinese Student Sample. *J. Res. Pers.* **2019**, *78*, 198–209. [CrossRef]
11. Naar, H. The Pursuit of Unhappiness: The Elusive Psychology of Well-Being. *Philos. Psychol.* **2012**, *25*, 307–310. [CrossRef]
12. Robinson, J.P.; Shaver, P.R. Measures of Social Psychological Attitudes. *Contemp. Sociol.* **1973**, *5*, 750.
13. Zheng, X.; Zhu, W.; Zhao, H.; Zhang, C. Employee Well-Being in Organizations: Theoretical Model, Scale Development, and Cross-Cultural Validation. *J. Organ. Behav.* **2015**, *36*, 621. [CrossRef]
14. Ram, R. Social Capital and Happiness: Additional Cross-Country Evidence. *J. Happiness Stud.* **2010**, *11*, 409–418. [CrossRef]
15. Thorbecke, E.; Babcock, H. Happiness and Economics. *J. Socio-Econ.* **2002**, *31*, 581–582. [CrossRef]
16. Diener, E.; Scollon, C. Subjective Well-Being Is Desirable, but Not the Summum Bonum. In *Interdisciplinary Workshop on Well-Being*; University of Minnesota: Minneapolis, MN, USA, 2003.
17. Gerdtham, U.G.; Johannesson, M. The Relationship between Happiness, Health, and Socio-Economic Factors: Results Based on Swedish Microdata. *J. Socio-Econ.* **2001**, *30*, 553–557. [CrossRef]
18. Clark, A.E.; Oswald, A.J. Unhappiness and Unemployment. *Econ. J.* **1994**, *104*, 648. [CrossRef]
19. Diener, E.; Biswas-Diener, R. Will Money Increase Subjective Well-Being? *Soc. Indic. Res.* **2002**, *57*, 119–169. [CrossRef]
20. Cramm, J.M.; Møller, V.; Nieboer, A.P. Individual- and Neighbourhood-Level Indicators of Subjective Well-Being in a Small and Poor Eastern Cape Township: The Effect of Health, Social Capital, Marital Status, and Income. *Soc. Indic. Res.* **2012**, *105*, 581–593. [CrossRef]
21. Knies, G.; Burgess, S.M.; Propper, C. Keeping Up with the Schmidts—An Empirical Test of Relative Deprivation Theory in the Neighbourhood Context. *SSRN Electron. J.* **2011**, *128*, 75–108. [CrossRef]
22. Knies, G. Income Comparisons Among Neighbours and Satisfaction in East and West Germany. *Soc. Indic. Res.* **2012**, *106*, 471–489. [CrossRef]
23. Ball, R.; Chernova, K. Absolute Income, Relative Income, and Happiness. *Soc. Indic. Res.* **2008**, *88*, 497–529. [CrossRef]
24. Dolan, P.; Peasgood, T.; White, M. Do We Really Know What Makes Us Happy? A Review of the Economic Literature on the Factors Associated with Subjective Well-Being. *J. Econ. Psychol.* **2008**, *29*, 94–122. [CrossRef]
25. Yip, W.; Subramanian, S.V.; Mitchell, A.D.; Lee, D.T.S.; Wang, J.; Kawachi, I. Does Social Capital Enhance Health and Well-Being? Evidence from Rural China. *Soc. Sci. Med.* **2007**, *64*, 35–49. [CrossRef]
26. Grootaert, C. Social Capital, Household Welfare and Poverty in Burkina Faso. *J. Afr. Econ.* **2002**, *11*, 4–38. [CrossRef]
27. Felix, R. Social Capital, Satisfaction and Quality of Life in the Workplace. *Soc. Indic. Res.* **2003**, *61*, 331–360.
28. Wilkinson, R.G.; Pickett, K.E. Income Inequality and Population Health: A Review and Explanation of the Evidence. *Soc. Sci. Med.* **2006**, *62*, 1768–1784. [CrossRef] [PubMed]
29. Chan, Y.K.; Lee, R.P.L. Network Size, Social Support and Happiness in Later Life: A Comparative Study of Beijing and Hong Kong. *J. Happiness Stud.* **2006**, *7*, 87–112. [CrossRef]
30. Gamble, A.; Gärling, T. The Relationships Between Life Satisfaction, Happiness, and Current Mood. *J. Happiness Stud.* **2012**, *13*, 31–45. [CrossRef]
31. Safi, M. Immigrants' Life Satisfaction in Europe: Between Assimilation and Discrimination. *Eur. Sociol. Rev.* **2009**, *26*, 159–176. [CrossRef]
32. Bartram, D. Happiness and 'Economic Migration': A Comparison of Eastern European Migrants and Stayers. *Migr. Stud.* **2013**, *1*, 156–175. [CrossRef]
33. Erlinghagen, M. Nowhere Better than Here? The Subjective Well-Being of German Emigrants and Remigrants. *Comp. Popul. Stud.* **2011**, *36*(4), 899–926. [CrossRef]
34. Sirgy, M.J.; Cornwell, T. How Neighborhood Features Affect Quality of Life. *Soc. Indic. Res.* **2002**, *59*, 79–114. [CrossRef]
35. Feijten, P.; Van Ham, M. Neighbourhood Change... Reason to Leave? *Urban Stud.* **2009**, *46*, 2103–2122. [CrossRef]
36. Hu, F. Homeownership and Subjective Wellbeing in Urban China: Does Owning a House Make You Happier? *Soc. Indic. Res.* **2013**, *110*, 951–971. [CrossRef]
37. Hu, M.; Ye, W. Home Ownership and Subjective Wellbeing: A Perspective from Ownership Heterogeneity. *J. Happiness Stud.* **2020**, *21*, 1059–1079. [CrossRef]
38. Zheng, X.; Yuan, Z.; Zhang, X. Does Happiness Dwell in an Owner-Occupied House? Homeownership and Subjective Well-Being in Urban China. *Cities* **2020**, *96*, 102404. [CrossRef]
39. Chen, J.; Qi, X.; Lin, Z.; Wu, Y. Impact of Governments' Commitment to Housing Affordability Policy on People's Happiness: Evidence from China. *Hous. Policy Debate* **2022**, *32*, 622–641. [CrossRef]
40. Liu, Y.; Zhang, F.; Liu, Y.; Li, Z.; Wu, F. The Effect of Neighbourhood Social Ties on Migrants' Subjective Wellbeing in Chinese Cities. *Habitat Int.* **2017**, *66*, 86–94. [CrossRef]
41. Zhao, Y. Causes and Consequences of Return Migration: Recent Evidence from China. *J. Comp. Econ.* **2002**, *30*, 376–394. [CrossRef]
42. Wang, W.W.; Fan, C.C. Success or Failure: Selectivity and Reasons of Return Migration in Sichuan and Anhui, China. *Environ. Planning. A* **2006**, *38*, 939–958. [CrossRef]
43. Lindstrom, D. Economic Opportunity in Mexico and Return Migration from the United States. *Demography* **1996**, *33*, 357–374. [CrossRef] [PubMed]
44. Spencer, H. *Social Statics: Together with The Man Versus the State*; Appleton, D. & Company, Ed.; American Psychological Association: Washington, DC, USA, 1892.

45. Meltzer, P.J. Using the Self-discovery Tapestry to Explore Occupational Careers. *J. Occup. Sci.* **2001**, *8*, 16–24. [CrossRef]
46. Wiedner, J.; Giesecke, J. Immigrant Men's Economic Adaptation in Changing Labor Markets: Why Gaps between Turkish and German Men Expanded, 1976–2015. *Int. Migr. Rev.* **2022**, *56*, 176–205. [CrossRef]
47. Irvine, J.; Firestone, J.; Ong, L.; Cribbie, R.; Dorian, P.; Harris, L.; Ritvo, P.; Katz, J.; Newman, D.; Cameron, D. A Randomized Controlled Trial of Cognitive Behavior Therapy Tailored to Psychological Adaptation to an Implantable Cardioverter Defibrillator. *Psychosom. Med.* **2011**, *73*, 226–233. [CrossRef]
48. Ang, S.; Van Dyne, L.; Koh, C.; Ng, K.Y.; Templer, K.J.; Tay, C.; Chandrasekar, N.A. Cultural Intelligence: Its Measurement and Effects on Cultural Judgment and Decision Making, Cultural Adaptation and Task Performance. *Manag. Organ. Rev.* **2007**, *3*, 335–371. [CrossRef]
49. Frey, B.S.; Stutzer, A. Happiness and Economics. In *Happiness and Economics*; Princeton University Press: Princeton, NJ, USA, 2010; ISBN 1400829267.
50. Chen, Y.; Wang, J. Social Integration of New-Generation Migrants in Shanghai China. *Habitat Int.* **2015**, *49*, 419–425. [CrossRef]

International Journal of
Environmental Research and Public Health

MDPI

Review

The Intellectual Structure of Research on Rural-to-Urban Migrants: A Bibliometric Analysis

Huichen Gao [1] and Shijuan Wang [2,*]

[1] School of Economics, Zhongnan University of Economics and Law, Wuhan 430073, China
[2] Faculty of Artificial Intelligence Education, Central China Normal University, Wuhan 430079, China
* Correspondence: wangshj143@ccnu.edu.cn

Abstract: As noted in the United Nations' Sustainable Development Goals 2030 agenda, sustainable cities "without leaving anyone behind" should take into consideration migrant groups, which may play only a marginal role but may be at the root of potential social conflicts. This study thereby promotes cross-disciplinary explorations of knowing and understanding the rural-to-urban internal migrants against the background of rapid urbanization. This study conducted a bibliometric analysis based on 2788 English language articles obtained from the Web of Science Core Collection database. As China's unique Hukou system highlights the divide between rural migrants and urban dwellers, migrant studies have extended to a diverse range of interests. We underlined the most productive sources and authors in this area and identified networks of collaboration among countries and institutions. Furthermore, we found trends in research themes and topics and research clusters through keyword-based analysis techniques. The results provide a rich source of information on the intellectual structure of the chosen domain of rural-to-urban migrants.

Keywords: rural-to-urban migrant; bibliometric analysis; performance analysis; science mapping; network analysis

Citation: Gao, H.; Wang, S. The Intellectual Structure of Research on Rural-to-Urban Migrants: A Bibliometric Analysis. *IJERPH* **2022**, *19*, 9729. https://doi.org/10.3390/ijerph19159729

Academic Editors: Jie Chen, Qian Zhou and Ting Zhang

Received: 30 June 2022
Accepted: 5 August 2022
Published: 7 August 2022

1. Introduction

In this era of accelerating globalization and rapid urbanization, cities and metropolitan areas play an essential role in pooling resources and providing opportunities for people to prosper both economically and socially. With a global share of the world population that is projected to reach 68% in 2050, urbanized areas are experiencing challenges in meeting the growing demand for public services while maintaining a sustainable environment for present and future generations [1]. Yet massive influxes of capital and preferential policies have created uneven economic development between rural and urban areas (as seen in China's dual economy), helping drive migration to cities [2–4]. As noted in the United Nations' Sustainable Development Goals (SDG) 2030 agenda, sustainable cities "without leaving anyone behind" should take into consideration migrant groups, which may play only a marginal role but may be at the root of potential social conflicts [5]. As a cross-cutting issue on the SDG 2030 agenda, migration is attracting the attention of researchers from multiple disciplines, and it poses novel challenges to the public and policymakers at both the national and international levels [6]. COVID-19 has sounded the alarm and drawn additional attention to unmet health needs within migrant communities [7]. Our research provides a lens to examine a particular group of migrants, namely, rural-to-urban internal migrants. Previous studies on migrant groups in urban wards cover a broad spectrum of themes and topics across disciplines, providing a vivid but fractional profile of this group of people [8,9]. Since the application of bibliometric methods in migration research is relatively new, we consider that it might be a good time to conduct an analysis with newly developed tools such as VOSviewer to interpret the intellectual structures of research on rural-to-urban migrants. This study thereby promotes cross-disciplinary explorations of knowing and understanding the migrant population against the background of rapid urbanization.

The article presents a bibliometric analysis aimed at sketching the outline of knowledge related to rural-to-urban migration at the initial stage (Sections 3.1 and 3.2). The social structure and collaboration patterns are then identified using network analysis based on co-authorship data (Section 3.3). Then, bibliometric analysis results allowed another analysis to be conducted to examine the coupling network of the documents and the co-citation network of references, which aids in mapping current areas of focus and landmark studies from the past (Section 3.4). This is followed by a keywords network analysis in Section 3.5, which briefly describes keyword frequency and three distinct subsections: keyword co-occurrence network analysis, thematic analysis, and conceptual structure analysis. Finally, the findings and policy implications are summarized.

2. Research Methodology

Researchers have applied this comprehensive science mapping approach to multiple domains, such as rural depopulation [10] and urban agriculture [11] since Aria and Cuccurullo [12] published the bibliometrix R-package. This one-of-a-kind open-source tool developed in R language offers a wide range of statistical and graphical techniques and a user-friendly web-interface application called Biblioshiny. As demonstrated by Rogers et al. [13], data collected for bibliometric analysis are typically massive. A bibliometric analysis of 200 papers appears to be a reasonable threshold to employ a bibliometric analysis. The bibliometric analysis applied in this research is conducted using the bibliometrix package (version 3.2.1), built in R (version 4.1.3). VOSviewer (version 1.6.18) is a well-developed visualization tool for building and viewing bibliometric networks [14]. When a "net" object is created in the R Programming Environment, VOSviewer functions using internal R routines.

The bibliographic data for this study were collected on 3 June 2022, from the Web of Science (WOS) Core Collection database, including indices of SCIE, SSCI, AHCI, ESCI, CPCI, BKCI and CCR&IC, provided by Clarivate within the indexed timespan from 1 January 2004 to 3 June 2022. Using the topic keyword "rural urban migrant" (the topic keywords are generated by Clarivate from the title, abstract, author keywords, and Keywords Plus) and filtering by English language and the document type "article," we obtained a total of 2790 publications in the first stage. After removing duplicates, 2788 papers remained. Each document's full record and cited references are exported for the bibliometric analysis.

3. Results and Discussion

3.1. Descriptive Bibliometric Analysis

As shown in Table 1, since 2004, 2788 articles have been published in this specific field in 1006 venues. Excluding 2022, the annual growth rate over this period is 13.61% (Figure 1). The total citations per article reached a peak of 68.1 in 2007, and the total number of references was 98860. Overall, 5626 author keywords and 3624 Keywords Plus were generated. As shown in Figure 1, the increase in publications since 2010 is noticeable, despite a slight decline in the years 2012–2013.

Statistical analysis was conducted based on Lotka's law, which measures the frequency distribution of scientific productivity [15]. Simply put, Lotka's Law states that there is a consistent ratio between the number of authors publishing a certain number of papers and the number of authors who publish a single one. The results show that the distribution of author frequency and number of publications follows Lotka's Law ($R^2 = 0.920$, p-value = 0.006). In all, 4546 authors contributed to one article each, accounting for 78.9% of all authors; of the remainder, 641 authors contributed to two articles (11.1%), 239 to three (4.1%), 113 to four (2.0%), and 222 to five or more articles (3.9%) regarding the topic addressed by this study. Figure 2 shows a Sankey diagram that presents a visualization of the connections between the main items of three fields, namely, authors, author keywords, and sources. We find that "China" and "Ghana" are two popular areas of research interest. A detailed description is given next.

Table 1. Primary information and summary of the dataset.

Description	Results
Timespan	1 January 2004–3 June 2022
Sources	1006
Documents	2788
Average years from publication	6.07
Average citations per document	17.05
Average citations per year per doc	2.123
References	98,860
DOCUMENT CONTENTS	
Keywords Plus	3624
Author's Keywords	5626
AUTHORS	
Authors	5761
Author Appearances	9167
Authors of single-authored documents	602
Authors of multi-authored documents	5159
AUTHORS COLLABORATION	
Single-authored documents	702
Documents per Author	0.484
Authors per Document	2.07
Co-Authors per Documents	3.29
Collaboration Index	2.47
International co-authorships %	38.2

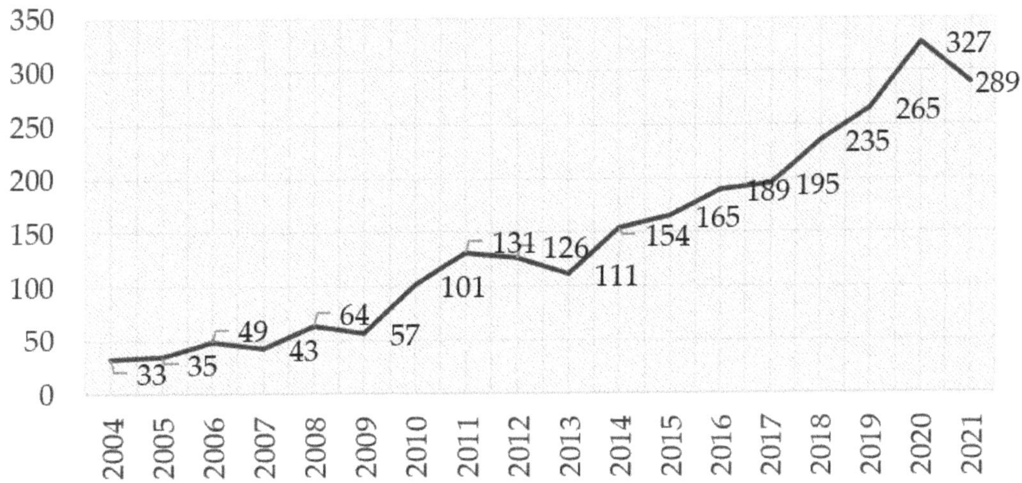

Figure 1. Number of articles published on the topic of rural-to-urban migrants from 2004 to 2021.

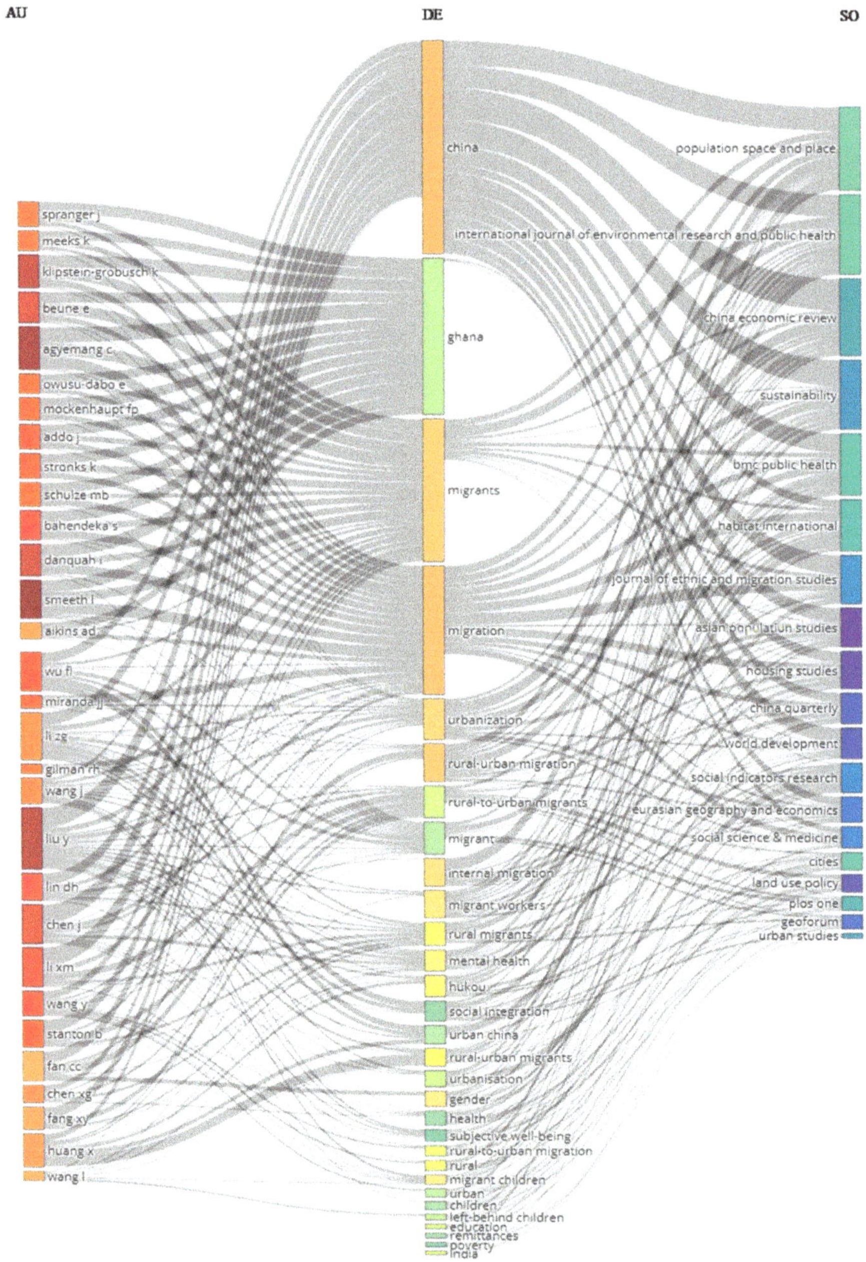

Figure 2. A Sankey diagram showing authors (AU), author keywords (DE), and sources (SO).

3.2. *Top Sources*

A Bradford analysis was conducted (Figure 3), and from 1006 sources, 37 core scientific journals were identified, marked as Zone 1 [16]. Zones 2 and 3 contain 203 and 766 sources, respectively. Each zone carries an equal number of citations.

The top 10 high-yield journals from Zone 1 are listed in Table 2, accounting for 17.8% of the total number of publications and 22% of the total citations. These are primarily international interdisciplinary journals covering multiple topics, such as occupational health and urban planning. H-indexes are not used to compare the sources in our analysis because different disciplines' citation traditions and methods vary.

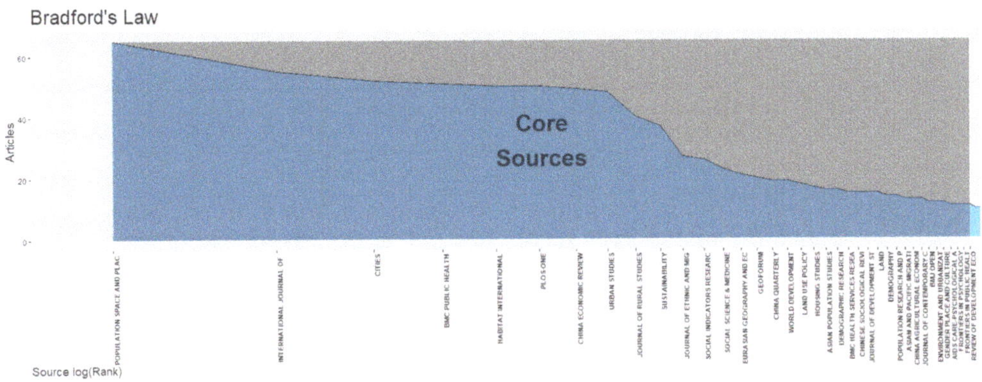

Figure 3. Core sources on the topic of rural-to-urban migrants (1 January 2004–3 June 2022).

Table 2. Top 10 journals with the most articles published on the topic of rural-to-urban migrants (1 January 2004–3 June 2022).

Journal	JCR Category	N. of Documents	Total Citations
POPULATION SPACE AND PLACE	- DEMOGRAPHY - GEOGRAPHY	65	1171
INTERNATIONAL JOURNAL OF ENVIRONMENTAL RESEARCH AND PUBLIC HEALTH	- PUBLIC, ENVIRONMENTAL and OCCUPATIONAL HEALTH - ENVIRONMENTAL SCIENCES	55	317
CITIES	- URBAN STUDIES	52	908
BMC PUBLIC HEALTH	- PUBLIC, ENVIRONMENTAL and OCCUPATIONAL HEALTH	51	1142
HABITAT INTERNATIONAL	- URBAN STUDIES - DEVELOPMENT STUDIES - REGIONAL and URBAN PLANNING - ENVIRONMENTAL STUDIES	50	2125
PLOS ONE	- MULTIDISCIPLINARY SCIENCES	50	946
CHINA ECONOMIC REVIEW	- ECONOMICS	49	1489
URBAN STUDIES	- URBAN STUDIES - ENVIRONMENTAL STUDIES	48	1420
JOURNAL OF RURAL STUDIES	- REGIONAL and URBAN PLANNING - GEOGRAPHY	40	806
SUSTAINABILITY	- ENVIRONMENTAL STUDIES - GREEN and SUSTAINABLE SCIENCE and TECHNOLOGY - ENVIRONMENTAL SCIENCES - TECHNOLOGY	37	123

3.3. Social Structure

3.3.1. Active Countries

Papers have been published by scholars from 76 countries (counting only the corresponding author's country) since 2004, and this number reaches 93 if co-authors are taken into account. Table 3 shows the countries with the highest output based on the frequency distribution of the corresponding author's affiliation country. China has the leading position, with 1035 papers, accounting for 37.4% of all published papers, followed by the United States (528 papers, 19.5%) and the United Kingdom (241 papers, 8.7%). The United Kingdom and the United States rank second (24.78) and third (23.64), respectively, in terms of average citations per article, while India has a relatively low frequency (7.35).

Table 3. Top 10 countries with the highest number of papers.

Country	Articles	Freq	SCP *	MCP **	MCP Ratio	Total Citations	Citations per Article
CHINA	1035	37.4%	657	378	0.365	14,878	14.37
USA	538	19.5%	328	210	0.390	12,720	23.64
UNITED KINGDOM	241	8.7%	132	109	0.452	5973	24.78
AUSTRALIA	137	5.0%	86	51	0.372	2416	17.64
NETHERLANDS	87	3.1%	35	52	0.598	1480	17.01
INDIA	71	2.6%	59	12	0.169	522	7.35
GERMANY	67	2.4%	46	21	0.313	1175	17.54
CANADA	62	2.2%	34	28	0.452	1171	18.89
SOUTH AFRICA	37	1.3%	27	10	0.270	593	16.03
SINGAPORE	34	1.2%	25	9	0.265	356	10.47
SWEDEN	34	1.2%	23	11	0.324	505	14.85

* SCP: Single Country Publication; ** MCP: Multiple Country Publication.

3.3.2. Active Institutions

Since 2004, 1973 institutions have engaged in the study of rural-to-urban migrants. Table 4 lists the top 10 high-yield institutions according to the number of publications, of which eight are from China. A collaboration network analysis is performed, using the affiliations of each co-author and corresponding author. The degree of centrality, the number of relational ties an objective has in a network, is calculated to enrich the bibliometric assessment of institutional cooperation [17]. The collaboration patterns among institutions presented in Figure 4 identify two major networks in this field: roughly defined, one is based in China and one is based in Europe. It should be noted that the large number of publications originating in China (1035, 37.4% of total) makes it a dominant player within the global network.

Table 4. Top 10 institutions in the field of rural-to-urban migrants (1 January 2004–3 June 2022).

Affiliations	Country	Articles
Sun Yat-sen University	China	124
Beijing Normal University	China	109
Peking University	China	97
Fudan University	China	83
London School of Hygiene and Tropical Medicine	UK	82
Chinese University of Hong Kong	China	81
University of Hong Kong	China	76
University of Amsterdam	The Netherlands	75
Renmin University of China	China	68
Zhejiang University	China	65

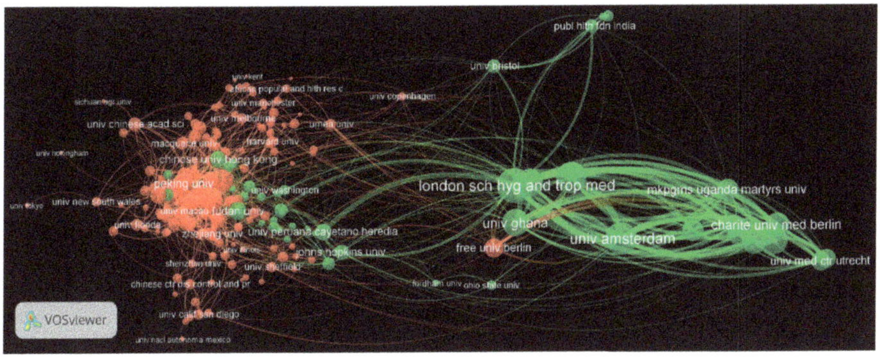

Figure 4. Network of institutional cooperation.

Moreover, a closer look at papers from the London School of Hygiene and Tropical Medicine, the fifth-ranking institution of origination, shows that its research interests are mainly centered on the health issues of residents of or migrants from sub-Saharan African countries. Work involving the Research on Obesity and Diabetes among African Migrants is an example of this (e.g., [18]). The League of European Research Universities, such as the University of Amsterdam and Utrecht University, can also be found within these networks, collaborating with African institutions, e.g., the University of Ghana and the University of the Witwatersrand.

3.3.3. Active Authors

Figure 5 shows 20 active authors in this field, including statistical data on the number of articles published per year by each and total citations each year. All of these authors have conducted long-term research on the topic of rural-to-urban migrants for 8–19 years. For example, Professor Liam Smeeth at the London School of Hygiene and Tropical Medicine has published papers on the topic (51 articles were identified in this study) since 2009; Professor Fulong Wu at University College London, whose interests include rural migrants in urban China, has maintained a productive research career (having published 27 articles found in this study) that spans the entire period covered by this study.

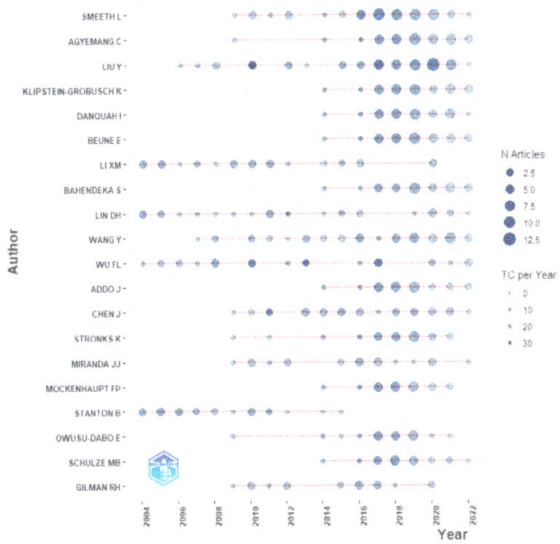

Figure 5. Top 20 authors' productivity on the topic of rural-to-urban migrants (1 January 2004–3 June 2022).

3.4. Most-Cited Articles

The analysis in this section uses the bibliometrix R-package to detect the historical roots of the set topic by examining each document's bibliography [19]. The results identify references as far back as the 18th century, e.g., [20]. The historical studies uncovered by this research explore regional imbalances, migration movements in the old times, and the spread of disease that accompanies the population flow [21–23].

Because the term for the articles retrieved from the WOS Core Collection database for this study is after 2004, the analysis of bibliographic coupling is of more help for mapping current fronts on which research is expanding than identifying schools of thought over time [24]. Thus, a co-citation analysis is provided to improve our understanding of any paradigm shift that lies in the references [25]. In simple terms, we analyze both the retrieved documents and their references to map current areas of focus and landmark studies from the past.

Table 5 shows the top 10 works for each category. In general, these are high-value nodes connected with other nodes in the coupling network or the co-citation network. Once again, studies of contemporary China have made a significant contribution to our understanding of urbanization and migration, raising concerns about the lack of a global perspective.

Table 5. Top 10 locally cited documents and references on the topic of rural-to-urban migrants (1 January 2004–3 June 2022).

	Cited Journal	LC *
Most Local Cited Documents		
Rural migrant workers in urban China: living a marginalized life [26]	International Journal of Social Welfare	123
China's floating population and their settlement intention in the cities: Beyond the Hukou reform [27]	Habitat International	92
Internal migration and health: re examining the healthy migrant phenomenon in China [28]	Social Science and Medicine	75
The Household Registration System and Migrant Labor in China: Notes on a Debate [29]	Population and Development Review	71
Circular migration, or permanent stay? Evidence from China's rural–urban migration [30]	China Economic Review	68
Migrants as second-class workers in urban China? A decomposition analysis [31]	Journal of Comparative Economics	66
Settlement Intention and Split Households: Findings from a Survey of Migrants in Beijing's Urban Villages [32]	China Review	65
The mental health status of Chinese rural–urban migrant workers [33]	Social Psychiatry and Psychiatric Epidemiology	59
The social networks of new-generation migrants in China's urbanized villages: A case study of Guangzhou [34]	Habitat International	58
Urban villages under China's rapid urbanization: Unregulated assets and transitional neighborhoods [35]	Habitat International	57
Most Local Cited References		
The Hukou System and Rural-Urban Migration in China: Processes and Changes [36]	China Quarterly	182
Contesting Citizenship in Urban China: Peasant Migrants, the State, and the Logic of the Market [37]	University of California Press	180
Is China Abolishing the Hukou System? [38]	China Quarterly	151
Rural migrant workers in urban China: living a marginalized life [26]	International Journal of Social Welfare	123
Migration, Unemployment and Development: A Two-Sector Analysis [39]	American Economic Review	120
The Two-Tier Labor Market in Urban China: Occupational Segregation and Wage Differentials between Urban Residents and Rural Migrants in Shanghai [40]	Journal of Comparative Economics	115
The Chinese Hukou System at 50 [41]	Eurasian Geography and Economics	110
The Elite, the Natives, and the Outsiders: Migration and Labor Market Segmentation in Urban China [42]	Annals of the American Association of Geographers	101
The settlement intention of China's floating population in the cities: recent changes and multifaceted individual-level determinants [43]	Population, Space and Place	98
The New Economics of Labor Migration [44]	American Economic Review	96

* LC: local citations.

3.5. *Keywords Network Analysis*

Keywords analysis is a core method in bibliometric analysis, due to the high degree of clarification and identification it provides, enabling a new approach to tracing the evolution of a discipline and determining the structure of a scientific field [45,46]. The results of the keywords network analysis are presented as follows.

3.5.1. Keyword Frequency

As shown in Figure 6, keyword frequency is measured and demonstrated using the word cloud technique. Given that the database was created through a topic search using "rural urban migrant" as a keyword phrase, we removed prominent high-frequency words that appear in or are closely related to this phrase (rural-to-urban, migrant, migration, etc.) to allow others to surface.

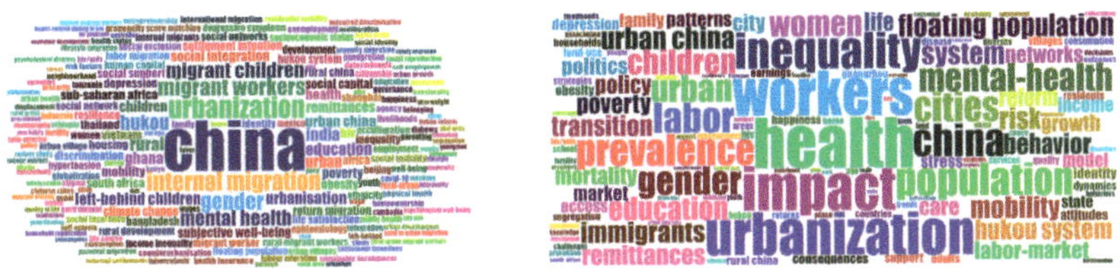

(a) (b)

Figure 6. Word cloud of ranking distribution with author keywords (**a**) and Keywords Plus (**b**).

Both figures indicate where the research focus falls, although the one derived from the author's keywords shows a higher concentration of research on China, a relatively high concentration, which is easy to understand, due to the rapid and widespread urbanization that has been taking place in China over the past couple of years. The word cloud derived from Keyword Plus indicates a diverse range of research interests, such as those regarding left-behind children, gender inequality, and mental health.

A keyword co-occurrence analysis (presented in Figure 7) using R and the visualization tool VOSviewer provides a co-occurrence network picture of the keyword universe and a much deeper understanding of the interaction dynamics of the field of migrant research [47,48]. Keyword Plus terms are used as inputs for the analysis because they are more broadly descriptive than author keywords [49]. Social inequality and physical and mental health are two major areas of migrant studies. A more detailed discussion of research clusters on rural-to-urban migrants is given in the following section, enhanced by a conceptual structure map.

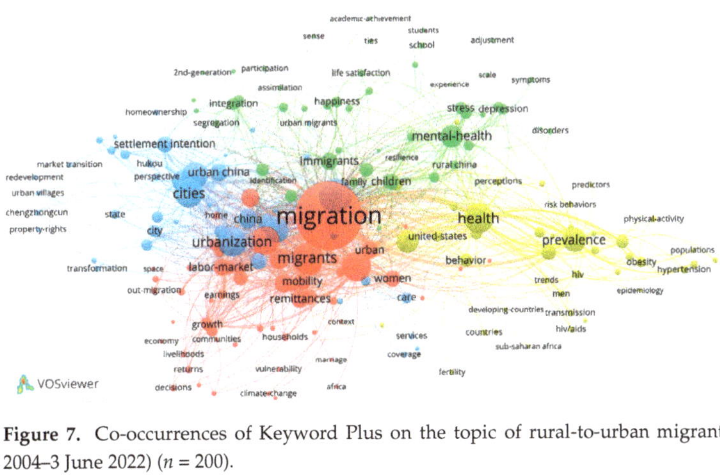

Figure 7. Co-occurrences of Keyword Plus on the topic of rural-to-urban migrants (1 January 2004–3 June 2022) ($n = 200$).

3.5.2. Trend Topics and Thematic Map

An analysis of trend topics provides further information on timelines and represents a knowledge transfer between topics at different periods [50]. Figure 8 presents a profile of research trajectories in the migrant research literature, from disease prevalence as the population moves, to labor market dynamics and interactions, and to settlement intention and social integration.

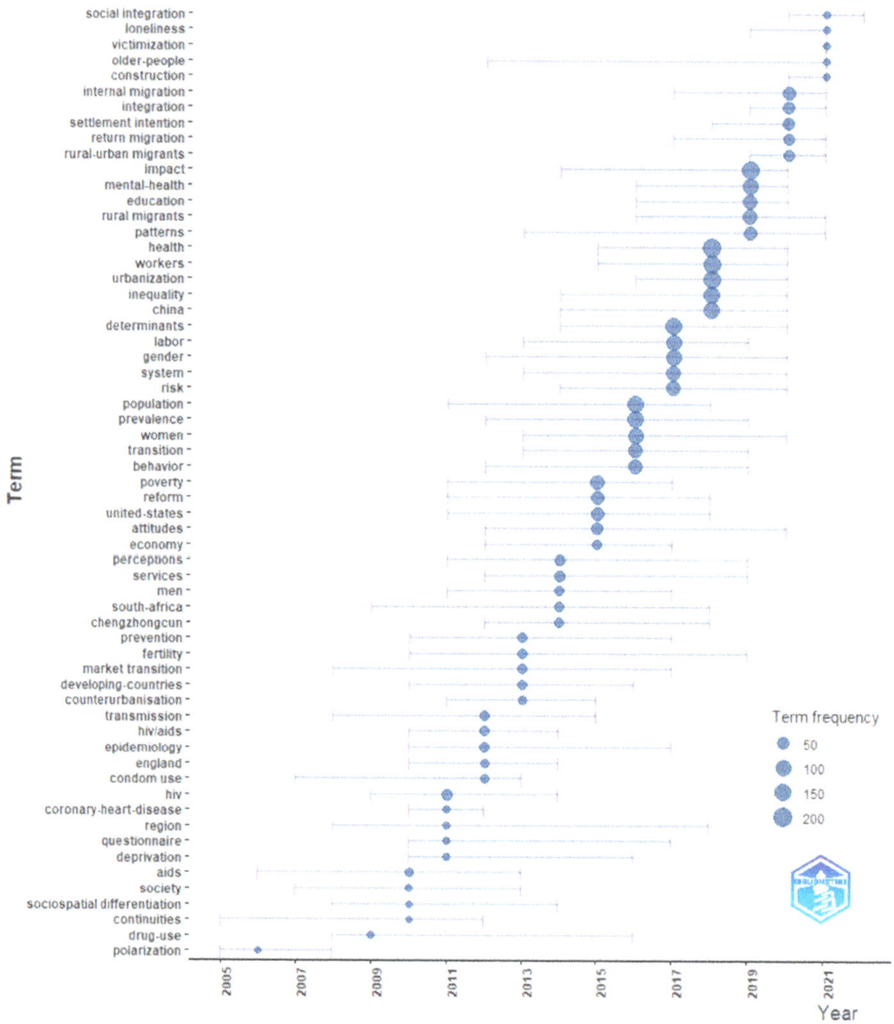

Figure 8. Trend topics of studies on rural-to-urban migrants (1 January 2004–3 June 2022).

Co-word analysis is performed across the entire period to detect and visualize specific themes, and bibliometric measures, such as the h-index, are used to evaluate the performance of each theme [51]. In other words, thematic evolution is examined by combining the performances of specific themes identified by co-word analysis at various subperiods. In the following step, two measures, Callon's centrality ($c = 10 \times \sum e_{kh}$ with e the equivalence index, k a local keyword, and h a keyword from other themes) and Callon's density ($d = 100 \sum \frac{e_{ij}}{w}$ with e the equivalence index, i and j both local keywords and w the number of keywords in the theme), are taken to measure the strength of external ties, that is, a theme to other themes and the internal strength of a particular theme, respectively [48,52]. Accordingly, we include a thematic analysis based on the frequency of co-occurrence of word pairs to examine the difficulties of specific research themes in this area and map them in a two-dimensional space based on their centrality and density.

As indicated in Figure 9, the diagram contains four quadrants: in the first, motor themes are recognized as developed and necessary with high centrality and density (Quadrant I); in the second, niche themes are developed and isolated from other themes (Quadrant II); in the third, emerging or declining themes show low centrality and density, or in other words, they are underdeveloped and marginal (Quadrant III); and in the fourth, basic themes appear that have a low degree of development (Quadrant IV) [53,54]. The themes of this study are mainly found in Quadrants I and III, reflecting two trends: (1) themes specifically related to the labor market are currently receiving less attention, while studies on gender and youth migration may emerge as a niche research field, e.g., [55], and (2) themes related to mental and physical health, as well as the acculturation and social integration of migrants and their family members, form the very essence of migrant studies. We argue that China's growing academic influence and its unique social structure play an essential role in shifting the center of collective intelligence and guiding both internal and external attention.

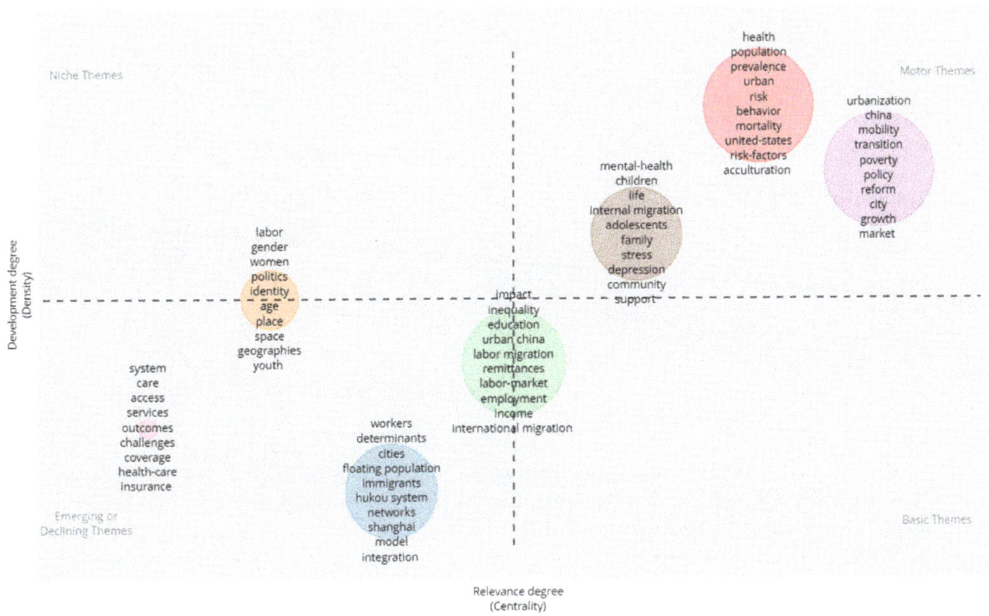

Figure 9. Thematic map of rural-to-urban migrant studies (1 January 2004–3 June 2022).

3.5.3. Conceptual Structure Map

The multiple correspondence analysis (MCA) method's built-in R was applied for the generation of a conceptual structure map (Figure 10) [56,57]. We set the minimum occurrences of author keywords to 15. The analysis identified four main clusters: (1) the green cluster, denoting China's Hukou system and its institutional impact; (2) the red cluster, indicating discrimination and social integration; (3) the blue cluster, which refers to health and well-being; and (4) the purple cluster, centering on epidemiology. The details of each cluster drawn from the documents that contain the highest contributions are provided as follows.

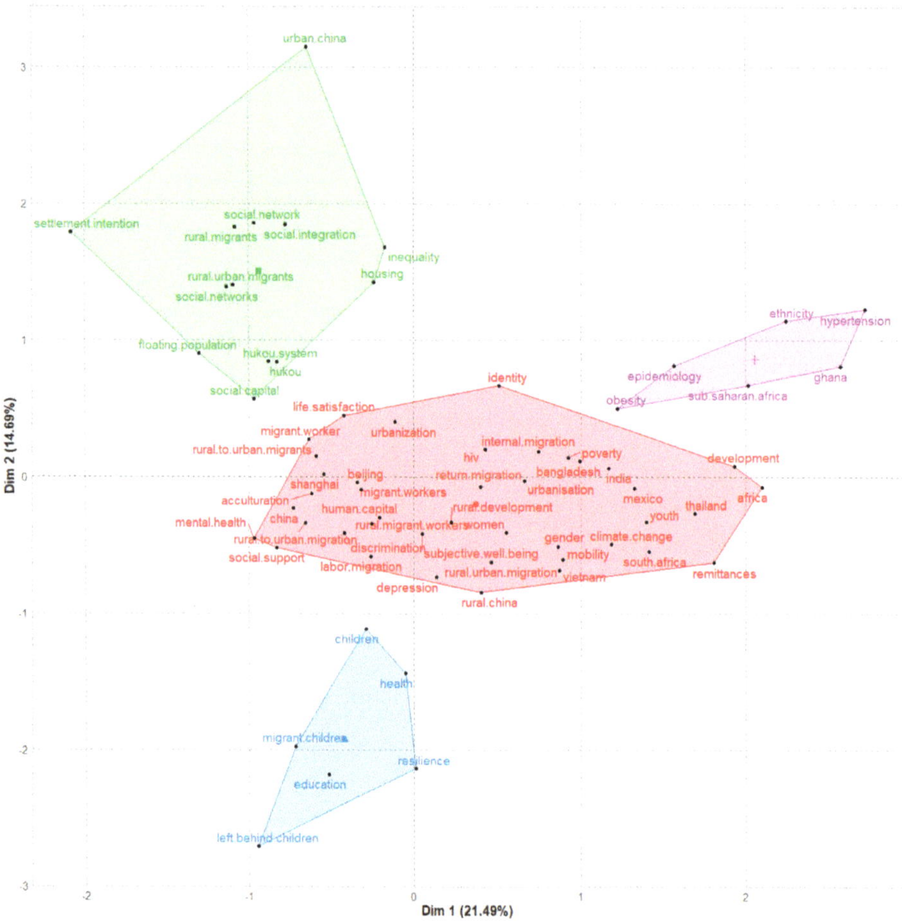

Figure 10. Conceptual structure map of rural-to-urban migrant studies (1 January 2004–3 June 2022).

Green cluster: China's Hukou system and its institutional impact. Attention was drawn to the urban development of China as millions of peasants migrated to its metropolises seeking employment and residence. The reasons for their decisions were studied by researchers working from diverse perspectives, such as analyzing the environmental differences between rural and urban localities, e.g., [58,59] and profiling migrants' demographic characteristics, e.g., [43]. When the Hukou system was established, a boundary was created between China's urban-dwelling migrants and its native urbanites. The Hukou classification scheme divides China's population by residential location and socioeconomic eligibility and features a birth-subscribed orientation [37]. These factors have made the conversion of Hukou registration far from a matter of personal choice [36,42,60].

The divide instituted by the state leads to parallel networks of urban rights and distribution of benefits to the urban peasants and their native urban neighbors [61]. Furthermore, a study found that migrant older people have less access to various well-being resources than urban residents due to residential segregation caused by Hukou's institutional constraints [62]. Concerns about socio-spatial inequalities are echoed in an air pollution study that reveals migrant groups bore a disproportionate share of Beijing's declining air quality from 2000 to 2010 [63]. As the burden of commuting differs between employees with and without a local Hukou, institutional discrimination arises; the former may exercise their right in terms of accommodation provided by the work unit. Individuals' housing and employment decisions reflect this inequality [64].

The disparity between the two groups might already have been present in the pre-market period due to the unequal educational opportunities available [31]. Despite the increasingly available option of converting to urban Hukou, migrants' intention to convert their Hukou remains at a low level for several reasons, not least of which is an unwillingness to abandon farmland [65].

Given that the Hukou system has long been China's central institutional mechanism for shaping the rural-urban and state-society relationships, its complexity was addressed in a range of studies. Topics are covered in multiple areas, including trends and developments, e.g., [41], reforms and changes, e.g., [29,38], and practical conditions and limitations, e.g., [27,66,67].

Red cluster: Discrimination and social integration. Findings on occupational segregation and wage differentials between rural migrants and urban residents imply the existence of discrimination against rural groups [40]. Furthermore, policing practices intended to ensure equal justice may lead to the mistreatment of rural migrants in an urban setting [68]. Social discrimination and unfair treatment even impact migrant children, who generally benefit from family unity in the city [69]. Nonetheless, according to Goodburn [70], migrant children in state schools face discrimination from classmates, teachers, and parents of local students. Meanwhile, private schools established by migrant communities face significant strain as a result of tensions between the state and China's emerging civil society. However, other factors that contribute to the rural–urban divide should not be overlooked, such as "distance from home," which makes the "digital invisible" circular migrants [71] and "irrational expectations," which lowers rural–urban migrant households' subjective well-being [72].

The term "floating population" emphasizes that a certain number of urban migrants consider their adventure in the city to be a temporary strategy, the result of multiple factors, such as the uncertainties of the temporary work labor market [27]. Studies of urban villages, a type of urban neighborhood containing urbanized villagers and migrant workers in various proportions, reinforce the notion that for migrant workers, the city is a workplace rather than a home [35,73]. Circulating between urban work and rural homes is a long-term practice among rural Chinese [32]. Non-kin resident ties (social ties between migrants and local urban residents) play an essential role in community integration [74,75]. In addition to social capital, cultural adaptability and financial resources are crucial for the integration of migrants' identity [76]. The choice of permanent migration often falls as an optimal combination of various options (distance from home, income stability, etc.) [30].

Generational factors should not be ignored when discussing settlement decisions, as the younger generation of migrants shows greater activity in speeding up their integration into the urban network [34]. Policymakers should recognize newcomers' needs across a broad spectrum of issues, including housing and social insurance; on the other hand, the role of an urban society, where multiple players such as nongovernment organizations can play their part in social integration [77,78].

Blue cluster: Health and well-being. The very nature of a floating labor force raises concerns about health risks to migrants, ranging from occupational disease and injury to infectious diseases and maternal health. Studies also found a positive correlation between high mobility and sexual risk among migrants, as well as an increase in cardiovascular disease, obesity, and diabetes associated with migration into urban areas [79–81]. Despite numerous health risks, migrant workers have a lower health insurance rate than the average due to disadvantaged socioeconomic status [82]. Meanwhile, various forms of abuse of female migrant workers can be found across nations [83,84].

Several studies have identified the importance of targeting mental health promotion and mental disorder prevention in the migrant population [28,85]. Taking a broader lens, Wong et al. [26] provide a deeper understanding of rural migrants' marginalized living experience and its psychosocial impacts on their lives. Attention to issues of mental health and risk perception is needed, due to the complex challenges that migrants are facing, especially younger migrants, known as the second-generation rural migrants, as "youth mining (conscious and unconscious trading of future ill health for present economic opportunities) is a prevalent behavior in migrant populations" [86] (p. 1718). Migration during childhood may contribute to an increased rate of first-episode psychosis [87]. Nevertheless, poor mental health is not necessarily a problem if everyone enjoys an equal likelihood of upward economic mobility, and social capital is relatively high within migrant communities [33].

On the other side, children left behind by one or both of their migrant parents, especially the mother, may suffer disadvantages expressed in their health behavior and school engagement [88,89]. According to studies, school-age children who are left behind experience more victimization and emotional distress, as well as higher anxiety and depression [90,91]. Unsurprisingly, left-behind wives and elders have a lower health-related quality of life [92,93]. Adhikari et al. [94] proposed understanding the differences in healthcare-seeking behavior between the elderly with children present and the elderly left behind to improve the elderly's physical health.

Purple cluster: Epidemiology. Health services are among the most crucial of all the resources designed to help maintain a growing urban population for the success of the system [95]. Migrating to urban areas generally means a better chance of getting healthcare. Yet a link between urbanization and extended epidemics was suggested, where migration might be the trigger [96]. Due to their demographic characteristics of high mobility, lack of education, and low socioeconomic status, migrant groups are considered to be vulnerable to epidemic diseases. During the coronavirus disease 2019 pandemic, Singapore's lessons highlight the high potential for disease transmission within migrant worker dormitories [97]. At the same time, the increasing populations of rural-to-urban migrants have put a heavy burden on epidemic control (e.g., tuberculosis control) in cities, and migrants' lack of perception of a need for treatment appears to be a barrier to disease control [98,99]. Apart from the vulnerability of the group itself, the low level of knowledge about epidemics among the general public also contributes to delays in seeking care [100]. However, an increasing number of circular labor migrants who become ill at work and return home to obtain care hints at a need to reconsider the distribution and allocation of healthcare resources [101].

The findings of the study highlight the importance of studying mental illness from an epidemiological standpoint. Saha et al. [102] argued that migrant status is an important risk factor for the increased prevalence of schizophrenia after reviewing 15 migrant studies from eight countries. Moreover, migrant adolescents who struggle to form culturally integrated friendships in school are more likely to have mental health problems [103]. Bhugra et al. [104] emphasized the importance of using epidemiological data to map cultural inconsistency and ethnic density.

Race and ethnicity play a role in epidemiologic studies, not only because people from different racial and ethnic minority groups have different health statuses and health outcomes but also because certain social determinants, such as inequalities and inequities, exist and pose a challenge to the delivery of better public health services [105,106].

As noted, at least four clusters were identified with the MCA method. However, these clusters were not isolated from each other but were entangled from different perspectives. The discussion is open to additional possibilities because the MCA graphics vary with different settings, such as in different keyword stemming fields, and any interpretation of the variables and their interactions must be subject to the author's limitations.

4. Conclusions

This study conducted a bibliometric analysis and had selected results mapped based on 2788 English articles obtained from the WOS Core Collection database. These results provide a rich source of information on the intellectual structure of the chosen domain of rural-to-urban migrants. Using the bibliometrix R-package and VOSviewer, our bibliometric analysis results allowed for network analysis, a document coupling analysis, a reference co-citation analysis, a co-occurrence network analysis, a thematic analysis, and a conceptual structure analysis based on keyword interactions. Efforts were made to promote cross-disciplinary explorations of knowing and understanding the migrant population against the background of fast-growing urbanization.

As China's unique Hukou system highlights the divide between rural migrants and urban dwellers, migrant studies have extended to a diverse range of interests. We underlined the most productive sources and authors in this area and identified networks of collaboration among countries and institutions among them. Furthermore, we found trends in research themes and topics and research clusters through keyword-based analysis techniques. From disease prevalence as the population moves to labor market dynamics and interactions, to settlement intention and social integration, research trajectories in the migrant research literature are profiled. The ups and downs of specific research themes in this area are examined, and four major cross-disciplinary clusters provide a comprehensive and detailed description of this group of people. The following are some suggestions for future study regarding rural-to-urban migrants:

- It should be noted that population registration systems such as the Hukou system in China are capable of serving multiple interests, that is, they do more than function as an administrative tool to monitor their residents;
- Migrants' decisions on whether to stay, circulate, or leave the city vary, creating a dynamic environment, and posing challenges for their family and community networks;
- More effort into researching the social determinants of migration and health is required.

Although migration studies may be subject to selection bias due to unobserved characteristics that vary over time and space, a bibliometric analysis may shed light on effective policy interventions to promote migrant livelihood improvement. Policymakers must recognize the value of families and communities in providing a support network for migrants and those who were left behind. Furthermore, occupation-specific medical policies and affordable health insurance are required, as is attention to the digital divide in the information age. Last but not least, potential institutional impacts must be assessed to prevent systemic discrimination and violence against migrant groups.

This study has several limitations. First, further analysis applied to data obtained from multiple sources, such as the Scopus database, could lead to a broader and deeper interpretation of this topic, as we only used data collected from the WOS Core Collection. Second, this study focuses on urban ward migrations, most of which occur in the domestic context, leaving the cross-border population (e.g., immigrants and refugees) out of the picture. Finally, a keyword-based conceptual analysis might only provide a broad but shallow interpretation of the intellectual structure, which could be enhanced by combining it with a systematic review approach.

Author Contributions: Conceptualization, H.G. and S.W.; methodology, H.G. and S.W.; software, H.G.; validation, H.G. and S.W.; formal analysis, H.G.; investigation, H.G.; resources, H.G.; data curation, H.G.; writing—original draft preparation, H.G.; writing—review and editing, H.G. and S.W.; visualization, H.G.; supervision, S.W.; project administration, H.G. and S.W.; All authors have read and agreed to the published version of the manuscript.

Funding: This research received no external funding.

Informed Consent Statement: Not applicable.

Data Availability Statement: The data that support the findings of this study are available from the corresponding author, S. Wang, upon reasonable request.

Conflicts of Interest: The authors declare no conflict of interest.

References

1. United Nations Department of Economics and Social Affairs. *World Urbanization Prospects: The 2018 Revision (ST/ESA/SER.A/420)*; United Nations: New York, NY, USA, 2019.
2. Chen, C.; LeGates, R.; Zhao, M.; Fang, C. The Changing Rural-Urban Divide in China's Megacities. *Cities* **2018**, *81*, 81–90. [CrossRef]
3. Seto, K.C. Exploring the Dynamics of Migration to Mega-Delta Cities in Asia and Africa: Contemporary Drivers and Future Scenarios. *Glob. Environ. Change* **2011**, *21*, S94–S107. [CrossRef]
4. Valerio Mendoza, O.M. Preferential Policies and Income Inequality: Evidence from Special Economic Zones and Open Cities in China. *China Econ. Rev.* **2016**, *40*, 228–240. [CrossRef]
5. Lin, Y.; Zhang, X.; Geertman, S. Toward Smart Governance and Social Sustainability for Chinese Migrant Communities. *J. Clean. Prod.* **2015**, *107*, 389–399. [CrossRef]
6. Mosler Vidal, E.; Laczko, F. *Migration and the SDGs: Measuring Progress*; Transnational Press: London, UK, 2022.
7. Machado, S.; Goldenberg, S. Sharpening Our Public Health Lens: Advancing Im/Migrant Health Equity during COVID-19 and Beyond. *Int. J. Equity Health* **2021**, *20*, 57. [CrossRef]
8. Bell, M.; Charles-Edwards, E.; Ueffing, P.; Stillwell, J.; Kupiszewski, M.; Kupiszewska, D. Internal Migration and Development: Comparing Migration Intensities around the World. *Popul. Dev. Rev.* **2015**, *41*, 33–58. [CrossRef]
9. Fellmeth, G.; Rose-Clarke, K.; Zhao, C.; Busert, L.K.; Zheng, Y.; Massazza, A.; Sonmez, H.; Eder, B.; Blewitt, A.; Lertgrai, W.; et al. Health Impacts of Parental Migration on Left-behind Children and Adolescents: A Systematic Review and Meta-Analysis. *Lancet* **2018**, *392*, 2567–2582. [CrossRef]
10. Rodriguez-Soler, R.; Uribe-Toril, J.; De Pablo Valenciano, J. Worldwide Trends in the Scientific Production on Rural Depopulation, a Bibliometric Analysis Using Bibliometrix R-Tool. *Land Use Policy* **2020**, *97*, 104787. [CrossRef]
11. Yan, D.; Liu, L.; Liu, X.; Zhang, M. Global Trends in Urban Agriculture Research: A Pathway toward Urban Resilience and Sustainability. *Land* **2022**, *11*, 117. [CrossRef]
12. Aria, M.; Cuccurullo, C. Bibliometrix: An R-Tool for Comprehensive Science Mapping Analysis. *J. Informetr.* **2017**, *11*, 959–975. [CrossRef]
13. Rogers, G.; Szomszor, M.; Adams, J. Sample Size in Bibliometric Analysis. *Scientometrics* **2020**, *125*, 777–794. [CrossRef]
14. van Eck, N.J.; Waltman, L. Software Survey: VOSviewer, a Computer Program for Bibliometric Mapping. *Scientometrics* **2010**, *84*, 523–538. [CrossRef] [PubMed]
15. Lotka, A.J. The Frequency Distribution of Scientific Productivity. *J. Washingt. Acad. Sci.* **1926**, *16*, 317–323.
16. Bradford, S.C. Sources of Information on Specific Subjects. *Engineering* **1934**, *137*, 85–86.
17. Donthu, N.; Kumar, S.; Mukherjee, D.; Pandey, N.; Lim, W.M. How to Conduct a Bibliometric Analysis: An Overview and Guidelines. *J. Bus. Res.* **2021**, *133*, 285–296. [CrossRef]
18. Agyemang, C.; Meeks, K.; Beune, E.; Owusu-Dabo, E.; Mockenhaupt, F.P.; Addo, J.; de Graft Aikins, A.; Bahendeka, S.; Danquah, I.; Schulze, M.B.; et al. Obesity and Type 2 Diabetes in Sub-Saharan Africans-Is the Burden in Today's Africa Similar to African Migrants in Europe? The RODAM Study. *BMC Med.* **2016**, *14*, 166. [CrossRef]
19. Marx, W.; Bornmann, L.; Barth, A.; Leydesdorff, L. Detecting the Historical Roots of Research Fields by Reference Publication Year Spectroscopy (RPYS). *J. Assoc. Inf. Sci. Technol.* **2014**, *65*, 751–764. [CrossRef]
20. Defoe, D. *A Journal of the Plague Year*; HarperCollins: London, UK, 1722.
21. Crymble, A.; Dennett, A.; Hitchcock, T. Modelling Regional Imbalances in English Plebeian Migration to Late Eighteenth-Century London. *Econ. Hist. Rev.* **2018**, *71*, 747–771. [CrossRef]
22. Davenport, R.; Schwarz, L.; Boulton, J. The Decline of Adult Smallpox in Eighteenth-Century London. *Econ. Hist. Rev.* **2011**, *64*, 1289–1314. [CrossRef]
23. Lambrecht, T.; Winter, A. An Old Poor Law on the Continent? Agrarian Capitalism, Poor Taxes, and Village Conflict in Eighteenth-Century Coastal Flanders. *Econ. Hist. Rev.* **2018**, *71*, 1173–1198. [CrossRef]
24. Kessler, M.M. Bibliographic Coupling between Scientific Papers. *Am. Doc.* **1963**, *14*, 10–25. [CrossRef]
25. Small, H. Co-Citation in the Scientific Literature: A New Measure of the Relationship between Two Documents. *J. Am. Soc. Inf. Sci.* **1973**, *24*, 265–269. [CrossRef]
26. Keung Wong, D.F.; Li, C.Y.; Song, H.X. Rural Migrant Workers in Urban China: Living a Marginalised Life. *Int. J. Soc. Welf.* **2007**, *16*, 32–40. [CrossRef]
27. Zhu, Y. China's Floating Population and Their Settlement Intention in the Cities: Beyond the Hukou Reform. *Habitat Int.* **2007**, *31*, 65–76. [CrossRef]
28. Chen, J. Internal Migration and Health: Re-Examining the Healthy Migrant Phenomenon in China. *Soc. Sci. Med.* **2011**, *72*, 1294–1301. [CrossRef]
29. Chan, K.W. The Household Registration System and Migrant Labor in China: Notes on a Debate. *Popul. Dev. Rev.* **2010**, *36*, 357–364. [CrossRef]
30. Hu, F.; Xu, Z.; Chen, Y. Circular Migration, or Permanent Stay? Evidence from China's Rural–Urban Migration. *China Econ. Rev.* **2011**, *22*, 64–74. [CrossRef]
31. Démurger, S.; Gurgand, M.; Li, S.; Yue, X. Migrants as Second-Class Workers in Urban China? A Decomposition Analysis. *J. Comp. Econ.* **2009**, *37*, 610–628. [CrossRef]

32. Fan, C. Settlement Intention and Split Households: Findings from a Survey of Migrants in Beijing's Urban Villages. *China Rev.* **2011**, *11*, 11–41.
33. Li, L.; Wang, H.; Ye, X.; Jiang, M.; Lou, Q.; Hesketh, T. The Mental Health Status of Chinese Rural–Urban Migrant Workers. *Soc. Psychiatry Psychiatr. Epidemiol.* **2007**, *42*, 716–722. [CrossRef]
34. Liu, Y.; Li, Z.; Breitung, W. The Social Networks of New-Generation Migrants in China's Urbanized Villages: A Case Study of Guangzhou. *Habitat Int.* **2012**, *36*, 192–200. [CrossRef]
35. Liu, Y.; He, S.; Wu, F.; Webster, C. Urban Villages under China's Rapid Urbanization: Unregulated Assets and Transitional Neighbourhoods. *Habitat Int.* **2010**, *34*, 135–144. [CrossRef]
36. Chan, K.W.; Zhang, L. The Hukou System and Rural-Urban Migration in China: Processes and Changes. *China Q.* **1999**, *160*, 818–855. [CrossRef] [PubMed]
37. Solinger, D.J. *Contesting Citizenship in Urban China: Peasant Migrants, the State, and the Logic of the Market*; University of California Press: Berkeley, CA, USA, 1999.
38. Chan, K.W.; Buckingham, W. Is China Abolishing the Hukou System? *China Q.* **2008**, *195*, 582–606. [CrossRef]
39. Harris, J.R.; Todaro, M.P. Migration, Unemployment and Development: A Two-Sector Analysis. *Am. Econ. Rev.* **1970**, *60*, 126–142.
40. Meng, X.; Zhang, J. The Two-Tier Labor Market in Urban China: Occupational Segregation and Wage Differentials between Urban Residents and Rural Migrants in Shanghai. *J. Comp. Econ.* **2001**, *29*, 485–504. [CrossRef]
41. Chan, K.W. The Chinese Hukou System at 50. *Eurasian Geogr. Econ.* **2009**, *50*, 197–221. [CrossRef]
42. Fan, C.C. The Elite, the Natives, and the Outsiders: Migration and Labor Market Segmentation in Urban China. *Ann. Assoc. Am. Geogr.* **2002**, *92*, 103–124. [CrossRef]
43. Zhu, Y.; Chen, W. The Settlement Intention of China's Floating Population in the Cities: Recent Changes and Multifaceted Individual-Level Determinants. *Popul. Space Place* **2010**, *16*, 253–267. [CrossRef]
44. Stark, O.; Bloom, D. The New Economics of Labor Migration. *Am. Econ. Rev.* **1985**, *75*, 173–178.
45. Peset, F.; Garzón-Farinós, F.; González, L.M.; García-Massó, X.; Ferrer-Sapena, A.; Toca-Herrera, J.L.; Sánchez-Pérez, E.A. Survival Analysis of Author Keywords: An Application to the Library and Information Sciences Area. *J. Assoc. Inf. Sci. Technol.* **2020**, *71*, 462–473. [CrossRef]
46. Tripathi, M.; Kumar, S.; Sonker, S.K.; Babbar, P. Occurrence of Author Keywords and Keywords plus in Social Sciences and Humanities Research: A Preliminary Study. *Collnet J. Sci. Inf. Manag.* **2018**, *12*, 215–232. [CrossRef]
47. Batagelj, V.; Cerinšek, M. On Bibliographic Networks. *Scientometrics* **2013**, *96*, 845–864. [CrossRef]
48. Callon, M.; Courtial, J.P.; Laville, F. Co-Word Analysis as a Tool for Describing the Network of Interactions between Basic and Technological Research: The Case of Polymer Chemsitry. *Scientometrics* **1991**, *22*, 155–205. [CrossRef]
49. Zhang, J.; Yu, Q.; Zheng, F.; Long, C.; Lu, Z.; Duan, Z. Comparing Keywords plus of WOS and Author Keywords: A Case Study of Patient Adherence Research. *J. Assoc. Inf. Sci. Technol.* **2016**, *67*, 967–972. [CrossRef]
50. Chen, B.; Tsutsui, S.; Ding, Y.; Ma, F. Understanding the Topic Evolution in a Scientific Domain: An Exploratory Study for the Field of Information Retrieval. *J. Informetr.* **2017**, *11*, 1175–1189. [CrossRef]
51. Coulter, N.; Monarch, I.; Konda, S. Software Engineering as Seen through Its Research Literature: A Study in Co-Word Analysis. *J. Am. Soc. Inf. Sci.* **1998**, *49*, 1206–1223. [CrossRef]
52. Cobo, M.J.; López-Herrera, A.G.; Herrera-Viedma, E.; Herrera, F. An Approach for Detecting, Quantifying, and Visualizing the Evolution of a Research Field: A Practical Application to the Fuzzy Sets Theory Field. *J. Informetr.* **2011**, *5*, 146–166. [CrossRef]
53. Della Corte, V.; Del Gaudio, G.; Sepe, F.; Sciarelli, F. Sustainable Tourism in the Open Innovation Realm: A Bibliometric Analysis. *Sustainability* **2019**, *11*, 6114. [CrossRef]
54. Sott, M.K.; Bender, M.S.; Furstenau, L.B.; Machado, L.M.; Cobo, M.J.; Bragazzi, N.L. 100 Years of Scientific Evolution of Work and Organizational Psychology: A Bibliometric Network Analysis From 1919 to 2019. *Front. Psychol.* **2020**, *11*, 598676. [CrossRef]
55. Awumbila, M.; Ardayfio-Schandorf, E. Gendered Poverty, Migration and Livelihood Strategies of Female Porters in Accra, Ghana. *Nor. Geogr. Tidsskr.-Nor. J. Geogr.* **2008**, *62*, 171–179. [CrossRef]
56. Greenacre, M.; Blasius, J. *Multiple Correspondence Analysis and Related Methods*; Chapman and Hall/CRC: London, UK, 2006; Volume 72. [CrossRef]
57. Nenadić, O.; Greenacre, M. Correspondence Analysis in R, with Two- and Three-Dimensional Graphics: The ca Package. *J. Stat. Softw.* **2007**, *20*, 1–13. [CrossRef]
58. Zhang, K.H.; Song, S. Rural–Urban Migration and Urbanization in China: Evidence from Time-Series and Cross-Section Analyses. *China Econ. Rev.* **2003**, *14*, 386–400. [CrossRef]
59. Zhao, Y. Leaving the Countryside: Rural-to-Urban Migration Decisions in China. *Am. Econ. Rev.* **1999**, *89*, 281–286. [CrossRef]
60. Cheng, T.; Selden, M. The Origins and Social Consequences of China's Hukou System. *China Q.* **1994**, *139*, 644–668. [CrossRef]
61. Song, Y. What Should Economists Know about the Current Chinese Hukou System? *China Econ. Rev.* **2014**, *29*, 200–212. [CrossRef]
62. Liu, Y.F.; Dijst, M.; Geertman, S. Residential Segregation and Well-Being Inequality between Local and Migrant Elderly in Shanghai. *Habitat Int.* **2014**, *42*, 175–185. [CrossRef]
63. Ma, J.; Liu, B.; Mitchell, G.; Dong, G. A Spatial Analysis of Air Pollution and Environmental Inequality in Beijing, 2000–2010. *J. Environ. Plan. Manag.* **2019**, *62*, 2437–2458. [CrossRef]
64. Liu, C.; Cao, M.Q.; Yang, T.R.; Ma, L.; Wu, M.L.; Cheng, L.; Ye, R.N. Inequalities in the Commuting Burden: Institutional Constraints and Job-Housing Relationships in Tianjin, China. *Res. Transp. Bus. Manag.* **2022**, *42*, 100545. [CrossRef]

65. Hao, P.; Tang, S. Floating or Settling down: The Effect of Rural Landholdings on the Settlement Intention of Rural Migrants in Urban China. *Environ. Plan. A* **2015**, *47*, 1979–1999. [CrossRef]
66. Liang, Z.; Ma, Z. China's Floating Population: New Evidence from the 2000 Census. *Popul. Dev. Rev.* **2004**, *30*, 467–488. [CrossRef]
67. Wu, W. Sources of Migrant Housing Disadvantage in Urban China. *Environ. Plan. A* **2004**, *36*, 1285–1304. [CrossRef]
68. Han, D. Policing and Racialization of Rural Migrant Workers in Chinese Cities. *Ethn. Racial Stud.* **2010**, *33*, 593–610. [CrossRef]
69. Lu, Y.; Yeung, J.W.J.; Liu, J.; Treiman, D.J. Migration and Children's Psychosocial Development in China: When and Why Migration Matters. *Soc. Sci. Res.* **2019**, *77*, 130–147. [CrossRef]
70. Goodburn, C. Learning from Migrant Education: A Case Study of the Schooling of Rural Migrant Children in Beijing. *Int. J. Educ. Dev.* **2009**, *29*, 495–504. [CrossRef]
71. Lloyd, A.D.; Antonioletti, M.; Sloan, T.M. Able but Not Willing? Exploring Divides in Digital versus Physical Payment Use in China. *Inf. Technol. People* **2016**, *29*, 250–279. [CrossRef]
72. Knight, J.; Gunatilaka, R. Great Expectations? The Subjective Well-Being of Rural–Urban Migrants in China. *World Dev.* **2010**, *38*, 113–124. [CrossRef]
73. Zheng, S.; Long, F.; Fan, C.C.; Gu, Y. Urban Villages in China: A 2008 Survey of Migrant Settlements in Beijing. *Eurasian Geogr. Econ.* **2009**, *50*, 425–446. [CrossRef]
74. Korinek, K.; Entwisle, B.; Jampaklay, A. Through Thick and Thin: Layers of Social Ties and Urban Settlement among Thai Migrants. *Am. Sociol. Rev.* **2005**, *70*, 779–800. [CrossRef]
75. Yue, Z.; Li, S.; Jin, X.; Feldman, M.W. The Role of Social Networks in the Integration of Chinese Rural–Urban Migrants: A Migrant–Resident Tie Perspective. *Urban Stud.* **2013**, *50*, 1704–1723. [CrossRef]
76. Wang, W.W.; Fan, C.C. Migrant Workers' Integration in Urban China: Experiences in Employment, Social Adaptation, and Self-Identity. *Eurasian Geogr. Econ.* **2012**, *53*, 731–749. [CrossRef]
77. Li, B. Floating Population or Urban Citizens? Status, Social Provision and Circumstances of Rural–Urban Migrants in China. *Soc. Policy Adm.* **2006**, *40*, 174–195. [CrossRef]
78. Song, Y.; Zenou, Y.; Ding, C. Let's Not Throw the Baby Out with the Bath Water: The Role of Urban Villages in Housing Rural Migrants in China. *Urban Stud.* **2008**, *45*, 313–330. [CrossRef]
79. Ebrahim, S.; Kinra, S.; Bowen, L.; Andersen, E.; Ben-Shlomo, Y.; Lyngdoh, T.; Ramakrishnan, L.; Ahuja, R.C.; Joshi, P.; Das, S.M.; et al. Indian Migration Study group. The Effect of Rural-to-Urban Migration on Obesity and Diabetes in India: A Cross-Sectional Study. *PLoS Med.* **2010**, *7*, e1000268. [CrossRef] [PubMed]
80. Li, X.; Fang, X.; Lin, D.; Mao, R.; Wang, J.; Cottrell, L.; Harris, C.; Stanton, B. HIV/STD Risk Behaviors and Perceptions Among Rural-To-Urban Migrants in China. *AIDS Educ. Prev.* **2004**, *16*, 538–556. [CrossRef]
81. Miranda, J.J.; Gilman, R.H.; Smeeth, L. Differences in Cardiovascular Risk Factors in Rural, Urban and Rural-to-Urban Migrants in Peru. *Heart* **2011**, *97*, 787–796. [CrossRef] [PubMed]
82. Chen, Y.; Parker, M.; Zheng, X.; Fang, X. Health Insurance Coverage of Migrant Workers in China. *Chin. Econ.* **2021**, *55*, 332–342. [CrossRef]
83. Castagna, P.; Ricciardelli, R.; Piazza, F.; Mattutino, G.; Pattarino, B.; Canavese, A.; Gino, S. Violence against African Migrant Women Living in Turin: Clinical and Forensic Evaluation. *Int. J. Leg. Med.* **2018**, *132*, 1197–1204. [CrossRef]
84. Pan, S.-M.; Yang, J.-T. Outsiders in the Family: Abuse of Migrant Domestic Workers in Taiwan. *Asian J. Womens Stud.* **2012**, *18*, 87–117. [CrossRef]
85. Zhong, B.-L.; Liu, T.-B.; Chan, S.S.M.; Jin, D.; Hu, C.-Y.; Dai, J.; Chiu, H.F.K. Prevalence and Correlates of Major Depressive Disorder among Rural-to-Urban Migrant Workers in Shenzhen, China. *J. Affect. Disord.* **2015**, *183*, 1–9. [CrossRef]
86. Hu, X.; Cook, S.; Salazar, M.A. Internal Migration and Health in China. *Lancet* **2008**, *372*, 1717–1719. [CrossRef]
87. Kirkbride, J.B.; Hameed, Y.; Ioannidis, K.; Ankireddypalli, G.; Crane, C.M.; Nasir, M.; Kabacs, N.; Metastasio, A.; Jenkins, O.; Espandian, A.; et al. Ethnic Minority Status, Age-at-Immigration and Psychosis Risk in Rural Environments: Evidence from the SEPEA Study. *Schizophr. Bull.* **2017**, *43*, 1251–1261. [CrossRef] [PubMed]
88. Liang, Z.; Chen, Y.P. The Educational Consequences of Migration for Children in China. *Soc. Sci. Res.* **2007**, *36*, 28–47. [CrossRef]
89. Wen, M.; Lin, D. Child Development in Rural China: Children Left Behind by Their Migrant Parents and Children of Nonmigrant Families. *Child Dev.* **2012**, *83*, 120–136. [CrossRef]
90. Zhou, Y.; Cheng, Y.; Liang, Y.; Wang, J.; Li, C.; Du, W.; Liu, Y.; Liu, Z. Interaction Status, Victimization and Emotional Distress of Left-behind Children: A National Survey in China. *Child. Youth Serv. Rev.* **2020**, *118*, 105348. [CrossRef]
91. Tomsa, R.; Jenaro, C. Children Left Behind in Romania: Anxiety and Predictor Variables. *Psychol. Rep.* **2015**, *116*, 485–512. [CrossRef] [PubMed]
92. Yi, J.; Zhong, B.; Yao, S. Health-Related Quality of Life and Influencing Factors among Rural Left-behind Wives in Liuyang, China. *BMC Women's Health* **2014**, *14*, 67. [CrossRef]
93. Yi, F.; Liu, C.; Xu, Z. Identifying the Effects of Migration on Parental Health: Evidence from Left-behind Elders in China. *China Econ. Rev.* **2019**, *54*, 218–236. [CrossRef]
94. Adhikari, R.; Jampaklay, A.; Chamratrithirong, A. Impact of Children's Migration on Health and Health Care-Seeking Behavior of Elderly Left Behind. *BMC Public Health* **2011**, *11*, 143. [CrossRef]
95. Cyril, S.; Oldroyd, J.C.; Renzaho, A. Urbanisation, Urbanicity, and Health: A Systematic Review of the Reliability and Validity of Urbanicity Scales. *BMC Public Health* **2013**, *13*, 513. [CrossRef]

96. Tian, H.; Hu, S.; Cazelles, B.; Chowell, G.; Gao, L.; Laine, M.; Li, Y.; Yang, H.; Li, Y.; Yang, Q.; et al. Urbanization Prolongs Hantavirus Epidemics in Cities. *Proc. Natl. Acad. Sci. USA* **2018**, *115*, 4707–4712. [CrossRef] [PubMed]
97. Chua, A.Q.; Tan, M.M.J.; Verma, M.; Han, E.K.L.; Hsu, L.Y.; Cook, A.R.; Teo, Y.Y.; Lee, V.J.; Legido-Quigley, H. Health System Resilience in Managing the COVID-19 Pandemic: Lessons from Singapore. *BMJ Glob. Health* **2020**, *5*, e003317. [CrossRef] [PubMed]
98. Tobe, R.G.; Xu, L.; Song, P.; Huang, Y. The Rural-to-Urban Migrant Population in China: Gloomy Prospects for Tuberculos is Control. *Biosci. Trends* **2011**, *5*, 226–230. [CrossRef] [PubMed]
99. Wang, Y.; Long, Q.; Liu, Q.; Tolhurst, R.; Tang, S. Treatment Seeking for Symptoms Suggestive of TB: Comparison between Migrants and Permanent Urban Residents in Chongqing, China. *Trop. Med. Int. Health* **2008**, *13*, 927–933. [CrossRef] [PubMed]
100. Long, Q.; Li, Y.; Wang, Y.; Yue, Y.; Tang, C.; Tang, S.; Squire, S.B.; Tolhurst, R. Barriers to Accessing TB Diagnosis for Rural-to-Urban Migrants with Chronic Cough in Chongqing, China: A Mixed Methods Study. *BMC Health Serv. Res.* **2008**, *8*, 202. [CrossRef]
101. Clark, S.J.; Collinson, M.A.; Kahn, K.; Drullinger, K.; Tollman, S.M. Returning Home to Die: Circular Labour Migration and Mortality in South Africa. *Scand. J. Public Health.* **2007**, *35* (Suppl. S2007), 35–44. [CrossRef]
102. Saha, S.; Chant, D.; Welham, J.; McGrath, J. A Systematic Review of the Prevalence of Schizophrenia. *PLoS Med.* **2005**, *2*, 0413–0433. [CrossRef]
103. Bhui, K.; Stansfeld, S.; Head, J.; Haines, M.; Hillier, S.; Taylor, S.; Viner, R.; Booy, R. Cultural Identity, Acculturation, and Mental Health among Adolescents in East London's Multiethnic Community. *J. Epidemiol. Community Health* **2005**, *59*, 296–302. [CrossRef]
104. Bhugra, D.; Gupta, S.; Bhui, K.; Craig, T.; Dogra, N.; Ingleby, J.D.; Kirkbride, J.; Moussaoui, D.; Nazroo, J.; Qureshi, A.; et al. WPA Guidance on Mental Health and Mental Health Care in Migrants. *World Psychiatry* **2011**, *10*, 2–10. [CrossRef]
105. Almeida-Filho, N.; Lessa, I.; Magalhães, L.; Araújo, M.J.; Aquino, E.; James, S.A.; Kawachi, I. Social Inequality and Depressive Disorders in Bahia, Brazil: Interactions of Gender, Ethnicity, and Social Class. *Soc. Sci. Med.* **2004**, *59*, 1339–1353. [CrossRef]
106. Detels, R.; Karim, Q.A.; Baum, F.; Li, L.; Leyland, A.H. *Oxford Textbook of Global Public Health*; Oxford University Press: Oxford, UK, 2021. [CrossRef]

International Journal of
Environmental Research and Public Health

MDPI

Article

The Effect of Environmental Policy Uncertainty on Enterprises' Pollution Emissions: Evidence from Chinese Industrial Enterprise

Dong Le [1], Fei Ren [1], Yiding Tang [2] and Yuke Zhu [1,*]

[1] Economics School, Zhongnan University of Economics and Law, Nanhu Avenue 182, Wuhan 430073, China
[2] School of Economics and Trade, Hunan University, Fenglin Road, Changsha 410006, China
* Correspondence: zhuyuke1994@163.com

Abstract: In response to the global call for emission reduction, China has assumed international responsibility for energy conservation and emission reduction by enacting several environmental policies to save energy and reduce consumption. However, it is debatable whether the increased uncertainty in environmental policies negatively affects firms' emission reduction. Few studies have examined this relationship based on micro-level data. Therefore, this study constructs a theoretical framework of environmental policy uncertainty affecting firms' pollution emissions. Based on comprehensive data from the Chinese Industrial Enterprise Database, the Chinese Industrial Enterprise Pollution Emission Database, and the Chinese Patent Database from 2002 to 2014, we empirically analyzed the impact of environmental policy uncertainty on firms' pollution emissions. The results show that (1) environmental policy uncertainty significantly aggravates the pollution emission intensity of industrial enterprises; (2) environmental policy uncertainty inhibits the improvement of enterprises' innovation capacity, reduces their human capital stock and foreign investment, and aggravates their pollution emission; (3) environmental policy uncertainty has significant heterogeneity on enterprise pollution emissions, that is, environmental policy uncertainty has a greater impact on non-export enterprises, large enterprises, young enterprises, capital-intensive enterprises, state-owned enterprises, and enterprises in polluting industries and central regions. This study provides a useful reference for the improvement of environmental policy and the green transformation of enterprises.

Keywords: environmental policy uncertainty; enterprise pollution emission; enterprise innovation; human capital; the foreign investment

Citation: Le, D.; Ren, F.; Tang, Y.; Zhu, Y. The Effect of Environmental Policy Uncertainty on Enterprises' Pollution Emissions: Evidence from Chinese Industrial Enterprise. *IJERPH* **2022**, *19*, 9849. https://doi.org/10.3390/ijerph19169849

Academic Editors: Jie Chen, Qian Zhou and Ting Zhang

Received: 30 June 2022
Accepted: 9 August 2022
Published: 10 August 2022

1. Introduction

Approximately four decades of economic growth made China the world's second-largest economy in 2010. However, this economic development brought in its wake serious resource constraints, high levels of pollution by enterprises, and the degradation of the ecosystem. According to the 2020 Report on China's Ecological and Environmental Conditions, only 59.9% of cities across the country have acceptable air standards, high pollution emissions cause 1.2–1.4 million deaths annually [1], and direct and indirect economic losses are pegged at 1–8% of China's GDP [2]. As the Central Committee of the Communist Party of China has proposed to strengthen socialist ecological civilization construction, the government has issued a series of rules and regulations to promote enterprise emission reduction, including the Action Plan for Air Pollution Prevention and Control (2013) [3], the Implementation Regulations of the Environmental Protection Tax Law of the People's Republic of China (2017), and the Guiding Opinions on Building a Modern Environmental Governance System (2020). Government regulations are an important measure to control the pollution discharge of enterprises. Given that the market is a dynamic process, environmental policies need to be dynamically adjusted in real time according to factors such as economic development and technological progress. These policies have, no doubt, effectively reduced the contradiction between economic development and enterprise emission reduction but have also increased the uncertainty of environmental policies. Research suggests that environmental policy uncertainty itself may lead to economic decline [4]. Currently, China's economy is in the transition phase, and environmental policy uncertainty is an important feature of this period. However, few studies have focused on whether an increase in environmental policy uncertainty impacts enterprise emission reduction. It is rarely mentioned in the existing literature. In the context of the green transformation development of enterprises, research on environmental policy uncertainty and enterprise emission reduction has immense theoretical and practical significance.

1.1. Literature Review

In the context of the green transformation and development of enterprises, enterprise pollution emission has become a hot topic in academia. Additionally, government regulation policy has an immense impact on enterprise pollution emission. If environmental policies are stringent or frequent, the technological progress of enterprises will be hindered, which will eventually lead to the development of enterprises [5]. Burtraw et al. [6] found that government energy-saving and consumption-reduction policies significantly promote enterprise emission reduction; additionally, they calculated the economic benefits generated by enterprise emission reduction. Oueslati [7] proposed that carbon emission trading rights and carbon taxes can significantly reduce carbon emissions; additionally, carbon emission trading rights can promote the improvement of low-carbon technologies of enterprises and enhance their market competitiveness [8].

1.1.1. Influencing Factors of Enterprise Pollution Discharge

Regarding the influencing factors of enterprise pollution discharge, the existing literature mainly focuses on technological innovation, human capital, and foreign investment. The development experience of developed countries shows that technological innovation can fundamentally solve the problem of excessive pollution emissions of enterprises and improve the competitiveness of enterprises' products, and the improvement of green innovation ability can help enterprises occupy market share [9]. When the intensity of environmental regulation increases, the innovation potential of enterprises will be stimulated to realize the coordinated development of environmental protection and the green development of enterprises [10]. Popp [11] proposed that government innovation support policies and enterprise innovation behavior can form a complementary situation. Government innovation support policies can motivate enterprises toward green production and improve enterprises' pollution discharge technology, in addition to promoting the reduction in enterprises' pollution emission intensity. Additionally, Porter [12] suggested that companies seek new technologies to reduce emissions and pollution costs.

Human capital—an important aspect of economic efficiency and green development—influences the maximization of resource utilization efficiency and breaking through the constraint of diminishing marginal returns. Investing in enterprise human capital enhances the quality of managers and laborers, thereby improving the energy utilization efficiency of enterprises. When enterprise human capital stock is high, it can significantly improve the absorption capacity and application ability of energy-saving technologies [13]. Kurtz et al. [14] used sample data from different countries to find that human capital can significantly improve the energy utilization efficiency of enterprises and reduce the unintended output in the production process. Lan et al. [15] identified that regional enterprises with low human capital are more prone to the "pollution paradise hypothesis." Lan and Munro [3] found that human capital transcends the constraint of diminishing marginal returns through positive externalities and reduces the intensity of enterprise pollution emission.

The influence of foreign investment on enterprises' pollution emissions has not been determined yet, and research has mainly focused on the "pollution paradise hypothesis" and "pollution halo hypothesis." The pollution paradise hypothesis holds that foreign-funded enterprises tend to move to countries with weak environmental regulations. Here, local enterprises engage in a vicious competition with transferring enterprises—most of which are pollution-intensive industries—reducing investment in green technology to save costs and increasing pollution emission intensity [16]. The pollution halo hypothesis holds that foreign investment reduces enterprise pollution emission intensity. On the one hand, when industrial transfer occurs in developed countries, foreign-funded enterprises often have more advanced pollution discharge technologies and better management systems. The competition encourages local enterprises to improve their own production technologies and management systems through imitation [17]. On the other hand, the products of foreign-funded enterprises are more environmentally friendly, and these enterprises require local suppliers to adopt green and efficient production technologies to guarantee their product advantage. At this time, foreign enterprises will provide advanced green production technology and a perfect management mode to local suppliers, so as to strengthen the spillover effect of advanced technology and reduce enterprise pollution emissions [18].

1.1.2. Discussion about Environmental Policy Uncertainty

Existing studies on environmental policy uncertainty focus on its connotations and impacts on enterprise investment, technological innovation, and economic development. Uncertainty implies that actors make decisions without access to complete information, and therefore, the specific impact of their decisions cannot be accurately predicted. When the object of uncertainty is environmental policy, then environmental policy uncertainty is formed [19]. Environmental policy uncertainty refers to the inability of economic entities to accurately predict when, how, and whether the government will change the current environmental policy. Since the central government proposed the comprehensive protection of the ecology and environment, local governments have frequently adjusted environmental regulations to reduce enterprise emission; so, the uncertainty of environmental policy has become the main feature of the economic transition period [20]. Environmental policy uncertainty is not a specific policy, but a measure of how often environmental policy changes. The greater the value of environmental policy uncertainty, the more frequent the government's environmental policy changes. The uncertainty of environmental policy has a negative impact on foreign investment, employment, and enterprise innovation. When the environment shows a dynamic trend of change, it is difficult for enterprises to predict future results, which increases the cost of enterprise decision making [21]. With the deepening of China's economic transformation, the influx of foreign capital, and stringent environmental regulations, Chinese enterprises are facing increasing uncertainty [22]. Increased environmental policy uncertainty raises financial risks and incentivizes risk avoidance, which pushes enterprises to reduce investment in pollution reduction and aggravates pollution emissions [23].

1.1.3. Summary

To date, studies have been conducted on enterprises' pollution emissions from the perspectives of government regulation policies, influencing factors, the connotations of environmental policy uncertainty, and its influence on foreign investment, employment, and enterprise innovation. However, little research has been performed on whether increasing environmental policy uncertainty impacts enterprise pollution emissions. Additionally, due to the lack of an effective micro-basis of macro-level research, the emission reduction path of the macro-level influence mechanism acting on micro-enterprises is not clear. In fact, how to deal with the increasing uncertainty of environmental policy is the basis and key to understand the relationship between policy fluctuation and emission reduction at the macro level. Therefore, based on the combined data of the China Industrial Enterprise Database, China Industrial Enterprise Pollution Emission Database, and China Patent Database from 2002 to 2014, this study illustrates the impact and mechanism of environmental policy uncertainty on enterprise pollution emissions from the perspective of micro-enterprises.

2. Materials and Methods

2.1. Theoretical Model

2.1.1. Environmental Policy Uncertainty Worsens Enterprise Pollution Emissions by Inhibiting Enterprise Innovation

Based on the research by Bloom, Bond, and Van Reenen [24], this study expounds how the uncertainty of environmental policy affects the pollution emission of enterprises. It is assumed that the production of enterprises in period t conforms to the Cobb–Douglas production function, and the specific function form is as follows:

$$F = A_t K_t^{\alpha} L_t^{\beta} G_t^{1-\alpha-\beta} \tag{1}$$

In Formula (1), A_t refers to the production conditions of the enterprise, mainly including its own production conditions and external factors; K_t is the capital stock of the enterprise; L_t is the labor stock of the enterprise; and G_t is the knowledge stock of the enterprise. It is assumed that G_t is proportional to the enterprise's innovation capability μ, so:

$$G_t = a\mu + \varepsilon \tag{2}$$

At this point, the demand function faced by the enterprise is:

$$D_t = B_t P^{-\frac{1}{\gamma}} \tag{3}$$

where B is the demand shock faced by the enterprise. Based on the relationship between demand and supply, the income function of the enterprise is as follows:

$$\begin{aligned} M(A_t, B_t, K_t, L_t, G_t) &= (A_t, K_t^{\alpha}, L_t^{\beta}, G_t^{1-\alpha-\beta})^{1-\gamma} B_t^{\lambda} \\ &= A_t^{1-\gamma} B_t^{\gamma} K_t^{\alpha(1-\lambda)} L_t^{\beta(1-\gamma)} G_t^{(1-\alpha-\beta)(1-\gamma)} \end{aligned} \tag{4}$$

We defined $X_t^{\varphi} = Z_t^{1-\gamma} B_t^{\gamma}$, where X indicates that the production and investment of enterprises are affected by the uncertainty of environmental policies, making $X_t^{\varphi} = f(\lambda) = (b\lambda + n)^{\varphi}$, $b > 0$. To judge the relationship between environmental policy uncertainty λ and innovation capability μ, we further simplified the model along with the research ideas of Bloom, Bond, and Van Reenen [24], assuming that capital K and labor L are completely flexible and their variable costs are 0. We substituted Formula (2) into Formula (4), and the return function is:

$$M(\lambda, \mu) = K(b\lambda + n)^{\varphi}(a\mu + m)^{1-\varphi} \tag{5}$$

To a homogeneous equation:

$$M = K\varphi(b\lambda + n) + (1 - \varphi)(a\mu + m) \tag{6}$$

The emission reduction in enterprise pollution is not only affected by the original pollutant discharge Q^* but is also closely related to the enterprise innovation ability. There is a positive correlation between enterprise innovation capacity and emission reduction. S is the influence coefficient of enterprise innovation capacity on enterprise emission reduction ($0 < s < 1$). Additionally, the technological innovation of enterprises reduces the cost of enterprises' pollution emission; e is the proportion of the impact of technological innovation on the cost of enterprises' emission reduction ($0 < e < 1$). Additionally, the innovation cost of enterprises is affected by the uncertainty of environmental policy and innovation capability.

Assume that the total cost of the enterprise is C, which mainly includes emission cost C_1 and innovation cost C_2, so:

$$C_1 = e\mu(Q^*(1 - s\mu)) \tag{7}$$

$$C_2 = \lambda\delta\mu \tag{8}$$

In Formula (8), δ measures the impact of environmental policy uncertainty on innovation capability ($\delta < 0$). Then, the total cost is:

$$C = C_1 + C_2 \tag{9}$$

$$C = e\mu(Q^*(1 - s\mu)) + \lambda\delta\mu \tag{10}$$

The total profit function of the enterprise is:

$$R = K\varphi(b\lambda + n) + (1 - \varphi)(a\mu + m) - e\mu(Q^*(1 - s\mu)) - \lambda\delta\mu \tag{11}$$

When profit is maximized, the first derivative of profit is 0, then:

$$\frac{\partial R}{\partial \mu^*} = a(1 - \varphi) - eQ^* + 2eQ^*s\mu^* - \delta\lambda = 0 \tag{12}$$

According to Formula (12), the relationship between environmental policy uncertainty λ and enterprise innovation μ is as follows:

$$\frac{\partial \lambda}{\partial \mu^*} = \frac{2esQ^*}{\delta} < 0 \tag{13}$$

According to Formula (13), the uncertainty of environmental policy will inhibit the improvement of enterprises' innovation ability, whereas the technological innovation of enterprises will promote the upgrading of industrial structure, improve energy utilization efficiency, and further reduce enterprises' pollution emissions [25,26]. Therefore, environmental policy uncertainty can inhibit enterprise innovation and aggravate enterprise pollution emissions.

2.1.2. Environmental Policy Uncertainty Increases Enterprise Pollution Emissions by Inhibiting the Increase in Human Capital Stock

The production function is adjusted on the basis of Formula (1), and the meaning of the letters remains unchanged. The specific function form is as follows:

$$F = A_t K_t{}^{\alpha} G_t^{\beta} L_t^{1-\alpha-\beta} \tag{14}$$

The larger the inflow of labor, the larger the stock of human capital [27]. The specific function form is as follows:

$$L_t = cl + \xi \tag{15}$$

There is a positive correlation between the stock of human capital and emission reduction, and s_1 is the influence coefficient of the stock of human capital on emission reduction ($0 < s_1 < 1$). Human capital can internalize technical knowledge to overcome the diminishing marginal returns of production and reduce the cost of enterprise pollution emission. e_1 is the proportion of human capital affecting enterprise emission reduction cost ($0 < e_1 < 1$). The cost of introducing human capital is affected by environmental policy uncertainty and the effect of human capital promoting emission reduction.

Assume that the total cost of the enterprise is C, which mainly includes emission cost C_1 and human capital introduction cost C_2, so:

$$C_1 = e_1 l(Q^*(1 - s_1 l)) \tag{16}$$

$$C_2 = \lambda\delta_1 l \tag{17}$$

δ_1 is to measure the impact of environmental policy uncertainty on the cost of introducing human capital ($\delta_1 < 0$). Through the derivation of Equations (9)–(12), it can be concluded that:

$$\frac{\partial \lambda}{\partial l^*} = \frac{2e_1 s_1 Q^*}{\delta_1} < 0 \tag{18}$$

According to Formula (18), the uncertainty of environmental policy will inhibit the improvement of enterprise human capital stock. The new economic growth theory states that human capital can overcome the law of diminishing marginal returns on means of production and then realize economic growth and enterprise emission reduction [28,29]. Therefore, environmental policy uncertainty can aggravate enterprises' pollution emission by inhibiting the increase in enterprises' human capital.

2.1.3. Environmental Policy Uncertainty Worsens Pollution Emissions by Inhibiting Foreign Investment

The production function is adjusted on the basis of Formula (1), and the meaning of the letters remains unchanged. The specific function form is as follows:

$$F = A_t G_t^{\alpha} L_t^{\beta} K_t{}^{1-\alpha-\beta} \tag{19}$$

As foreign investment will increase the production and working capital of enterprises, it is assumed that K_t is proportional to the foreign investment of enterprises, and the specific function form is as follows:

$$K_t = df + \zeta \tag{20}$$

The increase in foreign investment makes enterprises strict in the formulation of environmental standards, and most multinational companies will implement international environmental standards, thus reducing the pollution emissions of enterprises. The amount of foreign investment is positively correlated with emission reduction, and s_2 is the influence coefficient of foreign investment on emission reduction ($0 < s_2 < 1$). Foreign investment can expand the production scale of enterprises to produce scale effect and reduce the pollution emission cost of enterprises. e_2 ($0 < e_2 < 1$) is the proportion of foreign investment affecting enterprise emission reduction cost, which is affected by both environmental policy uncertainty and foreign investment income.

Assume that the total cost of the enterprise is C, which mainly includes emission cost C_1 and human capital introduction cost C_2, so:

$$C_1 = e_2 f(Q^*(1 - s_2 f)) \tag{21}$$

$$C_2 = \lambda \delta_2 f \tag{22}$$

$\delta_2 (\delta_2 < 0)$ is to measure the impact of environmental policy uncertainty on foreign investment returns. Through the derivation of Equations (9)–(12), it can be concluded that:

$$\frac{\partial \lambda}{\partial f^*} = \frac{2 e_2 s_2 Q^*}{\delta_2} < 0 \tag{23}$$

Increased foreign investment can significantly improve financial support for enterprises to reduce emissions. Additionally, foreign enterprises bring advanced emission reduction technologies that facilitate the implementation of international environmental standards in China. Moreover, by introducing green cleaning products from the home country, foreign investment has a clean technology spillover effect on its upstream and downstream industries, which is conducive to promoting emission reduction in domestic enterprises. Therefore, environmental policy uncertainty can inhibit foreign investment and aggravate the pollution emission of enterprises.

2.2. Mechanism Analysis

Currently, China's economy is in a transition phase, and the government's policy environment is experiencing significant fluctuations. The main feature of this phase is the increasing fluctuations and uncertainty of environmental policy. On the one hand, advanced production and pollution discharge technologies require enormous human and material investment, whereas the positive externality of technological innovation reduces the willingness of enterprises to invest in innovation. Additionally, environmental policy uncertainty intensifies the severe fluctuation of micro-enterprise performance, which increases the difficulty of operation. Enterprise managers will avoid the uncertainty of investment returns as much as possible because of their risk-averse and profit-oriented mindset and pay more attention to short-term investment and investment with definite returns. Then, they will reduce the investment in R&D [30]. Additionally, environmental policy uncertainty reduces the willingness of enterprise managers to invest in innovation, which lowers enterprise innovation ability [31]. On the other hand, the impact of such uncertainty on the production and earnings of enterprises is unknown. Enterprises' earnings will also fluctuate because of the increased uncertainty of environmental policies. When the fluctuation of enterprises' earnings is high, information asymmetry between enterprises and external investors increases accordingly, and creditors have difficulty predicting the likelihood of recovery and may reduce their risk by raising loan rates, demanding guarantees, or even not lending. Additionally, existing shareholders want to receive more cash dividends in the case of unexpected circumstances caused by uncertainty, and potential investors demand a higher risk premium, which leads to higher equity financing costs. Therefore, the increased uncertainty of environmental policies increases the financing difficulty of enterprises, forcing them to retain abundant cash to cope with the impact of environmental policy uncertainties. The lack of funds reduces enterprises' innovation investment willingness. Therefore, an increase in environmental policy uncertainty inhibits the improvement of enterprise innovation ability. Advanced green production technology can improve the energy efficiency of enterprises, help enterprises break the constraints of resources and environment, and promote the reduction in enterprise emissions. In summary, this study proposes Hypothesis 1.

Hypothesis 1 (H1). *Environmental policy uncertainty can inhibit the improvement of enterprises' innovation ability and aggravate enterprises' pollution emission.*

When the uncertainty of environmental policy increases, it induces enterprise managers to make investments with definite short-term benefits. The tendency of enterprises to choose investment projects with higher risks and less obvious short-term returns will be weakened. The human capital investment of enterprises has the characteristic of not having an obvious income effect, and relative to other factors of production, human capital adjustment cost is low [32]. In order to cope with the unknown situation brought by the uncertainty of environmental policies, enterprises are more inclined to keep more cash to withstand the unknown risks they may face, and enterprises will reduce the investment in human capital. Human capital input is mainly divided into employee training and employee health input. When enterprises reduce employee training input, it is difficult for employees to improve their working skills. At the same time, in order to reduce expenses, enterprises will also increase the labor supply time of employees. Employees are also faced with the risk of being fired and income reduction, which damages the physical and mental health of employees. As a result, the healthy human capital of employees is reduced. When the health of employees is damaged, their enthusiasm to participate in labor will also be reduced. Additionally, the more unstable the enterprise environment, the stronger the mobility of employees, which also makes the implementation of internal control more difficult. It is difficult to maintain the stock of human capital effectively and stably. As an important aspect of economic and efficient green development, human capital plays a significant role in breaking through the constraint of diminishing marginal returns and maximizes resource utilization efficiency. On the one hand, human capital can reduce the increase in pollution emissions caused by low-level labor. A high level of human capital can guide the transformation of a low-skilled labor force to a high-skilled labor force and optimize the human capital structure of enterprises [33]. On the other hand, it promotes technological innovation for emission reduction and gives full play to the energy-saving production advantages of products, thus maximizing resource utilization efficiency and reducing the enterprise pollution emission intensity [34]. In summary, this study proposes Hypothesis 2.

Hypothesis 2 (H2). *The uncertainty of environmental policy increases the pollution emission of enterprises by inhibiting the increase in human capital stock of enterprises.*

The fundamental purpose of foreign investments is profit. When the uncertainty of environmental policy increases, it becomes difficult to accurately predict the income of foreign investment. To maximize interests and avoid risks, investors tend to invest in enterprises with clear and stable returns; they may even reduce investments in domestic companies because it is difficult to accurately control the risk of investment returns. The uncertainty of environmental policies has aggravated the fluctuation of enterprise performance and raised the financing difficulty of enterprises, which has hindered the production and operation of domestic enterprises. In the case of uncertain returns, foreign enterprises further reduce investment to reduce risks, so the increase in environmental policy uncertainty reduces foreign investment. Foreign investment has been a key component of economic growth and an important means of transferring modern technology and providing employment to host countries. Especially in recent years, inflows of foreign investment have become more important than international trade [35]. Foreign investment can not only increase the formation of resources and capital, but more importantly, it is an important channel for transferring production technology, entering new international markets, improving production capacity, and reducing unemployment—these are even more important for developing countries. Increased foreign investment has made companies more stringent in setting environmental standards. Most multinational companies implement international environmental standards, which reduce their emissions. Moreover, foreign investment can expand the production scale of enterprises to produce a scale effect and reduce the cost of pollution emission. Therefore, with the increase in foreign investment resulting in the spillover of green production technology, the enterprise pollution emission intensity is reduced [36]. In conclusion, this study proposes Hypothesis 3.

Hypothesis 3 (H3). *Environmental policy uncertainty worsens pollution emissions by inhibiting foreign investment.*

2.3. Models, Variables, and Data

2.3.1. Research Model

To verify the impact of environmental policy uncertainty on enterprise productivity, the benchmark model is set as follows:

$$ei_{ijkt} = \beta_0 + \beta_1 epu_{ijkt} + \beta_2 X_{ijkt} + \lambda_i + \lambda_j + \lambda_k + \lambda_t + \varepsilon_{ijkt} \tag{24}$$

i indicates the enterprise, j indicates the industry, k indicates the region, and t indicates the year. The explained variable ei represents the pollution emission intensity of enterprises, and the core explanatory variable epu represents the uncertainty of environmental policy. X_{ijkt} is the control variable. λ_i represents the firm fixed effect, λ_j represents the industry fixed effect, λ_k represents the region fixed effect, and λ_t represents the year fixed effect. ε_{ijkt} is the random perturbation term.

2.3.2. Variable Selection

The Explained Variable Enterprise Pollution Emission Intensity

To measure the enterprise pollution emission intensity comprehensively and accurately, in this study, the comprehensive index method was used. Based on data availability and the harmfulness of pollutants, we mainly selected five individual indicators of industrial wastewater: chemical oxygen demand, industrial waste gas, sulfur dioxide, smoke, and dust emissions to measure the intensity of enterprise pollution emission [37]. First, the original data of these pollutant indicators are linearly standardized:

$$rpol_{nit} = \frac{pol_{nit} - \text{min}pol_{nit}}{\text{max}pol_{nit} - \text{min}pol_{nit}} \tag{25}$$

pol_{nit} represents the emission of pollutant n from enterprise i in phase t. Max and min indicate the maximum and minimum emissions of pollutant n by all enterprises each year. Second, the adjustment coefficient of enterprise i pollutant n is calculated:

$$w_{nit} = \frac{rpol_{nit}}{rpol_{nt}} \tag{26}$$

Then, $rpol_{nt}$ represents the average level of pollutant n discharged by all enterprises in China. Finally, by combining Equations (25) and (26), the comprehensive index of pollution emission of enterprise i can be obtained:

$$ei_{it} = \frac{1}{6}(\sum_{n} rpol_{nit} \times w_{nit}) \tag{27}$$

The higher the value of *ei*, the greater the pollution emission intensity of the enterprise.

Core Explanatory Variable

The change in both external and internal environment increases the uncertainty of environmental policy, which causes a fluctuation in the enterprise's sales revenue [38]. Therefore, the uncertainty of environmental policy can be measured by the fluctuation in the company's sales income, and the standard difference in sales income can be used to measure the uncertainty of environmental policy [39]. Ghosh and Olsen [40] used the standard deviation of a company's sales revenue to measure environmental policy uncertainty to eliminate the natural sales income's growth.

The ordinary least squares method was used in this study to estimate the abnormal sales income of enterprises in the past three years.

$$Sale = \varphi_0 + \varphi_1 Year + \varepsilon \tag{28}$$

Sale is the sales revenue of the enterprise and *Year* is the year. If the participation regression is the value of the past four years, then $Year = 1$; if participation regression is the value of the past three years, then $Year = 2$, and so on. The regression residual of Formula (28) is the abnormal sales revenue of the enterprise. The standard deviation of abnormal sales revenue for the past three years is calculated, and the standard deviation by is divided by the average sales revenue for the past three years to obtain the uncertainty of environmental policy without industry adjustment. The calculated environmental policy uncertainty is divided by the median of environmental policy uncertainty in the same industry to obtain the environmental policy uncertainty (*epu*).

Moderating Variables

The moderating variables are enterprise innovation, human capital, and foreign investment. Enterprise innovation (*iq*) is measured by the total number of patents granted per year; the existing literature suggests that employees without higher education are usually not considered within the scope of human capital [41]. However, the Chinese Industrial Enterprise Database only counted the educational level of employees in 2004, so the proportion of employees with college degrees in 2004 was used to measure the human capital of enterprises (*rlzb*). The amount of foreign investment in local enterprises (100 million) was selected to measure foreign investment (*fi*).

Other Variables

The selection of control variables mainly includes enterprise labor productivity (lp): to measure it, the total industrial value of the enterprise is divided by the total number of employees (10,000/person); wage level ($gzsp$): to measure it, enterprise wages and benefits are divided by the total number of employees (10,000/person); industrial structure (is): it is measured by the ratio of regional secondary industrial output value to total GDP; rationalization index ($hlhzs$): to measure it, the output value of each industry is divided by the corresponding number of people to obtain the per capita output value of each industry, and then the calculation results of each industry are added to obtain the rationalization index of each region; the dummy variable of state-owned enterprises ($sfgy$): 1 for absolute state-owned holding, 0 for other cases; import and export enterprise (ex): if the export delivery value of the enterprise is greater than 0, the ex value is 1; otherwise, 0; enterprise size ($qygm$): if the number of employees exceeds 1000, the value is 1 for large enterprises and 0 for small and medium enterprises; enterprise age (age): the enterprise age is calculated by subtracting the establishment year from the current year; capital labor ratio ($zbld$): to measure it, the total assets are divided by the number of workers (10,000/person); industry category dummy variable ($hyfl$): industry category 0 indicates polluting industry, and 1 indicates clean industry.

2.3.3. Data Source and Processing

The data source of this study was the combined data of the China Industrial Enterprise Database, China Industrial Enterprise Pollution Emission Database, and China Patent Database. The China Industrial Enterprise Database contains the information of all state-owned enterprises and non-state-owned enterprises with an annual output value of more than RMB five million in China, mainly including enterprise name, organization code, legal representative, holding status, main business income, etc. The annual data volume is as high as 340,000 pieces, and the content is detailed. The statistical output value of enterprises accounts for more than 90% of the total output value of Chinese enterprises. The pollution emission database of China's industrial enterprises is the most reliable data collected by the National Bureau of Statistics. It mainly collects statistics on enterprises with serious pollution discharge in each region. The table primarily includes the enterprise name, legal representative, organization code, wastewater, exhaust gas, and other pollution discharge indicators. For the purpose of research, this study merged the above two kinds of data. Firstly, the two kinds of data were processed according to the now commonly used processing methods [42]. Second, the company name and year were matched with patent data, and the matching data of the second and third steps were combined according to the organization code and year, and the duplicate values were removed. The combined data provided pollution emission information on enterprises with annual output values of more than RMB five million. Finally, certain enterprises with business status, state-owned status, enterprise size, industrial added value, or intermediate input missing, or negative values were deleted.

The State Intellectual Property Office is the authoritative source of China's Patent Database, which mainly collects statistics on enterprises' patent applications and authorization over the years. The content of China's Patent Database mainly includes the enterprise name, organization code, invention patent, utility model patent, and design patent. The data of the Chinese Patent Database, Chinese Industrial Enterprise Database, and Chinese Industrial Enterprise Pollution Emission Database were combined using the above-discussed matching method. Finally, the combined data of the Chinese Patent Database, Chinese Industrial Enterprise Database, and China Industrial Enterprise Pollution Emission Database were obtained. About 510,000 enterprises participated in the empirical analysis.

As the latest statistical year of the China Industrial Enterprise Database is 2014, this study used statistical data from 2002 to 2014 to conduct empirical regression. Table 1 shows the descriptive statistics of variables in this study. There is a significant difference in pollution emission intensity among enterprises, with the minimum value being 0.001 and the maximum value being 18.570. There is also substantial difference in environmental policy uncertainty faced by enterprises, with the minimum value being 0.152 and the maximum value being 16.350.

Table 1. Descriptive statistics of variables.

Variables	Std. Dev	Mean	Min	Max
ei	1.495	0.254	0.001	18.570
epu	1.877	1.589	0.152	16.350
lp	0.256	0.011	0.001	90.340
gzsp	1.002	0.048	0.001	261.200
is	0.220	0.816	0.494	3.662
hlhzs	0.139	0.216	0.017	0.932
iq	9.310	0.002	0.001	3093
rlzb	0.053	0.030	0.001	0.277
fi	0.173	0.155	0.001	0.718

3. Results

3.1. Basic Regression Results

Table 2 shows the results of stepwise regression. The uncertainty of environmental policy significantly aggravates the intensity of enterprise pollution emission. On the one hand, the increasing uncertainty of environmental policies aggravates the risks faced by enterprises, which then tend to keep more cash to cope with possible shocks [43]. Enterprise pollution investment needs to introduce a large amount of advanced purification equipment and environmental protection talents, but emission investment generally has the characteristics of low early return and high risk. This further dissuades enterprises from upgrading production emission technology and introducing human capital. On the other hand, the increasing uncertainty of environmental policies makes it difficult for foreign investors to accurately predict their investment returns. The operating and financial risks of enterprises increase significantly, leading to the reduction in foreign investment and the external financing ability of enterprises, and lowering the investment of enterprises in sewage discharge equipment. Finally, the increase in environmental policy uncertainty significantly intensifies the pollution emission intensity of enterprises.

Table 2. Stepwise regression results.

Variables	(1)	(2)	(3)	(4)	(5)
	ei	ei	ei	ei	ei
epu	0.017 ***	0.017 ***	0.017 ***	0.017 ***	0.017 ***
	(0.002)	(0.002)	(0.002)	(0.002)	(0.002)
lp		0.235 ***	0.302 ***	0.302 ***	0.302 ***
		(0.016)	(0.025)	(0.025)	(0.025)
gzsp			−0.017 ***	−0.017 ***	−0.017 ***
			(0.005)	(0.005)	(0.005)
is				0.191 ***	0.113 ***
				(0.029)	(0.031)
hlhzs					−0.615 ***
					(0.089)
Enterprise	Yes	Yes	Yes	Yes	Yes
Industry	Yes	Yes	Yes	Yes	Yes
Time	Yes	Yes	Yes	Yes	Yes
Reigon	Yes	Yes	Yes	Yes	Yes
Obs	204,355	204,318	200,585	200,585	200,585
R-squared	0.040	0.041	0.042	0.042	0.042

Note: *** denote the significance at 1% levels.

3.2. *Heterogeneity Analysis*

3.2.1. Enterprise Export Status Heterogeneity

We divided enterprises into exporting and non-exporting enterprises and investigated whether the impact of environmental policy uncertainty on enterprise pollution emissions is heterogeneous because of the different export statuses of enterprises. As can be seen from Columns (1) and (2) of Table 3, the environmental policy uncertainty of both export and non-export enterprises has a significant positive impact on enterprise pollution emission intensity; however, the influence coefficient of non-export enterprises is greater than that of export enterprises. On the one hand, export companies are forced to improve their pollution techniques because their products are subject to stricter inspections abroad. On the other hand, through "learning in export," export enterprises obtain more advanced sewage discharge technology and experience from abroad, which reduces the pollution emission intensity of export enterprises. Therefore, environmental policy uncertainty has little influence on the pollution emission intensity of export enterprises. However, the relatively backward pollution discharge technology of non-export enterprises leads to higher pollution discharge cost, and the pollution discharge of enterprises is significantly affected by environmental policies. Therefore, when the uncertainty of environmental policy increases, it impacts the pollution emission of non-export enterprises.

Table 3. Results of enterprise export status and size heterogeneity.

Variables	(1)	(2)	(3)	(4)
	Export Enterprises	Non-Export Enterprise	Big Companies	Small- and Medium-Sized Enterprises
	ei	ei	ei	ei
epu	0.013 ***	0.017 ***	0.039 ***	0.003 **
	(0.003)	(0.002)	(0.009)	(0.001)
Control variables	Yes	Yes	Yes	Yes
Enterprise	Yes	Yes	Yes	Yes
Industry	Yes	Yes	Yes	Yes
Time	Yes	Yes	Yes	Yes
Reigon	Yes	Yes	Yes	Yes
Obs	60,104	140,481	28,918	171,667
R-squared	0.020	0.051	0.115	0.038

Note: **, *** denote the significance at 5%, 1% levels, respectively.

3.2.2. Heterogeneity of Firm Size

Enterprises can be categorized as large- and small- and medium-sized enterprises based on whether the number of employees exceeds 1000 according to the classification standards of "Measures for The Classification of Statistically Large, Small and Medium-sized Enterprises (2017)." We aimed to investigate whether the impact of environmental policy uncertainty on enterprise pollution emissions is heterogeneous because of different enterprise sizes. Columns (3) and (4) of Table 3 show that environmental policy uncertainty has a greater impact on the pollution emission intensity of large enterprises. The pollution emission intensity of large enterprises is generally higher than that of small- and medium-sized enterprises. When the uncertainty of environmental policy increases, large enterprises reduce their investment in emission reduction technologies and reserve more cash to cope with possible shocks, because of which, their pollution emission increases. Therefore, the pollution emission of large enterprises is greatly affected by the uncertainty of environmental policy. Alternatively, small- and medium-sized enterprises have less pollution emissions, and the increase in environmental policy uncertainty has less impact on their pollution emissions.

3.2.3. Enterprise's Age Heterogeneity

Based on the median time of establishment, enterprises are divided into young and old enterprises. Columns (1) and (2) of Table 4 show that environmental policy uncertainty has a greater impact on the pollution emission intensity of young enterprises compared to old enterprises. The establishment period of young enterprises is relatively short, and they lack advanced sewage discharge equipment, abundant capital, and experience in dealing with environmental policy uncertainty. Alternatively, old enterprises have relatively better sewage discharge equipment, abundant sewage discharge capital, and greater experience in dealing with environmental policy uncertainty. So, the impact of environmental policy uncertainty on their pollution emission is less compared to that on young enterprises.

Table 4. Results of enterprise age and type heterogeneity.

Variables	(1)	(2)	(3)	(4)
	Younger Enterprises	**Older Enterprises**	**Labor-Intensive Enterprises**	**Capital-Intensive Enterprises**
	ei	**ei**	**ei**	**ei**
epu	0.018 ***	0.015 ***	0.002	0.031 ***
	(0.003)	(0.002)	(0.002)	(0.003)
Control variables	Yes	Yes	Yes	Yes
Enterprise	Yes	Yes	Yes	Yes
Industry	Yes	Yes	Yes	Yes
Time	Yes	Yes	Yes	Yes
Reigon	Yes	Yes	Yes	Yes
Obs	87,389	126,015	99,995	100,590
R-squared	0.026	0.058	0.031	0.048

Note: *** denote the significance at 1% levels.

3.2.4. Enterprise's Type Heterogeneity

Based on the median capital labor ratio of enterprises, they are categorized as labor-intensive and capital-intensive enterprises. Columns (3) and (4) of Table 4 show that environmental policy uncertainty has a significantly positive impact on enterprise pollution emission intensity in the case of capital-intensive enterprises, but not in the case of labor-intensive enterprises, in which environmental policy uncertainty has no significant impact on enterprise pollution emission intensity. As labor-intensive enterprises are mostly light industrial enterprises, their pollution emission intensity is relatively low. Alternatively, capital-intensive enterprises, which are mostly heavy industrial enterprises, have higher pollution emission intensity and are significantly affected by the uncertainty of environmental policy. Therefore, when environmental policy uncertainty changes, it has a greater impact on the pollution emission intensity of capital-intensive enterprises than labor-intensive enterprises.

3.2.5. Enterprise's Ownership Heterogeneity

Enterprises are divided into state-owned and non-state-owned enterprises depending on whether they are state holding enterprises or not. Columns (1) and (2) of Table 5 show that the uncertainty of environmental policy has a greater impact on the pollution emission intensity of state-owned enterprises, but a smaller impact on that of non-state-owned enterprises. As profits or emission reduction in state-owned enterprises are mostly affected by national policies, when the uncertainty of environmental policy changes, it has a significant impact on the pollution emission intensity of state-owned enterprises. Alternatively, non-state-owned enterprises are owned by private enterprises and foreign-funded enterprises, and their pollution emission intensity is less affected by environmental policy uncertainty.

Table 5. Results of enterprise ownership and industry category heterogeneity.

Variables	(1)	(2)	(3)	(4)
	State-Owned Enterprises	Non-State-Owned Enterprises	Clean Industry	Polluting Industries
	ei	ei	ei	ei
epu	0.044 ***	0.004 ***	0.016 ***	0.018 ***
	(0.007)	(0.002)	(0.005)	(0.002)
Control variables	Yes	Yes	Yes	Yes
Enterprise	Yes	Yes	Yes	Yes
Industry	Yes	Yes	Yes	Yes
Time	Yes	Yes	Yes	Yes
Reigon	Yes	Yes	Yes	Yes
Obs	35,504	165,079	36,518	164,067
R-squared	0.069	0.023	0.123	0.022

Note: *** denote the significance at 1% levels.

3.2.6. Industry Category Heterogeneity

Companies are divided into clean and polluting enterprises according to their industry. Columns (3) and (4) of Table 5 show that the uncertainty of environmental policy has a smaller impact on the pollution emission intensity of clean enterprises compared to polluting enterprises. As most clean enterprises are light industry and handicraft industry enterprises, their environmental pollution emission intensity is low; so, when the uncertainty of environmental policy increases, this has an insignificant impact on the pollution emission intensity of clean industry enterprises. However, the pollution emission intensity of enterprises in polluting industries is high. When the government's environmental regulation intensity is low, the pollution emission of enterprises is high, and when the government's environmental regulation intensity is high, enterprises reduce their pollution emission. Therefore, when the uncertainty of environmental policy increases, it has a greater impact on the pollution emission intensity of enterprises in polluting industries.

3.2.7. Region heterogeneity

China is divided into eastern, central, and western regions to study whether the environmental policy uncertainty in different regions has different effects on enterprises' pollution emission intensity. The results are shown in Table 6. Due to the better economic foundation in the eastern region, the government will force enterprises to update pollution equipment when the intensity of environmental regulation increases. Then, enterprises recruit a large number of scientific and technological innovative talents, so the enterprises' pollution emission technology in the eastern region is more advanced. At the same time, some polluting enterprises in the eastern region choose to migrate to the neighboring central region due to the increase in emission costs, so the enterprises' pollution emission intensity in the central region is more serious. When environmental uncertainty is increased due to the policy change, its impact on the enterprises' pollution emission intensity in the eastern region is low. On the one hand, the central region undertakes the transfer of polluting enterprises in the eastern region, so the enterprises' pollution emission intensity in the central region is higher. When the government's environmental regulation intensity is low, the pollution emission intensity increases. When the government's environmental regulation intensity increases, enterprises have to reduce the pollution emission intensity. Therefore, the change in environmental policy uncertainty in the central region has a greater impact on the pollution emission intensity. The development of the western region is relatively backward, and the economy mainly depends on resource extraction enterprises, which leads to high pollution emission intensity. Due to the inherent production nature and enterprises' development environment, it is difficult to reduce the pollution emission intensity in the western region. Therefore, when environment policy uncertainty increases, the change in pollution emission intensity in the western region is still low.

Table 6. Results of enterprise ownership and industry category heterogeneity.

Variables	(1)	(2)	(3)
	Eastern Region	Central Region	Western Region
	ei	ei	ei
epu	0.013 ***	0.031 ***	0.015 ***
	(0.002)	(0.006)	(0.007)
Control variables	Yes	Yes	Yes
Enterprise	Yes	Yes	Yes
Industry	Yes	Yes	Yes
Time	Yes	Yes	Yes
Reigon	Yes	Yes	Yes
Obs	127,373	38,521	34,691
R-squared	0.032	0.044	0.036

Note: *** denote the significance at 1% levels.

3.3. *Robustness Test*

3.3.1. Transform Core Explanatory Variables

In this section, the uncertainty of environmental policy is re-measured to verify whether its impact on enterprise pollution emission intensity is robust. The previous article mainly refers to the Ghosh and Olsen [40] algorithm. Environmental policy uncertainty is calculated based on abnormal sales income and standard deviation in the past three years. In this section, three years of calculation are raised to five years, and the same method is used to measure environmental policy uncertainty (*epu*1). Stepwise regression results are shown in Table 7. It can be seen that the environmental policy uncertainty still has a significant positive effect on the pollution emission intensity of enterprises, indicating that this study's conclusions are robust and reliable.

Table 7. Change the core explanatory variable—environmental policy uncertainty.

Variables	(1)	(2)	(3)	(4)	(5)
	ei	ei	ei	ei	ei
epu1	0.014 *	0.015 *	0.015 *	0.014 *	0.015 *
	(0.008)	(0.008)	(0.008)	(0.008)	(0.008)
lp		0.343 ***	0.316 ***	0.316 ***	0.315 ***
		(0.035)	(0.047)	(0.047)	(0.047)
gzsp			0.013	0.013	0.013
			(0.015)	(0.015)	(0.015)
is				0.152 ***	0.032
				(0.059)	(0.063)
hlhzs					−1.221 ***
					(0.226)
Enterprise	Yes	Yes	Yes	Yes	Yes
Industry	Yes	Yes	Yes	Yes	Yes
Time	Yes	Yes	Yes	Yes	Yes
Reigon	Yes	Yes	Yes	Yes	Yes
Obs	64,776	64,763	62,785	62,785	62,785
R-squared	0.038	0.040	0.041	0.041	0.041

Note: *, *** denote the significance at 10%, 1% levels, respectively.

3.3.2. Transform the Interpreted Variable

The pollution emission intensity of enterprises mentioned above was measured using the comprehensive index method. In this section, five single pollution emissions of enterprises are used to measure the pollution emission intensity of enterprises. The regression results are shown in Table 8. It can be seen that environmental policy uncertainty still significantly promotes the improvement of the pollution emission intensity of enterprises, indicating that the conclusions of this study are robust and reliable.

Table 8. Change the explained variable—pollution emission intensity of enterprises.

Variables	(1) Discharge of Industrial Wastewater	(2) Chemical Oxygen Demand Emissions	(3) Total Industrial Exhaust Emissions	(4) Sulfur Dioxide Emissions	(5) Smoke and Dust Emission
epu	1.312 ***	0.370 **	0.934 ***	1.188 ***	5.889 ***
	(0.337)	(0.180)	(0.172)	(0.204)	(1.713)
Control variables	Yes	Yes	Yes	Yes	Yes
Enterprise	Yes	Yes	Yes	Yes	Yes
Industry	Yes	Yes	Yes	Yes	Yes
Time	Yes	Yes	Yes	Yes	Yes
Reigon	Yes	Yes	Yes	Yes	Yes
Obs	177,652	192,764	82,159	191,119	147,529
R-squared	0.005	0.016	0.108	0.066	0.037

Note: **, *** denote the significance at 5%, 1% levels, respectively.

3.3.3. Eliminate the Sample of Entering and Exiting Enterprises

The entry and exit of enterprises in the sample period interferes with the impact of environmental policy uncertainty on enterprise pollution emissions. Therefore, this section deletes entering and exiting enterprises in the sample period for robustness tests. The regression results are shown in Column (1) of Table 9. The influence coefficient of environmental policy uncertainty on enterprise pollution emission intensity is significantly positive, indicating that the research conclusions in this study are robust and reliable.

Table 9. Regression results of eliminate the entry and exit samples, adjust the sample period and Winsor.

Variables	(1) Eliminate Entry Exit Sample	(2) 2012–2014	(3) Delete the Time Dummy Variable	(4) Winsor	(5) Add Variable L.ei
	ei	ei	ei	ei	ei
epu	0.008 ***	0.046 ***	0.017 ***	0.018 ***	0.018 ***
	(0.002)	0.004	(0.002)	(0.002)	(0.005)
Control variables	Yes	Yes	Yes	Yes	Yes
Enterprise	Yes	Yes	Yes	Yes	Yes
Industry	Yes	Yes	Yes	Yes	Yes
Time	Yes	Yes	Yes	Yes	Yes
Region	Yes	Yes	Yes	Yes	Yes
Obs	172,969	65,163	200,585	200,585	32,153
R-squared	0.048	0.031	0.042	0.047	0.039

Note: *** denote the significance at 1% levels.

3.3.4. Change Sample Period and Delete the Time Dummy Variable

In this study, macro-variables were controlled to eliminate the influence of time factor on empirical results, but time factors may still have had an impact on the results. Robustness was analyzed from two perspectives. (1) The sample period of this study was 2002–2014. The State Environmental Protection Administration set up six inspection centers in 2006. The Environmental Protection Law was introduced in 2008, and ecological progress was proposed at the 18th National Congress of the Communist Party of China in 2012. To control the influence of these factors, only samples from 2012 to 2014 are used for regression in this section. (2) We considered deleting the time dummy variable and substituting the rest of the dummy variables into the regression model to control the influence of the time effect. The results are shown in Columns (2) and (3) of Table 9. The influence coefficient of environmental policy uncertainty on enterprise pollution emission intensity is significantly positive, indicating that the conclusions of this study are robust and reliable.

3.3.5. Deleting Outliers

To eliminate the influence of outliers on regression results, variables were treated with Winsor at the level of 1%. The regression results are shown in Column (4) of Table 9. The influence coefficient of environmental policy uncertainty on enterprise pollution emission intensity is significantly positive, indicating that the research conclusions are robust and reliable.

3.4. Endogeneity Test

As environmental policy uncertainty is caused by the fluctuation of national macro-policy, and the micro-behavior of individual enterprises can hardly affect the macro-environmental policy, there is almost no reverse causality between enterprise pollution emissions and environmental policy uncertainty. Additionally, the fixed effects of enterprises, industries, regions, and years are strictly controlled in the empirical analysis of this study, which effectively avoids the endogenous problems caused by omitted variables. As eliminating the lag term of enterprise pollution emission intensity may affect the results, referring to Fang et al. (2015), this study added the variable *L.ei* into the regression Formula [43]; the results are shown in Column (5) of Table 9. The significance of the explanatory variables remains unchanged.

3.5. Mechanism Analysis

Based on the above theoretical analysis, environmental policy uncertainty can affect the pollution emission intensity of enterprises in three ways: enterprise innovation, human capital, and foreign investment. This section empirically tests the impact of environmental policy uncertainty on enterprise pollution emission intensity through these three channels. The specific model is as follows:

$$ei_{ijkt} = \beta_0 + \beta_1 epu_{ijkt} + \beta_2 iq_{ijkt} + \beta_3 epu_{ijkt} \cdot iq_{ijkt} + \beta_4 X_{ijkt} + \lambda_i + \lambda_j + \lambda_k + \lambda_t + \varepsilon_{ijkt} \quad (29)$$

$$ei_{ijkt} = \beta_0 + \beta_1 epu_{ijkt} + \beta_2 rlzb_{ijkt} + \beta_3 epu_{ijkt} \cdot rlzb_{ijkt} + \beta_4 X_{ijkt} + \lambda_i + \lambda_j + \lambda_k + \lambda_t + \varepsilon_{ijkt} \quad (30)$$

$$ei_{ijkt} = \beta_0 + \beta_1 epu_{ijkt} + \beta_2 fi_{ijkt} + \beta_3 epu_{ijkt} \cdot fi_{ijkt} + \beta_4 X_{ijkt} + \lambda_i + \lambda_j + \lambda_k + \lambda_t + \varepsilon_{ijkt} \quad (31)$$

Formula (29) shows that environmental policy uncertainty affects enterprise pollution emission intensity through firm innovation, Formula (30) shows that environmental policy uncertainty affects enterprise pollution emission intensity through human capital, and Formula (31) shows that environmental policy uncertainty affects enterprise pollution emission intensity through foreign investment. The regression results are shown in Table 10.

Table 10. Mechanism test results.

Variables	(1)	(2)	(3)
	ei	ei	ei
epu	0.017 ***	−0.002	0.021 ***
	(0.002)	(0.032)	(0.003)
iq	0.172 ***		
	(0.035)		

Table 10. *Cont.*

Variables	(1)	(2)	(3)
	ei	ei	ei
epu·iq	−0.017 *		
	(0.009)		
rlzb		5.088 ***	
		(1.445)	
epu·rlzb		−1.826 **	
		(0.710)	
fi			−0.248 ***
			(0.067)
epu·fi			−0.021 **
			(0.010)
Control variables	Yes	Yes	Yes
Enterprise	Yes	Yes	Yes
Industry	Yes	Yes	Yes
Time	Yes	Yes	Yes
Reigon	Yes	Yes	Yes
Obs	200,585	622	200,585
R-squared	0.043	0.140	0.043

Note: *, **, *** denote the significance at 10%, 5%, 1% levels, respectively.

3.5.1. Enterprise Innovation

The purpose of enterprise investment is profit maximization. With an increase in environmental policy uncertainty, the silent risk of enterprise investment and innovation also increases. Moreover, innovation investment is a project with high risk and a long cycle, so enterprise innovation investment needs sufficient capital guarantee. When the uncertainty of the environmental policy facing enterprises increases, the uncertainty of enterprise innovation investment income increases, and to reduce risks, enterprise managers decrease investment in innovation. This lowers the innovation capacity of enterprises. As can be seen from Column (1) of Table 10, the interaction coefficient between environmental policy uncertainty and enterprise innovation is significantly negative. It reveals that environmental policy uncertainty aggravates enterprises' pollution emission by inhibiting the improvement of enterprises' innovation ability. Thus, Hypothesis 1 is verified.

3.5.2. Human Capital

According to the classical financial theory, when an enterprise faces greater uncertainty in the external environment, it reserves more cash to cope with unknown shocks [44]. When the uncertainty of environmental policy increases, enterprises expect that financing in the capital market will be full of difficulties, the human capital input of enterprises has the characteristics of longer term and less obvious income, and the adjustment cost is lower than other factors of production. Therefore, enterprises decelerate the introduction of human capital to retain more cash to cope with unknown impacts of environmental policy uncertainty, which reduces the human capital stock of enterprises. Additionally, when the environmental uncertainty of enterprises increases, enterprises tend to reduce their operating costs in order to retain more cash to face possible future shocks. It is common for enterprises to lay off employees, increase the labor supply time of employees, and reduce salaries. Employees are faced with reduced income and increased labor intensity, which will further increase the incidence of disease, thus damaging the healthy human capital of employees. Column (2) of Table 10 shows that the interaction coefficient of environmental policy uncertainty and human capital is significantly negative, indicating that environmental policy uncertainty aggravates enterprise pollution emissions by inhibiting the increase in enterprise human capital stock. Thus, Hypothesis 2 is verified.

3.5.3. Foreign Investment

The change in external environment is an important factor affecting foreign investment, the main purpose of which is profit. When the uncertainty of investors' profit expectation increases, the opportunity cost of enterprise investment also increases, and foreign capital flows to projects with more definite investment returns. Therefore, the increased uncertainty of environmental policy reduces foreign investment expectations. Column (3) of Table 10 shows that the interaction coefficient between environmental policy uncertainty and foreign investment is significantly negative, indicating that environmental policy uncertainty aggravates enterprises' pollution emissions by inhibiting foreign investment. Thus, Hypothesis 3 is verified.

4. Discussion

Based on the combined data of the China Industrial Enterprise Database, China Industrial Enterprise Pollution Emission Database, and China Patent Database from 2002 to 2014, we empirically analyzed the impact of environmental policy uncertainty on enterprise pollution emission.

4.1. Contribution

The marginal contributions of this study are as follows: First, at the research level, the existing literature mainly discusses the impact of environmental regulations on regional environmental pollution emissions from a macro-perspective; the micro-viewpoint is the basis and key to understand the macro-perspective. From the perspective of micro-enterprises, this study was mainly based on the Chinese Industrial Enterprise Pollution Emission Database, and chemical oxygen demand, industrial waste gas, sulfur dioxide, smoke, and dust emissions were selected to measure the intensity of enterprise pollution emission. The composite index method makes the measurement result closer to the real enterprise pollution emission intensity. It also systematically discusses the influence of environmental policy uncertainty on enterprise pollution emissions to further refine the existing research and establishes the micro-basic cognition of the relationship between environmental policy uncertainty and enterprise pollution emissions. Thus, it makes up for the deficiencies of existing research in the field of micro-enterprises.

Second, in terms of research content and perspectives: (1) from the perspective of increasing environmental policy uncertainty, this article discussed the impact and mechanism of environmental policy uncertainty on enterprise pollution emissions and provides a new research perspective for enterprise pollution emissions; and (2) there is often summing bias in regional summing data, which may cover up or change the real relationship between variables in empirical tests, and as macro-research ignores the heterogeneity of enterprises, it is difficult to investigate how enterprises' emission reduction behaviors with different characteristics respond to environmental policy uncertainties. This article discussed the heterogeneity of enterprise export status, enterprise size, enterprise age, enterprise type, enterprise ownership, and enterprise industry category, which helps to form a comprehensive understanding of the relationship between environmental policy uncertainty and enterprise pollution emissions.

Third, regarding the mechanism of action, the existing literature on the mechanism of enterprise emission reduction is increasingly mature. However, from a new perspective of environmental policy uncertainty and micro level, the effectiveness of these mechanisms is questionable. Based on the theoretical model, this study revealed that environmental policy uncertainty affects enterprise pollution emissions through three channels: technological innovation, human capital, and foreign investment. It further deepened the understanding of the complete logical chain of environmental policy uncertainty to enterprise pollution discharge.

Forth, ordinary least squares was selected as the analysis method, and the interference of time, industry, region, and individual was controlled, so that the correlation coefficient between environmental policy uncertainty and enterprise pollution emission intensity was closer to the reality.

4.2. Limitations

The research still has certain limitations and should be further deepened. First, in view of the limitations of research methods, this paper selected panel data to analyze the heterogeneity of the Enterprise Pollution Emission Intensity and influencing factors in China; however, it lacked an analysis of the dynamic evolution of space. In the future, appropriate research methods will be selected to conduct a more in-depth spatial dynamic analysis of the Enterprise Pollution Emission Intensity. Second, since the latest data were only collected in 2014, if there are updated data in the future, we will further update the data in the following study.

5. Conclusions

Based on the combined data of the China Industrial Enterprise Database, China Industrial Enterprise Pollution Emission Database, and China Patent Database from 2002 to 2014, we empirically analyzed the impact of environmental policy uncertainty on enterprise pollution emission. The results show that:

First, the impact of environmental policy uncertainty on enterprise emission reduction was discussed theoretically and empirically. Second, the heterogeneity of environmental policy uncertainty on enterprise pollution emission was discussed from the perspectives of enterprise export status, enterprise size, enterprise age, enterprise type, enterprise ownership, enterprise industry category, and different region. Finally, we empirically examined whether environmental policy uncertainty can increase enterprise pollution emissions by inhibiting enterprise innovation, human capital, and foreign investment.

The conclusions of this study are as follows: (1) The uncertainty of environmental policy significantly intensifies the pollution emission intensity of enterprises and aggravates regional environmental pollution. (2) Environmental policy uncertainty intensifies enterprises' pollution emission intensity through three transmission channels: enterprise innovation, human capital, and foreign investment. In other words, environmental policy uncertainty intensifies enterprises' pollution emission intensity by inhibiting the improvement of their innovation ability, reducing their human capital stock, and discouraging foreign investment. (3) Environmental policy uncertainty has significant heterogeneity on enterprise pollution emissions, that is, environmental policy uncertainty has a greater impact on non-export enterprises, large enterprises, young enterprises, capital-intensive enterprises, state-owned enterprises, and enterprises in polluting industries and central regions.

Policy Enlightenment

The conclusions of this study have enlightening significance for the adjustment of environmental policy and enterprise green transformation. (1) The government should give full play to the decisive role of the market in resource allocation, strengthen macro-regulation, and reduce uncertainties in environmental policies. Currently, China needs enormous external capital, new talent, and green technology to promote economic transformation and upgradation. The government should build a stable economic environment to help enterprises acquire foreign capital, advanced technology, and new talents, and accelerate the transformation or elimination of high-pollution, high-consumption enterprises. (2) The government should construct a stable and efficient compound environmental regulation policy system. Although the government's environmental regulation measures can curb pollution emission by enterprises, the frequent introduction of environmental policies increases environmental policy uncertainty, which inhibits enterprise innovation, human capital, and foreign investment. Therefore, the government should maintain the sustainability of local environmental regulation policies, effectively promote the coordination and cooperation of heterogeneous environmental regulation tools, and reduce the negative impact of environmental policy uncertainty on enterprise emission reduction. (3) In the process of policy formulation and implementation, the government needs to further refine specific measures. Due to the significant heterogeneity of environmental policy uncertainty on enterprise pollution emission, the government needs to formulate detailed measures. As such, we will focus on monitoring pollution emissions of non-export enterprises and small enterprises, so as to minimize the negative impact of environmental policy uncertainty on enterprise emission reduction. In general, this study introduced a new research perspective and microscopic evidence for the green transformation development of Chinese enterprises.

Author Contributions: Conceptualization, D.L. and F.R.; data curation, Y.Z.; formal analysis, D.L., F.R., Y.T. and Y.Z.; funding acquisition, F.R. and Y.Z.; methodology, D.L., F.R., Y.T. and Y.Z.; software, Y.Z.; supervision, D.L. and Y.Z.; writing—original draft, D.L., Y.Z. and F.R.; writing—review and editing, D.L., F.R., Y.T. and Y.Z. All authors have read and agreed to the published version of the manuscript.

Funding: This research was funded by the Doctoral Research Innovation Project of Zhongnan University of Economics and Law [202110337]; the Philosophy and Social Science Fund project of Hunan Province [21YBQ079]; the Scientific Research Project of Hunan Education Department [19C0481]; the Postgraduate Scientific Research Innovation Project of Hunan Province [CX20210385].

Institutional Review Board Statement: Not applicable.

Informed Consent Statement: Not applicable.

Data Availability Statement: The Ministry of Ecology and Environment of the People's Republic of China (https://www.mee.gov.cn/, accessed on 15 March 2022); the National Bureau of Statistics (http://www.stats.gov.cn/, accessed on 16 March 2022); China National Intellectual Property Administration (https://www.cnipa.gov.cn/, accessed on 16 March 2022); China Patent Information Center (http://www.cnpat.com.cn, accessed on 17 March 2022). EPSDATA (https://www.epsnet.com.cn/index.html#/, Home, accessed on 17 March 2022).

Conflicts of Interest: The authors declare no conflict of interest. The funders had no role in the design of the study; in the collection, analyses, or interpretation of data; in the writing of the manuscript, or in the decision to publish the results.

References

1. Matus, K.; Nam, K.-M.; Selin, N.E.; Lamsal, L.N.; Reilly, J.M.; Paltsev, S. Health Damages from Air Pollution in China. *Glob. Environ. Chang.* **2012**, *22*, 55–66. [CrossRef]
2. Crane, K.; Mao, Z. *Costs of Selected Policies to Address Air Pollution in China*; RAND Corporation: Santa Monica, CA, USA, 2015.
3. Lan, J.; Munro, A. Environmental Compliance and Human Capital: Evidence from Chinese Industrial Firms. *Resour. Energy Econ.* **2013**, *35*, 534–557. [CrossRef]
4. Bloom, N. The Impact of Uncertainty Shocks. *Econometrica* **2009**, *77*, 623–685. [CrossRef]
5. Jaffe, A.B.; Newell, R.G.; Stavins, R.N. Technological Change and the Environment. In *Handbook of Environmental Economics*; Mäler, K.G., Vincent, J.R., Eds.; Elsevier: Amsterdam, The Netherlands, 2003. [CrossRef]
6. Burtraw, D.; Krupnick, A.; Palmer, K.; Paul, A.; Toman, M.; Bloyd, C. Ancillary Benefits of Reducing Air Pollution in the U.S. from Moderate Greenhouse Gas Mitigation Policies in the Electricity Sector. *J. Environ. Econ. Manag.* **2003**, *45*, 650–673. [CrossRef]
7. Oueslati, W. Environmental Tax Reform: Short-Term Versus Long-Term Macroeconomic Effects. *J. Macroecon.* **2014**, *40*, 190–201. [CrossRef]
8. Bergek, A.; Berggren, C. The Impact of Environmental Policy Instruments on Innovation: A Review of Energy and Automotive Industry Studies. *Ecol. Econ.* **2014**, *106*, 112–123. [CrossRef]
9. Rennings, K. Redefining Innovation—Eco-innovation Research and the Contribution from Ecological Economics. *Ecol. Econ.* **2000**, *32*, 319–332. [CrossRef]
10. Dechezleprêtre, A.; Sato, M. The Impacts of Environmental Regulations on Competitiveness. *Rev. Environ. Econ. Policy* **2017**, *11*, 183–206. [CrossRef]
11. Popp, D. Induced Innovation and Energy Prices. *Am. Econ. Rev.* **2002**, *92*, 168–180. [CrossRef]
12. Porter, M.E. America's GreenStrategy. *Sci. Am.* **1991**, *264*, 193–246.
13. Fu, X. China's Path to Innovation: Foreign Direct Investment, Absorptive Capacity and Regional Innovative Capabilities:Evi-Dence from China. *Oxf. Dev. Stud.* **2008**, *36*, 89–110. [CrossRef]
14. Kurtz, M.J.; Brooks, S.M. Conditioning the "Resource Curse": Globalization, Human Capital, and Growth in Oil-Rich Nations. *Comp. Pol. Stud.* **2011**, *44*, 747–770. [CrossRef]

15. Lan, J.; Kakinaka, M.; Huang, X. Foreign Direct Investment, Human Capital and Environmental Pollution in China. *Environ. Resour. Econ.* **2012**, *51*, 255–275. [CrossRef]
16. Levinson, A.; Taylor, M.S. Unmasking the Pollution Haven Effect. *Int. Econ. Rev.* **2008**, *49*, 223–254. [CrossRef]
17. Albornoz, F.; Cole, M.A.; Elliott, R.J.R.; Ercolani, M.G. The Environmental Actions of Firms: Examining the Role of Spillovers, Networks and Absorptive Capacity. *J. Environ. Manag.* **2014**, *146*, 150–163. [CrossRef]
18. Christmann, P.; Taylor, G. Globalization and the Environment: Determinants of Firm Self-Regulation in China. *J. Int. Bus. Stud.* **2001**, *32*, 439–458. [CrossRef]
19. Duncan, R.B. Characteristics of Organizational Environments and Perceived Environmental Uncertainty. *Admin. Sci. Q.* **1972**, *17*, 313–327. [CrossRef]
20. Gulen, H.; Ion, M. Policy Uncertainty and Corporate Investment. *Rev. Financ. Stud.* **2016**, *29*, 523–564. [CrossRef]
21. Waldman, D.A.; Javidan, M.; Varella, P. Charismatic Leadership at the Strategic Level: A New Application of Upper Echelons Theory. *Leadersh. Q.* **2004**, *15*, 355–380. [CrossRef]
22. O'Connor, N.G.; Vera-Munoz, S.C.; Chan, F. Competitive Forces and the Importance of Management Control Systems in E-Merging-Economy Firms:the Moderating Effect of International Market Orientation. *Acc. Organ. Soc.* **2011**, *36*, 246–266. [CrossRef]
23. Bonaime, A.; Gulen, H.; Ion, M. Does Policy Uncertainty Affect Mergers and Acquisitions? *J. Financ. Econ.* **2018**, *129*, 531–558. [CrossRef]
24. Bloom, N.; Bond, S.; Van Reenen, J.V. Uncertainty and Investment Dynamics. *Rev. Econ. Stud.* **2007**, *74*, 391–415. [CrossRef]
25. Kemfert, C. Induced Technological Change in a Multi-regional, Multi-sectoral, Integrated Assessment Model (WIAGEM). *Ecol. Econ.* **2005**, *54*, 293–305. [CrossRef]
26. Aghion, P.; Dechezleprêtre, A.; Hémous, D.; Martin, R.; Van Reenen, J.V. Carbon Taxes, Path Dependency and Directed Technical Change:Evidence from the Auto Industry. *J. Pol. Econ.* **2016**, *124*, 1–51. [CrossRef]
27. Xia, Y.; Lu, M. The Footprint of Human Capital Across Cities over Centuries: Historical Inheritance, Policy Shock and Contemporary Migration in China. *Econ. Res. J.* **2019**, *54*, 132–149. (In Chinese)
28. Grimaud, A.; Rouge, L. Carbon Sequestration, Economic Policies and Growth. *Resour. Energy Econ.* **2014**, *36*, 307–331. [CrossRef]
29. Poumanyvong, P.; Kaneko, S.; Dhakal, S. Impacts of Urbanization on National Transport and Road Energy Use:Evidence from Low, Middle and High Income Countries. *Energy Policy* **2012**, *46*, 268–277. [CrossRef]
30. Chen, H.; Guo, W.; Feng, X.; Wei, W.D.; Liu, H.B.; Feng, Y.; Gong, W.Y. The Impact of Low-Carbon City Pilot Policy on the Total Factor Productivity of Listed Enterprises in China. *Resour. Conserv. Recycl.* **2021**, *169*, 105457. [CrossRef]
31. Caggese, A. Entrepreneurial Risk, Investment and Innovation. *J. Financ. Econ.* **2012**, *106*, 287–307. [CrossRef]
32. Jung, B.; Lee, W.J.; Weber, D.P. Financial Reporting Quality and Labor Investment Efficiency. *Contemp. Acc. Res.* **2014**, *31*, 1047–1076. [CrossRef]
33. Moretti, E. Workers' Education, Spillovers, and Productivity: Evidence from Plant-Level Production Functions. *Am. Econ. Rev.* **2004**, *94*, 656–690. [CrossRef]
34. Merz, M.; Yashiv, E. Labor and the Market Value of the Firm. *Am. Econ. Rev.* **2007**, *97*, 1419–1431. [CrossRef]
35. Sapkota, P.; Bastola, U. Foreign Direct Investment, Income, and Environmental Pollution in Developing Countries: Panel Data Analysis of Latin America. *Energy Econ.* **2017**, *64*, 206–212. [CrossRef]
36. Al-Mulali, U.; Foon Tang, C.F. Investigating the Validity of Pollution Haven Hypothesis in the Gulf Cooperation Council (GCC) Countries. *Energy Policy* **2013**, *60*, 813–819. [CrossRef]
37. Su, D.; Sheng, B. Industrial Agglomeration, Agglomeration Externalities and Firm Emission Reduction—New Micro-evidence from China. *China Econ. Q.* **2021**, *21*, 1793–1816. (In Chinese)
38. Bergh, D.D.; Lawless, M.W. Portfolio Restructuring and Limits to Hierarchical Governance:the Effects of Environmental Uncertainty and Diversification Strategy. *Organ. Sci.* **1998**, *9*, 87–102. [CrossRef]
39. Cheng, J.L.C.; Kesner, I.F. Organizational Slack and Response to Environmental Shifts: The Impact of Resource Allocation Patterns. *J. Manag.* **1997**, *23*, 1–18. [CrossRef]
40. Ghosh, D.; Olsen, L. Environmental Uncertainty and Managers' Use of Discretionary Accruals. *Acc. Organ. Soc.* **2009**, *34*, 188–205. [CrossRef]
41. Barro, R.J.; Lee, J.W. International Comparisons of Educational Attainment. *J. Monet. Econ.* **1993**, *32*, 363–394. [CrossRef]
42. Brandt, L.; Van Biesebroeck, J.; Zhang, Y. Challenges of Working with the Chinese NBS Firm-Level Data. *China Econ. Rev.* **2014**, *30*, 339–352. [CrossRef]
43. Fang, L.H.; Lerner, J.; Wu, C. Intellectual Property Rights Protection, Ownership, and Innovation: Evidence from China. *Rev. Financ. Stud.* **2017**, *30*, 2446–2477. [CrossRef]
44. Almeida, H.; Campello, M. Financial Constraints, Asset Tangibility, and Corporate Investment. *Rev. Financ. Stud.* **2007**, *20*, 1429–1460. [CrossRef]

MDPI
St. Alban-Anlage 66
4052 Basel
Switzerland
Tel. +41 61 683 77 34
Fax +41 61 302 89 18
www.mdpi.com

International Journal of Environmental Research and Public Health Editorial Office
E-mail: ijerph@mdpi.com
www.mdpi.com/journal/ijerph

www.ingramcontent.com/pod-product-compliance
Lightning Source LLC
Chambersburg PA
CBHW061445220926
51850CB00004B/22
9783036560212